Transesophageal Echocardiography for Congenital Heart Disease

Pierre C. Wong • Wanda C. Miller-Hance
Editors

Transesophageal Echocardiography for Congenital Heart Disease

Springer

Editors
Pierre C. Wong, MD
Division of Cardiology
Children's Hospital Los Angeles
Department of Pediatrics
Keck School of Medicine
University of Southern California
Los Angeles, CA
USA

Wanda C. Miller-Hance, MD
Divisions of Pediatric Anesthesiology
and Pediatric Cardiology
Departments of Pediatrics and Anesthesiology
Texas Children's Hospital
Baylor College of Medicine
Houston, TX
USA

ISBN 978-1-4471-7127-0 ISBN 978-1-84800-064-3 (eBook)
DOI 10.1007/978-1-84800-064-3
Springer London Heidelberg New York Dordrecht

Softcover reprint of the hardcover 1st edition 2014

Printed on acid-free paper

Springer is part of Springer Science+Business Media (www.springer.com)

Preface

The inspiration for this book arose from several important observations. *First*, we have noted many specialists (both in pediatric and adult medicine) who feel uncomfortable with or incapable of performing a systematic transesophageal echocardiographic (TEE) examination in a patient with congenital heart disease (CHD), or interpreting such a study. Even some advanced practitioners who can adequately perform/interpret a transthoracic echocardiogram have difficulty with TEE because, despite the many similarities between the two echocardiographic modalities, competent performance of a TEE study in a patient with CHD requires both technical proficiency and specialized cognitive skills. Among these, one must be able to insert safely and manipulate the TEE probe, obtain a variety of cross-sectional views (particularly those pertinent to CHD), and then have the expertise to understand and interpret the echocardiographic information. *Second*, compared to other specialized forms of echocardiography for CHD (such as fetal cardiac imaging), comparatively little educational material is readily available regarding the use of this modality for the evaluation of CHD. Although good instructional materials on the subject exist, these are scattered among a number of different publications and across various websites. No currently available textbook or didactic source comprehensively and specifically focuses upon the subject, particularly in the pediatric age group. In fact, only one such textbook has ever been written, and its publication occurred well before the widespread availability of multiplane TEE imaging. *Third*, it is a well-recognized fact that, with improving outcomes and successes of congenital heart surgery, many children are now living well into adulthood. However unlike transthoracic examination in infants and young children, the echocardiographic imaging of adults with CHD often suffers from poor image quality and limited windows. Therefore alternative diagnostic modalities such as TEE assume a much more prominent role for the providers involved in the care of these patients. Thus, the need for a dedicated TEE resource to assist such specialists has become much more compelling.

The current textbooks that do discuss the applications of TEE assessment in CHD fall into two main categories. In one group are the large, comprehensive TEE textbooks written principally by adult cardiovascular specialists (mostly anesthesiologists), and all include chapters on the evaluation of CHD. Although they are excellent resources, the discussion of the subject is of necessity more limited in scope, and oriented primarily toward the adult with CHD, based upon well established and standardized guidelines intended primarily for the examination of the structurally normal adult heart. In the other category are the contemporary textbooks written specifically on the subject of pediatric echocardiography and CHD, authored mainly by pediatric and adult congenital heart specialists. These textbooks provide thorough, extensive coverage of the many unique aspects of CHD diagnosis by echocardiography. However, the discussions center primarily around transthoracic (and, to a lesser extent, fetal) imaging; the description of the TEE examination is usually brief (if it is given at all), with scant detail regarding specifics of techniques and views used to evaluate the various cardiac defects.

This textbook represents the first work of its kind to provide a comprehensive, modern, and integrated approach to the TEE evaluation for CHD. To this end, we have opted to combine the techniques and views detailed by adult TEE specialists with the unique diagnostic approach to CHD evaluation provided by leaders in the field. This textbook extensively describes the in-depth anatomic and physiologic TEE assessment of the many different forms of CHD, and includes approaches to certain types of defects that previously have not been reported or well described. While the pediatric patient represents a major focus of attention, the material in this textbook has equal application in operated and unoperated adult patients with CHD. One of our principal objectives was also to address the diagnostic needs of the burgeoning field of adult CHD.

Our goal is that *Transesophageal Echocardiography for Congenital Heart Disease* will prove an invaluable resource for those who utilize this imaging approach in the care of patients with CHD, both children and adults. It is directed toward individuals with all levels of expertise—cardiologists, surgeons, anesthesiologists, intensive care specialists, sonographers—as well as trainees wishing to acquire basic knowledge or advance their understanding of the field. We sincerely hope that our readers find this textbook both informative and practical; we encourage them to enjoy this book, and refer to it often.

Los Angeles, CA, USA Pierre C. Wong, MD
Houston, TX, USA Wanda C. Miller-Hance, MD

Acknowledgements

This textbook is the product of the collective experience and expertise of its many outstanding contributors. It has been crafted through numerous hours of writing, researching, revising, and discussion. The editors would like to thank the individual authors for their hard work and dedication; without your contributions, this unique textbook would not have been possible.

The editors would also like to thank our publisher, Springer, and particularly Grant Weston, Senior Editor of Medicine at Springer, for his firm yet gentle guiding hand throughout this whole project. We are greatly indebted to our wonderful developmental editor, Barbara Lopez-Lucio, whose guidance, support, patience, and encouragement helped keep us going even when the work seemed overwhelming, the end unattainable.

From Pierre C. Wong: Thanks to Mark Pearson for his valuable assistance in the preparation of the TEE view diagrams. Special thanks to my wife Yolanda and my son Michael for their unconditional love and support. You have always known how much this means to me, and how proud I am of it. Also my deepest appreciation to my father Thomas, an ageless wonder whose wisdom and vitality continue to inspire us all, and to my late mother Simone, who is still with me in so many ways. I can see you smiling right now. Of course, thanks to all my colleagues at CHLA for their tireless efforts and never-ending spirit of collaboration. Finally, thanks so very much to my co-editor, Wanda. Working with you has been a joy every step of the way, and you've taught me so much in the process.

From Wanda C. Miller-Hance: I wish to express my sincere gratitude to the special people in my life for their motivation, encouragement, unwavering support, and, above all, their never-ending patience and love. This project has been a dream come true! My deep appreciation goes to colleagues and mentors for their commitment to excellence and from whom I continue to learn every day. This book is my humble tribute to all the patients for whom I have had the privilege to provide care and who serve as inspiration for this work. A special thanks goes to my co-editor, Pierre, for his insight and vision in making this effort come to life.

Contents

Contributors

Jamil A. Aboulhosn, MD Departments of Medicine and Pediatrics, David Geffen School of Medicine at UCLA, Los Angeles, CA, USA

Nancy A. Ayres, MD Division of Cardiology, Department of Pediatrics, Texas Children's Hospital, Baylor College of Medicine, Houston, TX, USA

Louis I. Bezold, MD Department of Pediatrics, Kentucky Children's Hospital, University of Kentucky College of Medicine, Lexington, KY, USA

Qi-Ling Cao, MD Departments of Pediatrics and Internal Medicine, Rush Center for Congenital and Structural Heart Disease, Rush University Medical Center, Chicago, IL, USA

John S. Child, MD Department of Medicine, David Geffen School of Medicine at UCLA, Los Angeles, CA, USA

Nadine F. Choueiter, MD Department of Pediatrics, Albert Einstein College of Medicine, Children's Hospital at Montefiore, Bronx, NY, USA

Meryl S. Cohen, MD Division of Cardiology, Department of Pediatrics, The Children's Hospital of Philadelphia, Perelman School of Medicine at the University of Pennsylvania, Philadelphia, PA, USA

Vivian Wei Cui, MD Division of Pediatric Cardiology, Department of Pediatrics, Advocate Children's Hospital Heart Institute, Oak Lawn, IL, USA

Benjamin W. Eidem, MD, FACC, FAAP, FASE Division of Pediatric Cardiology and Cardiovascular Diseases, Departments of Pediatrics and Medicine, Mayo Clinic, Rochester, MN, USA

Mark K. Friedberg, MD Division of Cardiology, Department of Pediatrics, The Labatt Family Heart Center, The Hospital for Sick Children, University of Toronto, Toronto, ON, Canada

Peter C. Frommelt, MD Division of Pediatric Cardiology, Department of Pediatrics, Medical College of Wisconsin, Children's Hospital of Wisconsin, Milwaukee, WI, USA

Ziyad M. Hijazi, MD, MPH, FSCAI, FACC, FAAP Departments of Pediatrics and Internal Medicine, Rush Center for Congenital and Structural Heart Disease, Rush University Medical Center, Chicago, IL, USA

Ling Hui, MD, PhD Cardiac Fluid Dynamics and Imaging Laboratory, School of Medicine, Oregon Health and Science University, Portland, OR, USA

Peter R. Koenig, MD, FACC, FASE Department of Pediatric Cardiology, Ann & Robert H. Lurie Children's Hospital of Chicago, Northwestern University Feinberg School of Medicine, Chicago, IL, USA

Grace C. Kung, MD Division of Cardiology, Children's Hospital Los Angeles, Department of Pediatrics, Keck School of Medicine, University of Southern California, Los Angeles, CA, USA

Leo Lopez, MD Department of Pediatrics, Albert Einstein College of Medicine, Children's Hospital at Montefiore, Bronx, NY, USA

Gerald Ross Marx, MD Department of Cardiology, Boston Children's Hospital, Harvard School of Medicine, Boston, MA, USA

Laura M. Mercer-Rosa, MD, MSCE Division of Cardiology, Department of Pediatrics, The Children's Hospital of Philadelphia, Perelman School of Medicine at the University of Pennsylvania, Philadelphia, PA, USA

Wanda C. Miller-Hance, MD Divisions of Pediatric Anesthesiology and Pediatric Cardiology, Departments of Pediatrics and Anesthesiology, Texas Children's Hospital, Baylor College of Medicine, Houston, TX, USA

David A. Roberson, MD Division of Pediatric Cardiology, Department of Pediatrics, Advocate Children's Hospital Heart Institute, Oak Lawn, IL, USA

Isobel A. Russell, MD, PhD, FACC Department of Cardiovascular Anesthesiology, Kaiser Permanente, San Francisco, CA, USA

David J. Sahn, MD Division of Cardiology, Department of Pediatrics, Oregon Health and Science University, Portland, OR, USA

Norman H. Silverman, MD, DSc (Med), FACC, FASE, FAHA, FCP(SA) Division of Pediatric Cardiology, Department of Pediatrics, Lucile Packard Children's Hospital, Stanford University School of Medicine, Palo Alto, CA, USA

Theresa Ann Tacy, MD Division of Pediatric Cardiology, Department of Pediatrics, Lucile Packard Children's Hospital, Stanford University School of Medicine, Palo Alto, CA, USA

Roque Ventura, RCS Department of Pediatrics, Miami Children's Hospital, Miami, FL, USA

Pierre C. Wong, MD Division of Cardiology, Children's Hospital Los Angeles, Department of Pediatrics, Keck School of Medicine, University of Southern California, Los Angeles, CA, USA

List of Videos

Video 4.1 Sweep demonstrating slow withdrawal of the TEE probe in the lower esophageal position depicting hepatic veins entering into the inferior vena cava, as seen from the lower esophageal situs short axis view (multiplane angle 0°), and later in the clip, from the lower esophageal IVC long axis view (multiplane angle 71–79°)

Video 4.2 Mid esophageal bicaval view, obtained with a multiplane angle of about 90°. The entrance of the superior vena cava (SVC) into the right atrium is seen. With further probe advancement into the esophagus the entrance of the inferior vena cava (IVC) into the right atrium would be demonstrated. *LA* left atrium, *RA* right atrium, *RAA* right atrial appendage

Video 4.3 Sweep demonstrating a left superior vena cava (LSVC) returning to the coronary sinus. In this patient there is an absent right SVC, with the innominate vein (Inn V) returning to the LSVC, which then drains through a dilated coronary sinus (CS) to the right atrium. From the upper esophageal aortic arch short axis view (multiplane angle about 90°), the probe is turned to the left. It is then advanced to visualize the LSVC returning to the CS. The LSVC courses anterior to the left pulmonary artery (LPA). A catheter is seen in the Inn V and LSVC. *Ao* transverse aortic arch, *LA* left atrium, *LV* left ventricle, *PA* main pulmonary artery

Video 4.4 Right and left pulmonary veins returning to the left atrium, multiplane angle approximately 0°. From a mid esophageal four chamber view, the probe is withdrawn slightly and first rotated to the right, then to the left. For both sides, the lower veins take a more horizontal course (on the display) than the upper veins. On either side, a slight amount of probe advancing/withdrawal can be used to visualize the individual pulmonary veins. *LLPV* left lower pulmonary vein, *LUPV* left upper pulmonary vein, *RLPV* right lower pulmonary vein, *RUPV* right upper pulmonary vein

Video 4.5 Atrial septum as visualized from the mid esophageal view, using imaging and color flow Doppler. The first part of the video is from a mid esophageal four chamber view, multiplane angle 0°, with probe rotation toward the right. Slowly withdrawing and then advancing the probe performs a superior to inferior sweep of the septum. A catheter is seen in the superior vena cava. The second part shows a multiplane angle sweep from 0° to about 85–95°, producing the mid esophageal bicaval view. The right coronary artery can also be seen traversing the atrioventricular groove. *IVC* inferior vena cava, *LA* left atrium, *LV* left ventricle, *RA* right atrium, *RAA* right atrial appendage, *RV* right ventricle, *SVC* superior vena cava

Video 4.6 Atrial septum visualized from the mid-esophagus, with multiplane angle 0°. The probe is rotated to the right, showing both right atrium (RA) and left atrium (LA) and the thin atrial septum primum (*arrow*) located to the left of septum secundum. The right atrial appendage (RAA) is also visible. Withdrawal of the probe demonstrates the superior limbic band of septum secundum, along with the entrance of the superior vena cava (SVC) into the RA, just anterior to the entrance of the right upper pulmonary vein (RUPV) to the LA. *Ao* aorta, *RV* right ventricle

Video 4.7 Left atrial appendage (LAA) and left upper pulmonary vein (LUPV) as seen from a mid esophageal view with probe rotation toward the left, and multiplane angle of 20–30°. *LA* left atrium

Video 4.8 Mid esophageal bicaval view with leftward probe rotation demonstrating a small patent foramen ovale with left to right shunting. *LA* left atrium, *RA* right atrium, *RV* right ventricle

Video 4.9a Contrast injection into a central venous catheter to evaluate for occult atrial right to left shunting. Video shows no right to left shunt at the atrial level

Video 4.9b Contrast injection into a central venous catheter to evaluate for occult atrial right to left shunting. Video shows an occult right to left shunt

Video 4.10 Mid esophageal four chamber view (multiplane angle 0°) showing the atrioventricular valves both by two-dimensional imaging and color flow Doppler

Video 4.11 Mid esophageal mitral commissural view (multiplane angle 60–70°), showing the mitral valve. On the first portion of the video, P1 and P3 scallops of the posterior leaflet, as well as the A2 segment of anterior leaflet, are seen. On the second portion of the video, the papillary muscles can be seen as well as the mitral valve. *LA* left atrium, *LV* left ventricle

Video 4.12 Mid esophageal two chamber view (multiplane angle 94°) showing the mitral valve, left atrium, left ventricle, and left atrial appendage. The papillary muscles are also briefly visualized. At the end of the video, the circumflex coronary artery is also seen coursing along the atrioventricular groove

Video 4.13 Mid esophageal long axis view (multiplane angle 100–130°) showing the anterior leaflet (A2) and posterior (P2) of the mitral valve, as well as the left ventricular outflow tract and aortic valve. In this view, mitral to aortic fibrous continuity is readily seen. *Ao* aorta, *LA* left atrium, *LV* left ventricle, *RV* right ventricle

Video 4.14 Transgastric basal short axis view of the left ventricle in cross section with the mitral valve *en face*. The anterior (Ant leaflet) and posterior leaflets (Post leaflet) of the mitral valve are shown. This view is obtained with the TEE probe in the anteflexed position, using a multiplane angle between 0° and 20°

Video 4.15 Transgastric mid short axis view of the left ventricle (LV) and right ventricle (RV) in cross section. From the position in Video 4.14, the probe has been advanced further in the stomach (while maintaining anteflexion) to visualize the anterolateral (AL) and posteromedial (PM) papillary muscles as well as the more inferior portion of the LV

Video 4.16 Transgastric two-chamber view of the left atrium (LA) and left ventricle (LV). The probe has been advanced into the stomach to the level of the transgastric window, and anteflexed. Using a multiplane angle between 80 and 100°, the LA, LV, and mitral valve leaflets are visualized. The probe is then rotated slightly counterclockwise (to the left) and the multiplane angle changed to 100–110° to visualize the mitral valve chordae and LV papillary muscles

Video 4.17 Transgastric long axis view (multiplane angle 90–120°). The left atrium (LA), left ventricle (LV), mitral valve (MV), aortic valve (AoV), and ascending aorta (Ao) can all be seen. This view provides an excellent view of the LV outflow tract, enabling good color flow Doppler evaluation and providing a favorable angle for spectral Doppler assessment. There is also a limited view of the pulmonary valve seen anterior to the aortic valve

Video 4.18 Visualization of tricuspid valve inflow and right ventricular outflow using a mid esophageal probe position. This mid esophageal right ventricular inflow-outflow view can be obtained using a multiplane angle of 60–90°. *AO* aorta, *LA* left atrium, *MPA* main pulmonary artery, *RA* right atrium, *RV* right ventricle

Video 4.19 Modified transgastric mid/basal short axis view, with the probe anteflexed and turned toward the right (*clockwise*). By adjusting the multiplane angle between 0 and 50°, the tricuspid valve can be seen *en face*. All three tricuspid valve leaflets are visualized: anterior (A), posterior (P), and septal (S). *LV* left ventricle, *RV* right ventricle

Video 4.20 Development of the transgastric right ventricular inflow view. This video first starts with a modified transgastric basal/mid short axis, in which the probe is rotated to the right (*clockwise*) to visualize the right ventricle (RV) and tricuspid valve. The multiplane angle is then rotated from 0° to about 100°, producing the transgastric right ventricular inflow view. The tricuspid valve leaflets, as well as chordae and papillary muscles, are well seen. Slight leftward (*counterclockwise*) probe rotation then visualizes the apical RV and RV outflow tract (RVOT). With further leftward probe rotation, the left ventricular outflow tract (LVOT) is shown. If the probe were rotated even further, a transgastric long axis view might be obtainable, though additional forward rotation of the multiplane angle (to about 100°) might be necessary to achieve this view. *LV* left ventricle, *RA* right atrium

Video 4.21 Modified transgastric right ventricular inflow view. The probe is rotated slightly more rightward to visualize the inflow of superior vena cava (SVC) into the right atrium. Note the excellent angle for spectral interrogation of SVC inflow. *RA* right atrium, *RV* right ventricle

Video 4.22 Evaluation of the ventricular septum in multiple planes in the mid esophagus to display the inlet, membranous, and muscular portions. This assessment requires the use of multiple angles of interrogation from several transducer positions (see text for details). The views shown are obtained by rotating the imaging plane as well as flexing the probe anteriorly and posteriorly at the midesophageal level

Video 4.23 Left ventricular outflow tract as viewed from mid esophageal four chamber view (multiplane angle of 0°) as the probe is anteflexed (also known as the mid esophageal five chamber view), and mid esophageal aortic valve long axis view (multiplane angle about 120°). Both two dimensional imaging and color flow Doppler are used. *LA* left atrium, *LV* left ventricle, *LVOT* left ventricular outflow tract, *RA* right atrium, *RV* right ventricle

Video 4.24a Mid esophageal ascending aortic long axis view provides excellent visualization of the ascending aorta (Asc Ao) in a long axis as it courses anterior to the right pulmonary artery (RPA). This view is very useful for evaluation of supravalvar aortic stenosis, and also for quantitative measurements of the Asc Ao

Video 4.24b Mid esophageal ascending aortic long axis view. With slight leftward (*counterclockwise*) probe rotation, the main pulmonary artery (MPA) can be seen; this view is helpful for assessment of pathology in the supravalvar pulmonary area

Video 4.25 Mid esophageal ascending aortic short axis displays the ascending aorta (Ao) in cross-section. This view is also useful for visualizing the main pulmonary artery (MPA) and right pulmonary artery (RPA), and sometimes the pulmonary valve (*arrow*) can also be seen. *SVC* superior vena cava

Video 4.26 Deep transgastric long axis view with multiplane angle of 0–20°. The left ventricular outflow tract is well seen and there is an excellent angle for spectral Doppler evaluation. This particular image also shows a perimembranous ventricular septal defect. *Ao* aorta, *LA* left atrium, *LV* left ventricle, *RA* right atrium, *RV* right ventricle

Video 4.27 Deep transgastric sagittal view evaluating both right and left ventricular outflow tracts. Multiplane angle of about 90° simulates a transthoracic subcostal sagittal view. Note the favorable angles for spectral Doppler interrogation of flow across both outflow tracts. Some clockwise/counterclockwise (right/left) probe rotation can be helpful to visualize each individual outflow tract. *Ao* ascending aorta, *LV* left ventricle, *PA* main pulmonary artery, *RV* right ventricle

Video 4.28 Deep transgastric sagittal view that simulates a transthoracic subcostal sagittal view. The superior vena cava (SVC) is seen to enter the right atrium (RA), and the left atrium (LA) is also seen, as well as a small atrial septal defect (*arrow*). A catheter tip is present in the RA. Color flow Doppler shows SVC return and left to right flow across the atrial defect

Video 4.29a Aortic valve as viewed *en face* in the mid esophageal aortic valve short axis view, multiplane angle about 35°. Both coronary origins can be well-seen. *AoV* aortic valve, *LA* left atrium, *LCA* left coronary artery, *PA* main pulmonary artery, *RA* right atrium, *RCA* right coronary artery

Video 4.29b Mid esophageal sweep displaying the branches of the left main coronary artery. The sweep starts with a modified long axis view (multiplane angle about 100°) in which the right ventricular (pulmonary) outflow tract is seen and a small portion of the aortic valve. The left main coronary artery is briefly shown in cross section. As the probe is rotated leftward (counterclockwise) from this position, the left anterior descending coronary artery (LAD) is seen. With further leftward probe shaft rotation, the circumflex coronary artery comes into view coursing along the atrioventricular groove

Video 4.30 Mid and upper esophageal views of the great arteries, using a multiplane angle of 0°. Starting first at mid esophageal ascending aorta short axis view, the main pulmonary artery (MPA) and pulmonary valve (PV) are seen along with the ascending aorta (Asc Ao) in cross-section. Turning the probe to the right, the MPA is seen continuing to the right pulmonary artery (RPA), with the superior vena cava (SVC) anterior to the RPA. The probe tip is rotated back to midline and slightly leftward, and when the probe is gradually withdrawn, an upper esophageal aortic arch long axis view is obtained, showing Asc Ao and transverse aortic arch (ARCH). When the probe is advanced slightly and turned to the left, the upper esophageal pulmonary artery long axis view can often be obtained, showing the left pulmonary artery (LPA) just anterior to the aortic arch/descending aorta (Ao). If the probe were then turned back to midline, the MPA and RPA will be seen again, and sometimes the bifurcation of the branch pulmonary arteries

Video 4.31 Upper esophageal aortic arch short axis view (multiplane angle 90–100°). The probe is slowly turned from right to left, showing the innominate vein (Inn V), ascending aorta (Asc Ao), aortic arch (Ao), and main pulmonary artery (MPA). Note the position of the Inn V anterior and superior to the transverse aortic arch. Further leftward probe rotation and slight probe advancement displays the descending aorta (Desc Ao) and left pulmonary artery (LPA)

Video 4.32 Upper esophageal aortic arch short axis sweep (multiplane angle about 90°) used to display the aortic arch vessels, in a patient with a left aortic arch. The transducer is first turned to the right to visualize the ascending aorta (Asc Ao); in this view the innominate artery (Inn Artery) is first seen. As the transducer is rotated toward to the left (*counterclockwise*), the aortic arch (Ao) gives rise to the left common carotid artery (LCCA) and left subclavian artery (LSCA). Note the innominate vein (Inn Vein) seen in cross section (short axis), anterior and superior to the aortic arch. *LPA* left pulmonary artery, *MPA* main pulmonary artery

Video 4.33 Upper esophageal aortic arch long axis view in the patient from Video 4.3 with an absent right superior vena cava. The innominate vein (Inn V) is seen crossing anterior to the aortic arch (Ao) to connect with a left SVC (LSVC), which then drains via a dilated coronary sinus into the right atrium (not shown). A catheter is seen in the Inn V and LSVC

Video 4.34 Descending thoracic aorta views. In the mid esophageal window the probe is rotated to the left (*counterclockwise*) to visualize the aorta. A multiplane angle of 0° displays the descending thoracic aorta (AoDT) in cross section; changing the multiplane angle to 90–110° produces a long axis display of the vessel

Video 5.1a An 11 year old referred for surgical closure of moderate sized secundum atrial septal defect. (**a**) Preoperative mid esophageal four chamber view demonstrates mild right ventricular dilation with qualitatively normal systolic function. Normal left ventricular size and systolic function are also present. In this view the interatrial communication is not displayed

Video 5.1b An 11 year old referred for surgical closure of moderate sized secundum atrial septal defect. Transgastric image demonstrating a short axis view of the left and right ventricles. Note the mild right ventricular dilatation with normal qualitative systolic function. Normal left ventricular size and systolic function are demonstrated as well

Video 5.1c An 11 year old referred for surgical closure of moderate sized secundum atrial septal defect. Postoperative mid esophageal four chamber view demonstrates a smaller right ventricular size after atrial septal defect closure as compared to the preoperative examination (Video 5.1a) with qualitatively normal systolic function. A rhythm disturbance is noted

Video 5.1d An 11 year old referred for surgical closure of moderate sized secundum atrial septal defect. Transgastric image demonstrating a short axis view of the left and right ventricles. Note the normalized right ventricular size and normal biventricular systolic function

Video 5.1e An 11 year old referred for surgical closure of moderate sized secundum atrial septal defect. Postoperative imaging from a transgastric window demonstrating a short axis view of the left ventricle that may allow for quantitative M-mode assessment

Video 5.2a Same patient as Video 5.1. Postoperative mid esophageal four chamber view demonstrates normal right and left ventricular size and systolic function

Video 5.2b Same patient as Video 5.1. Video from transgastric orientation demonstrating a short axis view of the left and right ventricles. Note the normal right ventricular size and normal biventricular systolic function

Video 5.3a A 20 year old with history of tetralogy of Fallot and long-standing severe pulmonary regurgitation. (**a**) Preoperative mid esophageal four chamber demonstrates moderate right ventricular dilatation with qualitatively low normal right ventricular systolic function

Video 5.3b A 20 year old with history of tetralogy of Fallot and long-standing severe pulmonary regurgitation. Deep transgastric sagittal view demonstrating the ventricles. Note the moderate right ventricular dilation with qualitatively low normal systolic function. Normal left ventricular size and systolic function are noted

Video 5.3c A 20 year old with history of tetralogy of Fallot and long-standing severe pulmonary regurgitation. Deep transgastric imaging in the sagittal plane demonstrating the right ventricular outflow tract (RVOT). Note the severe pulmonary regurgitation (*red flow*) into the dilated right ventricle as detected by color flow Doppler. No RVOT obstruction is present (*laminar blue flow*)

Video 5.3d A 20 year old with history of tetralogy of Fallot and long-standing severe pulmonary regurgitation. Multiplane pre-operative imaging (42°) from the transgastric position demonstrating a short axis view of ventricles. Note the orientation of the left ventricle suitable for M-mode assessment

Video 5.3e A 20 year old with history of tetralogy of Fallot and long-standing severe pulmonary regurgitation. Postoperative mid esophageal four chamber view following pulmonary valve replacement demonstrates a lesser degree of right ventricular dilatation as compared to the preoperative examination (5.3a) with qualitatively mildly decreased systolic function

Video 5.3f A 20 year old with history of tetralogy of Fallot and long-standing severe pulmonary regurgitation. Postoperative deep transgastric view in a sagittal plane confirms a lesser degree of right ventricular dilatation as compared to the preoperative examination (5.3c) and qualitatively mild-moderately decreased systolic function

Video 6.1 Transesophageal echocardiographic image of the right atrium viewed in the mid-esophageal bicaval view. The superior vena cava is seen superiorly with a small amount of contrast, and the right pulmonary artery is seen in cross section as it courses behind the SVC. The broad-based right atrial appendage is seen anteriorly

Video 6.2 Image of the left atrium in the midesophageal two chamber view. The left upper pulmonary vein is seen, and directly anterior to this is the entrance of the narrow based left atrial appendage into the left atrium

Video 6.3 The hepatic veins can be seen entering the right atrium in a nearly coronal plane from a transgastric window

Video 6.4 In this view the TEE imaging probe is advanced to a low esophageal position to display the lower esophageal inferior vena cava long axis view as the probe angle is adjusted to the sagittal (90°) plane. The inferior vena cava (*IVC*) is demonstrated and a hepatic vein is seen joining the IVC anteriorly and superiorly

Video 6.5 In the midesophageal four chamber view the probe has been retroflexed within the esophagus to demonstrate the coronary sinus and its relation to the left atrium

Video 6.6 In this image at 0°, the probe has been withdrawn and rotated to the left (counter-clockwise) from the midesophageal four chamber view to demonstrate the relationship of the descending aorta (*DAO*), left pulmonary vein (*LPV*), and left atrial appendage (*LAA*) in a posterior to anterior position

Video 6.7 In this image at 0°, the probe has been rotated rightward (clockwise) in the mid-esophageal four chamber view and advanced slightly within the esophagus to demonstrate the entrance of the right lower pulmonary vein to the left atrium

Video 6.8 A view of the left pulmonary veins from the midesophageal position as they enter the left atrium using an imaging plane of approximately 125°

Video 6.9 A view of the right pulmonary veins from the midesophageal position, with color flow mapping as they join the left atrium. This view can be obtained with rightward rotation of the probe, using an imaging plane of approximately 30–50°

Video 6.10 Midesophageal two chamber view displaying the left atrium and left ventricle. A dilated coronary sinus is demonstrated in its short axis

Video 6.11 View of the coronary sinus in its longitudinal plane. This receives a left superior vena cava as demonstrated by color flow mapping. This view can be obtained by initially obtaining a short axis view of the coronary sinus and rotating the transducer to 60°–80°

Video 6.12 Midesophageal two chamber view demonstrating a coronary sinus atrial septal defect

Video 6.13 Midesophageal bicaval view demonstrates the commitment of a right superior vena cava to the left atrium. Color Doppler demonstrates flow from the superior vena cava entering both the left atrium (*red*) and right atrium (*blue*)

Video 6.14 Equivalent view as depicted in Video 6.4 in a patient with interrupted inferior vena cava with azygous continuation. In this view only the hepatic veins are seen

Video 6.15 In this view the TEE probe is in the low retrocardiac position, and has been rotated posteriorly in the sagittal plane. Two vascular structures are seen coursing adjacent to each other. Color Doppler demonstrates pulsatile flow directed caudally (the descending aorta) anteriorly and a second posterior structure, which has venous flow traveling towards cranially (the azygous vein)

Video 6.16 View of the azygous vein as it travels towards the superior vena cava. At 90°, the distal azygous vein can be seen coursing over the right pulmonary artery seen in its short axis. This is a modified view obtained at the level of the mid esophagus

Video 6.17 From the midesophageal ascending aortic short axis view (angle 0°) a teardrop shape of the superior vena cava indicates an anomalous pulmonary venous connection, in this case of a right upper vein to the superior vena cava

Video 6.18 Deep transgastric view in the sagittal plane demonstrating by color Doppler turbulent flow from a right lower pulmonary vein as it drains into the posterior aspect of the inferior vena cava above the level of the diaphragm

Video 6.19 Transesophageal echocardiogram in an infant with hypoplastic left heart syndrome in the midesophageal four chamber view demonstrating the usual appearance for the septum primum initially however as one withdraws the probe within the esophagus, the septum is seen shifting to a more leftwards position

Video 6.20 This view is oriented to identify the right pulmonary veins. Close relationship between pulmonary veins (red flow) and pulmonary arteries (blue flow) is evident here—the pulmonary artery being directly anterior and usually slightly superior to the pulmonary veins

Video 6.21 The video represents a representative sweep in an infant with total anomalous pulmonary venous connection to the left innominate vein. The exam is initiated at the midesophageal four chamber view. From this window, modified views at the level of the mid esophagus display the right upper and lower pulmonary veins (*RUPV*, *RLPV*) and left pulmonary veins (*LPVs*) are seen returning to a large horizontal confluence. A large vertical vein (*VV*) arises from the left side of the confluence and travels anteriorly and superiorly, coursing over the left pulmonary artery (*LPA*) to insert into the left innominate vein (*Inn V*). The length of the vertical vein is best seen in a sagittal plane, with the midesophageal ascending aortic and upper esophageal aortic arch short axis views, and leftward rotation of the probe. There is no obstruction at any point to pulmonary venous return. A catheter placed in the left internal jugular vein is seen in the vertical vein by two-dimensional imaging. On this video, prominent electrocautery and Doppler mirror image artifacts are seen

Video 6.22 In this midesophageal four chamber view a pulmonary venous confluence is shown adjacent to the left atrium (circular structure)

Video 6.23 Orthogonal view from that shown in Video 6.22. Color Doppler interrogation of pulmonary venous confluence in infant with total anomalous pulmonary venous connection as displayed in the long axis. The blue flow away from the transducer suggests an infradiaphragmatic course

Video 6.24 Mid esophageal four chamber view with clockwise transducer rotation demonstrating direct drainage of a right lower pulmonary vein to the right atrium

Video 6.25 In this midesophageal four chamber view a dilated coronary sinus is seen

Video 6.26 This is an image specifically examining the right pulmonary veins after direct anastomosis of the pulmonary venous confluence to the left atrium. Torsion of the anastomosis resulted in localized narrowing of the right upper pulmonary vein

Video 6.27 Corresponding image to that displayed in Video 6.26 with color flow Doppler across right upper pulmonary vein demonstrating narrowing resulting from torsion of the pulmonary venous confluence to the left atrial anastomosis

Video 6.28 In this midesophageal four chamber view the anastomotic site between the pulmonary venous confluence and left atrium is well seen. This appears widely patent by two-dimensional imaging

Video 6.29 Modified midesophageal bicaval view performed post repair of sinus venosus atrial septal defect. Flow disturbance was seen near the cardiac end of the superior vena cava suggestive of obstruction. This led to further investigation and revision of the repair

Video 7.1 Two-dimensional image of a mid esophageal four chamber view. This cross section represents a starting point in the evaluation of atrial septal defects as it adequately displays both atria, the interatrial septum, atrioventricular valves, and ventricular inflows. Right and left probe shaft rotation in this window optimizes structures of interest

Video 7.2 A centrally located secundum atrial septal defect is displayed in the mid esophageal four chamber view with rightwards probe rotation. Color flow Doppler interrogation demonstrates a moderate amount of left-to-right shunting across the defect (*blue signal*)

Video 7.3 Four chamber view in the mid esophagus (with slight rightwards probe rotation) demonstrates aliasing of color flow Doppler consistent with restrictive flow across a small secundum atrial communication. The interatrial septum bulges towards the right suggesting elevated left atrial pressures

Video 7.4 Sweep of the interatrial septum in a mid esophageal four chamber view with slight rightwards probe rotation. Note that the deficiency in the central aspect of the interatrial septum and the rims around the secundum defect are only seen in portions of this video. This emphasizes the importance of full sweeps when assessing communications at the atrial septum as well as many other defects

Video 7.5 Superior sinus venosus atrial septal defect as seen by withdrawal of the imaging probe above the level of the fossa ovalis from a mid esophageal position. Color Doppler interrogation demonstrates flow across the defect

Video 7.6 Color Doppler image displaying left-to-right shunting across a primum atrial septal defect in the mid esophageal four chamber view. Note the trivial-mild amount of associated right and left atrioventricular valve regurgitation

Video 7.7 Transesophageal view displaying the characteristic broad-based nature of the right atrial appendage. There is also a moderate to large secundum atrial septal defect present

Video 7.8 Cross-sections obtained by turning the imaging probe from the mid esophageal four chamber view clockwise to visualize right-sided structures. Color Doppler demonstrates an intact atrial septum and laminar tricuspid inflow in this video

Video 7.9 Mid esophageal view with clockwise probe shaft rotation to examine the right pulmonary venous connections into the left atrium

Video 7.10 Color flow Doppler in a similar plane as shown in Video 7.9 to assess drainage of the right upper pulmonary vein (*red color flow*) into the left atrium

Video 7.11 Mid esophageal four chamber view obtained with counterclockwise rotation of the imaging probe demonstrates a markedly dilated left atrium, in this case due to mitral regurgitation. Note the abnormal configuration of the interatrial septum from a volume loaded left atrium

Video 7.12 The courses of two left sided pulmonary veins into the left atrium are demonstrated in this sweep. Note the two different orientations of the pulmonary veins as they enter the left atrium

Video 7.13 Color Doppler interrogation as it assists in the characterization of pulmonary venous flow

Video 7.14 Video displays color Doppler imaging of the left upper pulmonary vein as it courses towards the left atrium. A concern for pulmonary vein stenosis was raised from the disturbed color flow signal superimposed on the two-dimensional images. This finding should prompt further evaluation that includes pulsed Doppler interrogation

Video 7.15 Video displays a dilated coronary sinus (seen in cross-section) below the left pulmonary venous inflow. This finding may indicate the presence of a persistent left superior vena cava

Video 7.16 Video obtained with transducer anteflexion as the imaging probe is withdrawn to a nearly mid esophageal aortic valve short axis plane. The left atrial appendage is seen just anterior to the left upper pulmonary vein

Video 7.17 Mid esophageal two chamber view demonstrating the anterior orientation of the left atrial appendage. A mildly dilated coronary sinus is seen posteriorly in cross-section

Video 7.18 Mid esophageal long axis view (multiplane angle 114°) corresponding to the same patient displayed in Video 7.11. This image confirms the large dimensions of the left atrium related to severe mitral regurgitation and displays the left ventricle and aortic root. A mild amount of prolapse of the anterior mitral leaflet is seen

Video 7.19 Video obtained after slightly advancing the probe from the mid esophageal four chamber view. The coronary sinus in seen in long axis as it courses along the atrioventricular groove to drain into the right atrium. This is not to be confused with a primum atrial septal defect

Video 7.20 Contrast echocardiogram obtained following injection of agitated saline into a left arm vein in a patient with a persistent left superior vena cava to coronary sinus connection. Contrast is seen along the dilated coronary sinus as this empties into the right atrium

Video 7.21 Mid esophageal bicaval view displaying the entire atrial septum. The flap valve of the foramen is well seen in this video

Video 7.22 Video of a mid esophageal bicaval view displaying a dilated left atrium with bulging of the interatrial septum towards the right atrium. The inferior vena cava as it enters the right atrium is well seen in this view

Video 7.23 Two-dimensional image of a superior sinus venosus defect as demonstrated in the mid esophageal bicaval view. The superior vena cava is seen straddling the interatrial septum. Color flow Doppler confirms atrial level left-to-right shunting (*blue flow*)

Video 7.24 Small secundum atrial septal defect as shown in the mid esophageal bicaval view. The right atrial appendage is intermittently seen in the video images

Video 7.25 Image demonstrates a high secundum atrial septal defect in the mid esophageal bicaval view by two-dimensional imaging and color flow Doppler

Video 7.26 Large secundum atrial septal defect with associated left-to-right shunting. Note the slightly more inferior location of this defect as compared to the atrial communication illustrated in a similar imaging plane in Video 7.25

Video 7.27 Mid esophageal bicaval view displaying a superior sinus venosus atrial septal defect by two-dimensional imaging (*left video*) and color flow interrogation (*right video*). Left-to-right shunting is seen across the defect (*blue flow*). Note the red color Doppler signal entering the area of the defect representing anomalous drainage of the right upper pulmonary vein. Video courtesy of Thomas M. Burch, MD

Video 7.28 Video of a mid esophageal right ventricular inflow-outflow view. This cross-section is useful in the comprehensive assessment of atrial septal defects as it displays the tricuspid valve, left atrium, right atrial and right ventricular sizes, right ventricular inflow and outflow tract, pulmonary valve, and proximal main pulmonary artery. In this example there is also a large secundum atrial septal defect. Mild tricuspid valve septal leaflet prolapse is also noted

Video 7.29 Transgastric mid short axis view demonstrating a large, volume loaded right ventricle in a patient with a large atrial septal defect

Video 7.30 Deep transgastric sagittal images of the atrial septum displaying two-dimensional and color information. The interatrial septum appears to be intact in this case

Video 7.31 Images obtained in the same cross-sections as shown in Video 7.30. In this example, the presence of a secundum atrial septal defect is demonstrated by two-dimensional imaging and color Doppler

Video 7.32 The video displays a modified plane in the deep transgastric window that also allows for echocardiographic assessment of the interatrial septum. This view is similar to a transthoracic subcostal echocardiographic view

Video 7.33 Video of an inferior sinus venosus atrial septal defect as obtained from a modified deep transgastric sagittal view (same view as shown in Videos 7.30 and 7.31). Note the deficiency in the lower aspect of the interatrial septum and the presence of left-to-right shunting across the defect by color Doppler imaging. The Eustachian valve is also seen. Additional planes in this window may provide information regarding associated anomalies of pulmonary venous drainage

Video 7.34 Mid esophageal images in orthogonal planes obtained with a three-dimensional imaging probe to assess right ventricular size and function. The images demonstrate right ventricular dilation with low normal systolic function

Video 7.35 Images demonstrate an aneurysm of the interatrial septum as shown by two-dimensional imaging (*left panel*), color flow mapping (*middle panel*), and contrast echocardiography (*right panel*). Injection of agitated saline into a lower extremity vein was performed to assess for the presence of a patent foramen ovale in a child with a history of multiple strokes

Video 7.36 Transesophageal imaging sequence capturing the steps involved during radiofrequency perforation of the interatrial septum in a critically ill infant with hypoplastic left heart syndrome and an intact atrial septum. The images were acquired in the mid esophageal bicaval view and modified cross-sections that allowed for transesophageal monitoring during the procedure as follows: (1) intact atrial septum with hypertensive left atrium (*LA*) and bulging of the interatrial septum towards the right atrium; (2) catheter advanced across inferior vena cava and positioned against atrial septum; (3) catheter perforation of interatrial septum (note image artifact during radiofrequency perforation and microbubbles in the LA once chamber is entered); (4) an exchange wire is advanced well into the LA; (5) a stent is positioned across the septum over a balloon and deployed straddling the interatrial septum; (6) color and spectral interrogation are performed to document flow thought the stent and confirm adequacy of the intervention

Video 7.37 Mid esophageal four chamber imaging with color flow Doppler interrogation to assess the results of the surgical intervention following patch closure of a secundum atrial septal defect. A trivial signal of tricuspid regurgitation (physiologic) is seen

Video 7.38 Video displays the post surgical evaluation of a secundum atrial septal defect in the mid esophageal bicaval plane. No residual shunting is detected across the patch

Video 7.39 Video depicts the abnormal orientation of the interatrial septum in the mid esophageal four chamber view in a patient with juxtaposed left atrial appendages

Video 7.40 Video displays the abnormal position of the right atrial appendage in the mid esophageal four chamber view as it extends to lie next to the left atrial appendage in left juxtaposition of the atrial appendages. The abnormal orientation of the interatrial septum is also appreciated in these images

Video 7.41 Deep transgastric long axis sweep performed to further assess the anatomy/orientation of the atrial appendages in the infant shown in Videos 7.39 and 7.40 with juxtaposition of the atrial appendages. Note that as the imaging plane moves posteriorly the left-deviated right atrial appendage is seen as it courses behind the great arteries to lie next to the left atrial appendage (left juxtaposition). Associated defects in this patient included double outlet right ventricle/malposed great arteries (Taussig Bing Anomaly). Note the prominent left coronary artery anterior to the right atrial appendage

Video 7.42 Cor triatriatum membrane as seen in the mid esophageal four and two chamber views by two-dimensional and color flow imaging. Although the membrane appears rather thick, the relatively laminar nature of the color Doppler signal does not suggest significant obstruction across this region

Video 7.43 In contrast to the images shown in Video 7.42, the cor triatriatum membrane in this patient was of an obstructive nature. Note the division of the left atrium by the membrane into proximal and distal portions. Color Doppler displays aliased flow across a small orifice for the egress of blood across the proximal atrial chamber. Spectral Doppler demonstrates lack of the normal phasic flow pattern across venous structures

Video 7.44 In this mid esophageal sweep it is seen that the left atrial appendage lies below the level of the membrane in cor triatriatum. This is in contrast to a supravalvar mitral ring where the appendage lies above the membrane

Video 7.45 Sweep across several planes at the mid esophageal level displaying a severely dilated left atrial chamber proximal to a cor triatriatum membrane. A small eccentric posteriorly located orifice is seen measuring 5.7 mm. Note the aliased color flow consistent with severe obstruction across this area

Video 8.1 Video displays a complete atrioventricular septal defect in the mid esophageal four chamber view. The atrial (*short arrow*) and ventricular (*long arrow*) communications are seen. *LA* left atrium, *LV* left ventricle, *RA* right atrium, *RV* right ventricle

Video 8.2 Deep transgastric view demonstrating a common atrioventricular valve *en face*. All the components of the common atrioventricular valve are seen in this view including the superior bridging leaflet with attachments to the crest of the septum (Rastelli type A)

Video 8.3 Deep transgastric images at 55° display *en face* view of common atrioventricular valve in a complete atrioventricular septal defect

Video 8.4 Transthoracic parasternal short axis image demonstrating a cleft in left atrioventricular valve pointing toward the inlet septum in an atrioventricular septal defect

Video 8.5 Transgastric basal short axis view demonstrating a cleft in left atrioventricular valve (*arrow*). *LV* left ventricle, *RV* right ventricle

Video 8.6 Mid esophageal long axis view displaying a cleft in the left-sided component of a common atrioventricular valve (*arrow*). This is associated with abnormal motion of this region of the valve as shown. In this defect the cleft points towards the septum. *Ao* aorta, *LA* left atrium, *LV* left ventricle, *RV* right ventricle

Video 8.7 Deep transgastric sagittal view in a child with a complete atrioventricular septal defect and double-orifice of the left component of the atrioventricular valve. In diastole, the common atrioventricular valve orifice is seen *en face* with its left (*arrows*) and right components. A separate valvar area of double orifice is seen over the left ventricle. *LV* left ventricle, *PA* pulmonary artery, *RV* right ventricle

Video 8.8 Mid esophageal four chamber view of an atrioventricular septal defect. Color Doppler depicts shunting across two atrial communications (ostium primum and ostium secundum defects). Shunting across a small ventricular septal defect is also seen. *LA* left atrium, *LV* left ventricle, *RA* right atrium, *RV* right ventricle

Video 8.9 A large secundum atrial septal defect is seen (*arrow*) in association with an atrioventricular septal defect. Color interrogation confirms atrial level left-to-right shunting. A turbulent color flow signal is identified in the left atrium corresponding to a jet of left atrioventricular valve regurgitation (not fully displayed in the video). *LA* left atrium, *LV* left ventricle, *RA* right atrium, *RV* right ventricle

Video 8.10 Video displays large ventricular component (*arrow*) of a complete atrioventricular septal defect. Note the right ventricular wall thickness reflecting the elevated pulmonary artery pressure that characterizes this type of lesion. *LA* left atrium, *LV* left ventricle, *RA* right atrium, *RV* right ventricle

Video 8.11 Deep transgastric long axis view depicting shunting across the ventricular component of an atrioventricular septal defect (*arrow*). *Ao* aorta, *LV* left ventricle, *RV* right ventricle

Video 8.12 Mid esophageal four chamber view depicting a ventricular septal defect of the 'atrioventricular canal-type'. In this defect separate atrioventricular valve orifices were present and the atrial communication was of the secundum-type. Several chordal attachments (*arrows*) are seen from the atrioventricular valves to the crest of the ventricular septum. Note the lack of normal offsetting of the atrioventricular valves. *LA* left atrium, *LV*, left ventricle, *RA* right atrium, *RV* right ventricle

Video 8.13 The 'goose neck' deformity of the left ventricular outflow tract that characterizes atrioventricular septal defects is shown in this deep transgastric sagittal view. *Ao* aorta, *LA* left atrium, *LV* left ventricle

Video 8.14 Modified mid esophageal four chamber view with anterior transducer angulation displaying chordal attachments of the left atrioventricular valve across the left ventricular outflow tract onto the interventricular septum (*arrow*). In some cases this can result in outflow tract obstruction. *Ao* aorta, *LA* left atrium, *LV* left ventricle

Video 8.15 The video displays unbalanced atrioventricular septal defects (right and left ventricular dominant types) as noted

Video 8.16 Mid esophageal four chamber view displays a tricuspid pouch lesion (*arrow*) in a patient with a partial atrioventricular septal defect. *LA* left atrium, *LV* left ventricle, *RA* right atrium, *RV* right ventricle

Video 8.17 The video displays a complete atrioventricular septal defect in different transesophageal echocardiographic cross-sections. Two-dimensional imaging depicts the anatomical features of the defect. Color flow mapping demonstrates interatrial and interventricular shunting in addition to a significant regurgitant jet across the left component of the common atrioventricular valve. The characteristics of the regurgitant jet are further defined by multiplane imaging, highlighting the importance of color Doppler interrogation in multiple views

Video 8.18 Preoperative mid esophageal four chamber view displaying a partial atrioventricular septal defect. The atrial ostium primum defect is well seen and tissue tags are noted on the right ventricular aspect of the septum (no evidence of ventricular level shunting seen). Color Doppler interrogation demonstrates two jets originating from the left ventricle. One jet is diverted by atrial septal tissue into both atria and a second one is directed from the left ventricle into the right atrium (left ventricular to right atrial shunt)

Video 8.19 The image shows preoperative color flow information obtained in a mid esophageal four chamber view using a pediatric biplane transesophageal probe in a small infant with a complete atrioventricular septal defect. Significant regurgitation is demonstrated from both the left and right atrioventricular valvar components, during systole

Video 8.20 Deep transgastric long axis view in infant with Down syndrome and 'tet-canal defect'. Note the free-floating superior bridging leaflet of the common atrioventricular valve (Rastelli type C defect). The characteristic aortic override in tetralogy of Fallot is well seen

Video 8.21 Postoperative transesophageal echocardiogram following repair of a complete atrioventricular septal defect. Color Doppler interrogation demonstrates two small jets of left atrioventricular valve regurgitation. The jet closest to the interatrial septum represents regurgitation across a residual cleft

Video 8.22 Mid esophageal long axis view displaying mitral valve stenosis resulting from cleft closure following repair of an atrioventricular septal defect. The left atrium appears dilated. Narrowing of the left ventricular outflow tract is also noted in association with multiple chordal attachments across the subaortic region onto the ventricular septum. Color flow information superimposed on the morphologic data shows a turbulent jet across the left ventricular inflow corresponding to mitral stenosis. The disturbed systolic color flow signal across the left ventricular outflow tract also confirms the subaortic obstruction. A small jet of aortic regurgitation is noted. The coronary sinus appears mildly dilated

Video 8.23 Preoperative transesophageal echocardiogram in an infant requiring reoperation to address a residual inlet ventricular septal defect as well as significant regurgitation across a large left atrioventricular valve cleft related to suture dehiscence Both lesions are well characterized by color flow imaging in the mid esophageal four chamber view

Video 8.24 Deep transgastric long axis view obtained following repair of an atrioventricular septal defect. The image displays interrogation of the left ventricular outflow tract using a combination of Doppler modalities (color flow mapping and spectral Doppler). No evidence of obstruction was demonstrated. Note the favorable angle for pulsed wave Doppler interrogation of the outflow tract in this view. *Ao* aorta, *LV* left ventricle, *RV* right ventricle

Video 8.25 Postbypass transesophageal echocardiogram obtained in the mid esophageal four chamber view demonstrates flow by color Doppler from the left atrium (LA) into the right ventricle (RV; blue jet). This communication, representing a left-to-right shunt, was inadvertently created during surgical repair of the defect. The echocardiographic findings led to revision of the repair. *LV* left ventricle, *RA* right atrium

Video 8.26 The initial portion of the video displays a mid esophageal four chamber view obtained immediately after separation from bypass following repair of a complete atrioventricular septal defect. Both atrial and ventricular septal patches are well seen. A contrast study was performed to evaluate a small color Doppler signal suggestive of residual ventricular level shunting (not shown). Agitated saline injected through a femoral venous catheter demonstrated opacification of the right atrium with unexpected almost immediate appearance of contrast in the superior aspect of the left atrium. The findings were thought to be suggestive of mistaken partial incorporation of inferior vena cava flow into the left atrium (right-to-left shunt). This was confirmed upon return to bypass and after surgical revision (postbypass #2) a similar contrast injection demonstrated the expected normal flow pattern and no residual shunts. *LA* left atrium, *LV* left ventricle, *RA* right atrium, *RV* right ventricle

Video 8.27 Three-dimensional image obtained by transesophageal echocardiography in an older child displaying *en face* view of a complete atrioventricular septal defect (Video by courtesy of David A. Roberson, M.D.)

Video 8.28 Mid esophageal four chamber view displaying an abnormal mitral valve. The mitral valve exhibits grossly abnormal leaflets with reduced diastolic excursion. Small ridges on the leaflets could be construed as a supravalvar mitral ring. Color Doppler imaging demonstrates a turbulent color jet across the mitral valve. The degree of flow velocity acceleration is significant, reaching the left ventricular apex before it turns round, while maintaining its dimensions until distorted by the apical wall. This finding indicates the significant severity of the obstruction. *LA* left atrium, *LV* left ventricle, *RA* right atrium, *RV* right ventricle

Video 8.29 Video displays a mid esophageal four chamber view in a child with a mitral stenosis. The distorted funnel-shaped mitral valve inflow is seen. A tiny ridge at the posterior annulus is suggestive of a supravalvar mitral ring. The left atrium appears substantially enlarged

Video 8.30 Transgastric imaging in the mid left ventricular short axis and two chamber views demonstrates a single posteromedial papillary muscle in a child with a parachute mitral valve deformity

Video 8.31 Transesophageal echocardiogram depicts a supravalvar mitral ring (*arrow*). The pathology is well seen in orthogonal views that display the mitral inflow (mid esophageal four chamber and two chamber views). Color Doppler demonstrates flow acceleration at the level of the mitral valve annulus and a small jet of mitral regurgitation. *LA* left atrium, *LV* left ventricle, *RA* right atrium, *RV* right ventricle

Video 8.32 The images display a supravalvar mitral ring as viewed from the mid esophageal mitral valve commissural view obtained at 60°. The supravalvar ridges (*arrows*) that characterize this lesion are shown. Note the dilated left atrium (LA). *LV* left ventricle (Video by courtesy of Louis I. Bezold, M.D.)

Video 8.33 Mid esophageal long axis view recorded from the same infant depicted in Video 8.32 demonstrates a supravalvar ring and reduced diastolic excursion of the mitral valve leaflets. Aliasing of the color flow signal at the mitral inflow confirms the obstruction. Associated lesions included aortic valve stenosis, a subaortic ridge, and, a perimembranous ventricular septal defect. *Ao* aorta, *LA* left atrium, *LV* left ventricle, *RV* right ventricle (Video by courtesy of Louis I. Bezold, M.D.)

Video 8.34 Mid esophageal four chamber view displaying flow convergence between the left atrium and left ventricle due to a supravalvar mitral ring. Additionally, two jets of mitral inflow in diastole are seen corresponding to two areas of stenosis in this abnormal mitral valve. A regurgitant mitral jet is also evident. A small amount of aortic regurgitation is also seen

Video 8.35 Transthoracic left ventricular parasternal short axis image depicting a double-orifice mitral valve

Video 8.36 Mid esophageal two chamber view depicting a double-orifice mitral valve. Two-dimensional imaging shows two distinct valvar orifices during diastole. Color flow appears more prominent across the more posterior valvar opening, which also displays a small jet of regurgitation. No evidence of obstruction is detected across the valve by color Doppler (confirmed by pulsed wave Doppler interrogation in the mid esophageal four chamber view)

Video 8.37 Transgastric basal short axis view displays the mitral valve *en face*. The cleft (*arrow*) is associated with mitral regurgitation as depicted by color Doppler imaging. *LV* left ventricle, *RV* right ventricle

Video 8.38 Multiplane imaging of the mitral valve demonstrating restricted diastolic valvar motion and marked thickening of the leaflets and support apparatus. The leaflets appear to insert directly into bulky subvalvar structures without definitive chordae, suggesting the presence of a mitral arcade (confirmed at surgery). Color Doppler demonstrates aliased flow across through an eccentric opening and a mitral regurgitant jet

Video 8.39 Transesophageal echocardiogram depicting a straddling mitral valve in a child with double outlet right ventricle. The sweep starts at the mid esophageal four chamber view. As the transducer is anteflexed from a posterior position a ventricular septal defect comes into view. At this level, chordal attachments from the mitral valve are seen to straddle the ventricular septum and insert on the right ventricular aspect near the crest of the ventricular septum. The abnormal, side-by-side spatial orientation of the great arteries is depicted. A secundum atrial septal defect is seen. The deep transgastric long axis view demonstrates abnormal mitral valve chordal structures along the pathway from the left ventricle to adjacent great artery (aortic root)

Video 8.40 Multiplane examination in the mid esophageal and transgastric views in infant with congenital mitral regurgitation. Two-dimensional imaging demonstrates the dysplastic and thickened valve leaflets with rolled edges that coapt poorly. A broad mitral regurgitant jet is seen coursing along the posterolateral aspect of the left atrium. Severe left atrial dilation is seen with shifting of the interatrial septum in the left to right direction consistent with left atrial hypertension

Video 8.41 The characteristic features of Ebstein anomaly are displayed in this mid esophageal four chamber view including: apical septal leaflet displacement, redundancy of the anterior leaflet, and atrialization of the right ventricle. The anterior, 'sail-like' leaflet prolapses mildly into the right atrium. Although the left ventricle is not well seen, the right ventricle appears to be the dominant ventricular chamber in this patient

Video 8.42 Mid esophageal four chamber view of severe form of Ebstein anomaly displaying adherence of the tricuspid septal leaflet to the underlying myocardium and tethering of chordal structures. The marked redundancy of the anterior leaflet is seen. The valvar coaptation point is displaced well into the apex of the right ventricle (*RV*). The deep transgastric sagittal view depicts the degree of atrialization of the right ventricle (*aRV*). Note the small size of the 'true' or 'functional' RV. *LA* left atrium, *LV* left ventricle, *RA* right atrium

Video 8.43 Mid esophageal four chamber view demonstrating bulging of the interventricular septum towards the left ventricle (*LV*), resulting in narrowing of the left ventricular outflow tract (LVOT; *arrow*) and a "pancaked" appearance of the LV. *Ao* aorta, *LA* left atrium, *RV* right ventricle

Video 8.44 Mid esophageal four chamber view displaying an abnormal tricuspid valve (thickened and dysplastic leaflets) with associated severe regurgitation. The images show an exaggerated degree of normal offset of the atrioventricular valves onto the septum suggesting a more likely diagnosis of Ebstein anomaly over that of tricuspid valvar dysplasia, where normally hinged leaflets are present. *LA* left atrium, *LV* left ventricle, *RA* right atrium, *RV* right ventricle

Video 9.1 Mid esophageal four chamber view (multiplane angle 0°) of a perimembranous ventricular septal defect partially occluded by tricuspid valve aneurysmal tissue, using both two dimensional imaging as well as and color flow Doppler

Video 9.2 Modified mid esophageal right ventricular inflow-outflow view, multiplane angle 53°, with anteflexion of the TEE probe. This view, which is comparable to an inverted transthoracic parasternal short axis view, shows a large perimembranous ventricular septal defect with aneurysmal tricuspid valve tissue, using both two dimensional imaging as well as color flow Doppler

Video 9.3 Mid esophageal four chamber view (multiplane angle 0°) of a large inlet ventricular septal defect, using both two dimensional imaging as well as color flow Doppler

Video 9.4a Transgastric mid short axis view (multiplane angle 0°) of a moderate size mid-muscular ventricular septal defect, using both two dimensional imaging as well as color flow Doppler

Video 9.4b Mid esophageal four chamber view (multiplane angle 0°) of a mid-muscular ventricular septal defect in a patient with D-transposition of the great arteries, using both two dimensional imaging as well as color flow Doppler. Note the flow by color Doppler from the right ventricle to the left ventricle

Video 9.5 Mid esophageal four chamber view (multiplane angle 0°) of a small apical ventricular septal defect which was difficult to appreciate by two dimensional imaging, but was easily seen with color flow Doppler

Video 9.6 Mid esophageal four chamber view (multiplane angle 0°) with probe retroflexion demonstrating two muscular ventricular septal defects, a large perimembranous/inlet muscular defect, and a smaller defect near the apex, as seen by two dimensional imaging as well as color flow Doppler. During the study, the probe is advanced and anteflexed to visualize the muscular defects

Video 9.7 Larger inlet/muscular and apical ventricular septal defects, as noted from the mid esophageal four chamber view (multiplane angle 0°) and retroflexion of the TEE probe. Both two-dimensional imaging and color flow Doppler are used

Video 9.8 Mid esophageal long axis view (105–122°) to modified mid esophageal right ventricular inflow-outflow view sweep of a perimembranous ventricular septal defect with attention to the right ventricular outflow tract. No outflow tract obstruction is present. With probe retroflexion and a multiplane angle of 25-30°, the ventricular septal defect is visible and appears partially covered by tricuspid valve tissue

Video 9.9 Mid esophageal 0° and 90° views of a supracristal ventricular septal defect, showing both two-dimensional imaging and color flow Doppler. The RV inflow-outflow view at 90° demonstrates deficiency of conal septum, and fibrous continuity between the aortic and pulmonary valves. Note the right coronary cusp of aortic valve protruding through the defect

Video 9.10 Mid esophageal modified aortic valve short axis (0°) and long axis (88–103°) views of a malalignment ventricular septal defect in a patient with tetralogy of Fallot. The aortic valve overrides the ventricular septum by approximately 50 % and forms the "roof" of the defect

Video 9.11 Deep transgastric sweep of a perimembranous ventricular septal defect from a long axis (0°) and Sagittal (90°) view, as noted by two dimensional imaging and color flow Doppler

Video 9.12 Double chambered right ventricle (RV) as seen first from a modified mid esophageal RV inflow-outflow view (multiplane angle 75°) and then from a deep transgastric sagittal view (multiplane angle about 70°). Note the prominent muscle bundles and mid-cavitary RV narrowing (shown by *). The mid esophageal view also shows left to right shunting across a perimembranous ventricular septal defect. *AoV* aortic valve, *LA* left atrium, *LV* left ventricle, *PA* pulmonary artery, *RVOT* right ventricular outflow tract

Video 10.1 Hypoplastic left heart syndrome, as viewed from the mid esophageal four chamber view. The hypoplastic left-sided cardiac structures and the atrial septum are well seen from this view. Rotation of the imaging plane to approximately 90° affords a long axis visualization of the ascending aorta

Video 10.2 Pulmonary atresia/intact ventricular septum, also known as hypoplastic right heart, as viewed from the mid esophageal position, multiplane angle rotated between 0° and 100°. The right ventricular cavity is small, muscular, and non-apex forming; there is an underdeveloped trabecular portion. The pulmonary valve is present but imperforate. By color flow Doppler, no antegrade flow is seen across the pulmonary valve. There is significant tricuspid regurgitation

Video 10.3 Tricuspid atresia, normally related great arteries, using a combination of mid and upper esophageal views, multiplane angle 0°. First, the equivalent of the mid esophageal four chamber view is obtained. There is no visible tricuspid valve, only a muscular shelf, and a hypoplastic right ventricular chamber. A small ventricular septal defect or bulboventricular foramen is noted, with turbulent left to right shunting. Withdrawal and slight anteflexion of the TEE probe demonstrates the aortic valve arising from the left ventricle, and with further withdrawal of the probe to the upper esophageal pulmonary artery long axis view, the main and left pulmonary arteries are seen arising from the hypoplastic right ventricle (the right pulmonary artery is not well-seen on this particular study). In this video there is a redundant, mobile atrial septum seen

Video 10.4 Tricuspid atresia with D-transposed great arteries, using the mid esophageal long axis view and a multiplane angle of 90°. This shows the aorta arising from a small anterior right ventricular outflow chamber. The bulboventricular foramen/ventricular septal defect (BVF/VSD) is noted by the *arrow*. *LA* left atrium, *LV* left ventricle, *PA* pulmonary artery, *RV* right ventricle, *Ao* Aorta

Video 10.5 Double inlet left ventricle, normally related great arteries (Holmes' heart) as viewed from the equivalent of the mid esophageal four chamber view. A multiplane angle of 30° is used to visualize both atrioventricular valves (mild regurgitation of both valves is identified by color Doppler). Rotation of multiplane angle to approximately 40° and probe tip anteflexion demonstrates the mid esophageal aortic valve short axis view, with the origin of the pulmonary artery from the right ventricle. Withdrawal of the probe (multiplane angle about 0°) and tip anteflexion produce the upper esophageal pulmonary artery long axis view. Aliased flow across a distally placed pulmonary artery band is present, and spectral Doppler interrogation documents a 51 mmHg gradient across this region

Video 10.6 Double inlet, double outlet right ventricle, obtained from the equivalent of the mid esophageal four chamber view. Both right and left atrioventricular valves drain into the right ventricle and insert into a large, bizarre papillary muscle in the mid esophageal four chamber view. There is a hypoplastic left sided left ventricle. As the probe is withdrawn into an upper esophageal position, both arterial roots are seen in short axis with the anterior vessel (aorta) giving rise to the left main coronary artery. As the multiplane angle is rotated to about 90°, the mid esophageal long axis view shows the abnormal ventriculo-arterial connection (double outlet) and spatial great artery relationship (parallel). These abnormalities are also confirmed in the deep transgastric sagittal views

Video 10.7 Double inlet left ventricle, D-transposed great arteries, following pulmonary artery band. The mid esophageal long axis view (multiplane angle 117°) demonstrates the long axis of both outflow tracts, as well as the ventricular septal defect/bulboventricular foramen. Flow across the pulmonary artery band is identified by color flow Doppler

Video 10.8 Pre-Fontan study in a patient with right isomerism (asplenia) and double outlet right ventricle/pulmonary atresia and unbalanced atrioventricular canal, right dominant. Withdrawal of the probe from lower esophageal situs short axis view to mid esophageal four chamber position (multiplane angle 0°) demonstrates that the inferior vena cava receives the right hepatic veins and returns to the right atrium. The pulmonary veins are also seen to return to the right sided atrium

Video 10.9 Separate entrances of the right and left hepatic veins (patient from Video 10.8). Withdrawal of the probe from lower esophageal situs short axis view to mid esophageal four chamber position (multiplane angle 0°) demonstrates that the inferior vena cava receives the right hepatic veins and returns to the right atrium in the normal manner; however, the left sided hepatic veins return separately and directly to the left sided atrium

Video 10.10 Right modified Blalock-Taussig shunt, visualized from upper esophageal pulmonary artery long axis view, multiplane angle 0°, showing continuous flow entering the small right pulmonary artery (MPG 3240 kb)

Video 10.11 Evaluation of pulmonary artery band in a patient with D-transposed great arteries and a ventricular septal defect. The band is well-seen using two-dimensional imaging and color flow Doppler, as seen from the mid esophageal long axis view (multiplane angle 80–110°) and deep transgastric long axis view (multiplane angle approximately 0°). The deep transgastric window provides for an excellent angle for Doppler interrogation across the pulmonary artery band, with a peak gradient of approximately 84 mmHg. *Ao* aorta, *PV* pulmonary valve

Video 10.12 Damus-Kaye-Stansel anastomosis as viewed from mid to upper esophageal view, multiplane angle 80–90°. The widely patent anastomosis (shown by the arrow) lies just above the semilunar valves. *Ao* native aorta, *PA* native pulmonary artery

Video 10.13 Problematic Damus-Kaye-Stansel (DKS) repair in a patient with situs inversus, congenitally corrected transposition of the great arteries and hypoplastic right ventricle, as viewed from the mid esophageal long axis view. The creation of the DKS anastomosis resulted in distortion of the native pulmonary valve, producing significant pulmonary regurgitation (posterior great artery) and trace aortic regurgitation (anterior great artery). The ventricular function was severely compromised. A large subepicardial hematoma occurred as the result of external cardiac massage

Video 10.14 Patient with hypoplastic left heart syndrome variant, following Norwood-Sano procedure. The anastomosis between a relatively good size native aorta (Ao) and native pulmonary artery (PA) is well seen from the mid esophageal view long axis view. A few frames showing pulsatile Sano conduit flow are seen toward the end of the study. Though not well-shown in this video, the Sano conduit is positioned in the typical location along the anterior aspect of the right ventricle (RV), arising from the RV outflow tract just below the neo-aortic valve (old pulmonary valve). *Ao* native aorta, *PA* pulmonary artery

Video 10.15 The Sano shunt (right ventricle to pulmonary artery conduit) shown from the upper esophageal pulmonary artery long axis view, multiplane angle approximately 0°. Color Doppler shows aliased to and fro flow seen in the Sano conduit (also shown on the spectral Doppler tracing); this flow is also seen in both branch pulmonary arteries

Video 10.16 Right bidirectional cavopulmonary (Glenn) anastomosis as viewed from the mid esophageal ascending aortic long axis view with rightward probe rotation, multiplane angle 95°. The anastomosis is well seen by imaging and color flow Doppler. *RPA* right pulmonary artery, *SVC* superior vena cava (MPG 5242 kb)

Video 10.17 Atriopulmonary Fontan, as seen from the mid esophageal four chamber view in a patient with double inlet left ventricle and L-malposed great arteries. Note the severely dilated right atrium with sluggish flow demonstrated as swirling (also known as spontaneous echo contrast). The atriopulmonary connection is shown by two-dimensional imaging and color flow Doppler, as the probe is rotated leftwards

Video 10.18 Atriopulmonary Fontan in a patient with tricuspid atresia, showing a severely dilated right atrium (*RA*) completely filled with thrombus. Note the dilated coronary sinus (CS). *LA* left atrium, *LV* left ventricle

Video 10.19 Lateral tunnel Fontan connection in a patient with double inlet left ventricle, as seen from the transgastric, lower and mid esophageal positions. With a multiplane angle of 0°, the lateral tunnel is seen in cross-section as a sweep is performed inferiorly to superiorly (a catheter is seen in the upper portion of the tunnel). Rotation of the multiplane angle to 90° shows the entire length of the tunnel and the Glenn anastomosis more superiorly. *LV* left ventricle

Video 10.20 Extracardiac Fontan with a patent fenestration, as viewed from 0° mid esophageal four chamber view. Right to left shunting is clearly seen by color flow Doppler into the physiologic "left" atrium

Video 10.21 Extracardiac Fontan conduit placed between a right sided IVC and the left pulmonary artery in a patient with heterotaxy and dextrocardia. TEE evaluation was performed as a sweep from lower to mid to upper esophageal positions, using a multiplane angle of 0°. As it passes to the left, the conduit compresses the pulmonary veins, causing pulmonary venous obstruction (mean gradient 8 mmHg) that had previously led to a low cardiac output state, and may have contributed to the development of thrombus within the conduit

Video 11.1a Deep transgastric long axis view at 0° showing the left ventricular outflow tract

Video 11.1b Deep transgastric sagittal view at 90° showing the right ventricular outflow tract

Video 11.2 Three-dimension mid esophageal aortic valve short axis view depicting the three-dimensional nature of a normal trileaflet aortic valve

Video 11.3 Mid esophageal aortic valve long axis view at 120° showing the left ventricular outflow tract

Video 11.4 Mid esophageal aortic valve short axis view at ~30° shows a true bicuspid aortic valve with only two leaflets (the right and left coronary leaflets) and absent non-coronary leaflet, giving a "fishmouth" appearance to the valve orifice. Color flow Doppler shows turbulence across the valve, as well as the origin of the left coronary artery seen posteriorly, and a brief glimpse of the right coronary artery seen anteriorly

Video 11.5 Mid esophageal aortic valve short axis view at 30° showing a bicuspid aortic valve with fusion or underdevelopment of the intercoronary commissure

Video 11.6 Mid esophageal aortic valve short axis view at 30° showing a bicuspid aortic valve with fusion or underdevelopment of the commissure between the right and non-coronary leaflets

Video 11.7 Mid esophageal aortic valve short axis view at 30° of a dysplastic aortic valve with thickened right and non coronary leaflets

Video 11.8 Mid esophageal aortic valve long axis view at 120° showing a dysplastic aortic valve associated with valvar aortic stenosis

Video 11.9 Transcatheter aortic valve replacement/implantation (TAVR/TAVI). This video, obtained from a mid esophageal aortic valve long axis view at 120–130° first shows the abnormal aortic valve, which is thickened and has restricted motion. A catheter and then the balloon-mounted valve are seen, with the balloon shown as it is expanded and the valve implanted in the aortic position. During balloon dilation, rapid ventricular pacing is performed to reduce ventricular ejection, thereby stabilizing the valve for placement. Following valve implantation, leaflet motion is seen and there are two jets of regurgitation seen—one central (transvalvular), one peripheral (paravalvular). *LM* left main coronary artery (Video provided courtesy of Siemens Medical Systems USA, Inc. © 2012–13 Siemens Medical Solutions USA, Inc. All rights reserved)

Video 11.10 Mid esophageal four chamber view with probe anteflexion to visualize the left ventricular outflow tract. This video shows a subaortic fibromuscular ridge associated with subvalvar aortic stenosis, depicting a steep aorto-septal angle and extension of the fibromuscular ridge to the anterior mitral leaflet. Color Doppler demonstrates flow aliasing originating at the region of the ridge or membrane

Video 11.11 Systolic anterior motion (SAM) of the mitral valve, in a patient with pronounced ventricular septal hypertrophy. This video, obtained from the mid esophageal four chamber, two chamber and long axis views, shows significant systolic displacement of the anterior mitral leaflet into the left ventricular outflow tract. SAM appears to be caused by a "drag" effect resulting from a hyperdynamic, underfilled left ventricle. The anterior leaflet is pulled into the left ventricular outflow tract and contributes to dynamic outflow tract obstruction. The SAM prevents the mitral valve from effective coaptation and produces significant mitral regurgitation, as noted by the color flow Doppler jet. The left ventricular outflow tract gradient can be very high; in this patient the peak velocity was measured at nearly 8 m/s, or 256 mmHg. Note the dagger-shaped spectral Doppler tracing

Video 11.12 Mid esophageal aortic valve long axis view at 120° showing a subaortic fibromuscular ridge and a dysplastic aortic valve resulting in combined subvalvar and valvar aortic stenosis in addition to a small membranous ventricular septal defect (the fibromuscular ridge is located at the crest of the muscular septum)

Video 11.13 Mid esophageal aortic valve long axis view at 120° showing discrete narrowing at the sino-tubular junction resulting in supravalvar aortic stenosis

Video 11.14 Deep transgastric long axis view at 30° with two-dimensional imaging and color flow Doppler showing discrete narrowing of the sino-tubular junction resulting in supravalvar aortic stenosis. Associated aortic regurgitation is seen

Video 11.15 Quadricuspid aortic valve as displayed from the mid esophageal aortic valve short axis view

Video 11.16a Ruptured non-coronary sinus of Valsalva aneurysm into the right atrium in a mid esophageal aortic valve short-axis view at 45°

Video 11.16b Ruptured non-coronary sinus of Valsalva aneurysm into the right atrium in a modified mid esophageal right ventricular inflow-outflow view at 90°

Video 11.17 Mid esophageal aortic valve long axis view at 120° showing a prosthetic aortic valve with motion of the prosthetic hemidisc leaflets

Video 11.18 Mid esophageal ascending aortic long axis view at 120° showing a markedly dilated aortic root and ascending aorta with associated aortic dissection along the anterior wall of the ascending aorta in a patient with Marfan syndrome

Video 11.19 Markedly dilated aortic root as seen from the mid esophageal four chamber and aortic valve short and long axis views, showing central aortic regurgitation

Video 11.20 Mid esophageal aortic valve long axis with counterclockwise probe rotation to demonstrate the right ventricular outflow tract followed by upper esophageal aortic arch short axis views at 90°. This video shows valvar pulmonary stenosis with thin but doming pulmonary valve leaflets, and post-stenotic dilation of the main pulmonary artery (along with swirling of flow) in association with a moderate secundum atrial septal defect (not shown). This study was done in the catheterization laboratory during closure of the defect; a catheter is seen in the left atrium

Video 11.21 Upper esophageal pulmonary artery long axis view at 0° showing the main pulmonary artery in the setting of mild valvar pulmonary stenosis, and minimal flow acceleration across the valve. In this video the bifurcation of the branch pulmonary arteries can also be seen

Video 11.22 Mid esophageal right ventricular inflow-outflow view at 60° showing a double-chambered right ventricle with prominent muscle bundles at the infundibular os separating the proximal right ventricular chamber from the well-developed right ventricular infundibular chamber and resulting in subvalvar pulmonary stenosis (the pulmonary annulus is within normal limits in size). Moderate tricuspid regurgitation is also seen.

Video 11.23 Deep transgastric sagittal view at 90° showing a double-chambered right ventricle with prominent muscle bundles at the infundibular os separating the proximal right ventricular chamber from the well-developed right ventricular infundibular chamber and resulting in subvalvar pulmonary stenosis (the pulmonary annulus is within normal limits in size); this is an ideal view to measure the gradient along the right ventricular outflow tract

Video 11.24 Mid esophageal right ventricular inflow-outflow view at 60° showing free pulmonary regurgitation in the setting of tetralogy of Fallot repair with a transannular right ventricular outflow tract patch

Video 12.1 Tetralogy of Fallot: Mid esophageal four chamber view showing right ventricular hypertrophy, the large malalignment ventricular septal defect, and overriding aorta. *LA* left atrium, *LV* left ventricle, *RV* right ventricle

Video 12.2 Tetralogy of Fallot: Modified mid esophageal right ventricular inflow-outflow view (multiplane angle about 90°) showing the malalignment ventricular septal defect (VSD), as well as the narrowing of right ventricular outflow due to a malaligned conal septum. *Ao* aorta, *MPA* main pulmonary artery, *PV* pulmonary valve, *RV* right ventricle

Video 12.3 Tetralogy of Fallot: Deep transgastric long axis and sagittal views that simulate transthoracic subcostal coronal and sagittal views, showing the anteriorly malaligned infundibular septum producing subpulmonary stenosis. The spectral Doppler tracing shows the typical "dagger" shape seen with subpulmonary stenosis. Color Doppler displays the aliased flow across the right ventricular outflow tract and right to left shunting across the ventricular septal defect. *Ao* aorta, *LV* left ventricle, *PA* pulmonary artery, *RA* right atrium, *RV* right ventricle

Video 12.4 Mid esophageal four chamber view demonstrating right ventricular hypertrophy in a patient with tetralogy of Fallot. Also note the presence of a ventricular septal defect patch, in good position

Video 12.5 Preoperative study in a patient with tetralogy of Fallot. A prominent anterior descending coronary artery (*arrows*) arises from the right coronary artery (*RCA*) and courses anterior to the right ventricular outflow tract, thereby precluding a transannular patch. *Ao* aorta, *PA* main pulmonary artery

Video 12.6 Modified mid esophageal long axis view, with multiplane angle 87° in a patient with tetralogy of Fallot demonstrating a residual ventricular septal defect. The defect is located in the superior aspect of the patch just under the aortic valve. Shunting is seen into the right ventricular outflow tract

Video 12.7 Patient with tetralogy of Fallot who underwent complete repair, including unifocalization of discontinuous pulmonary arteries. Modified mid esophageal long axis view shows a good size main pulmonary artery (*MPA*). From here, probe withdrawal yields the upper esophageal aortic arch short axis view that, with counterclockwise (*leftward*) rotation, demonstrates significant left pulmonary artery stenosis. Spectral continuous wave Doppler tracing shows the high gradient across the stenotic area, along with diastolic runoff that produces a continuous flow pattern. *Desc Ao* descending aorta, *LPA* left pulmonary artery, *MPA* main pulmonary artery, *RV* right ventricle

Video 12.8 Residual right ventricular outflow tract narrowing is seen in a patient after tetralogy of Fallot repair in a modified mid esophageal right ventricular inflow-outflow view, with slight probe withdrawal to display the outflow tract more clearly

Video 12.9 Mid esophageal aortic valve long axis view demonstrating an unobstructed left ventricular outflow tract after repair of tetralogy of Fallot

Video 12.10 Mid esophageal four chamber view with probe withdrawn to evaluate the left ventricular outflow tract demonstrates that there is no residual VSD seen by color Doppler interrogation after tetralogy of Fallot repair. In addition, flow is laminar into the left ventricular outflow tract

Video 12.11 Mid esophageal four chamber view in a patient who has undergone tetralogy of Fallot and atrioventricular canal repair. A large ventricular septal defect patch is seen. Minimal residual atrioventricular valve regurgitation is seen across the right and left atrioventricular valves

Video 12.12 Severe tricuspid regurgitation prompted tricuspid valve replacement in this adult long after tetralogy of Fallot repair. This is a short sweep that starts in a mid esophageal bicaval view, and as the probe is rotated counterclockwise (*leftwards*) to a modified mid esophageal right ventricular inflow-outflow view (multiplane angle 97°), the prosthetic valve appears in cross section

Video 12.13 Mid esophageal four chamber view in a patient with double outlet right ventricle, posterior malalignment of the conal septum, and subpulmonary ventricular septal defect, with the probe withdrawn towards the base of the heart. The aorta and pulmonary artery (PA) come into view, both arising from the right ventricle (RV). The PA is smaller than the aorta because of the conal septal malalignment and pulmonary outflow tract stenosis. Note that the ventricular septal defect appears to extend into the inlet portion of the ventricular septum

Video 12.14 Mid esophageal aortic valve long axis view in the patient in Video 12.13 with double outlet right ventricle, posterior malalignment of the conal septum with subpulmonary ventricular septal defect highlighting the posterior deviation of the conal septum resulting in severe subpulmonary stenosis. The conal septum is also hypertrophied

Video 12.15 Double outlet right ventricle with pulmonary outflow tract stenosis. Mid esophageal four chamber view shows a large ventricular septal defect (*arrow*). With probe withdrawal and anteflexion, the semilunar valves are visualized in a side-by-side orientation. However the pathway from left ventricle (LV) to aortic valve (AoV) is not clearly shown. Rotation of multiplane angle to about 90° and sweep from right to left shows right atrium (RA) and right ventricle (RV) as well as AoV, but it is still unclear whether the pathway from LV to AoV is unobstructed. The deep transgastric long axis view shows that this pathway is unobstructed; it also shows the origin of both great arteries from the RV. This patient successfully underwent patch closure of the ventricular septal defect and relief of pulmonary outflow tract stenosis. *LA* left atrium, *PV* pulmonary valve

Video 12.16 Left juxtaposition of the atrial appendages in a patient with double outlet right ventricle and pulmonary stenosis. This video was obtained with a mid esophageal aortic valve short axis view. Note how the right atrial appendage (RAA) crosses posterior to the great arteries to lie just anterior to the left atrial appendage (LAA). *AoV* aortic valve, *RA* right atrium, *PV* pulmonary valve

Video 12.17 Mid esophageal sagittal (90°) clockwise sweep (*from left to right*) in the patient from Videos 12.13 and 12.14 with double outlet right ventricle, posterior malalignment of the conal septum and subpulmonary ventricular septal defect after the Nikaidoh procedure (aortic translocation). The translocation of the aorta has placed the aortic valve closer to the left ventricle, improving left ventricle to aortic valve alignment and reducing the possibility of subaortic obstruction once the ventricular septal defect has been closed by a patch. This video demonstrates the "physiologic" repair achieved by baffling the ventricular septal defect to the aorta in its new position, and the right ventricle to pulmonary artery conduit

Video 12.18 Truncal valve seen *en face* from a modified mid esophageal aortic valve short axis view (angle 0°). This shows a quadricuspid truncal valve with thickened edges and a central area of noncoaptation associated with a small amount of valvar regurgitation

Video 12.19 Truncus arteriosus type "1½ ". From the mid esophageal ascending aortic short axis view, the right pulmonary artery (RPA) and left pulmonary artery (LPA) origins are seen immediately adjacent to each other, arising from the posterior aspect of the trunk (TRUN). Color Doppler demonstrates unobstructed flow across the origin of the branch pulmonary arteries. From the mid esophageal aortic valve long axis view the posterior origin of the pulmonary arteries is also seen (*arrow*) and the truncal valve shown to override the ventricular septal defect. Trace truncal valve regurgitation is demonstrated. *Ao* ascending aorta, *LA* left atrium, *LV* left ventricle, *RV* right ventricle

Video 12.20 Postop truncus repair, seen from mid esophageal four chamber view with probe anteflexion. The ventricular septal defect patch is shown by the *arrow*; no residual defect is present. A small amount of truncal valve regurgitation is seen. *LV* left ventricle, *RV* right ventricle

Video 12.21 Postop truncus arteriosus repair, seen from a modified mid esophageal aortic valve long axis view, multiplane angle of 75°, with imaging and color flow Doppler. The ventricular septal defect patch is seen as well as the takeoff of the conduit (COND) from the right ventricle (RV) to the pulmonary artery. *LV* left ventricle

Video 12.22 Transposition of the great arteries. Using a mid esophageal aortic valve short axis view, both semilunar valves are seen *en face*, with the aortic valve (AoV) anterior and rightward to the pulmonary valve (PV). *LA* left atrium, *RA* right atrium

Video 12.23 Origins of the right and left coronary arteries (*arrows*) from the corresponding sinuses facing the pulmonary artery, in transposition of the great arteries, as seen from the mid esophageal aortic valve short axis view. The left anterior descending and circumflex coronary arteries arise from the leftward facing sinus (not shown on the video). This coronary pattern is the most common type seen in this cardiac defect. *Ao* aorta, *PA* pulmonary artery

Video 12.24 Transposition of the great arteries, as viewed from the mid esophageal four chamber view. With anteflexion and slight probe withdrawal, both great arteries are seen in parallel, with the aorta (Ao) arising from the right ventricle (RV), and the pulmonary artery

(PA) from the left ventricle. Color flow Doppler shows continuous flow in the PA from ductal left-to-right shunting. During this sweep, a coronary artery (either left circumflex coronary artery, or left main coronary artery) can be briefly seen coursing posterior to the pulmonary artery, and anterior to the mitral valve

Video 12.25 Transposition of the great arteries, as viewed from a mid esophageal right ventricular inflow-outflow/long axis view, multiplane angle about 90°. Both great arteries are seen in parallel, with the aorta arising from the right ventricle, and the pulmonary artery from the left ventricle. Color flow Doppler shows unobstructed laminar flow across both semilunar valves, and mild turbulence (color aliasing) as flow enters the right branch pulmonary artery. *Ao* aorta, *LA* left atrium, *LV* left ventricle, *PA* pulmonary artery, *RA* right atrium, *RV* right ventricle

Video 12.26 Transposition of the great arteries, with a large ventricular septal defect and pulmonary outflow obstruction, as seen from modified mid esophageal four chamber, bicaval, and long axis views. A right to left sweep is performed from the bicaval to long axis view, showing the atrioventricular valves, ventricles, and ventricular septal defect. Posteriorly malaligned infundibular septum produces prominent subpulmonary narrowing, and turbulence is seen by color flow Doppler across the pulmonary outflow tract. Flow from a systemic to pulmonary artery shunt is seen in the main pulmonary artery. *Ao* aorta, *LA* left atrium, *LV* left ventricle, *PA* pulmonary artery, *PV* pulmonary valve, *RA* right atrium, *RV* right ventricle, *SVC* superior vena cava

Video 12.27 Postoperative study following arterial switch operation. From the mid esophageal long axis view, the neo-aortic valve is seen with a small amount of regurgitation. The aortic anastomosis is shown by the arrow. Withdrawal of the probe to the mid esophageal ascending aorta long axis view shows the pulmonary artery anastomosis (*arrow*); the branch pulmonary arteries arise just above (superior to) the anastomosis. In this video, the right pulmonary artery is seen. *Ao* aorta, *LA* left atrium, *LV* left ventricle, *MPA* main pulmonary artery, *RPA* right pulmonary artery, *RV* right ventricle

Video 12.28 Postoperative study following arterial switch operation, showing the branch pulmonary arteries from the upper esophageal pulmonary artery long axis view. A Lecompte maneuver was performed so that the main and branch pulmonary arteries are situated anterior to the aorta (Ao). Color flow Doppler demonstrates flow in both the main and branch pulmonary arteries. *LPA* left pulmonary artery, *RPA* right pulmonary artery

Video 12.29 Modified mid esophageal right ventricular inflow-outflow view with the probe advanced toward the liver in an adult who has undergone an atrial switch operation for transposition of the great arteries. The color interrogation demonstrates flow from the pulmonary venous channel to the systemic venous channel (*left to right shunt*)

Video 12.30 Mid esophageal right ventricular inflow-outflow view in the same patient in Video 12.29 with an atrial switch and a baffle leak. This video is obtained during device deployment to occlude the baffle leak. The image demonstrates an Amplatzer device just prior to release

Video 12.31 Modified mid esophageal four chamber view of a patient after atrial switch operation demonstrating the pulmonary venous channel as it makes its way to the tricuspid valve. In this patient, the pathway is unobstructed

Video 12.32 Mid esophageal bicaval view with probe turned clockwise. This image is from a patient who has superior systemic venous limb obstruction after an atrial switch operation. In this view, both inferior and superior limbs of the systemic venous channel are seen with the pulmonary venous channel coursing in between. Pacing wires are seen in the superior limb

Video 12.33 Modified mid esophageal right ventricular inflow-outflow view using color Doppler in the same patient as Video 12.32 after atrial switch operation, with superior limb obstruction. Aliasing of the color flow is seen in the superior limb of the channel

Video 12.34 Congenitally corrected transposition of the great arteries. A mid esophageal four chamber view shows inferior displacement of the septal leaflet of the left sided tricuspid valve, compared with the right sided mitral valve. Incomplete coaptation of this valve results in a mild to moderate degree of tricuspid insufficiency. *LA* left atrium, *LV* left ventricle, *RA* right atrium, *RV* right ventricle

Video 12.35 Congenitally corrected transposition of the great arteries. Using the mid esophageal long axis view, the left sided tricuspid valve is seen, with significant regurgitation. *Ao* aorta, *LA* left atrium, *PA* pulmonary artery, *RV* right ventricle

Video 12.36 Mid esophageal four chamber view shows a large perimembranous ventricular septal defect (*arrow*) in a patient with congenitally corrected transposition of the great arteries. Note the left sided tricuspid valve chordal attachment to the ventricular septum, as well as the presence of a moderator band in the left sided right ventricle (RV). *LA* left atrium, *LV* left ventricle, *RA* right atrium

Video 12.37 Congenitally corrected transposition of the great arteries. Transgastric mid short axis view shows the inverted ventricles in cross section. Note the smooth walled septal surface in the left ventricle (LV), and the prominent moderator band in the right ventricle (RV)

Video 12.38 Congenitally corrected transposition of the great arteries, as seen from the mid esophageal window in an approximately 90° sagittal plane. There is a "windsock" aneurysm of tissue (*arrow*) originating from the anterior leaflet of mitral valve and protruding into the pulmonary outflow tract, just below the pulmonary valve. In addition fibrous tissue from the mitral valve extends across the outflow tract and attaches to the ventricular septum. Neither of these was obstructive. A pulmonary artery band is seen in the main pulmonary artery, with flow acceleration noted across it. *LA* left atrium, *LV* left ventricle, *PA* pulmonary artery, *RA* right atrium

Video 12.39 Deep transgastric long axis view in a patient with congenitally corrected transposition of the great arteries and ventricular septal defect, in whom a pulmonary artery band (Band) was placed. The transducer first visualizes the right ventricle (RV) and ascending aorta (Ao). Further probe anteflexion and advancement is required to visualize the more posterior pulmonary artery (PA). Significant aliasing is noted across the band, and spectral Doppler calculated gradient is 84 mmHg. Note the excellent angle for Doppler interrogation across the band. *LV* left ventricle, *RA* right atrium, *RV* right ventricle

Video 12.40 Mid esophageal four chamber view in a patient with congenitally corrected transposition of the great arteries and ventricular septal defect. A sweep is performed in which the probe is simultaneously anteflexed and withdrawn to a view approximating a mid esophageal aortic valve short axis view. During this sweep, the aortic valve is seen to arise from the left sided right ventricle (RV), and there is subaortic conal muscle seen, along with discontinuity between the left sided tricuspid valve and aortic valve (AoV). At the same time, the pulmonary valve (PV), which arises from the right sided left ventricle (LV), is shown to have fibrous continuity with the right sided mitral valve. The coronary arteries are clearly seen arising from the anterior aorta. *LA* left atrium, *RA* right atrium

Video 12.41 Mid esophageal long axis view in congenitally corrected transposition of the great arteries, showing the parallel course of both aorta (Ao) and pulmonary artery (PA) as they arise from the heart. In this view, the ventriculoarterial discordance, and parallel arrangement of the great arteries, is very similar to that seen in D-transposition of the great arteries. Thus complementary views and sweeps are necessary to determine visceroatrial situs and atrioventricular connections. *LA* left atrium

Video 12.42 Deep transgastric long axis view in congenitally corrected transposition of the great arteries. With the probe advanced in the stomach to point the tip more posteriorly, the pulmonary artery (PA) is seen arising from the left ventricle (LV). The right atrium (RA) is also seen emptying into the LV. There is unobstructed flow across the pulmonary outflow tract. The probe is then withdrawn slightly, pointing the tip more anteriorly, to visualize the anterior aorta

(Ao) arising from the right ventricle (RV). Flow across the aorta is also unobstructed. Note the moderator band present in the RV

Video 12.43 Mid esophageal sagittal sweep in congenitally corrected transposition of the great arteries. Starting with the mid esophageal bicaval view, the left atrium (LA), right atrium (RA), mitral valve and left ventricle (LV) are noted. The transducer is rotated counterclockwise (*leftward*) to visualize further the LV and pulmonary artery (PA). With further leftward probe rotation, the LA, tricuspid valve, right ventricle (RV) and aorta (Ao) are visualized. During this sweep, some changes in multiplane angle are also performed to optimize imaging of the intracardiac structures. *RAA* right atrial appendage, *SVC* superior vena cava

Video 12.44 Same patient as Video 12.39. The pulmonary artery band is clearly seen well above the pulmonary valve, and color flow Doppler demonstrates significant aliasing across the band. *LV* left ventricle, *PA* pulmonary artery, *RA* right atrium, *RV* right ventricle

Video 13.1 Patent ductus arteriosus. Upper esophageal pulmonary artery long axis view demonstrating left-to-right shunting across a patent ductus arteriosus (PDA, *arrow*). *AO* aorta, *PA* main pulmonary artery

Video 13.2 Patent ductus arteriosus. Mid esophageal right ventricular inflow-outflow view depicts flow (*blue signal, arrow*) across a patent ductus arteriosus (PDA) into main pulmonary artery (MPA). *AO* aorta

Video 13.3 Patent ductus arteriosus. Upper esophageal aortic arch short axis view demonstrating aliased flow (between the arrows) corresponding to a restrictive patent ductus arteriosus. *Ao* aorta, *PA* pulmonary artery (Reproduced with permission from Russell et al. [131])

Video 13.4 Tricuspid regurgitation. Color Doppler interrogation of the tricuspid valve in two different planes demonstrates moderate regurgitation and a peak velocity of the regurgitant jet that reaches nearly 4 meters per second. The peak jet velocity predicts an elevated right ventricular and pulmonary artery systolic pressure in this infant. *Ao* aorta, *LA* left atrium, *LV* left ventricle, *RA* right atrium, *RV* right ventricle

Video 13.5 Left heart dilation resulting from a patent ductus arteriosus. Mid esophageal four chamber view obtained in a patient with a ductus arteriosus and left-to-right shunting. The left sided structures are dilated, particularly the left atrium, due to the volume overload. A tricuspid valve aneurysm is seen without evidence of ventricular level shunting. *LA* left atrium, *LV* left ventricle, *RA* right atrium, *RV* right ventricle

Video 13.6 Aortopulmonary window. Mid esophageal ascending aorta short axis view in infant with an aortopulmonary (AP) window. Note the echocardiographic drop out in the region between the arterial roots (*arrow*), corresponding to faulty aortopulmonary septation, and the shunting across this region by color Doppler. *AO* aorta, *PA* pulmonary artery

Video 13.7 Aortopulmonary window. View of the ascending aorta obtained at the upper esophageal level depicting an aortopulmonary (AP) window (*arrow*). The spectral Doppler tracing across the right pulmonary artery displays systolic flow and continuous forward flow during diastole as a result of the abnormal aortopulmonary connection. *AO* aorta, *PA* pulmonary artery, *RV* right ventricle

Video 13.8 Aortopulmonary window. Postoperative transesophageal echocardiogram in the mid esophageal ascending aortic long axis view depicts the bright region along the wall of the ascending aorta (*arrow*) corresponding to the pericardial patch placed to obliterate the abnormal communication. Color Doppler interrogation across the right pulmonary artery does not suggest concerning obstruction. *Ao* aorta, *MPA* main pulmonary artery, *RPA* right pulmonary artery

Video 13.9 Pulmonary artery sling. Upper esophageal pulmonary artery long axis view of a pulmonary artery sling in an infant. The abnormal origin of the left pulmonary artery from the right pulmonary artery is seen. Note the absence of the normal main pulmonary artery bifurcation, which should be seen in a more proximal relationship to the pulmonary valve. The course of the anomalous vessel with respect to the trachea (*asterisk*) is noted. In this patient there was associated pulmonary valve stenosis. *AO* aorta, *LPA* left pulmonary artery, *MPA* main pulmonary artery, *RPA* right pulmonary artery

Video 13.10 Pulmonary artery sling. Color Doppler image of the same cross-section depicted in Video 13.9 obtained in a zoom mode. Note flow into the left pulmonary artery (LPA) as it arises from the right pulmonary artery (RPA). *AO* aorta, *MPA* main pulmonary artery

Video 13.11 Main pulmonary artery bifurcation. Normal branching of the main pulmonary artery (MPA) into the right (RPA) and left (LPA) pulmonary arteries as imaged from the upper esophageal pulmonary artery long axis view. *AO* aorta

Video 13.12 Main pulmonary artery bifurcation. Modified deep transgastric long axis image obtained in an infant with double outlet right ventricle and a subaortic ventricular septal defect to demonstrate the normal main pulmonary artery bifurcation as seen in cross-section from this window. *AO* aorta, *LA* left atrium, *LPA* left pulmonary artery, *RA* right atrium, *RPA* right pulmonary artery

Video 13.13 Aortic origin of right pulmonary artery. Upper esophageal pulmonary artery long axis view displaying only the left pulmonary artery (LPA) as it arises from the main pulmonary artery (MPA). Note the absence of the normal pulmonary artery confluence in this patient, due to anomalous origin of the right pulmonary artery from the aorta (AO)

Video 13.14 Aortic origin of right pulmonary artery. Longitudinal plane imaging using a biplane transesophageal probe displaying anomalous origin (*arrow*) of the right pulmonary artery (RPA) from the aorta (AO). *LA* left atrium, *RA* right atrium, *RV* right ventricle

Video 13.15 Aortic origin of right pulmonary artery. Transverse plane sweep in same patient as depicted in Video 13.14 demonstrating anomalous origin of the right pulmonary artery (RPA) from the aorta (AO) by two-dimensional and color Doppler imaging. A catheter is seen in the superior vena cava. *MPA* main pulmonary artery, *RA* right atrium

Video 13.16 Anomalous origin of right pulmonary artery. Mid esophageal ascending aortic long axis view displaying anomalous origin of right pulmonary artery from the ascending aorta (AO). Note the more distal origin of the anomalous vessel (*arrow*) as compared to that seen in the patient shown in Videos 13.14 and 13.15. Flow into the anomalous pulmonary artery is demonstrated by color and spectral Doppler interrogation. A perimembranous ventricular septal defect is briefly seen in this video. *PA* main pulmonary artery

Video 13.17 Coarctation of the aorta. Mid esophageal descending aorta long axis view depicting narrowing at the level of the thoracic descending aorta (*arrow*) consistent with coarctation of the aorta. (Reproduced with permission from Russell et al. [131])

Video 13.18 Coarctation of the aorta. Sweep obtained from the upper esophageal window (upper esophageal short axis view) demonstrating the aortic arch in short axis (Arch), a large patent ductus arteriosus (PDA) and the left pulmonary artery (LPA). As the probe is slightly advanced and rotated to the left, the descending aorta (AoDT) is displayed longitudinally; the LPA is again seen in this view. A discrete area of narrowing is noted (*arrow*) corresponding to a coarctation. Color Doppler imaging displays turbulent flow across the region of obstruction. This video was obtained in an infant with a ductal-dependent coarctation.

Video 13.19 Interrupted aortic arch. Two-dimensional mid esophageal four chamber view and corresponding color flow mapping in an infant with interrupted aortic arch demonstrating a large posteriorly malaligned ventricular septal defect, hypoplastic subaortic region, aortic annulus, and ascending aorta. *AO* aorta, *LA* left atrium, *LV* left ventricle, *RV* right ventricle

Video 13.20 Interrupted aortic arch. Mid esophageal aortic valve long axis view obtained from the same infant as shown in Video 13.19 demonstrating the ventricular septal defect and marked discrepancy in the sizes of the arterial roots. *AO* aorta, *PA* main pulmonary artery

Video 13.21 Interrupted aortic arch. Deep transgastric long axis image with color flow mapping from the same patient as shown in Videos 13.19 and 13.20 demonstrating the ventricular septal defect and subaortic narrowing. *AO* aorta, *LA* left ventricle, *LV* left ventricle *RA* right atrium, *RV* right ventricle

Video 13.22 Interrupted aortic arch. Mid esophageal ascending aortic short axis view demonstrates a severely hypoplastic ascending aorta (AO). Note the dilated pulmonary artery (PA)

Video 13.23 Interrupted aortic arch. Intraoperative images from the mid esophageal four chamber view following aortic arch advancement, aortic (AO) augmentation, subaortic resection, and closure of the ventricular septal defect (VSD) in the infant with interrupted aortic arch shown in videos 13.19, 13.20, and 13.22. Note the large pericardial VSD patch and the relatively small subaortic area, aortic annulus, and aortic root. In the presence of moderately decreased left ventricular systolic function, no significant gradient was recorded across the left ventricular outflow tract. Note that a reasonable spectral Doppler tracing could be obtained of the outflow tract in this particular TEE view. *LA* left atrium, *LV* left ventricle, *RV* right ventricle

Video 13.24 Interrupted aortic arch. The same findings noted in Video 13.23 following surgical intervention are confirmed in the mid esophageal long axis view. Trace intermittent aortic regurgitation is seen. *AO* aorta, *LA* left atrium, *LV* left ventricle, *PA* main pulmonary artery, *RV* right ventricle, *VSD* ventricular septal defect

Video 13.25 Interrupted aortic arch. Postoperative, mid esophageal four chamber view demonstrating a dilated left ventricle (LV) with markedly decreased systolic function in the same infant depicted in prior videos (13.23 and 13.24). Moderate mitral valve regurgitation is also seen. *LA* left atrium, *LV* left ventricle

Video 14.1a Mid esophageal aortic valve short axis view in a patient with anomalous origin of the right coronary artery (*RCA*) from the left sinus of Valsalva and an intramural course of the anomalous vessel. The anomalous RCA can be seen arising from the left sinus of Valsalva (*L*) and coursing intramurally within the anterior aortic wall between the aorta and the right ventricular outflow tract before exiting the aortic wall from the right sinus of Valsalva (*R*). The non-coronary cusp (*N*) is seen posteriorly

Video 14.1b Color Doppler imaging in the mid esophageal aortic short axis view corresponding to the same patient shown in Video 14.1a demonstrates the linear diastolic flow of the anomalous right coronary artery within the anterior aortic wall; the blue color signal confirms anomalous coronary flow away from the transducer anteriorly, consistent with the RCA originating from the left sinus and coursing towards the more anteriorly positioned right sinus. The Nyquist limit has been lowered to 28 cm/s to enhance visualization of the low velocity diastolic coronary flow

Video 14.2 Mid esophageal right ventricular inflow-outflow view displays the aortic root in a patient with anomalous origin of the right coronary artery (*RCA*) from the left sinus of Valsalva and short intramural course of the anomalous coronary. The relationship between the aortic intercoronary commissure and the anomalous RCA origin can be seen in this sweep with the coronary arising from the rightward aspect of the left sinus of Valsalva near the commissure with a short intramural course before exiting the aortic wall from the right sinus of Valsalva. The short intramural course with the anomalous origin of the RCA near the aortic commissure is typical of this lesion

Video 14.3 Mid esophageal right ventricular inflow-outflow view through the aortic root in a patient with anomalous origin of the left coronary artery (*LCA*) from the right sinus of Valsalva. The relationship between the aortic commissure and the anomalous LCA origin can be seen in this sweep with the coronary arising from the mid-portion of the right sinus of Valsalva with a long intramural course within the anterior aortic wall before exiting the wall from the left sinus of Valsalva. The longer intramural course with the anomalous origin of the LCA from the middle of the right sinus is typical of this lesion, in contrast to the shorter intramural course and origin adjacent to the commissure with anomalous origin of the right coronary artery from the left sinus (as shown in Video 14.2)

Video 14.4a Mid esophageal right ventricular inflow-outflow view through the aortic root in the same patient shown in Video 14.3 with anomalous origin of the left coronary artery (*LCA*) from the right sinus of Valsalva. The imaging plane is angled slightly superiorly to better visualize the origin of both the anomalous LCA and the normally positioned right coronary as both arise from the right sinus of Valsalva. The long intramural course of the anomalous LCA within the anterior aortic wall is well visualized

Video 14.4b Mid esophageal right ventricular inflow-outflow view with color Doppler clip through the aortic root in the same patient shown in Video 14.3 with anomalous origin of the left coronary artery from the right sinus of Valsalva demonstrates the red linear diastolic flow signal in the intramural segment coursing posteriorly towards the left sinus (and the posteriorly positioned TEE transducer)

Video 14.5 Mid esophageal long axis view through the left ventricle in a patient with anomalous origin of the left coronary artery (*LCA*) from the opposite sinus with an interarterial course. The anomalous coronary LCA is seen coursing anterior to the aorta between the great arteries as a discreet circle; the probe is then rotated towards the patient's left (counterclockwise) to follow the course of the LCA as the intramural portion of the vessel exits the aortic wall and bifurcates into the left anterior descending and circumflex coronary branches

Video 14.6 Sweep from a deep transgastric long axis position through the left ventricle and aortic outflow from a patient with anomalous origin of the left coronary artery (*LCA*) from the right sinus of Valsalva with an intramural course. As the imaging plane is angled more anteriorly towards the right ventricular outflow tract, the intramural segment of the LCA and normal course of the right coronary along the anterior aspect of the aortic root are well imaged. The usual origin of the LCA from the left sinus, which is frequently well imaged from this view, is not seen

Video 14.7 Mid esophageal right ventricular inflow-outflow view displaying the aortic root in the same patient shown in Videos 14.3, 14.4a, and 14.4b with anomalous origin of the left coronary artery (*LCA*) from the right sinus of Valsalva after surgical unroofing. The long intramural course of the anomalous LCA within the anterior aortic wall has been removed, and the vessel now appears to arise normally from the left sinus of Valsalva, with an easily visualized neo-orifice from the appropriate sinus

Video 14.8a Mid esophageal aortic valve short axis TEE view of the anomalous insertion of the left main coronary artery (*LCA*) into the posterior aspect of the proximal main pulmonary artery (*PA*) in a patient with anomalous left coronary artery from the pulmonary artery (*ALCAPA*). The LCA is seen connecting to the PA through a short segment and then bifurcating into the left anterior descending and circumflex branches (*arrows*), clearly a long distance from the normal entrance into the aortic root (*Ao*)

Video 14.8b Video is color Doppler imaging in the same patient in Video 14.8a with anomalous left coronary artery from the pulmonary artery (*ALCAPA*). Color Doppler shows a blue color signal in the left coronary artery (*arrows*), consistent with coronary flow towards the pulmonary artery (*PA*). The prominent color Doppler signal in the PA represents retrograde flow of the anomalous coronary as it empties into the PA. *Ao* aortic root

Video 14.9 Modified mid esophageal view displaying the aortic root (*Ao*) and a dilated left coronary artery (*LCA*) in a child with anomalous origin of the right coronary artery (*RCA*) from the pulmonary artery; the LCA measured 3.5 mm at its origin, which is significantly abnormal for age. The LCA arises normally from the Ao; the anomalous RCA is not seen. The LCA is dilated because of the increased flow into the left coronary bed as it functions as the single coronary supplying the entire myocardium with steal of coronary flow from the anomalous RCA emptying into the low pressure pulmonary bed

Video 14.10 Mid esophageal right ventricular inflow-outflow view using color Doppler to identify the course of the anomalous vessel in the same patient as Video 14.9 with anomalous right coronary artery from the pulmonary artery (*PA*). The coronary is imaged anterior to the right aortic sinus of Valsalva taking a tortuous course (*arrows*) with the color Doppler signal demonstrating flow towards the PA. The coronary artery appears remote from its usual origin off the right aortic sinus

Video 14.11 Mid esophageal long axis view through the left ventricle (*LV*) in the same patient as Videos 14.9 and 14.10 with anomalous origin of the right coronary artery from the pulmonary artery (*ARCAPA*). There is a continuous color Doppler flow signal entering the pulmonary artery (*PA*) anteriorly above the right ventricular outflow tract (*RVOT*). A diastolic flow signal in the PA is seen because the anomalous vessel is supplied retrograde from the normally arising left coronary artery. The retrograde flow empties into the lower pressure PA. This coronary steal flow signal may be the first clue that there is an anomalous coronary artery arising from the PA, as direct visualization of a coronary entering the PA can sometimes be difficult to obtain

Video 14.12 Transgastric ventricular mid short axis view from a patient with a left coronary artery to right ventricular fistula. This video displays color Doppler imaging of the fistula as it empties into the right ventricle near the apex

Video 14.13a Modified mid esophageal view of the aorta (*Ao*) displaying the origin of the right coronary artery (*RCA*) in a patient with a RCA fistula. The coronary arises appropriately from the anterior aspect of the Ao and is markedly dilated (*arrows*) because of the increased flow into that vessel, which measured 5 mm in diameter proximally

Video 14.13b Video is color Doppler imaging in the same patient in Video 14.13a with right coronary artery (*RCA*) fistula. The continuous flow signal is easily appreciated by color Doppler without decreasing the Nyquist scale because of the high volume flow into the RCA from the fistula steal

Video 14.14a Deep transgastric sagittal view displaying the left ventricle (*LV*) and aortic outflow (*Ao*) in a longitudinal plane from the same patient shown in Video 14.13 with a right coronary artery (*RCA*) fistula. Because of the increased flow into the RCA to supply the fistula, the proximal RCA is easily seen by two-dimensional imaging and appears markedly dilated (*arrows*). The right ventricle is seen anteriorly (*RV*) and appears dilated, secondary to the fistula shunt

Video 14.14b Deep transgastric sagittal view displaying the left ventricle (*LV*) and aortic outflow (*Ao*) in a longitudinal plane from the same patient shown in Videos 14.13 and 14.14a with a right coronary artery (*RCA*) fistula. With color Doppler, continuous flow into the distal RCA is visualized, again reflecting the increased flow into the vessel secondary to the fistula steal. The distal termination site of the fistula into the right ventricle is not well visualized in this image

Video 16.1 Large vegetation on the anterior leaflet of mitral valve, resulting in chordal destruction and severe mitral regurgitation. Mid esophageal four chamber view, multiplane angle 0°

Video 16.2 Aortic valve endocarditis, seen from a mid esophageal aortic valve long axis view (multiplane angle 85°–116°). The aortic valve is significantly damaged and prolapses in diastole, and severe regurgitation is seen

Video 16.3 Endocarditis in a patient with a prosthetic aortic valve (St. Jude bileaflet tilting disk valve). The mid esophageal four chamber view demonstrates a perivalvar abscess that extends into the noncoronary cusp, causing a fistulous tract communicating with the right atrium. A large vegetation has developed in this area and shunting is seen into the right atrium. There is marked aortic regurgitation seen through several areas of valve dehiscence. A small jet of mitral regurgitation is also seen, likely due to endocarditis involving the anterior leaflet of mitral valve. Rotation of the multiplane angle to 90° shows the significant regurgitation resulting from valve dehiscence

Video 16.4 Infected sinus of Valsalva aneurysm from aortic valve endocarditis. The preoperative study, obtained from the mid esophageal aortic valve short axis and long axis views, shows a large vegetation of the aortic valve and erosion of the right sinus of Valsalva, with blood filling the aneurysm during diastole. Following aortic valve and aortic root surgery, no residual vegetation is seen and the aortic valve manifests normal function, with no insufficiency

Video 16.5 Infected pseudoaneurysm arising from ascending aorta, as seen from the upper esophageal aortic arch short axis view. This TEE was performed to evaluate the aortic valve in a patient with a previous aortic valve surgery and persistent fungemia. A large pseudoaneurysm (*arrow*) was discovered using the upper esophageal window, multiplane angle 60°. Note that the superior portion of aorta and innominate vein can be seen well in this patient by TEE

Video 16.6 Thrombus in the left ventricular apex of a patient with Duchenne muscular dystrophy and dilated cardiomyopathy. Mid esophageal four and two chamber views, multiplane angles 0° and 88°, respectively

Video 16.7 Thrombus in the superior vena cava, probably associated with a catheter, as seen from mid esophageal bicaval view, (multiplane angle 99°)

Video 16.8 Thrombus in the left atrial appendage, as viewed from a modified mid esophageal aortic valve short axis view with leftward rotation. There are mobile filamentous strands arising from the thrombus. *AoV* aortic valve, *LA* left atrium. Video courtesy of Siemens Medical Systems USA, Inc. © 2012–13 Siemens Medical Solutions USA, Inc. All Rights Reserved

Video 16.9 Example of spontaneous echo contrast in a patient after repair of D-transposition of the great arteries, with a pseudoaneurysm arising from a previous cannulation site in the aorta. Video obtained from the upper esophageal aortic arch long axis view. Note the visible swirling of flow due to red cell aggregation. The left pulmonary artery is being compressed by the pseudoaneurysm

Video 16.10 Wilms tumor invading the right atrium by direct extension from the inferior vena cava, as seen from the mid esophageal bicaval view, multiplane angle 113°. The multiplane angle is rotated to 55° and all four chambers are visualized. The tumor obstructs IVC inflow. At the end of the video, the extracted primary tumor is shown

Video 16.11 Multiple rhabdomyomas in a patient with tuberous sclerosis, including one that caused near complete obstruction of the left ventricular outflow tract. Mid esophageal four chamber view (multiplane angle 0°), and mid esophageal long axis view (multiplane angle 90°) show a large tumor in the outflow tract. Turbulent color flow Doppler is seen in this region

Video 16.12 Fibroma attached to the left ventricular free wall, visualized from mid esophageal four chamber and long axis views. The fibroma is very large, circumscribed, and has a heterogeneous appearance, studded with echolucent areas most likely representing cystic degeneration or necrosis

Video 16.13 Left atrial myxoma, seen from mid esophageal four chamber and long axis views. A large, lobulated myxoma is attached to the interatrial septum and left atrial wall, just posterior to the aortic root. Multiple fimbriations of the tumor are freely mobile

Video 16.14 Right atrial hemangioma as seen from the mid esophageal four chamber and mid esophageal right ventricular inflow-outflow views. Note the heterogeneous nature of the large mass in the right atrium. As can be seen by the rapid atrial rate, the patient had an atrial arrhythmia, probably chaotic atrial tachycardia, during the study

Video 16.15 Prosthetic mitral valve (bileaflet tilting disk). Mid esophageal mitral commissural view, multiplane angle 69°. The multiplane angle is rotated until both leaflets are profiled and open symmetrically in diastole. There is the usual color flow Doppler profile across the valve during diastole, and in systole the "normal" pivot point washing jets are seen

Video 16.16 Prosthetic mitral with a frozen leaflet, causing stenosis of the valve. Mid esophageal four chamber view, multiplane angle 0°

Video 16.17 Concentric pannus formation above the mitral valve prosthesis, causing significant supravalvar narrowing, seen during diastole. Mid esophageal mitral commissural view, multiplane angle 58°

Video 16.18 Prosthetic aortic valve (bileaflet tilting disk) viewed from deep transgastric position. At a multiplane angle of 25° the valve is seen from the side, and the usual pivot-point washing jets can be seen by color flow Doppler. The multiplane angle is then rotated (about 95°) until both leaflets are profiled and symmetric leaflet motion is noted in diastole and systole. This view affords a good edge-on view of leaflet motion and flow across the valve, and also provides an excellent angle for spectral Doppler evaluation

Video 16.19 Paravalvar regurgitation in a child who underwent mitral valve replacement with a mechanical bileaflet prosthesis (the patient previously underwent repair of an atrioventricular septal defect). This video was obtained from a mid esophageal four chamber view. The prosthesis was too large for the annulus and required insertion at an angle, which resulted both in a large area of paravalvular regurgitation (seen to the left of the prosthesis) as well as a very small effective orifice

Video 16.20 Transcatheter aortic valve replacement/implantation (TAVR/TAVI). This video, obtained from a mid esophageal aortic valve short axis view (28°) and then a mid esophageal long axis view (120°–130°) first shows the abnormal native aortic valve, which is thickened and has restricted motion. A catheter and then the balloon-mounted valve are seen, with the balloon shown as it is expanded and the valve implanted in the aortic position. During balloon dilation, rapid ventricular pacing is performed to reduce ventricular ejection, thereby stabilizing the valve for placement. Following valve implantation, leaflet motion is seen and there are two jets of regurgitation—one central (transvalvular), one peripheral (paravalvular). (Echocardiographic images were obtained from a Siemens SC 2000 platform and are courtesy of Siemens Medical Systems USA, Inc. © 2012–13 Siemens Medical Solutions USA, Inc. All Rights Reserved)

Video 16.21 Berlin Heart placement in a patient with dilated cardiomyopathy. Mid esophageal four chamber and long axis views. The cannula in the left ventricular apex withdraws blood returning from the left atrium. When the blood has sufficiently filled the chamber in the device, it is pumped into the ascending aorta, as shown from mid esophageal aortic valve long and short axis views

Video 16.22 Following heart transplantation, imaging in the mid esophageal four chamber view, multiplane angle 0°. The anastomosis of the donor left atrium to the cuff of the recipient left atrium creates an area of echogenicity that can be mistaken for thrombus. Unobstructed return of right and left pulmonary veins is also shown. The mid esophageal bicaval view then demonstrates unobstructed IVC and SVC anastomoses. *IVC* inferior vena cava, *LA* left atrium, *RA* right atrium, *SVC* superior vena cava

Video 16.23 Post-lung transplant, with thrombosis of the right pulmonary veins due to a large lymph node. Mid esophageal view, multiplane angle 0°. There is extensive thrombus in the right pulmonary veins. No flow was seen in the vessel by color flow Doppler. Normal flow is seen in the contralateral left pulmonary veins

Video 16.24 Dissection of the ascending and descending aorta (DeBakey Type I) in a patient with Marfan syndrome. The patient also had a dilated aortic root and significant aortic valve regurgitation. The intimal flap is clearly seen, as well as the true and false lumens. Upper esophageal aortic arch long axis view, multiplane angle 0°, shows the false lumen to be much larger than the true lumen in the ascending aorta and aortic arch. Retrograde diastolic flow reversal is seen only in the true lumen by color flow mapping. Mid esophageal descending aortic long axis view, multiplane angle 90° (probe rotated leftward) shows the dissection extending into descending aorta. *LA* left atrium, *LV* left ventricle, *LVOT* left ventricular outflow tract

Video 17.1 TEE monitoring during transcatheter occlusion of a secundum atrial septal defect. The sequence of events involved is outlined in Figs. 17.2 and 17.3 and Table 17.1. Note the variety of multiplane TEE angles used during this study to obtain optimal visualization of the defect, and to monitor and assess device placement

Video 17.2 TEE monitoring during transcatheter occlusion of a muscular ventricular septal defect. The sequence of events involved is outlined in Fig. 17.4 and Table 17.2

Video 18.1 Transesophageal echocardiogram at mid esophageal level, multiplane angle 0°, demonstrating a secundum atrial septal defect. The communication in the interatrial septum is centrally located. Septal rims are seen above and below the defect

Video 18.2 Color flow mapping demonstrating left-to-right atrial level shunting across a secundum atrial septal defect in same patient shown in Video 18.1

Video 18.3 Balloon sizing of secundum atrial septal defect during transcatheter device placement in a modified mid esophageal view

Video 18.4 Mid esophageal bicaval view (multiplane angle 57°) showing a small amount of left-to-right shunting between the discs of an Amplatzer atrial septal defect occluder device immediately after deployment. This is not an unusual finding

Video 18.5 Color Doppler flow imaging in the mid esophageal long axis view demonstrating a membranous ventricular septal defect with left-to-right shunting

Video 18.6 Pre and postoperative two-dimensional imaging and color Doppler flow mapping in an adult with double-chambered right ventricle as visualized from the mid esophageal right ventricular inflow-outflow view. The preoperative examination (early frames of the video) demonstrates severe narrowing at the mid ventricular level, functionally dividing the chamber into proximal and distal portions. Aliased flow across this region confirms the level and severity of the obstruction. The post-repair examination (later frames in the video) demonstrates no residual anatomic obstruction, confirmed by color flow interrogation

Video 18.7 Transgastric basal short axis view of the left ventricle showing a cleft in the anterior mitral leaflet in a patient with an ostium primum atrial septal defect

Video 18.8 Mid esophageal aortic valve long axis view demonstrating chordal attachments from the anterior mitral leaflet to the outflow septum causing subaortic stenosis in the setting of an atrioventricular canal defect

Video 18.9 Color flow mapping at a mid esophageal position demonstrating severe pulmonary regurgitation into the right ventricular outflow tract in a patient with a history of tetralogy of Fallot previously repaired using a transannular patch

Video 18.10 Mid esophageal short axis view of bicuspid aortic valve in a patient with a vegetation and clinical evidence of endocarditis. Fusion of the left-right intercoronary commissure is seen

Video 18.11 Transgastric long axis view of the left ventricle during transcatheter aortic balloon valvuloplasty of a stenotic bicuspid aortic valve

Video 18.12 Color flow Doppler interrogation post-balloon dilation of bicuspid aortic valve shown in Video 18.11 demonstrates a jet of aortic regurgitation that courses along the edges of the left ventricular outflow. There is reduced systolic excursion of the aortic valve leaflets consistent with residual obstruction

Video 18.13 Mid esophageal aortic valve long axis view demonstrating a membrane immediately underneath the aortic valve consistent with subaortic stenosis

Video 18.14 Mid esophageal four chamber view displaying the elongated, redundant, 'sail-like' anterior leaflet in Ebstein malformation of the tricuspid valve. The apical displacement of the septal leaflet is also seen. *LA* left atrium, *LV* left ventricle, *RA* Right atrium

Video 18.15 Mid esophageal four chamber view in a patient with congenitally corrected transposition of the great arteries. The left panel displays the characteristic appearance of atrioventricular discordance. Note the apical displacement (Ebsteinoid appearance) of the left sided systemic tricuspid valve. The right panel demonstrates associated severe regurgitation across the dysplastic valve

Video 18.16 This image was obtained in the mid esophageal long axis view (multiplane angle 86°) in a patient with congenitally corrected transposition of the great arteries. The abnormal atrioventricular connection is shown as the left atrium (*LA*) empties into the right ventricle (*RV*), and the abnormal ventriculoarterial connection is demonstrated as the RV connects and ejects into the aorta (*Ao*). A significant degree of tricuspid valve regurgitation (*TR*) is observed (*arrow*)

Video 18.17 Mid esophageal long axis view in a patient status-post Senning atrial baffle procedure for *d*-transposition of the great arteries. Two pacemaker leads traverse the systemic venous limb of the atrial baffle

Video 18.18 Color flow Doppler imaging in orthogonal mid esophageal planes obtained in a patient with *d*-transposition of the great arteries several years post Senning procedure demonstrating a communication (baffle leak) between the pulmonary and systemic venous baffles resulting in left-to-right (pulmonary baffle to systemic baffle) shunting

Video 18.19 Contrast injection into a central venous catheter in the patient shown in Video 18.18 results in initial opacification of the systemic venous limb of the baffle and subsequent egress of blood into the pulmonary venous aspect confirming the presence of a baffle leak

Video 18.20 Large thrombus in the inferior portion of the dilated right atrium in a patient with an atriopulmonary Fontan connection and history of intra-atrial reentrant tachycardia as seen from a mid esophageal 120° view

Video 18.21 Mid esophageal view at 44° in a patient with tricuspid atresia and a Bjork Fontan procedure (right atrial to right ventricular outflow tract connection). Spontaneous echo contrast is seen in the dilated right atrium

Video 18.22 Right-to-left atrial level shunting in same patient with Bjork Fontan connection as shown in Video 18.21 as depicted by color Doppler. Pulsed wave Doppler echocardiography and hemodynamic data obtained at cardiac catheterization confirmed a pressure gradient between the atria

Video 18.23 Mid esophageal image demonstrating a large thrombus during long axis interrogation of a lateral tunnel Fontan connection

Video 18.24 Color flow Doppler with a low Nyquist limit (set at 28 cm/s) in the same patient as shown in Video 18.23 demonstrates a small amount of flow around the thrombus without disturbance in this region

Video 18.25 Gigantic right coronary artery aneurysm in a patient with congenital coronary artery ectasia as shown during transesophageal imaging at a mid esophageal level, multiplane angle 60°

Video 19.1 Example of three-dimensional "live 3D" format in a patient with repaired tetralogy of Fallot and an abnormal aortic valve. A standard mid esophageal aortic valve long axis was used to position and orient the probe. Note that the front portion of the dataset displays the tomographic image similar to a standard two-dimensional (2D) image, which helps to orient the echocardiographer. The dataset is then rotated to show the wedge-shaped thickness of the volume, and then rotated the other direction (towards the apex of the heart) to show the aortic valve and left ventricular outflow tract more clearly

Video 19.2 Example of the three-dimensional full volume dataset in the patient from Video 19.1. Four subvolumes were collected and rapidly stitched together to form a pyramidal dataset. Now a significant portion of the heart, including the whole aortic valve, is contained in this volume. The volume is then cropped to reveal an image similar to that seen with the standard 2D image and also the live 3D image

Video 19.3 Example of a three-dimensional (3D) color flow Doppler dataset in the same patient described from Videos 19.1 and 19.2. Turbulent systolic flow is noted across the aortic valve, as well as aortic valve regurgitation. Some stitch artifact is visible on this video

Video 19.4 xPlane mode from the Philips X7-2t 3D TEE probe. Two different 2D planes are shown simultaneously in this patient with mild subaortic stenosis. On the left is a mid esophageal four chamber view, on the right a mid esophageal long axis view. The circle on the display indicates the relationship of the two planes

Video 19.5 Example of the three-dimensional (3D) full volume dataset in the patient from Videos 19.1 and 19.2. Cropping in one of the standard perpendicular (x, y, z) cropping planes is shown, followed by "anyplane" cropping from two different angles, and then rotation of the dataset in the other direction towards the apex of the heart, using a standard perpendicular cropping plane

Video 19.6 Left atrial view imaging the superior surfaces of the left atrioventricular valve in a 23 year old woman who had previous closure of a primum atrial septal defect and subsequently developed progressive left atrioventricular valve regurgitation. The aortic valve or superior aspect of the heart is to the left, and the anterior aspect, tricuspid valve, is to the top of the screen. During diastole a significant residual cleft in the anterior leaflet is easily seen, with thickened leaftet edges

Video 19.7a A 12-year-old with severe aortic regurgitation. Images were constructed to view the superior surface of the aortic valve as if looking from the aorta down onto the leaflets. To the top is the right coronary cusp, to the left the left coronary cusp, and to the right is the non coronary cusp. The video is pre-bypass and shows the marked lack of coaptation and resulting area of regurgitation due to the retracted, scarred non coronary cusp. 3D color flow Doppler verifies color protruding through the region on the regurgitant orifice area of the non coronary cusp

Video 19.7b This is a post-bypass video from the same patient in Video 19.7a. The patient had pericardial replacement of the non coronary leaflet, and pericardial extension of the right and left coronary leaflet. The resultant post bypass 3D echo shows excellent coaptation of all three leaflets

Video 19.8a Ebstein malformation of the tricuspid valve. This video is a four chamber view of the heart oriented anteriorly and shows a very large anterior leaflet and severely tethered septal leaflet. The second part of the video is a short axis plane oriented from the RV apex to base of the heart demonstrating a very large zone of non-coaptation

Video 19.8b The video is post-bypass in the same patient in Video 19.8a after cone reconstruction. The entire leaflet structure now folds together during systole without a region of non-coaptation

Video 19.9a Transcatheter device closure of atrial septal defect (*ASD*). The video is a full volume acquisition demonstrating an en-face view of a secundum ASD from the left atrium

Video 19.9b Transcatheter device closure of atrial septal defect (*ASD*). This video is a full volume acquisition of the ASD from the right atrial side demonstrating the relationship to the aorta and superior vena cava

Video 19.9c Transcatheter device closure of atrial septal defect (*ASD*). This video is a live acquisition from the left atrial view demonstrating the sheath placed through the defect and the left atrial disc deployed within the left atrium

Video 19.9d Catheterization device closure of ASD. This video is an *en face* view of the right atrial disc after being deployed

Video 19.10 *En face* view of large membranous ventricular septal defect from the left ventricle

Video 19.11 Cross sectional view of doubly committed subarterial VSD with prolapse of the right coronary cusp through the defect causing right ventricular outflow tract obstruction

Video 19.12 A Image of 7 year old child with severe subaortic stenosis. The *first part* of the video displays a slightly oblique long axis view showing the thickened subaortic membrane immediately below the aortic valve. The *second part* of the video is a short axis view oriented from the left ventricular apex to the aorta demonstrating the concentric nature of the subaortic membrane and corresponding small outflow area

Video 19.13 Quantitative assessment of left ventricular (LV) volume and systolic function using three-dimensional (3D) echocardiography. From a transthoracic 3D echocardiographic dataset of the LV, the endocardium can be traced, and a semi-automated border detection method utilized to build a 3D surface rendered LV volume that can be displayed with dynamic "real-time" motion (*top left* and *right panels*). The volumes throughout the cardiac cycle are calculated and displayed on a curve (not shown). Using the maximum and minimum volumes obtained from this curve, an ejection fraction can be calculated (*bottom right panel*). As well, the LV endocardium can be divided into segments for evaluation of LV endocardial dyssynchrony (an example of the 16 segment model is shown in the *bottom left panel*). The systolic dyssynchrony index is calculated using the 16 segment (SDI 16) and 17 segment (SDI 17) models (*bottom right panel*)

Video 19.14 Quantitative assessment of right ventricular (RV) volume and systolic function using three-dimensional (3D) echocardiography, using software from TomTec (4D RV-function©). From a full volume transthoracic 3D echocardiographic data set of the RV, the RV endocardium is manually traced in three orthogonal. The software utilizes a semi-automated border detection method to generate a dynamic model of the RV, which is displayed in the *top panel*. RV volume is displayed on a curve of volume over time throughout the cardiac cycle in the *lower left panel*. The RV stroke volume (SV) and ejection fraction (EF) are automatically calculated and displayed in the *lower right panel*

Video 19.15 Example of stitch artifact with a full volume dataset. This can occur as a result of irregularities in cardiac rhythm, and/or respiratory/patient movement

Video 20.1 Full volume 3D acquisition in a mid esophageal four chamber view obtained in a patient with cor triatriatum, dextrocardia, and multiple ventricular septal defects. The cor triatriatum membrane divides the left atrium into proximal and distal chambers

Video 20.2 3D color Doppler flow map obtained in the same patient displayed in Video 20.1 demonstrates turbulent flow through the cor triatriatum obstructive orifice from a posterior view

Video 20.3 Live 3D mid esophageal aortic valve short axis acquisition from a patient with a bicuspid aortic valve due to left and right leaflet fusion

Video 20.4 Live 3D mid esophageal aortic valve short axis acquisition from a patient with a bicuspid aortic valve due to right and non-coronary leaflet fusion

Video 20.5 Full volume 3D mid esophageal four chamber view of the hypoplastic and doming parachute mitral valve

Video 20.6 Live 3D color Doppler flow mapping image of muscular ventricular septal defect from a mid esophageal long axis view

Video 20.7 Perimembranous ventricular septal defect as seen from a mid esophageal four chamber view with slight rightward probe rotation using full volume 3D acquisition

Video 20.8 Multiple orifice secundum atrial septal defect obtained from a mid esophageal four chamber view using 3D zoom mode. A thin vertical band of septum primum divides the ASD into a large anterior orifice and small posterior orifice

Video 20.9 View of an Amplatzer device as seen from a deep transgastric modified view acquired using live 3D

Video 20.10 Full volume 3D acquisition showing a muscular ventricular septal defect device after transcatheter device closure. The images were obtained from the mid esophageal four chamber view

Video 20.11 Live 3D acquisition from the mid esophageal aortic valve long axis view demonstrating dehiscence of a bicuspid aortic valve leaflet augmentation repair in a patient with endocarditis. The leaflet augmentation material oscillates between the left ventricular outflow tract and aorta

Video 20.12 Mid esophageal aortic valve long axis full volume 3D acquisition of a Konno procedure and aortic valve replacement using a bioprosthetic valve. The ventricular septal defect patch and bioprosthetic aortic valve are demonstrated

Video 20.13 Mid esophageal short axis full volume 3D acquisition of the same patient shown in Video 20.12 following a Konno procedure and aortic valve replacement. The bioprosthetic aortic valve is seen

Video 20.14 Mid esophageal four chamber view acquired using full volume 3D from a patient with *D*-transposition of the great arteries, after a Mustard procedure. The systemic and pulmonary venous baffles are seen

Video 20.15 Deep transgastric live 3D acquisition from a patient with *D*-transposition of the great arteries after a Mustard procedure demonstrating stenosis in the left ventricular outflow tract beneath the pulmonary valve

Video 20.16 Three-dimensional image in a patient with a 'classic' Fontan operation (atriopulmonary connection) displaying an organized thrombus within the Fontan connection

Video 20.17 Image in a patient with an atriopulmonary Fontan connection demonstrating very dense spontaneous contrast (sludge)

Video 20.18 Transgastric mid left ventricular short axis live 3D view in a patient with hypertrophic cardiomyopathy demonstrating the hypertrophied left ventricle and a pericardial effusion after defibrillator lead perforation of the right ventricle. The lead is well seen in the pericardial space

Introduction

The past 30 years have witnessed a dramatic evolution in the technology and clinical use of transesophageal echocardiography (TEE). Initially embraced by anesthesiologists in the early 1980s, TEE was used primarily as an intraoperative monitoring tool in the adult. Major applications included the evaluation of cardiac function and ventricular filling, detection of myocardial ischemia, and investigation of the etiology of perioperative hemodynamic instability. During the next decade, rapid and significant advancements in transducer and ultrasound imaging technology catalyzed the development of TEE into an important imaging modality for evaluating both acquired and congenital heart disease (CHD). With the advent of single-plane imaging, followed by subsequent developments in biplane and omniplane/multiplane technology, TEE rapidly became recognized for its excellent imaging capabilities in adult patients. At the same time, TEE probe miniaturization, along with enhanced spatial and temporal resolution of ultrasonic imaging, led to the growth and development of TEE for the pediatric population. Since then, its use in both pediatric and adult patients with CHD has increased, and the safety and efficacy of this imaging approach—even in neonates—has been widely validated. Thus, TEE has developed into an important tool for the evaluation and management of CHD. With the ongoing refinements and recent advances in three-dimensional TEE, this modality has tremendous potential for further enhancing the assessment of congenital cardiovascular malformations.

TEE continues to play a prominent role in the intraoperative setting and is widely recognized as a mainstay for preoperative and postoperative assessment for CHD. Over the course of time, however, the use of TEE has grown well beyond the operating room environment. It is now used in both inpatient and outpatient settings as a diagnostic and evaluative modality for children and adults with CHD. Even with alternative noninvasive imaging techniques such as cardiac magnetic resonance imaging and multi-slice, high-speed computerized tomography of the heart readily available, TEE remains an important and highly useful imaging approach for evaluating CHD in numerous settings and disease conditions. Its utility likely will continue well into the future.

In this textbook, we have endeavored to provide a comprehensive, thorough, and unique reference on TEE, one dedicated exclusively to the many applications of this modality for a wide spectrum of congenital pathologies. Every chapter provides highly instructive textual material, including unique insights on TEE gleaned from the knowledge and experience of each author, and supplemented by numerous pictorial and video examples. This textbook is not intended to be an encyclopedic compendium covering every aspect of TEE, nor is it meant to supplant the excellent references available for the echocardiographic evaluation of pediatric and CHD patients. Rather, we seek to provide a work that focuses and expands upon the applications of TEE specifically in the setting of CHD, complementing other important resources. To this end, we have assembled the contributions of highly regarded specialists in the field in order to share their expertise with others engaged in the important discipline of TEE.

Science of Ultrasound and Echocardiography

1

Pierre C. Wong

Abstract

For anyone seeking to achieve proficiency in transesophageal echocardiography, it is important to have a solid understanding of the underlying science of ultrasound, along with knowledge of the instrumentation and equipment utilized for cardiac imaging. This chapter provides a review of all of these topics, particularly as they apply to echocardiography. Basic principles of sound will first be discussed, followed by the process of ultrasonic two-dimensional image formation. Principles of Doppler echocardiography (and its applications) will then be presented. Finally, echocardiography instrumentation, echocardiographic artifacts, and digital archiving/networking of echocardiographic studies will be discussed. Familiarity with the information in this chapter will provide readers a greater understanding of the many technical aspects of echocardiography, enabling them to optimize their cardiac ultrasound platforms so that the best possible information can be obtained.

Keywords

Ultrasound physics • B-mode imaging • Phased array transducers • Doppler echocardiography • Spectral Doppler • Color flow Doppler • DICOM

Introduction

This is a textbook on transesophageal echocardiography (TEE), specifically TEE for the evaluation of congenital heart disease (CHD). But what is TEE? It is a specialized form of echocardiography, which is itself a specialized form of ultrasonography focusing upon the heart and related vascular structures. Thus, anyone seeking to achieve proficiency in echocardiography and TEE needs to have a solid understanding of the underlying science of ultrasound, particularly its strengths and weaknesses as applied to the evaluation of the cardiovascular system.

P.C. Wong, MD
Division of Cardiology, Children's Hospital Los Angeles, Department of Pediatrics, Keck School of Medicine, University of Southern California, 4650 Sunset Blvd, Mailstop #34, Los Angeles, CA 90027, USA
e-mail: pwong@chla.usc.edu

This chapter reviews the physics and instrumentation of ultrasound and echocardiography. It is not intended to be an exhaustive review of the subject—that would require a separate textbook, and a number of excellent and comprehensive references have already been written on this topic [1–4]. Rather, its purpose is to provide an overview of the science of ultrasound, focusing on aspects that apply especially to modern day echocardiography and TEE technology, and touching upon details pertinent to the echocardiographic evaluation of CHD.

This chapter is divided into six major sections: (1) Physics of Sound and Ultrasound; (2) Important Principles of Echocardiographic Image Formation; (3) Doppler Echocardiography; (4) Overview of the Echocardiography Machine; (5) Artifacts; (6) Digital Imaging and DICOM. While knowledge of the material in earlier sections aids in the comprehension of later sections, readers should feel free to peruse the chapter in whatever order they find most applicable.

P.C. Wong, W.C. Miller-Hance (eds.), *Transesophageal Echocardiography for Congenital Heart Disease*,
DOI 10.1007/978-1-84800-064-3_1, © Springer-Verlag London 2014

Background

The concept of utilizing sound for the purposes of location and imaging has its origins in nature. It is well known that bats use ultrasound (high frequency sound above the range of human hearing) in order to fly and locate their prey, even in complete darkness. This capability, which evolved over millions of years, is known as "echolocation". Dolphins, porpoises, and toothed whales are also known to utilize ultrasound underwater for echolocation. In World War I, SONAR (**SO**und **NA**vigation and **R**anging) was developed, in which piezoelectric materials were formulated as senders and receivers of high frequency sound waves, and these were employed to detect enemy submarines underwater. This technology was further developed and put to good use in World War II, and is still widely utilized today in both the commercial and military nautical industry. Medical diagnostic ultrasound was first developed in the 1940s–1950s. Over the past 50–60 years, rapid advancements in computing and probe miniaturization technology have made possible the development of high resolution, real-time two-dimensional (2D) ultrasonography, leading to the ability to define precisely the anatomy and physiology of the heart by echocardiography [5].

Regardless of whether it is used in bats, SONAR, or medical imaging, the basic principle (known as the *pulse-echo* principle) remains the same. Sound waves of known frequency are generated and sent (*pulsed*) in a specific direction, with the intention that a target object (or objects) will reflect some or all of the sound waves back to the source (Fig. 1.1). The sender then "listens" for the returning signals (*echoes*) from the target object; these returning echoes carry important information that can be used to abstract details about the object, including distance, image, size, movement, etc.

The following sections discuss the physical process in which ultrasound, specifically through the use of the pulse-echo principle, is utilized to obtain detailed information for medical diagnostic imaging—particularly in regard to noninvasive cardiac evaluation by echocardiography, including TEE.

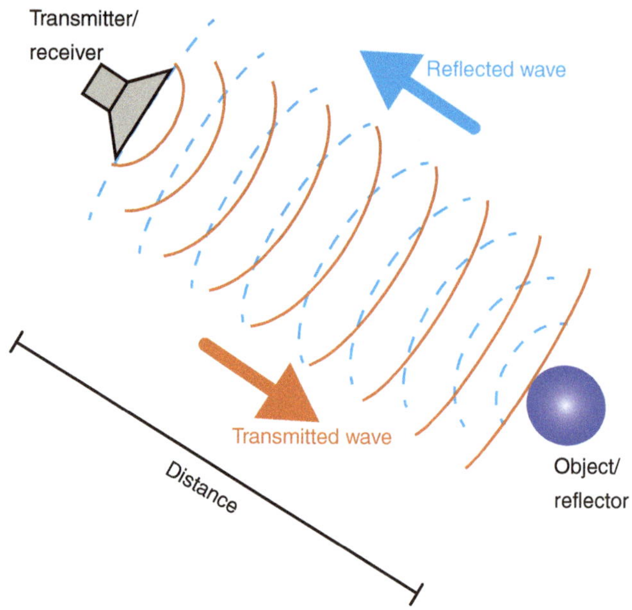

Fig. 1.1 Pulse-echo principle. A *pulse* of sound of known frequency is generated and emitted in a known direction. The *echoes* returning from an object can be used to derive information regarding the object, including distance, size, etc.

Physics of Sound and Ultrasound

Sound: Definition and Properties

Sound is a form of mechanical energy that requires a physical medium for transmission; this medium must contain molecules (such as air, water, etc.) that are used to propagate the sound. Unlike electromagnetic waves, which do not require a medium for propagation, sound cannot be transmitted in a vacuum. A sound wave is created when a discrete source—a vibrating or oscillating object—pushes and pulls adjacent molecules, causing them in turn to vibrate; this vibration spreads to adjacent molecules, and thus a disturbance is propagated away from the source in the form of a longitudinal wave characterized by a series of back and forth vibrations of molecules (Fig. 1.2). The direction of this back and forth vibration is parallel to the direction of wave propagation. The wave that is created represents a series of *compressions*, when the molecules are pushed together, and *rarefactions*, when the molecules are pulled apart (Fig. 1.2). If one could measure the instantaneous pressure at different points, the regions of compression, in which there is a greater density of molecules, would have a higher pressure than normal, and the regions of rarefaction (with a lesser density) would have a lower pressure than normal. Plotting a graph of pressure vs. distance from the source (along the line of propagation) would produce a curve in the shape of a sine wave (Fig. 1.2). The importance of this sine wave is that, like any wave, it has certain properties that can be used to describe it. The peak of one wave to the next peak (or valley to valley) represents one full wave or one complete cycle or period; the number of times per second that the cycle is repeated is termed the **frequency**, and the unit to measure this is cycles per second, or **Hertz** (**Hz**). This frequency is determined by the number of oscillations per second made by the sound source. The physical distance between two peaks (or valleys) is termed the **wavelength** and often designated by the symbol λ. This is the distance the sound wave travels in one complete cycle. The importance here is that frequency and

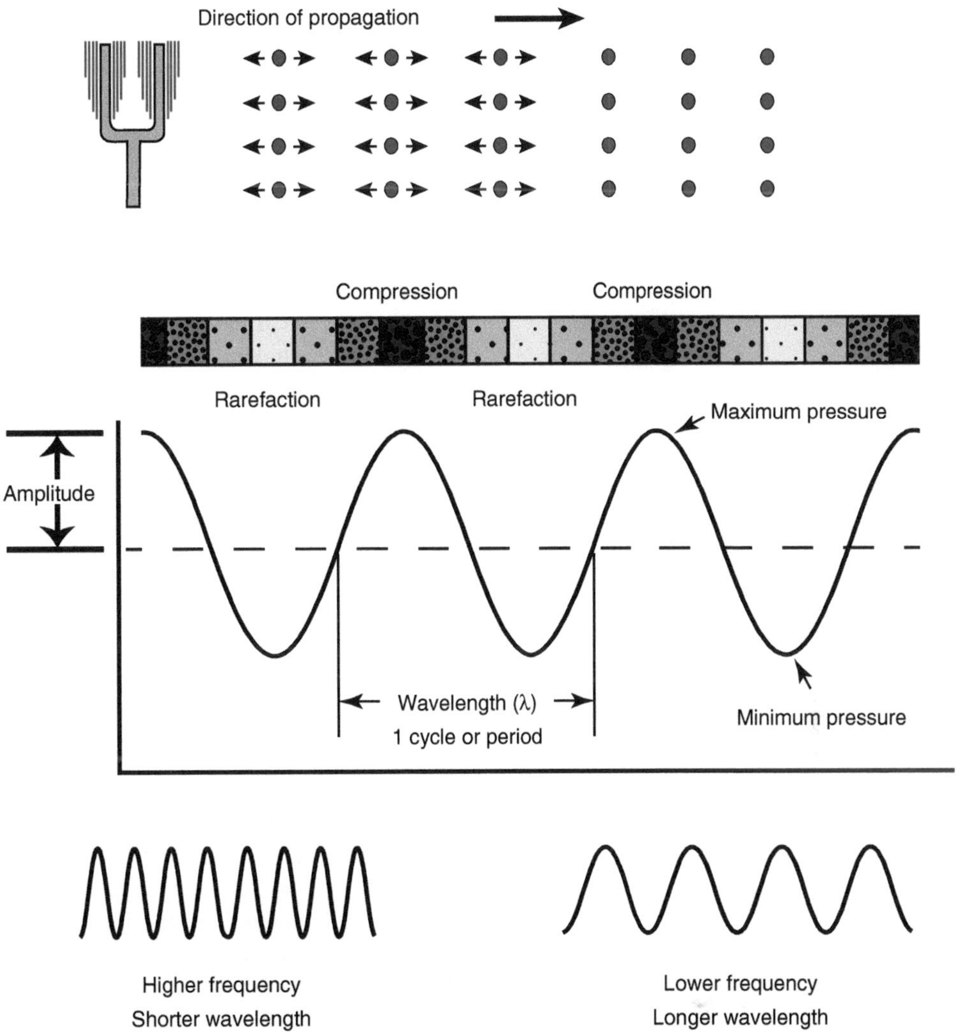

Fig. 1.2 Generation of a sound wave. A vibrating source (in this case, a tuning fork) causes adjacent air molecules to vibrate in a back-and-forth direction. This oscillating motion propagates away from the source in a series of compressions and rarefactions; when the air pressure at any one point is plotted as a function of time, a sine wave is obtained with a wavelength (λ) and pressure amplitude (P). Shorter wavelengths are associated with higher wave frequencies; longer wavelengths with lower frequencies. This example shows sound propagation in air, but the same principles apply in water or in the soft tissue of the human body

wavelength are inversely related, and their magnitude depends upon the speed of sound in the medium (Table 1.1A). The equation relating these three variables is given as follows:

$$\lambda = \frac{c}{f} \tag{1.1}$$

λ = wavelength
c = speed of sound in the medium
f = frequency in cycles/second

The speed of sound varies depending upon the medium: the denser the medium, the faster the speed of propagation. In biological systems, the speed of sound exhibits wide variation: it is lowest in the lungs, which are air-filled structures (about 600 m/s), and highest in bone (about 4,080 m/s) (Table 1.1A). In the soft tissues, the average speed of sound is about **1,540 m/s**, and this is the number generally used when calibrating the range-measuring circuits of most diagnostic ultrasound instrumentation [1]. As will be shown throughout this chapter, the speed of sound in the human body plays an important role in a number of considerations related to echocardiography.

The importance of Eq. 1.1 is that, by knowing the speed of sound in the medium, the wavelength can be calculated for a given sound frequency, and vice-versa. The range of sound frequencies audible by the human ear is between 20 and 20,000 Hz. However, if sound waves of these frequencies were transmitted in the body, the corresponding wavelengths would be far too large for use in the medical field. For diagnostic medical imaging, adequate resolution is possible only when the wavelength of the sound wave is comparable to the size of the smallest objects being imaged [6, 7]. For echocardiography, this translates to millimeters or less, which means that sound frequencies in the *millions* of Hertz (megahertz, or MHz) must be used. Note that these frequencies are extremely high, several orders of magnitude beyond the range of human hearing—hence the term *ultrasound*. Echocardiography generally utilizes frequencies between 1 and 15 MHz, which by Eq. 1.1 yields a wavelength between

Table 1.1 Physical properties of sound for various tissues in the human body

A. Speed of sound	
Material	*Speed of sound (m/s)*
Lung	600
Fat	1,460
Liver	1,555
Blood	1,560
Kidney	1,565
Muscle	1,600
Lens of eye	1,620
Skull bone	4,080
B. Acoustic impedance	
Tissue	*Acoustic impedance (Rayls × 10^{-4})*
Air	0.0004
Lung	0.18
Water	1.5
Brain	1.55
Blood	1.61
Liver	1.65
Kidney	1.62
Human soft tissue, mean	1.63
Muscle	1.71
Skull bone	7.8
C. Attenuation coefficient	
Tissue	*Attenuation coefficient (dB/cm)*
Water	0.0022
Blood	0.18
Brain	0.85
Liver	0.9
Fat	0.6
Kidney	1.0
Muscle	1.2
Skull bone	20
Lung	40

Source: Zagzebski [1]

For each table, measurements are listed from lowest to highest value

0.1 mm (15 MHz) and 1.54 mm (1 MHz). The higher the frequency, the smaller the wavelength, and the better the spatial resolution.

The other important property of a sound wave is its amplitude, which describes the strength of the wave, or maximum pressure elevation from baseline (Fig. 1.2). This corresponds to the "loudness" of the sound. This property, also known as **acoustic pressure**, is measured in **Pascals (P)**. The amplitude of the sound represents the energy associated with the sound wave: the more the energy, the "louder" the sound and the greater the amplitude. Another parameter used to express the "loudness" of the sound is known as **intensity**. This term is used to describe the energy flowing a cross-sectional area per second and is proportional to the square of acoustic pressure, as noted by the equation:

$$I = \frac{P^2}{2\rho c} \tag{1.2}$$

I = intensity
P = acoustic pressure in Pascals
ρ = density of the medium
c = speed of sound in the medium

Intensity is the parameter used to characterize the spatial distribution of ultrasound energy. As noted, it describes the amount of ultrasonic power per unit area (given in watts/square meter, or more commonly milliwatts per square centimeter), and can vary depending upon location. The difference between acoustical power and intensity can be illustrated in the following example: two beams (one focused, one unfocused) are emitted with the same acoustic power. While the unfocused beam has a more uniform distribution of energy; the focused beam will produce more concentrated energy in the area focused. Hence, the intensity is greater in that area. Intensity is also one of the parameters used to evaluate the biological effects of ultrasound. At sufficiently high intensities and long enough exposure times, ultrasound can produce a measurable effect on tissues, notably in the form of heating and cavitation (tiny bubbles from dissolved gases in the medium) [1]. The subject of the biological effects of ultrasound on human tissue is beyond the scope of this chapter. Suffice it to say that while no known ill effects have been noted from the intensity levels and scan times commonly used in diagnostic medical ultrasound, it is still important to be mindful of the remote possibility—particularly if equipment manufacturers were to increase output intensities to improve imaging [3, 8].

For medical imaging, a standard method for quantifying intensities or power levels is to use the decibel (dB) system. Instead of providing an absolute number, this method produces a value that represents a relative change (or ratio) between two amplitudes or two intensities. Using two echo signal intensities I_1 and I_2 or two echo signal amplitudes A_1 and A_2 (I_1 and A_1 representing the reference signal), the signal level in dB is calculated as follows:

$$\textit{Signal level} = 10\log\frac{I_2}{I_1} \text{ or } \textit{Signal level} = 20\log\frac{A_2}{A_1} \tag{1.3}$$

It is meaningless to use a dB level as an absolute value. Rather, the dB notation provides a value obtained when comparing a particular intensity or amplitude to a reference value. In diagnostic medical ultrasound, the transmitted signal generally serves as the reference value. Note that the dB represents a logarithmic scale, therefore an intensity change of +3 dB represents a doubling of intensity, and −3 dB a halving of intensity. The dB system is used to express output power, dynamic range, or ultrasonic attenuation in tissue (see below). It represents a simpler, more compact method to express large differences in power levels or intensity, and will be used throughout the remainder of this chapter.

Reflection: The Key to Ultrasonic Imaging

As an ultrasound wave propagates through the body, several different interactions are possible as it encounters the various tissues interfaces. These interactions, analogous to those occurring with light waves, include: (a) continued transmission, (b) reflection, (c) refraction, (d) absorption. Of these, **reflection** is the key interaction that makes possible the generation of ultrasonographic/echocardiographic information. As mentioned above, diagnostic medical ultrasound consists of emitting sound pulses in a known direction, and then collecting and processing the returning echo signals—that is, the signals that have been *reflected* from the various internal structures in the body (in the case of echocardiography, the heart, blood, and vascular structures). The differences in the strength of the returning signals enable the ultrasound machine to build an image of the various tissues, as well as the tissue-tissue and tissue-blood interfaces, and this forms the basis of echocardiographic imaging. What determines how echo signals are reflected, and the strength of these signals? A fundamental factor is **acoustic impedance**, an intrinsic property of tissue that characterizes its capacity for sound transmission. The acoustic impedance of a tissue is directly proportional to its underlying density—the denser the tissue, the higher the acoustic impedance. Each type of tissue has a different acoustic impedance: air has an extremely low impedance, bone has a very high impedance, and the various soft tissues have impedances that differ from each other but vary within a much narrower range (Table 1.1B). At a tissue interface, the degree of reflection vs. transmission of an incident sound wave depends upon the relative difference in acoustic impedance between the two tissues—that is, the degree of *impedance matching*. When there is a small impedance mismatch, most of the sound energy is transmitted, and only a small amount is reflected and returns to the source (transducer) to be used as imaging information (Fig. 1.3). As the transmitted energy continues further, some is reflected in a similar manner at more distant interfaces, yielding imaging information from deeper structures. This process continues along the length of the ultrasound beam. In this manner, ultrasonic information is progressively obtained, and imaging is possible to significant depths because the acoustic impedance differences are small for most soft tissue-soft tissue interfaces. However, if a significant impedance mismatch exists between two tissues, then virtually all sound is reflected, and very little transmitted. Almost no usable information is available beyond the interface (a phenomenon known as "acoustic shadowing"). This is the reason that lung

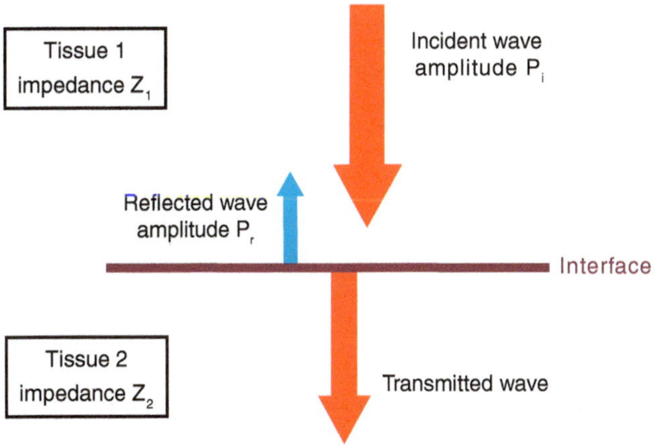

Fig. 1.3 Specular reflection. When an incident sound wave of amplitude P_i encounters a smooth interface perpendicular to the direction of propagation, some is reflected (amplitude P_r) and the remainder transmitted. The degree of transmission vs. reflection depends upon the relative differences in acoustic impedance between the two tissues (Z_1 and Z_2)—the greater the impedance mismatch, the greater the amount of sound reflected

interferes with ultrasonic imaging: it is not that ultrasound cannot propagate through lung, it is that the impedance mismatch is so great between lung and soft tissue that virtually all ultrasound energy is reflected. It is also the reason that ultrasonic gel is used with transthoracic imaging: to improve the acoustic coupling (impedance matching) between the transducer and the chest wall.

Acoustic impedance matching is important whenever a sound wave encounters an interface between two tissues, and it is particularly important for those interfaces that are much larger than the size of the ultrasound wavelength. When such interfaces are large and smooth, they are termed **specular reflectors** and they behave like a large acoustic mirror (*speculum* = mirror in Latin). If there is a sizable impedance mismatch, incident ultrasound beams will undergo a great deal of reflection. If the incident beam is directed perpendicular to the surface, the reflected sound waves return to the transducer as a well-defined, redirected beam (echo), leading to a very bright appearance on the display screen (Fig. 1.4). If the incident ultrasound beam strikes the specular reflector at an angle, the reflected portion will be directed at an angle θ_r which is equal to the incident angle θ_i but in the opposite direction. The remainder of the incident beam that is transmitted can be "bent" or **refracted**, with the amount of refraction depending upon the difference between the speed of sound between the two tissues, as given by Snell's Law (Fig. 1.5). The greater the difference in the speed of sound between the two tissues, the greater the degree of refraction. Again, this is analogous to the behavior of light waves. In general, refraction is not a major problem with diagnostic ultrasound because there is little variation in the speed of sound among the soft tissues in the human body.

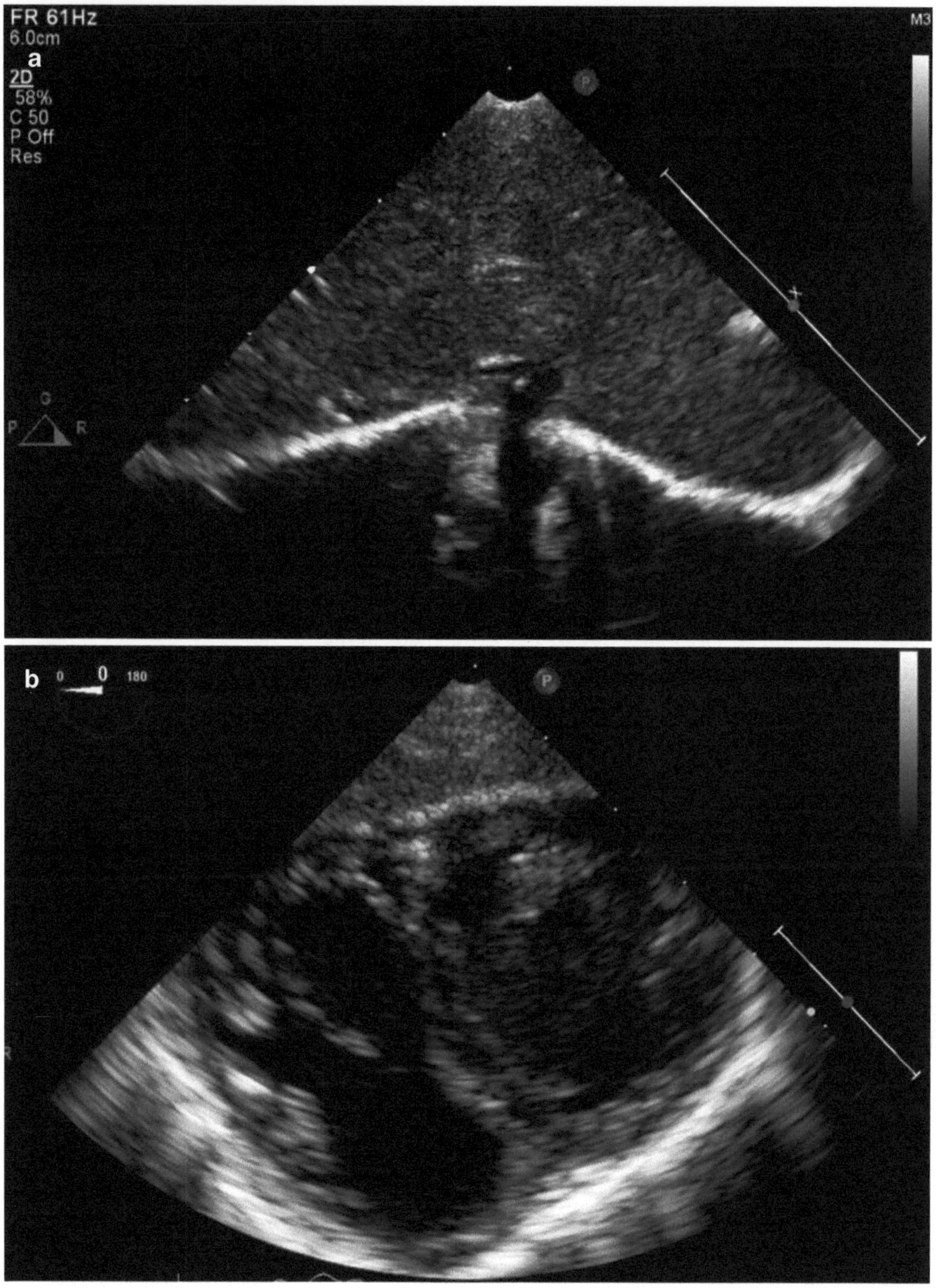

Fig. 1.4 Example of a large specular reflector (diaphragm) and acoustic scattering produced by imaging of the liver (**a**) and myocardium (**b**). Note that the echoes from the specular reflector have the largest amplitude (brightness) when the surface is perpendicular to the angle of insonation. In (**b**), the myocardium has the characteristic heterogeneous 2D appearance produced by natural acoustic reflections and interference patterns (scattering) from its various components, also known as "speckle"

However in certain situations, refraction can lead to image errors; this can be seen in the setting of interfaces between fat and soft tissue.

What if the large surface is not smooth, but rough? In this case the uneven surface causes incident energy to be reflected in a number of different directions. This is called **diffuse reflection** (Fig. 1.6). Such reflections can cause a loss of beam coherence and a weaker echo returning to the transducer. Some organ boundaries, as well as the walls of the heart chambers (irregular endocardial surfaces), fall within this category. At first glance, it would appear that that these signals, along with the nonperpendicular signals to a specular reflector (whether reflected at an angle or refracted) would not be as useful for imaging because they are not directed back to the transducer. However in practice, even these off-angle specular and diffuse reflectors are useful for ultrasonic imaging due to the range to different transducer positions that can be utilized. In addition, divergences of the ultrasound beam can result in sound waves that will be reflected back to the transducer [9]. In fact, echoes from diffuse reflectors, while weaker, can be useful because of the fact that they are not as sensitive to the orientation of the transducer.

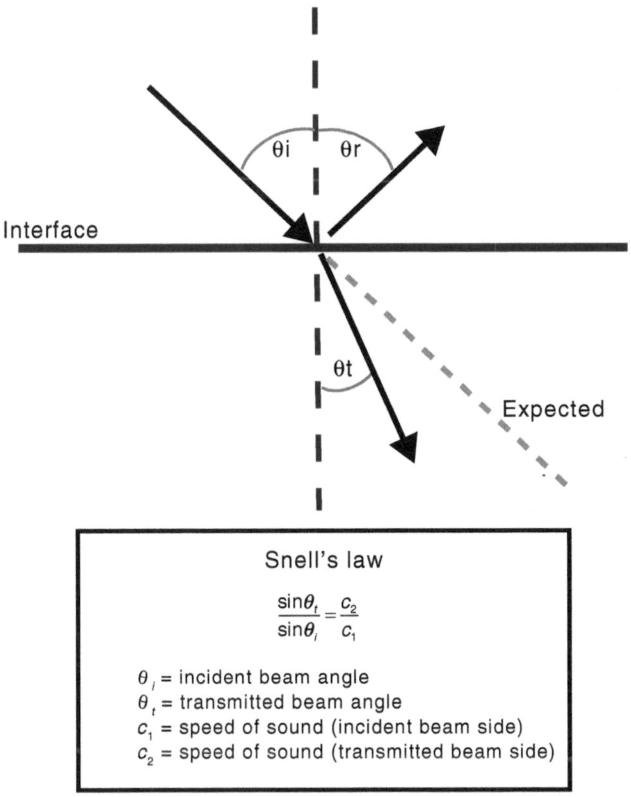

Fig. 1.5 Refraction and Snell's law. When the incident sound wave encounters a large specular reflector at a nonperpendicular angle θ_i (θ_i refers to the angle as measured from the perpendicular axis), the reflected beam travels off at an equivalent angle θ_r. The transmitted wave undergoes refraction or "bending". The amount of refraction can be predicted by Snell's law, which is itself based upon the difference in the speed of sound between the two tissues. The greater the difference, the greater the degree of refraction

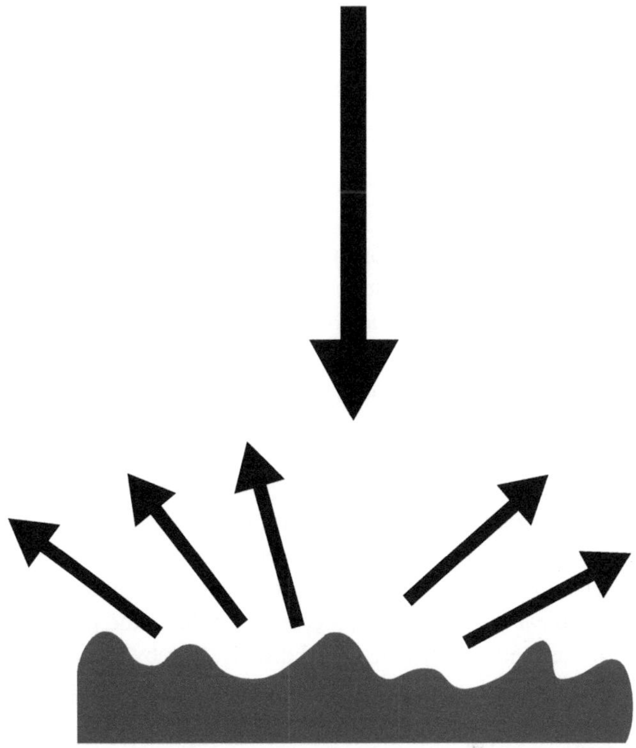

Fig. 1.6 Diffuse reflector. An incident beam striking a rough, uneven surface results in lower amplitude reflected waves that travel away from the reflector in multiple directions. This type of echo is not as dependent upon interface orientation as a specular reflector

The information from diffuse and specular reflectors is most useful at the boundaries of objects and organs, for example along the diaphragm or pericardium. However an even more important type of reflection accounts for much of the useful diagnostic information in ultrasonic imaging, including echocardiography. This type of reflection is called **acoustic scattering**, also known as *nonspecular reflection*. It refers to reflections from objects the size of the ultrasound wavelength or smaller. The parenchyma of most organs, including the heart, contains a number of objects (reflectors) of this size. The signals from these reflectors return to the transducer through multiple pathways. The sound from such reflectors is no longer a coherent beam; it is instead the sum of a number of component waves that produces a complex pattern of constructive and destructive interference. This interference pattern is known as "speckle" and provides the characteristic ultrasonic appearance of complex tissue such as myocardium (Fig. 1.4a) [7]. These signals tend to be weaker, and echo signal strength varies depending upon the degree of scattering. The degree of scattering is primarily based upon: (a) number of scatterers per unit volume; (b) acoustic impedance changes at the scatterer interfaces; (c) size of the scatterer—increased size produces increased scattering; (d) ultrasonic frequency—scattering increases with increasing frequency/decreasing wavelength [1]. The last point is important, because it contrasts to specular reflection, which is *frequency independent*. Therefore it is possible to enhance scattering selectively over specular reflection by using higher ultrasound frequencies. Also, because of the fact that scattering occurs in multiple directions, the incident beam angle/direction is not as important as with specular reflectors. This is why organ parenchyma (such as liver) can be readily viewed from a number of different transducer positions (Fig. 1.4b). Changes in scattering amplitude will result in brightness changes on the ultrasound image on the display, giving rise to the terms **hyperechoic** (increased scattering, brighter) and **hypoechoic** (decreased scattering, darker), and **anechoic** (no scattering, black appearance).

At the opposite extreme from the large specular reflectors are the very small reflectors whose dimensions are much less than the ultrasonic wavelength. Such reflectors also produce scattering, and are termed **Rayleigh scatterers**. This category most notably includes red blood cells, and the scattering that results from these gives rise to the echo signals from blood for Doppler and color flow imaging. Scattering from Rayleigh scatterers increases exponentially (to the fourth power) as frequency is increased.

Attenuation and Ultrasonic Imaging

As ultrasound travels through tissue, the amplitude and intensity of the signal decreases as a function of distance. This is known as **attenuation**, and is due to several mechanisms. The first mechanism is one in which acoustic energy is converted into another form of energy, principally heat; this is known as *absorption*. The second mechanism involves redirection of beam energy, by a number of different processes including *scattering*, *reflection*, *refraction*, *diffraction*, and *divergence* (the latter two processes result in a spreading of the sound beam). Scattering and reflection (and also refraction) were discussed above; while both play an essential role in diagnostic medical imaging, each process also reduces the intensity of ultrasound energy transmitted distally, thereby attenuating the transmitted signal. The third mechanism involves interaction between sound waves, known as *interference*. Wave interference occurs when two waves meet. It can be constructive or destructive, depending upon whether the two waves are in phase or out of phase. When in phase (constructive), an additive effect is produced, increasing amplitude; when out of phase (destructive), the waves can effectively cancel each other out. The degree of attenuation can be given as an *attenuation coefficient* (α) in decibels per centimeter (dB/cm), representing the reduction in signal amplitude or intensity as a function of distance. The amount of attenuation, as measured in decibels, can be calculated by the equation: Attenuation (dB) $= \alpha \times$ distance (cm). The attenuation coefficient varies with the type of medium through which the ultrasound is transmitted (Table 1.1C). As can be seen, there is little attenuation in blood, but significant attenuation in bone. Attenuation in muscle is twice that of other tissues such as liver. Another important determinant of attenuation is the frequency of the ultrasound beam. In most cases, attenuation increases approximately linearly with frequency: the higher the frequency, the greater the attenuation (Fig. 1.7).

However, as will be seen with much of ultrasound, there are tradeoffs. In this particular case, the tradeoff is depth. While higher frequencies provide enhanced spatial resolution, in soft tissue they are attenuated much more rapidly than lower frequencies, hence the depth of penetration is much less, and so the higher frequencies are not as useful for visualizing deeper structures. This is why higher frequency, higher resolution transthoracic imaging is much more feasible in pediatric compared to adult patients. It is also one of the reasons that TEE provides superior imaging compared to transthoracic imaging in larger patients: the proximity of the esophagus to the heart significantly reduces attenuation and enables the use of higher frequency ultrasonic imaging.

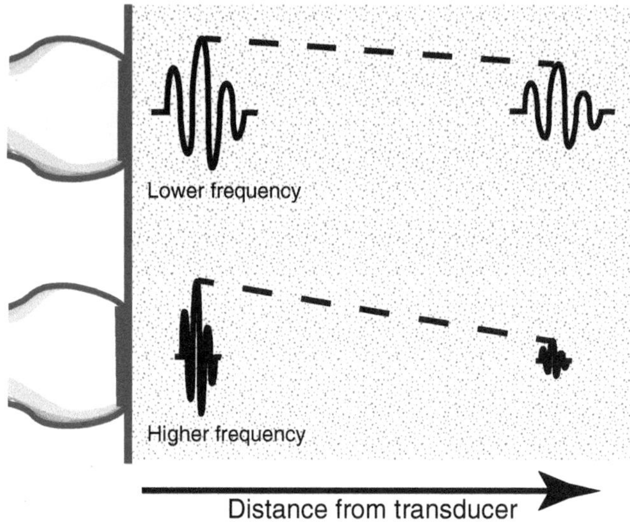

Fig. 1.7 Attenuation of ultrasound in parenchyma. As an ultrasound pulse travels through tissue, its amplitude and intensity decrease as a function of distance from the transducer. This is known as attenuation. Higher frequency sound waves are attenuated much more rapidly than lower frequencies

Important Principles of Echocardiographic Image Formation

At first glance, the basic premise behind 2D imaging in echocardiography seems relatively straightforward. Using the pulse-echo principle discussed above, an ultrasound pulse is emitted as a well-directed beam, and reflected echo signals are collected from the beam line. If this is continued while the ultrasound beam is swept in an arc (sector), a 2D image can be constructed, using echo arrival times and beam axis location to determine the precise location of reflectors within the sector (Fig. 1.8).

However, the actual process by which reflected ultrasound signals are converted into real-time, 2D echocardiographic images is deceptively complex, requiring sophisticated and technologically intricate hardware, along with highly advanced and powerful computing and digital signal processing capabilities. A number of different steps are involved: generation of high quality and well-directed ultrasound pulses, reception and digitization of the returning signals, multilayered digital signal processing, and conversion of these signals to a real-time 2D image of sufficient medical diagnostic quality (while at the same allowing operator manipulation and pre/post processing of the images). Moreover, for echocardiography and TEE the same process must be repeated rapidly and continuously in order to display the real time motion of the heart.

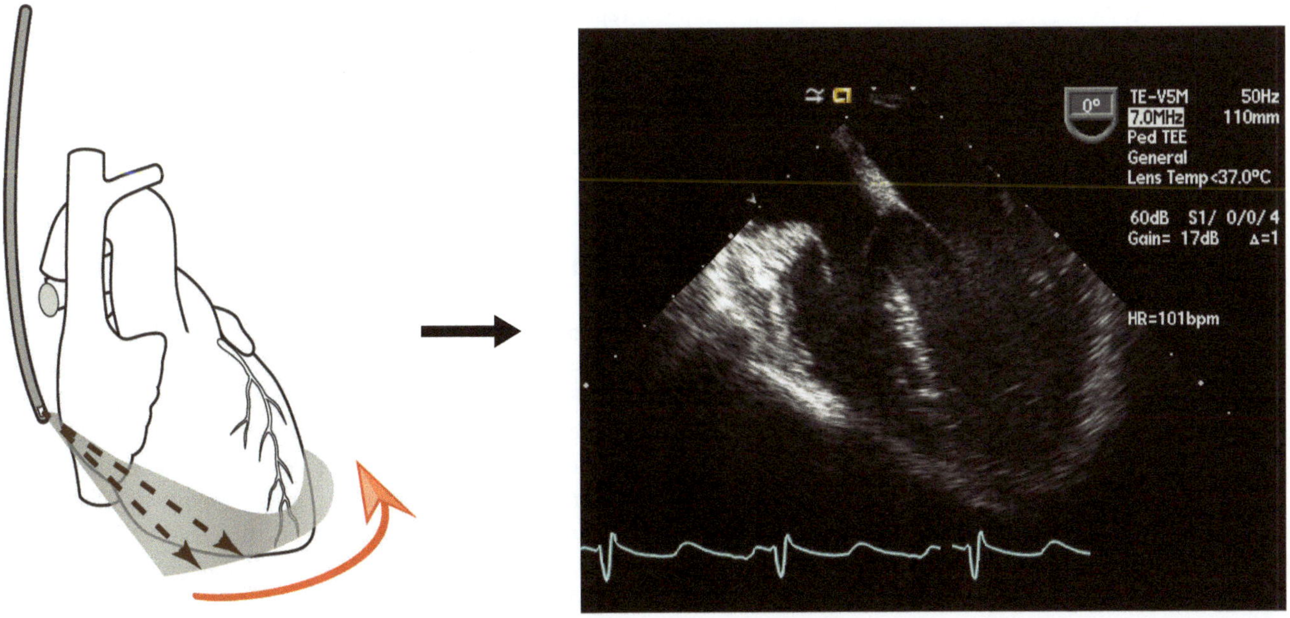

Fig. 1.8 Production of an ultrasound (echocardiographic) image. A pulse of ultrasound is transmitted in a well defined beam, and the transducer "listens" while echoes are received from the same beam path. These echoes appear as *dots* (brightness) corresponding to signal amplitude. During 2D imaging, the beam is swept across a sector (*red arrow*), and displaying all the beams along this sector results in a two-dimensional (B-mode) image. In this example, a transesophageal transducer is shown, but the same process occurs with transthoracic echocardiography

The sections that follow discuss the process by which ultrasound pulse generation leads to image formation, specifically as pertains to echocardiography. For simplicity's sake, the discussion will first cover basic ultrasound beam forming principles utilizing single element transducers. These principles will then be applied to array transducers, which form the basis for modern day echocardiography, including TEE.

Transducers

The first step in ultrasound imaging requires the creation and transmission of an appropriate sound wave; this is accomplished by the use of a **transducer**. Technically, the term transducer refers to any device that is used to convert one form of energy into another. The ultrasonic transducer converts electrical energy to mechanical (acoustic) energy in the form of sound waves that are then transmitted into the medium. When reflected sound waves return, the reverse process occurs: the transducer receives the acoustic energy and converts it into electrical signals for processing. Transducers in medical ultrasound achieve this conversion by the *piezoelectric* (PZE) effect. The PZE effect is a special property seen with certain types of crystals (quartz, ceramics, etc.). When an electrical signal is applied to such a crystal, it vibrates at a natural resonant frequency, sending a sound wave into the medium. Conversely, acoustic energy received by the crystal produces mechanical pressure or stress, which then causes the crystal to generate an electrical charge that can be amplified, yielding a useful electrical signal. Thus PZE transducers can serve as both detectors and transmitters of ultrasound. As noted previously, the signals must be appropriate for imaging of tissues in the human body—wavelengths must be no more than 1–2 mm, which means sound frequencies must be in the *millions* of Hertz. While several PZE crystals found in nature (e.g. quartz) have been used for ultrasonography, most present day ultrasound transducers utilize man-made PZE ceramic (such as lead zirconate titanate, also known as PZT) and composite ceramic elements. When excited, these PZE elements can produce the very high frequencies required for diagnostic medical imaging. A PZE transducer operates best at its natural resonance frequency, which corresponds to the crystal (element) thickness; however newer composite elements have wide frequency bandwidths and can operate at different frequencies, enabling generation of multiple frequencies from one transducer. In these instances, the native frequency, which usually represents the midpoint of the frequency distribution, is termed the "center" or "central carrier" frequency.

However, a transducer is not simply a housing surrounding a PZE element or collection of elements (see arrays below). While the PZE element serves as the most important component of an ultrasound transducer, a number of other essential components also reside in the transducer. These include backing (damping) material, electrodes, an insulating cover, housing, matching layer, and acoustic lens (in some transducers) (Fig. 1.9). The matching layer, which covers and attaches to the PZE element, is very important

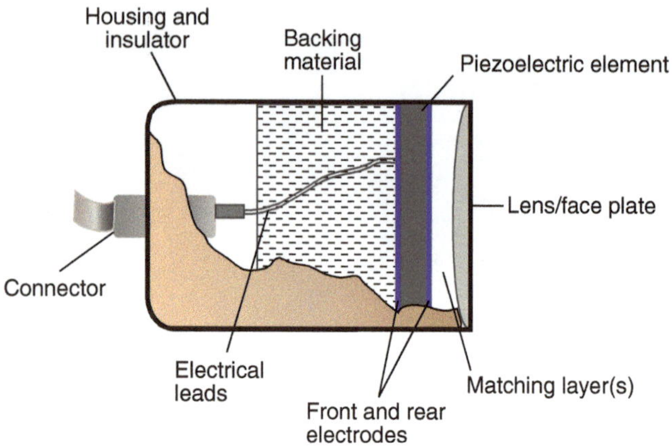

Fig. 1.9 Diagram of a single element transducer. The various components of the transducer are seen. In this example, there is a large, single piezoelectric crystal. For an array transducer, instead of a large single element, multiple elements would be laid in a single row, each with its own electrical connector. However the other parts of the transducer would be analogous to the single element transducer

because of the significant impedance mismatch that exists between the PZE element and surface (skin or esophagus). The matching layer contains an acoustic impedance intermediate between the two surfaces; this helps to match impedances from one surface to the other, allowing for efficient sound transmission between transducer element and soft tissue. In some transducers, multiple matching layers are used to facilitate transmission of a range of ultrasound frequencies. Also, newer composite PZE elements have acoustic impedances much closer to that of soft tissue.

The backing (damping) material also serves an important role. Pulse-echo ultrasound involves the transmission of a short pulse of sound, followed by a period in which the transducer "listens" for the returning echoes. As it turns out, for ultrasound imaging the transducer spends only a tiny fraction of time actually transmitting sound—this is known as the *duty factor*, and typically comprises less than 1 % of the total time. The rest of the time is spent listening for returning echoes. For this to occur, the transducer can emit only a very short pulse of acoustic energy, usually a small number of cycles in length. To produce these, short bursts of electrical energy cause the PZE element to vibrate or "ring", which generates the acoustic pulse. The length of the pulse train, also known as *pulse duration* or *spatial pulse length*, is truncated by *damping* the duration of the vibration as quickly as possible, and the backing material plays an important role here. An important point regarding pulse duration is that short pulses are desirable to optimize axial resolution, as will be discussed below. The typical pulse length is 1–3 cycles in length. Of note, a shorter pulse is a less "pure" tone, and contains a wider range of frequencies, also known as having a broader bandwidth (Fig. 1.10). This range of frequencies encompasses the labeled operating (center) frequency, which represents the midpoint of the frequency distribution. Wide bandwidth associated with short pulse duration is more desirable for imaging applications; narrower frequency bandwidth associated with longer pulse duration is more useful for pulsed Doppler applications.

Transducer Beam Formation and Geometry

When sound waves originate from a single, small point source whose size is similar to the wavelengths it produces (such as a bell), the waves radiate outward in all directions (Fig. 1.11a). However this results in an unfocused signal, unsuitable for medical imaging in which a directed, focused ultrasound beam becomes considerably more important. Diagnostic medical ultrasound transducers are designed to direct ultrasound pulses in a specific direction. A single element ultrasound source of large dimension (for example, a transducer face much larger than the wavelength of sound emanating from it) can produce equally spaced, linear wavefronts (Fig. 1.11b) also known as *planar wavefronts* [10]. Conceptually, these planar wavefronts can be described as a collection of multiple individual point sources, also known as *Huygen sources*, and the wavelets arising from these sources are known as *Huygen wavelets* [1]. Interference among wavelets results in the large planar waveform (Fig. 1.11c).

One of the important aspects of ultrasound beam formation concerns the geometry of the beam and its impact upon imaging. With a single element, unfocused ultrasound transducer, the individual wavelets from a transducer form a near parallel beam wave front, as noted in Fig. 1.11c. Two important zones develop in this beam. The first distance is the *near field*, or *Fresnel zone*. This area is characterized by many regions of constructive and destructive interference, leading to fluctuations in intensity. In this zone, the beam remains well collimated for a certain distance, and even narrows slightly (Fig. 1.12). Beyond the near field, the beam diverges, and some energy escapes along the periphery of the beam; this is known as the *far field* or *Fraunhofer zone* (Fig. 1.12). Fresnel (near-field) length is directly proportional to aperture of the transducer element and inversely proportional to transducer frequency, as given by the equation:

$$D_{Fresnel} = \frac{d^2}{4\lambda} \tag{1.4}$$

$D_{Fresnel}$ = Fresnel (near field) length
d = diameter, or aperture, of the transducer
λ = ultrasound wavelength

The importance of these two zones lies in the fact that lateral resolution is best before divergence of the beam, hence the best imaging and spatial detail are obtained within the Fresnel zone, or near-field. From Eq. 1.4, it becomes

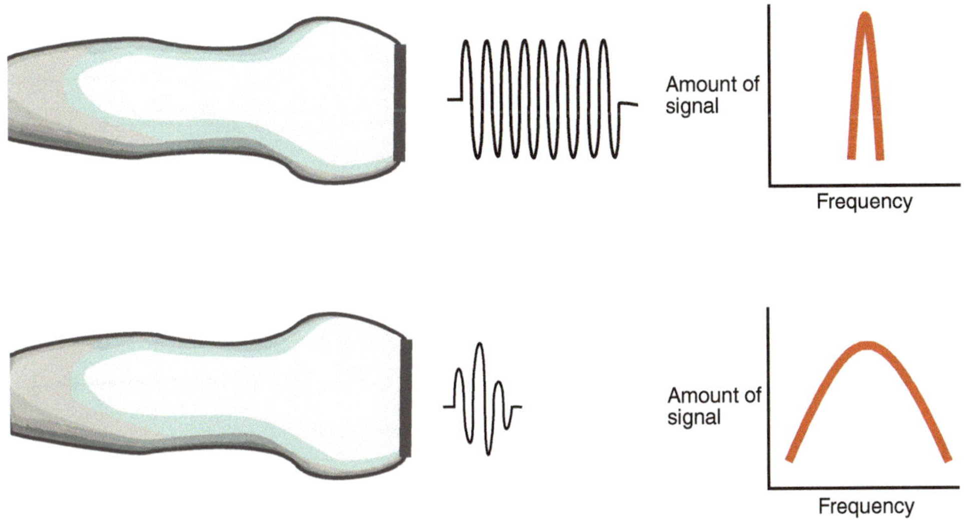

Fig. 1.10 Spatial pulse length. The top pulse has undergone less damping; therefore it has a longer duration, or spatial pulse length, and a purer "tone" with most of the sound at or near a certain frequency. Contrast this with the bottom pulse, which has undergone excellent damping that reduces the spatial pulse length. This type of pulse is characterized by a large frequency bandwidth

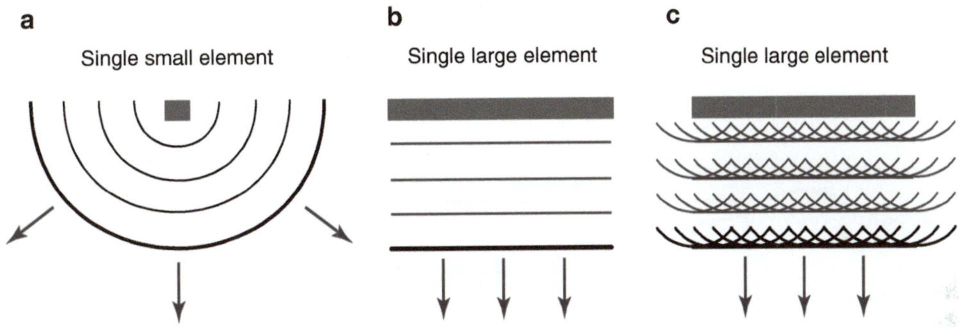

Fig. 1.11 Sound wave geometry. (**a**) A single small element has a size similar to the wavelength it produces. Sound from this element radiates in all directions. (**b**) The single element is much larger than the sound wavelengths it produces, resulting in equally spaced, planar wavefronts. These planar wavefronts can be thought of as a collection of individual point sources, each with its own wavelet. These are known as *Huygen wavelets* (**c**)

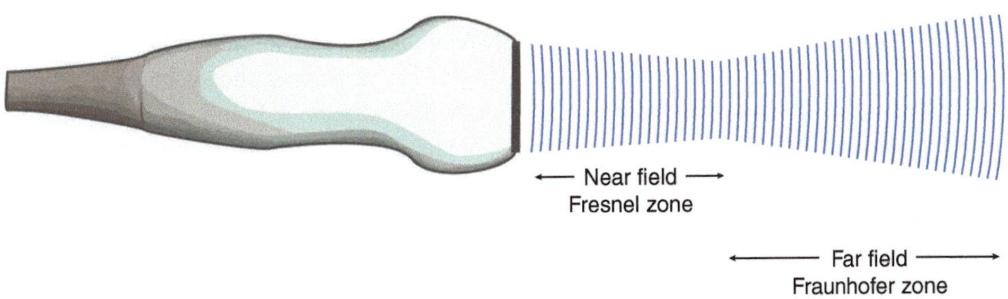

Fig. 1.12 Sound beam pattern from a single element, unfocused transducer. The near field is known as the *Fresnel zone*, the far field is known as the *Fraunhofer zone*. Note that the sound beam is well collimated in the near field and diverges in the far field

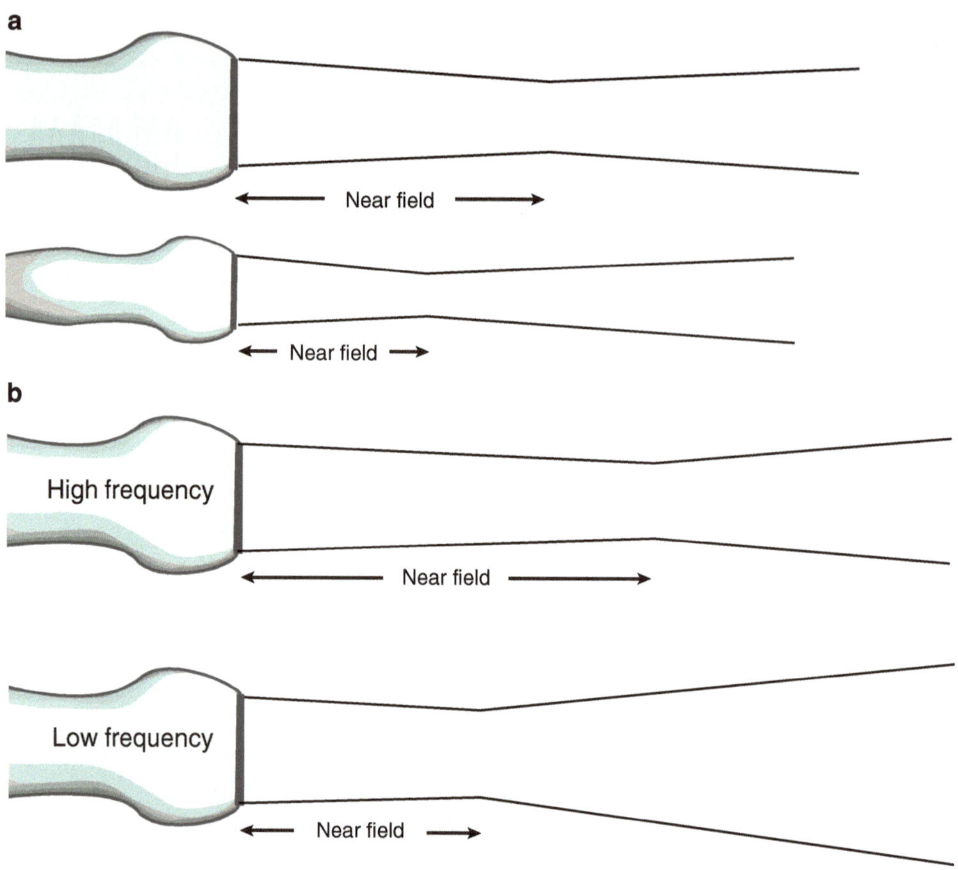

Fig. 1.13 Effect of transducer frequency and diameter on near field length. (**a**) Both transducers have the same frequency but the larger diameter transducer has a longer near field length, and less beam divergence. (**b**) Both transducers have the same diameter, but the transducer with the higher frequency has the longer near field length and less beam divergence

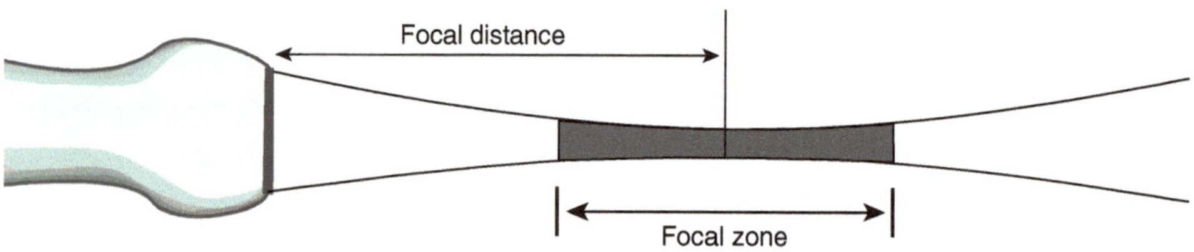

Fig. 1.14 Beam pattern for a focused transducer. The beam is narrowest at the focal distance, hence the best lateral resolution is within the focal zone. Focusing can either be done externally (e.g. acoustic lens) for a single element transducer or, in the case of an array transducer, focusing can be performed electronically and dynamically

apparent that a larger transducer diameter as well as higher frequencies (leading to shorter wavelengths) will increase the near field length and maximize image quality (Fig. 1.13). These have an immediate impact on lateral resolution.

The above considerations of frequency and transducer diameter were discussed in the context of a single element, unfocused transducer. It is clear that—even without beam focusing—it is desirable to perform imaging in the near field. However there is another very important aspect of beam geometry: that of *focusing* the beam, which has the effect of narrowing the beam profile. The narrowest portion of this beam is the *focal distance*, and the *focal zone* corresponds to the region over which the width of the beam is less than two times the beam width at the focal distance (Fig. 1.14). This is the area in which ultrasound intensity is highest, and also where the lateral resolution is best; whenever possible, imaging of key structures should be performed within this zone. As will be discussed below, a focused, narrow beam is desirable for 2D imaging. With single element transducers, this is performed by utilizing a curved PZE element or acoustic lens to focus and narrow the beam width; however in such cases the focal distance is generally fixed. Nonetheless in the past these focused, single element transducers formed the basis of the early mechanical sector echocardiography platforms. Obviously the ability to change a transmit focus dynamically would enhance the imaging capabilities of an ultrasound platform. The advent of array technology marked a significant advance in the field of echocardiography: variable beam

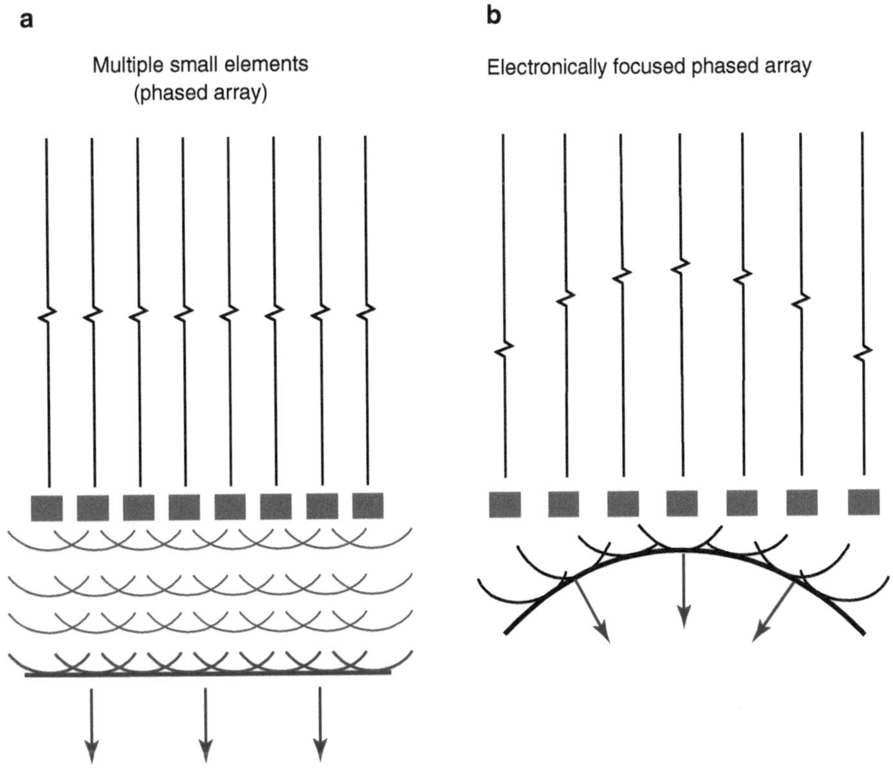

Fig. 1.15 Phased array transducer. When all elements are stimulated simultaneously, the waves from the individual elements act as Huygen point sources, merging to produce a large planar wavefront (**a**). With an array transducer, the beam can be focused by introducing time delays to the separate elements (**b**), producing beam geometry analogous to that obtained by an acoustic lens

focusing and beam shaping became a reality, adding a great deal of flexibility and versatility to echocardiographic imaging. Array technology is discussed in the next section.

Arrays

The foundation of current ultrasound transducer technology, particularly that used in echocardiography, is built upon the concept of transducer **arrays**. Rather than a single element, an array consists of a group of closely spaced PZE elements, each with its own electrical connection to the ultrasound machine. This enables the array elements to be excited individually or in groups. The resultant sound beam emitted by the transducer results from a summation of the sound beams produced by the individual elements. The wave from an individual element (which is quite small, often less than half a wavelength) is by itself broad and unfocused. However when a group of elements transmits simultaneously, there is reinforcement (constructive interference) of the waves along the beam direction, and cancellation (destructive interference) of the waves in other directions, yielding a more well-defined, planar ultrasound beam (Fig. 1.15a). The whole concept of arrays is based upon Huygens' principle, in which a large ultrasound beam wavefront can be divided into a large number of point sources (Huygen sources) from which small diverging waves (Huygen wavelets) merge to form a planar wavefront [1]. The resultant beam can also be focused electronically by introducing time delays to the separate elements, in a manner essentially the same as using a focusing lens or curved PZE element (Fig. 1.15b). Electronic beam steering can occur, in which beams can be swept across an imaged field without any mechanical motion in the transducer (unlike the older mechanical sector transducers). Moreover the focal distance is not fixed but dynamic, and can be adjusted by the operator. Furthermore, multiple transmit focal zones can be utilized to increase the focal zone of an instrument, thereby improving image quality throughout the sector (however this requires extra "pulses" and can result in a lower image frame rate). Thus the array transducer provides a tremendous amount of flexibility for imaging.

There are a number of different types of arrays available for ultrasonic imaging (linear, curvilinear, annular), but the **phased array** transducer is generally the one used for 2D transthoracic and transesophageal echocardiography. This type of array is smaller than linear and curvilinear arrays, thereby providing a transducer "footprint" that allows the transducers to be used with the smaller windows available for transthoracic (particularly pediatric) and transesophageal imaging. The number of PZE elements in a transthoracic phased array probe generally ranges between 64 and 256 (or more) elements. One of the important distinguishing characteristics of phased array transducers is that—unlike linear and curvilinear arrays—*all* elements of the phased array are excited during the production of one transmitted beam line (Fig. 1.16). The direction of the beam is steered electronically

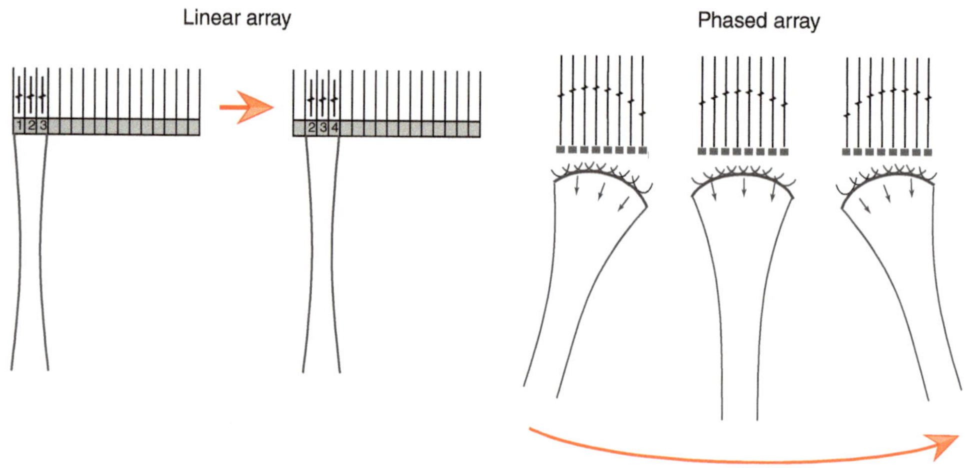

Fig. 1.16 Linear vs. phased array transducer. In the linear array, small groups of elements are stimulated to produce one beam line. Once the returning signals are received, a second adjacent group of elements is stimulated to produce the second beam line. This process continues sequentially down the length of the transducer. Not all elements are stimulated at one time. In contrast, the phased array transducer has a smaller footprint, and all elements are utilized to produce and steer every beam electronically. By varying the timing of pulses to the elements, sequential beam lines are generated and swept in an arc (*red arrow* under the right diagram)

by varying the timing sequence of excitation pulses; the term *phasing* describes the control of the timing of PZE element excitation in order to steer and focus the ultrasound beam. In this manner, timing sequence alterations allow successive beam lines to be generated (Fig. 1.16). Therefore in phased array transducers, the beam can be electronically swept in an arc, providing a wide field of view despite the relatively small footprint. In addition, the direction of echo reception ("listening") can be varied electronically. Returning echo signals from reflectors along each scan line are received by all the elements in the phased array; because of slightly different distances from a reflector to the individual elements, the returning signals will not be in phase and therefore electronic receive focusing must be performed to bring them back into phase to prevent destructive interference of returning signals. This is done by applying time delays to the individual element returning signals, analogous to the time delays used for transmission. In this way, the signals from the individual elements will be in phase when summed together to produce a single signal for each reflector. Receive focusing is adjusted dynamically and automatically by the ultrasound machine in order to compensate for different reflector depths.

An essential component of modern ultrasound systems that use array transducers is the *beam former*. This component of the system provides pulse-delay sequences to individual elements to achieve transmit focusing. In addition, it controls beam direction and dynamic focusing of received echoes, as well as other signal processing. It is located on the ultrasound system and electronically connected to the individual transducer PZE elements. Traditionally, beam formers have been analog, but most ultrasound manufacturers now utilize digital beam formers.

A newer type of array, the **matrix array**, has been developed for real-time three-dimensional (3D) transthoracic and transesophageal echocardiography. This consists of more than 2,500–3,000 elements laid out in a two-dimensional square array slightly larger than 50×50 elements [11] (Fig. 1.17). Analogous to 2D phased array, all elements in the matrix array are active during beam forming. Because of the large number of elements the process of beam forming is divided into two areas: (1) pre-beam forming by custom made integrated circuits within the transducer handle, and (2) traditional digital beam forming within the ultrasound system [12, 13]. The most important aspect of 3D beam forming is the ability to steer in both lateral and elevational directions, thereby providing a pyramidal 3D dataset. Three-dimensional technology and imaging (specifically in the context of 3D TEE) is discussed in Chap. 2 as well as Chaps. 19 and 20.

Transesophageal Echocardiographic Transducers

All current 2D TEE probes utilize phased array technology, usually in a row of 64 elements for current adult multiplane TEE probes (some pediatric probes have fewer elements—see Chap. 2). TEE probes are constructed similar to standard transthoracic transducers: they have a collection of piezoelectric elements, backing material, electrical connector, housing, and matching layer. In addition an acoustic lens is added below the matching layer to improve focusing. The important difference is that all the components, as well as the housing, are much smaller, and special cabling is required for anterior/posterior flexion (anteflexion/retroflexion) and (in some probes) right/left rotation (Fig. 1.18). In addition, with multiplane TEE probes the piezoelectric elements can be electronically or mechanically rotated by cables (Fig. 1.18), a rotor, or even a small motor housed in the probe tip, and attached to the elements, allowing the tomographic

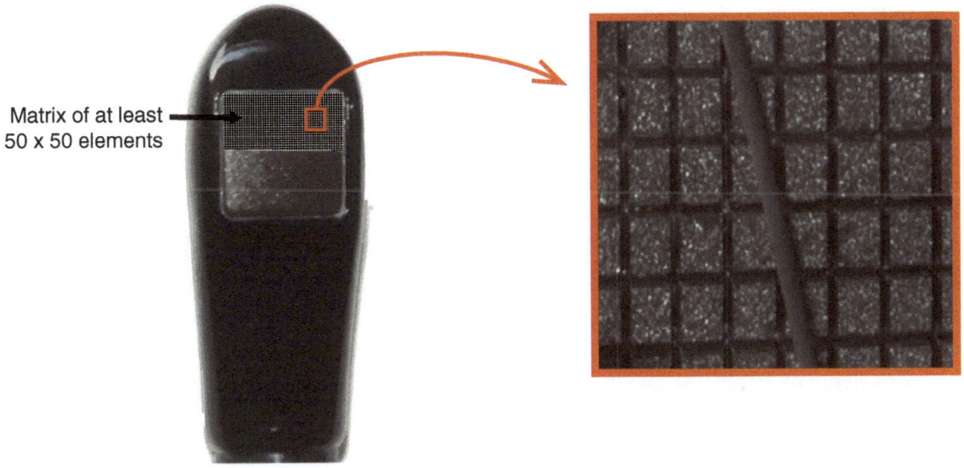

Fig. 1.17 Matrix array three-dimensional transesophageal echocardiography probe. The transducer is a square matrix of at least 50×50 elements (2,500–3,000 total elements). A pyramidal three dimensional dataset is produced from this. Each individual element is just larger than the diameter of a human hair (Photograph on the right, courtesy of Philips Medical Systems, Andover, MA)

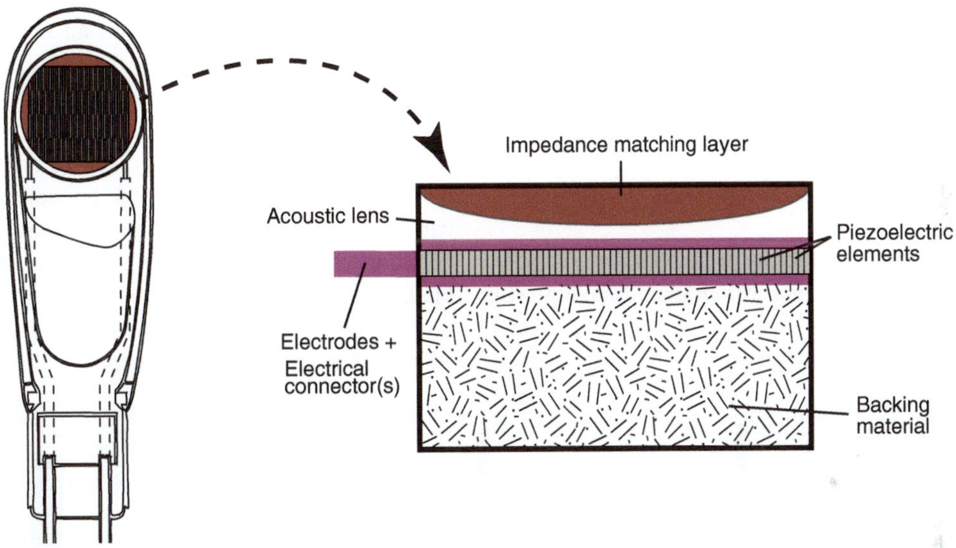

Fig. 1.18 Internal layout of model of a multiplane transesophageal echocardiographic (TEE) probe. The probe utilizes phased array technology; the transducer containing the array of elements is located at the probe tip and can be rotated between 0° and 180° by either an electronic or mechanical control in the probe handle. The principal transducer components (right diagram) are similar to those found in a transthoracic probe. Rotation of the transducer can be achieved using cables (as shown on left), a central rotor, or a small motor housed in the probe tip. The TEE probe itself is similar to a gastroscope, with controls in the probe handle (not shown, see Chap. 2) for tip movement anteriorly/posteriorly and right/left (Note: in some pediatric probes, the right/left control has been omitted)

plane to be varied between 0° and 180°. More detailed discussion of TEE technology is given in Chap. 2.

Pulse Repetition Frequency

Ultimately, one of the major factors determining the quality of information obtained by ultrasonic imaging, particularly that of echocardiography, is the speed of sound in tissue. This generally fixed value imposes certain restrictions on pulse-echo imaging as well as pulsed wave and color flow Doppler evaluation—specifically, it places limits on the at maximum rate at which ultrasound pulses can be emitted. A transducer cannot send and receive ultrasound pulses at the same time; once a pulse has been sent, the transducer must wait a certain period of time for returning echoes, with the round-trip time depending upon the depth of the reflector. The equation relating distance to time is:

$$T = \frac{2D}{c} \tag{1.5}$$

T = Time it takes a pulse of sound to travel to a reflector, and for an echo to return to the transducer (round-trip time)
D = Distance from the transducer
c = Speed of sound in the medium

Given a speed of sound in tissue of 1,540 m/s, the round-trip time is equivalent to **13 μs/cm of depth**, hence the time needed to collect all returning echoes from a scan line of depth D is equal to 13 μs × D. This time is also known as the *pulse repetition period*, and the reciprocal of this is known as the **pulse repetition frequency**, or **PRF**. This is a very important concept in echocardiography, because *the maximum PRF represents the maximum number of times a pulse can be emitted per second*. PRF will vary with the speed of sound in different media. However, assuming a constant speed of sound (as is seen with soft tissues in the human body), *PRF is totally dependent upon depth*: *the greater the depth, the less the maximum PRF*. In the soft tissues of the human body, maximum PRF calculates to **77,000/s/cm of depth** (roughly equivalent to 1 divided by 13 μs). Typically, PRF is expressed in units of Hz or kiloHz (kHz). For example, for a depth of 10 cm, the maximum PRF for one scan line will be 77,000 ÷ 10 cm, or 7,700/s (also given as 7,700 Hz or 7.7 kHz). In other words, for this particular depth, the maximum number of times a sound pulse can be transmitted and received is 7,700 times/s. As will be seen, the PRF plays an important role in determining the limits of temporal resolution for both 2D imaging as well as the maximum velocities measurable by pulsed wave and color flow Doppler.

Generation of an Echocardiographic Image

The pulse-echo principle serves as the fundamental concept underlying ultrasonic and echocardiographic imaging. This principle is based upon a predictable and reliable constant: the speed of sound in the soft tissues of the human body, which, as noted above, is 1,540 m/s. When an acoustic pulse is emitted by a transducer, the time delay between transmission and signal detection can be used to calculate distance from the transducer, by rearranging Eq. 1.5 above:

$$D = \frac{cT}{2} \qquad (1.6)$$

Thus for ultrasonography and echocardiography, it is axiomatic that *time equals distance*: the transmit/receive time (divided by 2) serves as the measurement for distance. Returning echoes along a scan line will have their various depths registered as a function of their time of return, as calculated by Eq. 1.6. In addition, these returning echoes will have different amplitudes that correspond to the different reflectors encountered. In the past, the amplitude of returning signals was displayed directly by an oscilloscope (known as "*A-mode*"). However, all modern-day echocardiography platforms convert the amplitude of returning echoes to a corresponding gray scale value for display on a computer monitor—this is known as brightness mode, or "*B-mode*". By plotting these varying brightness points as a function of distance from the transducer, one scan line can be displayed. If successive scan lines are rapidly swept across the object of interest, a 2D image can then be assembled, with echo signal location on the display corresponding to the reflector positions in relation to the transducer (Fig. 1.19). As discussed previously, this scan line sweep

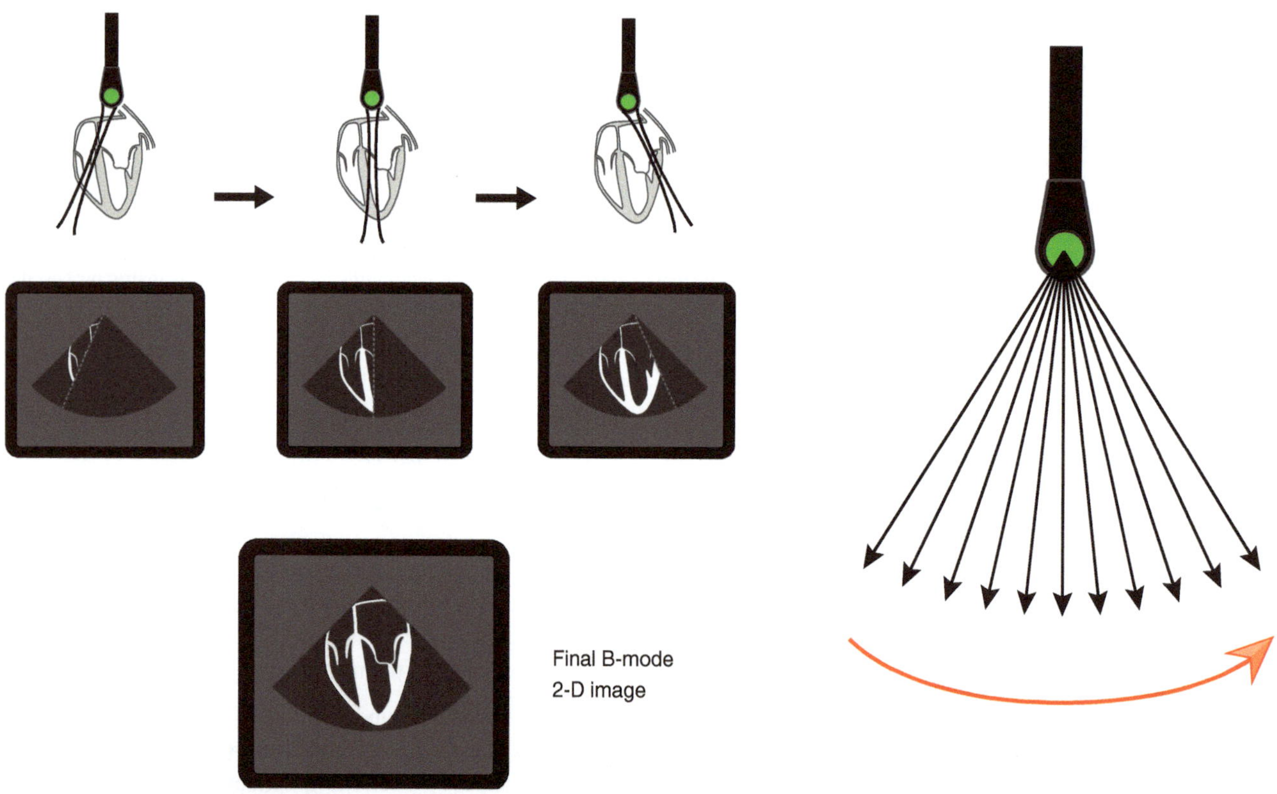

Fig. 1.19 Generation of a two dimensional (2D) echocardiographic image. The returning echo amplitudes from one scan line are converted to pixel gray scale brightness on a computer monitor. This is also known as "B-mode" (for brightness mode). If successive scan lines are obtained and rapidly swept across the sector, a 2D image can be generated (*red arrow* indicates the direction of the scan line sweep). This process must be repeated rapidly in order to depict accurate real-time cardiac motion

is performed electronically with a phased array transducer, using time delay sequences to vary the activation of the individual elements and sequentially "steer" the scan lines. Typically, 100–200 separate scan lines are used for a single 2D image [3]. For echocardiography, this process must be repeated rapidly in order to depict accurate, real-time cardiac motion.

The process whereby the reflected echoes are converted to real-time, 2D echocardiographic images requires highly specialized and advanced technology, as well as sophisticated digital signal processing capabilities. Returning echo signals from reflectors along each scan line are received by all the phased array elements in the transducer; as noted previously, electronic receive focusing is performed to bring returning signals into phase. Analog to digital conversion also occurs during this process. To compensate for different reflector depths, this receive focusing is adjusted dynamically and automatically by the digital beam former. These digital signals are then sent to a receiver in the ultrasound machine, where they undergo a number of preprocessing steps to "condition" the signal; these include signal preamplification and demodulation, as well as operator-adjustable time gain compensation (TGC), noise reduction (known as reject), and dynamic range/compression (that varies contrast). The TGC is a selective form of amplification used to compensate for the weaker, attenuated signals from increased depths. Some of this can be performed by the operator, but modern echocardiography machines now incorporate an adaptive TGC that automatically adjusts the TGC in real-time [3]. The operator-adjusted TGC controls will be discussed in a separate section below.

Once the signals have been amplified and processed, they are sent to a **scan converter**, which is a digital imaging matrix used to store and buffer returning signal information. In the process, the returning echo signal locations are converted from polar to Cartesian coordinates—in other words, angle and depth information are converted to a matrix format for display on a computer monitor. A common setup is a matrix of 512×512 pixels, with each pixel having 8 bits of storage allowing 256 levels of gray scale (though other types of setup are possible) (Fig. 1.20). Location information is

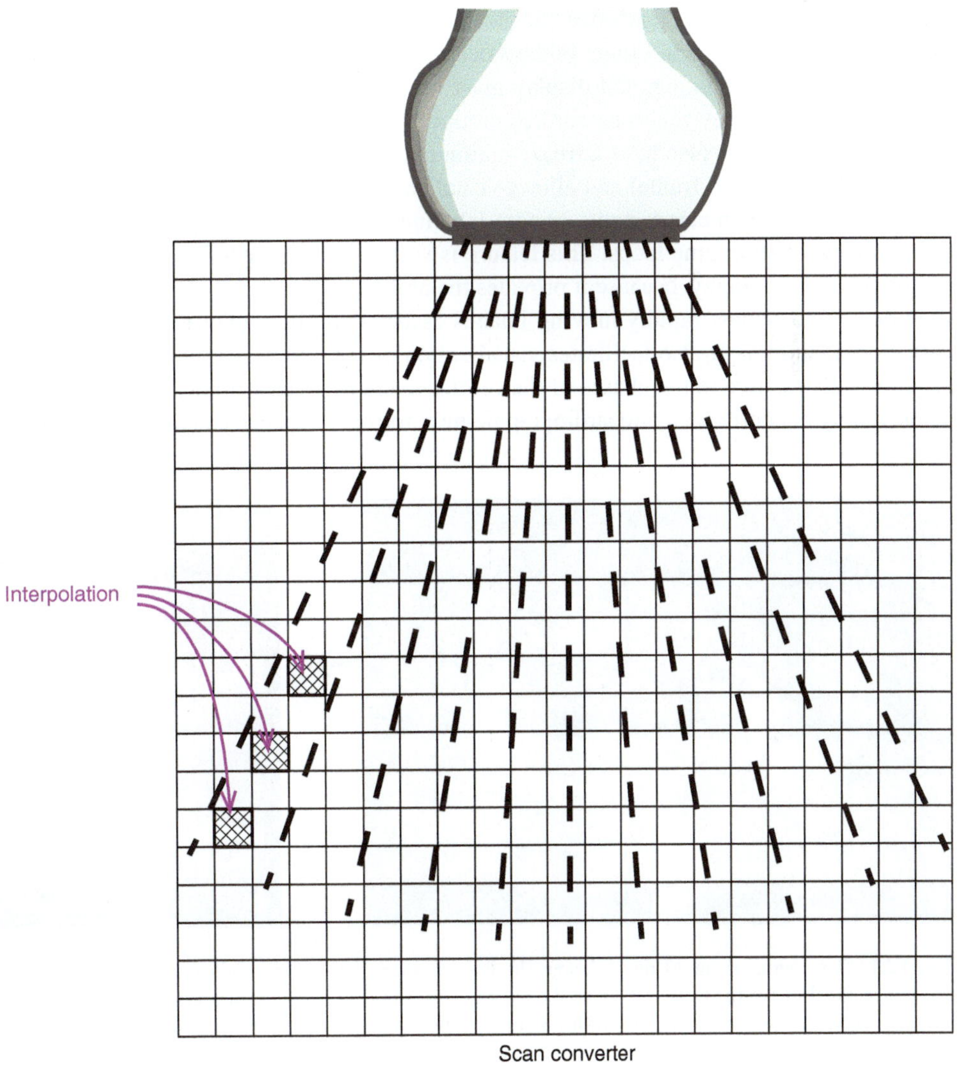

Fig. 1.20 Scan converter. The scan lines are converted from polar to Cartesian coordinates, and the information placed in a scan converter matrix, and used to construct a two dimensional image that can be visualized on a computer monitor. A common setup is a 525×525 pixel matrix, with each pixel having 8 bits of storage allowing 256 levels of gray scale. However, other matrix sizes and bits/pixels are possible. Interpolation is performed for those pixels in which no scan line information is available

obtained from: (a) angle of the scan line in relation to a reference axis, which is parallel to the surface of the array elements; (b) distance from the scan line to the reflector, as calculated from Eq. 1.6 above. These two coordinates are then converted into Cartesian x and y coordinates, which can then be placed into a large rectangular matrix suitable for pixel mapping on a 2D computer display. What becomes apparent during this conversion process is that, when the scan lines are superimposed upon the matrix, adjacent scan lines will not sample all of the pixels in the matrix. To fill in these areas, a process of *interpolation* is performed in which an averaged signal from nearby pixels is used to fill in the value of the blank (unsampled) pixel (Fig. 1.20).

In the scan converter, image data can be held in memory and continuously updated with new echo data. At the same time, information is continuously read out to a video buffer to provide real-time visualization of the scanned images on a video monitor. Most echocardiography systems now use a large digital computer monitor, generally one based upon liquid crystal display (LCD) technology. Various postprocessing techniques can also be performed on the digital image data stored in the computer memory; these techniques include contrast and edge enhancement, as well as smoothing and B-mode color. For echocardiography, image acquisition, updating, and display must occur in a rapid fashion to portray real-time cardiac motion. Almost all ultrasound systems also have a freeze option that stops image acquisition (still frame) and allows visualization of a single image (for measurements or text labeling), and also a review of short cine loops. This feature is very useful for echocardiography, because it provides the ability to slow down and review rapidly moving images associated with cardiac motion. It also facilitates visualization of the acquired data relative to the phases of the cardiac cycle as displayed by concurrent electrocardiographic monitoring.

Instead of sweeping a B-mode scan line in an arc to obtain a 2D image, a simpler (and less processor-intensive) method can be used to display the B-mode data. If the scan line remains fixed, and instead a continuous recording of the line is made over time, then an *M-mode* tracing is obtained—the M stands for motion (Fig. 1.21). This type of display was the principal form of echocardiography used in the 1970s and early 1980s. Because only one scan line is involved, a high PRF can be used and therefore this mode has excellent temporal resolution. Frame rates of 1,000–2,000 lines/second are possible, significantly increased compared to standard frame rates of 30–120 frames/second for 2D imaging. Axial resolution is also excellent, making M-mode ideal for linear and time measurements. For example, M-mode measurements are very useful for assessment of left ventricular dimensions and function, such as calculation of left ventricular end diastolic dimension and shortening fraction. Since there are published normal ranges and values for M-mode measurements, these measurements serve as an important method of distinguishing normal vs. abnormal cardiac size and function (discussed in Chap. 5). However, M-mode does not provide a real-time 2D display of cardiac anatomy, making interpretation more difficult, and limiting its effectiveness with CHD. Thus M-mode imaging has largely been supplanted by 2D and 3D echocardiography. While still available on modern echocardiography machines, it generally comprises a very small fraction of a total examination.

Image Resolution

Resolution is a term commonly used to describe the quality of an ultrasonic image. With ultrasonic imaging, and specifically with echocardiography, there are three major types of resolution: spatial, contrast, and temporal. These will be discussed below.

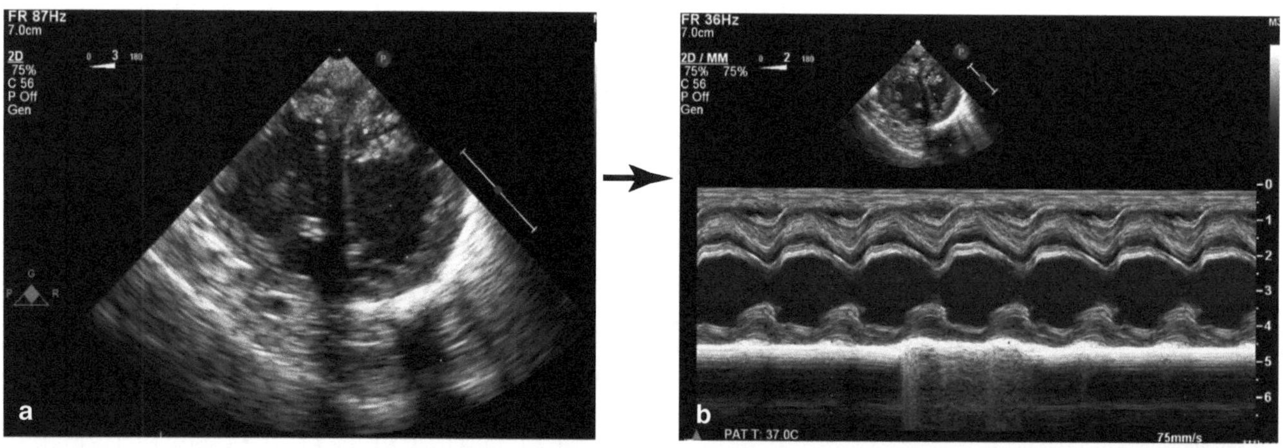

Fig. 1.21 Generation of an M-mode image. In this instance, the two-dimensional image (**a**) is used to guide the placement of the scan line (*dotted line*) for M-mode assessment (**b**). Real-time information is then obtained along the single scan line, plotted as time vs. depth from the transducer. M-mode imaging is characterized by excellent axial and temporal resolution

Spatial Resolution

Spatial resolution refers to the ability to discriminate objects in space, and applies specifically to 2D imaging. It is defined as the ability to distinguish two discrete objects located in close proximity to each other—in other words, the ability to resolve them as separate as opposed to overlapping structures. There are three types of spatial resolution: axial, lateral and elevational, representing the x, y, and z planes of a 2D ultrasonic/echocardiographic image (Fig. 1.22). Axial and lateral resolutions affect the two planes readily seen on a 2D image; elevational resolution refers to the "hidden" plane perpendicular to the other two planes, and not as apparent on 2D imaging. Factors affecting the resolution in each plane are discussed below.

Axial Resolution

Axial resolution describes the ability to discriminate two objects located along the axis of the sound beam (i.e. the scan line). It is determined principally by the transmitted ultrasonic pulse duration. The pulse duration is itself determined by two major factors: the number of cycles in the pulse, and the wave period (which is the inverse of frequency). In order to distinguish two separate objects along the axis of the sound beam, it is necessary that there be a short pulse duration (Fig. 1.10)—specifically, the time gap between the arrival of two pulses from two separate reflectors should be greater than the length (duration) of each pulse. Otherwise, there will be overlap of the two pulses and the two reflectors will not be resolved (Fig. 1.23). To improve axial resolution, the pulse duration should be decreased. This can be achieved by two methods. One is to use a higher frequency transducer, which decreases wavelength and wave period. The other is to improve damping of the "ringing" of the transducer so that each pulse will have fewer cycles. Broad bandwidth, high frequency transducers will provide the best axial resolution

The typical axial resolution for most modern ultrasound systems is between 0.3 and 2.0 mm; a rule of thumb is that the axial resolution of a system is 1.5 times the wavelength of the system. Therefore for a 7.5 MHz transducer, axial resolution is 0.3 mm [14]. In general, axial resolution tends to be the best of all the three dimensions. It is fairly constant with depth, though signal attenuation plays a role with the higher frequency transducers.

Lateral Resolution

Lateral resolution refers to the ability to distinguish two closely spaced reflectors positioned perpendicular to the axis of the ultrasound scan line. This is determined by two factors. The first is *beam width*: if the width of the beam is less than the distance between the two reflectors, then they can be resolved. Otherwise, if the beam is too wide, the images merge together and the two reflectors cannot be resolved (Fig. 1.24). Beam width changes with distance from the transducer; optimal beam width occurs within the near field (Fresnel) zone, prior to beam divergence. A long near field is therefore preferable for ultrasonography and echocardiography, and as noted previously in Eq. 1.4, the depth of the Fresnel zone is equal to $d^2/4\lambda$. Two important observations can be gleaned from this equation. First, lateral resolution can be improved by using a larger transducer aperture (diameter), which extends the depth of focus and lengthens the near field. Second, using a higher transmitted frequency will also extend the length of the near field, thereby improving lateral resolution further along the scan line (Fig. 1.25). However this latter point must be balanced by the greater attenuation of higher frequency sound waves, which can limit the depth of penetration. Focusing a beam (mechanically or electronically) will also enhance lateral

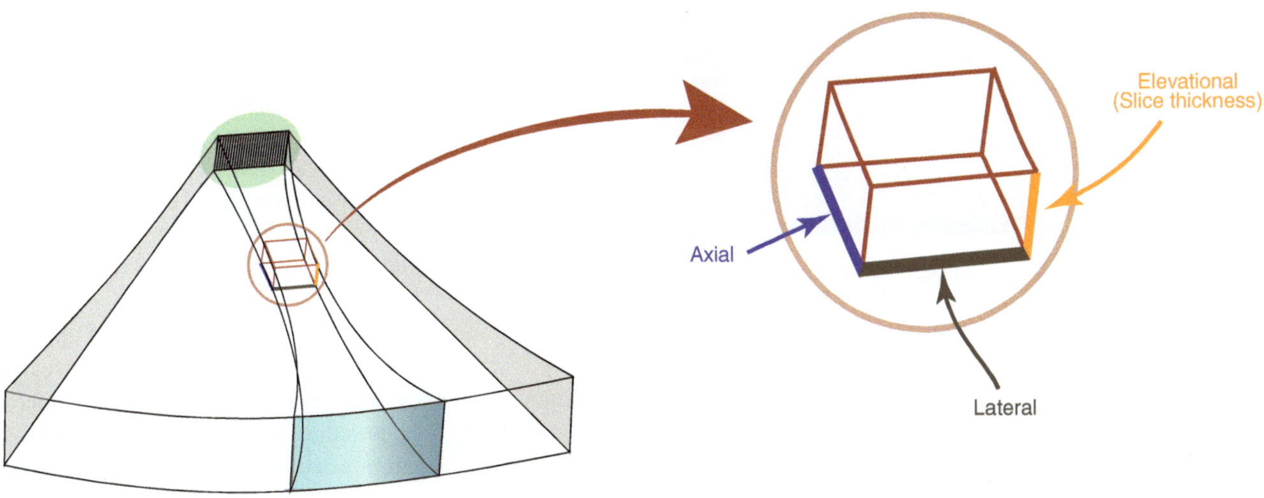

Fig. 1.22 The three spatial resolution planes: axial, lateral, and elevational (slice thickness)

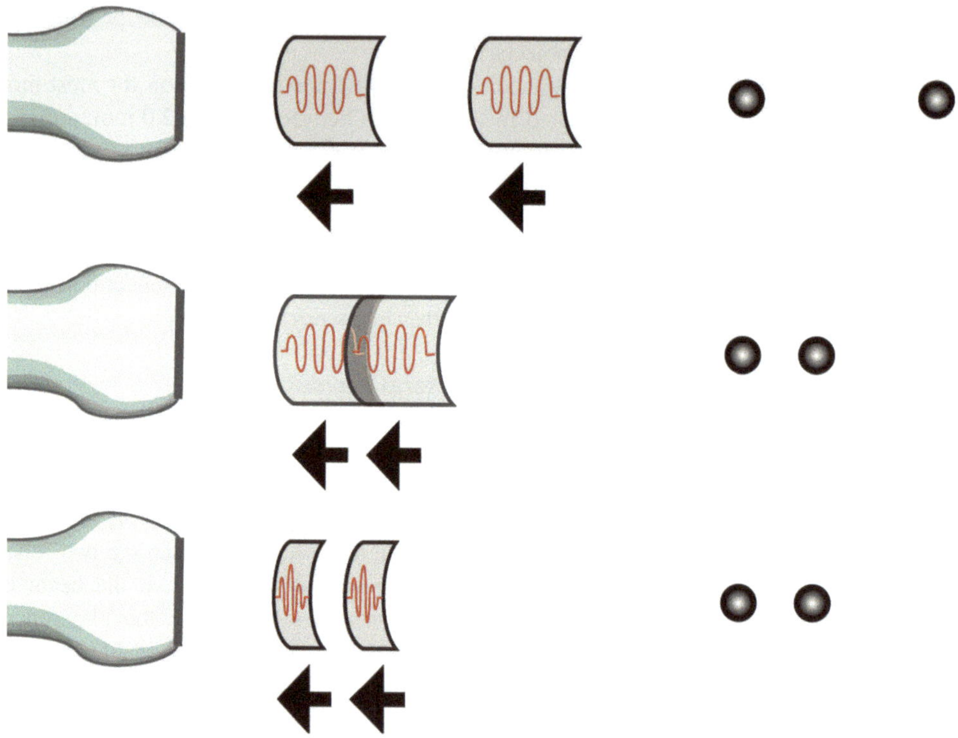

Fig. 1.23 Axial resolution. This diagram illustrates the effect of pulse duration on axial resolution. Each panel shows two pulses from two separate reflectors. In the *top panel*, the pulse duration is longer (which can be due to lower frequency, more cycles/pulse, or both). However because the two reflectors are spaced further apart, the longer pulses are still able to distinguish them as separate objects. In the *middle panel*, the reflectors are closely spaced and the long pulses are no longer able to distinguish the objects as separate; the two pulses overlap and appear to be one on the monitor. In the *bottom panel*, the two reflectors are still closely spaced (as in the *middle panel*) but pulse duration has been shortened by the use of a higher frequency and/or decreased number of cycles/pulse. The shorter pulse duration enables the two objects to be shown as separate objects on the screen, hence axial resolution has been enhanced

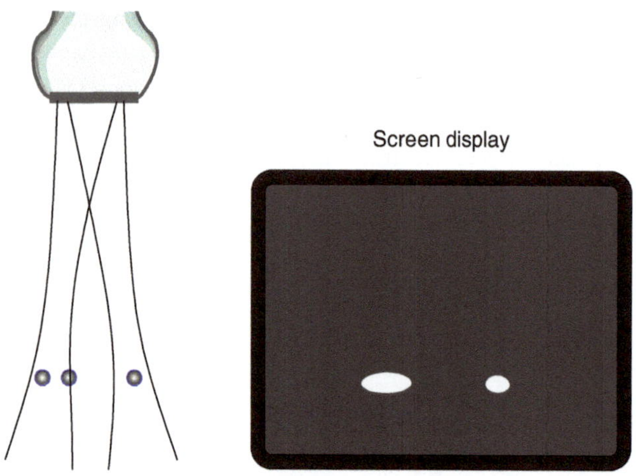

Fig. 1.24 Lateral resolution. This diagram illustrates the effect of beam width on lateral resolution. Two reflectors can be distinguished separately when the beam width is less than the lateral distance between two reflectors. When the beam is wider than this distance, the two objects cannot be resolved as separate reflectors

resolution by narrowing the beam width; the best resolution occurs within the focal zone, where the beam is narrowest (Fig. 1.14). With phased array transducers, dynamic adjusting of the focal zone to the desired depth can be performed to optimize the lateral resolution for that level.

The other important factor affecting lateral resolution is especially pertinent to echocardiography. This involves *line spacing or line density*. As will be discussed in the section on temporal resolution, the frame rates for real-time 2D imaging depend upon the depth of scanning as well as the number of scan lines per imaging sector. To improve frame rates, the number of scan lines can be reduced, with the result being less scanning time required per sector, but increased spacing between scan lines. This can reduce lateral resolution because even with a narrow beam width, if the line spacing is greater than the distance between two closely spaced objects, the objects still might be not be resolved as separate reflectors.

Typically, at a depth of 10 cm, a beam width of approximately 2 mm is achieved (obviously this will be affected by signal frequency and transducer size). Thus lateral resolution tends to be less than axial resolution, and unlike axial resolution, it exhibits depth-dependence. Nonetheless lateral resolution is a major factor determining the quality of ultrasound images. For this reason, modern

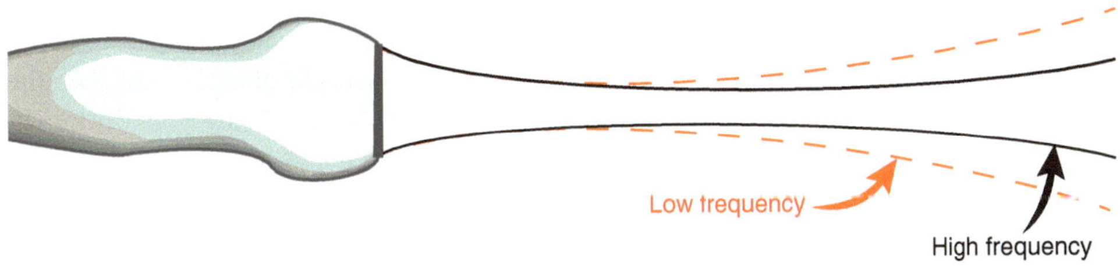

Fig. 1.25 Effect of frequency on near field length and beam width. In this diagram both beams have been focused. However even with a focused beam, using a higher frequency transducer lengthens the focal zone and near field, and there is less divergence in the far field

echocardiography manufacturers attempt to enhanced lateral resolution by utilizing combinations of time-delayed firing and changing beam aperture—available with phased array technology—to optimize focusing at different depths (also known as multiple focal zones). This effectively lengthens the focal zone. However as noted above, it requires multiple pulse sequences, which can reduce temporal resolution.

Elevational Resolution

Contrary to appearances, a 2D tomographic image is not flat. It is in fact a slice, and this slice has a thickness aspect, which is known as the elevational plane with an axis perpendicular to the imaging plane (Fig. 1.22). Similar to lateral resolution, slice thickness depends upon beam size—that is, the size of the beam in the elevational plane. However unlike lateral resolution, in most standard 2D transducers there is no electronic focusing available in this plane; a fixed focal length acoustic lens generally determines beam width in this dimension. Slice thickness is minimal closest to the focal zone, and widens beyond that point. As with lateral resolution, a higher frequency transducer improves the elevational resolution by lengthening the near field. Slice thickness is also determined by the width of the beam in the elevational plane.

What is the importance of elevational resolution? While the elevational plane is not displayed in a conventional 2D image, objects that exist within the slice can overlap with the 2D image being displayed, potentially causing slice thickness artifacts.

Of the three types of resolution, the elevational resolution is usually the worst. In most phased array transducers, elevational slice thickness ranges between 3 mm (near the focal zone) and 10 mm as the beam diverges [15]. While little information is available regarding elevational resolution in TEE transducers, slice thickness artifacts are likely to be minimized due to a several factors: (a) higher frequencies of the transducer; (b) some focusing from the transducer's acoustic lens; (c) reduced transducer depth, usually about 5–10 cm in the vast majority of patients for most TEE views except for the deep transgastric views.

Optimizing Spatial Resolution

From the above discussion it becomes apparent that *the best spatial resolution occurs in the near field and focal zone of the transducer*. Beyond this area, lateral and elevational resolution decrease as the beam diverges. Use of higher frequency transducers improves axial resolution and lengthens the near field, thereby improving lateral and elevational resolution. Focusing of the beam further decreases beam width at the focal zone, thereby improving lateral and elevational resolution. However focusing can increased beam divergence, and lateral/elevational resolution are reduced in the far field. While axial resolution does not change with depth, with greater depths there is reduced penetration of higher frequency ultrasound, thus lower frequencies must sometimes be used for imaging of more distant structures, leading to reduced resolution.

Therefore for echocardiographic 2D imaging, as a rule it is desirable to position the transducer as close as possible to the object of interest, and to use the highest frequency transducer possible. Fortunately these conditions can be achieved with most TEE imaging, as the close proximity between esophagus and heart (from most TEE windows) enables the optimization of all three types of spatial resolution.

Contrast Resolution

Contrast resolution refers to the ability to differentiate between body tissues that have slightly different properties, and therefore different acoustic impedances, using different shades of gray on the display. There are two components to contrast resolution. The first is the intrinsic contrast, and how this is encoded in the stored pixel values in the image memory. Intrinsic contrast depends upon the different tissue interfaces/acoustic impedances, as well as acquisition parameters (beam width, pulse shape) and processing (compression, edge enhancement). It also depends in part on how gray scale is encoded in the process of analog to digital conversion of the amplified voltage signal: the larger the number of bits per pixel, the larger the number of gray scale shades available. Extrinsic contrast translates these pixel values into brightness levels on the monitor, and is dependent upon operator-adjustable contrast and brightness controls. During this process, the *compression* can be adjusted by the operator to vary the dynamic range of the signal amplitude. Increasing the dynamic range increases the range of gray scale and decreases contrast; decreasing the dynamic range does the opposite. It should be noted that improving the contrast often improves the ability to distinguish structures, thereby enhancing spatial resolution.

Temporal Resolution

Temporal resolution refers to the ability to visualize smooth real-time motion, and is related to image refresh speed, also known as frame rate. Frame rate is dictated by four factors: the speed of sound, sampling depth, the number of separate transducer beam lines used to form an image, and the number of focal zones. The equation relating these variables is given as follows:

$$F = \frac{c}{2DNn} \tag{1.7}$$

F = frame rate
c = speed of sound
D = sampling depth
N = number of sampling lines per frame
n = number of focal zones used to produce one image

Pulse repetition period and PRF play an integral role here. As noted previously, a small time period is required for a pulse to be transmitted and for collection of all echoes emerging from that scan line. The round-trip time per scan line in soft tissue (pulse repetition period) is 13 μs/cm of depth. Therefore for an image sector 10 cm deep (from the transducer), the pulse repetition period per scan line is 130 μs. If the image sector is composed of 100 scan lines, the time for one image equals 13 ms, thus the maximum frame rate is approximately 77 frames/s. This is with a single focal zone; if multiple transmit focal zones are used (advantageous for improving lateral resolution), then frame rate decreases because multiple pulse sequences must be generated per scan line. *What becomes apparent is that frame rate is principally affected by sampling depth and number of scan (beam) lines.* Deeper scanning depths as well as wider imaging sectors (requiring more scan lines) will appreciably lower frame rates. To improve frame rates, a smaller depth should be used. The number of scan lines can be decreased in one of two ways: (a) decreasing the number of scan lines while maintaining the same size imaging sector (however this increases lateral line spacing, thereby reducing lateral resolution); (b) narrowing the imaging sector while maintaining the same line spacing (which maintains lateral resolution but decreases the field of view) (Fig. 1.26). Of course, any combination of these maneuvers can further improve temporal resolution. In addition, newer technologies are now being employed including parallel processing, which allows more scan lines to be acquired at one time, thereby reducing the total time require to acquire the image.

In the realm of diagnostic medical ultrasound, temporal resolution considerations are especially applicable for echocardiography because of one simple fact: the heart is in constant motion. For visualizing a rapidly moving structure such as the heart, the image must be refreshed a minimum number of times per second to produce the appearance of smooth, real-time cardiac motion; otherwise a "strobe" effect is created and motion no longer appears smooth and can be difficult to interpret. The minimum frame rates needed to present smooth real-time motion will vary depending upon heart rate—the faster the heart rate, the greater the necessary frame rate. While no published standard exists, for visualizing cardiac motion it is generally desirable to have a frame rate that allows for at least 10 samplings (frames) per cardiac cycle; 20–30 frames/cycle will usually provide good temporal resolution. Conversely, when the rate decreases to less than five frames/cardiac cycle, cardiac motion ceases to be smooth and important information can be lost because of the inadequate sampling rate. Thus for a heart rate of 100/min, a frame rate of 50 frames/s will yield 30 frames/cardiac cycle, thereby providing acceptable temporal resolution. However a frame rate of 10 frames/s yields only 6 frames/cardiac cycle, which is barely adequate for most cardiac imaging. In such instances the operator should attempt to boost frame rates by using the maneuvers outlined above. Obviously one should strive for the highest frame rates possible, which will permit more detailed analysis of cardiac motion and function; this is especially pertinent given the higher heart rates found in young children. Very high frame rates are also desirable for precise evaluation of myocardial mechanics using methods such as tissue Doppler evaluation and strain/strain rate imaging.

Fortunately, with TEE the close proximity of the transducer to the heart means that smaller distances are needed to visualize the cardiac structures. Hence excellent temporal resolution is generally possible, even while at the same time being able to use higher ultrasound frequencies to optimize axial and lateral resolutions.

Tissue Harmonic Imaging

Tissue harmonic imaging is a technique used to enhance 2D imaging, particularly in patients with poor echocardiographic windows. It is based upon the detection of *harmonic frequencies* generated by beam propagation through tissue. It relies upon the fact that a relatively high-pressure amplitude sound wave changes shape during propagation, a phenomenon known as nonlinear wave propagation. The sinusoidal shape becomes distorted, and this change in shape corresponds to a change in frequency components of the sound wave—harmonic frequencies are generated from the original sound wave. These intensify with distance from the transducer as the waveform becomes more distorted. The harmonic components occur as multiples of the fundamental frequency: if the fundamental frequency is 2.5 MHz, the second harmonic is 5.0 MHz, the third

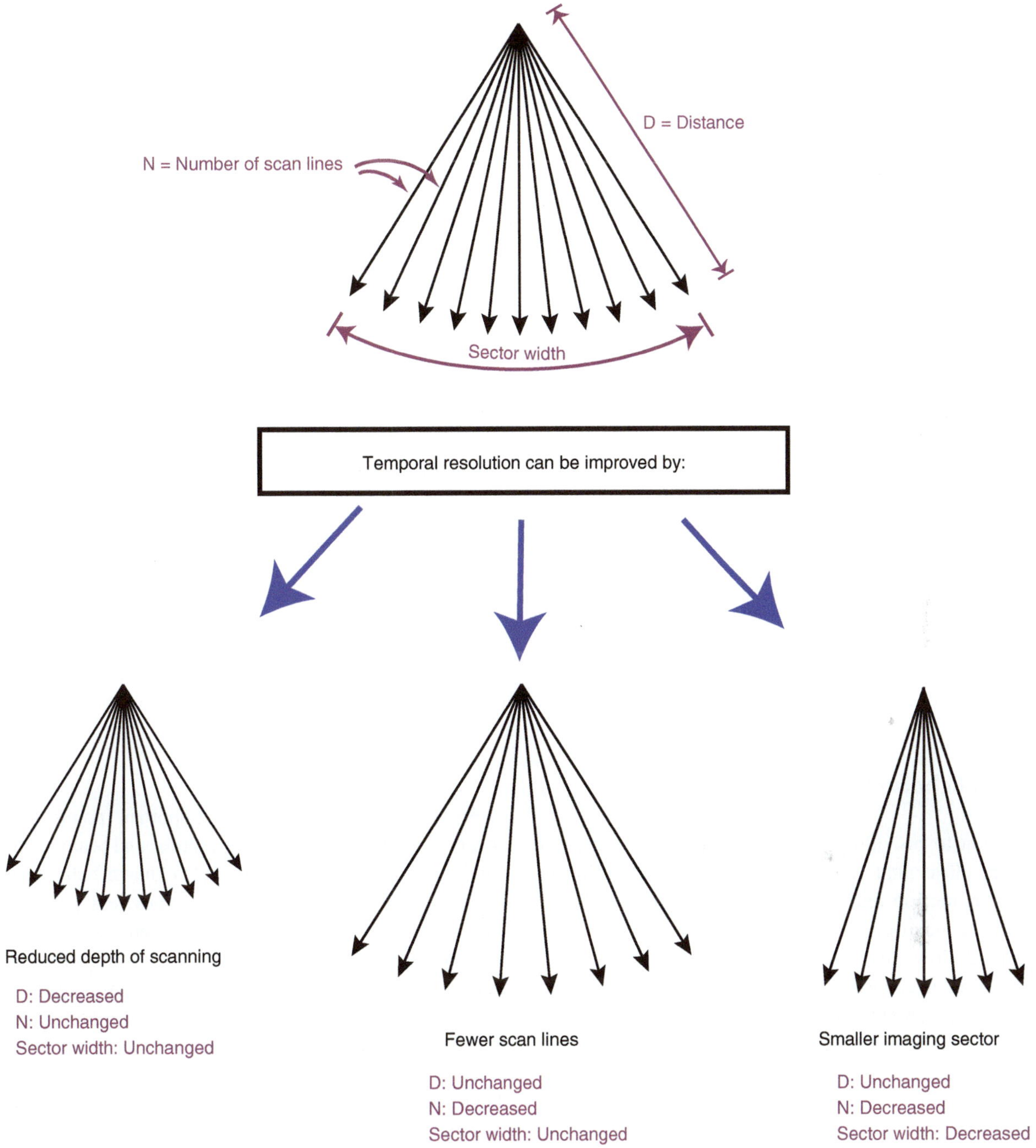

Fig. 1.26 Enhancement of temporal resolution. Temporal resolution is dependent upon sector depth and number of beam lines. It can be improved by several methods, including: (**a**) reducing sector depth (*leftward panel*); (**b**) reducing the number of scan lines without changing sector width, effectively reducing line density (*middle panel*); (**c**) narrowing the sector width, which also has the effect of decreasing the number of scan lines while maintain line density (*rightward panel*). Any combination of these maneuvers can be performed to enhance temporal resolution further

harmonic 7.5 MHz, etc. However the third and higher harmonics have weak amplitudes and therefore harmonic imaging is confined principally to the second harmonic frequency.

Tissue harmonic imaging relies upon the detection of this second harmonic frequency. The ultrasound machine can be configured to isolate this component for image formation. The advantage of this type of imaging is that artifacts are reduced or eliminated because they arise from the fundamental frequency, which is suppressed with tissue harmonic imaging. Thus signal to noise ratio is increased, and contrast resolution and border delineation are enhanced. Moreover the width of the main beam is effectively narrower than the main beam at the fundamental frequency, thus lateral resolution can be enhanced. The drawbacks of harmonic imaging depend upon the methods used for second harmonic isolation. One method, known as harmonic band filtering, utilizes longer spatial pulse length to narrow transmission bandwidth and enhance separation of fundamental and harmonic frequencies. However, the longer spatial pulse length can lead to poorer axial resolution. The other method, known as pulse phase inversion, utilizes a two-pulse sequence in which the second pulse is shifted 180° in phase. With standard sinusoidal waveforms, summation of these two returning pulses would cancel each other out. However with nonlinear propagation, the returning harmonic components that are generated are not identical in amplitude, thus summation of the returning signals will isolate the harmonic frequency that has been produced. Broadband transmitted pulses with short spatial pulse length can be used, so this method preserves axial resolution; however, using the multiple pulse technique can reduce temporal resolution and produce motion artifacts [16].

Harmonic imaging has found great utility in transthoracic echocardiographic imaging of adult patients with poor windows, and occasionally it proves beneficial in selected pediatric patients because of its improvements in contrast resolution. It has less applicability with TEE because of the close proximity and generally excellent imaging afforded by the proximity of the esophagus to the heart [17].

Doppler Echocardiography

In addition to providing information about anatomy and function, ultrasound can also furnish important information about motion and velocity. This is particularly relevant in echocardiography, where knowledge of cardiac and blood flow velocities—made possible through the use of Doppler echocardiography—can be used to derive a wealth of noninvasive information on cardiac physiology. This section discusses the science of Doppler echocardiography.

The Doppler Principle

The Doppler effect was discovered and first described by the Austrian physicist Christian Doppler in 1842. While studying the light from the stars, he discovered that the colored appearance of moving stars was caused by their motion relative to the earth. The motion resulted in either a red or blue shift of the light's frequency, depending upon the direction of motion. Doppler mathematically described the shift that occurred, and also correctly surmised that the same type of perceived frequency shifts would occur for a stationary observer listening to sound waves produced from a moving source. The perceived frequency of sound would be higher (compared to the emitted frequency) for an approaching object, and lower for a retreating object (Fig. 1.27).

The Doppler principle can also be applied to ultrasonography, and specifically to echocardiography. The ultrasound transducer serves as the stationary observer, and emits a sound of known frequency toward a moving target. The signal reflected from the moving target will return with a different frequency (the Doppler shift), and this change in frequency is proportional to the velocity of the reflector. The velocity of the moving reflector can be calculated using the **Doppler equation**:

$$f_D = \frac{2 f_0 V \cos\theta}{c} \tag{1.8}$$

f_D = the Doppler frequency shift = $f_r - f_0$
f_0 = the transmitted frequency of sound
f_r = the received frequency of sound
V = reflector velocity
θ = the intercept angle between the ultrasound beam and the direction of blood flow
c = the velocity of sound

If this equation is rearranged to derive the reflector velocity from the frequency shift between transmitted and received ultrasonic signals, the following equation is obtained:

$$v = \frac{f_r - f_0}{\cos\theta} \times \frac{c}{2 f_0} \tag{1.9}$$

From these equations, three important points become apparent. First, the angle (θ) of the ultrasound beam relative to the direction of reflector motion (also known as the angle of insonation) is important—as θ becomes less parallel and changes from 0° to 90°, the Doppler frequency shift (f_d) is reduced by the factor cosine θ. When the direction of the beam is perpendicular to reflector motion, cosine 90° = 0 and no frequency shift is detected. Table 1.2 shows the reduction in calculated velocity (as compared to actual velocity) for a reflector moving at 1 m/s, as θ increases from 0° to 90°. Angles greater 30° result in significant decreases in calculated velocity. The message here is simple and straightforward: *when evaluating for a Doppler velocity, the angle of insonation must be as parallel as possible to the direction of motion.*

The second important point is that the Doppler frequency shift depends upon the frequency of the incident beam—for a given reflector velocity, the higher the incident frequency, the higher the Doppler shift. As will be seen, the incident frequency, and the magnitude of this frequency shift, are important in determining the limits of pulsed and color flow Doppler evaluation.

The third important point is that reflector direction of motion can be determined. As is evident from Fig. 1.27, the Doppler frequency shift incorporates directionality: approaching objects increase the returning frequency of the

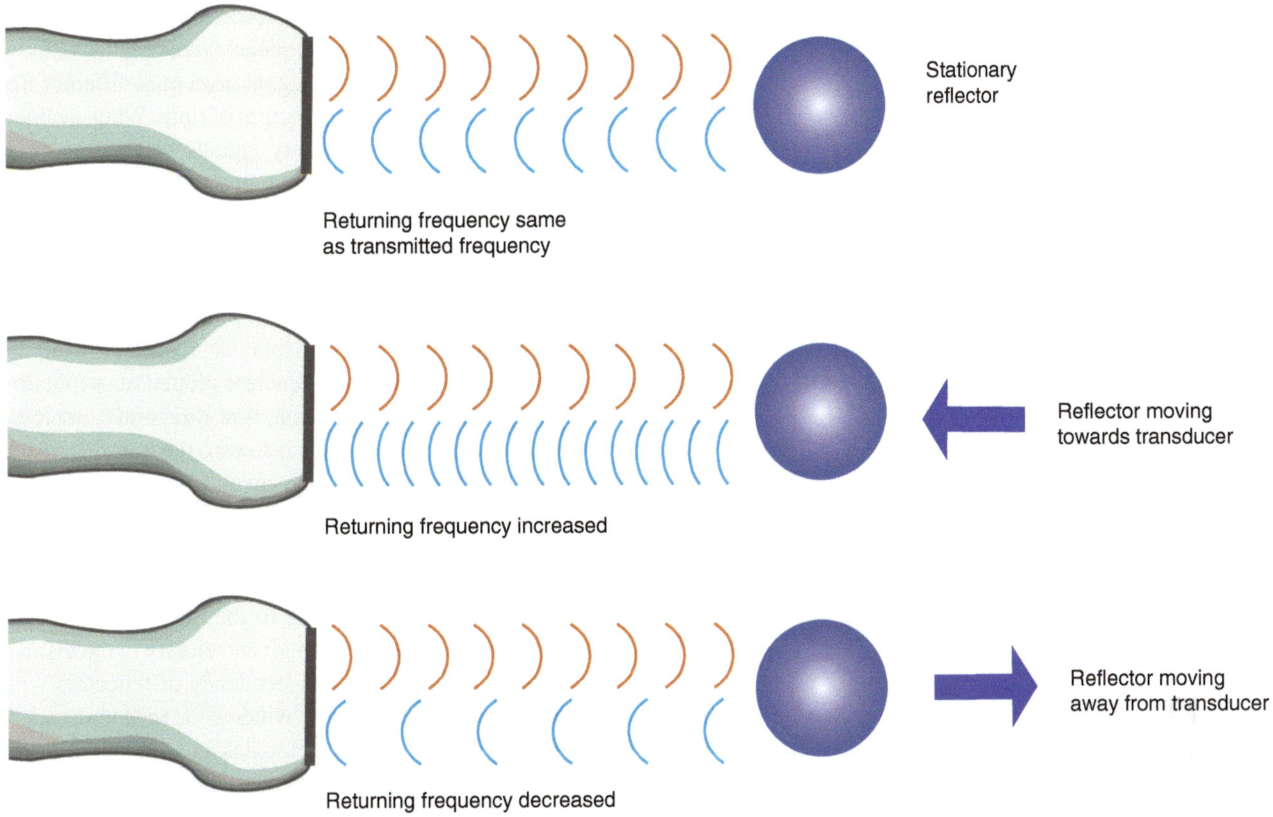

Fig. 1.27 The Doppler principle. When an ultrasound pulse of known frequency is transmitted, the returning pulse from a stationary reflector will have an identical frequency. However, the pulse returning from a reflector moving *towards* the transducer will have an *increased* frequency, and if the reflector is moving *away* from the transducer, the pulse will have a *decreased* frequency. The change between incident and reflected frequencies is known as the Doppler frequency shift, and from this shift, the reflector velocity can be calculated

Table 1.2 Doppler angle and velocities for a reflector velocity of 1 m/s, using a 5 MHz transducer

Doppler angle (degrees)	Doppler shift (kHz)	Actual velocity (cm/s)	Calculated velocity (cm/s)
0	6,494	100	100
30	5,624	100	87
45	4,592	100	71
60	3,248	100	50
75	1,681	100	26
90	0	100	0

signal, and retreating objects decrease the frequency. While the process in which the echocardiography machine determines reflector direction is not as straightforward as might appear from Eq. 1.9, the fact remains that reflector direction of motion is another important piece of information that can be extracted from the returning echo signal.

Doppler echocardiography plays a major role in the noninvasive hemodynamic evaluation of the cardiovascular system, primarily for the assessment of blood flow in the arterial and venous systems. Because red blood cells (Rayleigh scatterers) reflect ultrasound, blood flow evaluation by Doppler can readily be performed, and from this a great amount of hemodynamic information can be derived. In addition, myocardial motion can also be assessed by Doppler, yielding important information about myocardial systolic and diastolic function and mechanics.

There are several methods in which Doppler information can be displayed by echocardiography: spectral, color flow Doppler, and audible Doppler. These will be presented below.

Spectral Doppler

In the example given above, a single velocity was used to characterize a moving object. However it is a simplistic notion to view flow in the human blood vessel as a constant river or stream of one single velocity; in fact, quite the opposite is true. In the human body, blood flow in the heart, arteries and veins is not steady, and exhibits considerable variation during the cardiac cycle, especially given the pulsatile nature of cardiac output. Blood flow also varies with external factors such as inspiration/expiration. Moreover, even in the normal flow through a vessel, at any one point there is a distribution of velocities, with a much higher velocity in the

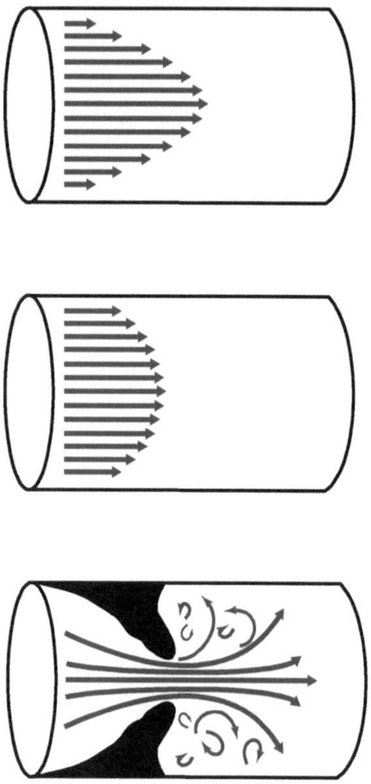

Fig. 1.28 Laminar vs. turbulent flow in a blood vessel. In normal vessels, the blood cells move fastest along the central axis of the vessel, and the velocity decreases virtually to zero next to the vessel wall. While blood flow direction is still orderly and well-organized, there is a parabolic appearance to the flow in the vessel (*top panel*). In larger vessels, this flow takes on a more blunt profile, with less variation in velocities in the center of the vessel (*middle panel*). When turbulence occurs, such as when blood passes through an area of obstruction, a disordered and chaotic flow pattern is produced (*lower panel*)

center of the vessel compared to flow near the periphery (adjacent to the vessel wall). This is known as *laminar* flow, and is due to the friction between layers, resulting in the lowest velocities along the wall, and the highest velocities centrally. Thus the velocity profile assumes a rounded or parabolic configuration, as noted in Fig. 1.28. A laminar flow pattern is characterized by a smooth, organized and orderly appearance. With higher blood flow velocities, such as those encountered with vessel or valve stenosis, there is a loss of orderliness in blood flow. This is known as *turbulence*. The blood flow pattern presents a chaotic picture, with flow orientation in a number of different directions, and considerable dispersion in detectable blood flow velocities (Fig. 1.28).

Whether laminar or turbulent, the returning Doppler signal from blood is seen as a complex wave representing a combination of frequency shifts produced by different velocities. Doppler **spectral analysis** is the process whereby this complex signal is broken down into simpler frequency components for analysis. In echocardiography, the process most commonly used is known as *Fourier analysis*, and the device used to perform the analysis is called a fast Fourier transform analyzer. A spectral analyzer then records the relative amount of signal for several discrete frequency "bins". This analysis allows the amount of Doppler signal present at different frequencies to be displayed as a function of time. When evaluating blood flow, the low velocity signals originating from myocardial motion are filtered. At any given time point, the distribution of velocities is shown on the y axis; for each velocity, pixel brightness corresponds to the quantity of red blood cells with that velocity. By obtaining successive signals, a continuous spectral display of velocity vs. time is obtained. In essence, a visual display is created showing the breakdown of velocities (frequencies) plotted as a function of time (Fig. 1.29). By convention, flow direction is depicted as above the baseline when flow is toward the transducer, and below the baseline when flow is away from the transducer (Fig. 1.30). When there is a narrow range of velocities present, such as that seen with smooth laminar flow, the spectral envelope displays a small band along the top edge of the spectral envelope corresponding to the range of velocities. The brightness of the pixels of a given velocity in the display corresponds to the number and frequency of reflectors with that velocity. A darker spectral "window" is seen underneath this band because no other velocities are present. With a wider range of velocities sampled, such as turbulent blood flow or with continuous wave Doppler, the spectral window becomes "filled in". This is also known as spectral broadening (Fig. 1.31).

Spectral Doppler evaluation represents the fundamental basis for quantitative noninvasive hemodynamic assessment. From the spectral curves, a number of important parameters can be used for analysis including peak velocity, mean velocity as calculated using the time-velocity integral (represented by the area under the curve for a single cardiac cycle), and acceleration. Applications for these will be discussed in subsequent portions of this chapter, and also in other chapters of this textbook.

There are two principal methods of spectral Doppler analysis: *continuous wave* and *pulsed wave* Doppler. These two methods will be discussed below. What will become apparent is that these two methods are complementary—each has its own strengths and weaknesses, but the strengths of one complement the weaknesses of the other, and ideally the two should be used together for a full Doppler evaluation.

For transthoracic, fetal, and transesophageal echocardiography, modern phased array transducers have the capability of performing B-mode imaging and spectral Doppler evaluation (such systems are sometimes called "duplex scanners"). These transducers can rapidly alternate between imaging and spectral Doppler evaluation. The transducer "time-shares" between both, displaying the spectral Doppler tracing while at the same time periodically updating the 2D image to verify location of the Doppler cursor. Broadband phased array transducers can also be optimized for both

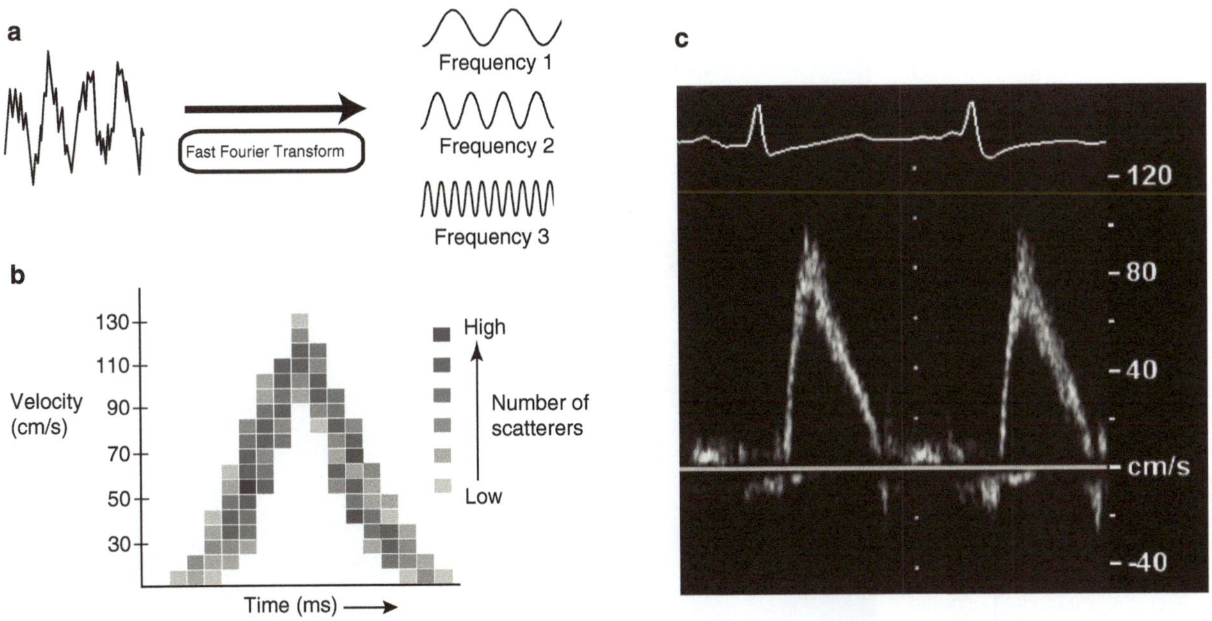

Fig. 1.29 Spectral Doppler display. The returning Doppler velocity profile is complex, and contains a range of different Doppler frequencies that can be analyzed into simpler frequency components by the use of a fast Fourier transform (FFT) analyzer (**a**). A spectral analyzer then produces a record showing the relative amount of signal within each of several discrete bins corresponding to the relative amount of each signal. The Doppler spectral display (**b**) provides a readout of velocity vs. time, with the pixel brightness reflecting the relative amount of scatterers with that velocity at that point in time. In this way, a spectral Doppler tracing is obtained (**c**)

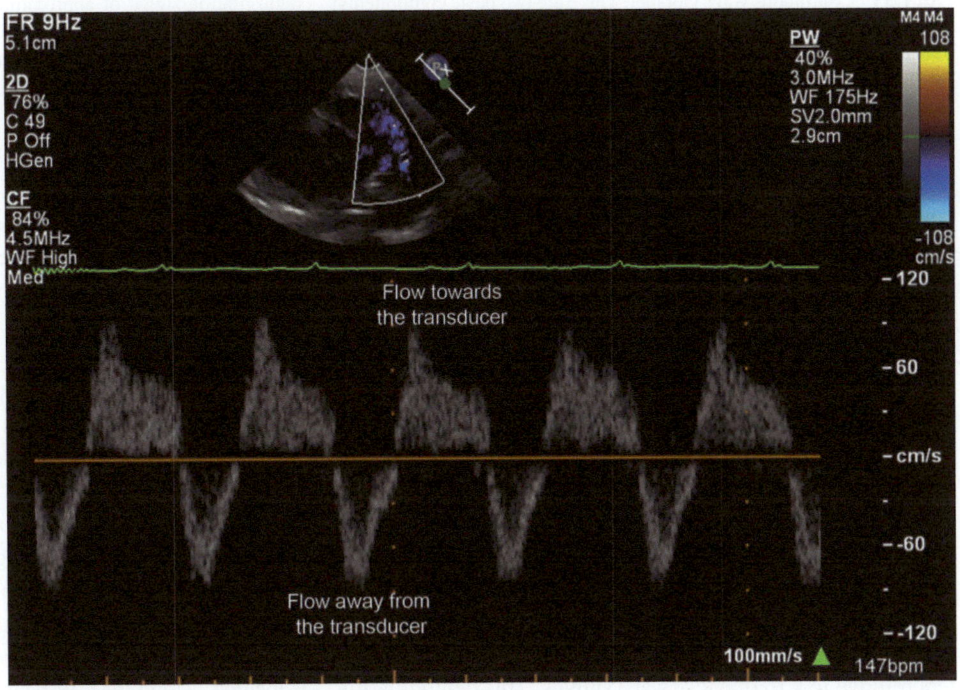

Fig. 1.30 Spectral Doppler from a transthoracic echocardiogram displaying flow directionality in this patient with to and fro flow across a patent ductus arteriosus. Flow below the baseline represents flow away from the transducer; flow above the baseline represents flow towards the transducer

modes—they can operate at lower frequencies in Doppler mode to optimize detectability of velocities at increased depths, and high frequency in imaging mode to optimize spatial resolution. In addition, these highly sophisticated transducers also have the capability of performing M-mode imaging, tissue Doppler imaging, and (in some instances) more advanced technologies such as 3D and strain imaging/speckle tracking.

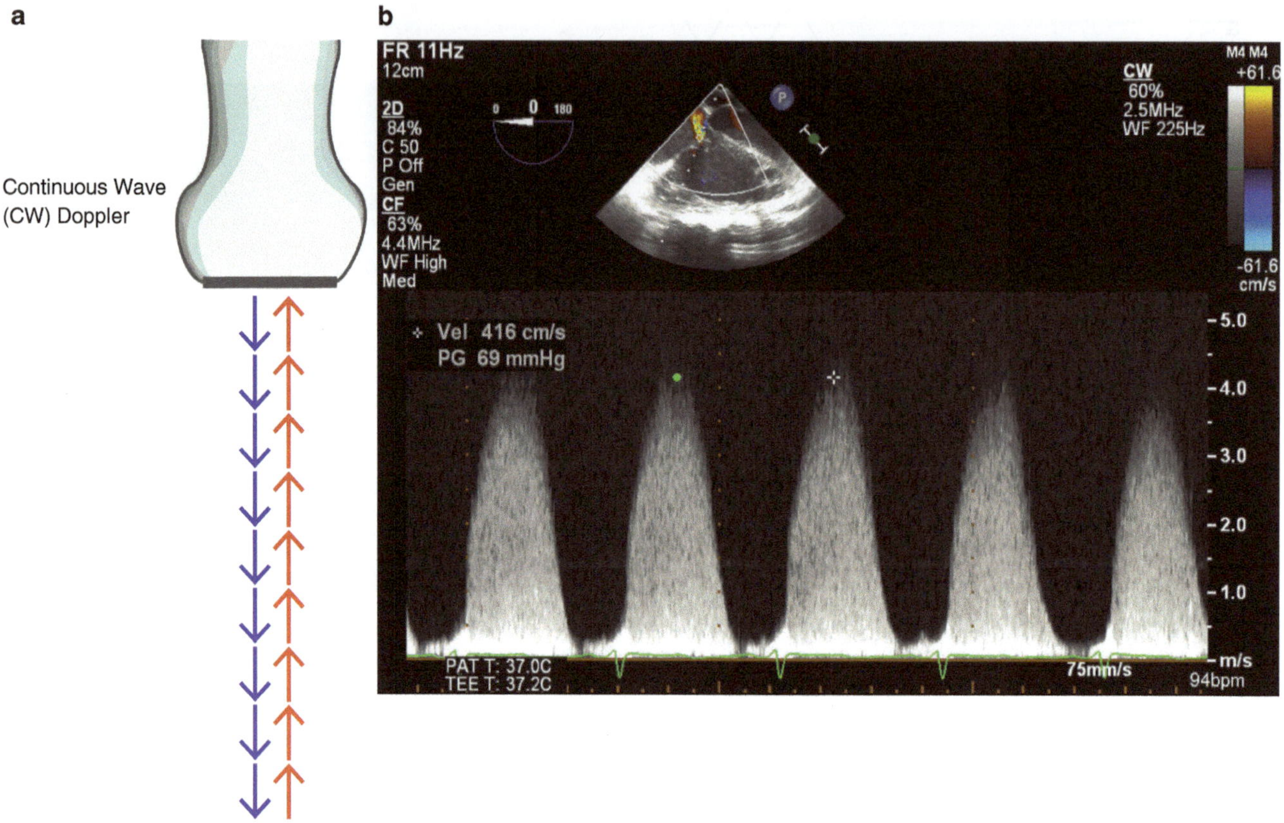

Fig. 1.31 Continuous wave Doppler. There are two basic components: a transmitter that continuously sends sound waves of known frequency, and a separate receiver that continuously receives all returning signals (**a**). The "difference frequency" is plotted as a function of time, yielding a spectral display with a wide dispersion of frequencies and significant spectral broadening (**b**). In this example, a high velocity tricuspid regurgitation signal of approximately 4.2 m/s is obtained. This study was performed with a transesophageal echocardiographic probe with broadband capabilities: B-mode imaging was performed at a frequency of 7 MHz; color flow Doppler at 4.4 MHz, and a frequency of 2.5 MHz was used for the continuous wave Doppler evaluation

Continuous Wave Doppler

Continuous wave (CW) Doppler is the simpler of the two spectral Doppler methods. The transducer is essentially divided into two separate elements: a transmitter and receiver. Two elements are needed because both operate continuously: the transmitter continuously excites the transducer to produce a reference signal of known frequency f_0 (Fig. 1.31a) The signals returning from reflection and scattering are amplified and combined with the reference (transmitted) signal to create a complex Doppler signal which is then demodulated to obtain the "difference" or "beat" frequency, which is equal to the Doppler frequency shift corresponding to the velocities of the reflectors. The beat signal is amplified, low pass filters remove high frequency signals, and high pass filters remove low frequency (wall) signals. This demodulation yields the Doppler shift, but gives no information regarding directionality. To obtain information about flow direction, a commonly used signal processing technique known as *quadrature detection* is used. This method sends the echo signal to two demodulators, and the phase relationship of the two resultant signals can be used to determine whether the Doppler shift is positive or negative. A spectral tracing of velocities vs. time is then created in the manner described above. In practice, many moving interfaces reflect signals to the receiver, thus many beat frequencies are produced. Because of this wide mixture of velocities being sampled, there is significant spectral broadening of the CW Doppler signal (Fig. 1.31b).

The advantage of CW Doppler is its ability to measure very high blood flow velocities, in excess of 6–7 m/s (or higher). Because the signal is continuously emitted and sampled, the spectral tracing will not be subject to aliasing (discussed below). This gives it great utility when evaluating areas of stenosis. However the disadvantage of this technique is a complete lack of depth specificity, also known as *range ambiguity*. A high velocity might be detected, but based upon the CW tracing alone, it is impossible to determine at what depth this velocity is located. Along the CW beam line, *all* velocities will be sampled and displayed in one spectral tracing. Therefore if there are several levels of obstruction, for example if high velocities are present along the line from two (or more) separate locations, it might be very difficult to separate the different velocities.

Pulsed Wave Doppler

Pulsed wave (PW) Doppler is used for the evaluation of Doppler signals at a specific range or depth. Using the

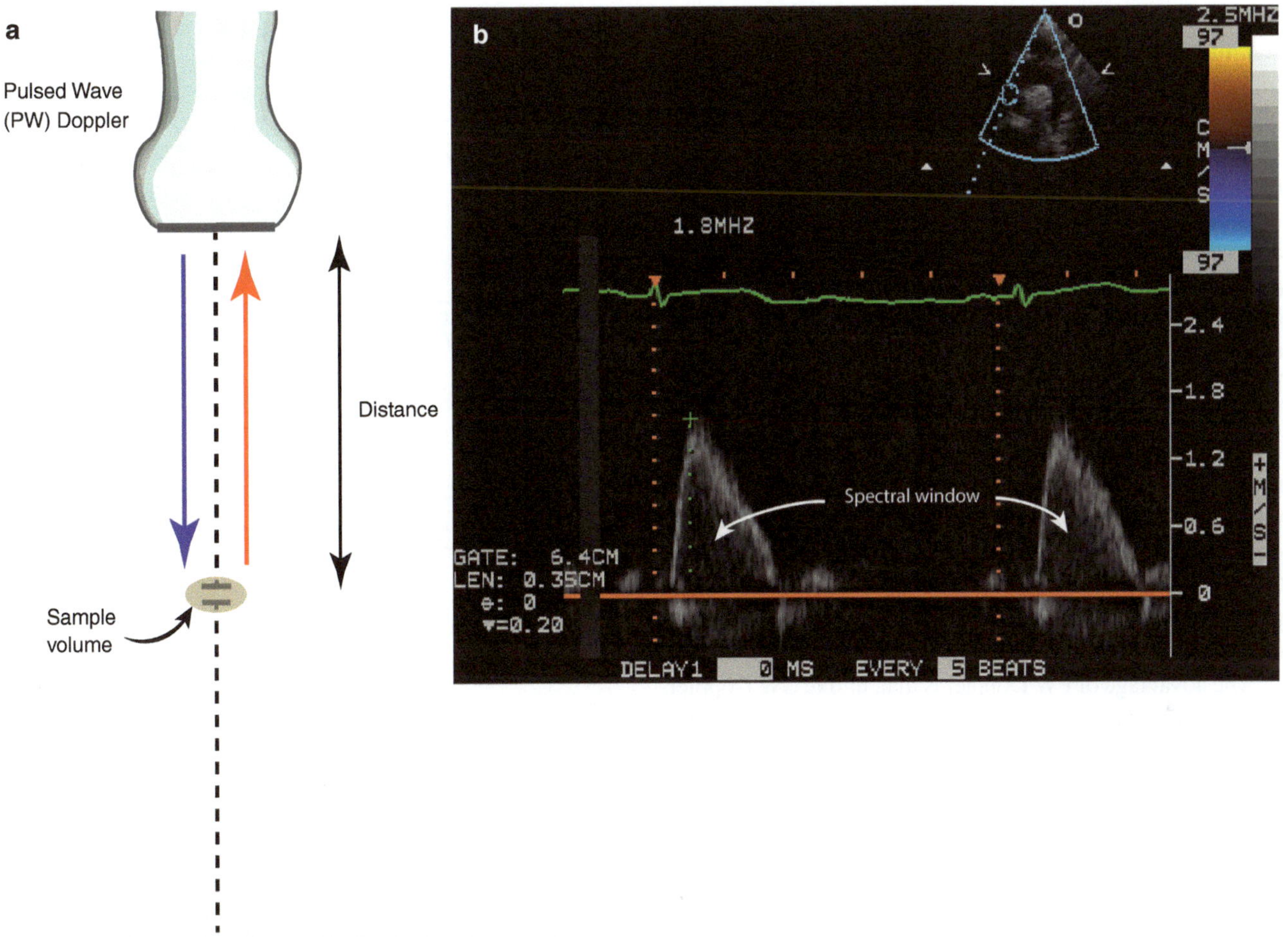

Fig. 1.32 Pulsed wave Doppler. This is used to evaluate Doppler signals at a specific range or depth, and relies upon the pulse-echo principle to determine which signals to sample. A sample volume is placed in the area where Doppler evaluation is desired (**a**). Pulses are transmitted over a beam line along which the sample volume is located; however only echoes returning in a time window equivalent to sample volume depth (depth ∝ (round-trip echo time/2)) are collected. The resultant signals are processed and a spectral display generated (**b**), in this example a spectral Doppler recording has been obtained by transthoracic echocardiography from the ascending aorta. Note that normal blood flow has a narrow range of blood flow velocities displayed as a band of *gray scale brightness*. This creates an open area underneath known as a "spectral window"

principle of pulse-echo 2D imaging, PW Doppler involves emitting a signal of known frequency, and by selecting transmission/reception time in conjunction with the speed of sound in soft tissue, returning signals originating from a specific depth can be isolated and evaluated. However unlike 2D imaging, the important information evaluated by PW Doppler is not signal amplitude, but rather the *Doppler frequency shift* of the returning signal, which can then be used to calculate reflector velocity and direction.

To perform PW Doppler evaluation, it is necessary to have updated 2D image information so that the desired region of interrogation can be selected; this region is designated on the image by the use of a *sample volume*, which is usually a pair of small parallel lines orthogonal to a visible scan line on the display. This sample volume can be adjusted for depth and position anywhere within the image (Fig. 1.32a). The sample volume or gate size can also be adjusted for size; increasing the gate size accepts Doppler signals from a longer axial region. Like pulse-echo imaging, the same PZE element serves as both transmitter and received of ultrasound pulses. These pulses tend to be longer in duration (spatial pulse length 5–25 cycles) to produce a narrow frequency bandwidth pulse and improved sensitivity, though this comes at the expense of poorer axial resolution and greater acoustic exposure. As previously noted, only the echoes returning during a specified time window (corresponding to the desired depth, as given in Eqs. 1.5 and 1.6) are selected for analysis. These echoes undergo the same processes of amplification, demodulation and filtering that are utilized with CW Doppler, yielding a velocity and directionality of the moving reflector. The signals are stored in a sample and hold unit, and held there awaiting the results of another transmit pulse. Subsequent ultrasound pulses are transmitted as soon as the previous pulses are received; the maximum frequency of transmission is the maximum PRF, which, as discussed earlier, is completely dependent upon the depth of the sample volume. In general, a PRF of 4,000–12,000 Hz is utilized with PW Doppler [1]. With each pulse transmission-reception, the incoming signals are processed, resulting in the construction of the Doppler signal. The spectral tracing displays the range of velocities over time, with pixel brightness corresponding to the number of reflectors with a specific velocity. With laminar flow, there is a much narrower range of velocities displayed as a small band along the edge of the spectral envelope, and a spectral "window" underneath (Fig. 1.32b). This band broadens slightly with peak flow rates as a more parabolic shape of velocities occurs. As noted previously, turbulence results in a wider range of velocities and "fill-in" of the spectral window, also known as spectral broadening.

With current phased array transducer technology, 2D imaging and Doppler capabilities are all present on one transducer. For PW Doppler, the 2D image information is utilized for precise placement of the sample volume in the desired location. During the periods when the transducer is "listening" for the returning Doppler information, image pulses can be sent. Therefore an intermittent image update can occur even during the PW spectral Doppler display.

The advantage of PW Doppler is that, unlike CW Doppler, the sample volume can be precisely located anywhere within the field of view, enabling collection of velocity information from a specific location. However, this comes with a tradeoff—for PW Doppler there is an upper limit to the maximum velocity that can be measured unambiguously, and this limit varies with depth. This is discussed in the section below.

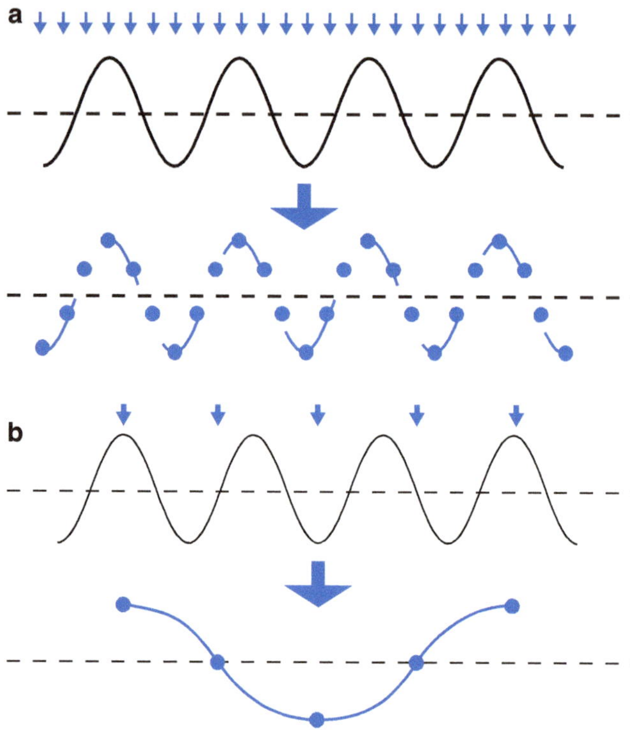

Fig. 1.33 Examples of adequate and inadequate signal sampling. To describe a wave accurately, there must be adequate sampling of the signal. The greater the sampling frequency, the better the signal is rendered. At the very minimum, sampling needs to occur at twice the frequency of the wave being sampled. Otherwise, *aliasing* will occur. (**a**) A sine wave is sampled frequently (*arrows*), allowing for an accurate rendering of the signal. (**b**) The sampling frequency of the same wave is inadequate, leading to aliasing and the erroneous rendition of a lower frequency wave

Aliasing and the Nyquist Limit

Unlike CW Doppler, sampling with PW Doppler cannot be performed continuously. The echo pulse transmit/reflect time must be used to determine sample volume distance, which means that one complete pulse must be sent and received before the next is sent. Therefore a Doppler signal must be sampled at discrete intervals. The greater the sampling frequency, the better the construction of the signal (Fig. 1.33a). For PW Doppler, the sampling frequency is equal to the pulse repetition frequency (PRF). The upper limit of the sampling frequency is given by the maximum PRF, which in turn is dictated by the distance from the transducer: the farther the distance between sample volume and transducer, the less the maximum PRF.

To provide an accurate measurement of a reflector's velocity by PW Doppler, at minimum the PRF needs to be high enough to sample the Doppler frequency shift unambiguously at least *twice* per wave cycle. If not, a phenomenon known as **aliasing** occurs in which the reported frequency shift will appear to be erroneously low (Fig. 1.33b) [18]. This is akin to the well-known example in movies of a rapidly spinning wheel—if the movie frame rate is not twice the frequency of the spinning wheel, aliasing occurs in which the wheel appears to be spinning slowly in the other direction. For PW Doppler, the minimum PRF needed to avoid aliasing is twice the Doppler shift frequency (f_d), as given by the equation: Minimum PRF = $2f_d$. When viewed in another manner, the maximum frequency shift (f_d)—which equates to the maximum nonaliased velocity measurable by a PW Doppler—is equal to PRF/2. This is known as the **Nyquist limit**. Doppler frequency shifts below the Nyquist limit can be determined accurately; those above the Nyquist limit result in aliasing and the erroneously production of a waveform of lower frequency. Aliasing of PW Doppler is manifest as a "wrapping around" of the signal from the top to the bottom on the spectral display (Fig. 1.34).

As an example, consider blood coming directly toward the transducer at 1 m/s. Using PW Doppler with a 5 MHz transmission frequency will result in a Doppler frequency shift of 6,490 Hz for the returning signal. If the sample volume is located 5 cm from the transducer, the maximum PRF at that point is 77,000 ÷ 5 or 15,400 Hz. This is more than twice the Doppler frequency shift of 6,490 Hz, hence at this distance the velocity can be determined accurately, without aliasing. However if the sample volume were located at 10 cm, the maximum PRF of 7,700 Hz (77,000 ÷ 10) is less than twice the Doppler frequency shift, and aliasing would occur at this level.

The Nyquist limit will vary both with sample volume depth as well as the frequency of the signal. The equation for calculation of maximum reflector velocity without aliasing is given as follows:

$$V_{\max} = \frac{c^2}{8 f_0 D \cos\theta} \tag{1.10}$$

V_{max} = the maximum measurable velocity of blood
c = the velocity of sound in tissue
f_0 = the transmitted frequency of sound
D = depth of interest
θ = the intercept angle between the ultrasound beam and the direction of blood flow

As previously mentioned, greater depth reduces PRF, thereby reducing the Nyquist limit for a given transducer. However, from Eq. 1.10 it is evident that, in addition to distance, there is an inverse relationship between transmitted ultrasound frequency and maximum detectable velocity using PW Doppler. Lower ultrasound frequencies enable detection of higher velocities than do higher frequencies, because the Doppler shifts are lower for the same reflector

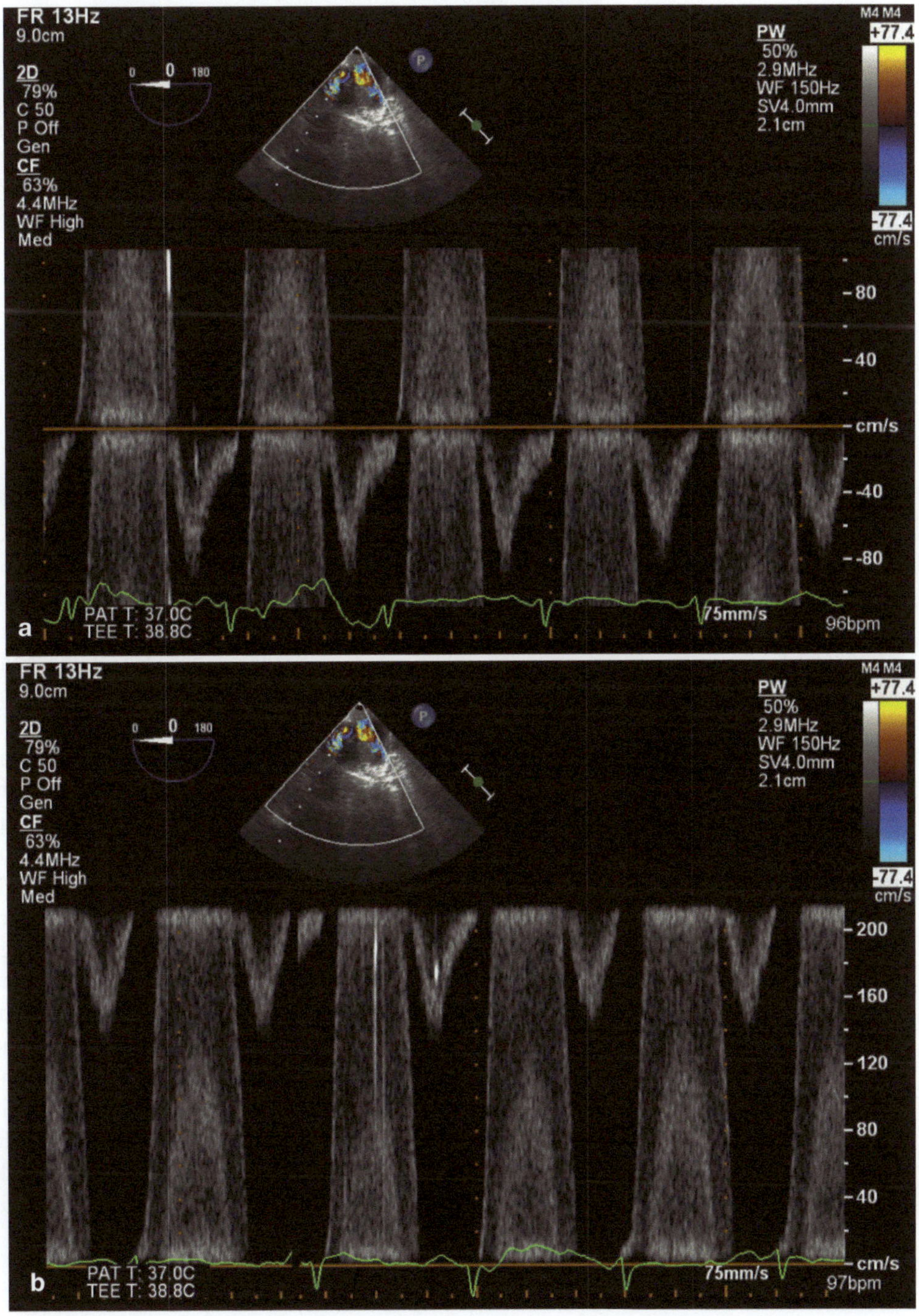

Fig. 1.34 Spectral display of aliasing by pulsed wave Doppler echocardiography in a patient with pulmonary conduit stenosis. The display "wraps around" so that the Doppler tracing is cut off at the top and appears to arise from the bottom of the screen, protruding through the baseline and up into the same wave (**a**). Even moving the baseline down to allocate the entire frequency range to the signal still results in an aliased signal (**b**). This indicates that the Doppler frequency of the signal is higher than the Nyquist limit for this particular transducer (operating at 2.9 MHz). When continuous wave Doppler evaluation is performed, a high velocity of over 4 m/s is measured, adequately resolved by this modality (**c**)

Fig. 1.34 (continued)

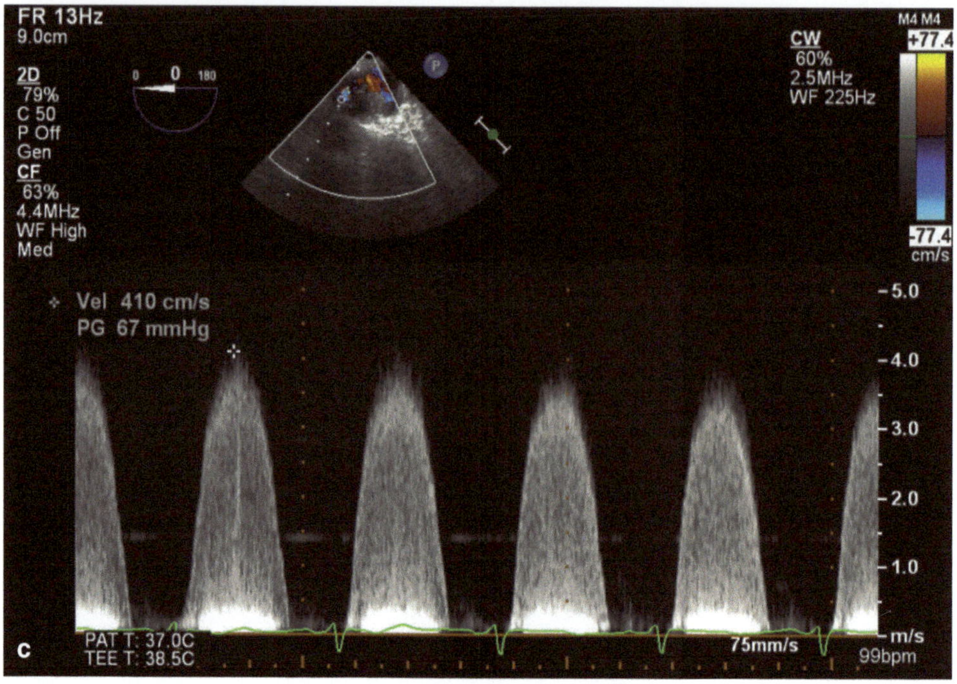

velocity. This is well shown on Fig. 1.35, which displays a graph of depth vs. calculated maximum detectable velocity for different transmitted ultrasound frequencies (assumed angle of insonation of 0°).

In summary, to maximize PW Doppler evaluation and minimize aliasing, several techniques can be performed:

- Increase the velocity scale, which increases PRF.
- Adjust the spectral baseline to the top or bottom. This allocates the entire frequency range to the maximum PRF available on the machine, though directional discrimination is lost.
- Use a lower frequency transducer.
- If possible, decrease the depth to the sample volume.

Some echocardiography machines provide a "high PRF" option for PW Doppler. This feature enables the use of a PRF higher than that allowed for the prescribed depth. This means that echoes are obtained from more than one sample volume, which in turn can lead to range ambiguity. Obviously if range ambiguity is not a concern, then CW Doppler should be used for the most accurate quantification of high velocities.

Combining the Spectral Doppler Modalities

With PW Doppler, precise depth information is available for localization, but there is a limit to the maximum measurable velocity due to the possibility of aliasing, particularly with deeper sample volumes. Conversely, CW Doppler has no such velocity limit but it can become difficult to determine the precise location of a high velocity signal. In practice, the two should be used in combination: PW Doppler for localization and quantification of blood flow through most structures, CW Doppler for quantification of high velocity jets such as stenotic valves and tricuspid regurgitant jets (as demonstrated in Fig. 1.34).

Avoidance of Artifacts with Spectral Doppler

Proper technique is important when performing spectral Doppler evaluation. As noted previously, the angle of insonation should be as parallel as possible to the direction of blood flow. With TEE, this can become even more challenging because of the confinement of the probe to the esophagus. In such cases, the different TEE positions and views (discussed in Chap. 4, as well as multiple chapters in this textbook) should be explored to determine an optimal Doppler angle of insonation—for example, the transgastric and deep transgastric views for evaluation of the left ventricular outflow tract. Visual assessment by color flow Doppler can be very useful to optimize this evaluation. Also, it is important to obtain a high quality Doppler signal with a well-demarcated, bright, and easily visualized spectral envelope. In some instances the signal is incomplete or weak, and increasing the gain settings results in significant artifact. "Feathering" (artifactual echo signals beyond the main spectral envelope) can also result in overestimation of the velocities [19]. During evaluation of flow across atrioventricular valves, some short, prominent valve closure signals can be mistaken for valvar regurgitation, resulting in erroneous estimation of regurgitant velocities. The operator should be well aware of all of these potential pitfalls.

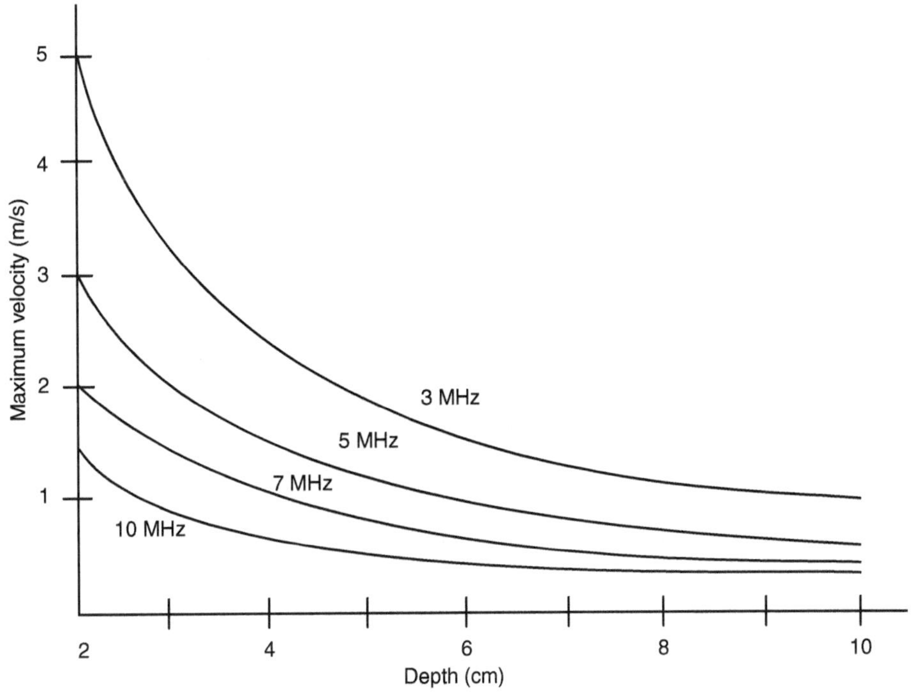

Fig. 1.35 Maximum detectable velocity without aliasing using pulsed wave Doppler, as plotted against depth of the sample volume. Four different transducer frequencies are plotted using the Nyquist equation (Equation 1.10) and assuming a 0° angle of insonation. Note that, for any given depth, lower transducer frequencies yield higher maximum detectable velocities

Spectral Doppler for Hemodynamic and Myocardial Assessment

Spectral Doppler serves as the basis for quantitative assessment of hemodynamics by echocardiography, and it is also useful for the evaluation of myocardial function. Using real-time spectral Doppler tracings that display velocity over time, important physiologic data can be derived in regard to pressure, flow, and function. These are discussed below.

Pressure Gradients and Intracardiac Pressures

This represents one of the most common and important applications of spectral Doppler. The calculation of pressure gradients is based upon Newton's law of conservation of energy, which states that the total amount of energy within a system must remain constant. Thus as blood flows through a stenotic orifice, kinetic energy (proportional to square of velocity) increases while potential energy decreases, and past the area of stenosis, some potential energy "recovers" while kinetic energy decreases. Using blood velocity as obtained by spectral Doppler (either PW or CW Doppler), the pressure gradient can be derived by using the Bernoulli equation:

$$\Delta P = \frac{1}{2}\rho\left(V_2^2 - V_1^2\right) + \rho\int_1^2 \frac{DV}{DT}DS + R\left(V\right) \quad (1.11)$$

Convective acceleration (Kinetic)	Flow acceleration (Inertial)	Viscous friction (Shear stress)

ΔP = pressure difference across an obstructive orifice (in mmHg)
V_1 = flow velocity proximal to the obstruction
V_2 = flow velocity distal to the obstruction
ρ = mass density of blood
DV = change in velocity over time (DT)
DS = distance over which change in pressure occurs
R = viscous resistance in blood vessel
V = velocity of blood flow

The first term corresponds to kinetic energy resulting from acceleration through the stenosis; the second term represents energy loss from blood flow acceleration/deceleration; the third term represents energy loss due to viscous friction. Obviously the complete Bernoulli equation is quite complicated and requires the input of a number of different variables. However in clinical practice, the Bernoulli equation can be simplified because generally the effects of flow acceleration and viscous friction can be ignored when evaluating flow across a discrete area of stenosis. The value of $\frac{1}{2}\rho$ in blood is 4, thus yielding the *modified* Bernoulli equation: $\Delta P = 4(V_2^2 - V_1^2)$. In most clinical situations, V_2 is much greater than V_1 and therefore V_1 can be discounted and V_2 used by itself, yielding a simpler version of the modified Bernoulli equation often called the *simplified* Bernoulli equation: $\mathbf{\Delta P = 4V^2}$ (V is equal to the measured spectral Doppler velocity). For example, when the maximal instantaneous velocity across a stenotic valve is 3.5 m/s, the calculated pressure gradient = $4 \times (3.5)^2$ or 49 mmHg. Either PW or CW Doppler can be used, though in many situations,

Table 1.3 Noninvasive hemodynamic assessment by spectral Doppler

Pressure	Equation	Useful TEE view(s) for velocity measurement
RV/PA systolic pressure	4 [V(**TR**)]2 + CVP/RAp	ME 4 Ch ME RV In-Out TG RV In
RV/PA systolic pressure (VSD and left to right shunt present)	Systolic BP – 4[**V(VSD)**]2	ME 4 Ch ME RV In-Out ME AV SAX ME LAX
PA systolic pressure (PDA and left to right shunt present)	Systolic BP – 4[**V(PDA)**]2	UE PA LAX UE Ao Arch SAX
PA mean pressure	4 [**V(early PR)**]2 + CVP/RAp	ME RV In-Out DTG Sagittal
PA diastolic pressure	4 [**V(late PR)**]2 + CVP/RAp	ME RV In-Out DTG Sagittal
LA pressure	Systolic BP – 4 [V(**MR**)]2	ME 4 Ch ME 2 Ch ME LAX
LA pressure (ASD and left to right shunt present)	CVP/RAp + **mean gradient across ASD**a	ME 4 Ch ME Bicaval DTG LAX DTG Sagittal
LV end diastolic pressure	Diastolic BP – 4 [V(**AR**)]2	ME AV LAX DTG LAX DTG Sagittal TG LAX

Note: For each derived pressure, the velocity measured by spectral Doppler in shown in **bold**. All estimated pressures in mm Hg

[a]Mean pressure gradient is the Bernoulli-derived pressure gradient averaged over a selected period of time (e.g. one cardiac cycle), obtained by tracing the spectral Doppler envelope

Abbreviations: Ao aortic, ASD atrial septal defect, AR aortic regurgitation jet, AV aortic valve, BP blood pressure, Ch chamber, CVP mean central venous pressure, DTG deep transgastric, In inflow, LA left atrium, LV left ventricle, LAX long axis, ME mid esophageal, MR mitral regurgitation jet, Out outflow, PA pulmonary artery, PDA patent ductus arteriosus, PR pulmonary regurgitation jet, RAp right atrial mean pressure, RV right ventricular, SAX short axis, TG transgastric, TR tricuspid regurgitation jet, UE upper esophageal, V velocity, VSD ventricular septal defect. See Chap. 4 for a description of the individual transesophageal echocardiographic (TEE) views

particularly with the evaluation of stenosis, CW Doppler is needed due to the high velocities that cause aliasing with PW Doppler.

A few caveats are important regarding the simplified Bernoulli equation. First, as with all Doppler evaluation, the angle of insonation should be as parallel as possible in order to obtain an accurate Doppler gradient. Second, the simplified equation becomes less accurate when there is a long, tubular stenosis (such as a Blalock-Taussig shunt). In such cases, the effect of viscous friction becomes significant, and the simplified Bernoulli equation can underestimate the pressure gradient. Third, by changing the mass density (ρ) of blood, anemia and polycythemia can have an effect upon the gradient. Finally, in some clinical situations such as hypoplastic aortic arch/coarctation of the aorta, V_1 could become significant and therefore should be accounted for, i.e. the modified Bernoulli equation should be used.

The modified/simplified Bernoulli equations have many uses: evaluation of pressure gradients across stenotic valves or outflow tracts, derivation of ventricular chamber pressures using the velocity across ventricular septal defects, calculation of gradients in the great arteries (e.g. coarctation, ductus arteriosus), etc. In the absence of pulmonary outflow or pulmonary artery obstruction, a tricuspid regurgitant velocity can be used to calculate systolic pulmonary artery pressure using the simplified Bernoulli equation. Other chamber and blood vessel pressures can be also be derived noninvasively, sometimes with the use of additional information such as arterial blood pressure or central venous pressure. Some of these hemodynamic calculations are listed in Table 1.3. Most, if not all, of these measurements can be obtained from TEE. The modified and simplified Bernoulli equations have a wide variety of applications in CHD evaluation, and their various applications will be discussed in multiple sections of this book.

Cardiac Flow

Stroke volume and cardiac output can be calculated using spectral Doppler. Stroke volume is calculated from echocardiography by the equation:

$$Q = TVI \times CSA \tag{1.12}$$

Q = volumetric flow (stroke volume)
TVI = time velocity integral
CSA = cross sectional area of the area that velocity is measured

Assuming a circular cross sectional area, the cardiac stroke volume can then be calculated from the diameter measured at the selected area. For left sided cardiac output, the left ventricular outflow tract diameter, represented by aortic valve annulus diameter, can be best obtained from the mid esophageal aortic valve long axis view. Cross sectional area (in cm^2) is then calculated by the formula $\pi \times (\text{diameter}/2)^2$. The time velocity integral (in cm) is calculated by manual tracing of the spectral Doppler tracing, which for the aortic valve is best obtained from a deep transgastric long axis or sagittal view, or a transgastric long axis view (see Chap. 4 for description of individual views). Once the stroke volume is obtained, cardiac output (C.O.) can be calculated as follows:

$$C.O. = HR \times Q \qquad (1.13)$$

HR = heart rate (beats/min)
Q = stroke volume (from Equation 1.12)

Cardiac index (C.I.), in $l/min/m^2$, is calculated as follows:

$$C.I. = C.O./BSA\ (m^2) \qquad (1.14)$$

It should be noted that this calculation should be performed when there is laminar, not turbulent, blood flow across the area in question. Also, the aortic valve is best used for this measurement because of its circular cross section, which does not vary significantly throughout the cardiac cycle.

A similar principle of volume assessment can be applied to the calculation in the calculation of aortic valve area (in the case of aortic valve stenosis), using the *continuity equation*. This equation is based upon the principle of conservation of mass, which stipulates that volumetric flow remains equal as it passes from one site through another. Hence the continuity equation is given as follows:

$$CSA_1 \times TVI_1 = CSA_2 \times TVI_2 \qquad (1.15)$$

In this case, the CSA_1 and TVI_1 are obtained from the left ventricular outflow tract below the aortic valve, using the method noted above. The spectral velocity tracing across the outflow tract is obtained by PW Doppler. The TVI_2 can then be calculated from the CW Doppler spectral tracing, and from these variables, the equation can be solved for CSA_2, which is the aortic valve area. It should be noted that this equation is predicated upon the assumption of a circular cross-sectional area of the left ventricular outflow tract. However recent 3D literature has suggested that the cross-sectional geometry of the outflow tract is more likely elliptical than circular [20, 21].

The continuity equation serves as the basis for the calculation of valve regurgitant orifice area as measured by the proximal isovelocity surface area (PISA) method. PISA is not widely used with congenital valve disease; it is utilized to a greater extent in adult cardiology, particularly with mitral valve disease [22, 23]. The continuity equation is also discussed in several other sections in this book, for example its use in adults with prosthetic heart valves for the calculation of valve effective orifice area (discussed in further detail in Chap. 16).

Myocardial Function

Doppler echocardiography plays an integral role in the assessment of myocardial mechanics, particularly as regards diastolic function. Spectral Doppler assessment of ventricular filling, as well as pulmonary and systemic venous Doppler waveforms, are methods used to evaluate left ventricular and left atrial diastolic properties. In addition, newer methods such as tissue Doppler imaging (also known as Doppler tissue imaging) utilize direct spectral Doppler evaluation of myocardial motion for assessment of ventricular diastolic function. This modality evaluates the low velocity, high amplitude signals of the myocardium that are filtered out by conventional spectral and color flow Doppler evaluation of blood flow (Fig. 1.36). A discussion of these methods is provided in Chap. 5.

Tissue Doppler imaging can also be used for strain analysis, one of the newer methods of myocardial functional assessment. Strain measures the extent of myocardial deformation, and strain rate measures the rate of change of this deformation. Tissue Doppler imaging was the initial technique used to evaluate these parameters—strain rate was derived from the gradient of the velocity over a sampling distance, and strain obtained as the integral of this. However the major limitation is that, like all Doppler techniques, strain could only be evaluated in one dimension—the direction along the scan line (i.e. longitudinal strain). Since myocardial strain occurs in several other directions (radial and circumferential), an alternative methodology of strain analysis has emerged to evaluate these other types of strain—that of speckle tracking. This is a 2D method that tracks a matrix of myocardial speckles corresponding to minute tissue structures. Using speckle tracking, strain can be tracked in any direction. While this method currently appears to be the preferred method of strain evaluation, tissue Doppler is still utilized. The discussion of strain evaluation is beyond the scope of this chapter; the reader is referred to Chap. 5 and other sources that provide more in-depth discussion of deformation analysis [24–26].

Color Flow Doppler

Color flow Doppler is one of the most important echocardiographic tools available, particularly for the assessment of CHD. This modality provides a visual depiction of Doppler

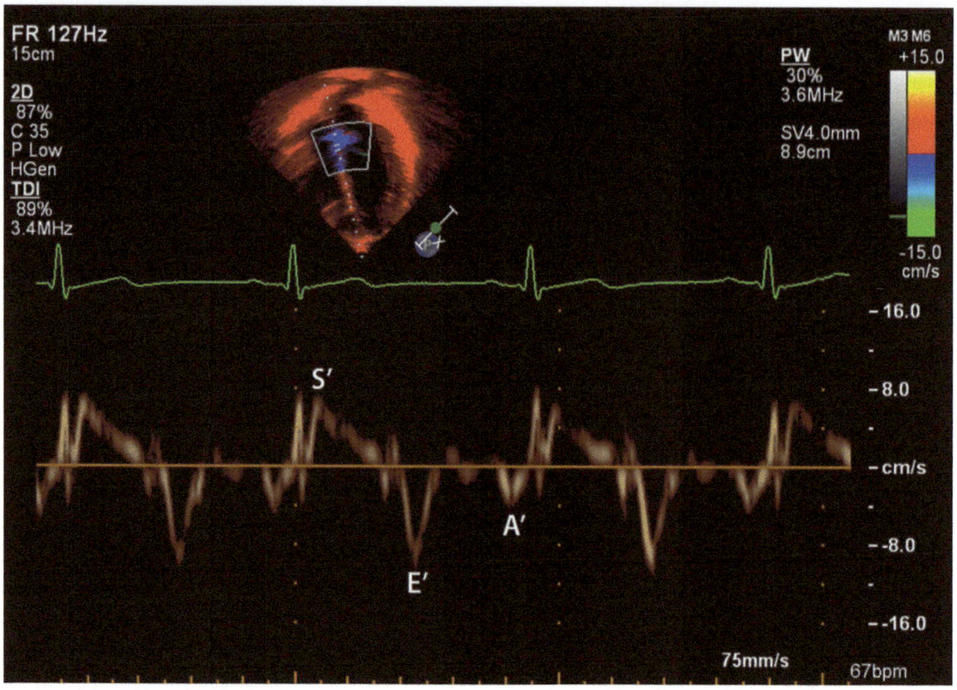

Fig. 1.36 Tissue Doppler imaging. This tracing is taken from a transthoracic echocardiogram apical four chamber view. The sample volume is placed at the level of the medial mitral valve annulus, and a pulsed wave spectral Doppler tracing is recorded. The E′ and A′ waves correspond to early and late diastolic filling (the E and A waves of mitral valve inflow), and the S′ wave corresponds to ventricular systole. Note the low tissue velocities (less than 10 cm/s), much lower than those normally found in blood pool

information for multiple reflectors and scatterers in motion—in general, these represent blood flow within the heart and arteries/veins. Doppler information is encoded as a color map, and overlaid upon the corresponding B-mode images, whether 2D, 3D, or M-mode displays. Thus real-time blood flow visualization and flow characteristics can be seen with a wide range of different physiologic situations and conditions.

The acquisition of color flow data is an extension of pulse-echo gray scale imaging, but instead of echo amplitudes, reflector velocities are determined. For each image, multiple scan lines are utilized, and multiple receiver "gates" are present for each scan line (Fig. 1.37). Ultrasound pulses are transmitted along the scan lines; these pulses are slightly longer in length than standard B-mode imaging to improve Doppler processing. Image (B-mode) data are acquired as outlined previously for 2D imaging. However in contrast to B-mode imaging, in which only one pulse-echo sequence is necessary per scan line, multiple pulse-echo sequences (known as a *pulse packet*) are sent along each beam line. Often 8–10 pulses are sent in one packet. The first returning signals, both from moving and stationary reflectors, are stored in a Doppler processing unit, in a series of registers corresponding to depth. The second set of returning signals are compared to the first set. Stationary reflectors will have identical signals and are therefore eliminated from further processing using a "stationary echo canceler". Moving reflectors will have different signals, and the differences are used to determine reflector velocities and direction. Several techniques can be used to estimate reflector velocity, but the best known is a mathematical technique termed *phase shift autocorrelation*, in which the change in phase from one transmit pulse to the next is compared, and a velocity calculated. Over the course of multiple pulses, an average or *mean* velocity is calculated. This process is repeated for all the pulses in a packet. There is a tradeoff here: the more pulses

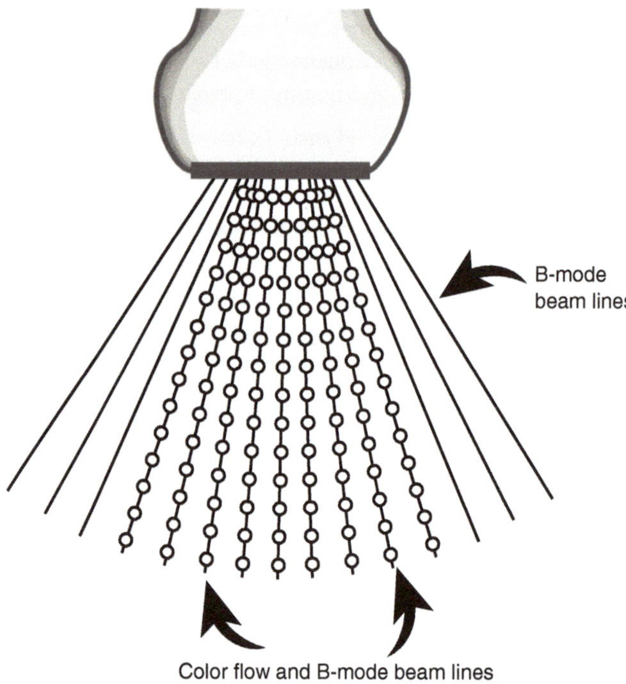

Fig. 1.37 Diagram of color flow Doppler. Both B-mode imaging and color flow Doppler are combined; the *scan lines* represent B-mode beam lines, and the *small circles* represent the multiple receiver "gates" located along the beam lines for color flow Doppler (these are combined color flow and B-mode beam lines). In general, only part of the imaging sector is used for color flow Doppler

in a packet, the better the estimates of reflector velocities but the longer the acquisition time, which slows frame rates.

Once the data from all pulse packets in one scan line have been obtained, the next scan line is evaluated. This process continues in sequence for each scan line, acquiring both color flow as well as B-mode image data, until the entire color Doppler sector has been acquired (a color flow sector tends to be smaller than the underlying B-mode imaging area). Like B-mode imaging, a sweep of the sector is continually repeated and rapidly processed to achieve real-time scan rates. Nonetheless, there are tradeoffs with color flow Doppler in both temporal and spatial resolution. Frame rates for color flow Doppler are inherently lower than B-mode imaging due to the multiple pulse sequences per packet. Increased frame rates can be achieved by reducing color sector depth, and/or reducing the total number of scan lines by either narrowing the color sector or reducing scan line density. This is analogous to the options available to improve B-mode temporal resolution, as discussed previously. Spatial resolution of color flow Doppler is also less than B-mode imaging. Because of the longer spatial pulse lengths used for Doppler evaluation, axial resolution is reduced. Also, a reduced number of scan lines (to improve temporal resolution) will reduce lateral resolution.

There are several ways in which information is displayed visually by color flow Doppler. Direction of flow is indicated by hue: by convention, red typically indicates flow *towards* the transducer, blue indicates flow *away* from the transducer (also known as "BART"—blue away, red towards). The brightness or saturation of the color can be used to indicate flow velocity, with brighter or whiter color indicating higher flow rates (Fig. 1.38). Some color flow mapping schemes include a *variance* mode in which wider variability among velocities in a single packet is indicated by a green or yellow color (Fig. 1.39a). Being a form of pulse-echo, color flow Doppler is subject to aliasing, which is displayed as color reversal or as a mosaic of multiple colors such as yellow, orange, green, etc. (Fig. 1.39a, b). With color flow Doppler, the velocity scale shown is for mean velocities; nonetheless the Nyquist limit is lower and aliasing will occur at lower velocities than PW Doppler due to the significant computational demands associated with color flow processing.

It should be noted that the method of signal processing used by color flow Doppler is fundamentally different from that used for CW and PW Doppler. This is because the fast Fourier transform methods utilized for spectral evaluation are more time-consuming and, if performed for multiple scan lines and reflectors in a designated sector, the rapid processing needed for display of real-time images could not be achieved.

Importance of Color Flow Doppler

Color Doppler echocardiography plays a vital role in the noninvasive evaluation of cardiac disease. No other imaging modality provides, in real-time, the rich variety of physiologic and functional information offered by this technique. This is particularly true with CHD, in which color flow Doppler interrogation has become indispensable for echocardiographic evaluation. Its importance cannot be overstated; in a number of instances color flow information is equally as important, if not more so, than standard 2D imaging. This is due to its exquisite sensitivity for abnormal flow velocities in

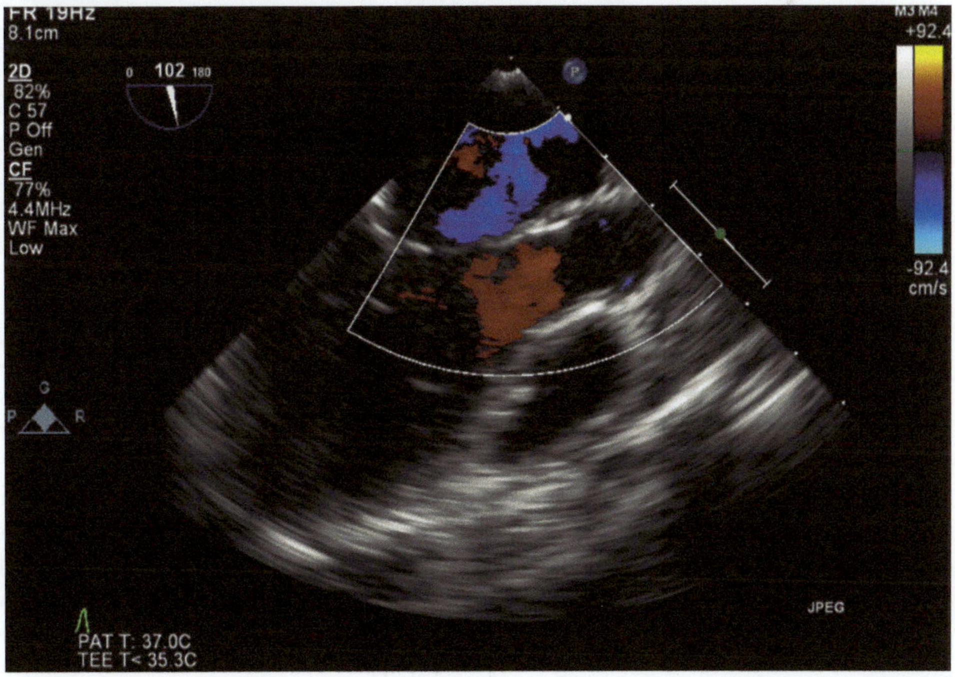

Fig. 1.38 Transesophageal echocardiogram, mid esophageal long axis view during systole showing color flow Doppler. The red flow represents normal flow velocity in the left ventricular outflow tract, the blue flow represents pulmonary venous blood returning to the left atrium

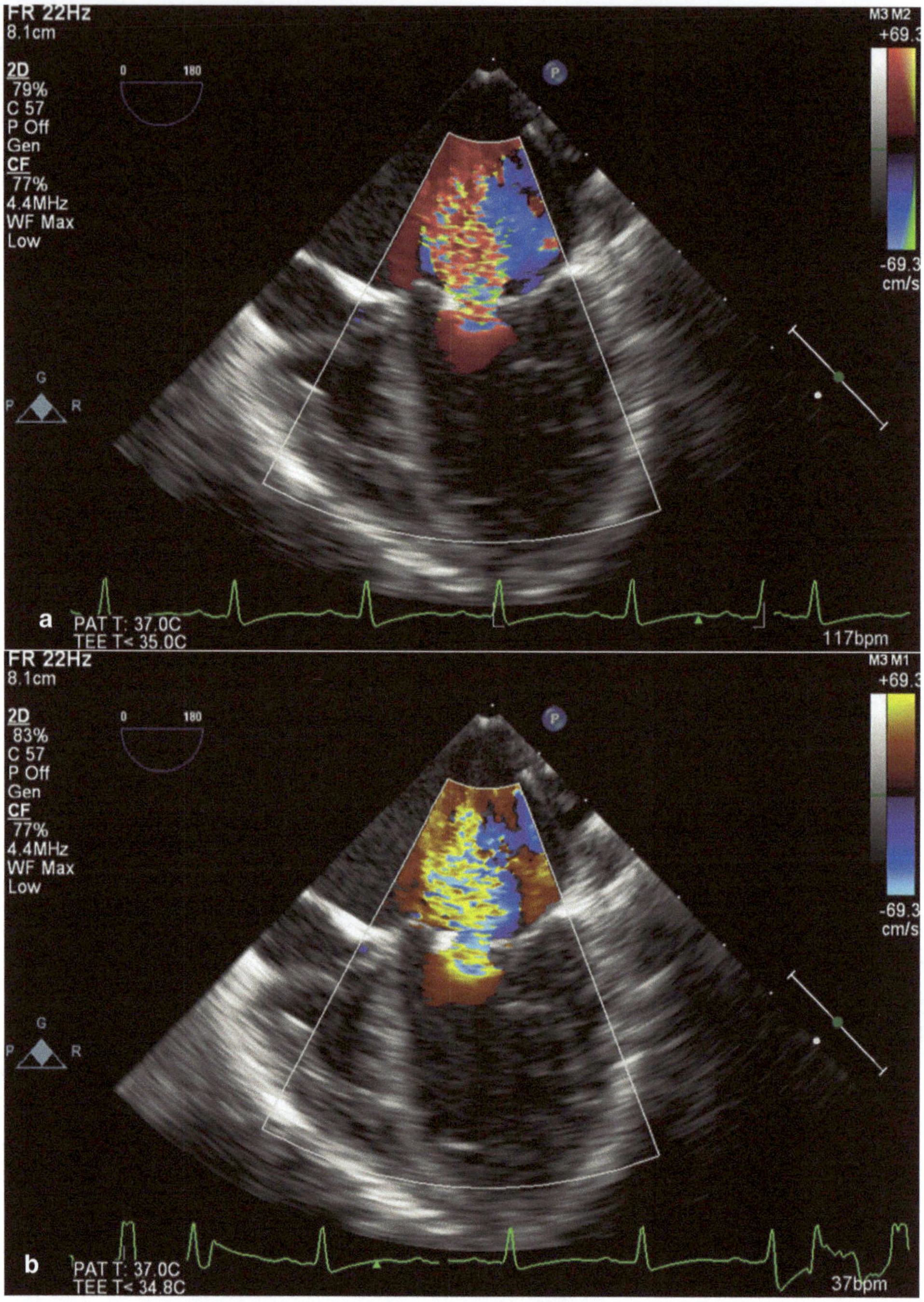

Fig. 1.39 Transesophageal echocardiogram, mid esophageal four chamber view in a patient with significant mitral insufficiency, obtained during systole, showing different color flow Doppler maps. (**a**) Shows the regurgitant jet using variance mode, (**b**) Shows the same jet using brightness mode

many different forms of congenital cardiac pathology. There are a number of congenital cardiac defects that cannot be fully assessed until color flow Doppler evaluation is performed—in some cases the pathology is incompletely seen or not even visible by 2D imaging alone (despite the superior spatial resolution of 2D imaging). Color Doppler is an essential part of the evaluation of shunts, vascular anomalies, and any pathology involving the atrioventricular and/or semilunar valves. It provides an important visual assessment of the location(s), extent, and severity of valvular stenosis or regurgitation and is very useful in directing the spectral Doppler evaluation of a stenotic/regurgitant jet by providing the optimal location and angle for spectral Doppler interrogation.

Color flow Doppler also has utility for a number of congenital heart defects typified by low velocity blood flow states. Examples of this include evaluation of Glenn and Fontan evaluation, and anomalous systemic and pulmonary venous pathways/connections. In these instances, the PRF is reduced (and wall filter settings can also be reduced) to decrease the velocity scale and improve color flow brightness/detectability for lower velocity reflectors. However the lower PRF results in a decreased frame rate.

In fact, color flow Doppler has become such an integral part of the echocardiographic examination that sometimes its potential shortcomings and limitations are not fully considered. As a form of Doppler evaluation, color flow Doppler is subject to the same limitations as PW Doppler. Like PW Doppler, aliasing will occur when the Nyquist limit is exceeded by the Doppler frequency shift of moving reflectors, and this will be reflected in the color flow reversal or mosaic patterns described above. Lower frequency transducers enable higher PRFs and Nyquist limits. Furthermore, the color (Doppler) signals will vary depending the angle of insonation; the more perpendicular the angle, the lower the Nyquist limit. As with any Doppler modality, whenever feasible, one should strive to utilize a color Doppler angle of interrogation as parallel to the intended flow as possible.

Another important reminder: it is easy to perform and record too much color flow Doppler. Because the color map is superimposed upon the real-time image, the examiner can also see the underlying anatomy while the color flow is being displayed. What can result is a study dominated by color flow Doppler evaluation and color flow Doppler recorded clips. However for a number of reasons, it is important to ensure that adequate B-mode imaging is performed. With color flow Doppler, the spatial and temporal resolution of the underlying B-mode images will be inferior to that of imaging alone; at times the disparity is striking, particularly the reduction in temporal resolution when color flow Doppler is activated. Also, the overlying color flow Doppler map has the potential to obscure important anatomic details, especially smaller structures. For this reason, the observer must be conscious of the need to strike a balance between adequate 2D imaging and judicious and proper use of color flow evaluation.

The other important fact to remember about color flow Doppler is that it is a map of mean velocities, and thus it is representative of blood in motion. It is not a map of blood or blood volume itself. This consideration applies particularly to valvular regurgitation, in which the color flow Doppler depiction of a regurgitant jet is often used as a visual estimate of the actual volume of the jet. However it is important to note that this jet can be made to appear larger or smaller due to a number of factors. Instrument settings can change the appearance of the jet size: the jet size can appear larger when the color gain setting is increased, and also when the PRF is decreased (i.e. the Nyquist limit is lowered). If the pressure in the receiving chamber is high (e.g. the left atrium with mitral regurgitation), the pressure gradient decreases more rapidly. This can lead to lower jet velocities and a smaller color flow jet area. Furthermore the extent and geometry of the regurgitant jet will vary depending upon whether it is central or adjacent to a cardiac boundary or wall (a "wall-hugging" jet). Even with the same regurgitant orifice, a jet next to a wall cannot entrain adjacent fluid, and therefore will appear smaller than the same jet seen in the center of the valve. Finally, color flow jets do not have the same degree of spatial resolution as the B-mode image, and often color flow jet or shunt margins are imprecise and tend to "bleed" over the 2D boundaries, thus the measurement of color flow jet diameter across, for example, a ventricular septal defect can overestimate the true defect diameter.

Audible Doppler

While ultrasound frequencies are measured in millions of Hz (or MHz), the Doppler shift produced by moving structures in the body generally falls within audible frequency range. For example, if a 5 MHz signal is sent towards a reflector moving straight towards the transducer at 1.0 m/s (a typical velocity for normal blood flowing through the great arteries), the Doppler shift would be 6,490 Hz (6.49 kHz), well within the human audible range of 20–20,000 Hz. Most echocardiography machines provide a sound system that can amplify and play these signals as audio. Using this signal is a useful method to guide spectral Doppler assessment—by listening for the pitch (frequency) and loudness of the signal, one can determine the optimal position for spectral Doppler evaluation, and also detect areas of turbulence/stenosis. Prior to the widespread availability of color flow Doppler, listening to the audio component served as an important part of Doppler evaluation. It was particularly helpful in screening for occult high velocity flow signals such as small ventricular septal defects that were not obvious by 2D imaging: the echocardiographer would pass a pulsed wave Doppler sample volume across the entire ventricular septum, listening for high frequency signals that might indicate a possible defect. This is a technique still used by some experienced echocardiographers. However, for many practitioners color flow Doppler has largely replaced audio because of its sensitivity and efficient evaluation of large volumes of real-time Doppler information.

Overview of the Echocardiography Machine

Competent performance of an echocardiogram requires an understanding and familiarity with all of the equipment. In the case of TEE, this includes not just the transducer and associated controls on the handle, but the cardiac ultrasound machine as well. Given the time constraints of many TEE studies, particularly those performed intraoperatively, it is essential that one proceed in a rapid and efficient manner. This requires the operator to have a thorough working knowledge of all aspects of the imaging system.

The layout of the echocardiography machine and its multiple controls/functions will vary with each manufacturer. Nonetheless, certain features are common to every current system, and lend a certain degree of familiarity no matter what platform is used. All machines have a large high-resolution screen with which to view the live images. Most current machines now have "hard" keys assigned to certain unchanging functions and "soft" keys that can vary depending upon the mode of scanning performed (B-mode, color Doppler, etc.) (Fig. 1.40a). Most new machines incorporate these "soft" keys into touch screens with menus that will change and update depending upon the mode of scanning; each set of menus contains multiple options to optimize imaging and/or Doppler settings. There will also be a keyboard used for inputting of patient information as well as annotation/labeling in specific images; a trackball is also present and used for many functions including selection of specific images, movement of the cursor on the screen, etc. Other important features common to all echocardiography machines include a digital loop acquisition button, freeze frame/cine looping function that allows the user to scroll

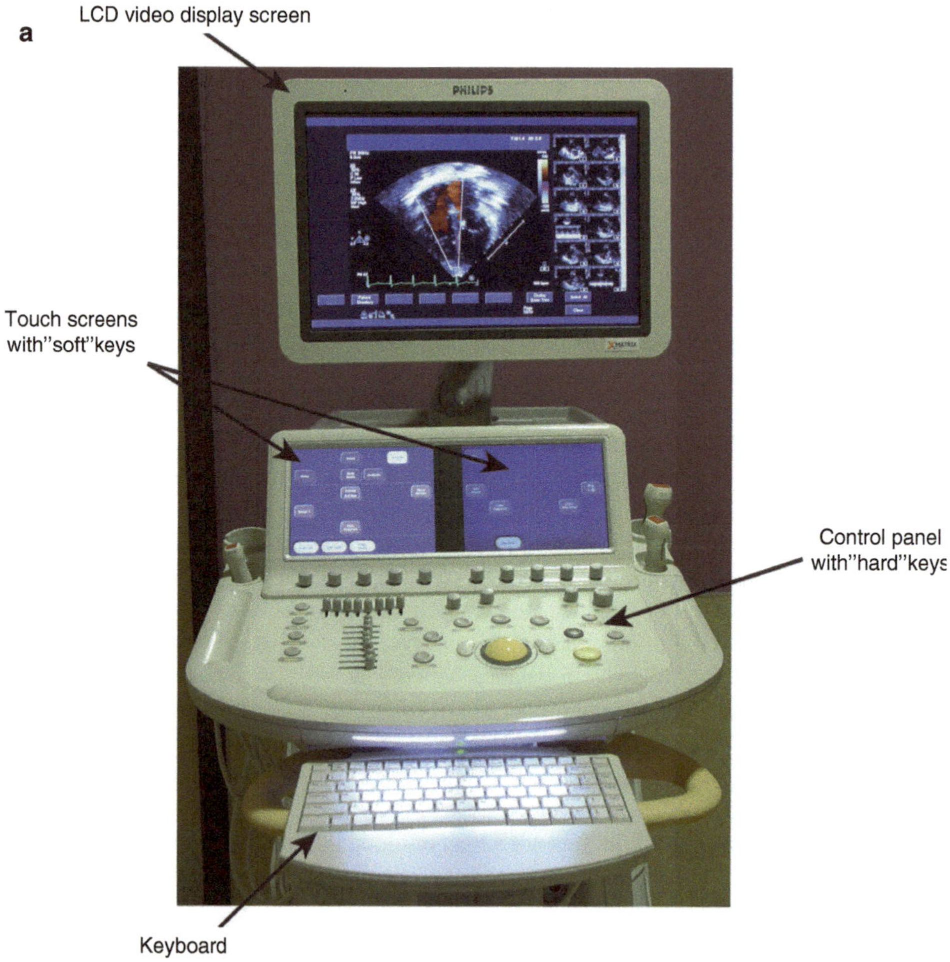

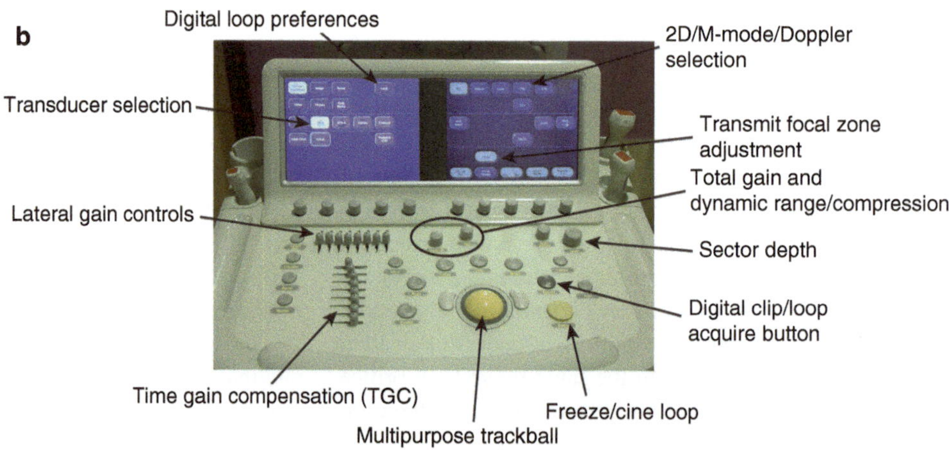

Fig. 1.40 Photograph of a standard echocardiography machine (Philips IE-33). The major components of an echocardiography machine are shown in (**a**). (**b**) The control panel and touch screen are shown in more detail, along with a number of important controls detailed in the text

through a loop frame by frame (very useful for fast heart rates), as well as calipers available for making measurements directly upon the screen (Fig. 1.40b). In addition, there are specific ultrasonic features common to all echocardiographic machines, some of which are listed below:

- **Transmit power**. Most machines allow the operator to adjust the output power, thereby providing higher intensity pulses with greater amplitude of the transmitted echo signals. This will improve visualization of the echo signal from weaker reflectors, but will also increase the exposure of the patient to greater acoustic energy (which can produce more heat). This control is variously labeled output, power, dB, or transmit. Thus during procedures that require continuous TEE monitoring (such as monitoring of cardiac function during surgery), it is advisable to decrease the output power to reduce the potential amount of heat generated. To help gauge the potential level of acoustic exposure, two standardized indices can be found on the display of the contemporary echocardiography machines from most manufacturers. It should be noted that these are calculated indices, based upon conservative assumptions, and represent "worse case" situations. The first, *Thermal Index (TI)*, relates to the possibility of tissue heating due to absorption of ultrasound energy, and represents the ratio of acoustic power produced by the transducer to the power required to raise the temperature of tissue by 1 °C. There are several calculations used, depending upon whether bone is encountered along the ultrasound path; the measurement is called TIS when only soft tissue is encountered, TIB if bone is at or near the focal zone of the transducer (e.g. fetal scans), and TIC if bone is close to the transducer. The other index, known as *Mechanical Index (MI)*, is related to the likelihood of cavitation produced by acoustic energy. As transmit power output increases, both the TI and MI will be noted to increase. These indices have been established to help guide echocardiographers in minimizing acoustic exposure, and standardization allows them to be used and compared across a number of different echocardiography platforms, regardless of manufacturer.
- **Temperature sensor**. Many TEE transducers have a built-in temperature sensor to monitor the patient temperature, and automatic shutoff if the temperature exceeds a predefined threshold. Nonetheless, if the probe temperature and/or local patient temperature (adjacent to the probe) is noted to increase significantly, transmit power should be reduced to decrease acoustic energy output.
- **Transmit frequency adjustment**. As has been previously noted, broadband frequency transducers (which include TEE transducers) provide the ability for the operator to alter transmit frequency to accommodate the particular clinical imaging needs. The transducer's default frequency is generally its center frequency, but the frequency can be increased for greater resolution (less penetration), or decreased for improved penetration (with less resolution). For TEE, given the generally excellent imaging afforded by most TEE views and windows, it is rare that significant frequency adjustment is necessary. The exception might be the deep transgastric views (see Chap. 4), in which the great distance from the transducer to certain cardiac structures could necessitate the use lower frequencies, particularly in larger patients.
- **Gain control**. This adjusts the amplification of the received signal in order to increase or increase the sensitivity of the instrument. It should be noted that this control, unlike transmit power, does not increase the acoustic exposure to the patient. It only increases the amplification of the received signal. There are several types of gain control. The first control is the *Overall Gain Control* and increases amplification at all depths. The second is are the TGCs, or *Time Gain Compensation* controls. These are the individual slider bars that provide adjustment of receiver gain at specific depth ranges. They are used to compensate for the attenuation of signals that occur at greater depths—in other words, a "slope" of TGCs occurs, with progression from less to more gain as the depth increases. Presently, most machines now provide an internal TGC feature that automatically corrects for depth, obviating the need for some manual adjustment of TGCs. Also, because a brief pulse of ultrasound contains a range of frequencies, manufacturers now provide a *dynamic frequency tracking* feature in which the transducer responds most effectively to higher frequencies arising from shallower depths, and to lower frequencies for greater depths. This feature capitalizes on the greater penetration of lower frequency signals, and the better resolution (but lesser penetration) of the higher frequency signals. Finally, some machines also offer lateral gain control settings as well. These adjust amplification along individual beam lines (laterally), but do not adjust for depth.
- **Dynamic range and compression**. Most machines have a control that varies the range of gray scale that can be displayed. In essence, it affects the contrast and contrast resolution on the monitor—low dynamic range produces higher contrast, and vice-versa. On some scanners, reducing dynamic range also eliminates low-level echo signals, thereby producing the effect of reducing overall gain. This control is also called compression, log compression, or dynamic range.
- **Transmit focus (focal zone)**. This is a feature of phased array systems, and enables operator adjustment of the focal zone to various depths, based upon the timing of pulses from the individual elements. This feature helps to optimize lateral resolution.
- **Image invert**. Images can be presented with the apex of the sector at the top (the default setting for most systems) or inverted "up-down" so that the image is rotated 180° along its horizontal axis, and the apex of the sector is

located at the bottom of the screen. As will be discussed in Chap. 4, almost all TEE views in this book are presented with the apex of the sector at the top of the screen, with the exception of the deep transgastric views, which are inverted to display structures in their anatomic relationship. Of note, images can also be inverted "left-right" 180° along their vertical axis, though this is rarely (if ever) necessary, and can be very confusing.

- **Doppler invert**. Both color flow and spectral Doppler scales can be inverted so that the direction of flow can be reversed 180°. For color flow Doppler, this means that blue is flow towards the transducer, and red away from the transducer. For spectral Doppler, this means flow above the line is away from the transducer, and below the line is flow towards the transducer. It is rarely necessary to perform Doppler invert, and in fact it can be potentially confusing. Image and Doppler invert are performed independent of each other.
- **Image freeze/cine loop**. The image freeze/cine loop allows the user to "freeze" a short cine loop, which can then be scrolled backwards and forwards, frame by frame, enabling acquisition and storage of selected single images. Cine loop also enables measurements to be performed on appropriate images (these can also be stored). It should be noted that, while in freeze, the TEE transducer does not emit any ultrasound, therefore this mode should be selected when it is desirable to avoid heating adjacent tissues (for example, if the TEE probe is kept in a patient's esophagus between pre and postoperative studies).
- **Digital loop preferences**. Preferences for digital loop acquisition are generally available as a secondary menu, sometimes selected with one of the soft keys. Clip duration can be selected as a prescribed number of beats (if an ECG is present), or alternatively as a defined time period (number of seconds). In addition, some systems provide the choice of capturing clips prospectively or retrospectively.
- **Sector depth**. The depth of scanning can be reduced, which has the effect of improving frame rates, and also increasing the size of the structures visualized.
- **Sector size and line density**. These are controls available for imaging and color flow Doppler. Decreasing sector size, depth and line density can increase frame rates. However decreased sector size will reduce the field of view; decreased line density will reduce lateral resolution.
- **Zoom**. This is a function that allows a selected area of imaging sector to be magnified and expanded. There are two types of zoom: read and write. Read zoom takes the image data already existing in the scan converter and magnifies the existing pixels so that the selected zoom area fills the whole screen. This can be done on a frozen image. However, the existing data can appear coarse and pixelated. In contrast write zoom allows the operator to select the zoom area first, then transducer rescans only that area and writes only the data from the zoom area to the scan converter. Theoretically, this method can result in better image detail than the read zoom function because all scan converter pixels are assigned to the zoom area. However in practice, imaging improvements will ultimately still be limited by beam width and spatial pulse length (i.e. lateral and axial resolution).
- **Sweep speed**. The speed of certain displays such as M-mode and spectral Doppler can be varied; the usual settings are between 25 and 100 mm/s. Slower speeds allow display of more information and variation of information over time (for example, to visualize Doppler velocity variation with respiration, or spectral Doppler signals during bradycardic heart rates). Faster speeds allow more precise quantitative measurements, such as measurement of a Doppler waveform TVI.
- **Reject**. This is a form of electronic noise reduction in which low-level echoes and "noise" are eliminated from the display. It applies both to image as well as Doppler displays.

There are of course many other controls available, some of which focus primarily upon one mode of imaging. Again, the soft keys seen will change depending upon mode selected, and there will be variation in both terminology and layout depending upon the manufacturer. It is important that the operator become very familiar with the operational aspects of whichever machine is being used.

Artifacts

The nature of ultrasonic imaging is such that artifacts will inevitably be encountered. Artifacts are structures and features on an image that are either spurious, or whose displayed position does not correspond to the actual position of the object being scanned [27]. Ultrasound artifacts are can be produced by the changes in sound wave direction that occur while traveling through the body (i.e. reflection, refraction) as well as the use of reflector transmit/receive time as the proxy for reflector distance. A number of different artifacts are possible, many more than can be discussed in this section. For a complete discussion the reader is referred to several references [1–3]. Nonetheless it is important for the echocardiographer to be aware of some of the more common artifacts that might be seen. A few will be discussed below.

Mirror Image Artifacts

Mirror image artifacts arise from regions where an object is located next to a very strong reflector such as diaphragm.

When a transmit pulse encounters the object, it is reflected back to the transducer, producing the first image. However some sound is transmitted through the object and then continues to the interface beyond the object. The sound that returns from that interface undergoes partial reflection at the object, and this secondary echo returns back to the interface, where it is reflected again, giving rise to a secondary object that appears to be beyond the interface and appears as a mirror image. This is shown in Fig. 1.41. Mirror image artifacts can also occur with color flow Doppler. One such example is with the descending aortic long axis view, in which a color flow signal can be seen posterior to the aorta.

Mirroring can also be seen with the Doppler spectral display. This is different from the mirror image artifacts described above. A complete mirroring of the spectral tracing is seen on the opposite side of the baseline. This can be produced by a 90° angle between Doppler beam and direction of blood flow, or sometimes with too high a Doppler gain setting (Fig. 1.42).

Reverberation Artifacts

Reverberation artifacts occur when there is a fairly large impedance mismatch between interfaces (soft tissue-gas, fat-muscle, etc.). If the interface is oriented perpendicular to the direction of propagation, the reflected sound creates a strong echo. Some of this reflected sound is received by the transducer (creating an initial image), but some is also reflected from the transducer face back toward the interface, which then reflects back toward the transducer. This process can continue several times—in essence, sound "bounces" between the two surfaces. Each time, some of the returning sound is received and registered at an increased depth due to the perceived additional transmit-receive time (Fig. 1.43). Reverberation signals can be detrimental in that they can partially obscure actual echo signals on the display, and also produce additional "acoustic noise".

Another type of reverberation artifact is when multiple internal reflections occur within a small but highly reflective object, often a metallic object such as a needle, clip, or staple. This creates a series of echoes "ringing" within the object; some of the sound returns to the transducer, resulting in a number of small bands, known as **comet tails**. These produce a distinctive image on the display. Comet tails can also be seen distal to a strong reflector (Fig. 1.41).

Side Lobes and Grating Lobes

There are two important artifacts associated with transducer beams. The first is *side lobe* artifacts, which are secondary low intensity projections of ultrasound energy adjacent to the mean beam. They result from radial vibrations of the PZE elements, as opposed to the longitudinal vibrations used to generate the main beam. Side lobes can create imaging artifacts and noise in the image that can degrade lateral resolution. These artifacts tend to be of low intensity, but if a side lobe encounters a highly reflective surface outside the main beam, the object will appear to be incorrectly positioned as an image along the path of the main beam (Fig. 1.44). These artifacts can be recognized by their

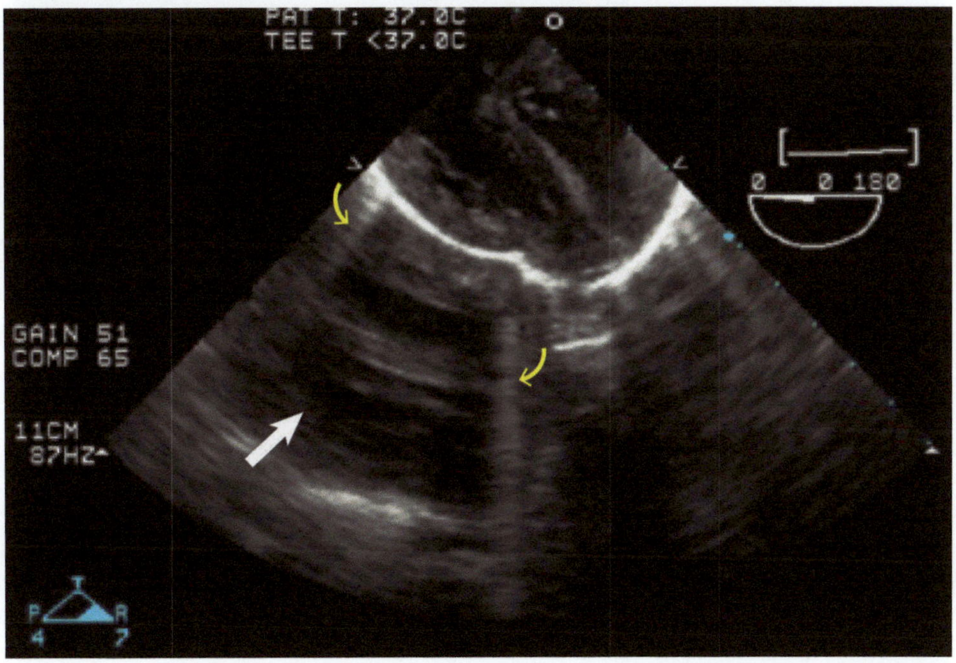

Fig. 1.41 Example of a mirror image artifact (*white arrow*) from a transesophageal echocardiogram in a mid esophageal four chamber view. The mirror image is seen on the opposite side of a large specular reflector, in this case, pericardium. Comet tail artifacts (*yellow arrows*) are also seen

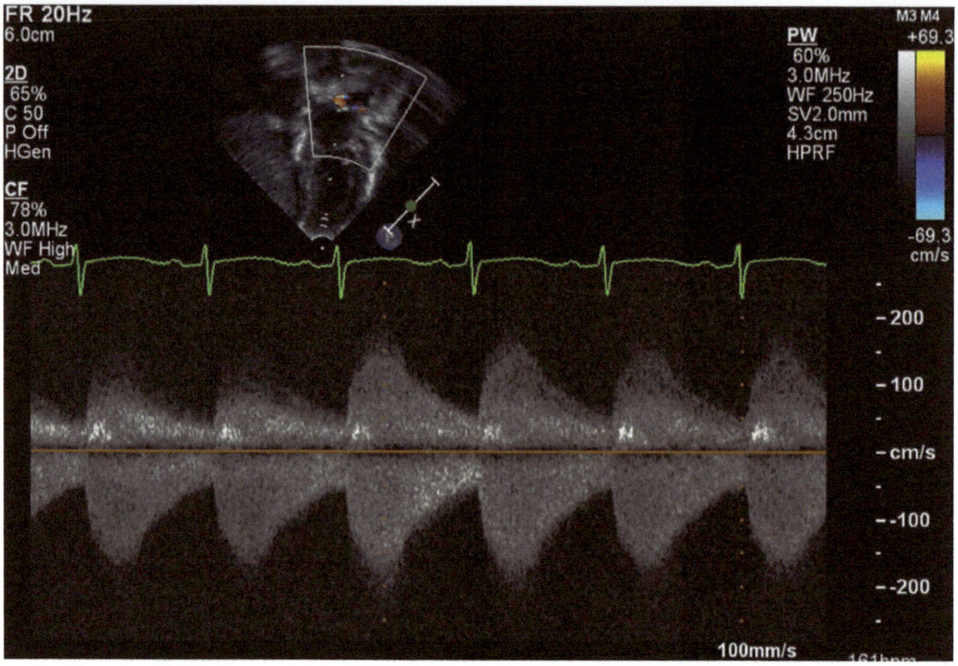

Fig. 1.42 Example of a spectral Doppler mirror image artifact in a patient with a patent ductus arteriosus. In this case the transducer was nearly perpendicular to the direction of blood flow, producing the artifact. Spectral broadening is also seen

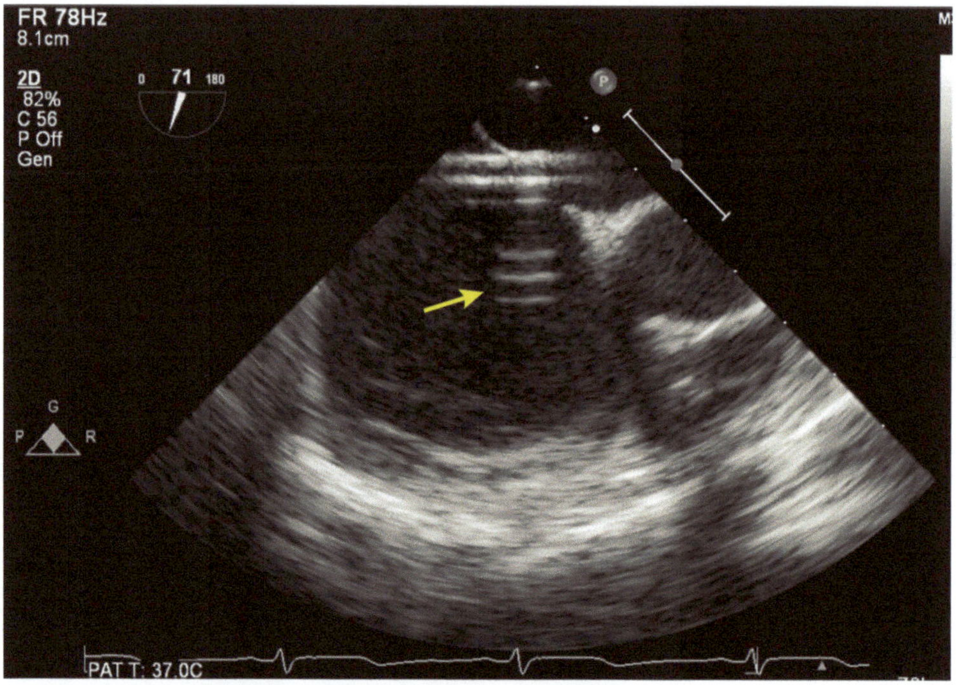

Fig. 1.43 Example of a reverberation artifact in a patient undergoing transcatheter closure of an atrial septal defect. The catheter sheath in the left atrium presents a large impedance mismatch; at the points perpendicular to the ultrasound path, reverberations are seen (*arrow*)

appearance of crossing anatomic borders such as cardiac walls (Fig. 1.45). They have an inconstant appearance; with adjustment of sector depth or transducer angle, they can disappear. The other type of artifact is *grating lobes*, which are a by-product of array transducers. These are multiple low intensity accessory beams that appear near the transducer face, but at large angles from the main beam. Ghost images can occur. These grating lobes can also degrade lateral resolution. Grating lobes can be eliminated by using very thin, closely spaced elements.

Acoustic Shadowing

When an interface is encountered with significant acoustic impedance mismatching, virtually all incident sound is reflected and none is transmitted. Thus, no imaging information is available past the interface. This leads to shadowing beyond the interface, characterized by a dark, anechoic area (Fig. 1.46). Acoustic shadowing is typically seen at the interface between blood/soft tissue and very dense objects such as metal or calcium; however it can also

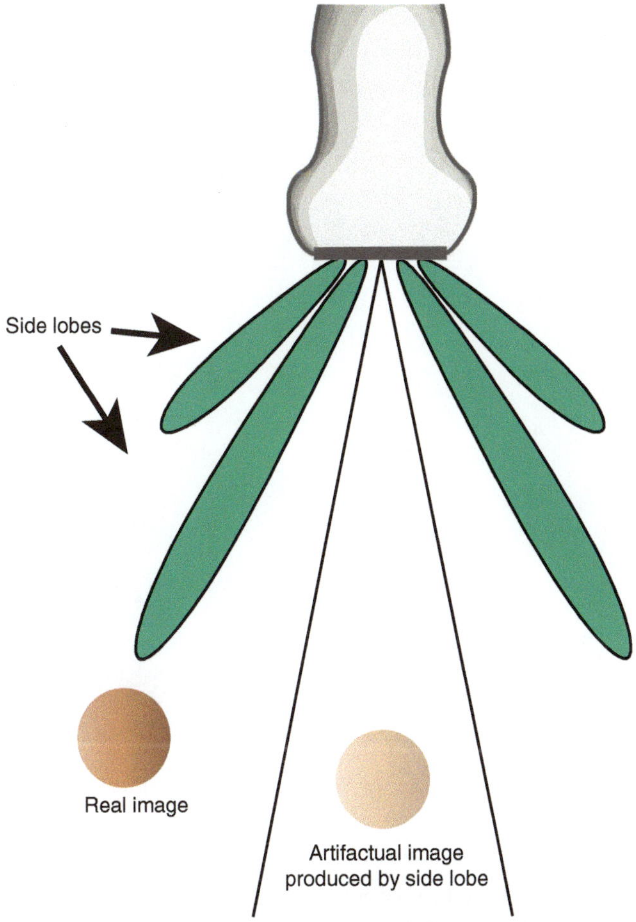

Fig. 1.44 Diagram of side lobes and the artifact that is can be produced. In this case an object encountered by one of the side lobes appears to be incorrectly positioned in the path of the main beam

be seen at soft tissue/lung interface. Whenever shadowing is encountered, other transducer positions should be attempted (if available) to circumvent the interface and visualize the area beyond it.

Digital Image Storage and DICOM

For a number of reasons, proper, secure recording and storage of echocardiographic information is imperative. First, all of the images, Doppler tracings, measurements and calculations obtained by echocardiography represent patient-related information, and need to be stored permanently as part of the medical record. Second, it is vital for the different medical/surgical subspecialists to have access to the actual echocardiographic images and data, not just the reports, when making decisions about medical/surgical therapy. Third, access to the actual data from past echocardiographic studies is useful in many ways: for comparing new information to older studies, for quality control, for research and education, and for medical-legal reasons.

Virtually all current echocardiographic machines and systems now store their information digitally in accordance with DICOM, the universal open standard created to ensure imaging intercompatibility among all medical imaging vendors and imaging modalities, including ultrasound, computerized tomography, magnetic resonance imaging, angiography, and radiography. It was expressly created to avoid proprietary, closed technology developed by different vendors. DICOM, which stands for **D**igital **I**maging and **CO**mmunications in **M**edicine, is not merely a file format, but rather an extensive

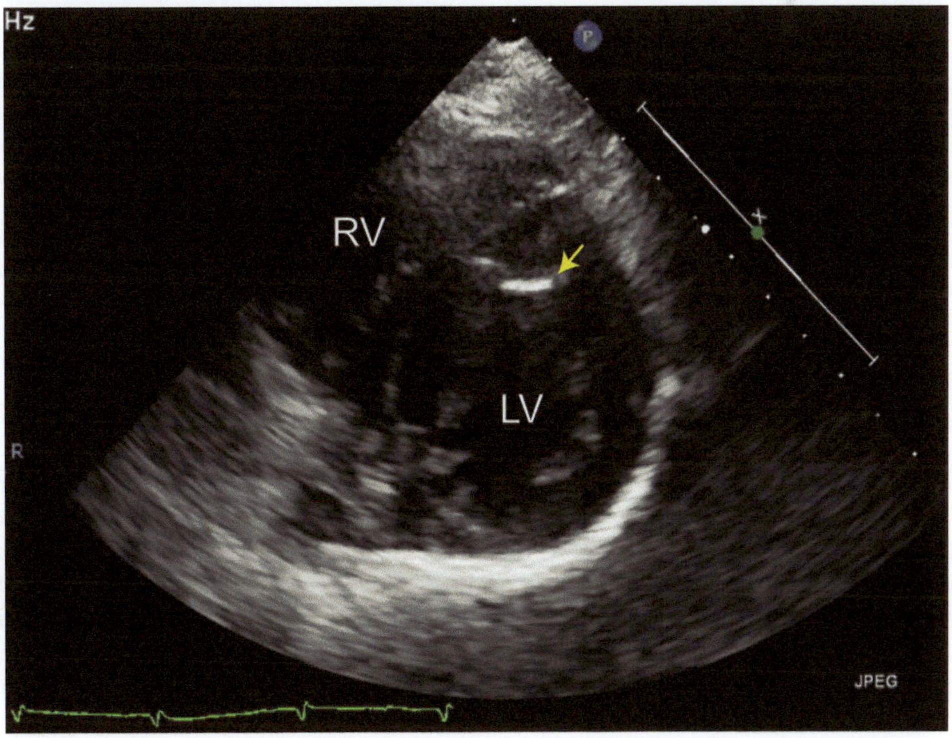

Fig. 1.45 Example of side lobe artifact, as shown with a transthoracic echocardiogram obtained from a standard parasternal short axis window, which was used to image the left ventricle (LV) and right ventricle (RV). The patient was known to have a central venous line in the right atrium. However on this image, the artifactual catheter tip (*arrow*) appeared to be located between ventricular septum and left ventricular cavity. This is due to side lobe energy giving the appearance of the catheter tip within the main beam

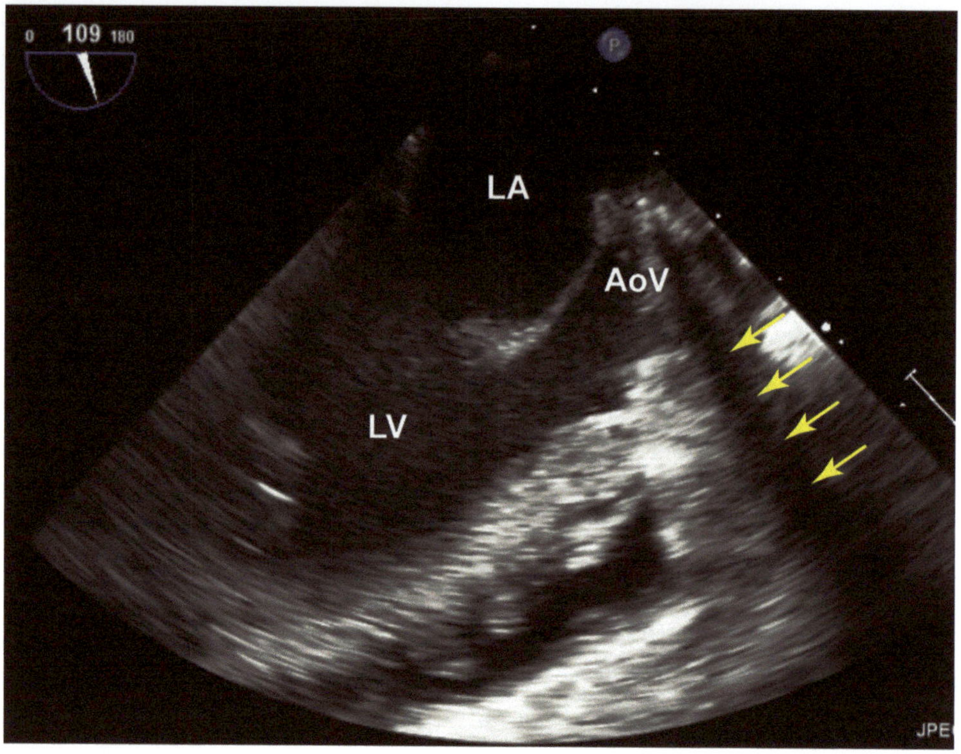

Fig. 1.46 Acoustic shadowing in a patient with a mechanical prosthetic aortic valve (AoV), as viewed from the transesophageal mid esophageal long axis view. The metal prosthetic ring causes significant acoustic impedance mismatching, such that no sound is transmitted beyond that point and a *dark*, anechoic wedge of shadowing is produced (*yellow arrows*). Reverberation is also present. *LA* left atrium, *LV* left ventricle

set of rules and protocols written in a number of separate sections, and crafted to specify the terminology, rules, equipment, file formats, image compression standards, hardware, and structured reporting that facilitate exchange of medical images [28–30]. The individual sections in the DICOM standard include networking standards based on Transmission Control Protocol/Internet Protocol (TCP/IP) to allow communication and transfer of information within an imaging network, also known as a PACS (**P**icture **A**rchiving and **C**ommunication **S**ystems) network. Other sections define a syntax and commands that can be used for the exchange of information. The use of these standards allows the integration of number of different devices (printers, scanners, workstations, servers, and storage devices) and imaging modalities on the same PACS network. Moreover, the stored images can be read on any computer or other device equipped with DICOM reading software. A DICOM file not only contains images, but a wealth of other information including patient information, study information, calibration information for the images (allowing offline measurements and adjustments to be made), etc. To assure intercompatibility, each vendor must publish a DICOM conformance statement. The DICOM standard is regularly reviewed and updated by the National Electrical Manufacturers Association (NEMA); new supplements and sections (parts) are routinely being added to keep the standard current with technology advances in the industry. As of this writing, the DICOM standard consists of 18 parts (Table 1.4), with more parts undoubtedly to follow in the future. Further information regarding DICOM can be obtained from the DICOM/NEMA website, http://medical.nema.org.

Table 1.4 DICOM standard (2011)

PS 3.1	Introduction and overview
PS 3.2	Conformance
PS 3.3	Information object definitions
PS 3.4	Service class specifications
PS 3.5	Data structures and encoding
PS 3.6	Data dictionary
PS 3.7	Message exchange
PS 3.8	Network communication support for message exchange
PS 3.10	Media storage and file format for data interchange
PS 3.11	Media storage application profiles
PS 3.12	Media formats and physical media for data interchange
PS 3.14	Grayscale standard display function
PS 3.15	Security profiles
PS 3.16	Content mapping resource
PS 3.17	Explanatory Information
PS 3.18	Web access to DICOM persistent objects (WADO)
PS 3.19	Application hosting
PS 3.20	Transformation of DICOM to and from HL7 standards

Source: DICOM/NEMA website—http://medical.nema.org

When recording an echocardiographic study, it is important for the operator to be aware of the need to record images carefully and adequately. In the videotape (analog) era, this was a simpler process—the recording could be started with the press of a button, and large portions of the study could be taped continuously without heed to storage space requirements. The paradigm changed with digital recording. Digital studies are superior in so many ways—improved image quality, nonlinear viewing capabilities, instantaneous accessibility from multiple networked sites, as well as the tremendous amount of additional information (aside from the images) contained in a recorded study. However the modern digital DICOM study is not recorded continuously with the simple press of a button, but rather as a series of individual clips/loops that can be as short as one beat in length. A typical transthoracic study for CHD can vary widely between 30 and 150 separate clips/loops, depending upon study complexity. It is an active process: the operator must regularly press the "capture" button (or its equivalent) in order to record a clip, and at times the clip length must be adjusted several times during a study. However recording must be performed assiduously, otherwise it is easy to produce a digital recording that contains only a small number of images and therefore an inadequate record of the entire study. This can be true especially with TEE, in which a rapid study is sometimes necessary due to the limited time available, particularly in the intraoperative setting. When ongoing monitoring is performed, the operator must be selective about the information acquired so as not to accumulate repetitive images. With CHD, sweeps are often necessary to develop a 3D appreciation of the anatomy, and a longer capture (3–5 s or more) might be necessary to record the desired information [29]. With modern echocardiography machines, the captured loop/sweep can be reviewed immediately to determine whether the information is adequate recorded, or whether more clips/loops are necessary. With TEE, it is even more important to record enough sweeps and clips, as there might not be another opportunity to repeat the study.

When a report is generated for the TEE study, it should be constructed with an eye toward readability and completeness. The report should provide an accurate, complete description and interpretation of the information contained within the images. Ideally, the report should contain essential elements including important patient demographic information, indications for the study, a description of study findings, any quantitative measurements, and a summary of pertinent positive and negative findings [31, 32].

Summary

This chapter provides a concise summary of the many important aspects regarding the science of ultrasound and echocardiography, as well as the use and control of the echocardiographic machine. Knowledge of the different technical aspects is important for all who perform echocardiography and TEE. By understanding the important concepts presented in this chapter, echocardiographers will have a solid foundation of knowledge, which will give them the necessary tools to optimize their echocardiographic imaging and Doppler evaluation of CHD. They will also have an appreciation of the many strengths, as well as the limitations and potential pitfalls, associated with echocardiography.

References

1. Zagzebski JA. Essentials of ultrasound physics. St. Louis: Mosby; 1996.
2. Hendee WR, Ritenour ER. Medical imaging physics. 4th ed. New York: Wiley; 2002.
3. Hedrick WR, Hykes DL, Starchman DE. Ultrasound physics and instrumentation. 4th ed. St. Louis: Mosby; 2004.
4. Gibbs V, Cole D, Sassano A. Ultrasound physics and technology: how, why and when. Edinburgh/New York: Churchill Livingstone/Elsevier; 2009.
5. Feigenbaum H. History of echocardiography. In: Feigenbaum's echocardiography. 7th ed. Philadelphia: Wolters Kluwer Health/Lippincott Williams & Wilkins; 2010. p. 1–8.
6. Denny MW. Air and water: the biology and physics of life's media. Princeton: Princeton University Press; 1993.
7. Hendee WR, Ritenour ER. Ultrasound waves. In: Medical imaging physics. 4th ed. New York: Wiley; 2002. p. 303–16.
8. Shankar H, Pagel PS. Potential adverse ultrasound-related biological effects: a critical review. Anesthesiology. 2011;115:1109–24.
9. Gauvin A, Cloutier G, Germain M. Principles of ultrasound. In: Denault AY, Couture P, Vegas A, Buithieu J, Tardif J-C, editors. Transesophageal echocardiography multimedia manual: a perioperative transdisciplinary approach. 2nd ed. New York/London: Informa Healthcare; 2011. p. 1–18.
10. Hendee WR, Ritenour ER. Ultrasound transducers. In: Medical imaging physics. 4th ed. New York: Wiley; 2002. p. 317–29.
11. Prager RW, Ijaz UZ, Gee AH, Treece GM, Wells PNT. Three-dimensional ultrasound imaging. Proc Inst Mech Eng H J Eng Med. 2010;224:193–223.
12. Rabben SI. Technical principles of transthoracic three-dinensional echocardiography. In: Badano LP, Lang RM, Zamorano JL, editors. Textbook of real-time three dimensional echocardiography. London: Springer; 2011. p. 9–24.
13. Salgo IS. 3D transesophageal echocardiographic technologies. In: Badano LP, Lang RM, Zamorano JL, editors. Textbook of real-time three dimensional echocardiography. London: Springer; 2011. p. 25–32.
14. Maslow A, Perrino AC. Principles and technology of two-dimensional echocardiography. In: Reeves ST, editor. A practical approach to transesophageal echocardiography. 2nd ed. Philadelphia/London: Lippincott Williams & Wilkins; 2008. p. 3–23.
15. Erb J. Basic principles of physics in echocardiographic imaging and Doppler techniques. In: Feneck RO, Kneeshaw J, Ranucci M, editors. Core topics in transesophageal echocardiography. Cambridge/New York: Cambridge University Press; 2010. p. 13–33.
16. Hedrick WR, Hykes DL, Starchman DE. Real-time ultrasound instrumentation. In: Ultrasound physics and instrumentation. 4th ed. Philadelphia: Elsevier Mosby; 2005. p. 129–54.
17. Bulwer BE, Shernan SK, Thomas JD. Physics of echocardiography. In: Savage RM, Aronson S, editors. Comprehensive textbook of perioperative transesophageal echocardiography. 2nd ed. Philadelphia: Lippincott Williams & Wilkins; 2010. p. 3–41.
18. Evans DH, McDicken WN. Doppler ultrasound: physics, instrumentation, and signal processing. 2nd ed. Chichester/New York: Wiley; 2000.
19. Lopez L, Colan SD, Frommelt PC, et al. Recommendations for quantification methods during the performance of a pediatric echocardiogram: a report from the Pediatric Measurements Writing

Group of the American Society of Echocardiography Pediatric and Congenital Heart Disease Council. J Am Soc Echocardiogr. 2010;23:465–95.
20. Gaspar T, Adawi S, Sachner R, et al. Three-dimensional imaging of the left ventricular outflow tract: impact on aortic valve area estimation by the continuity equation. J Am Soc Echocardiogr. 2012;25(7):749–57.
21. Saitoh T, Shiota M, Izumo M, et al. Comparison of left ventricular outflow geometry and aortic valve area in patients with aortic stenosis by 2-dimensional versus 3-dimensional echocardiography. Am J Cardiol. 2012;109:1626–31.
22. Otto CM, Bonow RO. Valvular heart disease: a companion to braunwald's heart disease. 3rd ed. Philadelphia: Saunders Elsevier; 2009.
23. Armstrong WF, Ryan T. Hemodynamics. In: Armstrong WF, Ryan T, Feigenbaum H, editors. Feigenbaum's Echocardiography. 7th ed. Philadelphia: Wolters Kluwer Health/Lippincott Williams & Wilkins; 2010. p. 217–40.
24. Armstrong WF, Ryan T. Evaluation of systolic function of the left ventricle. In: Armstrong WF, Ryan T, Feigenbaum H, editors. Feigenbaum's Echocardiography. 7th ed. Philadelphia: Wolters Kluwer Health/Lippincott Williams & Wilkins; 2010. p. 123–57.
25. Chassot P-G, Toussignant C. Basic principles of Doppler ultrasound. In: Denault AY, Couture P, Vegas A, Buithieu J, Tardif J-C, editors. Transesophageal echocardiography multimedia manual: a perioperative transdisciplinary approach. 2nd ed. New York/London: Informa Healthcare; 2011. p. 19–49.
26. Gorcsan J, Tanaka H. Echocardiographic assessment of myocardial strain. J Am Coll Cardiol. 2011;58:1401–13.
27. Zagzebski JA. Image characteristics and artifacts. In: Essentials of ultrasound physics. St. Louis: Mosby; 1996. p. 123–47.
28. Thomas JD. The DICOM image formatting standard: what it means for echocardiographers. J Am Soc Echocardiogr. 1995;8: 319–27.
29. Thomas JD, Adams DB, Devries S, et al. Guidelines and recommendations for digital echocardiography. J Am Soc Echocardiogr. 2005;18:287–97.
30. Pianykh OS. Digital Imaging and Communications in Medicine (DICOM): a practical introduction and survival guide. Berlin: Springer; 2008.
31. Evangelista A, Flachskampf F, Lancellotti P, et al. European Association of Echocardiography recommendations for standardization of performance, digital storage and reporting of echocardiographic studies. Eur J Echocardiogr. 2008;9:438–48.
32. Picard MH, Adams D, Bierig SM, et al. American Society of Echocardiography recommendations for quality echocardiography laboratory operations. J Am Soc Echocardiogr. 2011;24: 1–10.

Instrumentation for Transesophageal Echocardiography

2

Ling Hui and David J. Sahn

Abstract

Though transesophageal echocardiography (TEE) first started with single crystal devices and motor driven sector scanners, ultrasound instrumentation using phased array technology has now been universally adopted for the use of TEE in patients with congenital heart disease, including applications in neonates and infants. This chapter reviews the history, technology, methods, and instrumentation related to TEE utilized during support of surgical and interventional catheterization procedures, particularly in regard to the treatment and diagnosis of congenital heart disease. The instruments to be reviewed include miniaturized fully functional phased array probes and their utlity for cardiac imaging from transesophageal, epicardial, and intracardiac imaging locations. An important theme of this chapter is the role of miniaturization: the smaller and more versatile the probes, the better adapted they will be for use in children, especially neonates born with serious forms of congenital heart disease.

Keywords

Biplane transesophageal echocardiography • Multiplane transesophageal echocardiography • Intracardiac echocardiography • Intravascular ultrasound • Three-dimensional transesophageal echocardiography

In the 1970s, echocardiographers were keenly interested in finding better echocardiographic windows for defining the two-dimensional anatomy of the heart. In many adult patients, emphysema, chronic obstructive pulmonary disease, obesity, and other conditions prevented optimal imaging of cardiac anatomy from the standard transthoracic echocardiographic views. Thus, transesophageal echocardiography (TEE) developed into an alternative method for evaluating the heart.

The origin of TEE dates back to 1976. Frazin et al. described their initial experience with a single-crystal ultrasound transducer attached to a coaxial cable that was passed into the esophagus [1]. They placed an M-mode transducer at the tip of a transesophageal probe and demonstrated how they could obtain an M-mode recording of the heart from the esophagus. Although Frazin and his colleagues [1] were the first Americans to describe TEE, the first major breakthrough came outside the United States in the early 1980s. Initially, the devices for real-time two-dimensional (2D) imaging were mechanical and developed by the Japanese investigators Hisanaga et al. [2] and Matsuzaki et al. [3]. They later became electronic phased array devices. TEE using a steerable single crystal probe was invented by Schluter and Hanrath [4] from Europe; they showed how clinically useful this echocardiographic

L. Hui, MD, PhD
Cardiac Fluid Dynamics and Imaging Laboratory,
School of Medicine, Oregon Health and Science University,
3181 SW Sam Jackson Park Road,
Portland, OR 97239, USA

D.J. Sahn, MD (✉)
Division of Cardiology, Department of Pediatrics,
Oregon Health and Science University,
3181 SW Sam Jackson Park Road, Portland, OR 97239, USA
e-mail: sahnd@ohsu.edu

P.C. Wong, W.C. Miller-Hance (eds.), *Transesophageal Echocardiography for Congenital Heart Disease*,
DOI 10.1007/978-1-84800-064-3_2, © Springer-Verlag London 2014

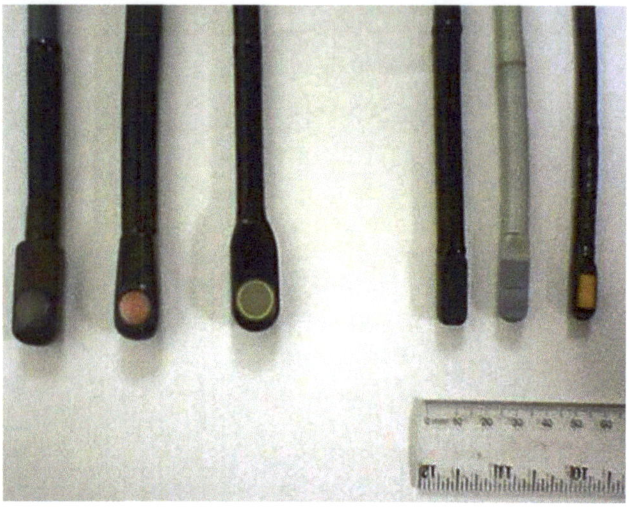

Fig. 2.1 Adult multiplane transesophageal echocardiography transducers (*on the left*) and pediatric biplane transducers. (*on the right*) available 10–15 years ago

approach could be in adult patients, when used with a small probe to scan in the transverse plane. Not long afterward, pediatric cardiologists recognized the utility of this technique. Most of the early clinicians that demonstrated the utility of TEE were Europeans [5–7]. Engineers such as Souquet et al. in 1982 made major contributions to the use of phased array transesophageal electronic sector scan probes [7]. Although several early devices used a rotating mechanical scanner, phased array transducers connected to more flexible endoscopes were also introduced and made even smaller [5–8].

After the initial monoplane (single plane) probes that allowed scanning in one (transverse) image plane, early biplane probes were developed. These devices had two separate ultrasound transducers with a perpendicular orientation of the two image planes. The second (longitudinal) image plane markedly improved scanning, particularly of the more vertically oriented structures that are important in congenital heart disease (CHD), such as the superior vena cava, interatrial septum, ascending aorta, atrial appendages, right ventricular outflow tract, and left ventricular long axis [9–11]. In the 1990s, adult biplane and multiplane transducers with color flow and Doppler capabilities were introduced and refined, and a concurrently selection of pediatric single plane and biplane transducers gradually became available. However during this time period, devices for intraoperative use in children under 15 kg did not yet offer the capability for multiplane imaging. Figure 2.1 features a collection of adult multiplane and pediatric biplane TEE transducers, which were the only devices commercially available approximately 10–15 years ago.

In the last 10 years, multiplane TEE probes have become widely available for both adult and pediatric patients, allowing stepwise study of an area of interest by fine mechanical or electronic rotation of the scanning plane through 180° [12–17]. With advances in technology, multiplane TEE probes have gradually decreased in size from 16 to 14, to 13, 10, and even 7.5 mm. These devices include phased array technology, with the array on a rotating turntable at the tip of the probe engineered to steer the ultrasound-examining plane through a 180° arc. This technology effectively provides a 360° "panoramic" image of the heart, but requires a flexible ribbon connector to the array probe to allow its rotation. All standard echocardiographic modalities discussed, including M-mode, color flow Doppler imaging, spectral Doppler (pulse and continuous wave), and color M-mode, typically can be obtained with a modern multiplane transesophageal scanner.

Probes for TEE

The early TEE probes were actually modified gastroscopes with fiberoptic visualization and suction ports. In contrast, modern transesophageal probes have been specifically manufactured for echocardiographic purposes only. The ultrasound beam is propagated from the transducer and the returning signals are processed in a manner identical to that used for transthoracic echocardiography. However, the transducer face is smaller than the transthoracic probe and there are fewer channels available for transmission.

The modern TEE probes cover multiple frequencies, typically ranging from 3 to 10 MHz. Today, all adult TEE probes as well as the smaller pediatric TEE probes are fully equipped with two-dimensional imaging, M-mode, and complete Doppler capabilities. In view of the unobstructed window for interrogation and the intrinsically high frequencies, the potential benefit of tissue harmonic imaging for TEE is probably less than that for transthoracic imaging. Table 2.1 gives a summary of the most widely available pediatric and adult size TEE probes in North America, including selected probe information, produced by the three largest echocardiography manufacturers.

The pediatric TEE probes provide high frequency, high quality imaging. Their small size and greater probe flexibility make them well suited for use in children and infants; however the same features so advantageous for the pediatric age group can limit their usefulness in adults. Specifically, the smaller probe size and greater flexibility can lead to difficulty maintaining constant wall contact in a larger (adult-size) esophagus, and the higher probe frequencies can reduce the effective depth useful for two-dimensional and color flow

Table 2.1 Currently available transesophageal echocardiography probes (adult and pediatric)

	Tip dimensions (Width × Height × Length, mm)	Shaft dimensions (Width × Length, mm)	Number of elements	Imaging frequencies (MHz)
Philips (Hewlett Packard/Agilent)				
Pediatric biplane (21366A)	9.3 × 8.8 × 27	8 × 80	64	5.5–7.5
Pediatric mini-multiplane (T6207/S7–3t)	10.7 × 7.2 × 25.4	7.4 × 70	48	4.0–7.0
Pediatric micro-multiplane (S8–3t)	7.5 × 5.5 × 18.5	5.2 × 85	32	3.0–8.0
Adult multiplane (Omni III)	14.5 × 11.2 × 42	10.5 × 100	64	4.0–7.0
Adult 3D TEE (X7–2t)	16 × 12 × 40	10 × 106	2,500+ (Matrix)	2.0–7.0
Siemens (Acuson)				
Pediatric biplane (V7B)	9.5 × 8.5 × 31	8.5 × 85	48	5.0–8.0
Pediatric mini-multiplane (V7M)	10.7 × 7.2 × 25.4	7.4 × 70	48	4.0–8.0
Adult multiplane (V5M)	14.5 × 11.5 × 45	10.5 × 110	64	3.5–7.0
General electric (Vingmed)				
Pediatric multiplane (9T, MPTE, 9Tc/9T-RS)	10.9 × 8.4 × 35.2	7 × 70	48	3.0–10.0
Adult multiplane (6T/6TV, 6Tc-RS/6Tc-RS)	14 × 12.5 × 45	10.5 × 110	64	3–8.0
Adult 4D TEE (6VT-D)*	14.3 × 12.7 × 45	10.5 × 110	2,500 (Matrix)	3.0–8.0

Note: Imaging frequency may vary with each individual manufacturer
*Information courtesy of GE Healthcare, used with permission

Doppler imaging. For these reasons, the pediatric TEE probes have limited utility in adult patients, though in some adults they can be used to image structures in the near to mid field [18].

History of TEE Probe Development for Children

The 1982 report of the first phased array TEE probe by Hanrath's group included an example of an ostium secundum atrial septal defect [6]. Nonetheless, in its early stages the application of TEE for evaluation of CHD was limited due to several factors: (a) the large sizes of the early TEE probes precluded their use in patients less than 20 kg, i.e. infants and children in whom the vast majority of cardiac disease was congenital; (b) color flow and spectral Doppler evaluation, integral tools for CHD evaluation, were not yet available; (c) only a single TEE plane could be used, limiting optimal visualization of a number of cardiac structures. It was only after important technological advances in TEE probe and imaging technology in the late 1980s and early 1990s that the use of TEE for evaluation of CHD began to grow. Following the availability of higher resolution imaging and color flow Doppler mapping, Sutherland and colleagues [19] as well as other investigators [20, 21] demonstrated the ability of TEE to evaluate CHD using an adult size TEE probe. However the use of TEE for CHD evaluation remained limited until the development of a smaller TEE probe that could be used in pediatric size patients.

Single-Plane Probes

Single-plane TEE for pediatric patients was developed in the late 1980s. The first transesophageal probe for use in children, developed in 1988 by Omoto and colleagues, consisted of a single-plane, phased array, 24 element, 5 MHz unit mounted on an pediatric gastroscope measuring 6.8 mm in diameter [22]. This TEE probe produced a single, transverse scan plane and could only be used in patients who weighed more than 3.0 kg [23]. However, single plane TEE for pediatric patients was superseded by the rapid technological advances in the 1990s that made possible the development of small biplane and multiplane transesophageal probes appropriate for use in infants and small children with CHD [24–26].

Biplane Probes

In the biplane transesophageal probe for children, there are two sets of transducers, 48 × 48 or 64 × 64 elements mounted perpendicular to each other, one above the other, at the tip of the probe (Fig. 2.2). The centers of the transverse palette and the longitudinal palette are separated by less 1.0 cm

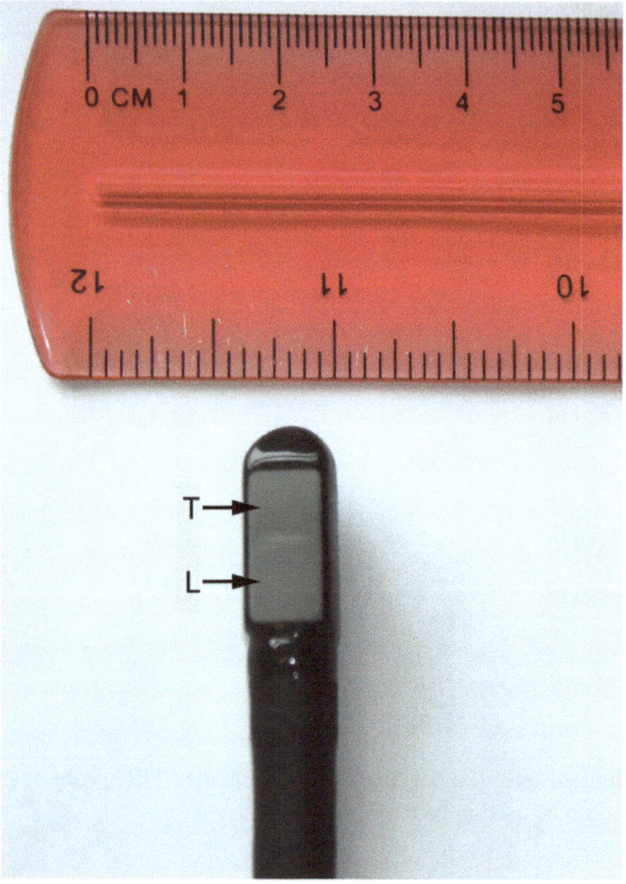

Fig. 2.2 Pediatric biplane probe tip. There are two sets of transducers, each imaging in a separate plane. The transverse plane (*T*) images at 0°, the longitudinal plane (*L*) at 90°, thus the two planes are orthogonal to each other

depending upon the transducer size. Commercially available biplane transesophageal probes are about 7–10 mm in diameter. With biplane transesophageal imaging, one transducer set imaged in a transverse plane (0°), the other set imaged in a longitudinal scan plane (90°) orthogonal to the transverse plane. For these probes, the patients needed to weigh more than 3.0 kg as well, similar to single-plane probes [27–29]. While biplane adult TEE probes are no longer actively used (having been replaced by multiplane TEE probes), pediatric biplane probes are still available and used in some institutions. In some instances, these probes can be used when the slightly larger mini-multiplane probe (discussed below) cannot be inserted into the esophagus.

Multiplane Probes

Multiplane transesophageal transducer technology consists of a single array of crystals that is electronically or mechanically rotated about the long axis of the sound beam in a 180° arc, producing a circular continuum of tomographic, two-dimensional images [30]. Multiplane TEE probes were first introduced in early 1990s [12, 13, 16, 17]. Because of the 64 imaging elements and cabling needed to generate multiplane imaging, the early multiplane TEE probes were large, with diameters anywhere from 14 to 18 mm (Fig. 2.3), which limited their use to pediatric patients who weighed more than 20–30 kg (or even larger). Continued technological improvements, however, soon led to the development of multiplane TEE transducers suitable for small children, infants, and even neonates.

Mini-multiplane

With the evolving approach of pediatric cardiac surgery to perform one-stage repairs in newborns or infants with CHD under the age of 3 months, the need for smaller TEE probes became clear and compelling. In the early 1990s, Dr. Charles Lancée of Erasmus University in Rotterdam and his team produced a prototype of a mini-multiplane TEE probe [31]. It involved 48 elements, 5 MHz and the smallest introduction diameter of 9.5–10 mm. This device subsequently went into original equipment manufacturer distribution, and was used by GE/VingMed, Philips, and Siemens (Fig. 2.4) as their main pediatric TEE product. It remains the mainstay of the pediatric TEE imaging systems for both Philips and Siemens (GE subsequently developed its own pediatric multiplane probe). This mini-multiplane probe produces very high quality images, and it can be used in weight ranges down to about 2.5–3.0 kg, which is adequate for many 90–95 % neonates requiring surgery (although some have used it successfully in neonates down to 2 kg in weight). For diagnosis and post-operative evaluation, the mini-multiplane was a liberating invention for neonates and infants with CHD (Figs. 2.5, 2.6, and 2.7). Its efficacy and durability have been documented in multiple studies, and it remains, up to the time of this writing, the predominant pediatric multiplane TEE probe in use [32, 33].

Micro-multiplane

If one were to design a multiplane TEE probe that could safely be used in a wide range of neonates of different weights, what might be its specifications? The ideal device would be 7.5 MHz, and 8 mm or smaller, to allow safe probe placement even in neonates under 2 kg. It was on this basis that the high frequency array technology was developed, eventually becoming the micro-multiplane TEE probe. The micro-multiplane TEE probe, however, sets a specification of element size at 100-μm spacing and interconnects density in order to wire the array. This requires technology to achieve an adequate yield rate for 85 % or more of array pallets to be incorporated successfully into fully wired TEE probes, and to maintain their integrity for more than 2 years. As such, the specifications of the micro-multiplane TEE probe are a 6 MHz center frequency, 32 elements and 7.5 mm maximum tip diameter (Fig. 2.8). The probe offers full TEE ultrasound capabilities, including 2D imaging, color flow, pulsed and continuous wave Doppler, M-mode and color flow M-mode.

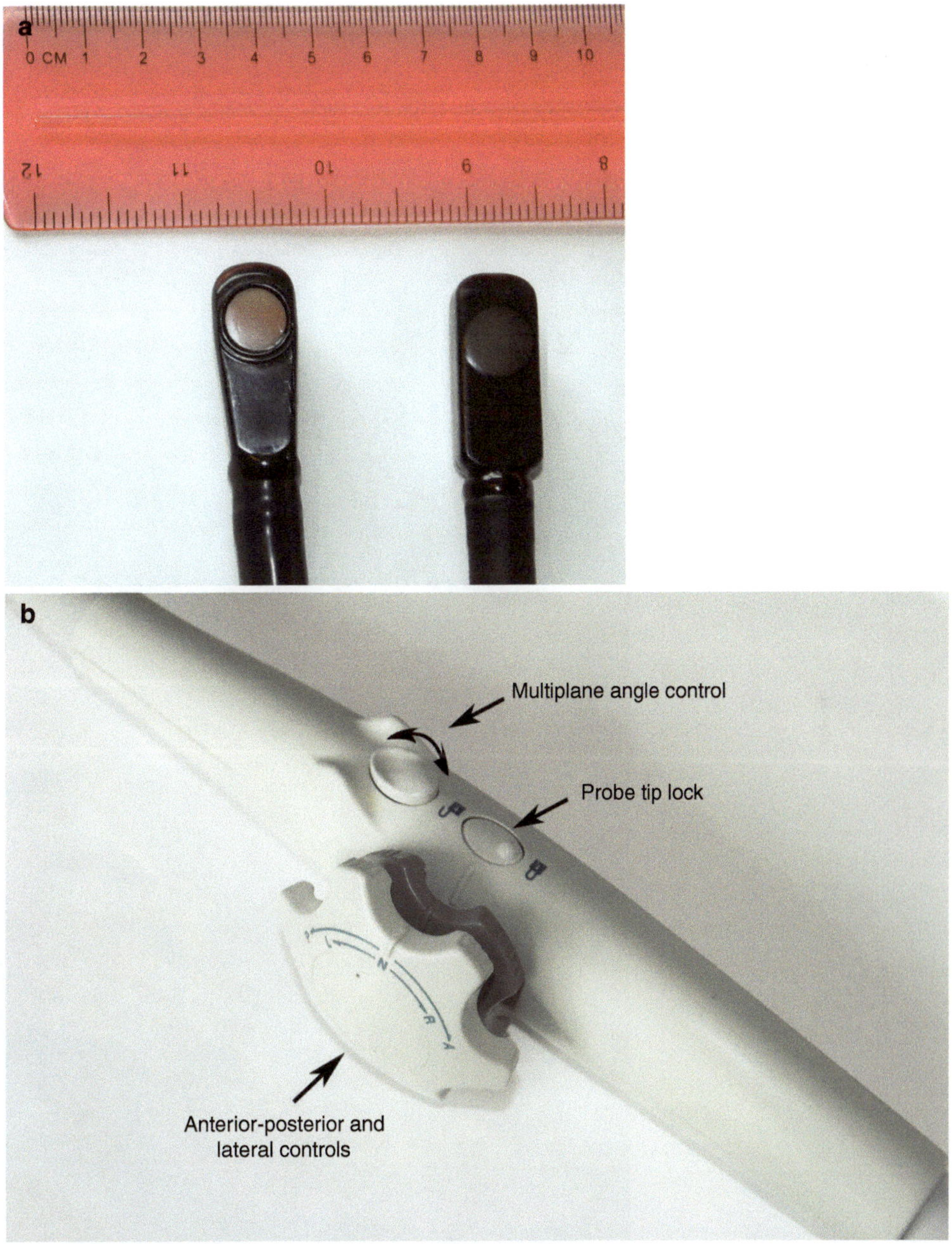

Fig. 2.3 Adult multiplane probes, tip and handle. (**a**) Shows two adult multiplane transesophageal echocardiography transducers. There is a single array of crystals that can be rotated in a 180° arc. Note that the large size of these transducers precludes their use in children under 20–25 kg. (**b**) Shows the probe handle, which includes controls for probe tip movements (anterior-posterior, right-left), multiplane angle rotation, and locking of the probe tip (one of the two probe tip locks on this probe is located on the other side of handle, and therefore not visible on this photograph)

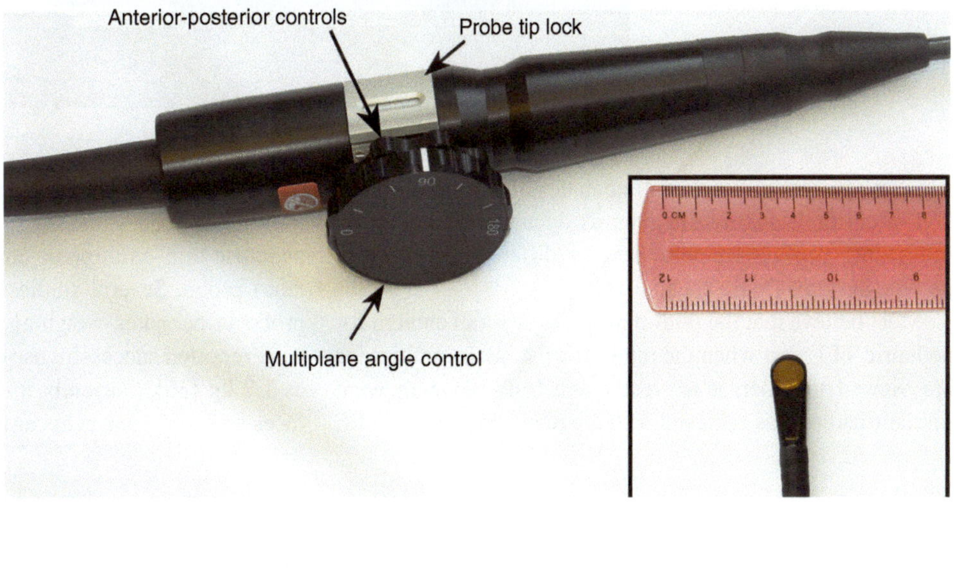

Fig. 2.4 Mini-multiplane transesophageal echocardiography probe and handle. The small probe size (*inset*) allows it to be inserted into neonates and young infants. The single array of crystals is rotated manually (mechanically) using the large outer dial, enabling adjustment of multiplane angle between 0° and 180°. The probe can flex only in an anterior-posterior direction, using the inner dial on the handle; lateral controls are not available on this probe. The probe tip can be locked/unlocked by the silver latch (shown in the diagram)

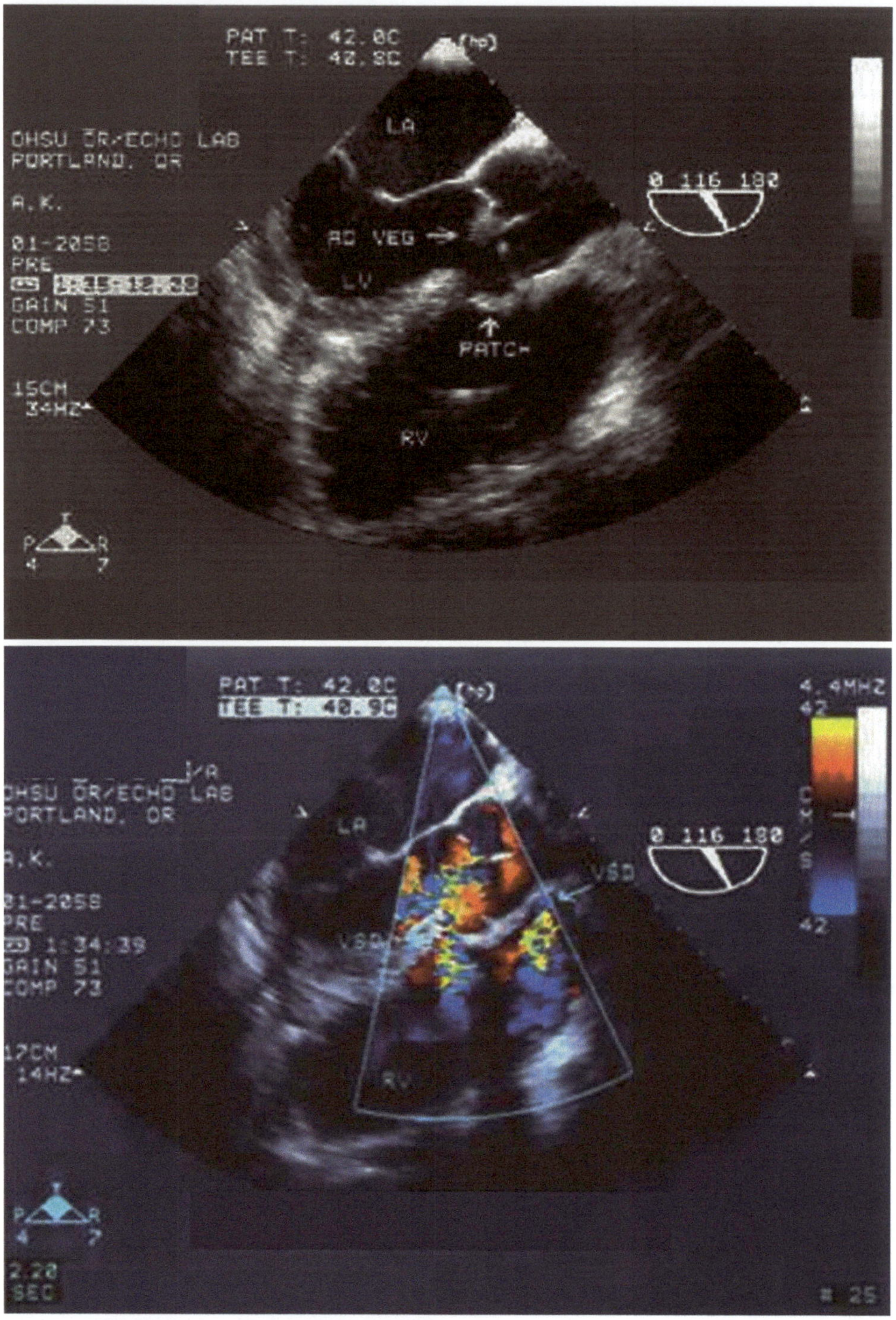

Fig. 2.5 Aortic valve endocarditis with subaortic ventricular septal defect (VSD), as seen from the mid esophageal aortic valve long axis view. This patient had undergone patch closure of the VSD. A vegetation is present on the aortic valve (*top panel*), and color flow Doppler shows a small amount of aortic valve regurgitation (*bottom panel*). In addition, a small residual VSD is seen at the inferior margin of the patch. *Ao veg* vegetation on aortic valve, *LA* left atrium, *LV* left ventricle, *RV* right ventricle

It can be placed in very small neonates and young infants, and offers high quality imaging, as documented in studies interfacing this device with several different echocardiographic systems (Figs. 2.9 and 2.10) [34].

Most believe that the mini-multiplane is small enough for pediatric TEE; but when the mini- and the micro-multiplane are viewed together, it is clearly and truly amazing what miniaturization has achieved with the micro-multiplane TEE probe. Figure 2.8 shows the relative sizes of three available multiplane probes: the micro-multiplane (arrow) next to the pediatric mini-multiplane and the adult multiplane (omniplane) probe. Several studies have validated the use of this probe in neonates weighing 2.5 kg [35–37]; some authors have reported successful use of the probe in patients as small as 1.7 kg [36]. Currently the micro-multiplane probe interfaces with only one echocardiography platform.

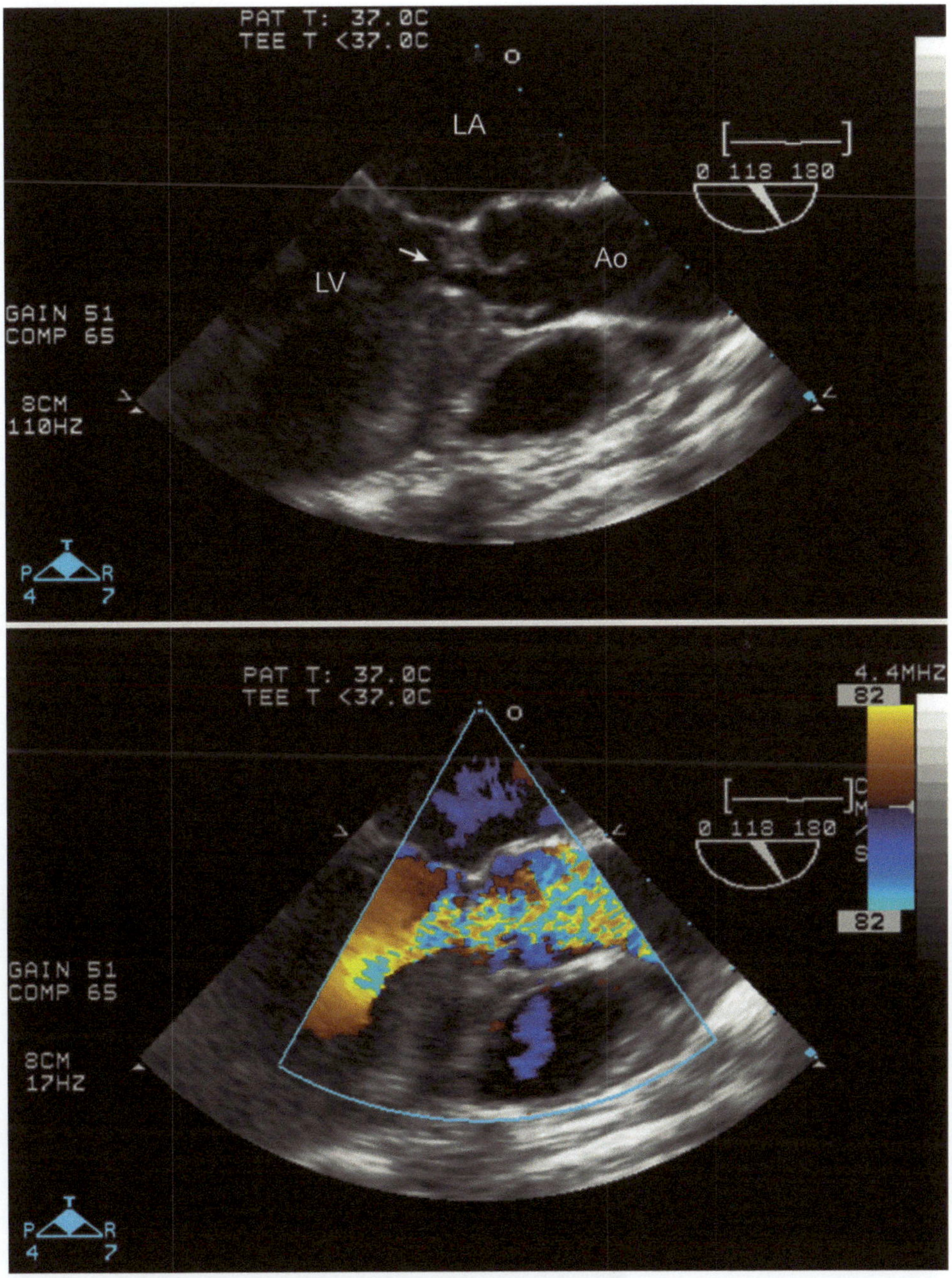

Fig. 2.6 Subaortic stenosis, as viewed with a preoperative transesophageal echocardiogram, using a mid esophageal aortic valve long axis view. Marked fibromuscular subaortic narrowing (*arrow*) is noted just below the aortic valve. There is also considerable ventricular septal hypertrophy (*top panel*). Color flow Doppler shows aliasing that begins at subaortic level (*bottom panel*). *Ao* ascending aorta, *LA* left atrium, *LV* left ventricle

Clinical Experience—TEE for Children with CHD

In the early clinical experience with TEE for pediatric CHD patients, the major challenge was the lack of probes suitable for use in small infants. The first small probes used in children with CHD in the intraoperative setting were made available through Professor Ryozo Omoto [9]. These were single or biplane devices of 7 mm tip width. Maximal introduction diameter for these was kept up to 7 mm, with 24×24 or 32×32 element biplane configurations. Once multiplane imaging became available, it was obvious, from the feedback of our adult cardiology colleagues, that multiplane imaging provided flexibility that would be especially important in the TEE evaluation of CHD [38–40]. Early work with epicardial scanning by surgeons and subsequent TEE imaging during surgery for CHD demonstrated that intraoperative echocardiography positively affected patient outcome [41–44].

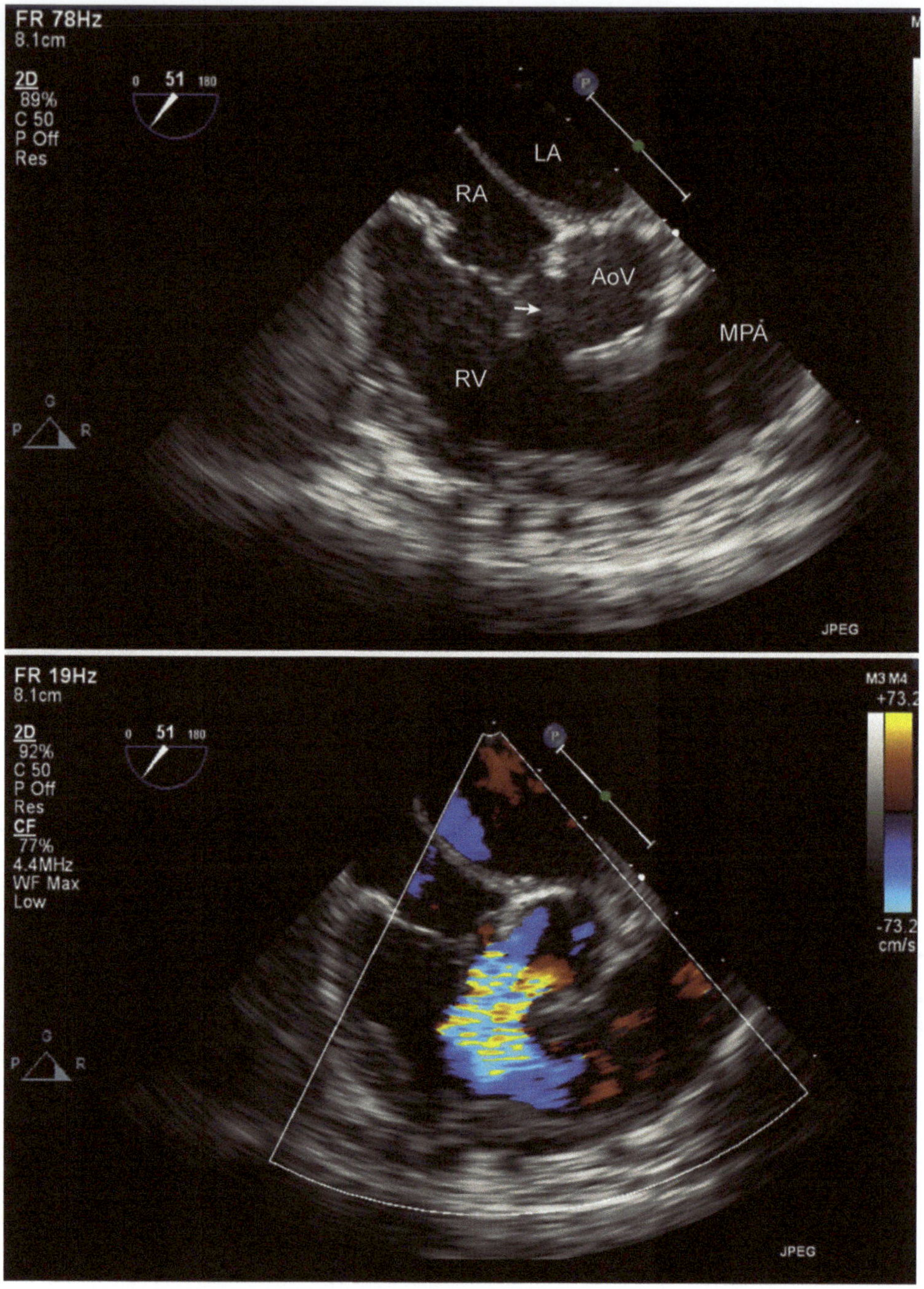

Fig. 2.7 Large perimembranous ventricular septal defect (VSD), as noted from a modified right ventricular inflow-outflow view, multiplane angle 51°. A large ventricular septal defect is seen in the top panel (*arrow*). Left to right shunting is shown across the VSD by color Doppler (bottom panel). *AoV* aortic valve, *LA* left atrium, *MPA* main pulmonary artery, *RA* right atrium, *RV* right ventricle

Over the past 20 years, the utility of TEE in the pediatric patient with congenital and acquired pathology has been well documented [32, 45–51]. Nonetheless despite the fact that TEE provides excellent detail of cardiac anatomy and hemodynamics in pediatric patients, the indications for TEE are more limited in scope, due to its semi-invasive nature [52, 53]. The most common application of TEE in children is for monitoring surgical and interventional procedures in CHD (see Chap. 3).

Multiple studies have documented the benefits of intraoperative TEE for surgical correction or palliation of CHD, noting its ability to alter patient management by visualizing virtually all areas of the heart, thereby allowing a highly accurate diagnosis for the majority of anatomic cardiac problems [54–57]. The benefits of intraoperative TEE include: (1) identification of additional anatomic or other diagnostic information preoperatively that alters the surgical repair or approach; (2) identification of significant residual anatomic abnormalities postoperatively that require additional surgical intervention, often with a return to cardiopulmonary bypass; and (3) identification of postoperative functional abnormalities, which require additional medical support, re-initiation of cardiopulmonary bypass, or use of other devices to support the circulation [58].

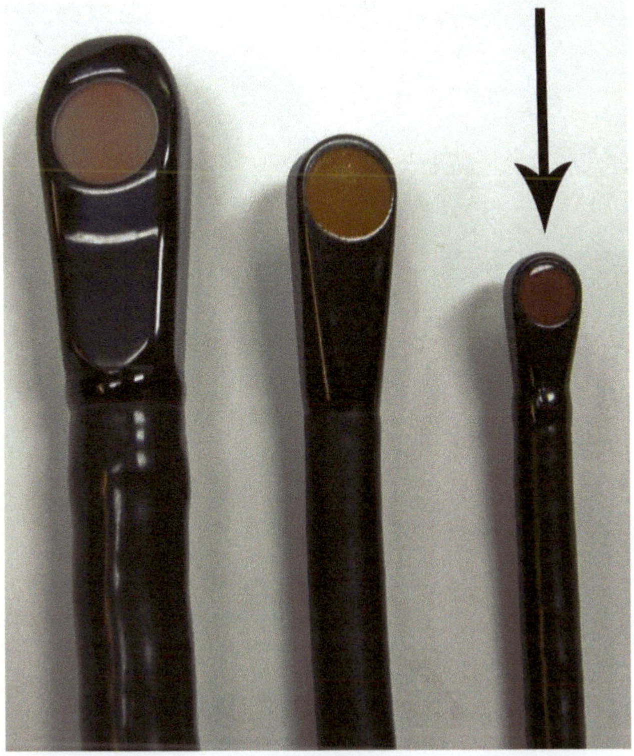

Fig. 2.8 Comparison of three different sized TEE probes. Adult multiplane (omniplane) 14.5 mm probe on the left, compared with a mini-multiplane 9.5 mm probe (center) and micro-multiplane 7.5 mm probe on the right (*arrow*). All three probes interface with the same echocardiographic platform from a single vendor

The combination of high resolution scanning and unobstructed visualization make TEE an ideal technique for identifying fine anatomic detail such as small congenital cardiac defects, valve chordae, vegetations in patients with suspected endocarditis, left atrial appendage thrombus, and evaluation of the thoracic portions of the aorta. As noted above, TEE serves as an important intraoperative tool to review the patient's anatomy just prior to the surgical procedure, and an immediate reassurance to the surgeon of a good repair [59]. In addition to surgical intervention of patients for CHD, TEE has also been beneficial for interventional procedures in the cardiac catheterization laboratory [60], especially for those patients undergoing catheter-delivered atrial septal defect closure devices [51, 61–63], and ventricular septal defect closure either by transcatheter delivery [64–68] or by perventricular approach [69–73].

Three-Dimensional TEE

The early steps toward three-dimensional (3D) TEE are found in works by Steve Smith, Olaf von Ramm, Hanrath and Moser from Freiburg [74]. Initially 3D echocardiography relied upon a reconstructive approach, in which a sequential set of 2D tomographic planes was obtained using defined, discrete, incremental changes in the position of the image plane. The data from these planes was then reassembled into a 3D volume dataset, from which a volume-rendered 3D image could be extracted, as well as other

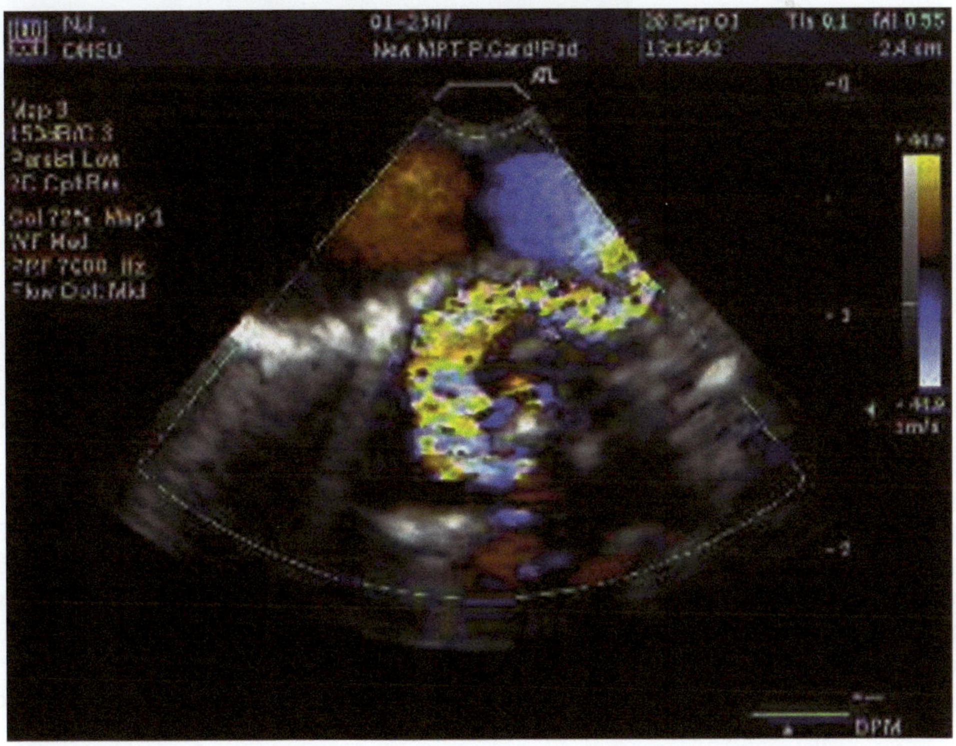

Fig. 2.9 Pulmonary atresia with ventricular septal defect. Intraoperative imaging of bronchial collateral vessels, by color Doppler (top panel), spectral assessment (middle panel), and evaluation of flow across a secundum atrial septal defect (bottom panel) using the micro-multiplane probe

Fig. 2.9 (continued)

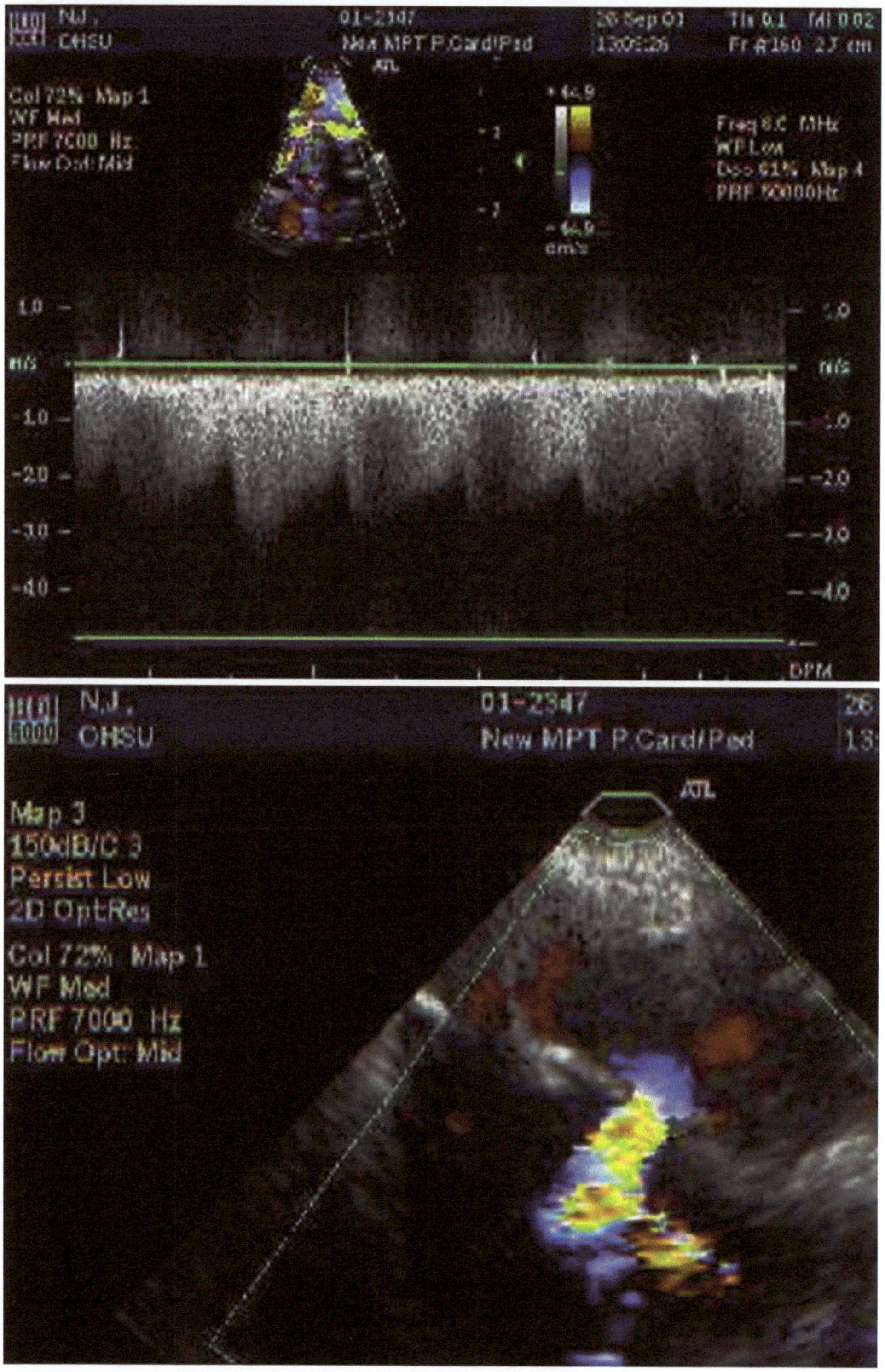

user-defined 2D tomographic planes [75]. The reconstructive method capitalized on the rotational ability of the multiplane TEE transducer and the electronic steering of the rotating array. From the transesophageal approach, the probe position remained fixed, and the planar array was automatically rotated forward by 2–5° increments; at each increment new imaging data were collected. After a full stepwise collection of data through 180°, the images were assembled offline into a 3D, cone-shaped dataset, from which a 3D rendering could be generated of the cardiac structures within the dataset. It was obviously important that the transducer position and orientation within the esophagus remain absolutely stable. Even a slight motion of the transducer, due either to patient or operator motion,

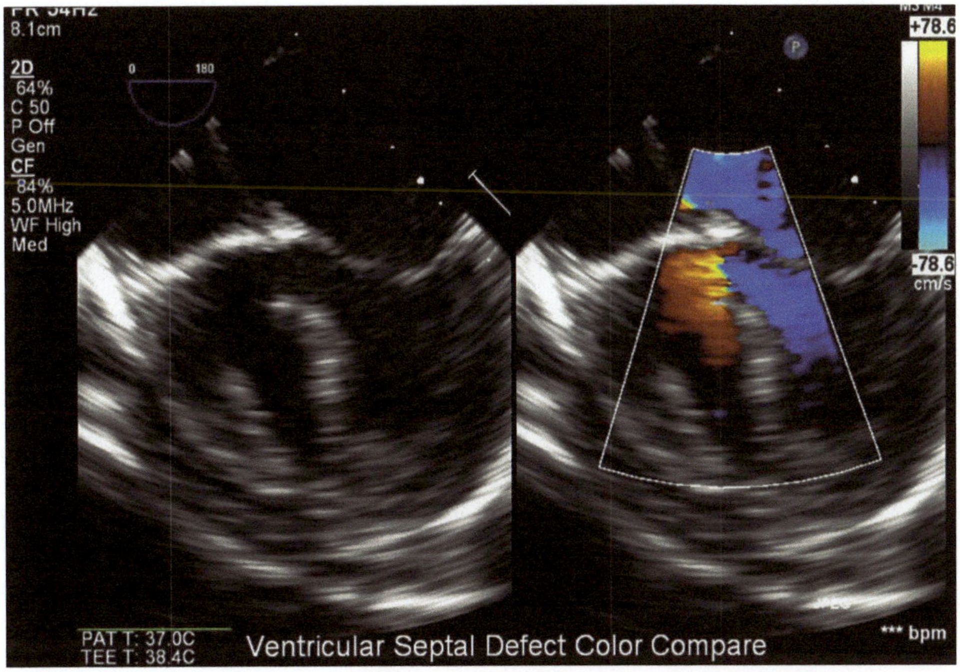

Fig. 2.10 Ventricular septal defect viewed from mid esophageal four chamber view. These images were obtained with the micro-multiplane probe

resulted in marked deterioration of imaging quality. Typically, 3–7 min were required to obtain a complete 3D dataset with this approach. For 3D echocardiography obtained via transthoracic imaging, a similar approach was undertaken by mounting the rotating TEE probe on a hand-held transthoracic device that could be used to acquire a 3D dataset in exactly the same manner as that for 2D TEE.

In the early 2000s, real-time 3D echocardiographic imaging was introduced; initially this technology was available only for transthoracic transducers [76, 77]. However in 2007 a real-time 3D TEE probe (X7–2t, Philips Medical Systems, Andover, Massachusetts) became available for clinical use [78]. This 3D TEE probe provides a real-time, 3D display of cardiac anatomy, along with all of the modalities mentioned above including standard 2D imaging, spectral and color flow Doppler, M-mode, and Doppler tissue imaging (Fig. 2.11). The method of acquisition of 3D echocardiographic data is volumetric imaging. The transducer is constructed with a matrix array of transmitting and receiving crystals in a square grid, containing a total of about 2,500 elements. This allows for collection of a pyramidal image data set. This new generation ultrasound platform provides a true, real-time 3D image. For acquisition of a complete volume of cardiac data, sequential cardiac cycles (from 4 to 7) are typically captured and added together ("stitched") to create a complete volume of information for full volumetric scanning [79, 80]. However, newer software allows acquisition of a full volume while performing live 3D imaging; this is known as "single beat" full volume scanning, and does not require ECG-gating. The development of 3D TEE is increasing: recently, a second adult-sized 3D TEE probe has been introduced as part of another cardiac ultrasound platform (6VT-D as part of Vivid E9 BT-12 system, GE Healthcare, Wauwatosa, Wisconsin) (Fig. 2.12).

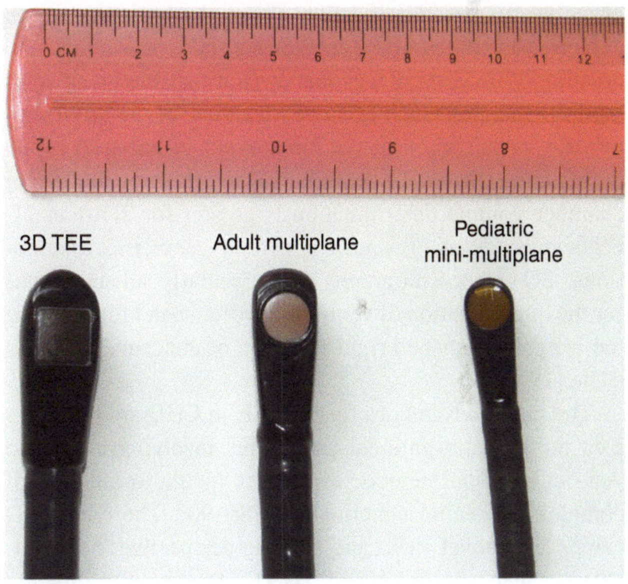

Fig. 2.11 Three-dimensional transesophageal echocardiography (3D TEE) probe on *left*, compared side by side with an adult two-dimensional (2D) multiplane probe (*center*), and pediatric mini-multiplane probe (*right*). Despite the fact that the 3D TEE matrix array has over 2,500 elements, the probe size is not much larger than the standard 2D adult multiplane probe (All probes from Philips Healthcare, Andover, Massachusetts)

Currently, 3D echocardiography is the newest TEE technology available. The new generation real-time 3D TEE probes avoids, the intermediate steps of "image reconstruction" and provide the option for simultaneous acquisition of true real-time biplane 2D imaging (X-plane).

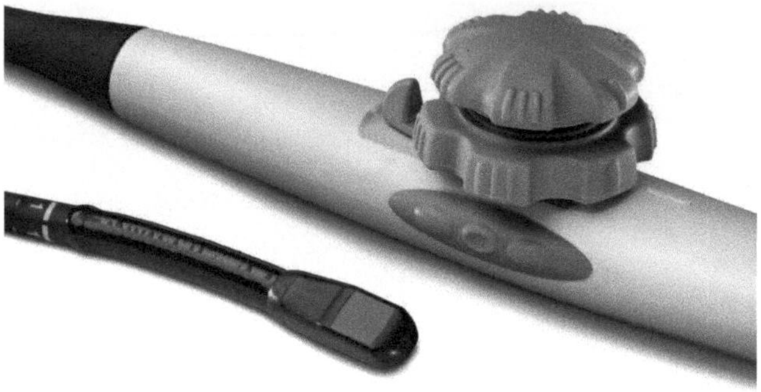

Fig. 2.12 Four-dimensional transesophageal echocardiography recently introduced by GE Healthcare, as part of the Vivid E9 BT-12 cardiac ultrasound system. Like the 3D TEE probe shown in Fig. 2.11, this TEE probe also has a matrix array containing 2,500 elements (Photograph courtesy of GE Healthcare, used with permission)

Although 2D TEE is still the predominant form of imaging used clinically, 3D provides a more complete spatial orientation. The additive value of 3D TEE has been well-documented in the evaluation of atrioventricular and semilunar valve disease in adult patients [81–85]. In addition, it can prove useful for identification of small ventricular septal defects, assessment of the size of an atrial septal defect, and creation of imaging planes that are not feasible using standard 2D imaging–such as an *en face* view of the atrial septum for visualization of the fossa ovalis or an atrial septal defect (See Chaps. 19 and 20). Quantitative accuracy for chamber volume determination is greater for 3D than 2D echocardiography. Because it avoids geometric assumptions, 3D echocardiography is particularly advantageous for the quantification of ventricular volume and function for the irregularly shaped right ventricle or abnormal left ventricle [79].

The major advantages for 3D TEE in CHD are best realized during interventional procedures involving atrial and ventricular septal defects, as well as for the evaluation of complex congenital abnormalities [86–90]. The use of 3D can provide novel views and imaging perspectives not available by the more conventional 2D TEE tomographic imaging planes. The applications for 3D TEE in CHD will be discussed further in Chapters. 19 and 20.

Care and Maintenance of TEE Probes

The TEE probe is a precision medical instrument with a number of components, including multiple moving parts. As with any mechanical device, some degree of wear and tear is inevitable. Thus the TEE probe must undergo routine and regular inspection and periodic testing to ensure probe integrity and continuing high-level functionality. A TEE probe is expensive and represents a considerable financial investment. It should be treated and handled carefully, especially the TEE probe tip because the piezoelectric elements are particularly susceptible to damage from physical trauma. Every TEE probe manufacturer provides detailed instructions regarding TEE probe care and maintenance; these should be reviewed and implemented. Regular preventative maintenance can help to avert or limit major problems. The more frequently a probe is used, the more careful the probe maintenance must be. Regular, rigorous probe care will help to maximize the life and utility of a TEE probe.

TEE Probe Handling During the Study

During the TEE study, a bite guard should be used if the patient is conscious to avoid biting and laceration of the probe housing. Anesthetic sprays and other chemicals should not be applied directly to any part of the TEE probe. The TEE probe should not be dropped or knocked against other objects during handling, transportation, and storage. Although the TEE probe tip and shaft are waterproof, the control housing (handle), cable and connector are not, so care should be taken not to spill fluids on these parts.

Cleaning, Disinfection and Storage

After the TEE probe has been removed from the patient, it must be cleaned and disinfected prior to its next use. Again, the following instructions pertain only to the TEE probe tip and shaft, *not* to the control housing, cable and connector. Once the probe is removed, it should right away be wiped and rinsed in lukewarm running water for about 1 min. Some TEE probe manufacturers recommend cleaning the probe by immersing it in an enzymatic cleaner (Klenzyme, Cidezyme) for a short period of time; the cleaning process, including soak times and dilution rates, should strictly follow the instructions of the enzymatic cleaner's manufacturer. If this step is performed, the probe must then be rinsed once again for about 1 min in lukewarm running water to remove residual cleaner, and then wiped dry. The next step is disinfection. The probe tip and shaft should be immersed in a glutaraldehyde-based (Cidex, Omnicide) or non-glutaraldehyde (Cidex OPA, Perasafe) disinfectant solution for 20–30 min. Again, the chemical manufacturer's instructions should be following regarding dilution rates and soak times, and the probe should not be left for longer than 1 h in the disinfectant, because probe damage could occur. Once the probe is removed from the disinfectant it should be rinsed thoroughly in running water for at least 1 min, then dried completely and stored in a clean, dry place. Many manufacturers recommend storing the probes vertically when not in use. TEE probes should never be sterilized with autoclave, ultraviolet, gamma radiation, gas, steam or heat sterilization techniques. These can result in severe damage to the probe.

TEE Probe Maintenance

Probe maintenance should be performed regularly to optimize and maintain TEE probe functionality, and also to assure patient safety. This testing should be performed in

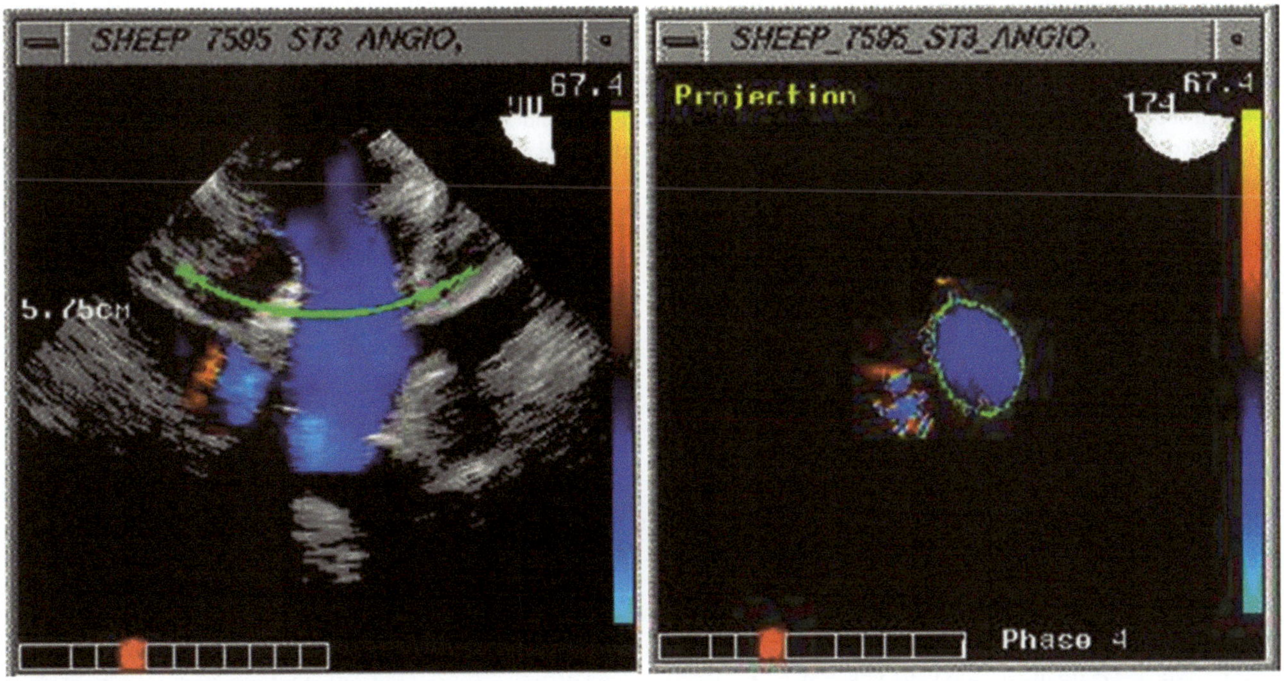

Fig. 2.13 (**a**) Rotational acquisition and (**b**) perpendicular Gaussian surface processing of three-dimensional stroke volume flow. This view is comparable to the TEE deep transgastric long axis view

accordance with the manufacturer's specifications, and includes the following:

- *Electrical leakage testing*. This is a very important procedure that should be performed regularly, using appropriate testing equipment (sometimes supplied by the TEE probe manufacturer). Electrical leakage signifies a break in the integrity of the probe housing/insulation, which could potentially be harmful for the patient, and also could lead to leakage of fluids and subsequent damage to the interior of the TEE probe.
- Regular visual inspection of the probe and shaft housing for breaks, bite marks, etc.
- Inspection and testing of the connector for bent pins, cracks, etc.
- Evaluation of the integrity of the connecting cable
- Regular testing of the probe's articulation mechanism (knobs on control handle)

It is highly recommend that, for each separate TEE probe, a regularly updated probe maintenance and inspection log be maintained.

Other Techniques Applicable to TEE, Intraoperative and Intraprocedural Imaging

Three-Dimensional Flow Quantification Methods

Three-dimensional flow quantification methods involving implementation of a digital 3D laminar flow stroke volume calculation method have been developed by the authors [91]. This is an accurate method for calculation of stroke volume. The 3D flow data is sectioned along an arc perpendicular to the direction of flow, and integrated over a Gaussian surface as pixels with a value of cm/s, over an area in cm^2 to yield cm^3/s as the value of the color disk shown. These discs are then integrated over the heart cycle to yield stroke volume/beat (Fig. 2.13). This method avoids the geometric assumptions behind spectral Doppler determination of cardiac output based upon 2D echocardiographic methods, such as the assumption of a circular cross-sectional area in the left ventricular outflow tract. In the operating room, this method of rotational acquisition during color Doppler imaging of an outflow tract, for instance from the deep transgastric views, could allow for estimation of stroke volume and cardiac output.

Epicardial Echocardiography

In the late 1980s-early 1990s, epicardial echocardiography gained prominence as a method for real-time ultrasonic cardiac imaging in the perioperative setting [41, 92]. The epicardial approach required a standard transthoracic imaging probe encased in a sterile wrapping, and then placed directly upon the beating heart by the surgeon, who performed all probe manipulations. The surgeon or cardiologist could then monitor the images on the screen. While image quality was routinely excellent, the procedure was found to be logistically cumbersome for several reasons: (1) surgeons required a large number of cases (>200) to become proficient with the echo probe [43]; (2) since the surgeon needed to perform the scanning, the study interrupted the course of the operation, thereby prolonging surgery; (3) undesirable cardiac side effects (arrhythmias, hypotension) could occur with pressure of the probe upon the beating heart [93]. Thus as TEE technology evolved, it was not surprising that surgeons, anesthesiologists, and cardiologists alike expressed a preference for this method of intraoperative cardiac imaging, particularly as reports surfaced that TEE imaging quality and accuracy were comparable to that obtained by epicardial imaging [93, 94]. Though epicardial echocardiography still provided superior imaging of certain intracardiac structures such as the anterior ventricular septum and right ventricular outflow tract, TEE enabled a longer, more complete postoperative study, provided continuous imaging, and most importantly, did not interfere with the surgical field or the course of surgery. Thus TEE largely replaced epicardial echocardiography as the preferred modality for intraoperative echocardiographic imaging.

Nonetheless, epicardial echocardiography maintains a small but important role in the intraoperative/interventional setting. Guidelines published by the American Society of Echocardiography/Society of Cardiovascular Anesthesiologists specifically delineate training requirements, method of examination, and imaging planes for epicardial echocardiography [95]. These guidelines were subsequently endorsed by the Society of Thoracic Surgeons [96]. In adult patients, epicardial echocardiography provides important additional information in regard to the aortic valve and aorta [97–103] and pulmonary arteries [104]. For CHD evaluation, epicardial echocardiography can be helpful in those instances in which TEE cannot be performed due to small patient size or when there are congenital or acquired esophageal abnormalities. In pediatric patients, epicardial echocardiography can also be useful for the evaluation of extracardiac vascular abnormalities such as branch pulmonary artery and Glenn anastomosis obstruction [105]. It can also be helpful when performing hybrid interventional procedures [106–108]. Epicardial echocardiography has been reported with the use of a pediatric transthoracic 3D probe for the evaluation of mitral and aortic valves in adult patients [109, 110]. Comparable applications of epicardial 3D echocardiography for CHD have yet to be developed.

Intravascular Ultrasound and Intracardiac Echocardiography

Intravascular ultrasound (IVUS) and intracardiac echocardiography (ICE) are technologies that have undergone rapid changes and improvements since catheter-based ultrasound was first developed by Cieszynski in 1960 [111]. Bruce et al. broadly defined IVUS as the navigation and visualization of small blood vessels, such as coronary arteries, while the definition of ICE is the navigation and visualization of large blood-filled cavities or vessels in the cardiovascular system such as the right ventricle or pulmonary arteries [112]. Both IVUS and ICE use a catheter-mounted transducer to image the cardiac system.

Currently, IVUS and ICE catheter shafts vary in size from 2.5 French (0.8 mm diameter) to 10 French (3.2 mm diameter). The smaller IVUS catheters are typically mounted with high-frequency (20–30 MHz) transducers, while the larger ICE catheters are usually mounted with lower frequency (9–10 MHz) transducers. The two most popular imaging transducer designs for IVUS and ICE are rotational/mechanical and phased array devices.

The IVUS devices produce a radial 360° circular display around the catheter, which is located in the center of the display. Because of the very high frequencies (20–30 MHz) at which these devices operate, the depth of penetration is low, usually 1 cm or less. Moreover most devices provide only anatomic imaging and no Doppler information. Given the small size and higher frequency probes used by IVUS, this modality is more suitable for high-resolution evaluation of structures close to the catheter. The majority of clinical applications for IVUS have been in the evaluation of the arterial and pulmonary vascular systems [113–115], predominantly the coronary arteries in adults [116]. Specific coronary artery applications in adults include evaluation of coronary atherosclerosis [79, 117], surveillance/assessment of coronary vasculopathy in heart transplant patients [118, 119], and evaluation of anomalous coronary artery origin from the aorta [120]. However IVUS has been used for a broad spectrum of other cardiac applications [121] such as for the evaluation of the cardiac valves [122], ventricles [123], and great vessels, as well as the guidance of electrophysiological procedures in the adult patient [124]. It should be noted that newer technologies are currently available that might eventually supplant IVUS in the evaluation of blood vessel wall microstructure. One such technology is optical coherence tomography, which is also catheter-based and intravascular. It utilizes light in the near infrared range instead of ultrasound to provide a cross sectional image similar to that seen by IVUS; it provides higher resolution of approximately 10 μm. However penetration depth is limited, ranging from 0.1 to 2.0 mm [125, 126].

For CHD, the major application of IVUS has been in the hands of the pediatric interventional cardiologist. Experience using IVUS at the authors' institution shows that imaging patients with certain types of CHD can be very useful. IVUS can be used to detect thrombus formation in the pulmonary arteries [127]; this is applicable to patients who have had Fontan procedures and are at high risk of thrombus formation. Another use for IVUS is the assessment of pulmonary vascular disease [128, 129], and also for coronary artery changes in patients with Kawasaki disease [130, 131].

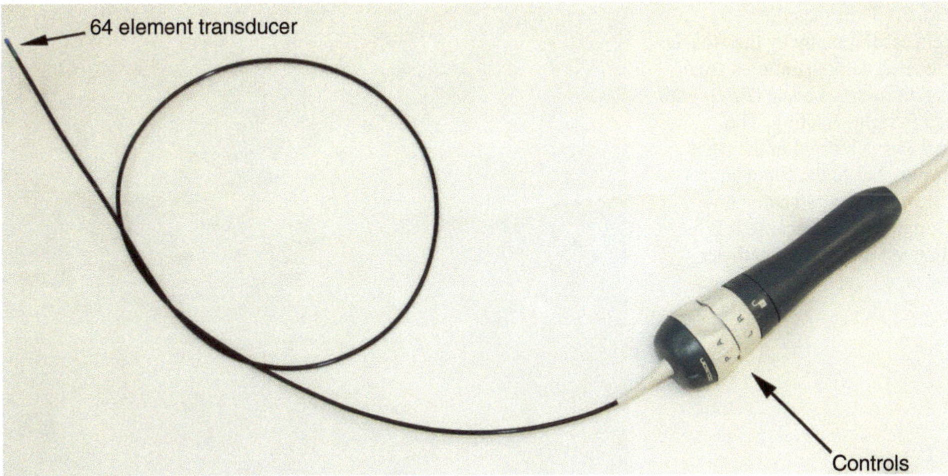

Fig. 2.14 AcuNav (Siemens Medical) intracardiac echocardiography probe showing the 64-element transducer and controls

The use of IVUS can be helpful in defining anatomy and wall stiffness/distensability in coarctation of the aorta [132, 133], as well as the results of dilation such as coarctation of the aorta or recoarctation [134]. IVUS can also be useful in assessing balloon dilation and stent placement in those patients with branch or peripheral pulmonary artery stenosis [135], and baffle obstruction in patients with postoperative atrial switch procedures [136].

In contrast to IVUS, ICE catheters offer imaging and functionality much more akin to transthoracic and transesophageal imaging. As an alternative to TEE, ICE is not new [137, 138]. Both mechanical and phased array probes are available. The mechanical rotational probes operate at 9–12.5 MHz and project a radial display similar to a standard IVUS catheter. Penetration depth is about 4 cm. This greater depth allows for visualization of a number of intracardiac structures. Imaging quality is reasonably good, however these probes do not adequately suffice for intracardiac imaging because they do not perform multi-pulse sequences, which are needed for color or tissue Doppler mapping. This requires miniature phased-array technology to adequately guide surgery or interventional catheterization procedures. The availability of a high-frequency 5–10 MHz steerable linear array (although side-looking by design) has facilitated this application. This system utilizes a multifrequency (5.5–10 MHz) phased array consisting of 64 elements, and mounted on either an 8 or 10 French catheter (Fig. 2.14). In addition to multifrequency imaging, the catheter also has full color and spectral Doppler capabilities. While it images only in a longitudinally oriented monoplane, the catheter tip has both anteroposterior and lateral flexion controls, permitting visualization of cardiac structures from a number of tomographic planes [139]. The depth of penetration is approximately 12 cm. Thus this catheter is well suited for visualizing intracardiac anatomy, and it has been used for a number of applications in interventional electrophysiology and interventional catheterization. For CHD, it is particularly useful for monitoring percutaneous closure of atrial septal defects (Fig. 2.15), atrial septal puncture, cannulation/dilation of stenotic pulmonary veins, pulmonary valve replacement, as well as other interventions [112, 121, 140–143]. A number of interventional catheterization laboratories use ICE instead of TEE for intraprocedural monitoring of atrial septal defect closure [144, 145]. This type of ICE catheter has also been used effectively in the intraoperative setting in neonates who are too small for a standard TEE probe; the catheter is inserted into the esophagus and manipulated in the same manner as a TEE probe (Fig. 2.16). Images and Doppler information are high quality, and frame rates are excellent, although the lack of a transverse (0°) plane limits its effectiveness in certain forms of CHD [146, 147]. Other types of intraprocedural applications have been described, such as guidance of myocardial biopsy in transplant patients [148]. For interventional electrophysiology, ICE has already become established as a useful tool for guiding arrhythmia therapy, particularly as regards to testing, electrode placement, and monitoring of complications [149–151]. An important development with interventional electrophysiology is the use of 3D ICE for assistance in arrhythmia mapping and ablation. This has been described primarily using reconstructed 2D ICE images that have been merged with other imaging data such as 3D computed tomography or rotational angiography [152–155]. However, recently a novel real-time 3D ICE catheter has been developed, to be used in conjunction with C-arm computed tomography for guidance of invasive electrophysiology procedures [156]. This technology has potential application for other types of interventions, particularly where multiple imaging tools are used [153].

It is interesting to speculate that future intraprocedural imaging devices might incorporate a combination of different features. For example, an imaging catheter might incorporate some combination of features including side-looking, which would be ideal for intracardiac imaging, and near-field optimized and forward-looking would also be useful for

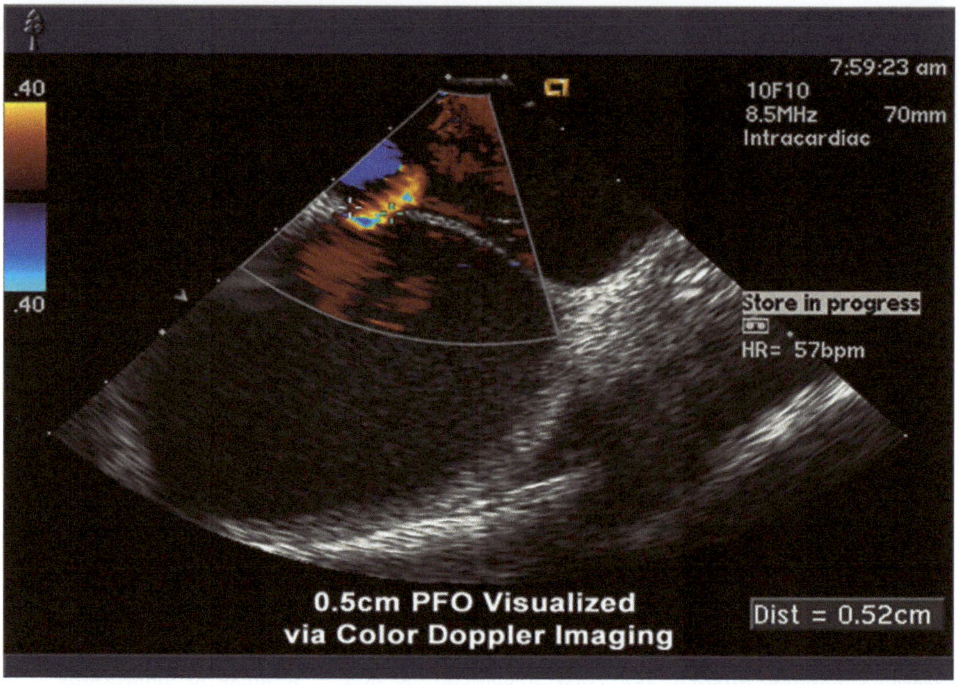

Fig. 2.15 Intracardiac echocardiography by the AcuNav catheter, demonstrating a small patent foramen ovale (*PFO*) with left to right shunting. The catheter is located in the right atrium, hence the shunt across the PFO has a *red color* flow Doppler signal because it is directed towards the catheter

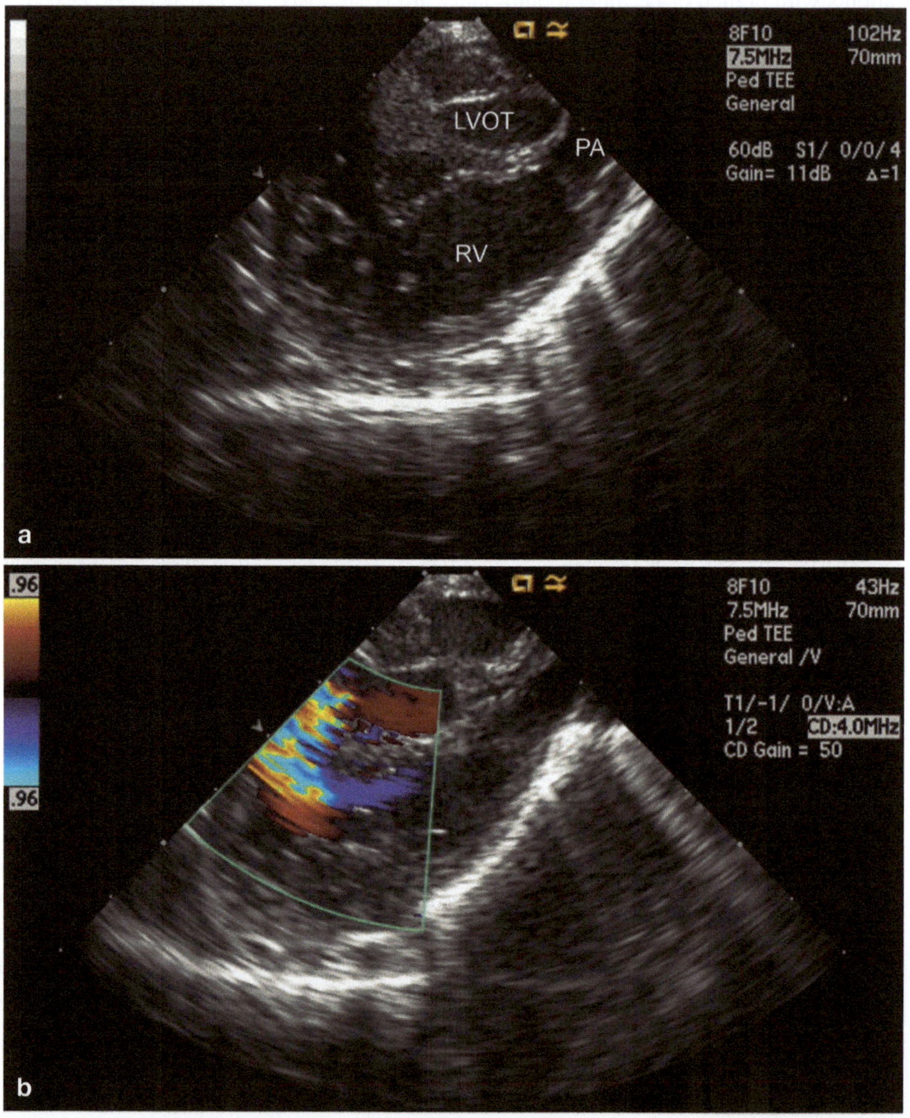

Fig. 2.16 Transesophageal echocardiography using an intracardiac echocardiography (ICE) probe in a very asmall neonate with Ebstein anomaly of the tricuspid valve. Both high quality imaging (**a**) and color flow Doppler (**b**) are seen; however only one plane is available. *LVOT* left ventricular outflow tract, *PA* pulmonary artery, *RV* right ventricle

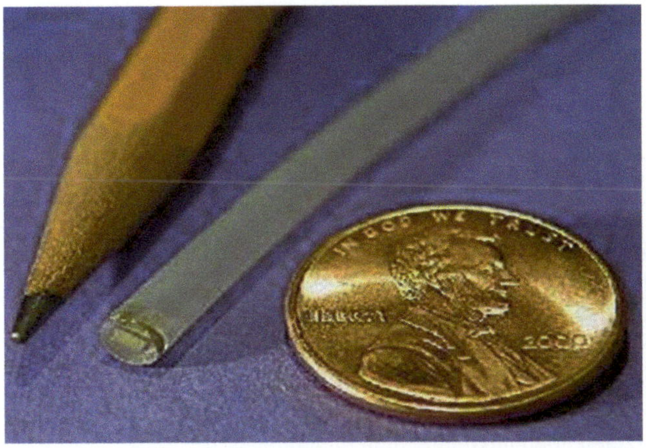

Fig. 2.17 Forward-looking intracardiac imaging catheter developed by our technology partnership

monitoring limited access surgery especially when performed with robotic assistance. Another example of a combination device, developed in our laboratory, incorporates a forward-looking microlinear phased array for ICE, along with electrophysiologic mapping and ablation electrodes mounted on the side of the catheter (Figs. 2.17, 2.18, and 2.19).

The Future

Clearly, all of the technology currently available for TEE imaging has room for improvement. This includes increasing capabilities for partitioning piezoelectric materials into smaller element sizes and high-density interconnections. In addition, smaller coaxial cables or, as an alternative, multi-

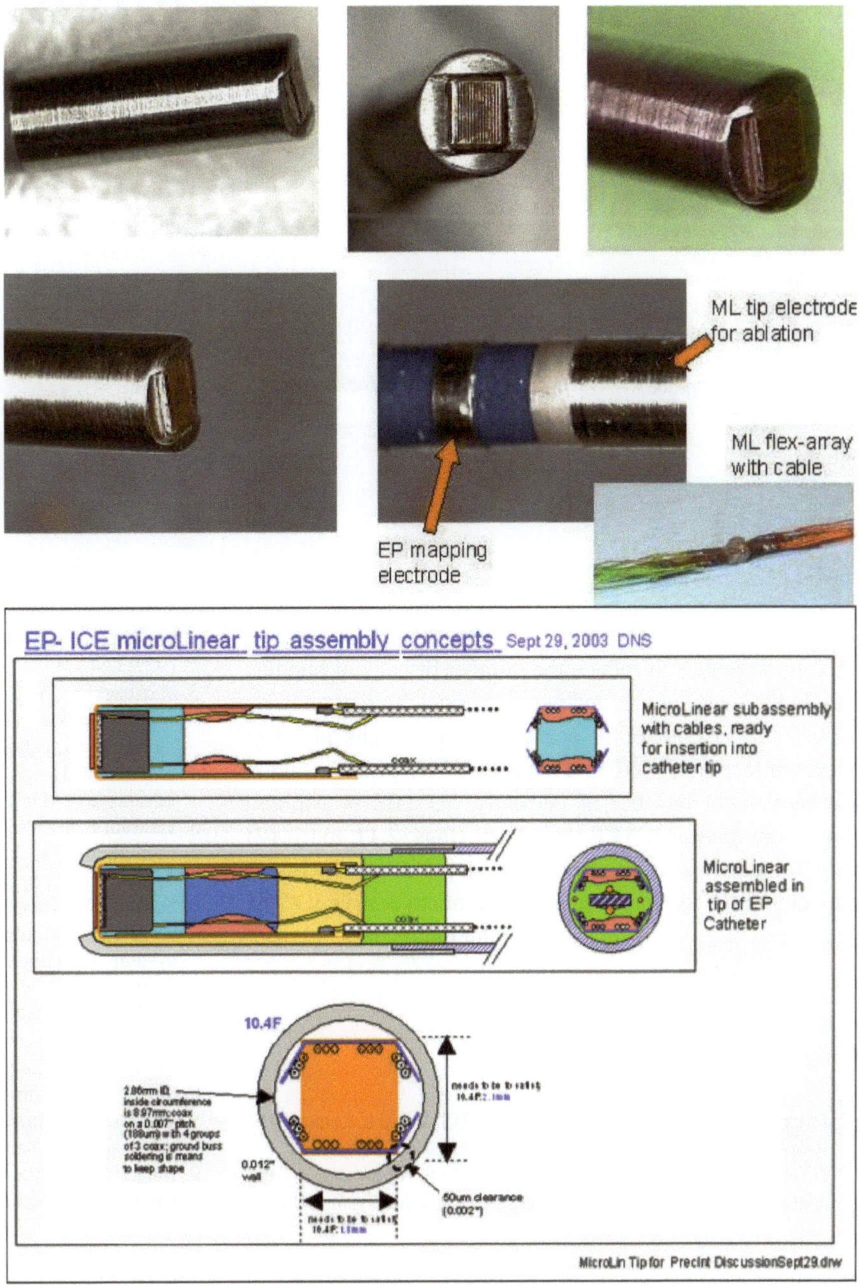

Fig. 2.18 The microlinear (*ML*) intracardiac echocardiography (*ICE*) probe and its construction. This probe, designed for invasive electrophysiology (*EP*), has electrodes for EP mapping as well as a ML tip electrode for ablation

Fig. 2.19 Microlinear array for the intracardiac imaging catheter shown in Fig. 2.18

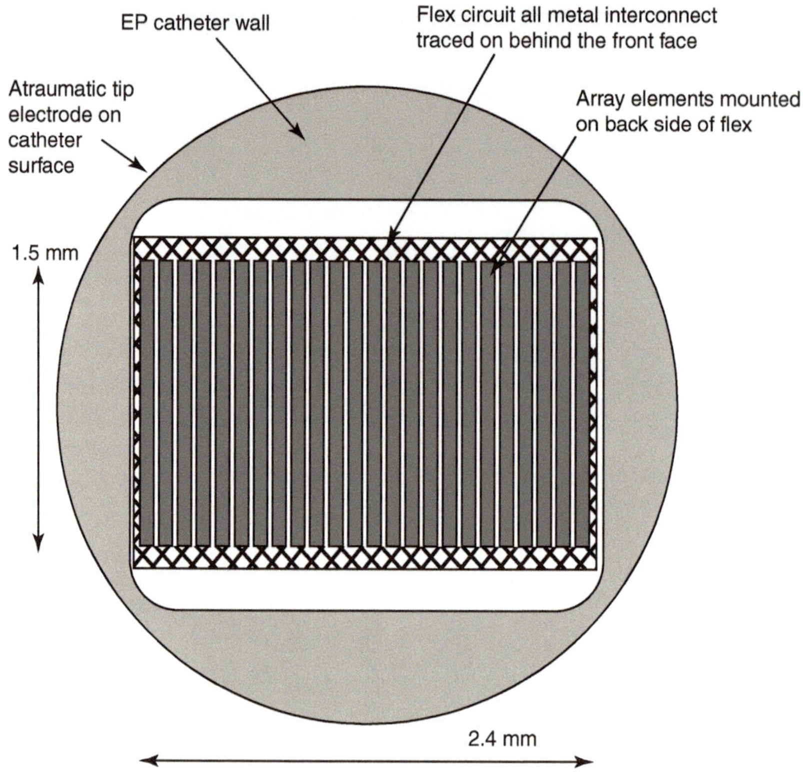

Fig. 2.20 Schematic for a novel investigational pediatric micro matrix three-dimensional transesophageal echocardiography probe

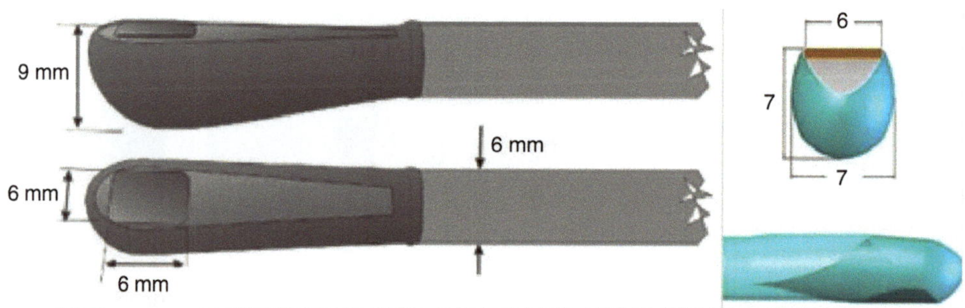

plexing strategies to reduce the number of coaxial bundles, should facilitate smaller and more agile steerable or rotatable probes for TEE, ICE, or epicardial applications in CHD. Meanwhile, a small pediatric matrix 3D TEE probe would be the next major advance as currently, 3D TEE is available only as an adult size TEE transducer (Figs. 2.11 and 2.12). Ongoing efforts, including work being performed by one of the authors (DJS) on a novel pediatric micro matrix 3D TEE probe (Fig. 2.20), hold promise for the future.

References

1. Frazin L, Talano JV, Stephanides L, Loeb HS, Kopel L, Gunnar RM. Esophageal echocardiography. Circulation. 1976;54:102–8.
2. Hisanaga K, Hisanaga A, Nagata K, Yoshida S. A new transesophageal real-time two-dimensional echocardiographic system using a flexible tube and its clinical applications. Proc Jpn J Med Ultrason. 1977;32:43–4.
3. Matsuzaki M, Shimizu M, Nomoto R, et al. Assessment of left ventricular anterior wall motion: a new application of esophageal echocardiography. J Cardiogr. 1978;8:113–24.
4. Schluter M, Hanrath P. Transesophageal echocardiography: potential advantages and initial clinical results. Pract Cardiol. 1983;9:149–51.
5. Hanrath P, Schlüter M, Langenstein BA, et al. Detection of ostium secundum atrial septal defects by transoesophageal cross-sectional echocardiography. Br Heart J. 1983;49:350–8.
6. Schlüter M, Langenstein BA, Polster J, et al. Transoesophageal cross-sectional echocardiography with a phased array transducer system. Technique and initial clinical results. Br Heart J. 1982; 48:67–72.
7. Souquet J, Hanrath P, Zitelli L, Kremer P, Langenstein BA, Schlüter M. Transesophageal phased array for imaging the heart. IEEE Trans Biomed Eng. 1982;29:707–12.
8. Schlüter M, Hinrichs A, Thier W, et al. Transesophageal two-dimensional echocardiography: comparison of ultrasonic and anatomic sections. Am J Cardiol. 1984;53:1173–8.
9. Bansal RC, Shakudo M, Shah PM. Biplane transesophageal echocardiography: technique, image orientation, and preliminary expe-

rience in 131 patients. J Am Soc Echocardiogr. 1990;3: 348–66.
10. Omoto R, Kyo S, Matsumura M, Shah PM, Adachi H, Matsunaka T. Biplane color Doppler transesophageal echocardiography: its impact on cardiovascular surgery and further technological progress in the probe, a matrix phased-array biplane probe. Echocardiography. 1989;6:423–30.
11. Seward JB, Khandheria BK, Edwards WD, Oh JK, Freeman WK, Tajik AJ. Biplanar transesophageal echocardiography: anatomic correlations, image orientation, and clinical applications. Mayo Clin Proc. 1990;65:1193–213.
12. Daniel WG, Pearlman AS, Hausmann D, et al. Initial experience and potential applications of multiplane transesophageal echocardiography. Am J Cardiol. 1993;71:358–61.
13. Flachskampf FA, Hoffmann R, Verlande M, Schneider W, Ameling W, Hanrath P. Initial experience with a multiplane transoesophageal echo-transducer: assessment of diagnostic potential. Eur Heart J. 1992;13:1201–6.
14. Nanda NC, Pinheiro L, Sanyal R, Rosenthal S, Kirklin JK. Multiplane transesophageal echocardiographic imaging and three-dimensional reconstruction. Echocardiography. 1992;9:667–76.
15. Omoto R, Kyo S, Matsumura M, Yamada E, Matsunaka T. Variomatrix—a newly developed transesophageal echocardiography probe with a rotating matrix biplane transducer. Technological aspects and initial clinical experience. Echocardiography. 1993;10:79–84.
16. Pandian NG, Hsu TL, Schwartz SL, et al. Multiplane transesophageal echocardiography. Imaging planes, echocardiographic anatomy, and clinical experience with a prototype phased array OmniPlane probe. Echocardiography. 1992;9:649–66.
17. Roelandt JR, Thomson IR, Vletter WB, Brommersma P, Bom N, Linker DT. Multiplane transesophageal echocardiography: latest evolution in an imaging revolution. J Am Soc Echocardiogr. 1992;5:361–7.
18. Helmcke F, Mahan EF, Cooper JW, Nanda NC, Sanyal R. Use of the smaller pediatric transesophageal echocardiographic probe in adults. Echocardiography. 1990;7:727–37.
19. Sutherland GR, Van Daele MERM, Stumper OFW, Hess J, Quaegebeur J. Intraoperative echocardiography in congenital heart disease: an overview. In: Erbel R, Khanderia BK, Brennecke R, Meyer J, Seward JB, Tajik AJ, editors. Transesophageal echocardiography: a new window to the heart. Berlin: Springer; 1989.
20. Cyran SE, Kimball TR, Meyer RA, et al. Efficacy of intraoperative transesophageal echocardiography in children with congenital heart disease. Am J Cardiol. 1989;63:594–8.
21. Sreeram N, Stümper OF, Kaulitz R, Hess J, Roelandt JR, Sutherland GR. Comparative value of transthoracic and transesophageal echocardiography in the assessment of congenital abnormalities of the atrioventricular junction. J Am Coll Cardiol. 1990;16: 1205–14.
22. Kyo S, Koike K, Takanawa E, et al. Impact of transesophageal Doppler echocardiography on pediatric cardiac surgery. Int J Card Imaging. 1989;4:41–2.
23. Sahn DJ, Moises V, Cali G, Valdes-Cruz LM, Mazzei W, Mitchell M. Important roles of transesophageal color Doppler flow mapping studies (TEE) in infants with congenital heart disease [Abstract]. J Am Coll Cardiol 1990;15:204A.
24. Cromme-Dijkhuis AH, Djoa KK, Bom N, Hess J. Pediatric transesophageal echocardiography by means of a miniature 5-MHz multiplane transducer. Echocardiography. 1996;13:685.
25. Piel JE, Lewandowski RS, Lorraine PW, Smith LS, Shiota T, Sahn DJ. 7.5-MHz pediatric phased array transesophageal endoscope. Echocardiography. 1996;13:677–84.
26. Sloth E, Hasenkam JM, Sørensen KE, et al. Pediatric multiplane transesophageal echocardiography in congenital heart disease: new possibilities with a miniaturized probe. J Am Soc Echocardiogr. 1996;9:622–8.
27. Gentles TL, Rosenfeld HM, Sanders SP, Laussen PC, Burke RP, van der Velde ME. Pediatric biplane transesophageal echocardiography: preliminary experience. Am Heart J. 1994;128: 1225–33.
28. O'Leary PW, Hagler DJ, Seward JB, et al. Biplane intraoperative transesophageal echocardiography in congenital heart disease. Mayo Clin Proc. 1995;70:317–26.
29. Omoto R, Kyo S, Matsumura M, Maruyama M, Yokote Y. Future technical prospects in biplane transesophageal echocardiography: use of adult and pediatric biplane matrix probes. Echocardiography. 1991;8:713–20.
30. Seward JB, Khandheria BK, Freeman WK, et al. Multiplane transesophageal echocardiography: image orientation, examination technique, anatomic correlations, and clinical applications. Mayo Clin Proc. 1993;68:523–51.
31. Djoa KK, De Jong N, Cromme-Dijkhuis AH, Lancée CT, Bom N. Two decades of transesophageal phased array probes. Ultrasound Med Biol. 1996;22:1–9.
32. Sundar S, DiNardo JA. Transesophageal echocardiography in pediatric surgery. Int Anesthesiol Clin. 2008;46:137–55.
33. Hanna BM, El-Hewala AA, Gruber PJ, Gaynor JW, Spray TL, Seliem MA. Predictive value of intraoperative diagnosis of residual ventricular septal defects by transesophageal echocardiography. Ann Thorac Surg. 2010;89:1233–7.
34. Shiota T, Lewandowski R, Piel JE, et al. Micromultiplane transesophageal echocardiographic probe for intraoperative study of congenital heart disease repair in neonates, infants, children, and adults. Am J Cardiol. 1999;83:292–5, A7.
35. Scohy TV, Gommers D, Jan ten Harkel AD, Deryck Y, McGhie J, Bogers AJJC. Intraoperative evaluation of micromultiplane transesophageal echocardiographic probe in surgery for congenital heart disease. Eur J Echocardiogr. 2007;8:241–6.
36. Zyblewski SC, Shirali GS, Forbus GA, et al. Initial experience with a miniaturized multiplane transesophageal probe in small infants undergoing cardiac operations. Ann Thorac Surg. 2010;89: 1990–4.
37. Pushparajah K, Miller OI, Rawlins D, Barlow A, Nugent K, Simpson JM. Clinical application of a micro multiplane transoesophageal probe in congenital cardiac disease. Cardiol Young. 2012;22:170–7.
38. Faletra F, De Chiara F, Corno R, Passini L. Additional diagnostic value of multiplane echocardiography over biplane imaging in assessment of mitral prosthetic valves. Heart. 1996;75:609–13.
39. Warner JG, Nomeir AM, Salim M, Kitzman DW. A prospective, randomized, blinded comparison of multiplane and biplane transesophageal echocardiographic techniques. J Am Soc Echocardiogr. 1996;9:865–73.
40. Yvorchuk KY, Sochowski RA, Chan KL. A prospective comparison of the multiplane probe with the biplane probe in structure visualization and Doppler examination during transesophageal echocardiography. J Am Soc Echocardiogr. 1995;8:111–20.
41. Ungerleider RM, Greeley WJ, Sheikh KH, Kern FH, Kisslo JA, Sabiston DC. The use of intraoperative echo with Doppler color flow imaging to predict outcome after repair of congenital cardiac defects. Ann Surg. 1989;210:526–33; discussion 533–4.
42. Ungerleider RM, Greeley WJ, Sheikh KH, et al. Routine use of intraoperative epicardial echocardiography and Doppler color flow imaging to guide and evaluate repair of congenital heart lesions. A prospective study. J Thorac Cardiovasc Surg. 1990;100: 297–309.
43. Ungerleider RM, Greeley WJ, Kanter RJ, Kisslo JA. The learning curve for intraoperative echocardiography during congenital heart surgery. Ann Thorac Surg. 1992;54:691–6; discussion 696–8.
44. Ungerleider RM. The use of intraoperative epicardial echocardiography with color flow imaging during the repair of complete atrioventricular septal defects. Cardiol Young. 1992;2:56–64.

45. Fyfe DA, Kline CH. Transesophageal echocardiography for congenital heart disease. Echocardiography. 1991;8:573–86.
46. Ritter SB. Transesophageal real-time echocardiography in infants and children with congenital heart disease. J Am Coll Cardiol. 1991;18:569–80.
47. Stümper OF, Elzenga NJ, Hess J, Sutherland GR. Transesophageal echocardiography in children with congenital heart disease: an initial experience. J Am Coll Cardiol. 1990;16:433–41.
48. Muhiudeen Russell IA, Miller-Hance WC, Silverman NH. Intraoperative transesophageal echocardiography for pediatric patients with congenital heart disease. Anesth Analg. 1998;87: 1058–76.
49. Miller-Hance WC, Silverman NH. Transesophageal echocardiography (TEE) in congenital heart disease with focus on the adult. Cardiol Clin. 2000;18:861–92.
50. Stevenson JG. Utilization of intraoperative transesophageal echocardiography during repair of congenital cardiac defects: a survey of North American centers. Clin Cardiol. 2003;26:132–4.
51. Kamra K, Russell I, Miller-Hance WC. Role of transesophageal echocardiography in the management of pediatric patients with congenital heart disease. Paediatr Anaesth. 2011;21:479–93.
52. Rice MJ, McDonald RW, Reller MD, Sahn DJ. Pediatric echocardiography: current role and a review of technical advances. J Pediatr. 1996;128:1–14.
53. Weintraub R, Shiota T, Elkadi T, et al. Transesophageal echocardiography in infants and children with congenital heart disease. Circulation. 1992;86:711–22.
54. Dan M, Bonato R, Mazzucco A, et al. Value of transesophageal echocardiography during repair of congenital heart defects. Ann Thorac Surg. 1990;50:637–43.
55. Muhiudeen I, Silverman N. Intraoperative transesophageal echocardiography using high resolution imaging in infants and children with congenital heart disease. Echocardiography. 1993;10:599–608.
56. Rosenfeld HM, Gentles TL, Wernovsky G, et al. Utility of intraoperative transesophageal echocardiography in the assessment of residual cardiac defects. Pediatr Cardiol. 1998;19:346–51.
57. Stevenson JG, Sorensen GK, Gartman DM, Hall DG, Rittenhouse EA. Transesophageal echocardiography during repair of congenital cardiac defects: identification of residual problems necessitating reoperation. J Am Soc Echocardiogr. 1993;6:356–65.
58. Frommelt MA, Frommelt PC. Advances in echocardiographic diagnostic modalities for the pediatrician. Pediatr Clin North Am. 1999;46:427–39, xi.
59. Ungerleider RM. Biplane and multiplane transesophageal echocardiography. Am Heart J. 1999;138:612–3.
60. Stümper O, Witsenburg M, Sutherland GR, Cromme-Dijkhuis A, Godman MJ, Hess J. Transesophageal echocardiographic monitoring of interventional cardiac catheterization in children. J Am Coll Cardiol. 1991;18:1506–14.
61. Hellenbrand WE, Fahey JT, McGowan FX, Weltin GG, Kleinman CS. Transesophageal echocardiographic guidance of transcatheter closure of atrial septal defect. Am J Cardiol. 1990;66:207–13.
62. Magni G, Hijazi ZM, Pandian NG, et al. Two- and three-dimensional transesophageal echocardiography in patient selection and assessment of atrial septal defect closure by the new DAS-Angel Wings device: initial clinical experience. Circulation. 1997; 96:1722–8.
63. Diab KA, Cao Q-L, Bacha EA, Hijazi ZM. Device closure of atrial septal defects with the Amplatzer septal occluder: safety and outcome in infants. J Thorac Cardiovasc Surg. 2007;134:960–6.
64. Lim DS, Forbes TJ, Rothman A, Lock JE, Landzberg MJ. Transcatheter closure of high-risk muscular ventricular septal defects with the CardioSEAL occluder: initial report from the CardioSEAL VSD registry. Catheter Cardiovasc Interv. 2007;70:740–4.
65. Carminati M, Butera G, Chessa M, Drago M, Negura D, Piazza L. Transcatheter closure of congenital ventricular septal defect with Amplatzer septal occluders. Am J Cardiol. 2005;96:52L–8.
66. Arora R, Trehan V, Thakur AK, Mehta V, Sengupta PP, Nigam M. Transcatheter closure of congenital muscular ventricular septal defect. J Interv Cardiol. 2004;17:109–15.
67. Chessa M, Carminati M, Cao Q-L, et al. Transcatheter closure of congenital and acquired muscular ventricular septal defects using the Amplatzer device. J Invasive Cardiol. 2002;14:322–7.
68. Holzer R, Balzer D, Cao Q-L, Lock K, Hijazi ZM. Amplatzer Muscular Ventricular Septal Defect Investigators. Device closure of muscular ventricular septal defects using the Amplatzer muscular ventricular septal defect occluder: immediate and mid-term results of a U.S. registry. J Am Coll Cardiol. 2004;43:1257–63.
69. Pedra CAC, Pedra SRF, Chaccur P, et al. Perventricular device closure of congenital muscular ventricular septal defects. Expert Rev Cardiovasc Ther. 2010;8:663–74.
70. Xing Q, Pan S, An Q, et al. Minimally invasive perventricular device closure of perimembranous ventricular septal defect without cardiopulmonary bypass: multicenter experience and mid-term follow-up. J Thorac Cardiovasc Surg. 2010;139:1409–15.
71. Gan C, Lin K, An Q, et al. Perventricular device closure of muscular ventricular septal defects on beating hearts: initial experience in eight children. J Thorac Cardiovasc Surg. 2009;137: 929–33.
72. Gan C, An Q, Lin K, et al. Perventricular device closure of ventricular septal defects: six months results in 30 young children. Ann Thorac Surg. 2008;86:142–6.
73. Bacha EA, Cao QL, Galantowicz ME, et al. Multicenter experience with perventricular device closure of muscular ventricular septal defects. Pediatr Cardiol. 2005;26:169–75.
74. Meyer RA. History of ultrasound in cardiology. J Ultrasound Med. 2004;23:1–11.
75. Mumm B, Nanda NC, Sorrell VL. Technical background and current and future aspects of three-dimensional echocardiography. In: Atlas of three-dimensional echocardiography. Armonk: Futura Publishing Company, inc.; 2002. p. 1–20.
76. Sugeng L, Weinert L, Lang RM. Left ventricular assessment using real time three dimensional echocardiography. Heart. 2003;89 Suppl 3:iii29–36.
77. Chan K-L, Liu X, Ascah KJ, Beauchesne LM, Burwash IG. Comparison of real-time 3-dimensional echocardiography with conventional 2-dimensional echocardiography in the assessment of structural heart disease. J Am Soc Echocardiogr. 2004;17:976–80.
78. Skubas NJ, Mahmood F, Shook DC, Shernan SK. Perioperative applications of new modalities: strain echocardiography and three-dimensional echocardiography. In: Savage RM, Aronson S, editors. Comprehensive textbook of perioperative transesophageal echocardiography. 2nd ed. Philadelphia: Lippincott Williams & Wilkins; 2010. p. 694–724.
79. Armstrong WF, Ryan T. Specialized echocardiographic techniques and methods. In: Feigenbaum's echocardiography. 7th ed. Philadelphia: Wolters Kluwer Health/Lippincott Williams & Wilkins; 2010. p. 39–66.
80. Vegas A, Meineri M, Jerath A. Real-time three-dimensional transesophageal echocardiography: a step-by-step guide. New York: Springer; 2012.
81. Sugeng L, Shernan SK, Weinert L, et al. Real-time three-dimensional transesophageal echocardiography in valve disease: comparison with surgical findings and evaluation of prosthetic valves. J Am Soc Echocardiogr. 2008;21:1347–54.
82. Gripari P, Tamborini G, Barbier P, et al. Real-time three-dimensional transoesophageal echocardiography: a new intraoperative feasible and useful technology in cardiac surgery. Int J Cardiovasc Imaging. 2010;26:651–60.

83. Horton KD, Whisenant B, Horton S. Percutaneous closure of a mitral perivalvular leak using three dimensional real time and color flow imaging. J Am Soc Echocardiogr. 2010;23:903.e5–7.
84. La Canna G, Arendar I, Maisano F, et al. Real-time three-dimensional transesophageal echocardiography for assessment of mitral valve functional anatomy in patients with prolapse-related regurgitation. Am J Cardiol. 2011;107:1365–74.
85. Lang RM, Tsang W, Weinert L, Mor-Avi V, Chandra S. Valvular heart disease the value of 3-dimensional echocardiography. J Am Coll Cardiol. 2011;58:1933–44.
86. Cao Q, Radtke W, Berger F, Zhu W, Hijazi ZM. Transcatheter closure of multiple atrial septal defects. Initial results and value of two- and three-dimensional transoesophageal echocardiography. Eur Heart J. 2000;21:941–7.
87. Acar P, Abadir S, Aggoun Y. Transcatheter closure of perimembranous ventricular septal defects with Amplatzer occluder assessed by real-time three-dimensional echocardiography. Eur J Echocardiogr. 2007;8:110–5.
88. Balzer J, Kühl H, Rassaf T, et al. Real-time transesophageal three-dimensional echocardiography for guidance of percutaneous cardiac interventions: first experience. Clin Res Cardiol. 2008;97: 565–74.
89. Baker GH, Shirali G, Ringewald JM, Hsia TY, Bandisode V. Usefulness of live three-dimensional transesophageal echocardiography in a congenital heart disease center. Am J Cardiol. 2009;103:1025–8.
90. Shirali GS. Three-dimensional echocardiography in congenital heart disease. Echocardiography. 2012;29:242–8.
91. Irvine T, Li XN, Mori Y, et al. A digital 3-dimensional method for computing great artery flows: in vitro validation studies. J Am Soc Echocardiogr. 2000;13:841–8.
92. Sreeram N, Kaulitz R, Stümper OF, Hess J, Quaegebeur JM, Sutherland GR. Comparative roles of intraoperative epicardial and early postoperative transthoracic echocardiography in the assessment of surgical repair of congenital heart defects. J Am Coll Cardiol. 1990;16:913–20.
93. Muhiudeen IA, Roberson DA, Silverman NH, Haas G, Turley K, Cahalan MK. Intraoperative echocardiography in infants and children with congenital cardiac shunt lesions: transesophageal versus epicardial echocardiography. J Am Coll Cardiol. 1990;16: 1687–95.
94. Stümper O, Kaulitz R, Sreeram N, et al. Intraoperative transesophageal versus epicardial ultrasound in surgery for congenital heart disease. J Am Soc Echocardiogr. 1990;3:392–401.
95. Reeves ST, Glas KE, Eltzschig H, et al. Guidelines for performing a comprehensive epicardial echocardiography examination: recommendations of the American Society of Echocardiography and the Society of Cardiovascular Anesthesiologists. J Am Soc Echocardiogr. 2007;20:427–37.
96. Glas KE, Swaminathan M, Reeves ST, et al. Guidelines for the performance of a comprehensive intraoperative epiaortic ultrasonographic examination: recommendations of the American Society of Echocardiography and the Society of Cardiovascular Anesthesiologists; endorsed by the Society of Thoracic Surgeons. J Am Soc Echocardiogr. 2007;20:1227–35.
97. Wilson MJ, Boyd SY, Lisagor PG, Rubal BJ, Cohen DJ. Ascending aortic atheroma assessed intraoperatively by epiaortic and transesophageal echocardiography. Ann Thorac Surg. 2000;70:25–30.
98. Rosenberger P, Shernan SK, Löffler M, et al. The influence of epiaortic ultrasonography on intraoperative surgical management in 6051 cardiac surgical patients. Ann Thorac Surg. 2008;85: 548–53.
99. Ibrahim KS, Vitale N, Tromsdal A, Kirkeby-Garstad I, Fraser AG, Haaverstad R. Enhanced intra-operative grading of ascending aorta atheroma by epiaortic ultrasound vs echocardiography. Int J Cardiol. 2008;128:218–23.
100. Sylivris S, Calafiore P, Matalanis G, et al. The intraoperative assessment of ascending aortic atheroma: epiaortic imaging is superior to both transesophageal echocardiography and direct palpation. J Cardiothorac Vasc Anesth. 1997;11:704–7.
101. Suvarna S, Smith A, Stygall J, et al. An intraoperative assessment of the ascending aorta: a comparison of digital palpation, transesophageal echocardiography, and epiaortic ultrasonography. J Cardiothorac Vasc Anesth. 2007;21:805–9.
102. Hilberath JN, Shernan SK, Segal S, Smith B, Eltzschig HK. The feasibility of epicardial echocardiography for measuring aortic valve area by the continuity equation. Anesth Analg. 2009;108: 17–22.
103. Taneja R, Quaghebeur B, Stitt LW, et al. The role of epicardial echocardiography in the measurement of transvalvular flow velocities during aortic valve replacement. J Cardiothorac Vasc Anesth. 2009;23:292–7.
104. Allyn JW, Lennon PF, Siegle JH, Quinn RD, D'Ambra MN. The use of epicardial echocardiography as an adjunct to transesophageal echocardiography for the detection of pulmonary embolism. Anesth Analg. 2006;102:729–30.
105. Dragulescu A, Golding F, Van Arsdell G, et al. The impact of additional epicardial imaging to transesophageal echocardiography on intraoperative detection of residual lesions in congenital heart surgery. J Thorac Cardiovasc Surg. 2011;143(2):361–7.
106. Schmitz C, Esmailzadeh B, Herberg U, et al. Hybrid procedures can reduce the risk of congenital cardiovascular surgery. Eur J Cardiothorac Surg. 2008;34:718–25.
107. Chojnicki M, Haponiuk I, Jaworski R, et al. Intraoperative imaging of hybrid procedure for muscular ventricular septal defects closure with Amplatzer Duct Occluder II (Polish). Kardiol Pol. 2011;69:1280–1.
108. Li S, Chen W, Zhang Y, et al. Hybrid therapy for pulmonary atresia with intact ventricular septum. Ann Thorac Surg. 2011;91:1467–71.
109. De Castro S, Salandin V, Cavarretta E, et al. Epicardial real-time three-dimensional echocardiography in cardiac surgery: a preliminary experience. Ann Thorac Surg. 2006;82:2254–9.
110. Salandin V, De Castro S, Cavarretta E, et al. Epicardial real-time 3-dimensional echocardiography with the use of a pediatric transthoracic probe: a technical approach. J Cardiothorac Vasc Anesth. 2010;24:43–50.
111. Cieszynski T. Intracardiac method for the investigation of structure of the heart with the aid of ultrasonics. Arch Immunol Ther Exp (Warsz). 1960;8:551–7.
112. Bruce CJ, Packer DL, Belohlavek M, Seward JB. Intracardiac echocardiography: newest technology. J Am Soc Echocardiogr. 2000;13:788–95.
113. Mintz GS, Painter JA, Pichard AD, et al. Atherosclerosis in angiographically "normal" coronary artery reference segments: an intravascular ultrasound study with clinical correlations. J Am Coll Cardiol. 1995;25:1479–85.
114. Pandian NG, Weintraub A, Kreis A, Schwartz SL, Konstam MA, Salem DN. Intracardiac, intravascular, two-dimensional, high-frequency ultrasound imaging of pulmonary artery and its branches in humans and animals. Circulation. 1990;81:2007–12.
115. Weissman NJ, Mendelsohn FO, Palacios IF, Weyman AE. Development of coronary compensatory enlargement in vivo: sequential assessments with intravascular ultrasound. Am Heart J. 1995;130:1283–5.
116. Nissen SE, Yock P. Intravascular ultrasound: novel pathophysiological insights and current clinical applications. Circulation. 2001;103:604–16.
117. Mintz GS, Nissen SE, Anderson WD, et al. American College of Cardiology Clinical Expert Consensus Document on Standards

for Acquisition, Measurement and Reporting of Intravascular Ultrasound Studies (IVUS). A report of the American College of Cardiology Task Force on Clinical Expert Consensus Documents. J Am Coll Cardiol. 2001;37:1478–92.
118. Zimmer RJ, Lee MS. Transplant coronary artery disease. JACC Cardiovasc Interv. 2010;3:367–77.
119. Lee MS, Finch W, Weisz G, Kirtane AJ. Cardiac allograft vasculopathy. Rev Cardiovasc Med. 2011;12:143–52.
120. Angelini P, Flamm SD. Newer concepts for imaging anomalous aortic origin of the coronary arteries in adults. Catheter Cardiovasc Interv. 2007;69:942–54.
121. Foster GP, Picard MH. Intracardiac echocardiography: current uses and future directions. Echocardiography. 2001;18:43–8.
122. Isner JM, Losordo DW, Rosenfield K, et al. Catheter-based intravascular ultrasound discriminates bicuspid from tricuspid valves in adults with calcific aortic stenosis. J Am Coll Cardiol. 1990; 15:1310–7.
123. Schwartz SL, Pandian NG, Hsu TL, Weintraub A, Cao QL. Intracardiac echocardiographic imaging of cardiac abnormalities, ischemic myocardial dysfunction, and myocardial perfusion: studies with a 10 MHz ultrasound catheter. J Am Soc Echocardiogr. 1993;6:345–55.
124. Chu E, Kalman JM, Kwasman MA, et al. Intracardiac echocardiography during radiofrequency catheter ablation of cardiac arrhythmias in humans. J Am Coll Cardiol. 1994;24:1351–7.
125. Tearney GJ, Regar E, Akasaka T, et al. Consensus standards for acquisition, measurement, and reporting of intravascular optical coherence tomography studies: a report from the International Working Group for Intravascular Optical Coherence Tomography Standardization and Validation. J Am Coll Cardiol. 2012;59: 1058–72.
126. Tsimikas S, DeMaria AN. The clinical emergence of optical coherence tomography: defining a role in intravascular imaging. J Am Coll Cardiol. 2012;59:1090–2.
127. Ricou F, Nicod PH, Moser KM, Peterson KL. Catheter-based intravascular ultrasound imaging of chronic thromboembolic pulmonary disease. Am J Cardiol. 1991;67:749–52.
128. Scott PJ, Essop AR, al-Ashab W, Deaner A, Parsons J, Williams G. Imaging of pulmonary vascular disease by intravascular ultrasound. Int J Card Imaging. 1993;9:179–84.
129. Day RW, Tani LY. Pulmonary intravascular ultrasound in infants and children with congenital heart disease. Cathet Cardiovasc Diagn. 1997;41:395–8.
130. Sugimura T, Kato H, Inoue O, et al. Intravascular ultrasound of coronary arteries in children. Assessment of the wall morphology and the lumen after Kawasaki disease. Circulation. 1994;89: 258–65.
131. Iemura M, Ishii M, Sugimura T, Akagi T, Kato H. Long term consequences of regressed coronary aneurysms after Kawasaki disease: vascular wall morphology and function. Heart. 2000;83: 307–11.
132. DeGroff CG, Rice MJ, Reller MD, Shiota T, Sahn DJ. Intravascular ultrasound can assist angiographic assessment of coarctation of the aorta. Am Heart J. 1994;128:836–9.
133. Xu J, Shiota T, Omoto R, et al. Intravascular ultrasound assessment of regional aortic wall stiffness, distensibility, and compliance in patients with coarctation of the aorta. Am Heart J. 1997;134:93–8.
134. Sohn S, Rothman A, Shiota T, et al. Acute and follow-up intravascular ultrasound findings after balloon dilation of coarctation of the aorta. Circulation. 1994;90:340–7.
135. Nakanishi T. Balloon dilatation and stent implantation for vascular stenosis. Pediatr Int. 2001;43:548–52.
136. Chintala K, Forbes TJ, Karpawich PP. Effectiveness of transvenous pacemaker leads placed through intravascular stents in patients with congenital heart disease. Am J Cardiol. 2005;95:424–7.
137. Hardy BG, Silka MJ, Sahn DJ. Journeys inside the heart: fantastic voyages, but what will their impact be? Mayo Clin Proc. 1996;71:719–20.
138. Valdes-Cruz LM, Sideris E, Sahn DJ, et al. Transvascular intracardiac applications of a miniaturized phased-array ultrasonic endoscope. Initial experience with intracardiac imaging in piglets. Circulation. 1991;83:1023–7.
139. O'Leary PW. Intracardiac echocardiography in congenital heart disease: are we ready to begin the fantastic voyage? Pediatr Cardiol. 2002;23:286–91.
140. Rigatelli G, Dell' Avvocata F, Cardaioli P, et al. Five-year follow-up of intracardiac echocardiography-assisted transcatheter closure of complex ostium secundum atrial septal defect. Congenit Heart Dis. 2012;7:103–10.
141. Barker PCA. Intracardiac echocardiography in congenital heart disease. J Cardiovasc Transl Res. 2009;2:19–23.
142. Chessa M, Butera G, Carminati M. Intracardiac echocardiography during percutaneous pulmonary valve replacement. Eur Heart J. 2008;29:2908.
143. Huber CH, Hurni M, Tsang V, Segesser LKV. Valved stents for transapical pulmonary valve replacement. J Thorac Cardiovasc Surg. 2009;137:914–8.
144. Hijazi Z, Wang Z, Cao Q, Koenig P, Waight D, Lang R. Transcatheter closure of atrial septal defects and patent foramen ovale under intracardiac echocardiographic guidance: feasibility and comparison with transesophageal echocardiography. Catheter Cardiovasc Interv. 2001;52:194–9.
145. Bartel T, Konorza T, Neudorf U, et al. Intracardiac echocardiography: an ideal guiding tool for device closure of interatrial communications. Eur J Echocardiogr. 2005;6:92–6.
146. Bruce CJ, O'Leary P, Hagler DJ, Seward JB, Cabalka AK. Miniaturized transesophageal echocardiography in newborn infants. J Am Soc Echocardiogr. 2002;15:791–7.
147. Cannesson M, Hénaine R, Metton O, et al. Images in cardiovascular medicine. Intraoperative transesophageal echocardiography using a miniaturized transducer in a neonate undergoing Norwood procedure for hypoplastic left heart syndrome. Circulation. 2008;117:702–3.
148. Sheikh I, Kumar D, Liu Z, et al. Novel uses of intracardiac echocardiography with a phased-array imaging catheter. J Am Soc Echocardiogr. 2003;16:1073–7.
149. Ren J-F, Marchlinski FE. Utility of intracardiac echocardiography in left heart ablation for tachyarrhythmias. Echocardiography. 2007;24:533–40.
150. Wazni OM, Tsao H-M, Chen S-A, et al. Cardiovascular imaging in the management of atrial fibrillation. J Am Coll Cardiol. 2006;48:2077–84.
151. Dravid SG, Hope B, McKinnie JJ. Intracardiac echocardiography in electrophysiology: a review of current applications in practice. Echocardiography. 2008;25:1172–5.
152. Khaykin Y, Skanes A, Whaley B, et al. Real-time integration of 2D intracardiac echocardiography and 3D electroanatomical mapping to guide ventricular tachycardia ablation. Heart Rhythm. 2008;5:1396–402.
153. Kim SS, Hijazi ZM, Lang RM, Knight BP. The use of intracardiac echocardiography and other intracardiac imaging tools to guide noncoronary cardiac interventions. J Am Coll Cardiol. 2009;53:2117–28.
154. Bunch TJ, Weiss JP, Crandall BG, et al. Image integration using intracardiac ultrasound and 3D reconstruction for scar mapping and ablation of ventricular tachycardia. J Cardiovasc Electrophysiol. 2010;21:678–84.

155. Nölker G, Gutleben K-J, Asbach S, et al. Intracardiac echocardiography for registration of rotational angiography-based left atrial reconstructions: a novel approach integrating two intraprocedural three-dimensional imaging techniques in atrial fibrillation ablation. Europace. 2011;13:492–8.

156. Wein W, Camus E, John M, et al. Towards guidance of electrophysiological procedures with real-time 3D intracardiac echocardiography fusion to C-arm CT. Med Image Comput Comput Assist Interv. 2009;12:9–16.

3 Indications and Guidelines for Performance of Transesophageal Echocardiography in Congenital Heart Disease and Pediatric Acquired Heart Disease

Wanda C. Miller-Hance and Nancy A. Ayres

Abstract

Transesophageal echocardiography (TEE) represents a specialized application of ultrasound with significant benefits in the anatomic, functional, and hemodynamic assessment of patients with congenital heart disease (CHD). This imaging modality is also known to play an important role in the management of children with acquired heart disease. The indications for transesophageal imaging in children with conditions or diseases of the cardiovascular system as well as in adults with CHD have evolved over the years. In general, in the current medical era the indications can be categorized into those related to diagnostic evaluation, perioperative assessment, and monitoring during interventions. As the technology has advanced and the use of this imaging approach has become widespread, guidelines for training and performance of TEE in these patient groups have been developed.

This chapter reviews the evolution of indications and current guidelines regarding the use of TEE in CHD and pediatric acquired heart disease. Safety considerations, complications, and contraindications relevant to the TEE assessment in this patient population are also addressed.

Keywords

Transesophageal Echocardiography • Congenital Heart Disease • Pediatric Acquired Heart Disease • Indications • Guidelines • Complications • Contraindications

Introduction

Transesophageal echocardiography (TEE) plays an important role in the anatomic, functional, and hemodynamic assessment of patients with congenital heart disease (CHD). This imaging approach has been applied to both children and adults over a wide range of congenital cardiovascular malformations. In the pediatric age group, the applications of this imaging modality are not limited to those with structural defects, but also include children with acquired heart disease. Extensive clinical experience documents significant contributions of TEE, particularly in the perioperative setting. In fact, in the current medical era many consider this technology an essential adjunct to perioperative management in CHD. This chapter reviews indications for TEE related primarily to diagnostic evaluation, perioperative assessment, and monitoring during interventions. Guidelines are addressed regarding cognitive/technical skills and training requirements for performing TEE in this particular patient group. Finally, safety concerns, potential complications, and contraindications relevant to the TEE assessment in this patient population are discussed.

W.C. Miller-Hance, MD, FACC, FASE (✉)
Divisions of Pediatric Anesthesiology and Pediatric Cardiology, Departments of Pediatrics and Anesthesiology, Texas Children's Hospital, Baylor College of Medicine, 6621 Fannin, Suite W17417, Houston, TX 77030, USA
e-mail: wmh@bcm.edu

N.A. Ayres, MD
Division of Cardiology, Department of Pediatrics, Texas Children's Hospital, Baylor College of Medicine, 6621 Fannin, Suite W17417, Houston, TX 77030, USA

P.C. Wong, W.C. Miller-Hance (eds.), *Transesophageal Echocardiography for Congenital Heart Disease*, DOI 10.1007/978-1-84800-064-3_3, © Springer-Verlag London 2014

Indications for Transesophageal Echocardiography in Congenital Heart Disease and Pediatric Acquired Heart Disease

Evolution of Indications

The recognition of TEE as a specialized application of ultrasound in the 1980s resulted in collective multispecialty efforts in the 1990s addressing the indications for the use of this modality [1, 2]. The explosive use of this imaging approach led in 1992 to the generation of guidelines by the American Society of Echocardiography regarding training of physicians and sonographers providing these services [3]. At the time the most common indications in adult patients were noted as follows:

- Technically inadequate transthoracic images
- Evaluation of prosthetic valves
- Evaluation of native valves for disruption and/or vegetation
- Identification and assessment of masses and tumors

It was the consensus that in general TEE should not be performed prior to the completion of a comprehensive transthoracic examination. In regards to the applications of TEE in the intraoperative setting, it was recognized that this modality could serve as an on-line monitor, being potentially valuable in patients at high risk for cardiovascular complications. Additional merits of TEE included the detection of intravascular and intracardiac air, the evaluation of valvular surgery, and the assessment of complex CHD in the adult. TEE was also noted to potentially benefit the care of critically ill patients during the postoperative period.

Hardware miniaturization and evolving technological advances expanded the applications of TEE to the pediatric population. A report published in 1992 specifically addressed the use TEE in children [4]. This was an effort by the Committee on Standards for Pediatric TEE at the request of the Society for Pediatric Echocardiography to propose indications and guidelines for the optimal performance of TEE in this age group.

The pediatric TEE indications were listed as follows:

1. *Patients not known to have CHD*:
   Those with an unsatisfactory transthoracic examination with known or suspected pathology, and in which the study could provide valuable diagnostic information.
2. *Patients known to have CHD*:
   For preoperative evaluation when a transthoracic study failed to characterize relevant cardiovascular anatomy.
3. *Intraoperative or postoperative repair*:
   During surgical interventions for cardiac defects to determine if significant residual abnormalities were present.
4. *Postoperative examinations*:
   Those with an inadequate transthoracic examination and either residual hemodynamic compromise, suspected residual defects, or physiological abnormalities.
   Those requiring investigation for foci of endocarditis or thrombus formation.
   For evaluation of relevant regions of the heart in order to overcome challenges presented by prosthetic valves or other materials.
5. *Cardiac catheterizations*:
   For continuous evaluation during selected procedures/interventions.

As technology continued to evolve and the use of intraoperative echocardiography became widespread, in 1996 the American Society of Anesthesiologists and the Society of Cardiovascular Anesthesiologists generated practice guidelines regarding the perioperative applications of TEE [5]. These evidence-based recommendations, intended primarily for anesthesiologists, focused on the indications for performing TEE in the operative setting. Among indications supported by the strongest evidence or expert opinion "*the intraoperative use of TEE during congenital heart surgery for most lesions requiring cardiopulmonary bypass*" was listed. The task force believed that the use of TEE in the perioperative assessment of CHD likely improved clinical outcomes. Epicardial echocardiography was suggested as an alternate imaging approach when TEE was not feasible.

Following this report, an update of prior guidelines for the clinical application of echocardiography was published by the American College of Cardiology and American Heart Association (endorsed by the American Society of Echocardiography) in 1997 [6]. In contrast to the original document [2], the updated guidelines addressed indications for the use of TEE in pediatric patients. The following were considered class I indications, where there was evidence and/or general agreement that TEE was useful or effective for a given procedure or treatment.

- *Any patient with congenital or acquired heart disease, when the transthoracic echocardiogram is not considered diagnostic.*
- *Monitoring and guidance during procedures with risk for residual shunting, valvular obstruction, regurgitation, or myocardial dysfunction.*
- *Guidance of catheter/device placement during interventional catheterization/radiofrequency ablation in patients with CHD.*
- *Study of patients with intra-atrial baffle in whom the potential for thrombus is of concern.*
- *Patients with long-term placement of intravascular devices or prosthetic valves in whom thrombus or vegetation is suspected.*
- *Any patient with suspected endocarditis and inadequate transthoracic acoustical window.*

A subsequent statement published in 2003 by the American College of Cardiology/American Heart Association/American College of Physicians addressing clinical competence in echocardiography included the evaluation of a variety of congenital heart defects in both children and adults as one of the indications for TEE [7].

Table 3.1 Indications for transesophageal echocardiography in the patient with CHD

Diagnostic indications	Patient with suspected CHD and nondiagnostic TTE
	Presence of PFO and direction of shunting as possible etiology for stroke
	Evaluation of intra or extracardiac baffles following the Fontan, Senning, or Mustard procedure
	PFO evaluation with agitated saline contrast to determine possible right-to-left shunt, prior to transvenous pacemaker insertion
	Aortic dissection (Marfan syndrome, Marfan-like syndrome, blunt trauma to chest)
	Intracardiac evaluation for vegetation or suspected abscess
	Evaluation for intracardiac thrombus prior to cardioversion for atrial flutter/fibrillation
	Pericardial effusion or cardiac function evaluation and monitoring postoperative patient with open sternum or poor acoustic windows
	Evaluating status of prosthetic valve
	Blunt chest trauma and suspected acquired heart disease
	Evaluation of ventricular assist devices
Perioperative indications	Immediate preoperative definition of cardiac anatomy and function
	Postoperative surgical results and function
TEE guided interventions	Guidance for placement of ASD or VSD occlusion device
	Guidance for blade or balloon atrial septostomy
	Catheter tip placement for valve perforation and dilation in catheterization laboratory
	Guidance during radiofrequency ablation procedure
	Results of minimally invasive surgical incision or video assisted cardiac procedure

Reprinted from Ayres et al. [9]; with permission from Elsevier
ASD atrial septal defect, *CHD* congenital heart disease, *PFO* patent foramen ovale, *TTE* transthoracic echocardiography, *VSD* ventricular septal defect

An appropriateness review for transthoracic echocardiography (TTE) and TEE conducted by the American College of Cardiology Foundation and the American Society of Echocardiography in conjunction with key specialty and subspecialty societies was published in 2007 [8]. The criteria developed assumed adult patients and was based on common clinical applications or anticipated use of these imaging modalities. The assessment of known or suspected adult CHD either in unoperated patients or following repair/operation was considered among the indications for TTE/TEE.

Current Indications and Applications

In 2005, the Pediatric Council of the American Society of Echocardiography updated the previous statement published in 1992 and reviewed clinical indications for the performance of TEE in pediatric patients with acquired or congenital cardiovascular disease (group collectively referred to as "the patient with CHD") [9]. Indications for TEE were subdivided into the following primary categories (Table 3.1):

- Diagnostic assessment
- Perioperative evaluation
- Related to interventions

The American Society of Echocardiography and Society of Cardiovascular Anesthesiologists in recently published guidelines for performing a comprehensive TEE examination reiterated these indications in the adult patient with CHD [10].

The specific applications of TEE in both children and adults with CHD, as well as the benefits of the technology in pediatric acquired heart disease, are discussed in detail throughout this textbook. The sections that follow provide an overview of the use of TEE in these patient groups.

Diagnostic Assessment

Echocardiography is the diagnostic modality of choice in the initial and serial evaluation of most types of pediatric heart disease. In infants and young children in general, high-resolution transthoracic imaging allows for excellent definition of cardiovascular anatomy, assessment of hemodynamics, and evaluation of ventricular performance. When the transthoracic examination or other studies have not successfully elucidated the necessary clinically relevant information, TEE is able to provide diagnostic details in the majority of cases. By overcoming limitations related to poor windows, suboptimal image quality, or lung interference, TEE facilitates morphologic, hemodynamic, and functional assessment of congenital and acquired cardiac abnormalities. This is of particular relevance in individuals with limited acoustic windows, such as those who have undergone multiple cardiothoracic interventions, adults, or patients with a significant amount of soft tissue/body fat.

TEE is considered superior to transthoracic imaging in the adolescent or adult for the evaluation of certain suspected pathologies such as a patent foramen ovale, specific types of atrial septal defects, anomalous pulmonary venous connections, and complex cardiac malformations [11–13]. This modality has been also shown to be of benefit when confirming or excluding diagnoses of major clinical relevance such as atrial baffle pathology (leak or obstruction) following interventions for transpositions, Fontan obstruction or related venous thrombus, as well as acquired conditions such as intracardiac vegetations, aortic dissection, and aortic root abscess [14–18]. Other settings in which TEE has been applied include the evaluation of potential intracardiac thrombus prior to cardioversion of atrial rhythm disturbances and the assessment of prosthetic valve function [19]. As the technology for mechanical circulatory support has evolved, TEE has been used to monitor cannula placement, confirm adequacy of atrial and ventricular volume as required (decompression, venting, filling), assessment of aortic valve opening, hemodynamic stabilization, and surveillance of potential complications [20, 21].

Perioperative Evaluation

During Cardiovascular Surgery

Intraoperative evaluation currently represents the most common indication for TEE in patients with CHD and children with acquired cardiovascular disorders. Indications for intraoperative TEE include settings where there exists potential for significant residual pathology and/or myocardial dysfunction related to cardiovascular interventions.

It is recommended that all patients undergo a complete preoperative TTE prior to TEE. The study should be reviewed by the echocardiographer prior to initiating the intraoperative TEE assessment. TEE should be considered a complementary imaging modality, rather than a substitute for a comprehensive TTE. This is in recognition of the inherent limitations associated with transesophageal imaging such as the inability to evaluate certain cardiovascular structures, suboptimal conditions for imaging, and other challenges.

The benefits of the preoperative TEE study are many, including:

- Baseline evaluation
- Confirmation of preoperative diagnoses
- Identification of new or different pathology
- Exclusion of additional or suspected defects
- Influence on surgical plan
- Influence on anesthetic management

The exam provides a baseline evaluation of the underlying cardiac abnormalities and serves as a framework for later comparison in the postsurgical assessment. Also, the study can be used to address any important remaining preoperative concerns regarding intracardiac anatomy and physiology, questions in which TEE has a reasonable expectation of providing accurate and useful information. Important goals of the examination include the confirmation and/or exclusion of preoperative diagnoses, assessment of cardiac pathology, and the immediate preoperative evaluation of hemodynamics and ventricular function. TEE demonstrates in real-time the cardiac abnormalities to the perioperative providers prior to the intervention. The examination allows for refinements or modifications in the surgical plan and facilitates anesthetic care. Several reports have documented the many contributions of preoperative TEE including, for example, guidance during placement of intravascular and intracardiac catheters [22]. Performing a complete study (Chap. 4) should be an objective during the preoperative period; however, a focused examination might be necessary due to patient-related issues or unanticipated intraoperative problems/complications that could limit this assessment.

The benefits of the postsurgical TEE examination are also well recognized and include:

- Ensuring the adequacy of cardiac de-airing
- Evaluation of ventricular preload
- Monitoring of ventricular function
- Identification of problems associated with weaning from cardiopulmonary bypass
- Assessment of the adequacy of the surgical intervention
- Guidance during revision of the surgical repair
- Influence on anesthetic and medical managements
- Planning and optimizing postoperative care

Numerous publications have documented the impact of this imaging approach in patients with congenital cardiovascular defects and in children with acquired cardiovascular pathology [23–35]. While weaning from cardiopulmonary bypass, TEE ensures the adequacy of cardiac de-airing [36] and allows for assessment of ventricular function and loading conditions [37, 38]. Changes in inotropic strategy and volume replacement have also been reported as a direct result of intraoperative TEE [39, 40]. The postoperative study encompasses a complete analysis of the surgical results, hemodynamics, and functional status. The clinical condition, in conjunction with the TEE findings and other available hemodynamic information, are considered in the determination of whether the surgical repair is acceptable or if there is a need for reinstitution of cardiopulmonary bypass to revise the repair or address unsatisfactory results. In some cases, an "acceptable" result must be distinguished from a "perfect" result. The main goal of intraoperative TEE is the assessment of hemodynamically significant residual defects that may need reintervention prior to leaving the operating room, in order to improve overall clinical outcomes.

Additional settings where TEE has been shown to be useful in these patient groups include: during minimally invasive surgery when adequate visualization of structures may be limited [41–44], in the postoperative patient with suboptimal transthoracic windows or an open sternum [45, 46], in the critical care setting, and in the management of patients undergoing mechanical circulatory support [47]. These applications are discussed in further detail later in this chapter.

Over the past several decades, the contributions of TEE have accounted for improved perioperative care, by limiting morbidity and likely reducing mortality in many patients. The experience has been so compelling that the technology has been incorporated into standard clinical practice by many centers that care for patients with CHD and children with acquired cardiovascular pathology, despite the lack of rigorous scientific scrutiny of the impact of TEE on patient outcome.

During Noncardiac Surgery

Several practice guidelines have addressed the applications of TEE during noncardiac surgery in the adult. These indicate that TEE should be used during noncardiac procedures when the patient has known or suspected cardiovascular pathology that might result in hemodynamic, pulmonary, or neurologic compromise [48]. This indication, also applicable to the adult with CHD, has been emphasized in more recent recommendations.

Although the role of TEE during noncardiac surgery has not been extensively documented in children, nor adults with CHD, the limited experience suggests that this approach may facilitate perioperative management in selected patient groups [49–51]. High-risk individuals that may benefit from TEE during noncardiac surgery include those with untreated or palliated CHD, single ventricle physiology, or other complex structural abnormalities. In addition, TEE is likely to assist in the care of patients with residual hemodynamic abnormalities, myocardial dysfunction, cardiomyopathies, or pulmonary hypertension undergoing noncardiac operative procedures where significant fluid shifts are anticipated, or perturbations may result in hemodynamic compromise.

An executive summary regarding perioperative cardiovascular evaluation and care for noncardiac surgery was published as a joint effort of the American College of Cardiology and American Heart Association in 2007. In reference to CHD this indicated that certain postoperative patients may be at higher risk during noncardiac surgery [52]. As limited information is available for perioperative risk assessment in these patients, specific recommendations for intraoperative management, including monitoring, were not made. It was pointed out at the time the guidelines were developed that there was insufficient evidence to support the routine use of TEE during noncardiac surgery.

Guidance During Interventions

Interventional procedures have become increasingly employed in the non-surgical management of CHD. TEE allows for safer and more effective application of catheter-based approaches and may reduce radiation exposure, amount of contrast material administered, and duration of the interventional procedure. Major contributions during catheter-based interventions include: (1) acquisition of detailed anatomic and hemodynamic data prior to and during the procedure, (2) real-time evaluation of catheter placement across valves, vessels, and cardiac structures, (3) immediate assessment of the results, and (4) monitoring and detection of complications associated with the interventions [53–59]. The refinements in interventional cardiac catheterization techniques coupled with advances in TEE now allow for a high success rate of these procedures along with a low incidence of complications.

In the cardiac catheterization laboratory TEE has been applied to the closure of atrial septal defects [60–68], ventricular septal defects [69, 70], and occlusion of patent ductus arteriosus [71, 72], as well as communications such as Fontan baffle leaks and fenestrations [73, 74]. Additional procedures suitable for TEE monitoring/guidance include: balloon/blade atrial septostomy [75–77], stenting of restrictive atrial communications or other cardiovascular structures [78], balloon valvuloplasty [79, 80], radio frequency perforation of atretic valve or atrial septum, endomyocardial biopsy [81], pericardiocentesis [82, 83], and retrieval of devices/foreign bodies [84] (Chap. 17). TEE is also used to facilitate guidance of percutaneous ventricular septal defect closure and other interventions performed by combining catheter techniques and operative procedures, otherwise known as hybrid approaches [85, 86].

Applications in the Ambulatory and Critical Care Settings

Ambulatory (Outpatient) Setting

In adults, TEE is routinely and regularly utilized in the ambulatory setting. This is due in large part to the more difficult transthoracic windows and marginal imaging quality encountered in many adults, which limits the amount of information obtainable by TTE. However it also reflects the fact that ambulatory TEE is easier to perform in adult patients, because in most cases it can be done with moderate sedation.

In contrast, ambulatory TEE is less likely to be used in the pediatric setting. As indicated previously, transthoracic imaging generally provides high-quality diagnostic images in pediatric patients, particularly neonates, infants, and young children. Rarely does TEE provide any significant advantage compared to transthoracic imaging in the younger age-group; in addition, the greater availability of transthoracic windows means that a more comprehensive evaluation of the heart and adjacent cardiovascular structures can be performed, including those areas not consistently imaged by TEE (e.g. the branch pulmonary arteries, aortic arch). The other important deterrent is that ambulatory TEE is generally more involved in younger patients from the practical aspects. Even with sedation, children and adolescents are rarely able to cooperate and lie still. This not only can compromise patient safety but adds the potential for damage to the TEE probe. Thus, deep sedation or general anesthesia is necessary in most patients particularly in those with significant cyanosis, myocardial dysfunction, or potential ventilatory abnormalities [87].

When standard TTE imaging is unsatisfactory, the need for ambulatory TEE must be ascertained after a risk versus benefit analysis. This involves consideration of the type of information required and alternative diagnostic imaging modalities along with their attendant risk and benefits. Despite a good safety profile, TEE is a semi-invasive procedure with important potential risks and relative/absolute contraindications. Cardiac catheterization, cardiac magnetic resonance imaging, and chest tomography each provide certain types information (i.e., hemodynamic measurements, aortic arch imaging) that cannot be obtained by TEE. Nonetheless, there are a number of instances in which ambulatory TEE can provide superior diagnostic information in the patient with CHD, even compared to other imaging modalities. Abnormal atrioventricular valves, for example, are much better evaluated by TEE than other diagnostic approaches, as are prosthetic valves (Chap. 16). Subaortic membranes and subaortic stenosis are clearly shown by TEE, as are atrial septal defects, particularly those of the superior sinus venosus type. Other examples (by no means inclusive) include ventricular septal defect morphology, aortic valve pathology, proximal coronary artery anatomy, and relationship of ventricular defects to the semilunar valves (e.g. in complex malpositions of the heart). There are certain types of postoperative cardiac defects in which TEE is extremely useful, i.e. in patients who have undergone atrial baffles (Mustard/Senning procedures), Fontan, or Rastelli procedures. It is also well documented that TEE plays an important role in the evaluation of endocarditis and other infectious pathologies.

Critical Care Setting

The critical care setting is one area in which TEE can provide significant benefit. While TTE remains the first modality of choice for noninvasive cardiac assessment, a number of factors associated with the nature of the intensive care unit (ICU) can significantly limit the effectiveness of TTE. These factors include mechanical ventilation, tenuous hemodynamic and respiratory status, inability to alter patient positioning, and in some cases, recent cardiac and/or thoracic surgery. Such factors often contribute to poor or nonexistent conditions for TTE imaging. Indeed, in the adult experience the percentage of successful diagnostic TTE examinations approximates only about 50 % [88, 89], whereas TEE examination yields adequate results in >90 % of cases [90]. Thus, TEE now plays an increasing role in the diagnostic evaluation of adult patients in the critical care unit, particularly for indications unique to that setting including unexplained hypotension, suspected pulmonary embolism, unexplained hypoxemia, suspected endocarditis, prosthetic valve assessment, central line placement, and complications of cardiothoracic surgery [91, 92]. For pediatric patients in the ICU, indications for TEE are similar to those in adults but there are additional considerations pertinent to the child and young adult with CHD [93]. First, since patients are younger and tend to have better echocardiographic windows, TTE tends to provide more satisfactory imaging in general as previously mentioned, although image quality can vary significantly. Second, the semi-invasive nature of the TEE procedure necessitates careful consideration, particularly in the younger or more unstable patient. As in the ambulatory setting, TEE in the younger patient is optimally performed under conditions of deep sedation/endotracheal intubation. In the unintubated patient, a determination must be made as to whether the potential additional information gleaned from TEE warrants the small additional risk associated with the examination, particularly as compared to alternate diagnostic modalities. Third, the examiner must have a thorough understanding of the patient's previous history and underlying cardiac anatomy, as well as the specific indications for the TEE study. Common indications for TEE in the critical care setting include:

- Evaluation of underlying cardiovascular anatomy
- Evaluation of valvar function, particularly prosthetic valves
- Evaluation of myocardial function and hemodynamics
- Evaluation of results of cardiothoracic surgery
- Investigation of possible occult shunts (right-to-left, left-to-right)
- Evaluation for infective endocarditis and associated complications
- Assessment of intracardiac thrombus, mass, indwelling lines
- Evaluation of mechanical circulatory assist devices/weaning from circulatory support

Guidelines for Training and Performance of Transesophageal Echocardiography in Congenital Heart Disease and Pediatric Acquired Heart Disease

Knowledge Base, Skills, and Training Guidelines

The American Society of Echocardiography Committee for Physician Training in Echocardiography published guidelines for training in TEE in 1992 [3]. The recommendations were aimed at physicians in general wishing to provide TEE services either in the operating room environment or other nonoperative settings. The report suggested that individuals using TEE should have:

- *Thorough knowledge of cardiac disease and the hemodynamic alterations associated with acquired and congenital disorders*
- *Understanding of ultrasonic image formation and Doppler assessment of intracardiac blood flow*
- *Familiarity with the range of normal structural findings and the echocardiographic manifestations of a large number of cardiac disorders*

Initial practice guidelines specifically addressing the use of perioperative TEE were published in 1996 [5]. Subsequently, task forces by the American Society of Echocardiography and Society of Cardiovascular Anesthesiologists have documented guidelines for physician training on the subject [10, 93, 94]. In these reports, different levels of expertise in echocardiography are recognized and level-specific recommendations for training outlined. In addition to the training objectives suggested for basic level perioperative TEE practice, the advances level assumes comprehensive cognitive and technical skills to allow for the full potential applications of the TEE technology. TEE practice in pediatric patients and those with CHD is considered within the advanced pathway. Training requirements with respect to this application include detailed knowledge of the techniques, advantages, disadvantages, and potential complications of commonly used cardiac surgical procedures for the treatment of acquired and CHD.

In regards to training elements for the practice of advanced perioperative echocardiography, guidelines focusing mostly on adult applications suggest the following [10]:

- *Minimum number of TEE examinations: 300*
- *Minimum number of TEE examinations personally performed: 150*
- *Program director qualifications: Advanced perioperative echocardiography training in addition to atleast 150 additional perioperative TEE examinations*
- *Program qualifications: Full spectrum of perioperative applications of echocardiography*

A task force by the American College of Cardiology/American Heart Association/American College of Physicians-American Society of Internal Medicine in collaboration with other professional societies focused on clinical competence in echocardiography and published a statement on the subject in 2003 [7]. The document distinguished between training requirements and documentation of competence.

Regarding competence with respect to CHD, cognitive skills required for TEE included knowledge of alterations in cardiovascular anatomy that result from congenital pathology and their specific appearance on TEE.

Skills necessary to perform perioperative echocardiography in patients with CHD were listed under the category of advanced level and specified:

- *Knowledge of the echocardiographic manifestations of CHD*
- *Ability to utilize TEE to evaluate congenital heart lesions*
- *Ability to assess surgical intervention in CHD*

The guidelines underscored the requirement for additional training in CHD. In regards to training requirements for performance and interpretation of TEE, for individuals in a formal cardiology fellowship training program the guidelines indicated the following:

- *Need for attainment of at least level 2 experience in general TTE*
- *Performance of approximately 25 TEE probe placements*
- *Performance of approximately 50 diagnostic TEE examinations under supervision, including review, interpretation and reporting of study findings*

The task force emphasized that in certain specialized clinical settings even this training may be not be adequate for independent TEE practice and cited the assessment of complex CHD as one of these situations.

It is acknowledged that physicians from different specialties must attain comparable expertise in perioperative echocardiography while requiring different training to reach this goal. It is also recognized that trainees from different disciplines would use their time in training somewhat differently, depending on their varying backgrounds.

Although several publications delineate guidelines for perioperative echocardiography in general, it is well known that competent performance of TEE in pediatric patients with congenital or acquired heart disease, or adult patients with CHD, requires specialized knowledge, skills, and training. The guidelines for performance of TEE in these patient groups differ in many respects from those for TEE in the general adult population.

In recognition of the unique aspects and evolving applications of TEE, the statement of the Pediatric Council of the American Society of Echocardiography issued in 2005 outlined guidelines for performance of TEE in these particular patient groups [9]. Regarding knowledge base and skills the recommendations can be summarized as follows:

- *Fundamental knowledge, experience, and familiarity with the diagnosis of congenital cardiac abnormalities and acquired pediatric cardiovascular pathology are required. This assumes an understanding of normal cardiovascular anatomy, variants, spectrum of CHD, acquired diseases, associated hemodynamic perturbations, surgical options, etc.*
- *A thorough knowledge of two-dimensional echocardiography is necessary in order to recognize normal and abnormal anatomic findings, in addition to using the color and spectral Doppler modalities to define both normal intracardiac flow velocities and patterns, as well as correctly interpreting flow disturbances.*
- *In addition to being able to accurately interpret the information, under at times the most challenging circumstances, the ability to communicate the findings and other relevant information to appropriate health care providers (surgeons, interventionalists, other physicians) is essential.*
- *Technical skills include competency in probe placement, transducer manipulation to achieve suitable views for interrogation, and optimization of the two-dimensional image and Doppler settings by instrument control adjustments.*
- *Experience is necessary in a variety of clinical settings (operating room, cardiac catheterization laboratory, intensive care unit, and outpatient setting).*

Specific recommendations regarding guidelines for training and maintenance of proficiency in the performance of

Table 3.2 Guidelines for training and maintenance of competence in transesophageal echocardiography for congenital heart disease

Component	Objective	Duration	Number of cases
Echocardiography (Level 2) [3, 4, 7]	Prior experience in performing/ interpreting TTE	6 months or equivalent	400: ≥ 200 < 1 year
Esophageal intubation	TEE probe insertion	Variable	25 cases (12 < 2 years)
TEE exam	Perform and interpret with supervision	Variable	50 cases
Ongoing TEE experience (Level 3) [3, 4, 7]	Maintenance of competency	Annual	50 cases; or achievement of laboratory-established outcomes variables

Reprinted from Ayres et al. [9]; with permission from Elsevier
TEE Transesophageal echocardiography, *TTE* transthoracic echocardiography

TEE in this patient population were made as indicated in Table 3.2. In addition to prerequisite experience in TTE, a minimum number (25 cases) of esophageal intubations were suggested, as well as performance and interpretation of examinations under supervision. For physicians without formal training in pediatric cardiology or without a focus on TEE, acquisition of medical/echocardiographic knowledge base and practical skills equivalent to those acquired during pediatric cardiology specialty training were recommended in order to perform TEE independently. Required cognitive skills included knowledge of cardiac anatomy, congenital and acquired cardiac pathology, pathophysiology, differential diagnosis, and alternative diagnostic modalities.

The issue of who should be responsible for the intraoperative TEE interpretation in patients undergoing interventions for CHD and the respective roles of the specialized perioperative providers has been the subject of raging controversy [96–101]. To ensure quality of the evaluation, interpretation of findings, and to promote patient safety, expertise is required. The availability of a second appropriately trained individual in echocardiography or cardiovascular anesthesiology has been suggested when intraoperative echocardiography is being performed by a cardiovascular anesthesiologist. In their statement the Pediatric Council of the American Society of Echocardiography indicated that there was no intent in their guidelines of excluding physicians from performing TEE in pediatric patients. Ideally, intraoperative imaging should be collaboration between pediatric cardiologists, anesthesiologists, and cardiothoracic surgeons.

Safety Considerations and Complications

The safety of TEE has been the focus of various reports. A number of studies comprising large numbers of patients, and following an extensive clinical experience in the adult population (including relatively high-risk patient groups), have documented an overall extremely favorable safety profile for this modality [102–106].

Data in the pediatric age group likewise demonstrates a high margin of safety and low incidence of TEE-related complications in the range of 1–3 %. The use of TEE has been successfully reported in very small infants under 3.0 kg in weight, however extreme caution must be exercised in view of potential procedure-related respiratory or hemodynamic compromise [107].

Stevenson prospectively examined the incidence and severity of complications during TEE in 1650 pediatric cases (mean age of 3.6 years, mean weight of 17.2 kg) [108]. The complication rate was reported to be low, occurring in 2.4 % of the patient group (failure of probe placement excluded). Problems, when encountered, were mostly related to the respiratory system or vascular compression. No significant bleeding, arrhythmias, esophageal injuries, or deaths occurred.

Other studies addressing the use of TEE in children and/or during surgery for CHD have reported upon safety and the low incidence of complications. Randolph and associates did not identify major complications among 1,002 patients that comprised both children and adults with CHD [109]. Minor complications were noted in 1 % of the cases, most often observed in infants less than 4 kg in weight. A 10-year experience that examined 580 TEE studies during pediatric cardiac surgery observed a 2.7 % incidence of complications and the absence of any prolonged problems or morbidity secondary to TEE [110]. Others have reported similar results [111].

Andropoulos and colleagues evaluated the impact of TEE on ventilation and hemodynamic variables in small infants undergoing cardiac surgery [112, 113]. No significant changes in several measured parameters of gas exchange and pulmonary mechanics were observed in relation to probe insertion. The investigation noted that hemodynamic complications from TEE, although possible, were rare in this patient group. These data provided reassurance to those involved in intraoperative TEE imaging of very young infants.

Evidence linking anticoagulation with a significant risk for bleeding during a TEE examination is lacking. However, since minor trauma to oropharyngeal structures may occur at the time of probe placement and/or removal, it may be prudent for these maneuvers to be performed during times when patients are not expected to be fully heparinized for cardiopulmonary bypass.

Although rarely observed, the most frequently encountered complications relate to trauma to the oropharynx and/or esophagus, resulting in symptomatology such as pharyngeal discomfort, odynophagia, and dysphagia. The use of direct laryngoscopic guidance during TEE probe placement has been examined in adult patients in an effort to minimize potential oropharyngeal mucosal injury [114]. Whether this may also be the case in children remains to be determined. An interesting investigation proposed that head positioning to the side rather than the midline facilitated esophageal intubation with the TEE probe in children under 10 kg of body weight. The study theorized that anatomic changes in the hypopharynx associated with head turning would favor probe passage, which in their experience was confirmed by turning the head to the left [115].

Less likely problems related to TEE are respiratory difficulties or hemodynamic changes. Reported complications include: accidental tracheal extubation, ventilatory compromise related to impingement of the esophageal probe on the tracheobronchial tree, and alterations of cardiac rhythm [116–122]. Compression of adjacent cardiovascular structures by the probe has been reported resulting in circulatory derangement [123]. Compression of an aberrant subclavian artery may lead to a dampened radial artery blood pressure tracing [124]. Descending aortic compression may manifest as a change in the contour of a lower extremity arterial tracing or pulse oximeter signal. Serious complications such as esophageal perforation, inadvertent gastric incision during sternotomy, and subglottic stenosis have been described although, fortunately, these have been extremely rare [108, 125, 126].

One particular circumstance deserves further discussion. A cause for concern in infants undergoing intraoperative evaluation of total anomalous pulmonary venous drainage has been the potential for hemodynamic compromise resulting from compression of the pulmonary venous confluence by a TEE probe [127]. The issue was addressed in a case series that included 28 infants (ages 1 day to 7 months) with various types of anomalous pulmonary venous connections [128]. The study demonstrated the utility of TEE in the recognition of residual pulmonary venous obstruction and other pathology that deserved intraoperative attention, validating the benefits of the TEE examination in this subset of patients. However, nearly a third of the cohort developed acute hypotension and hypoxemia following probe insertion, prompting probe withdrawal. No changes in these parameters were recorded upon probe reinsertion after sternotomy. This approach was suggested in order to improve the margin of safety of TEE imaging in these infants. Clinical experience indicates that when TEE imaging is used in this group of patients, closed observation for possible hemodynamic compromise is warranted.

Trauma to the esophagus during TEE may be due to probe insertion, manipulation, or direct ultrasound energy transmission resulting in thermal injury. A few publications have addressed the subject of esophageal morbidity related to TEE in pediatric patients. A study by Greene and associates described findings upon flexible endoscopic examination in 50 children following cardiac surgery where TEE imaging was performed [129]. Children ranged from 4 days to 10 years of age, with a mean weight of 12.6 kg. Thirty-two of 50 patients (64 %) were found to have abnormal findings on the endoscopic examination. These occurred more frequently in those under 9 kg of body weight. Abnormalities included erythema, edema, and hematoma. Less frequently, mucosal erosion and petechiae were seen. No long-term feeding or swallowing difficulties were identified among the perioperative survivors. In view of the mild mucosal injury detected, it was suggested that meticulous care must be exercised in the insertion and manipulation of TEE probes in all patients, but particularly in the smallest of infants. To reduce the potential risk of thermal energy damage, the TEE probe should be advanced into the stomach and remain in a neutral position, non-imaging (frozen) mode when not interrogating the heart.

Kohr and coworkers investigated the incidence of dysphagia in pediatric patients following the use of TEE during cardiac surgery [130]. A significant proportion of the cohort was under 3 years of age. Among study patients, a high prevalence of complex cardiovascular disease was present. Dysphagia was found in 9 of the 50 patients (18 %). Risks factors included age less than 3 years, preoperative endotracheal intubation, longer duration of endotracheal intubation, and interventions for left-sided obstructive lesions. According to the authors, the presence of dysphagia affected postoperative recovery and contributed to major morbidity.

Recently a retrospective study was undertaken to evaluate risk factors for TEE probe insertion failure in neonates (<4 kg) undergoing cardiac surgery [131]. The imaging devices examined included the pediatric TEE biplane and pediatric minimultiplane probes. Factors associated with failure to insert these probes (defined as inability to advance TEE device into the mid esophagus or change in ventilatory or hemodynamic status) included lower weight, prematurity, abnormal craniofacial anatomy, and 22q11 deletion. Based on these findings an algorithm was proposed for either attempting or avoiding TEE placement in this patient group.

Despite the rare potential for morbidity and higher likelihood of complications in small infants, the overall experience supports that the benefit/risk assessment significantly favors the use TEE in the pediatric age group. The recent further miniaturization of imaging probes may provide for even safer applications of this modality in the smallest of infants.

Contraindications

In the task force report addressing guidelines for the performance of TEE in pediatric patients with congenital or acquired cardiovascular disease several contraindications were noted [9]. These were categorized into relative and absolute as listed in Table 3.3.

Table 3.3 Contraindications for transesophageal echocardiography

Absolute contraindications	Relative contraindications
Unrepaired tracheoesophageal fistula	History of prior esophageal surgery
Esophageal obstruction or stricture	Esophageal varices or diverticulum
Perforated hollow viscus	Gastric or esophageal bleeding
Poor airway control	Vascular ring, aortic arch anomaly with or without airway compromise
Severe respiratory depression	Oropharyngeal pathology
Uncooperative, unsedated patient	Severe coagulopathy
	Cervical spine injury or anomaly

Reprinted from Ayres et al. [9]; with permission from Elsevier

In general terms, patients with the potential for injuries related to probe insertion and/or manipulation include those with intrinsic esophageal abnormalities. High-risk conditions are congenital tracheoesophageal fistula, esophageal stricture, esophageal varices or diverticulum, or a history of prior esophageal surgery. The presence of Down syndrome in some cases has been associated with difficult TEE probe placement [132]. This may be related to a relatively large tongue or potential intrinsic narrowing of hypopharyngeal structures in these children. Individuals with Down syndrome are known to be at risk for cervical spine instability that may threaten spinal cord integrity. Although no consensus or evidence-based guidelines exist, nor specific recommendations regarding this issue in patients with Down syndrome, it may be prudent to exert gentle care to the neck during probe placement [133, 134]. Another consideration in these children is the potential for sinus bradycardia and in very rare cases, sinus arrest, presumably related to vagal stimulation during probe placement. Some practitioners anecdotally advocate the prophylactic administration of anticholinergic agents to prevent excessive bradycardia leading to hemodynamic alterations.

Surgical procedures that address isolated aortic arch anomalies, such as vascular rings, generally do not benefit significantly from TEE. In fact, TEE probe insertion in these cases, may lead to respiratory compromise since the trachea and esophagus are restricted to a confined space by the surrounding vascular structures.

Although the safety of TEE has not been formally examined following gastrostomy tube/button placement with or without Nissen fundoplication, it may be reasonable if a TEE examination is warranted to restrict the imaging planes to those obtained via the esophageal views and exclude interrogation from the transgastric and deep transgastric windows. It is unclear how long after these procedures should TEE imaging be undertaken, or whether the risk varies according to the exact nature of the procedure (percutaneous versus open gastrostomy tube placement).

Previously published practice guidelines for perioperative TEE by a task force of the American Society of Anesthesiologists and Society of Cardiovascular Anesthesiologists addressed contraindications to TEE imaging in the adult [48]. These are summarized in Table 3.4. Although there was some disagreement regarding the conditions considered to represent a contraindication for the use of TEE between members of the American Society of Anesthesiologists and consultants, the recommendation was that "TEE may the be used for patients with oral, esophageal, or gastric disease, if the expected benefit outweighs the potential risk, provided the appropriate precautions are applied."

We would recommend that if, after a careful assessment the use of TEE is favored, the following approaches may be considered in order to minimize potential problems: a focused examination to address important/critical issues, limiting unnecessary probe handling/manipulation, and restricting the examination to individuals with the highest level of expertise. In patients at potentially increased risk, considerations should be given for the use of alternate intraoperative imaging modalities, such as epicardial echocardiography.

Risk of Bacteremia and Endocarditis Prophylaxis

It has been documented that gastrointestinal endoscopic procedures can be associated with bacteremia [135]. The frequency of bacteremia has been linked to specific interventions performed. However, in general the overall incidence of bacteremia as a result of upper gastrointestinal endoscopy is considered small [136]. Although endocarditis temporally related to the TEE examination has been reported, the incidence of positive bacterial blood cultures immediately following TEE has been found to be very low, near 2 % or within the expected rate of false positive results [137, 138].

In the past, based on the low likelihood of endocarditis related to TEE, the routine administration of antibiotic prophylaxis was not recommended but could be considered optional in very high-risk individuals. Most recent American Heart Association guidelines, however, do not support the administration of antibiotics solely to prevent endocarditis for patients who undergo gastrointestinal tract procedures

Table 3.4 Contraindications for the use of transesophageal echocardiography as reported by perioperative practice guidelines

Conditions considered as ***absolute*** *contraindications by both ASA members and consultants*
Esophagectomy
Esophagogastrectomy
Conditions considered as ***absolute*** *contraindications, in addition to the above conditions, by some ASA members and consultants*
Esophageal stricture
Tracheoesophageal fistula
Postesophageal surgery
Esophageal trauma
Conditions that ***do not represent*** *absolute contraindications by both ASA members and consultants*
Barrett esophagus
Hiatal hernia
Large descending aortic aneurysm
Unilateral vocal cord paralysis
Conditions considered ***equivocal*** *as absolute contraindications by both ASA members and consultants*
Esophageal varices
Postradiation therapy
Previous bariatric surgery
Conditions with ***conflicting*** *opinions*
Zenker diverticulum
Colonic interposition
Dysphagia

ASA American Society of Anesthesiologists

[139]. The implication is that this also applies to esophageal instrumentation related to TEE.

Summary

High-resolution TEE imaging allows for comprehensive anatomic, hemodynamic, and functional evaluation in patients with CHD and pediatric acquired heart disease. The extensive benefits of TEE in the perioperative period and other non-surgical settings has led to its recognition as a critical tool and incorporation into several aspects of the standard of care by many CHD centers and those that specialize in the care of children with cardiovascular disease. It is anticipated that further refinements in ultrasound technology in the future will continue to expand the applications of TEE and add to the already significant contributions of this imaging modality in the management of these patients.

References

1. Schiller NB, Maurer G, Ritter SB, et al. Transesophageal echocardiography. J Am Soc Echocardiogr. 1989;2:354–7.
2. ACC/AHA guidelines for the clinical application of echocardiography. A report of the American College of Cardiology/American Heart Association Task Force on Assessment of Diagnostic and Therapeutic Cardiovascular Procedures (Subcommittee to Develop Guidelines for the Clinical Application of Echocardiography). J Am Coll Cardiol. 1990;16:1505–28.
3. Pearlman AS, Gardin JM, Martin RP, et al. Guidelines for physician training in transesophageal echocardiography: recommendations of the American Society of Echocardiography Committee for Physician Training in Echocardiography. J Am Soc Echocardiogr. 1992;5:187–94.
4. Fyfe DA, Ritter SB, Snider AR, et al. Guidelines for transesophageal echocardiography in children. J Am Soc Echocardiogr. 1992;5:640–4.
5. Practice guidelines for perioperative transesophageal echocardiography. A report by the American Society of Anesthesiologists and the Society of Cardiovascular Anesthesiologists Task Force on Transesophageal Echocardiography. Anesthesiology. 1996;84:986–1006.
6. Cheitlin MD, Alpert JS, Armstrong WF, et al. ACC/AHA guidelines for the clinical application of echocardiography: executive summary. A report of the American College of Cardiology/American Heart Association Task Force on practice guidelines (Committee on Clinical Application of Echocardiography). Developed in collaboration with the American Society of Echocardiography. J Am Coll Cardiol. 1997;29:862–79.
7. Quinones MA, Douglas PS, Foster E, et al. ACC/AHA clinical competence statement on echocardiography: a report of the American College of Cardiology/American Heart Association/American College of Physicians-American Society of Internal Medicine Task Force on Clinical Competence. J Am Coll Cardiol. 2003;41:687–708.
8. Douglas PS, Khandheria B, Stainback RF, et al. ACCF/ASE/ACEP/ASNC/SCAI/SCCT/SCMR 2007 appropriateness criteria for transthoracic and transesophageal echocardiography: a report of the American College of Cardiology Foundation Quality Strategic Directions Committee Appropriateness Criteria Working Group, American Society of Echocardiography, American College of Emergency Physicians, American Society of Nuclear Cardiology, Society for Cardiovascular Angiography and Interventions, Society of Cardiovascular Computed Tomography, and the Society for Cardiovascular Magnetic Resonance endorsed by the American

College of Chest Physicians and the Society of Critical Care Medicine. J Am Coll Cardiol. 2007;50:187–204.
9. Ayres NA, Miller-Hance W, Fyfe DA, et al. Indications and guidelines for performance of transesophageal echocardiography in the patient with pediatric acquired or congenital heart disease: report from the task force of the Pediatric Council of the American Society of Echocardiography. J Am Soc Echocardiogr. 2005;18:91–8.
10. Hahn RT, Abraham T, Adams MS et al. Guidelines for performing a comprehensive transesophageal echocardiographic examination: recommendations from the American Society of Echocardiography and the Society of Cardiovascular Anesthesiologists. J Am Soc Echocardiogr. 2013;26:921–64.
11. Schneider B, Zienkiewicz T, Jansen V, et al. Diagnosis of patent foramen ovale by transesophageal echocardiography and correlation with autopsy findings. Am J Cardiol. 1996;77:1202–9.
12. Siostrzonek P, Zangeneh M, Gossinger H, et al. Comparison of transesophageal and transthoracic contrast echocardiography for detection of a patent foramen ovale. Am J Cardiol. 1991;68:1247–9.
13. Acar P, Dulac Y, Roux D, et al. Comparison of transthoracic and transesophageal three-dimensional echocardiography for assessment of atrial septal defect diameter in children. Am J Cardiol. 2003;91:500–2.
14. Fyfe DA, Kline CH, Sade RM, et al. Transesophageal echocardiography detects thrombus formation not identified by transthoracic echocardiography after the Fontan operation. J Am Coll Cardiol. 1991;18:1733–7.
15. Fyfe DA, Kline CH, Sade RM, et al. The utility of transesophageal echocardiography during and after Fontan operations in small children. Am Heart J. 1991;122:1403–15.
16. Lam J, Neirotti R, Becker AE, et al. Thrombosis after the Fontan procedure: transesophageal echocardiography may replace angiocardiography. J Thorac Cardiovasc Surg. 1994;108:194–5.
17. Leung DY, Cranney GB, Hopkins AP, et al. Role of transoesophageal echocardiography in the diagnosis and management of aortic root abscess. Br Heart J. 1994;72:175–81.
18. Stumper O, Sutherland GR, Geuskens R, et al. Transesophageal echocardiography in evaluation and management after a Fontan procedure. J Am Coll Cardiol. 1991;17:1152–60.
19. Horenstein MS, Karpawich PP, Epstein ML, et al. Transthoracic echocardiography for precardioversion screening during atrial flutter/fibrillation in young patients. Clin Cardiol. 2004;27:413–6.
20. Miyake Y, Sugioka K, Bussey CD, et al. Left ventricular mobile thrombus associated with ventricular assist device: diagnosis by transesophageal echocardiography. Circ J. 2004;68:383–4.
21. Scohy TV, Gommers D, Maat AP, et al. Intraoperative transesophageal echocardiography is beneficial for hemodynamic stabilization during left ventricular assist device implantation in children. Paediatr Anaesth. 2009;19(4):390–5.
22. Andropoulos DB. Transesophageal echocardiography as a guide to central venous catheter placement in pediatric patients undergoing cardiac surgery. J Cardiothorac Vasc Anesth. 1999;13:320–1.
23. Stumper OF, Elzenga NJ, Hess J, et al. Transesophageal echocardiography in children with congenital heart disease: an initial experience. J Am Coll Cardiol. 1990;16:433–41.
24. Ungerleider RM. The use of intraoperative echocardiography with Doppler color flow imaging in the repair of congenital heart defects. Echocardiography. 1990;7:289–304.
25. Stumper O, Kaulitz R, Elzenga NJ, et al. The value of transesophageal echocardiography in children with congenital heart disease. J Am Soc Echocardiogr. 1991;4:164–76.
26. Sutherland GR, Stumper OF. Transoesophageal echocardiography in congenital heart disease. Acta Paediatr Suppl. 1995;410:15–22.
27. Ungerleider RM, Kisslo JA, Greeley WJ, et al. Intraoperative echocardiography during congenital heart operations: experience from 1,000 cases. Ann Thorac Surg. 1995;60:S539–42.
28. Stevenson JG. Role of intraoperative transesophageal echocardiography during repair of congenital cardiac defects. Acta Paediatr Suppl. 1995;410:23–33.
29. Muhiudeen Russell IA, Miller-Hance WC, Silverman NH. Intraoperative transesophageal echocardiography for pediatric patients with congenital heart disease. Anesth Analg. 1998;87:1058–76.
30. Miller-Hance WC, Silverman NH. Transesophageal echocardiography (TEE) in congenital heart disease with focus on the adult. Cardiol Clin. 2000;18:861–92.
31. Bettex DA, Schmidlin D, Bernath MA, et al. Intraoperative transesophageal echocardiography in pediatric congenital cardiac surgery: a two-center observational study. Anesth Analg. 2003;97: 1275–82.
32. Stevenson JG. Utilization of intraoperative transesophageal echocardiography during repair of congenital cardiac defects: a survey of North American centers. Clin Cardiol. 2003;26:132–4.
33. Russell IA, Rouine-Rapp K, Stratmann G, et al. Congenital heart disease in the adult: a review with internet-accessible transesophageal echocardiographic images. Anesth Analg. 2006;102:694–723.
34. Sundar S, DiNardo JA. Transesophageal echocardiography in pediatric surgery. Int Anesthesiol Clin. 2008;46:137–55.
35. Kamra K, Russell I, Miller-Hance WC. Role of transesophageal echocardiography in the management of pediatric patients with congenital heart disease. Paediatr Anaesth. 2011;21:479–93.
36. Al-Rashidi F, Landenhed M, Blomquist S, et al. Comparison of the effectiveness and safety of a new de-airing technique with a standardized carbon dioxide insufflation technique in open left heart surgery: a randomized clinical trial. J Thorac Cardiovasc Surg. 2011;141:1128–33.
37. Leung JM, Schiller NB, Mangano DT. Transesophageal echocardiographic assessment of left ventricular function. Int J Card Imaging. 1989;5:63–70.
38. Nishimura RA, Abel MD, Housmans PR, et al. Mitral flow velocity curves as a function of different loading conditions: evaluation by intraoperative transesophageal Doppler echocardiography. J Am Soc Echocardiogr. 1989;2:79–87.
39. Reich DL, Konstadt SN, Nejat M, et al. Intraoperative transesophageal echocardiography for the detection of cardiac preload changes induced by transfusion and phlebotomy in pediatric patients. Anesthesiology. 1993;79:10–5.
40. Ninomiya J, Yamauchi H, Hosaka H, et al. Continuous transoesophageal echocardiography monitoring during weaning from cardiopulmonary bypass in children. Cardiovasc Surg. 1997;5:129–33.
41. Lavoie J, Burrows FA, Gentles TL, et al. Transoesophageal echocardiography detects residual ductal flow during video-assisted thoracoscopic patent ductus arteriosus interruption. Can J Anaesth. 1994;41:310–3.
42. Sardari FF, Schlunt ML, Applegate 2nd RL, et al. The use of transesophageal echocardiography to guide sternal division for cardiac operations via mini-sternotomy. J Card Surg. 1997;12:67–70.
43. Ho AC, Tan PP, Yang MW, et al. The use of multiplane transesophageal echocardiography to evaluate residual patent ductus arteriosus during video-assisted thoracoscopy in adults. Surg Endosc. 1999;13:975–9.
44. Ho AC, Chen CK, Yang MW, et al. Usefulness of intraoperative transesophageal echocardiography in the assessment of surgical repair of pediatric ventricular septal defects with video-assisted endoscopic techniques in children. Chang Gung Med J. 2004;27:646–53.
45. Marcus B, Wong PC, Wells WJ, et al. Transesophageal echocardiography in the postoperative child with an open sternum. Ann Thorac Surg. 1994;58:235–6.
46. Scott PJ, Blackburn ME, Wharton GA, et al. Transoesophageal echocardiography in neonates, infants and children: applicability and diagnostic value in everyday practice of a cardiothoracic unit. Br Heart J. 1992;68:488–92.

47. Scheinin SA, Radovancevic B, Ott DA, et al. Postcardiotomy LVAD support and transesophageal echocardiography in a child. Ann Thorac Surg. 1993;55:529–31.
48. American Society of Anesthesiologists and Society of Cardiovascular Anesthesiologists Task Force on Transesophageal Echocardiography. Practice guidelines for perioperative transesophageal echocardiography. An updated report by the American Society of Anesthesiologists and the Society of Cardiovascular Anesthesiologists Task Force on Transesophageal Echocardiography. Anesthesiology. 2010;112:1084–96.
49. Bouch DC, Allsager CM, Moore N. Peri-operative trans-oesophageal echocardiography and nitric oxide during general anaesthesia in a patient with Eisenmenger's syndrome. Anaesthesia. 2006;61:996–1000.
50. Catena E, Mele D. Role of intraoperative transesophageal echocardiography in patients undergoing noncardiac surgery. J Cardiovasc Med (Hagerstown). 2008;9:993–1003.
51. Neira VM, Gardin L, Ryan G, et al. A transesophageal echocardiography examination clarifies the cause of cardiovascular collapse during scoliosis surgery in a child. Can J Anaesth. 2011;58:451–5.
52. Fleisher LA, Beckman JA, Brown KA, et al. ACC/AHA 2007 Guidelines on Perioperative Cardiovascular Evaluation and Care for Noncardiac Surgery: Executive Summary: A Report of the American College of Cardiology/American Heart Association Task Force on Practice Guidelines (Writing Committee to Revise the 2002 Guidelines on Perioperative Cardiovascular Evaluation for Noncardiac Surgery) Developed in Collaboration With the American Society of Echocardiography, American Society of Nuclear Cardiology, Heart Rhythm Society, Society of Cardiovascular Anesthesiologists, Society for Cardiovascular Angiography and Interventions, Society for Vascular Medicine and Biology, and Society for Vascular Surgery. J Am Coll Cardiol. 2007;50:1707–32.
53. Stumper O, Witsenburg M, Sutherland GR, et al. Transesophageal echocardiographic monitoring of interventional cardiac catheterization in children. J Am Coll Cardiol. 1991;18:1506–14.
54. van der Velde ME, Perry SB, Sanders SP. Transesophageal echocardiography with color Doppler during interventional catheterization. Echocardiography. 1991;8:721–30.
55. Tumbarello R, Sanna A, Cardu G, et al. Usefulness of transesophageal echocardiography in the pediatric catheterization laboratory. Am J Cardiol. 1993;71:1321–5.
56. Tong AD, Rothman A, Shiota T, et al. Interventional cardiac catheterization under transesophageal echocardiographic guidance. Am Heart J. 1995;129:827–31.
57. Van Der Velde ME, Perry SB. Transesophageal echocardiography during interventional catheterization in congenital heart disease. Echocardiography. 1997;14:513–28.
58. Cheung YF, Leung MP, Lee J, et al. An evolving role of transesophageal echocardiography for the monitoring of interventional catheterization in children. Clin Cardiol. 1999;22:804–10.
59. Rigby ML. Transoesophageal echocardiography during interventional cardiac catheterisation in congenital heart disease. Heart. 2001;86 Suppl 2:II23–9.
60. Hellenbrand WE, Fahey JT, McGowan FX, et al. Transesophageal echocardiographic guidance of transcatheter closure of atrial septal defect. Am J Cardiol. 1990;66:207–13.
61. Minich LL, Snider AR. Echocardiographic guidance during placement of the buttoned double-disk device for atrial septal defect closure. Echocardiography. 1993;10:567–72.
62. Elzenga NJ. The role of echocardiography in transcatheter closure of atrial septal defects. Cardiol Young. 2000;10:474–83.
63. Zhu W, Cao QL, Rhodes J, et al. Measurement of atrial septal defect size: a comparative study between three-dimensional transesophageal echocardiography and the standard balloon sizing methods. Pediatr Cardiol. 2000;21:465–9.
64. Latiff HA, Samion H, Kandhavel G, et al. The value of transesophageal echocardiography in transcatheter closure of atrial septal defects in the oval fossa using the Amplatzer septal occluder. Cardiol Young. 2001;11:201–4.
65. Mazic U, Gavora P, Masura J. The role of transesophageal echocardiography in transcatheter closure of secundum atrial septal defects by the Amplatzer septal occluder. Am Heart J. 2001;142:482–8.
66. Figueroa MI, Balaguru D, McClure C, et al. Experience with use of multiplane transesophageal echocardiography to guide closure of atrial septal defects using the amplatzer device. Pediatr Cardiol. 2002;23:430–6.
67. Lin SM, Tsai SK, Wang JK, et al. Supplementing transesophageal echocardiography with transthoracic echocardiography for monitoring transcatheter closure of atrial septal defects with attenuated anterior rim: a case series. Anesth Analg. 2003;96:1584–8.
68. Kleinman CS. Echocardiographic guidance of catheter-based treatments of atrial septal defect: transesophageal echocardiography remains the gold standard. Pediatr Cardiol. 2005;26:128–34.
69. van der Velde ME, Sanders SP, Keane JF, et al. Transesophageal echocardiographic guidance of transcatheter ventricular septal defect closure. J Am Coll Cardiol. 1994;23:1660–5.
70. Cao QL, Zabal C, Koenig P, et al. Initial clinical experience with intracardiac echocardiography in guiding transcatheter closure of perimembranous ventricular septal defects: feasibility and comparison with transesophageal echocardiography. Catheter Cardiovasc Interv. 2005;66:258–67.
71. Lam J, Tanke RB, van Oort A, et al. The use of transesophageal echocardiography monitoring of transcatheter closure of a persistent ductus arteriosus. Echocardiography. 2001;18:197–202.
72. Martin-Reyes R, Lopez-Fernandez T, Moreno-Yanguela M, et al. Role of real-time three-dimensional transoesophageal echocardiography for guiding transcatheter patent foramen ovale closure. Eur J Echocardiogr. 2009;10:148–50.
73. Gomez C, Lloyd T, Mosca R, et al. Fontan fenestration closure in the catheterization laboratory—echocardiographic evaluation of residual right to left shunts. Am J Cardiol. 1998;82(1304–6):A10–1.
74. Wang JK, Lin SM, Tsai SK, et al. Transesophageal echocardiography for recurrent aorto-left ventricular tunnel: transcatheter closure with an Amplatzer duct occluder. Echocardiography. 2006;23:258–9.
75. Kipel G, Arnon R, Ritter SB. Transesophageal echocardiographic guidance of balloon atrial septostomy. J Am Soc Echocardiogr. 1991;4:631–5.
76. Boutin C, Dyck J, Benson L, et al. Balloon atrial septostomy under transesophageal echocardiographic guidance. Pediatr Cardiol. 1992;13:176–7.
77. Walayat M, Cooper SG, Sholler GF. Transesophageal echocardiographic guidance of blade atrial septostomy in children. Catheter Cardiovasc Interv. 2001;52:200–2.
78. Ge S, Shiota T, Rice MJ, et al. Images in cardiovascular medicine. Transesophageal ultrasound imaging during stent implantation to relieve superior vena cava-to-intra-atrial baffle obstruction after mustard repair of transposition of the great arteries. Circulation. 1995;91:2679–80.
79. Weber HS, Mart CR, Myers JL. Transcarotid balloon valvuloplasty for critical aortic valve stenosis at the bedside via continuous transesophageal echocardiographic guidance. Catheter Cardiovasc Interv. 2000;50:326–9.
80. Hussain A, al Faraidi Y, Abdulhamed J, et al. Transesophageal echocardiography-guided transventricular balloon dilation of congenital critical aortic stenosis in the neonate and young infant. J Cardiothorac Vasc Anesth. 2002;16:766–72.
81. Kawauchi M, Gundry SR, Boucek MM, et al. Real-time monitoring of the endomyocardial biopsy site with pediatric transesophageal echocardiography. J Heart Lung Transplant. 1992;11:306–10.

82. Kronzon I, Tunick PA, Freedberg RS. Transesophageal echocardiography in pericardial disease and tamponade. Echocardiography. 1994;11:493–505.
83. Chen TH, Chan KC, Cheng YJ, et al. Bedside pericardiocentesis under the guidance of transesophageal echocardiography in a 13-month-old boy. J Formos Med Assoc. 2001;100:620–2.
84. Kamalesh M, Stokes K, Burger AJ. Transesophageal echocardiography assisted retrieval of embolized inferior vena cava stent. Cathet Cardiovasc Diagn. 1994;33:178–80.
85. Bacha EA, Hijazi ZM, Cao QL, et al. Hybrid pediatric cardiac surgery. Pediatr Cardiol. 2005;26:315–22.
86. Bacha EA, Cao QL, Galantowicz ME, et al. Multicenter experience with perventricular device closure of muscular ventricular septal defects. Pediatr Cardiol. 2005;26:169–75.
87. Marcus B, Steward DJ, Khan NR, et al. Outpatient transesophageal echocardiography with intravenous propofol anesthesia in children and adolescents. J Am Soc Echocardiogr. 1993;6:205–9.
88. Parker MM, Cunnion RE, Parrillo JE. Echocardiography and nuclear cardiac imaging in the critical care unit. JAMA. 1985;254:2935–9.
89. Heidenreich PA, Stainback RF, Redberg RF, et al. Transesophageal echocardiography predicts mortality in critically ill patients with unexplained hypotension. J Am Coll Cardiol. 1995;26:152–8.
90. Oh JK, Seward JB, Khandheria BK, et al. Transesophageal echocardiography in critically ill patients. Am J Cardiol. 1990;66:1492–5.
91. Font VE, Obarski TP, Klein AL, et al. Transesophageal echocardiography in the critical care unit. Cleve Clin J Med. 1991;58:315–22.
92. Heidenreich PA. Transesophageal echocardiography (TEE) in the critical care patient. Cardiol Clin. 2000;18:789–805, ix.
93. Wolfe LT, Rossi A, Ritter SB. Transesophageal echocardiography in infants and children: use and importance in the cardiac intensive care unit. J Am Soc Echocardiogr. 1993;6:286–9.
94. Cahalan MK, Stewart W, Pearlman A, et al. American Society of Echocardiography and Society of Cardiovascular Anesthesiologists task force guidelines for training in perioperative echocardiography. J Am Soc Echocardiogr. 2002;15:647–52.
95. Mathew JP, Glas K, Troianos CA et al. American Society of Echocardiography/Society of Cardiovascular Anesthesiologists recommendations and guidelines for continuous quality improvement in perioperative echocardiography. J Am Soc Echocardiogr. 2006;19:1303–13.
96. Fyfe D. Transesophageal echocardiography guidelines: return to bypass or to bypass the guidelines? J Am Soc Echocardiogr. 1999; 12:343–4.
97. Fyfe DA. Intraoperative transesophageal echocardiography in children with congenital heart disease: how, not Who! J Am Soc Echocardiogr. 1999;12:1011–3.
98. Russell IM, Silverman NH, Miller-Hance W, et al. Intraoperative transesophageal echocardiography for infants and children undergoing congenital heart surgery: the role of the anesthesiologist. J Am Soc Echocardiogr. 1999;12:1009–14.
99. Stevenson JG. Adherence to physician training guidelines for pediatric transesophageal echocardiography affects the outcome of patients undergoing repair of congenital cardiac defects. J Am Soc Echocardiogr. 1999;12:165–72.
100. Stevenson JG. Performance of intraoperative pediatric transesophageal echocardiography by anesthesiologists and echocardiographers: training and availability are more important than hats. J Am Soc Echocardiogr. 1999;12:1013–4.
101. Graydon C, Wilmshurst S, Best C. Transesophageal echocardiography (TEE) for pediatric cardiac surgery should routinely be performed and interpreted by a pediatric cardiac anesthetist: Moderator: Soriano S. Paediatr Anaesth. 2011;21:1150–8.
102. Daniel WG, Erbel R, Kasper W, et al. Safety of transesophageal echocardiography. A multicenter survey of 10,419 examinations. Circulation. 1991;83:817–21.
103. Stoddard MF, Longaker RA. The safety of transesophageal echocardiography in the elderly. Am Heart J. 1993;125:1358–62.
104. Kallmeyer IJ, Collard CD, Fox JA, et al. The safety of intraoperative transesophageal echocardiography: a case series of 7200 cardiac surgical patients. Anesth Analg. 2001;92:1126–30.
105. Garimella S, Longaker RA, Stoddard MF. Safety of transesophageal echocardiography in patients who are obese. J Am Soc Echocardiogr. 2002;15:1396–400.
106. Hilberath JN, Oakes DA, Shernan SK, et al. Safety of transesophageal echocardiography. J Am Soc Echocardiogr 2010;23:1115–27.
107. Mart CR, Fehr DM, Myers JL, et al. Intraoperative transesophageal echocardiography in a 1.4-kg infant with complex congenital heart disease. Pediatr Cardiol. 2003;24:84–5.
108. Stevenson JG. Incidence of complications in pediatric transesophageal echocardiography: experience in 1650 cases. J Am Soc Echocardiogr. 1999;12:527–32.
109. Randolph GR, Hagler DJ, Connolly HM, et al. Intraoperative transesophageal echocardiography during surgery for congenital heart defects. J Thorac Cardiovasc Surg. 2002;124:1176–82.
110. Bettex DA, Pretre R, Jenni R, et al. Cost-effectiveness of routine intraoperative transesophageal echocardiography in pediatric cardiac surgery: a 10-year experience. Anesth Analg. 2005;100:1271–5.
111. Sloth E, Pedersen J, Olsen KH, et al. Transoesophageal echocardiographic monitoring during paediatric cardiac surgery: obtainable information and feasibility in 532 children. Paediatr Anaesth. 2001;11:657–62.
112. Andropoulos DB, Ayres NA, Stayer SA, et al. The effect of transesophageal echocardiography on ventilation in small infants undergoing cardiac surgery. Anesth Analg. 2000;90:47–9.
113. Andropoulos DB, Stayer SA, Bent ST, et al. The effects of transesophageal echocardiography on hemodynamic variables in small infants undergoing cardiac surgery. J Cardiothorac Vasc Anesth. 2000;14:133–5.
114. Na S, Kim CS, Kim JY, et al. Rigid laryngoscope-assisted insertion of transesophageal echocardiography probe reduces oropharyngeal mucosal injury in anesthetized patients. Anesthesiology. 2009;110:38–40.
115. Mart CR, Rosen KL. Optimal head position during transesophageal echocardiographic probe insertion for pediatric patients weighing up to 10 kg. Pediatr Cardiol. 2009;30:441–6.
116. Gilbert TB, Panico FG, McGill WA, et al. Bronchial obstruction by transesophageal echocardiography probe in a pediatric cardiac patient. Anesth Analg. 1992;74:156–8.
117. Lunn RJ, Oliver WCJ, Hagler DJ, et al. Aortic compression by transesophageal echocardiographic probe in infants and children undergoing cardiac surgery. Anesthesiology. 1992;77:587–90.
118. Muhiudeen I, Silverman N. Intraoperative transesophageal echocardiography using high resolution imaging in infants and children with congenital heart disease. Echocardiography. 1993;10:599–608.
119. Stevenson JG, Sorensen GK. Proper probe size for pediatric transesophageal echocardiography. Am J Cardiol. 1993;72:491–2.
120. Bensky AS, O'Brien JJ, Hammon JW. Transesophageal echo probe compression of an aberrant right subclavian artery. J Am Soc Echocardiogr. 1995;8:964–6.
121. Zestos MM, Chehade M, Mossad E. A transesophageal echocardiography probe causes airway obstruction in an older child. J Cardiothorac Vasc Anesth. 1998;12:65–6.
122. Casta A, Brown DW, Yuki K. Induction of supraventricular tachycardia during transesophageal echocardiography: an

unusual complication. J Cardiothorac Vasc Anesth. 2008;22: 592–3.
123. Preisman S, Yusim Y, Mishali D, et al. Compression of the pulmonary artery during transesophageal echocardiography in a pediatric cardiac patient. Anesth Analg. 2003;96:85–7.
124. Koinig H, Schlemmer M, Keznickl FP. Occlusion of the right subclavian artery after insertion of a transoesophageal echocardiography probe in a neonate. Paediatr Anaesth. 2003;13: 617–9.
125. Liu JH, Hartnick CJ, Rutter MJ, et al. Subglottic stenosis associated with transesophageal echocardiography. Int J Pediatr Otorhinolaryngol. 2000;55:47–9.
126. Muhiudeen-Russell IA, Miller-Hance WC, Silverman NH. Unrecognized esophageal perforation in a neonate during transesophageal echocardiography. J Am Soc Echocardiogr. 2001;14: 747–9.
127. Frommelt PC, Stuth EA. Transesophageal echocardiographic in total anomalous pulmonary venous drainage: hypotension caused by compression of the pulmonary venous confluence during probe passage. J Am Soc Echocardiogr. 1994;7:652–4.
128. Chang YY, Chang CI, Wang MJ, et al. The safe use of intraoperative transesophageal echocardiography in the management of total anomalous pulmonary venous connection in newborns and infants: a case series. Paediatr Anaesth. 2005;15:939–43.
129. Greene MA, Alexander JA, Knauf DG, et al. Endoscopic evaluation of the esophagus in infants and children immediately following intraoperative use of transesophageal echocardiography. Chest. 1999;116:1247–50.
130. Kohr LM, Dargan M, Hague A, et al. The incidence of dysphagia in pediatric patients after open heart procedures with transesophageal echocardiography. Ann Thorac Surg. 2003;76:1450–6.
131. Wellen SL, Glatz AC, Gaynor JW, Montenegro LM, Cohen MS. Transesophageal echocardiography probe insertion failure in infants undergoing cardiac surgery. Congenit Heart Dis. 2013: 8:240–5.
132. Bezold LI, Pignatelli R, Altman CA, et al. Intraoperative transesophageal echocardiography in congenital heart surgery. The Texas Children's Hospital experience. Tex Heart Inst J. 1996;23:108–15.
133. Hata T, Todd MM. Cervical spine considerations when anesthetizing patients with Down syndrome. Anesthesiology. 2005;102:680–5.
134. Ali FE, Al-Bustan MA, Al-Busairi WA, et al. Cervical spine abnormalities associated with Down syndrome. Int Orthop. 2006;30:284–9.
135. Botoman VA, Surawicz CM. Bacteremia with gastrointestinal endoscopic procedures. Gastrointest Endosc. 1986;32:342–6.
136. Byrne WJ, Euler AR, Campbell M, et al. Bacteremia in children following upper gastrointestinal endoscopy or colonoscopy. J Pediatr Gastroenterol Nutr. 1982;1:551–3.
137. Foster E, Kusumoto FM, Sobol SM, et al. Streptococcal endocarditis temporally related to transesophageal echocardiography. J Am Soc Echocardiogr. 1990;3:424–7.
138. Melendez LJ, Chan KL, Cheung PK, et al. Incidence of bacteremia in transesophageal echocardiography: a prospective study of 140 consecutive patients. J Am Coll Cardiol. 1991;18:1650–4.
139. Wilson W, Taubert KA, Gewitz M, et al. Prevention of infective endocarditis: guidelines from the American Heart Association: a guideline from the American Heart Association Rheumatic Fever, Endocarditis, and Kawasaki Disease Committee, Council on Cardiovascular Disease in the Young, and the Council on Clinical Cardiology, Council on Cardiovascular Surgery and Anesthesia, and the Quality of Care and Outcomes Research Interdisciplinary Working Group. Circulation. 2007;116:1736–54.

Structural Evaluation of the Heart by Transesophageal Echocardiography

4

Pierre C. Wong

Abstract
It is well-known that the echocardiographic evaluation of congenital heart disease (CHD) can present challenges due to a number of factors: the multiplicity of the different forms of CHD, the variations in anatomy and physiology associated with each class of cardiac lesion, and the complex (and unique) three-dimensional anatomy seen with many of the individual cardiac defects. These challenges have been well documented with transthoracic and fetal echocardiography, and they are equally daunting, if not more so, with transesophageal echocardiography (TEE) due to the limited availability of echocardiographic windows afforded by the esophageal/gastric location of the probe. Nonetheless, in most patients with CHD, an excellent and comprehensive TEE study can be performed using a variety of probe manipulations and views as well as a systematic approach to evaluation. The goal of this chapter is to discuss the general aspects of structural evaluation of CHD by TEE. The standard American Society of Echocardiography/Society of Cardiovascular Anesthesiologists (ASE/SCA) TEE views and probe manipulations will be detailed, along with their specific application (and modifications) for CHD evaluation. Throughout this textbook, these guidelines will be used for the assessment of the various cardiac defects. This chapter also presents a methodology for a comprehensive, systematic, and segmental approach to the TEE evaluation of a patient with CHD.

Keywords
Heart defects • Congenital • Echocardiography • Transesophageal echocardiography • Pediatric cardiac surgery • Child • Infant • Intraoperative care • Intraoperative monitoring

Introduction

The inherent three-dimensional (3D) complexity of many forms of congenital heart disease (CHD) can present significant challenges in their anatomic depiction and diagnosis by two dimensional (2D) imaging modalities. Typically, the approach to 2D echocardiographic evaluation of CHD utilizes the principle that collection and display of images from multiple 2D tomographic planes enables the examiner to develop a mental 3D representation of the underlying cardiac anatomy. This is the fundamental underpinning of both fetal and transthoracic echocardiography for CHD, and it applies equally to transesophageal echocardiography (TEE). The TEE examination for CHD must be organized, methodical, and systematic; each cardiac structure should be explored carefully, with judicious use of 2D imaging and color flow/spectral Doppler to perform as thorough an examination as possible. In fact, a meticulous and well-organized approach assumes even

P.C. Wong, MD
Division of Cardiology, Children's Hospital Los Angeles, Department of Pediatrics, Keck School of Medicine, University of Southern California,
4650 Sunset Blvd, Mailstop #34, Los Angeles, CA 90027, USA
e-mail: pwong@chla.usc.edu

The online version of this chapter (doi:10.1007/978-1-84800-064-3_4) contains supplementary material, which is available to authorized users.

P.C. Wong, W.C. Miller-Hance (eds.), *Transesophageal Echocardiography for Congenital Heart Disease*,
DOI 10.1007/978-1-84800-064-3_4, © Springer-Verlag London 2014

greater importance for TEE because of several inherent limitations with the technique. First, unlike transthoracic echocardiography, TEE does not have the luxury of multiple echocardiographic windows from different sites of the thorax and abdomen—available TEE views are more limited due to the probe's confinement to the esophagus. Therefore not all cardiac structures can be depicted optimally, and Doppler interrogation of certain structures is sometimes limited or even impossible to perform. Second, TEE is a semi-invasive procedure, often requiring deep sedation or general anesthesia (particularly in the child), and with important potential risks. This generally precludes the ability to perform repeated, serial studies, and therefore the examiner should expect to collect all of the important information in one setting. This also underscores the need for accurate and complete recording of the TEE study. Third, the completeness of the examination will in part depend upon the conditions of the examination. For example, the rapid perioperative TEE evaluation of an unstable neonate or infant necessitates a brief and focused examination, and not every structure can be evaluated in detail.

For the above reasons, TEE is generally performed in patients with CHD as an adjunct to other diagnostic imaging modalities (e.g. transthoracic echocardiography), and often in a limited manner to provide targeted information (e.g. in the operating room setting). In most instances, previous diagnostic imaging has been performed and the TEE study provides complementary or confirmatory information; it is not meant to supplant or substitute for other diagnostic testing. Nonetheless, situations do arise in which diagnostic transthoracic images are either unavailable or of poor quality, and therefore TEE is necessary to provide more definitive (or sometimes missing) information. In these situations, a complete TEE examination can serve as the primary diagnostic study: using an organized and systematic approach, a tremendous amount of diagnostic anatomic and physiologic information can be obtained.

This chapter presents a methodology for a comprehensive, systematic, and segmental approach to the TEE evaluation of a patient with CHD. Nomenclature for TEE probe manipulation and image display—modified from the 1999 guidelines published by the American Society of Echocardiography/Society of Cardiovascular Anesthesiologists (ASE/SCA) [1]—will be defined. This nomenclature will be used throughout the remainder of the textbook.

Approach to Structural Evaluation

General Principles for CHD Assessment

The approach to the structural evaluation of CHD can best be summarized as follows: the TEE study should be systematic and thorough, and sweeps should be utilized to build a 3D understanding of the cardiac anatomy. Using this method, a comprehensive study can be performed in most patients with CHD—particularly those with complex anatomy. This approach incorporates the following principles:

1. When performing a complete anatomic assessment, a segmental approach should be utilized. The segmental approach to CHD, first proposed by Van Praagh and colleagues [2–4], has been detailed in a number of publications [4–10].[1] It derives from the embryologic development of the heart, in which the intracardiac anatomy is evaluated as a series of independent, yet interconnected, segments: the three main segments (atria, ventricles, great arteries), and two connecting segments (atrioventricular junction, conus arteriosus/infundibulum or ventriculo-arterial junction) [5, 11, 12]. Fundamental to this approach is the understanding that the anatomic layout of one segment is independent of the other levels, thus a right atrium does not necessarily connect to a right ventricle, nor does the right ventricle necessarily connect to the pulmonary artery, etc. Each segment must be analyzed individually. The approach is also termed "sequential", in that it proceeds in a blood flow sequence from atria to ventricles to great arteries [12]. The segmental approach facilitates a complete and organized approach to TEE evaluation, and encourages a thorough, step-by-step examination of all structures. It is particularly useful when dealing with complex CHD [13]. While the original segmental approach focuses primarily upon the three main and two connecting segments, the principles embodied can be applied to evaluation at all levels of the heart. An example of a modified stepwise approach to segmental analysis is given in Fig. 4.1.
2. When performing a TEE evaluation for CHD, particularly in patients with unknown or incompletely diagnosed anatomy, an organized methodology is essential so that all of the important information is obtained, and none is omitted.

[1]There are two major schools of thought regarding segmental evaluation of the heart, one led by Richard Van Praagh, MD, and the other by Robert Anderson, MD While a number of elements are common to both schools, there also exist important differences that have engendered some controversy among CHD specialists, particularly in regard to nomenclature, shorthand notation, and taxonomy. One important difference is that the Van Praagh school utilizes a shorthand method to record the three main cardiac segments of any given heart as a set, enclosed in braces. Individual letters are used to represent the different possibilities for each segment, listed in venoarterial sequence or blood flow order, as follows: {atria, ventricles, great arteries}. For example, a normal heart (situs solitus) would comprise the segmental set {S,D,S}, situs inversus/mirror image dextrocardia{I,L,I}, complete transposition {S,D,D}, etc. This shorthand method is rather elaborate, and while well known and widely used, it has not been universally adopted. A detailed exposition of this system, along with other similarities and differences between the two schools, is beyond the scope of this chapter. Instead, a simpler and more unified segmental approach is presented that, in the author's opinion, represents an integration of the best, most easily understandable elements from both schools. For further details, readers are referred to the references at the end of this chapter.

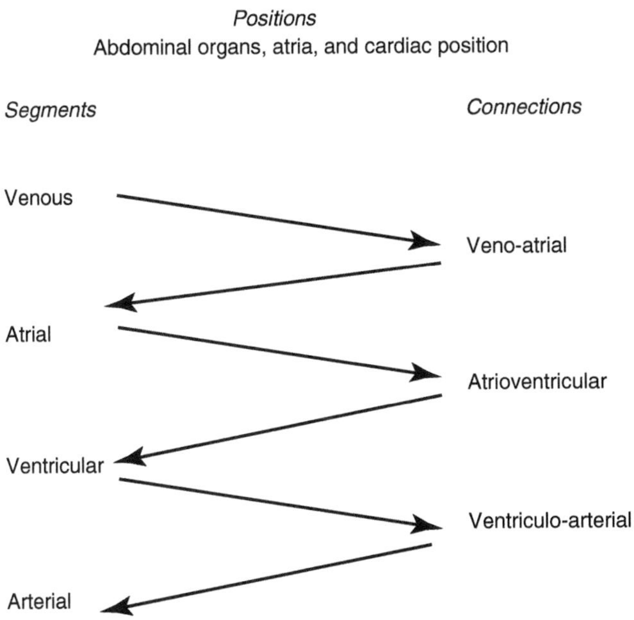

Fig. 4.1 Segmental approach to congenital heart disease (Reprinted with permission from O'Leary [7])

Whenever possible, it is preferable to perform as complete a study as possible, beginning each study in the same manner, and proceeding with a predefined and preplanned order of evaluation. However, this is not always feasible. In some instances, the exact order of examination will vary, first concentrating upon the most important information required, and then completing the remainder of the study. In other instances, a complete examination is not possible, or even necessary, and a more directed study is performed that focuses solely upon specific questions. Nevertheless, whether performing a focused or complete study, the examiner should always have in mind a mental checklist of the information required. Moreover, during the TEE examination, the examiner will note that, at any one time, a number of cardiac structures can often be visualized simultaneously. With so much information, some important details can easily be overlooked. This makes it even more important that the examiner maintain a mentally organized approach so that all essential information is obtained as methodically as possible.

3. Sweeps are especially useful in the evaluation of complex CHD, as they provide important spatial information about the cardiac structure(s) in question. With transthoracic echocardiography, sweeps are routinely performed by probe angulation (left to right, superior to inferior, anterior to posterior, etc.). With TEE, different manipulations must be used to perform sweeps. These sweeps incorporate the basic manipulations of the TEE probe, e.g. advancing/withdrawing the probe slowly to/from the esophagus, rotating the probe shaft slowly in a clockwise/counterclockwise (right/left) direction, anteflexion/retroflexion of the probe tip, and rotation of the multiplane angle (see below). As with transthoracic echocardiography, the use of sweeps in TEE helps to build an understanding of the 3D anatomy of individual cardiac structures, as well as the complex interrelationships that sometimes exist between these structures. Many of the video examples in this chapter demonstrate various TEE sweeps.

Probe Orientation and Manipulation

After the TEE probe has been inserted into the esophagus, it can be manipulated in several different directions. For this description it is assumed that the patient is lying supine, with the examiner situated just superior to the patient's head and facing the dorsum of the patient's feet. Regarding orientation, *superior* is towards the patient's head, *inferior* towards the stomach/feet, *posterior* towards the spine, *anterior* towards the sternum, and *right* and *left* towards the patient's right and left sides, respectively.

The TEE probe can be manipulated as follows (Fig. 4.2). Pushing the probe more inferiorly (towards the stomach) is termed *advancing* the probe, pulling the probe more superiorly is called *withdrawing* the probe. Rotating the probe clockwise is called *turning rightward* or *to the right*, and counterclockwise is called *turning leftward* or *to the left*. Flexing the tip of the probe anteriorly (using the anteroposterior control wheel) is called *anteflexion*; flexing the tip posteriorly is called *retroflexion*. If there is a second control wheel for lateral tip movement, flexing the tip to the patient's right and left is called *flexing to the right* and *flexing to the left*, respectively (right and left lateral movement controls are not as useful in pediatric patients, and not even included in many of the current pediatric TEE multiplane probes). Axial rotation of the multiplane angle of the probe (using either a mechanical or electronic control on the TEE probe handle) is described as *rotating forward* or *back* to *x degrees*, where *x* represents the multiplane angle. The multiplane angles will be shown as follows: at a multiplane angle of 0° (also known as the "horizontal" or "transverse" plane in biplane TEE imaging), the patient's right side appears on the left of the image display (Fig. 4.3a). Rotating the multiplane angle forward to 90° results in an orthogonal plane also known as the "vertical" or "longitudinal" plane in biplane TEE imaging. This plane provides tomographic sections of the heart oriented in the patient's sagittal plane. In this image, the left side of the screen is now the more inferior aspect (i.e. toward the patient's feet), and the right side of the screen is the more anterior/superior aspect (Fig. 4.3b). Rotation beyond 90° continues to provide important and useful information, but eventually results in a mirror image of 0° at 180°, with the patient's left side on the left of the screen (Fig. 4.3c). In general, the most useful TEE multiplane angles are obtained between 0° and 130°; it is rarely necessary (and potentially confusing) to use larger multiplane angles.

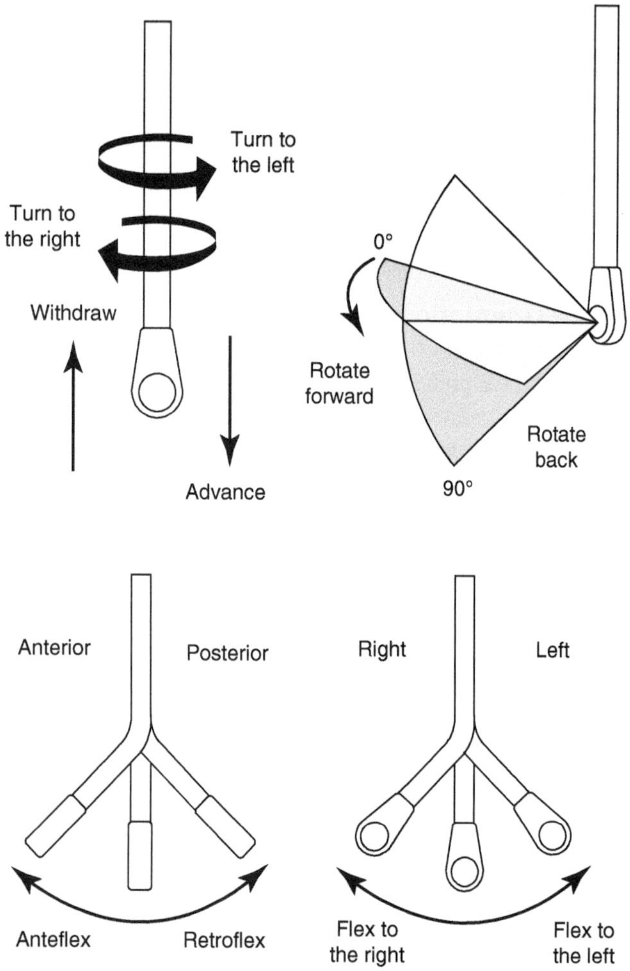

Fig. 4.2 Basics of probe manipulation during transesophageal echocardiography (TEE) (From Shanewise et al. [1], with permission from Elsevier)

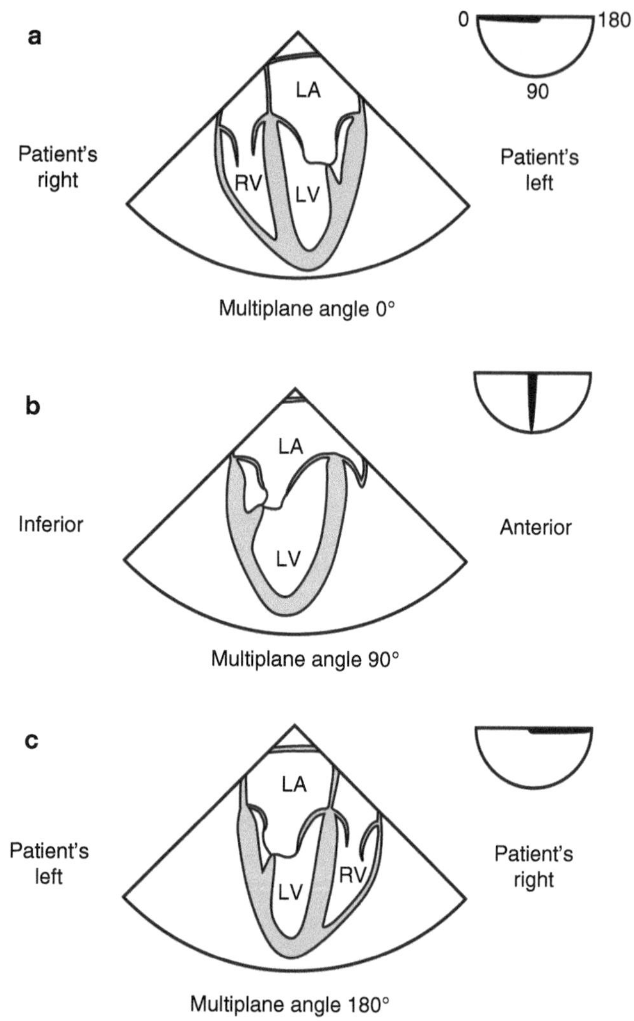

Fig. 4.3 Image orientation with multiplane angles of 0°, 90°, and 180°. Transducer location and near field (*narrow portion* of image sector) of the image sector are at the *top* of the display; far field (*wide portion* of image sector) is at the *bottom*. (**a**) Multiplane angle of 0°; (**b**) Multiplane angle of 90°; (**c**) Multiplane angle of 180°. *LA* left atrium, *LV* left ventricle, *RV* right ventricle (From Shanewise et al. [1], with permission from Elsevier)

Cross-Sectional TEE Views for CHD Evaluation

While a standardized nomenclature has been well established for the transthoracic echocardiographic views and windows used in the evaluation of pediatric patients, specifically as pertains to CHD evaluation [6, 14], the same cannot be said for TEE. Only one previous textbook (published in 1994) exclusively addressed TEE evaluation of CHD [15]. At the time, this textbook served as an excellent resource, elaborating upon TEE views and techniques specifically applicable for CHD. However, it was written in the early era of biplane TEE imaging, while the technology was still evolving, and prior to the availability of multiplane TEE transducers for pediatric applications. In fact most of the examples in that textbook were obtained from single plane (transverse) imaging. As biplane TEE became more widespread, several subsequent journal articles expanded upon its use in CHD evaluation [16–18]. With the increasing adoption of multiplane TEE imaging for adult patients, in 1999 the American Society of Echocardiography/Society of Cardiovascular Anesthesiologists (ASE/SCA) published guidelines for a standardized nomenclature pertinent to multiplane TEE probe manipulation, orientation and imaging. A series of 4 principal transducer locations (windows) and 20 anatomically directed cross-sectional tomographic views were defined [1]. These guidelines represented a significant contribution, and have since become widely accepted and employed for the standard performance of TEE [19]. While thorough and very extensive, they were nonetheless written primarily for the examination of the adult patient with an anatomically normal heart, with a focus upon evaluation of left ventricular function and mitral valve anatomy/function. However, since widespread availability of pediatric multiplane TEE probes did not occur until several years after the guidelines were published, comparable standardized guidelines have not been written specifically for the multiplane TEE evaluation of CHD, although several excellent articles have discussed the use of the ASE/SCA views/nomenclature for this purpose [20–22]. Of note, even the ASE guidelines for TEE in pediatric patients with congenital or acquired heart disease—authored by the ASE pediatric council—mentioned the ASE/SCA guidelines but gave no specific recommendations regarding the TEE views and methods needed for CHD evaluation. This article acknowledged the fact that no uniform consensus exists on standardized views and planes to be used for the TEE examination in the pediatric patient [20].

In this chapter, we present the ASE/SCA guidelines as they are suitable for the evaluation of CHD. In addition, we will expand upon the guidelines by presenting a modified version of the terminology/images and transducer windows that are essential or may complement the examination in this unique patient group. These modifications were designed and organized to facilitate their use for CHD evaluation. In this way, readers of the textbook will have a standardized "toolbox" of terms, views, and nomenclature that can be used as a reference for subsequent chapters in the textbook.[2]

TEE Transducer Locations and Views Used Throughout This Textbook

We define five principal TEE transducer locations, or windows—the upper esophageal, mid esophageal, lower esophageal, transgastric and deep transgastric, as shown in Fig. 4.4. These windows correspond to those used in the ASE/SCA guidelines, with the exception of the lower esophageal window, which was added for this textbook. For each of these windows, there are several typical or common views, each with a name describing the type of structure or view imaged, and some accompanied by the designation of "short" vs. "long" axis orientation (Fig. 4.5). Table 4.1 provides a listing of the individual cross-sectional views shown in Fig. 4.5, along with the abbreviation for each view, multiplane angle range, and structures imaged. We have also included several additional views that are not part of the original ASE/SCA guidelines—views that are useful for the evaluation of CHD. These additional views are designated with an asterisk. The specific images in Table 4.1 and Fig. 4.5, and their application, will be discussed in greater detail below.

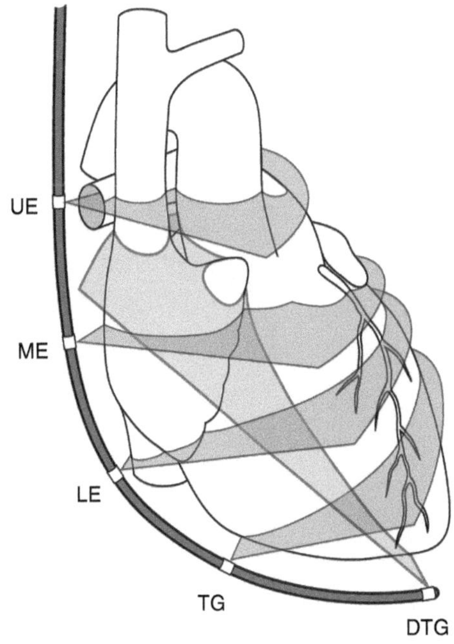

Fig. 4.4 The five basic windows for TEE evaluation. For simplicity, each view is shown with the multiplane angle at 0°. *UE* upper esophagus, *ME* mid esophagus, *LE* lower esophagus, *TG* transgastric, *DTG* deep transgastric

Image Display Conventions Used Throughout This Textbook

The reader will note that several TEE views are comparable to those obtained by standard transthoracic evaluation, and they are displayed in a similar manner (e.g. the four chamber view). However other TEE views are unique and/or oriented quite differently from their transthoracic counterparts. It is important to acknowledge that some variation exists among different CHD centers as to how these views should be displayed (e.g. some centers display, anterior structures at the top of the screen and inferior ones at the bottom), and this has led to some controversy. To minimize confusion and facilitate reader comprehension, images in this textbook will be displayed as per the convention of the ASE/SCA guidelines: with posterior anatomic structures closer to the imaging probe

[2] At the time of this textbook's final pre-publication editing, a revised set of ASE/SCA guidelines was released. While still primarily adult-based, these revised guidelines are much more extensive in scope compared to the previous document; they present a good deal of new information including TEE training recommendations, additional TEE views, and suggested 3D TEE evaluation protocols. Also, a brief section has been added that addresses adult CHD evaluation. While this textbook centers upon an approach to structural TEE evaluation based upon the previous ASE/SCA guidelines and additional modified views, the editors want to acknowledge the updated 2013 document and provide it as an important additional reference. The updated guidelines can be found in: Hahn RT, Abraham T, Adams MS, et al. Guidelines for performing a comprehensive transesophageal echocardiographic examination: recommendations from the American Society of Echocardiography and the Society of Cardiovascular Anesthesiologists. J Am Soc Echocardiogr 2013;26:921–964.

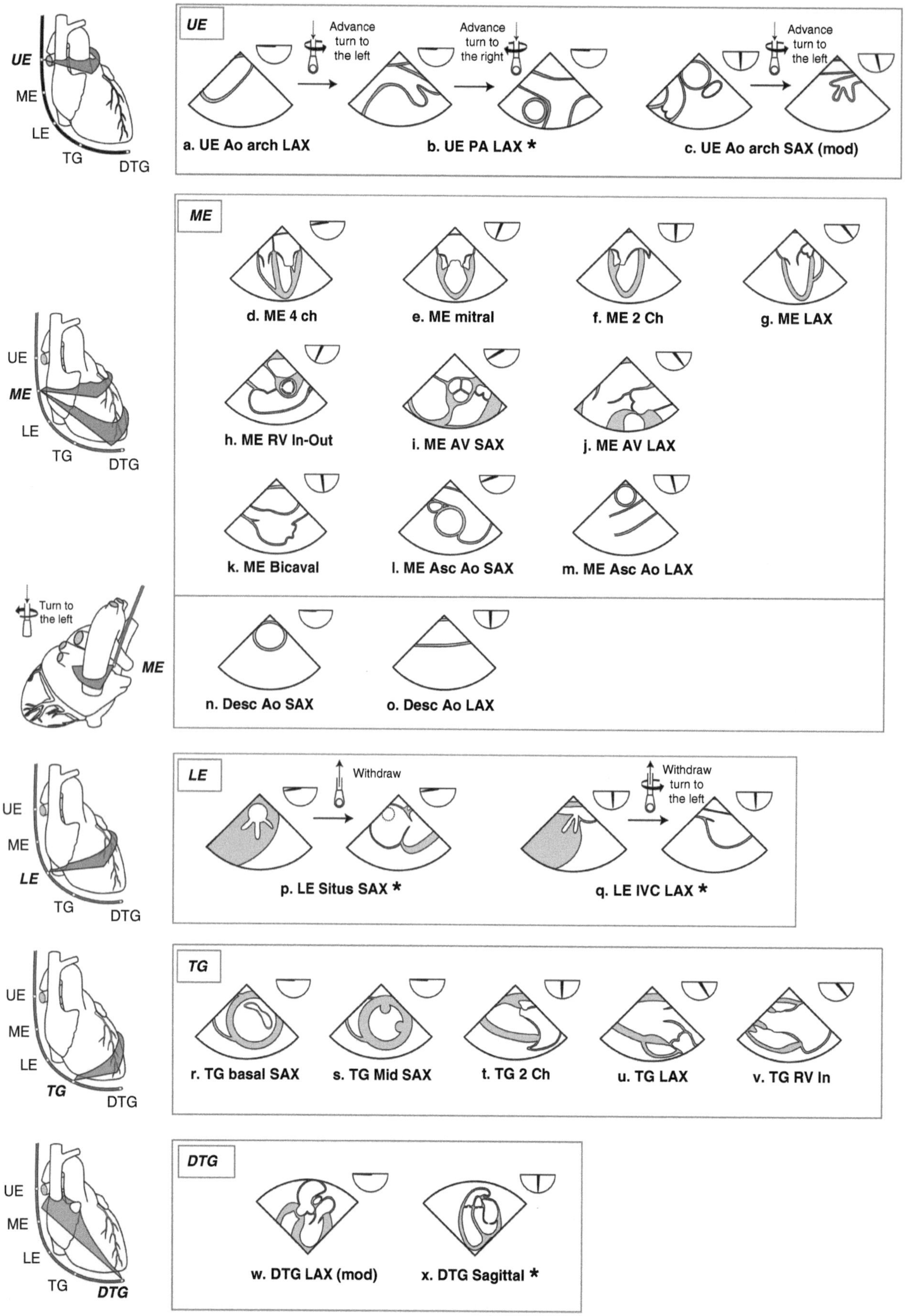
UE
ME
LE
TG
DTG
Advance turn to the left
Advance turn to the right
Advance turn to the left
a. UE Ao arch LAX
b. UE PA LAX *
c. UE Ao arch SAX (mod)
d. ME 4 ch
e. ME mitral
f. ME 2 Ch
g. ME LAX
h. ME RV In-Out
i. ME AV SAX
j. ME AV LAX
k. ME Bicaval
l. ME Asc Ao SAX
m. ME Asc Ao LAX
Turn to the left
n. Desc Ao SAX
o. Desc Ao LAX
Withdraw
Withdraw turn to the left
p. LE Situs SAX *
q. LE IVC LAX *
r. TG basal SAX
s. TG Mid SAX
t. TG 2 Ch
u. TG LAX
v. TG RV In
w. DTG LAX (mod)
x. DTG Sagittal *

Table 4.1 Recommended transesophageal echocardiography cross sections

Window	Cross section (see Fig. 4.5)	Abbreviation	Multiplane angle range	Structures imaged
Upper esophageal (UE)	Aortic arch long axis (a)	UE Ao Arch LAX	0°	Aortic arch, Inn v
	Pulmonary artery long axis (b)*	UE PA LAX	0°	PA bifurcation, LPA, RPA, PDA
	Aortic arch short axis (c)◊	UE Ao Arch SAX	90–100°	Aortic arch, MPA, LPA, PDA, PV, Inn v
Mid esophageal (ME)	Four chamber (d)	ME 4 Ch	0–20°	LV, LA, LAA, RV, RA, RAA, MV, TV, IAS, AV, CS
	Mitral commissural (e)	ME Mitral	60–70°	MV, LV, LA
	Two chamber (f)	ME 2 Ch	80–100°	LV, LA, LAA, MV, CS
	Long axis (g)	ME LAX	100–130°	LV, LA, AV, LVOT, MV, Asc Ao, IVS
	RV inflow-outflow (h)	ME RV In-Out	60–90°	RV, RA, TV, RVOT, PV, MPA, IVS
	AV short axis (i)	ME AV SAX	30–60°	AV, IAS, coronary origins, LVOT, PV
	AV long axis (j)	ME AV LAX	90–130°	AV, LA, LV, LVOT, MV, prox Asc Ao, RPA
	Bicaval (k)	ME Bicaval	80–110°	RA, RAA, SVC, IVC, IAS, LA
	Asc aortic short axis (l)	ME Asc Ao SAX	0–60°	Asc Ao, SVC, MPA, RPA
	Asc aortic long axis (m)	ME Asc Ao LAX	90–120°	Asc Ao, RPA, MPA
	Desc aorta short axis (n)	Desc Ao SAX	0°	Desc thoracic Ao, left pleural space
	Desc aorta long axis (o)	Desc Ao LAX	90–110°	Desc thoracic Ao, left pleural space
Lower esophageal (LE)	Situs short axis (p)*	LE Situs SAX	0–10°	IVC, Eustachian valve, RA, CS
	IVC long axis (q)*	LE IVC LAX	70–100°	Hepatic veins to IVC, RA, Eustachian valve, lower portion of IAS
Transgastric (TG)	Basal short axis (r)	TG Basal SAX	0–20°	LV, MV, RV, TV
	Mid short axis (s)	TG Mid SAX	0–20°	LV, RV, pap mm, IVS
	Two chamber (t)	TG 2 Ch	80–100°	LV, MV, LA, LAA, chordae, pap mm, CS
	Long axis (u)	TG LAX	90–120°	LVOT, AV, MV, Asc Ao
	RV inflow (v)	TG RV In	100–120°	RA, RV, TV + chordae, pap mm, SVC inflow
Deep transgastric (DTG)	Long axis (w)◊	DTG LAX	0–20° (anteflexion)	LVOT, AV, Asc Ao, IAS, IVS, MV, TV, RA, LA, RV, LV, RVOT, PV
	Sagittal (x)*	DTG Sagittal	80–110° (anteflexion)	LVOT, RVOT, AV, PV, MPA, MV, TV, IAS, IVS, RV, LV, RA, LA, SVC inflow (modified)

Views not part of the original ASE/SCA statement, and added as additional views for this textbook, are denoted with an asterisk (*). Existing ASE/SCA views that have been modified from the original are denoted with a diamond (◊).
Abbreviations: *Ao* aorta, *Asc* ascending, *AV* aortic valve, *CS* coronary sinus, *Desc* descending, *Inn v* Innominate vein, *IAS* interatrial septum, *IVC* inferior vena cava, *IVS* interventricular septum, *LV* left ventricle, *LA* left atrium, *LAA* left atrial appendage, *LPA* left pulmonary artery, *LVOT* left ventricular outflow tract, *MPA* main pulmonary artery, *MV* mitral valve, *prox* proximal, *pap mm* papillary muscles, *PDA* patent ductus arteriosus, *PV* pulmonic valve, *RA* right atrium, *RAA* right atrial appendage, *RPA* right pulmonary artery, *RV* right ventricle, *RVOT* right ventricular outflow tract, *SVC* superior vena cava, *TV* tricuspid valve (Modified with permission from: Shanewise et al. [1])

Fig. 4.5 Representative cross-sectional views showing the main structures displayed from each of the five principal windows. Approximate multiplane angle is indicated by the icon adjacent to each view. Views modified from the original ASE/SCA statement are given the designation (mod). Views not part of the original ASE/SCA statement, and added as additional views for this textbook, are denoted with an *. In some views, two images are shown depicting the changes that occur with probe manipulation; the specific probe maneuvers are shown in between the images. See text and Table 4.1 for further details. *Ao* aorta, *Asc* ascending, *AV* aortic valve, *Desc* descending, *DTG* deep transgastric, *In-Out* inflow-outflow, *IVC* inferior vena cava, *LAX* long axis, *LE* lower esophageal, *ME* mid esophageal, *PA* pulmonary artery, *RV* right ventricle, *SAX* short axis, *TG* transgastric, *UE* upper esophageal (Modified from Shanewise et al. [1], with permission from Elsevier) and in the near field (narrow portion or apex of the image sector) at the top of the screen, and the far field structures (wide portion of the image sector) at the bottom [1]. The only exceptions to this image display are the deep transgastric views, which will be shown inverted, with the apex of the heart at the bottom of the screen (right/left orientation remains the same), thereby presenting an "anatomically correct" image of the heart [23, 24].

Structural Evaluation of CHD by TEE

What follows below is a suggested methodology for a comprehensive TEE study that can be performed in most patients, utilizing both the ASE/SCA standard views as well as the additional modified views and nomenclature outlined above. This approach yields a detailed anatomic assessment of the heart, guided by the principles of segmental analysis. For each area of the heart, suggested probe position and view(s) are given in order to provide an optimal assessment of the structure(s) in question. It should be noted that subsequent chapters in this textbook will provide further details and elaboration of the TEE assessment discussed below, specifically pertaining to the normal and abnormal anatomy covered in that particular chapter.

The TEE examples shown in this chapter are taken almost exclusively from patients with normal cardiac position (levocardia) and normal cardiac anatomy, but the principles of examination embodied in these examples apply equally to any patient with simple or complex CHD. Obviously, the individual views given in Table 4.1 and Fig. 4.5 should be considered only as a starting point, or point of reference, for CHD evaluation. During the course of a study a number of modifications in probe position, probe rotation, and multiplane angle will generally be required to visualize different cardiac structures, particularly in patients with complex anatomy, cardiac malposition, or unusual relation of the esophagus to the heart. In some cases, optimal visualization of a given cardiac structure will require deviation (sometimes significant) from the multiplane angle and image views listed in Table 4.1; some images will bear little, if any, resemblance to the views presented in Fig. 4.5. As readers peruse this textbook, they will undoubtedly encounter sections in which the layout of the specific anatomy being discussed does not fully comport with the named views defined in this chapter—for example, using a "mid esophageal *four* chamber view" in a patient with double inlet left ventricle (only *three* main chambers), or a "mid esophageal aortic valve long axis view" when the patient has aortic valve atresia. What is most important for the reader to recognize is that CHD evaluation is a *structure-based*, not view-based, approach, and that it is the information contained within a view—not its name—that must be understood. With this in mind, throughout the textbook we will continue to utilize, as much as possible, the nomenclature and views as defined in this chapter. Maintaining a consistent approach and terminology will, we believe, assist the reader in fully understanding the specific methods of TEE evaluation described by the authors in their respective chapters. We strongly encourage the reader to become familiar with all of the views and nomenclature presented herein, and to refer to this chapter frequently if clarification is needed.

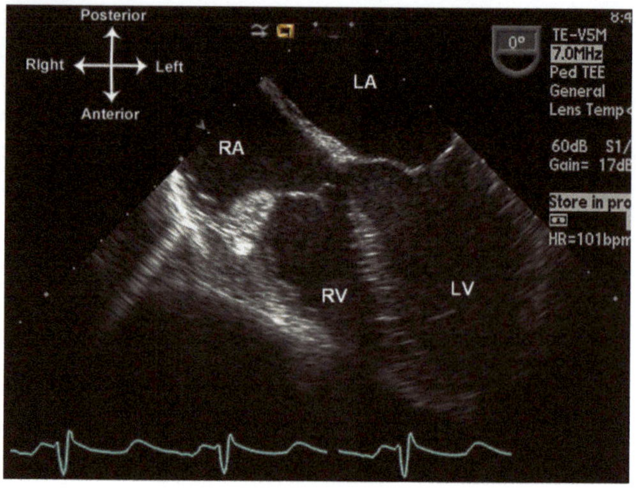

Fig. 4.6 Mid esophageal four chamber, or "home base" view. Multiplane angle is 0–10°. *LA* left atrium, *LV* left ventricle, *RA* right atrium, *RV* right ventricle

As mentioned previously, the confinement of the TEE probe to the esophagus leads to inherent limitations in the imaging of certain intra and extracardiac structures. Simply put, there are some structures and defects that TEE images well, and some that it does not. These limitations will be noted in this and subsequent chapters.

Initiation of TEE Study, Establishment of Atrial Situs and Systemic/Pulmonary Venous Return

This approach starts the TEE study with the probe in a neutral position facing anteriorly, in the mid esophageal position, with a multiplane angle of 0–10°. This produces the *mid esophageal four chamber view* (ME 4 Ch), which is the TEE equivalent of a standard transthoracic apical four chamber view (Figs. 4.5d and 4.6). Since it is readily recognizable, this view can be used for orientation, thereby serving as the "home base" view for the examination. The ME 4 Ch also serves to identify the base to apex orientation of the heart: levocardia (apex to the left), mesocardia (apex midline), and dextrocardia (apex to the right). Because of the esophageal location for TEE, it can be difficult to ascertain the exact position of the heart in the thorax, but in many cases the base to apex orientation corresponds with

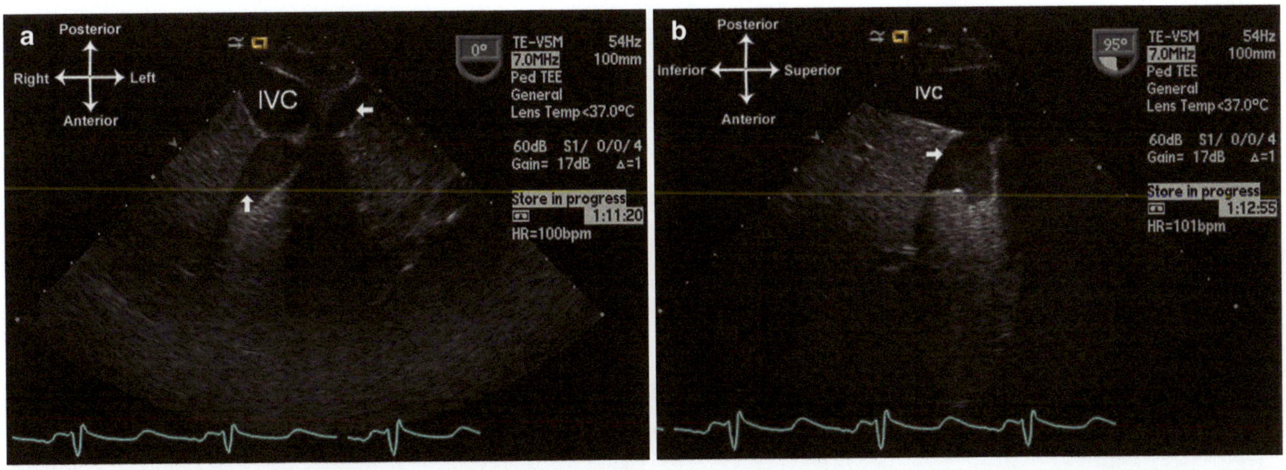

Fig. 4.7 Hepatic veins entering into the inferior vena cava (*IVC*) from the lower esophageal situs short axis view with a multiplane angle of 0° (**a**) and the lower esophageal IVC long axis view with a multiplane angle of 95° (**b**). The *arrows* show hepatic veins entering the IVC

the cardiac position [9]. It is important to verify the right/left orientation of the image display and confirm this with rotation of the probe to the right and left; an incorrect setting can complicate the examination, for example by making a patient with levocardia appear to have dextrocardia. Once this view is obtained and the examiner oriented, image settings can be optimized, and the study commences. If the examiner becomes disoriented by movement of the probe to an unfamiliar location, and/or by visualization of unfamiliar structures, the TEE probe can be returned to this "home base" position for reorientation.

The TEE study should begin with an evaluation of visceroatrial situs. This is an important and often overlooked part of the TEE examination for CHD. Visceral and atrial situs are almost always concordant [12], so atrial situs evaluation can be used. Atrial situs is either solitus, inversus, or ambiguous. In situs solitus (normal), the morphologic right atrium (RA) is located to the right of the morphologic left atrium (LA). In situs inversus, there is left-right reversal of the two, and in situs ambiguous (heterotaxy) there is atrial isomerism. By TEE, atrial situs can be determined by several methods. The characteristic features of the atrial appendages serve to distinguish the morphologic RA and LA. The right atrial appendage is typically triangular and broad based, while the left atrial appendage is long and tubular, with a narrow base [8]. In cases of atrial isomerism (heterotaxy, or situs ambiguous), two atrial appendages of the same morphology will usually be seen, presenting as mirror images of each other. Atrial appendage morphology can be readily identified by TEE [25]; the individual appendages can be seen using a combination of mid esophageal views including the mid esophageal bicaval, four and two chamber views (described below). Another important atrial structure, the atrial septum, can also help to establish atrial situs. The atrial septum is comprised of two individual components: the thicker septum secundum (comprised of superior and inferior limbic bands, or limbus), and the thinner septum primum, also known as the valve of the foramen ovale. The septum secundum forms the right atrial surface of the atrial septum, and the septum primum forms the left atrial surface. Therefore in normal atrial situs (solitus), the septum secundum should be located to the right of septum primum; the reverse holds true with atrial situs inversus (the atrial septum is often very deficient in situs ambiguous). When an atrial septum is present, its two components are readily visualized by several mid esophageal TEE views, as will be discussed below.

Atrial situs can also be established by visualization of the suprahepatic portion of inferior vena cava (IVC) and coronary sinus (CS) drainage. These two structures, when present, usually drain into the morphologic RA [26, 27]. Given the postero-inferior position of both structures, the best method to image these is by using a lower esophageal/transgastric window. Therefore from the "home base" (ME 4 Ch) position, the TEE probe is advanced into the stomach and anteflexed, using a multiplane angle of approximately 0° and slight rightward turning of the probe. The hepatic veins (HVs) can be visualized, as well as IVC. The probe is slowly withdrawn, and the HVs will be seen to drain into the IVC in the view that we will refer to as the *lower esophageal situs short axis view* (LE Situs SAX, Figs. 4.5p and 4.7a). In the same probe location, rotating the multiplane angle to 80–100° and turning the probe rightward (clockwise) visualizes the lengthwise extent of the IVC as it courses through the liver in the *lower esophageal IVC long axis view* (LE IVC LAX, Figs. 4.5q and 4.7b). This view is useful to distinguish the IVC from prominent HVs, which in some views can mimic the appearance of the IVC. The length of the Eustachian valve can be seen in this view. Rotating back to a multiplane angle of 0°, the probe is withdrawn further (continuing anteflexion to maintain contact with the stomach wall and

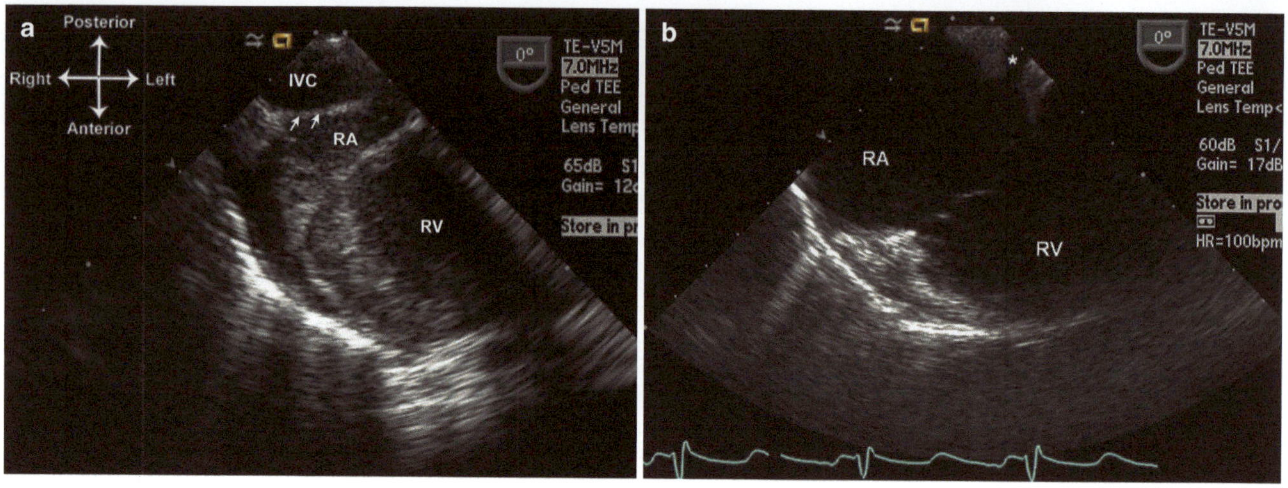

Fig. 4.8 Entrance of inferior vena cava (IVC) (**a**) and coronary sinus (*) (**b**) into the right atrium using lower esophageal situs short axis view. *Arrows* in (a) point to the Eustachian valve. *RA* right atrium, *RV* right ventricle

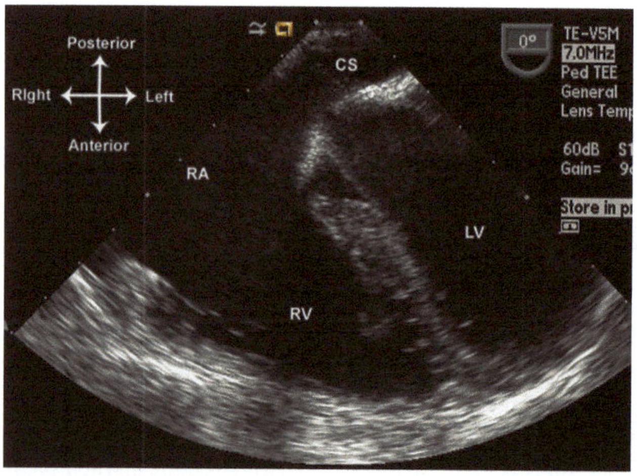

Fig. 4.9 Dilated coronary sinus seen from the mid esophageal four chamber view. *CS* coronary sinus, *LV* left ventricle, *RA* right atrium, *RV* right ventricle

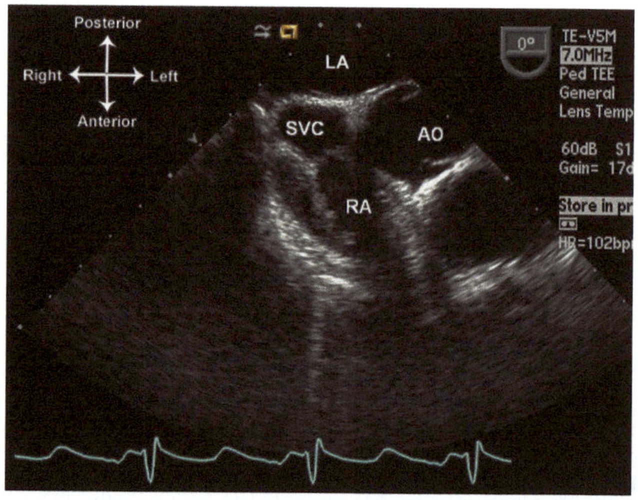

Fig. 4.10 Superior vena cava (*SVC*) entrance into the right atrium (*RA*) as seen from the mid esophageal level, multiplane angle of 0° and with rightward turning of the probe. *AO* Aorta; *LA* left atrium

esophagus), and the IVC can then be seen entering into the right atrium (Fig. 4.8a). Video 4.1 demonstrates this short sweep using nearly orthogonal multiplane angles between 0° and 90°. At this point, or with a small amount of probe withdrawal and retroflexion, the CS can be seen entering into the RA (Fig. 4.8b). Eustachian valve tissue is often seen at the mouth of the IVC, sometimes in continuity with the Thebesian valve of the coronary sinus. The diameter of the coronary sinus opening into the RA is often quite small, except in the presence of a left superior vena cava (LSVC) draining into the CS. The CS is located posteriorly and inferiorly in the heart, and therefore best visualized in its long axis from the lower esophageal window (LE Situs SAX) or the ME 4 Ch view, using a multiplane angle of 0°. Retroflexion of the probe sometimes enables the entire length of the CS to be seen. When the CS is dilated, its margins might not be as well defined, and sometimes a large CS can be confused for a large primum or secundum atrial septal defect. However the CS is more posterior and inferior than either of these defects. A dilated CS is mainly seen when an LSVC is present and drains to the CS; however it can be seen in other conditions as well. A lengthwise view of the dilated CS is best displayed with a multiplane angle of 0–10° (Fig. 4.9).

Once the TEE probe is back in the mid esophageal position, further evaluation of systemic and pulmonary venous return can be undertaken. To visualize a right-sided superior vena cava (the normal position for this vessel in situs solitus, abbreviated as SVC in this chapter), the probe is withdrawn further using slight anteflexion and turning to the right, with a multiplane angle of 0–10° (Fig. 4.10). The entrance of the SVC to the right atrium can be seen in cross section. With further probe withdrawal, more superior portions of the SVC can be seen although this area is not consistently visualized in all patients. Returning to right atrial level, rotation of the multiplane angle to 80–100° yields a sagittal view known as the

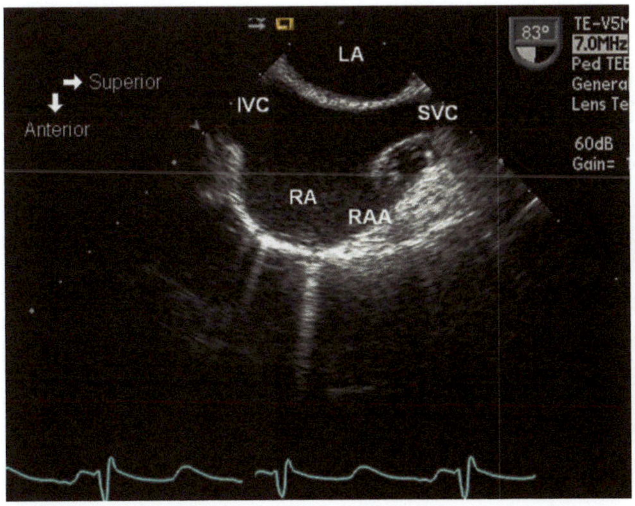

Fig. 4.11 Mid esophageal bicaval view, obtained with a multiplane angle between 80° and 90°. *IVC* inferior vena cava, *LA* left atrium, *RA* right atrium, *RAA* right atrial appendage, *SVC* superior vena cava

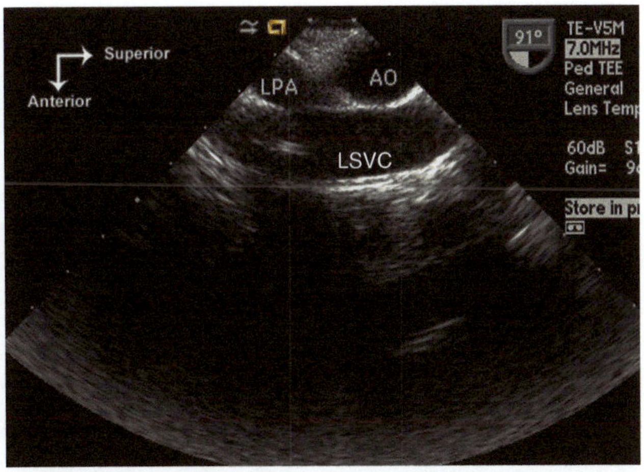

Fig. 4.12 Left superior vena cava (*LSVC*) returning to the coronary sinus. The LSVC courses anterior to the left pulmonary artery (*LPA*). The probe tip is located between mid and upper esophageal window, turned to the left, and the multiplane angle is approximately 90°. In this patient there is an absent right SVC, with the innominate vein returning to the right atrium via the LSVC and dilated coronary sinus. A catheter is seen in the LSVC. *Ao* transverse aortic arch

mid esophageal bicaval view (ME Bicaval, Figs. 4.5k and 4.11, Video 4.2), showing the SVC and IVC entrances to the RA as well as the right atrial appendage. If an LSVC is present, it can also be visualized at this level by rotating the probe leftward (counterclockwise), while maintaining a multiplane angle of 80–100°. This provides a lengthwise, long axis view of the LSVC (Fig. 4.12, Video 4.3). Keeping the probe in the same position and rotating the multiplane angle to 0–10° produces a cross-sectional, short axis view of the LSVC. In both long and short axis views, the LSVC can sometimes be visualized quite superiorly, at the level of the upper esophagus. From this position, by advancing the TEE probe from the upper to mid esophageal position, a superior to inferior sweep of the LSVC can be performed as it descends to its insertion into the dilated CS (Video 4.3). It should be remembered that a LSVC, when present, generally drains through a dilated CS to the RA. However, occasionally it can return directly to the LA, and in these instances the CS will usually not be dilated.

Evaluation of pulmonary venous drainage is one of the strengths of TEE. The close proximity of the LA and pulmonary veins to the esophagus not only provides superior imaging, but also an excellent Doppler color flow signal and favorable angles for spectral Doppler analysis. It is often helpful to utilize color flow mapping to aid assessment of the pulmonary veins. However, lowering of the Nyquist limit (to 30–60 cm/s) is sometimes necessary to visualize an optimal color flow signal.

The individual right and left pulmonary veins can be separately assessed by TEE, although slightly different views and techniques are required for each side [28, 29]. The right pulmonary veins are best evaluated using the ME 4 Ch view, turning the TEE probe to the right to visualize the lateral border of the RA. Advancing the probe and turning to the right enables visualization of right lower pulmonary vein, which takes a more horizontal course on the display (Fig. 4.13a, Video 4.4). With slow withdrawal and slight turning of the probe to the left, the right upper (and sometimes right middle) vein can be readily seen; these veins take a more vertical course on the display as they enter the RA (Fig. 4.13b, Video 4.4). The left pulmonary veins have a slightly different drainage pattern. There are generally two left pulmonary veins (upper and lower), and their sites of return to the LA are usually very close together (or even the same site). The left pulmonary veins can be identified by the ME 4 Ch view, with a multiplane angle of 0–10° and leftward (counterclockwise) turning of the probe. With these settings, slight advancing and withdrawing of the probe is necessary to visualize the individual pulmonary veins. Like the right pulmonary veins, the left lower pulmonary vein has a slightly more horizontal course on the display, and the left upper vein takes a more vertical course (Fig. 4.14a, b, Video 4.4). Both the right and left pulmonary veins can also be visualized from an orthogonal, sagittal (longitudinal) view, effectively a ME Bicaval view with the probe multiplane angle anywhere between 50° and 100°. With this type of evaluation, it is best to visualize first the LA and then rotate the probe rightward or leftward (clockwise/counterclockwise) to visualize the pulmonary veins on either side (Fig. 4.15a, b). These views provide an excellent display of the individual lobar veins as they enter the LA.

It is important to remember that, due to the frequency of anomalous pulmonary venous drainage anomalies seen with CHD, pulmonary venous drainage cannot be relied upon to determine atrial situs. Abnormalities of pulmonary venous drainage are discussed in Chap. 6.

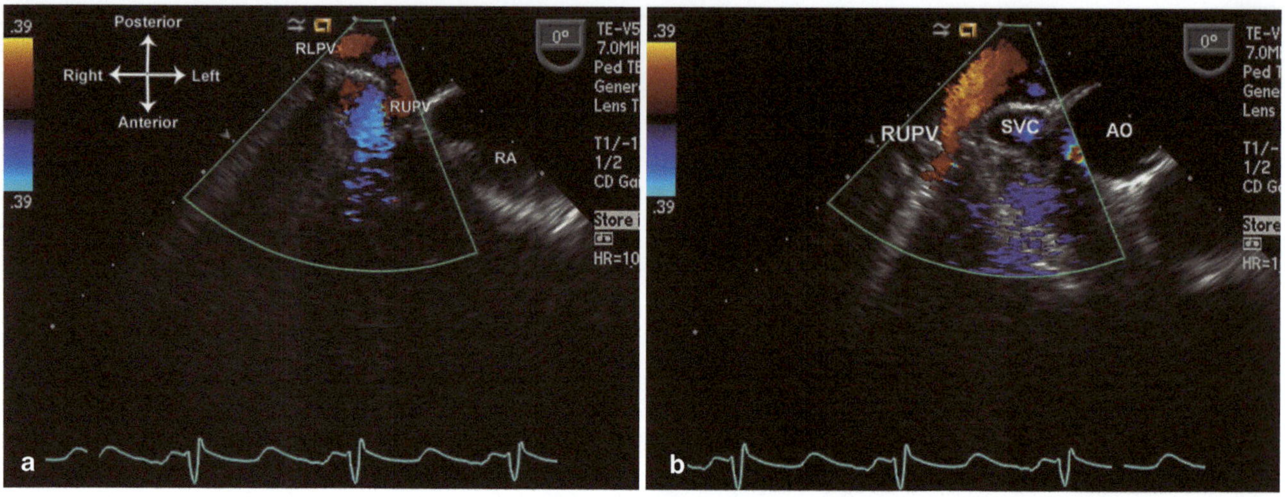

Fig. 4.13 Right pulmonary veins displayed by color Doppler as they enter into the left atrium. The lower (**a**) and upper pulmonary veins are seen (**a**). The right upper pulmonary vein is depicted as it courses in longitudinal fashion behind the superior vena cava (**b**). These images were obtained at a multiplane angle of 0° with probe turned slightly to the right. The Nyquist limit was lowered to optimize identification of these structures. *AO* aorta, *RLPV* right lower pulmonary vein, *RUPV* right pulmonary vein, *SVC* superior vena cava

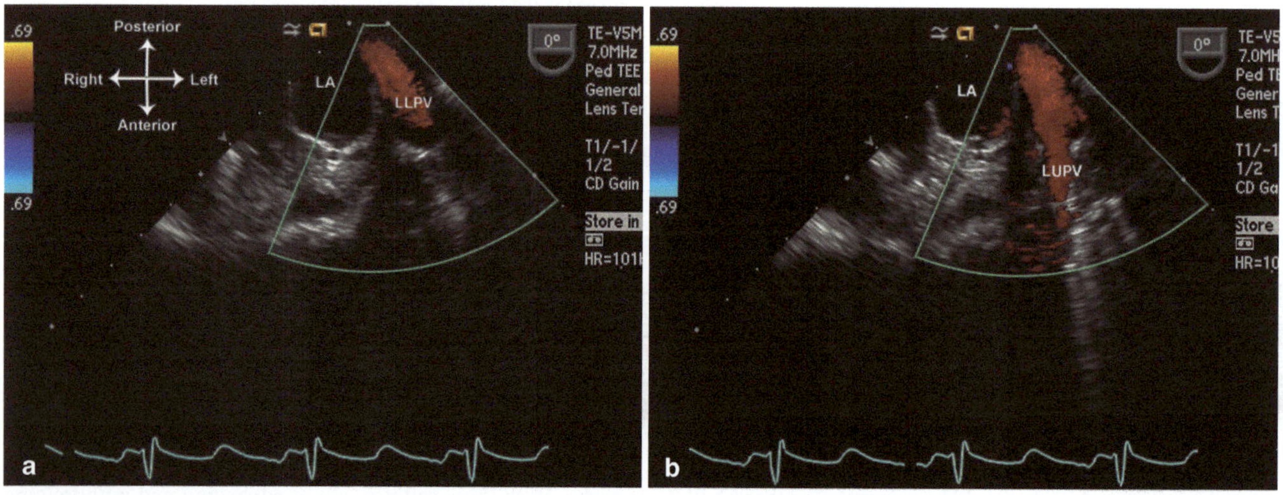

Fig. 4.14 Left lower (**a**) and upper (**b**) pulmonary veins shown as these return to the left atrium. Images obtained at a multiplane angle of 0°, probe turned slightly to the left. *LA* left atrium, *LLPV* left lower pulmonary vein, *LUPV* left upper pulmonary vein

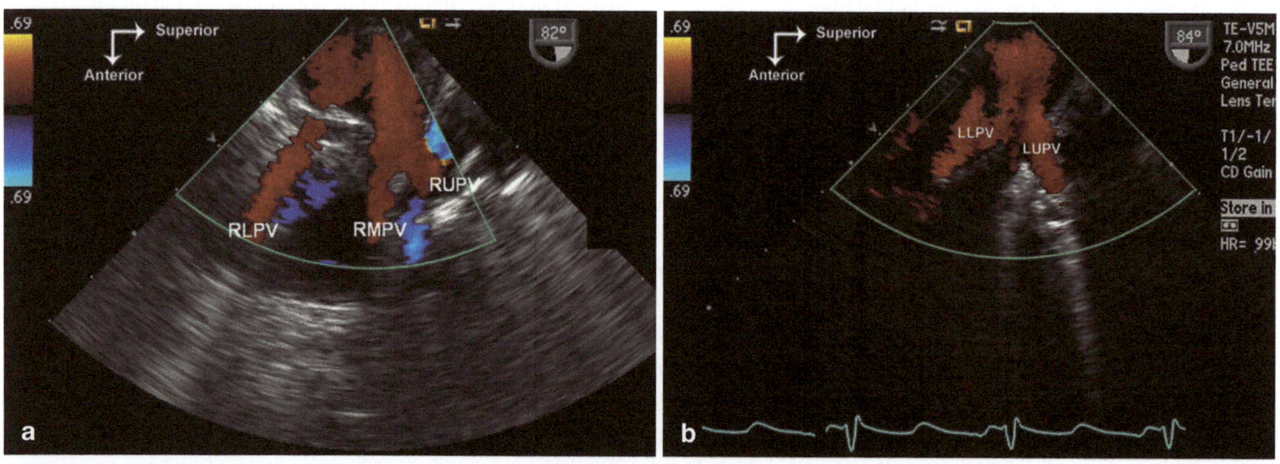

Fig. 4.15 Right and left pulmonary veins returning to the left atrium as viewed from a sagittal (90°) plane. The probe tip is at mid esophageal level, first turning to the right to visualize the right pulmonary veins (**a**), and then to the left to visualize the left pulmonary veins (**b**). *LLPV* left lower pulmonary vein, *LUPV* left upper pulmonary vein, *RLPV* right lower pulmonary vein, *RMPV* right middle pulmonary vein, *RUPV* right upper pulmonary vein

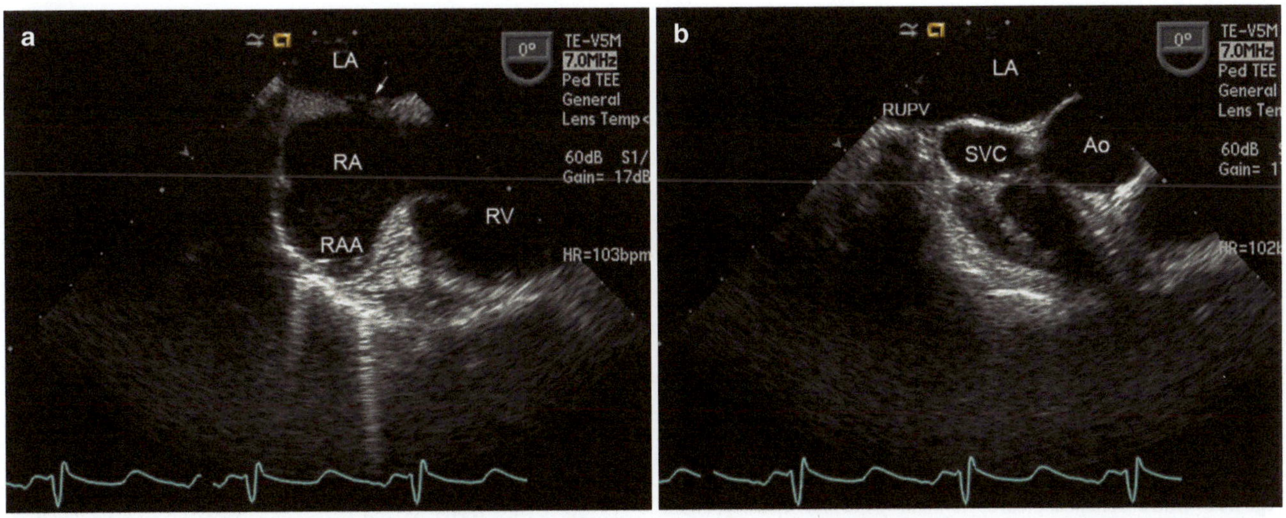

Fig. 4.16 Atrial septum visualized from the mid esophagus, with multiplane angle 0°. In (**a**) the probe is rotated to the right, showing both right atrium (*RA*) and left atrium (*LA*) and the thin atrial septum primum (*arrow*) located to the left of septum secundum. The right atrial appendage (*RAA*) is also visible. In (**b**) withdrawal of the probe demonstrates the superior limbic band of septum secundum, along with the entrance of the superior vena cava (*SVC*) into the RA, just anterior to the entrance of the right upper pulmonary vein (*RUPV*) to the LA. *Ao* aorta, *RV* right ventricle

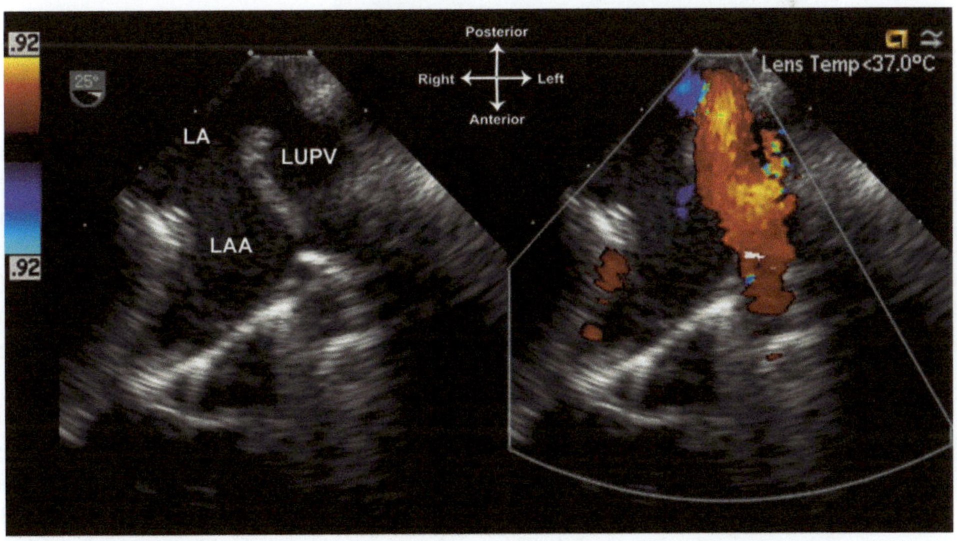

Fig. 4.17 Visualization of the left atrial structures. In the mid-esophageal view, with leftward turning of the probe as well as slight anteflexion and a multiplane angle of 25°, the left atrium (*LA*), left atrial appendage (*LAA*), and left upper pulmonary vein (*LUPV*) are seen. Color Doppler facilitates the identification of the left pulmonary veins

Atria and Atrial Septum

The atria and atrial septum are best visualized from the lower and mid esophageal views. A combination of sweeps is generally used. The first sweep begins in the lower esophagus, with a multiplane angle of 0° and a view of the mouth of the IVC entrance to the right atrium. The probe is gradually withdrawn so that the CS and inferior limbic band of atrial septum secundum come into view. Any defects in the posterior atrial septum can be visualized. With further probe withdrawal to the mid esophagus, both atria are well seen, as well as the thin atrial septum primum, and with slightly more rightward rotation, the right atrial appendage (Fig. 4.16a, Video 4.5). As the probe is withdrawn further, superior limbic band of septum secundum becomes visible, as well as the entrance of the SVC into the RA (Fig. 4.16b, Videos 4.5 and 4.6). The right pulmonary veins can be shown returning to the LA (as described above), along with their relationship to the atrial septum. From here, leftward probe rotation and slight probe anteflexion, as well as variation of the multiplane angle between 0° and 60°, will display the left atrial appendage (with its typical finger-like shape) just anterior to the left upper pulmonary vein (Fig. 4.17, Video 4.7).

An orthogonal, sagittal sweep is then performed by setting the multiplane angle to 80–90° and obtaining the ME Bicaval view. The SVC and IVC entrances to the RA, the posterior LA, as well as the right atrial appendage, are well seen (Fig. 4.11, Video 4.5). Rightward turning of the probe visualizes the right pulmonary veins (as noted above); slow leftward turning of the probe back to the ME Bicaval view visualizes

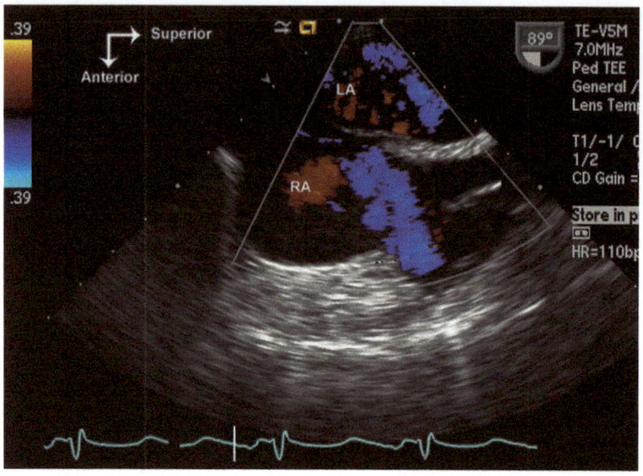

Fig. 4.18 Mid esophageal bicaval view shows the thin septum primum component of the atrial septum, located posterior and to the left of the thicker atrial septum secundum. *LA* left atrium, *RA* right atrium

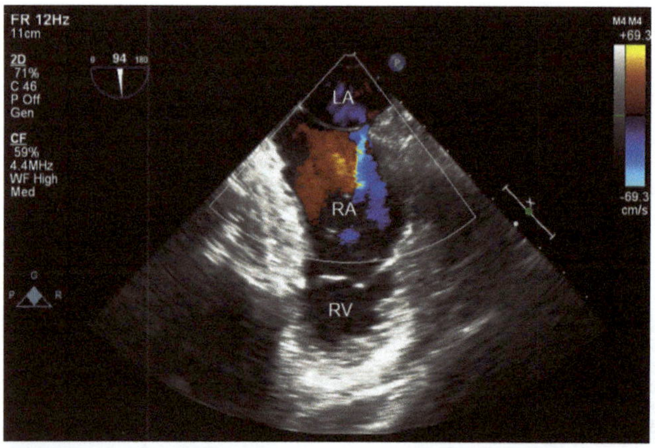

Fig. 4.19 Mid esophageal bicaval view with leftward probe rotation demonstrating a small patent foramen ovale with left to right shunting. *LA* left atrium, *RA* right atrium, *RV* right ventricle

the return of these veins back to the LA. The atrial septum is also very well shown with this sweep (Figs. 4.11 and 4.18, Videos 4.2 and 4.5). A patent foramen ovale, when present, is usually seen as a small flap in the atrial septum between its two components of septum secundum and septum primum. Atrial shunting can be confirmed by color flow Doppler (Fig. 4.19, Video 4.8). With further leftward turning of the probe, the remainder of atrial septum (including posterior rim) is visualized, and eventually the entire LA is displayed. A cross section of the CS is then visualized inferiorly. With even more leftward turning, the left atrial appendage and left pulmonary veins come into view (as described above).

If the atrial septum appears intact but atrial shunting is still suspected, a contrast injection can be performed through a peripheral or central vein, using agitated saline [30–32]. Contrast injection can often uncover small, occult right to left atrial level communications. Video 4.9a shows no right to left shunt atrial level shunt, Video 4.9b shows an occult right to left atrial shunt. However, it should be remembered that even with contrast injection, some atrial communications with potential for shunting could still go undetected [33, 34]. In older patients in whom TEE is performed under conscious sedation, provocative maneuvers such as a Valsalva maneuver [30] or coughing [31, 35] have been recommended in conjunction with contrast injection. In patients who are intubated, a simulated Valsalva maneuver can be performed by manually inflating the lungs with positive inspiratory pressure to about 25 mmHg for 10 s [36], maintaining inflation while injecting contrast, and then allowing the lungs to deflate as contrast is seen filling the heart.

Abnormalities of the atria and atrial septum are very well visualized by TEE. For this reason, TEE is widely used to evaluate atrial septal defects (including during transcatheter closure), atrial septal aneurysms, atrial masses and atrial/left atrial appendage thrombi. These applications will be discussed in subsequent chapters of this textbook.

Atrioventricular Valve Evaluation

Evaluation of the atrioventricular (AV) junction represents a key aspect of segmental analysis. Because the atrial and ventricular segments are independent of each other, different combinations can occur in the connection between the atria and ventricles [5, 12]. Normally, the RA empties into the morphologic right ventricle (RV) and LA into the morphologic left ventricle (LV), and this is termed AV *concordance.* However, when the RA empties into LV and LA into RV, there is AV *discordance*—as seen in congenitally corrected transposition of the great arteries (CCTGA). With two good-sized AV valves and ventricles, the general rule is that the AV valves arise from (and are associated with) their ventricle of entry, not the atrium of exit [37, 38]. Thus the AV valve associated with the morphologic LV is generally the mitral valve, and with the morphologic RV, the tricuspid valve. However, abnormalities of AV connection can occur that cause deviations from this rule, including override or straddling of one AV valve into another chamber, and connection of both AV valves to one ventricle (double inlet ventricle). In addition, other abnormalities can also occur such as absence of an AV valve (tricuspid/mitral atresia), and a common AV valve (AV septal or canal defect) [5, 8, 37]. When evaluating CHD, it is important for the TEE examiner to be mindful of these different possibilities. Nonetheless, the evaluation of the AV connections can be distilled into several important components. The first is, of course, correct morphologic identification of the individual atria (discussed above) and ventricles (discussed below) [8]. Once this is established, details of the AV connections can be determined, including: AV valve

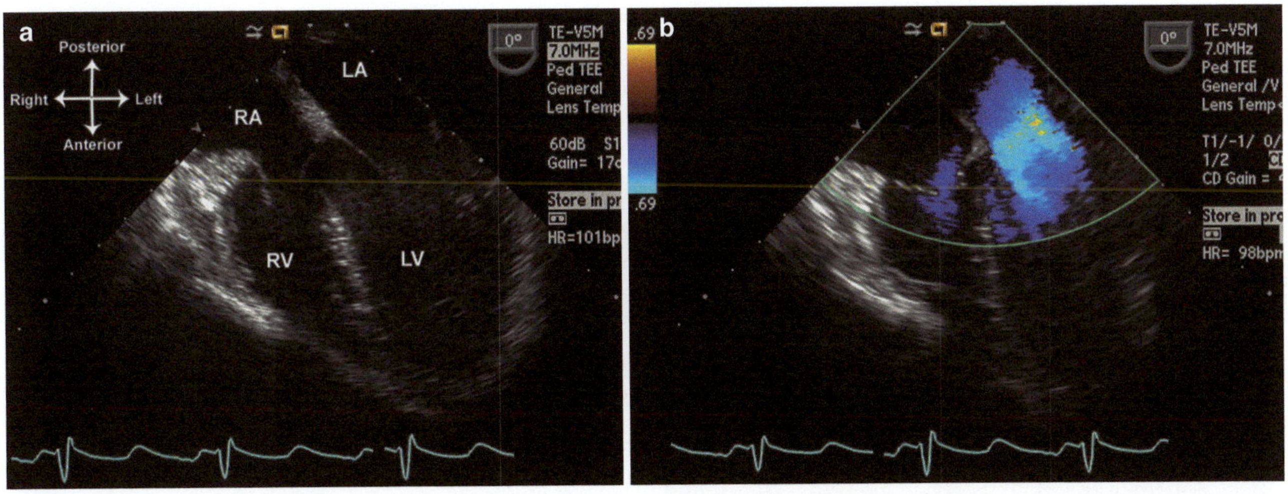

Fig. 4.20 Mid esophageal four chamber view (multiplane angle 0°) showing the atrioventricular valves open in diastole (**a**), along with diastolic inflow as noted by color flow Doppler (**b**). *LA* left atrium, *LV* left ventricle, *RA* right atrium, *RV* right ventricle

identification and number (one vs. two), how the atria and ventricles are connected, any possible override/straddling of the AV valves, and whether AV valve stenosis and/or insufficiency is present. For this type of evaluation, TEE generally provides excellent information.

From the "home base" (ME 4 Ch) view, the AV valves are displayed with a multiplane angle of 0–20°. The probe should be kept in a neutral position, or retroflexed to provide unforeshortened long axis images of the AV valves (Fig. 4.20a) Using this view, a number of details can be evaluated about the valves: relative sizes of the two valves and valve annuli, chordal attachments and (if present) chordal straddling, chordal length, and valve motion. Color flow Doppler (Fig. 4.20b, Video 4.10) provides evaluation of flow across both AV valves, and valvar stenosis or regurgitation is readily identified; valve stenosis or regurgitant jet velocities can be quantified using spectral Doppler.

As noted above, the mitral valve is associated with the morphologic LV. It has two leaflets—a deep anterior and a shallow posterior leaflet—and both leaflets have attachments to each of two prominent LV papillary muscles arising from the free wall. In the normal heart, typically there is fibrous continuity between the anterior leaflet and aortic valve. For the mitral valve, further anatomic and functional characterization can be performed using either of two principal anatomic nomenclature systems, as described by Carpentier and Duran [1, 39]. The more commonly used system is based upon the Carpentier nomenclature, and recommended by the ASE/SCA [1, 40]. It is outlined briefly as follows. The anterior and posterior leaflets are each divided into three parts, known as "thirds" for the anterior leaflet and "scallops" for the posterior leaflet, and numbered in ascending order from lateral to medial (A1–A2–A3 for the anterior leaflet, P1–P2–P3 for posterior leaflet) (Fig. 4.21a) The individual scallops and corresponding opposing segments can be visualized from the mid esophageal views when the LA and LV are centered on the image, and the rotational axis of the TEE transducer is placed in the center of the anterior leaflet, as shown in Fig. 4.21b. From the standard ME 4 Ch view, depending upon the amount of probe anteflexion/retroflexion, the scallops of the posterior leaflet are shown to the right of the display, and apposing components of the anterior leaflet to the left. Probe anteflexion will display more anterior portions of the mitral valve (A1 and P1), a neutral position will show the middle segments (A2 and P2), and probe retroflexion will demonstrate the most posterior portions (A3 and P3). Rotation of the multiplane angle to 60–70° yields the *mid esophageal mitral commissural view* (ME Mitral, Figs. 4.5e and 4.22, Video 4.11). This view demonstrates a lengthwise view of the papillary muscles, as well as the P1 (to the right of the display) and P3 (to the left of the display) scallops of the posterior leaflet and details of the anterior leaflet (particularly A2) wedged between the posterior leaflet scallops. Further mitral valve evaluation can be performed from the *mid esophageal two chamber view* (ME 2 Ch, Fig. 4.5f), with the multiplane angle rotated to 80–100° (Fig. 4.23, Video 4.12). In this view, the posterior leaflet (P3) is seen to the left of the display, and anterior leaflet (A1, A2, sometimes A3) to the right. Finally, the *mid esophageal long axis view* (ME LAX, Figs. 4.5g and 4.24, Video 4.13) is obtained from a multiplane angle of 100–130°; P2 scallop of posterior leaflet is seen to the left of the display, and anterior leaflet (A2) to the right [1, 41]. It should be noted the Carpentier nomenclature might have less application in CHD, given that the pathologies that commonly affect the mitral valve in adults (e.g. mitral valve prolapse) significantly differ from those seen in children. Nonetheless in some cases of congenital pathology that affect the mitral valve, or acquired pathology

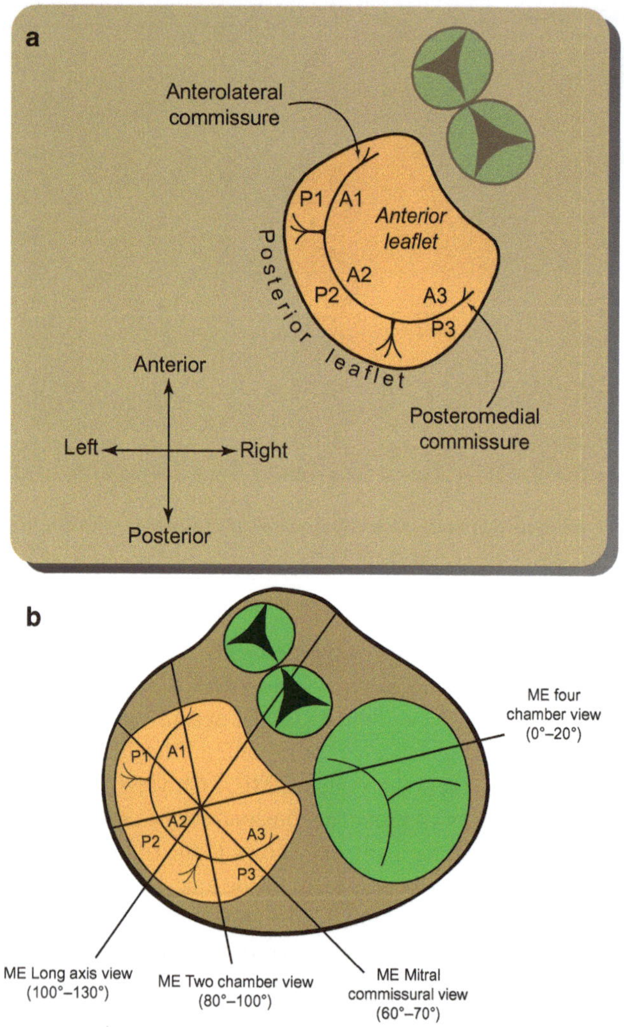

Fig. 4.21 Anatomy of the mitral valve leaflets as viewed from the left atrium, based on the Carpentier (ASE/SCA) classification. (**a**) The nomenclature. Both leaflets are divided into thirds, as noted in the diagram, with each third carrying a distinct label. (**b**) The various mid esophageal (*ME*) TEE views that display the different portions of the mitral valve. *A1* lateral third of anterior leaflet, *A2* middle third of anterior leaflet, *A3* medial third of anterior leaflet, *P1* lateral scallop of posterior leaflet, *P2* middle scallop of posterior leaflet, *P3* medial scallop of posterior leaflet

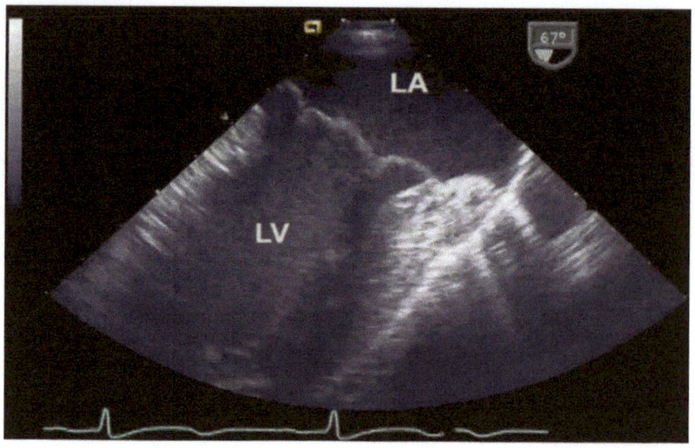

Fig. 4.22 Mid esophageal mitral commissural view (multiplane angle 60–70°), showing the mitral valve and the antero-lateral papillary muscle of the left ventricle (*LV*). The P1 and P3 scallops of the posterior leaflet can be seen to the right and left of the display respectively, and the A2 segment of anterior leaflet is wedged between the two posterior leaflet scallops. *LA* left atrium

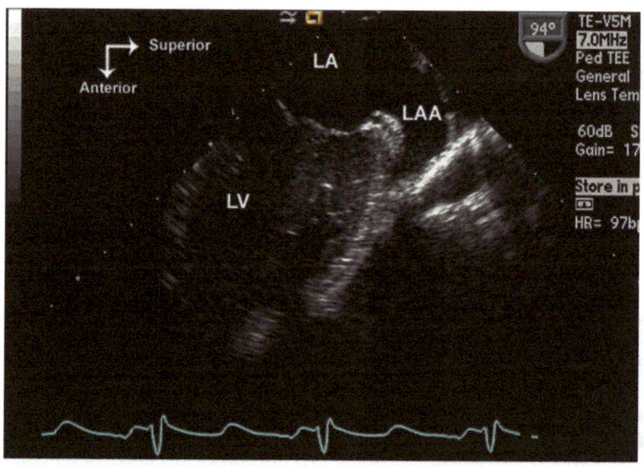

Fig. 4.23 Mid esophageal two chamber view (multiplane angle 80–100°) showing the mitral valve, left atrium (*LA*), left ventricle (*LV*), and left atrial appendage (*LAA*). For the mitral valve, the posterior leaflet (P3 scallop) is seen to the left of the image, and anterior leaflet (A1, A2, A3 segments) to the right

within the context of CHD, familiarity with this nomenclature and characterization of corresponding abnormalities by TEE is helpful in communicating the findings to the surgical team.

The mitral valve can also be evaluated with the transgastric views (Fig. 4.5r–u). These are obtained by advancing the probe into the stomach just past the gastro-esophageal junction and anteflexing, using various multiplane angles between 0° and 120°. Using a multiplane angle of 0–20°, an *en face* view of the mitral valve is afforded using the *transgastric basal short axis view* (TG Basal SAX, Figs. 4.5r and 4.25, Video 4.14). When available, this view can provide details of abnormalities such as mitral valve clefts. Using the same multiplane angle, further probe advancement displays the *transgastric mid short axis view* (TG Mid SAX, Figs. 4.5s and 4.26, Video 4.15), a view that enables assessment of the mitral support apparatus and characterization of papillary muscle detail such as number and spacing. This is also an important view for ventricular functional assessment, as regions supplied by the three main coronary arteries are depicted (Chap. 5). While still in the transgastric position, rotating the multiplane angle to 80–120° yields an orthogonal, longitudinally oriented visualization of the mitral valve and its tensor apparatus using the *transgastric two chamber view* (TG 2 Ch, Figs. 4.5t and 4.27, Video 4.16) and *transgastric long axis view* (TG LAX,

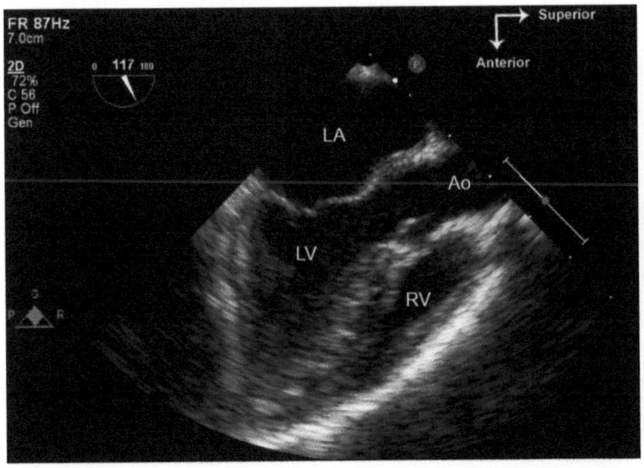

Fig. 4.24 Mid esophageal long axis view (multiplane angle 100–130°) showing the anterior leaflet (A2 segment) and posterior leaflet (P2 scallop) of the mitral valve, as well as the left ventricular outflow tract and aortic valve. In this view, mitral to aortic fibrous continuity is readily seen. *Ao* aorta, *LA* left atrium, *LV* left ventricle, *RV* right ventricle

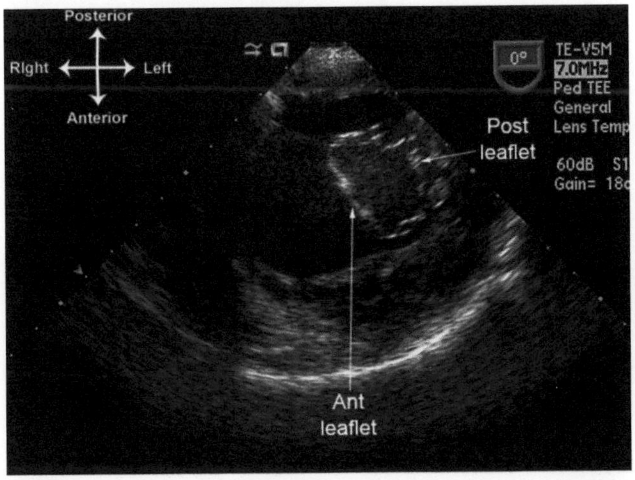

Fig. 4.25 Transgastric basal short axis view of the left ventricle in cross section with the mitral valve *en face*; the valve is open during diastole. The anterior leaflet (*Ant leaflet*) and posterior leaflets (*Post leaflet*) of the mitral valve are shown. This view is obtained with the TEE probe in the anteflexed position, using a multiplane angle between 0° and 20°

Fig. 4.5u). The TG LAX view also provides very good visualization of the LV outflow tract, including a good angle for spectral Doppler interrogation of this area (Fig. 4.28, Video 4.17).

The tricuspid valve is associated with the morphologic RV. It typically has three leaflets (anterior, posterior/inferior, septal), with the anterior leaflet being the most prominent. Unlike the mitral valve, the tricuspid valve has less well-defined papillary musculature, and usually the individual leaflets do not significantly "share" chordae among all of the different papillary muscles. The most prominent

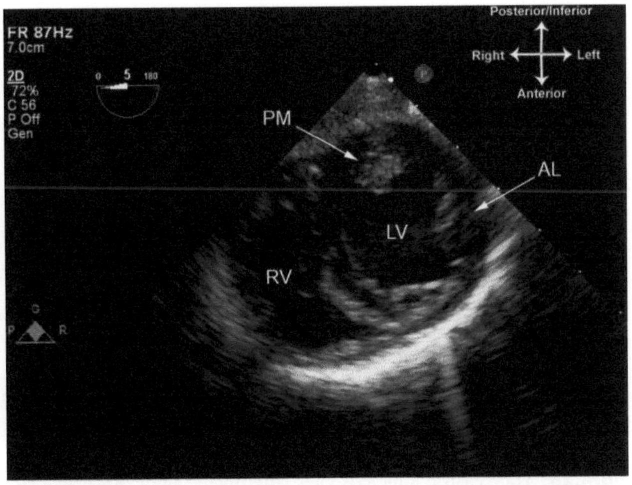

Fig. 4.26 Transgastric mid short axis view of the left ventricle (*LV*) and right ventricle (*RV*) in cross section. From the position in Fig. 4.25, the probe has been advanced further in the stomach (while maintaining anteflexion) to visualize the anterolateral (*AL*) and posteromedial (*PM*) papillary muscles as well as the more inferior portion of the *LV*

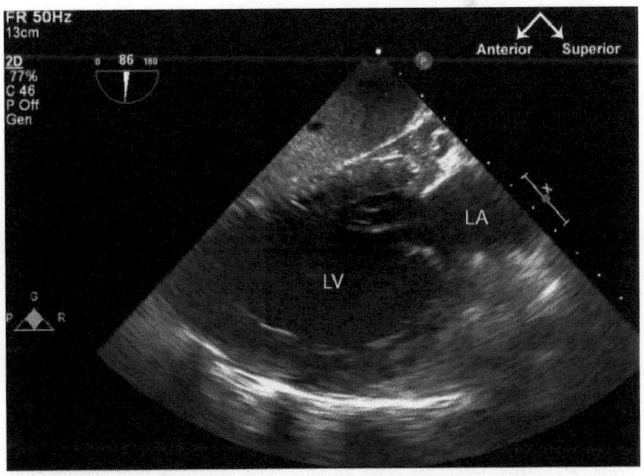

Fig. 4.27 Transgastric two chamber view of the left atrium (*LA*) and left ventricle (*LV*). The probe has been advanced into the stomach to the level of the transgastric window, and anteflexed. Using a multiplane angle between 80° and 100°, the LA, LV, and mitral valve leaflets are visualized

RV papillary muscle is the anterolateral papillary muscle with chordae attaching primarily (and sometimes exclusively) to the anterior leaflet [42]. The posterior/inferior leaflet has one to three smaller papillary muscles arising from the inferior RV surface, and the septal leaflet has multiple chordae attaching directly to more rudimentary papillary muscles on the ventricular septum [43]. By TEE, the tricuspid valve is best evaluated at the mid esophageal and transgastric levels (Fig. 4.29) [44]. Initial assessment of tricuspid inflow can be performed with the ME 4 Ch view, as shown on Fig. 4.20a, b and Video 4.10. This view typically

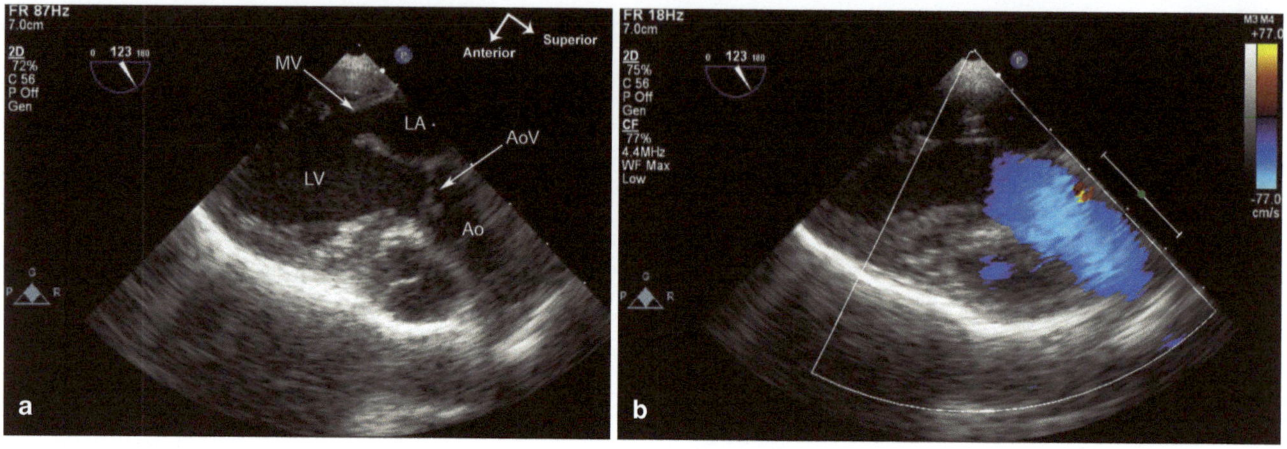

Fig. 4.28 Transgastric long axis view (multiplane angle 90–120°). (**a**) The left atrium (*LA*), left ventricle (*LV*), mitral valve (*MV*), aortic valve (*AoV*), and ascending aorta (*Ao*) can all be seen. This view provides an excellent view of LV outflow tract, enabling excellent color flow Doppler evaluation (**b**) and providing a good angle for spectral Doppler assessment

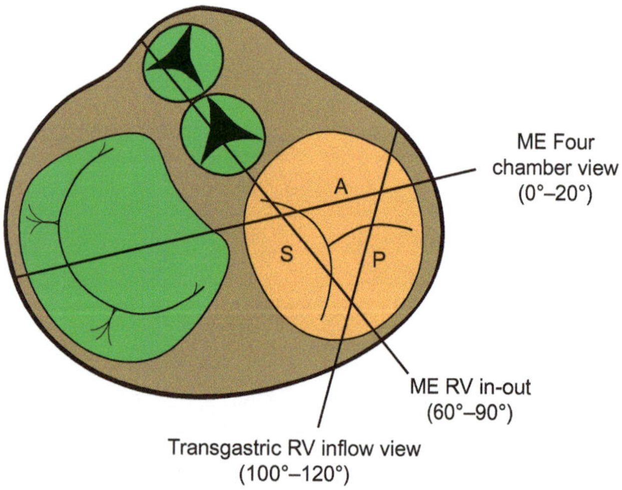

Fig. 4.29 Anatomy of the tricuspid valve leaflets as viewed from the atrial perspective. The three tricuspid valve leaflets—anterior (*A*), posterior (*P*), septal (*S*)—are seen *en face*. The common mid esophageal and transgastric views that visualize the individual tricuspid valve leaflets are shown

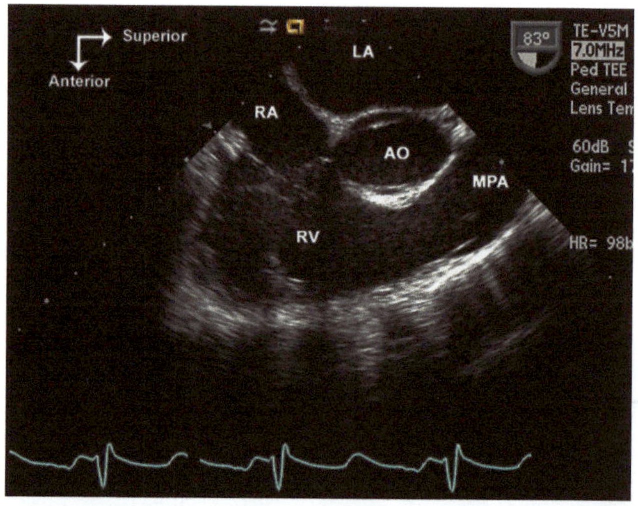

Fig. 4.30 Visualization of tricuspid valve inflow and right ventricular outflow using a mid esophageal probe position. This mid esophageal right ventricular inflow-outflow view can be obtained using a multiplane angle of 60–90°. *AO* aorta, *LA* left atrium, *MPA* main pulmonary artery, *RA* right atrium, *RV* right ventricle

demonstrates the anterior leaflet laterally, adjacent to the RV free wall, and septal leaflet medially, adjacent to the ventricular septum [44]. Additional views that provide anatomic detail, and allow for color flow and spectral Doppler evaluation, include a modified ME Bicaval view (visualizing anterior as well as posterior/septal leaflets). From the ME 4 Ch or Bicaval views, if the transducer is rotated toward the mid-portion of the RV and the multiplane angle set between 60° and 90° the *mid esophageal right ventricular inflow-outflow view* (ME RV In-Out, Figs. 4.5h and 4.30, Video 4.18) is obtained, visualizing posterior and septal leaflets as well as the inflow and outflow portions of the RV. For transgastric evaluation of the tricuspid valve, once the TEE probe is advanced into the transgastric position, anteflexion is performed to obtain the TG Mid and Basal SAX views, as described above (Fig. 4.5r, s). The TEE probe is then rotated slightly clockwise (to the right), and/or rightward flexion is performed in those probes with a lateral probe tip control. A multiplane angle between 0° and 50° can be applied to provide an *en face visualization* of all three tricuspid valve leaflets (Fig. 4.31, Video 4.19) [44]. While still in this position, the multiplane angle is turned to 100–120° to obtain the *transgastric right ventricular inflow view* (TG RV In, Figs. 4.5v and 4.32a, Video 4.20), which shows the anterior and posterior leaflets of the tricuspid valve as well as chordal apparatus and papillary muscles [44, 45]. If the probe is then turned leftward (counterclockwise), the trabecular and outflow portions of the

RV will become visible, as will a portion of the LV outflow tract (Video 4.20). A useful modification of the TG RV In view is obtained when the TEE probe is turned to the right from this view and advanced slightly; this provides visualization of SVC return to the right atrium by 2D and color flow Doppler, as well as a very good angle for spectral Doppler evaluation of SVC inflow (Fig. 4.32b, Video 4.21).

All of the above TEE views serve to visualize the tricuspid valve and its tensor apparatus from a number of different perspectives. They are meant to complement each other, allowing for enhanced anatomic evaluation of pathology that in some cases might not be evident from a single view.

If there is a common AV valve, as seen in a complete AV septal defect (complete or common AV canal), the relative

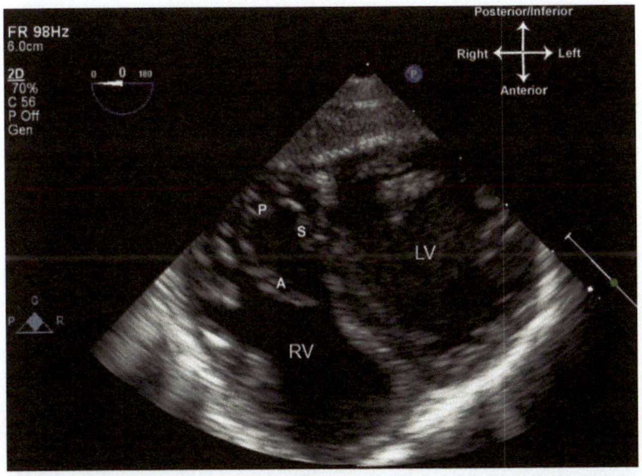

Fig. 4.31 Modified transgastric mid/basal short axis view, with the probe anteflexed and turned toward the right (*clockwise*). By adjusting the multiplane angle between 0° and 50°, the tricuspid valve can be seen *en face*. All three tricuspid valve leaflets are visualized: anterior (*A*), posterior (*P*), and septal (*S*). *LV* left ventricle, *RV* right ventricle

sizes of atrial and ventricular septal defects, as well as the balance of the valve above the ventricles, are well seen in the ME 4 Ch view. Transducer sweeps from anterior to posterior planes (retroflexion to anteflexion) facilitate this evaluation. The transgastric views discussed above, as well as the deep transgastric views (to be discussed below) can also be helpful. Evaluation of AV valves is discussed in detail in Chap. 8.

Ventricles and Ventricular Septum

An important part of CHD evaluation is the determination of ventricular morphology, looping, shape and size. Each ventricle can be identified by its distinctive morphologic characteristics. The RV has a crescenteric, triangular shape, coarse apical trabeculations, a moderator band near the apex, a prominent infundibulum (outflow), a trileaflet AV (tricuspid) valve, and attachments of the tricuspid valve to the ventricular septum (a "septophilic" valve). In contrast, the morphologic LV has an elliptical shape, fine apical trabeculations and a smooth ventricular septal surface, a bileaflet AV (mitral) valve, and no mitral valve attachments to the ventricular septum (a "septophobic" valve) [27]. When viewed from a four chamber view, the septal origin of anterior leaflet of mitral valve is located slightly more superior to that of the septal leaflet of tricuspid valve [4, 21, 46]. All of these morphologic features serve to differentiate RV from LV. Although in most cases a transthoracic echocardiographic evaluation allows for this assessment, it is important to highlight that all these features can also be discerned by TEE.

Starting from the "home base" position (ME 4 Ch), a multiplane angle of 0–10° is used to display the inflow of both ventricles, although in some cases of cardiac malposition,

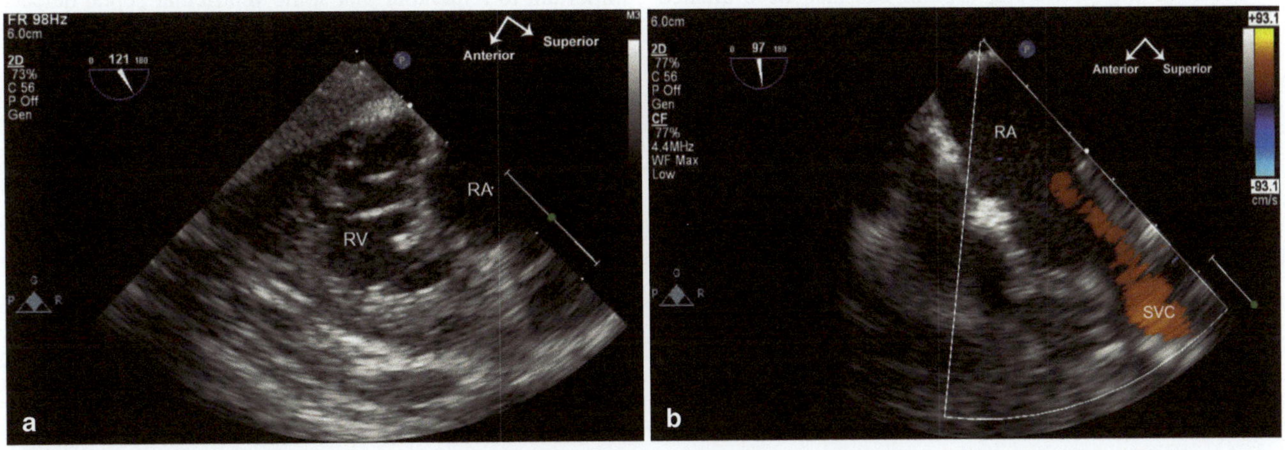

Fig. 4.32 Transgastric right ventricular inflow view, using a multiplane angle between 100° and 120°. The probe is rotated slightly to the right (*clockwise*). (**a**) A long axis view of the tricuspid valve, including the anterior/posterior leaflets and tensor apparatus. (**b**) The probe is rotated slightly more rightward to visualize the inflow of superior vena cava (*SVC*) into the right atrium. Note the excellent angle for spectral interrogation of SVC inflow. *RA* right atrium, *RV* right ventricle

the multiplane angle must be rotated to provide a suitable four chamber view. The TEE evaluation of the LV parallels that of the mitral valve (described above). Multiple cross-sections of the LV can be obtained with the ME 4 Ch and ME 2 Ch, as well as the ME Mitral and ME LAX views (Figs. 4.20, 4.22, 4.23, and 4.24, Videos 4.10, 4.11, 4.12, and 4.13). Important information and sweeps of the LV can also be obtained from the transgastric views: cross sectional views of the LV from the TG Basal and TG Mid SAX (Figs. 4.25 and 4.26, Videos 4.14 and 4.15), and long axis views from the TG 2 Ch and TG LAX (Figs. 4.27 and 4.28, Videos 4.16 and 4.17). Papillary muscle origins and mitral valve detail can be evaluated in the manner described above. In addition, the deep transgastric views (described below), obtained by advancing the imaging probe into the fundus of the stomach, may facilitate this evaluation.

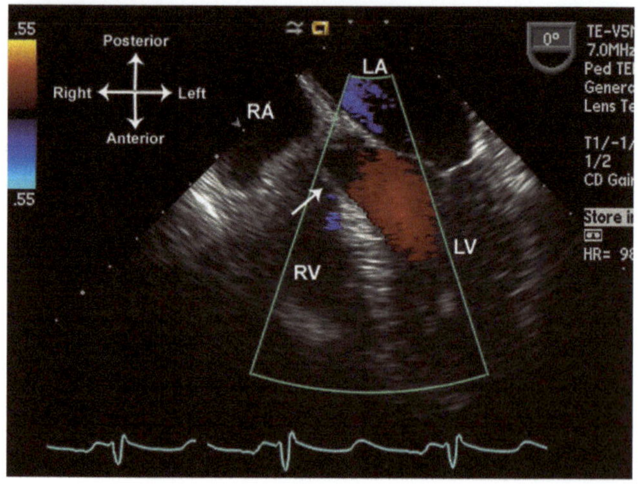

Fig. 4.33 Membranous and muscular ventricular septum viewed from the mid esophageal four chamber view, with slight TEE probe anteflexion. The *arrow* points to the thin membranous septum; seen more inferiorly is the thicker muscular or trabecular septum. *LA* left atrium, *LV* left ventricle, *RA* right atrium, *RV* right ventricle

The RV, with its triangular shape, can be divided into inflow, apical trabecular, and outflow (infundibular) portions. The inflow portion is best visualized using the same views for tricuspid valve evaluation. Using the, ME 4 Ch view (Fig. 4.20, Video 4.10), the TEE probe can be retroflexed to visualize the entire length of the right ventricular inflow and the moderator band. The TG RV In view also provides good visualization of the inflow and trabecular portions of the RV as well as some imaging of the RV outflow (Fig. 4.32a, Video 4.20). The RV trabecular and outflow portions can be seen with a ME 4 Ch view and probe anteflexion producing a ("ME five chamber view"), though this maneuver foreshortens the structures and provides more of a cross-sectional sweep of RV outflow. A better view to provide long axis visualization of the outflow (infundibular) portion of the RV is the ME RV In-Out view, using multiplane angles between 60° and 90° (Fig. 4.30, Video 4.18). The deep transgastric views (described below) can also provide additional detail of the RV outflow tract.

Much of the ventricular septum can also be evaluated from the ME 4 Ch view (0–10°). A sweep of the ventricular septum can be performed first starting at the membranous portion in the region of the septal leaflet of the tricuspid valve (Fig. 4.33), and then retroflexing the probe to visualize the inlet and more posterior portions of the muscular septum. While this sweep provides adequate visualization of the apical muscular septum, additional views of the apex can also be obtained by advancing the probe into the stomach (transgastric position) while maintaining probe anteflexion, to obtain the TG Basal SAX and TG Mid SAX views. Withdrawal of the probe to the mid esophageal position and anteflexion allow visualization of the more anterior portions of trabecular ventricular septum. Because the ventricular septum curves at the level of the infundibulum, or *crista supraventricularis,* full visualization of the infundibular (conal) septum is best performed with the probe tip approximately at the level of the semilunar valves, rotating the multiplane angle between 30° and 60° to obtain the *mid esophageal aortic valve short axis* view (ME AV SAX, Figs. 4.5i and 4.34a). This view simulates an inverted transthoracic parasternal short axis view, and is helpful for distinguishing perimembranous from outlet (supracristal) ventricular septal defects (see Chap. 9). Further views of the infundibular septum are provided by the ME RV In-Out view (multiplane angle rotation 60–90°), and by further rotating the multiplane angle between 90° and 110°, a modified ME LAX view (Fig. 4.34a, b). These views provide excellent imaging of the infundibular septum as well as its relationship to the semilunar valves. Video 4.22 demonstrates a typical sweep of the ventricular septum from multiple TEE views. Given the complex nature of the ventricular septum, it is important to remember that some ventricular septal defects will be seen on certain views, but not others. Thus, evaluation of the ventricular septum requires a comprehensive assessment, often utilizing multiple TEE views (discussed in Chap. 9).

In CHD evaluation, assessment of ventricular size and shape plays an important role. This can be done with the views outlined above. In particular cases, it may be important to determine whether both ventricles are "apex-forming", whether papillary musculature is normal, or whether the three parts of the RV are present and normal in size. The individual mitral and tricuspid valve annulus diameters should be measured. Abnormalities of ventricular shape should also be noted. For example, the RV should have a thin, crescenteric shape when viewed from the TG Basal and Mid SAX views (Fig. 4.5r, s). Dilation of the RV and flattening of the ventricular septum could signify abnormal loading conditions and/or abnormal RV function.

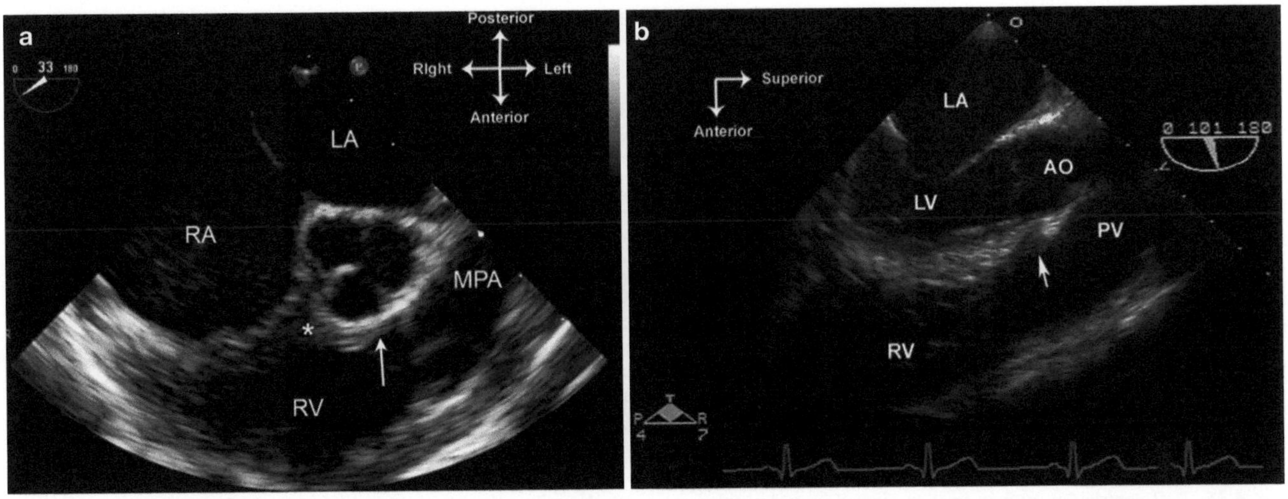

Fig. 4.34 Ventricular septum as viewed from two mid esophageal views. (**a**) The mid esophageal aortic valve short axis view displays the aortic valve *en face*, with all three leaflets seen. This view also shows the membranous (*asterisk*) and infundibular (*arrow*) portions of ventricular septum; it closely resembles an inverted transthoracic parasternal short axis view. Rotation of the multiplane element to about 100° shows a modified mid esophageal long axis view (**b**), displaying both right and left ventricular outflow tracts as well as the infundibular septum (*arrow*). *AO* aorta, *LA* left atrium, *LV* left ventricle, *MPA* main pulmonary artery, *RA* right atrium, *RV* right ventricle

Determination of ventricular looping (ventricular situs) is also an important element of CHD segmental analysis. There are three types of ventricular looping: D, L, and X (indeterminate looping). The normal cardiac looping is a 'D' loop, in which, during embryologic development, looping of the straight heart tube places the bulbus cordis to the *right* of the primitive ventricle, thus the morphologic RV lies to the *right* of the morphologic LV. In contrast, an 'L' loop occurs when the looping places the bulbus cordis to the left of the primitive ventricle, and the morphologic RV lies to the *left* of the morphologic LV. Most congenital cardiac defects are seen with a D-looped RV; however with some complex forms of CHD such as CCTGA and visceral-atrial situs inversus or ambiguous (heterotaxy), the RV is L-looped (or in some cases looping is indeterminate). Van Praagh et al first introduced the notion of *chirality* to characterize and differentiate 'D' vs. 'L' loops [47]. Chirality is used in chemistry to describe stereoisomeric forms of a given molecule; it refers to two objects that are nonsuperimposable mirror images of each other, such as the right and left hands. Van Praagh et al characterized the morphologic D-looped RV as having the same layout of a right hand: the thumb being inflow, fingers being outflow, palm being RV septal surface, dorsum being RV free wall. In the same manner, an L-looped RV has the layout of a left hand [47]. The importance of chirality is in the recognition that both D and L looped RVs maintain their distinctive shapes and are identifiable irrespective of their position in space; this can be valuable in the identification and analysis of certain complicated forms of CHD such as CCTGA and criss-cross heart [12, 47]. Identification of ventricular looping can have important clinical implications, for such factors as coronary artery pattern, conduction system, ventricular organization, and (in the case of CCTGA) possible Ebsteinoid malformation of the left sided AV valve [9]. As with other features of ventricular morphology, ventricular looping can readily be discerned both by transthoracic as well as TEE imaging. However it is important to remember that, given the independence of the individual segments from each other, ventricular looping should not be considered in isolation. Rather, it must be evaluated in conjunction with the rest of the segmental anatomy.

Outflow Tracts and Semilunar Valves

As the third major segment, the great arteries must be evaluated carefully, along with the connecting segment between the ventricles and great arteries, which gives rise to the left and right ventricular outflow tracts (LVOT and RVOT respectively). This portion of the anatomy, variously termed as the ventriculo-arterial (V-A) junction by Anderson [8] or subsemilunar infundibulum (conus) by Van Praagh [9, 38, 48], requires the careful assessment of several major features. First, the identity of each great artery must be established. The semilunar valves cannot be used for this purpose; unlike the AV valves, the semilunar valves are anatomically identical, and no specific characteristics differentiate a pulmonary from an aortic valve. Thus, the great arteries are identified by searching for the origin of the coronary arteries, and/or recognizing the characteristic anatomic features of branch pulmonary arteries or an aortic arch. Second, the relationship of the great arteries to the ventricles and any ventricular septal defect (if present) must be delineated. There are four principal types of V-A connection: (a) V-A *concordance*, in which RV

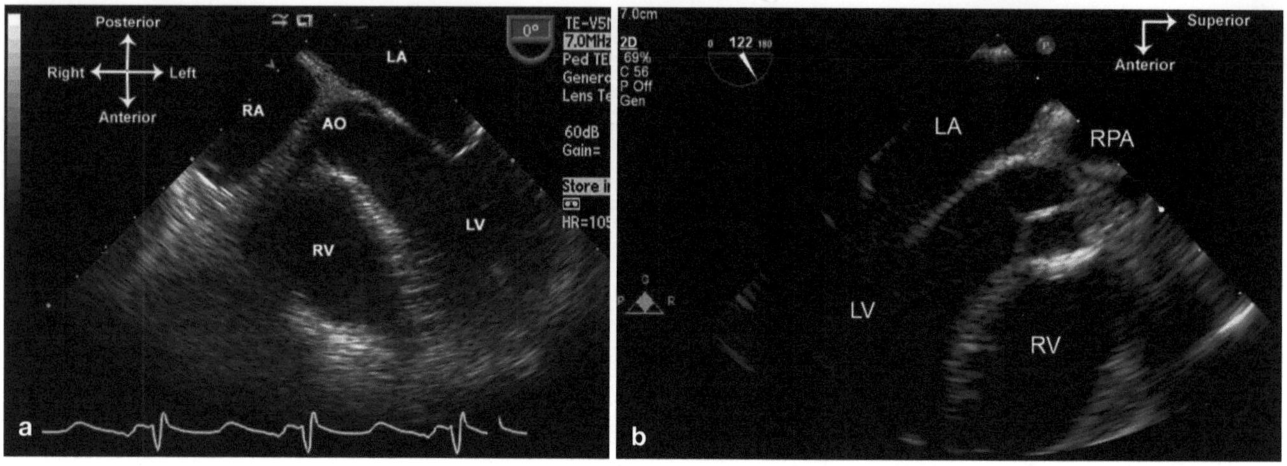

Fig. 4.35 Left ventricular outflow tract as viewed in mid esophageal four chamber view, with multiplane angle of 0° and probe anteflexion (also known as the mid esophageal five chamber view) (**a**), and mid esophageal aortic valve long axis view, multiplane angle approximately 120° (**b**). *AO* aorta, *LA* left atrium, *LV* left ventricle, *PV* pulmonary valve, *RA* right atrium, *RPA* right pulmonary artery, *RV* right ventricle

is connected to pulmonary artery, LV to aorta; (b) V-A *discordance*, in which LV is connected to pulmonary artery, RV to aorta; (c) Double outlet, in which both great arteries arise predominantly (at least 50 % of their semilunar valve circumference) or totally from one ventricle, either RV or LV; (d) Single outlet, in which only one great artery is seen to arise from the ventricles (either due to truncus arteriosus or atresia of one great artery) [8, 49]. Third, the relationship of the great arteries must be determined. Normally related great arteries are oriented at about 30–45° to each other, with the aorta posterior and rightward, the pulmonary artery leftward and anterior, subpulmonary conal muscle separating pulmonary from tricuspid valves, and lack of subaortic conal muscle allowing mitral to aortic fibrous continuity. However there are a number of congenital cardiac defects in which the great arteries are malposed or transposed, leading to an altered spatial relationship of the two vessels both in the anterior-posterior and right-left planes, often with a more parallel orientation of both great arteries, and variable amounts of conal (infundibular) musculature below one, both, or (less commonly) neither semilunar valve. Fourth, a determination of the presence/absence of outflow tract obstruction (to either great artery) must be made. Outflow tract obstruction, when present, can be subvalvar (often due to conal/outlet septal malalignment), valvar (abnormal and/or hypoplastic semilunar valve), supravalvar, or any combination of these levels. The above features can present a complicated evaluation for TEE, one in which a combination of different TEE windows and views (mid and upper esophageal, transgastric and deep transgastric) should be used for complete and optimal assessment. Abnormalities of the V–A junction are seen with many types of CHD. These are discussed in further detail in Chaps. 11 and 12.

Both the LVOT and RVOT can be visualized readily by TEE. The LVOT is best imaged from the ME 4 Ch view, with slight withdrawal/anteflexion of the TEE probe. The multiplane angle can then be steered between 0° and 130° to provide a complete anatomic assessment of the area (Fig. 4.35a, b, Video 4.23). In the ME 4 Ch view, probe anteflexion will visualize the LVOT (Fig. 4.35a); this view is often called the "mid esophageal five chamber view". Rotating the multiplane angle forward to 90–130° yields the *mid esophageal aortic valve long axis* (ME AV LAX) view (Figs. 4.5j and 4.35b, Video 4.23), which is a very important and useful view for the assessment of the LVOT and aortic valve/aortic root. This view enables detailed evaluation of aortic valve excursion and measurement of annular dimensions; it provides excellent visualization of pathology involving the subaortic and immediate supravalvar aortic region. From here, slight probe withdrawal, mild anteflexion of the TEE probe, and rotation of the multiplane angle to 30–50° will produce the ME AV SAX view (Fig. 4.34a). The three aortic valve cusps (or leaflets) can be seen *en face,* and aortic valve morphology and motion are well shown. If aortic valve pathology exists, color flow Doppler evaluation can be performed at this probe location from a number of multiplane angles (0–130°) to determine the location of the flow disturbance, and the characteristics of the aortic stenosis and/or aortic regurgitant jet.

For further evaluation of supravalvar aortic pathology, the *mid esophageal ascending aortic long axis* view (ME Asc Ao LAX) is useful. This view, obtained by withdrawal and slight rightward turning of the TEE probe from the ME AV LAX position, displays the ascending aorta in long axis as it passes anterior to the right pulmonary artery (Figs. 4.5m and 4.36a, Video 4.24a).

The RVOT is best evaluated from the ME RV In-Out view (a view that can be difficult to obtain with a biplane TEE probe). As noted previously, this view opens the entire right

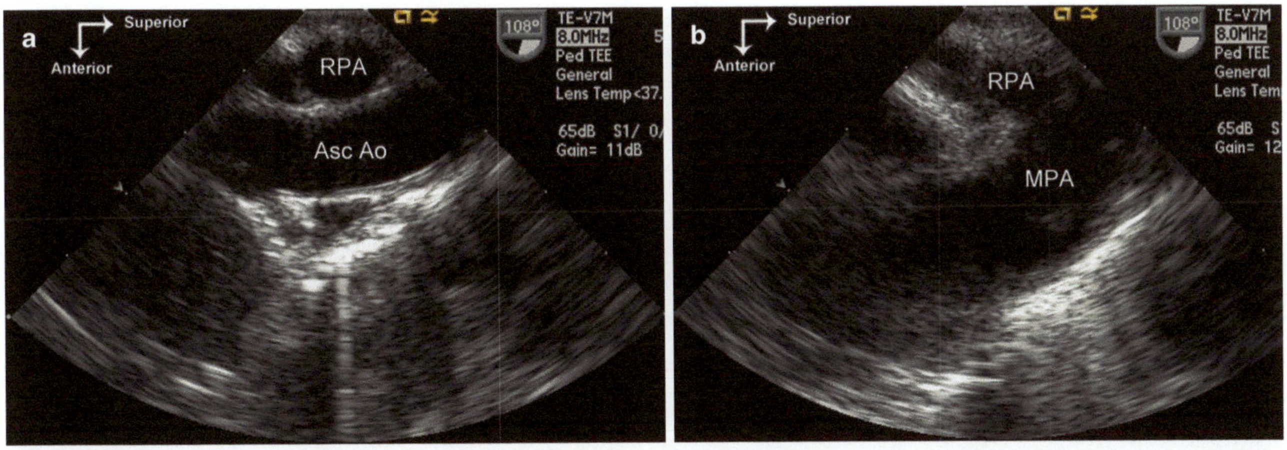

Fig. 4.36 Mid esophageal ascending aortic long axis (**a**) provides excellent visualization of the ascending aorta (*Asc Ao*) in a long axis as it courses anterior to the right pulmonary artery, seen in cross section (*RPA*). This view is very useful for evaluation of supravalvar aortic stenosis, and also for quantitative measurements of the Asc Ao. With slight leftward (*counterclockwise*) probe rotation, the main pulmonary artery (*MPA*) can be seen (**b**); this view is helpful for assessment of pathology in the supravalvar pulmonary area

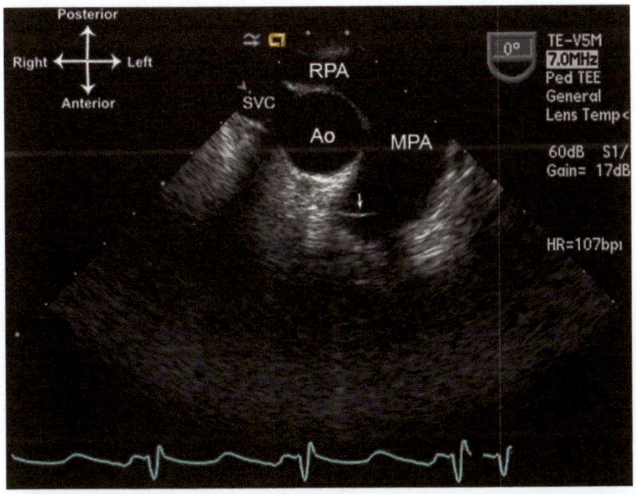

Fig. 4.37 Mid esophageal ascending aortic short axis displays the ascending aorta (*Ao*) in cross-section. This view is also useful for visualizing the main pulmonary artery (*MPA*) and right pulmonary artery (*RPA*), and sometimes the pulmonary valve (*arrow*) can also be seen. *SVC* superior vena cava

ventricular outflow tract from the right ventricular apex to the pulmonary valve (Fig. 4.30, Video 4.18). Because of the anterior position of the outflow tract, slight probe anteflexion is sometimes necessary to visualize the area. Withdrawal of the probe and rotation of the multiplane angle closer to about 90° facilitate visualization of the pulmonary valve from a more sagittal or long axis orientation, enabling measurement of the pulmonary valve annulus. The ME RV In-Out view provides excellent visualization of pathology involving the subpulmonary and immediate supravalvar pulmonary area. It also enables detailed color Doppler evaluation of flow characteristics across the pulmonary valve and adjacent areas along the pulmonary outflow tract. For further assessment of the supravalvar area, the ME Asc Ao LAX can be used, with slight leftward rotation of the TEE probe to view the main pulmonary artery (Fig. 4.36b, Video 4.24b). While keeping the TEE probe in the ME Asc Ao LAX position, rotation of the multiplane angle to 0–10° will give the *mid esophageal ascending aortic short axis* view (ME Asc Ao SAX), which shows the supravalvar pulmonary area as well as main pulmonary artery, right pulmonary artery, along with the ascending aorta and SVC in cross section (Figs. 4.51 and 4.37, Video 4.25). The pulmonary valve can also be seen in this view, although visualization might be variable. Another useful view for visualizing the supravalvar pulmonary area is the *upper esophageal aortic arch short axis* view (UE Ao Arch SAX). This view, which also provides an excellent angle for spectral Doppler interrogation of the pulmonary valve and supravalvar pulmonary region, will be discussed below.

The deep transgastric views are especially useful for evaluation of the LVOT and RVOT, particularly the subsemilunar portions of the ventricular outflow tracts. They are obtained as follows. From the mid or lower esophageal position, the probe is advanced slowly. Once the diaphragm and liver have been passed and the probe is free in the stomach, it should be anteflexed and, if contact is lost, withdrawn slightly. If a TG Mid SAX image is obtained, the probe is still too superior and needs to be advanced further while maintaining anteflexion. At times, slight and subtle manipulations of advancing and withdrawing the probe are required to maximize contact with the stomach. Once in the proper position, the image should be inverted so that the apex of the imaging sector is at the bottom of the screen, to obtain an anatomically "correct" view of the cardiac anatomy [23, 24]. The multiplane angle can be maintained at 0–20° to obtain the *deep transgastric long axis* view (DTG LAX, Fig. 4.5w), which can simulate a

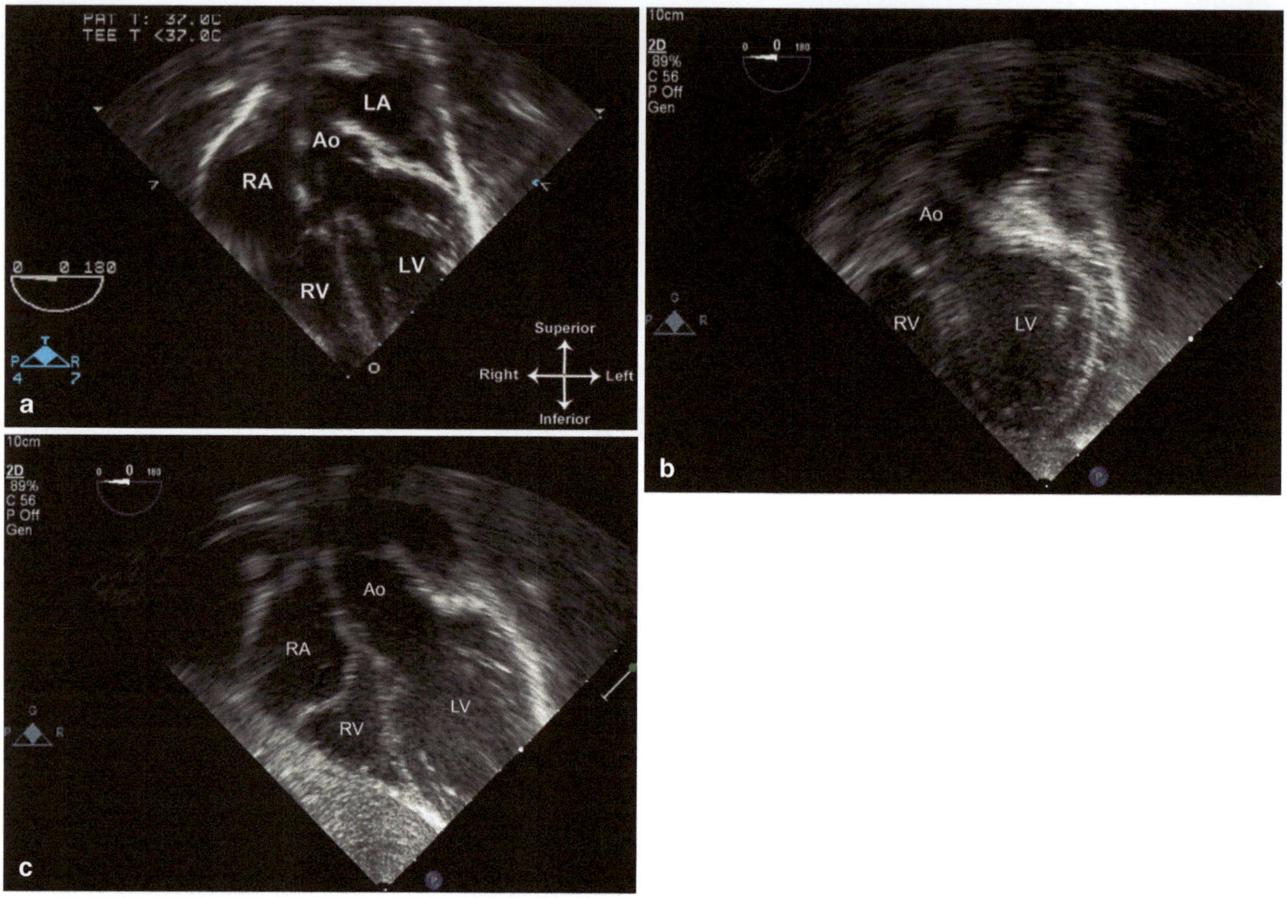

Fig. 4.38 Deep transgastric long axis views, as shown from different probe positions. (**a**) The left ventricular outflow tract is very well seen and there is an excellent angle for spectral Doppler evaluation. Mitral and tricuspid valve inflow are also well seen in this view. This particular image also shows a perimembranous ventricular septal defect. (**b**) The probe tip is closer to the apex and simulates a transthoracic apical view; (**c**) the probe was rotated to the right and more closely approximates a subcostal coronal view. Both (**b**) and (**c**) were obtained at nearly the same time from the same patient. *Ao* aorta, *LA* left atrium, *LV* left ventricle, *RA* right atrium, *RV* right ventricle

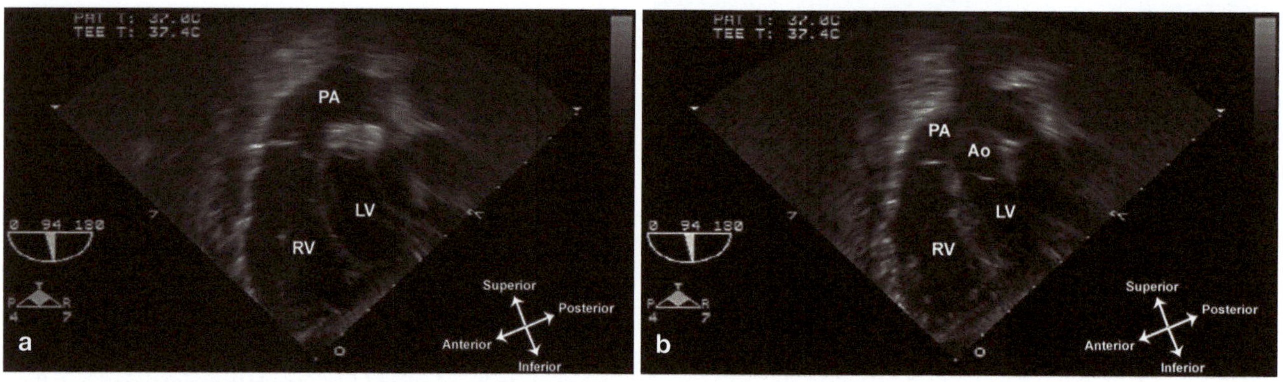

Fig. 4.39 Deep transgastric sagittal views (**a**, **b**) evaluating both right and left ventricular outflow tracts. The multiplane angle of approximately 90° simulates a transthoracic subcostal sagittal view. Note the favorable angles for spectral Doppler interrogation of flow across both outflow tracts. *Ao* aorta, *LV* left ventricle, *PA* pulmonary artery, *RV* right ventricle

transthoracic apical 4/5 chamber or subcostal coronal view, depending upon where the probe is located in relation to the heart (Fig. 4.38, Video 4.26). With this view, the outflow tracts can be visualized, as well as AV valve inflows [23]. In the same TEE probe position, rotation of the multiplane angle to 80–110° produces the *deep transgastric sagittal* view (DTG Sagittal, Fig. 4.5x), which simulates a transthoracic subcostal sagittal view. As the probe is advanced,

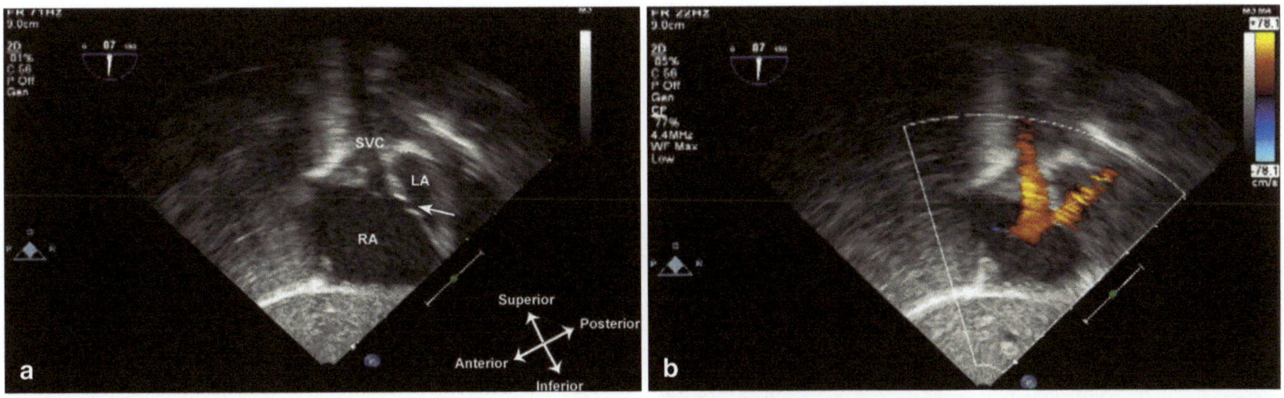

Fig. 4.40 Deep transgastric sagittal view that simulates a transthoracic subcostal sagittal image. (**a**) The superior vena cava (*SVC*) is seen to enter the right atrium (*RA*), and the left atrium (*LA*) is also seen, as well as a small atrial septal defect (*arrow*). (**b**) Color flow Doppler shows SVC return and left to right flow across the atrial defect

usually the RVOT is first visualized (Fig. 4.39a). To visualize the LVOT, the probe must be advanced further, while continuing significant anteflexion (to maintain contact with the stomach), in order to point the probe more posteriorly (Fig. 4.39b). Also, a small amount of rightward/leftward probe rotation can help to improve imaging of each outflow tract. Video 4.27 shows an example of outflow tract interrogation with color Doppler from the DTG Sagittal position, multiplane angle approximately 90°. With both the DTG LAX and Sagittal views, it should be emphasized that, to visualize the more posterior structures (e.g. LVOT), the TEE probe should be gently *advanced* while maintaining anteflexion to keep contact with the stomach.

In addition to their utility with the Doppler assessment of the outflow tracts, the DTG views can provide a great deal of additional information about other cardiac structures, such as the atrial septum and SVC inflow (Fig. 4.40, Video 4.28). Because they are similar to standard transthoracic subcostal views [6, 23, 24, 50], they can be particularly helpful for the evaluation of ventricular morphology and ventriculo-arterial relationships in outflow tract and conotruncal malformations (discussed in Chaps. 11 and 12) [21]. They can also serve as alternative views to evaluate ventricular shape and size and to examine the ventricular septum for possible mid and apical muscular defects, using color flow Doppler (discussed in Chap. 9). Inflow and outflow characteristics of both ventricles are often very well seen from the DTG perspective.

When evaluating obstruction across the LVOT and RVOT, different approaches must be used depending upon the level of obstruction. For optimal quantitative spectral Doppler interrogation, it is essential to obtain views that allow for alignment of the angle of insonation as parallel as possible to the direction of blood flow. The spectral Doppler interrogation of the LVOT is best performed by the TG LAX and deep transgastric views. Both of these windows provide optimal Doppler cursor alignment with the direction of blood flow in the LVOT. These views also provide additional anatomic detail of the LVOT, and they are helpful in the qualitative assessment of aortic valve regurgitation, thus complementing the mid esophageal views. For pulmonary valve stenosis, as well as supravalvar aortic and pulmonary valve stenosis, the mid and upper esophageal windows (ME AV LAX, ME AV SAX, ME Asc Ao LAX, ME Asc Ao SAX, UE Ao Arch SAX) can be utilized for assessment. However, for evaluation of subpulmonary stenosis (e.g. tetralogy of Fallot or double chamber RV), the utility of these views for Doppler interrogation can become problematic, as the Doppler angle can vary from one patient to another. In many instances of aortic valve stenosis, as well as RVOT and LVOT narrowing, the mid esophageal window becomes more unreliable because of a nearly perpendicular angle of interrogation for spectral Doppler. In these instances, Doppler evaluation of the outflow tracts is greatly enhanced from the deep transgastric position. These views, when available, generally provide excellent angles for spectral Doppler interrogation.

Coronary Artery Evaluation

For evaluation of the coronary arteries, the mid esophageal views are the most useful. Specifically, the ME AV SAX view displays the normal origins of the right and left coronary arteries from their respective sinuses (Fig. 4.41, Video 4.29a). Variation of the multiplane angle between 0° and 40° produces optimal visualization of each individual coronary artery origin, and in some cases the bifurcation of the left main coronary artery can be seen with leftward TEE probe rotation. With rotation of the multiplane angle to 90–130° to obtain a ME AV LAX view, and leftward probe rotation, it is sometimes possible to visualize the left main coronary artery bifurcating into the left anterior descending and circumflex coronary arteries (Video 4.29b). A number of congenital coronary artery anomalies can be evaluated by TEE, as will be discussed in Chap. 14.

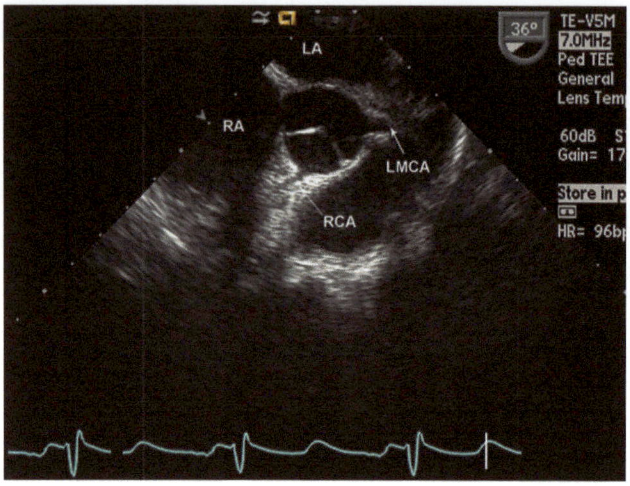

Fig. 4.41 Aortic valve as viewed *en face* in the mid esophageal aortic valve short axis view, multiplane angle about 35°. Both coronary origins can be well seen. *LA* left atrium, *LMCA* left main coronary artery, *RA* right atrium, *RCA* right coronary artery

Main and Branch Pulmonary Arteries, Aortic Arch

To evaluate the great arteries and more superior venous structures, the mid and upper esophageal positions are primarily utilized. Some probe anteflexion is generally necessary, and color flow Doppler is often helpful to identify blood flow direction and pulsatility. As noted previously, the ME Asc Ao SAX displays the main pulmonary artery and ascending aorta in cross section as they arise from the heart (Figs. 4.51 and 4.37, Video 4.25). Although this view was classified along with other mid esophageal cross sections in the standard TEE exam, its display requires further withdrawal of the probe above the level of the ME AV SAX. With rightward (clockwise) rotation of the probe, the right pulmonary artery can then be seen along its long axis as it courses posterior to the aorta. Maintaining a multiplane angle of 0°, a left aortic arch is shown with leftward (counterclockwise) rotation as

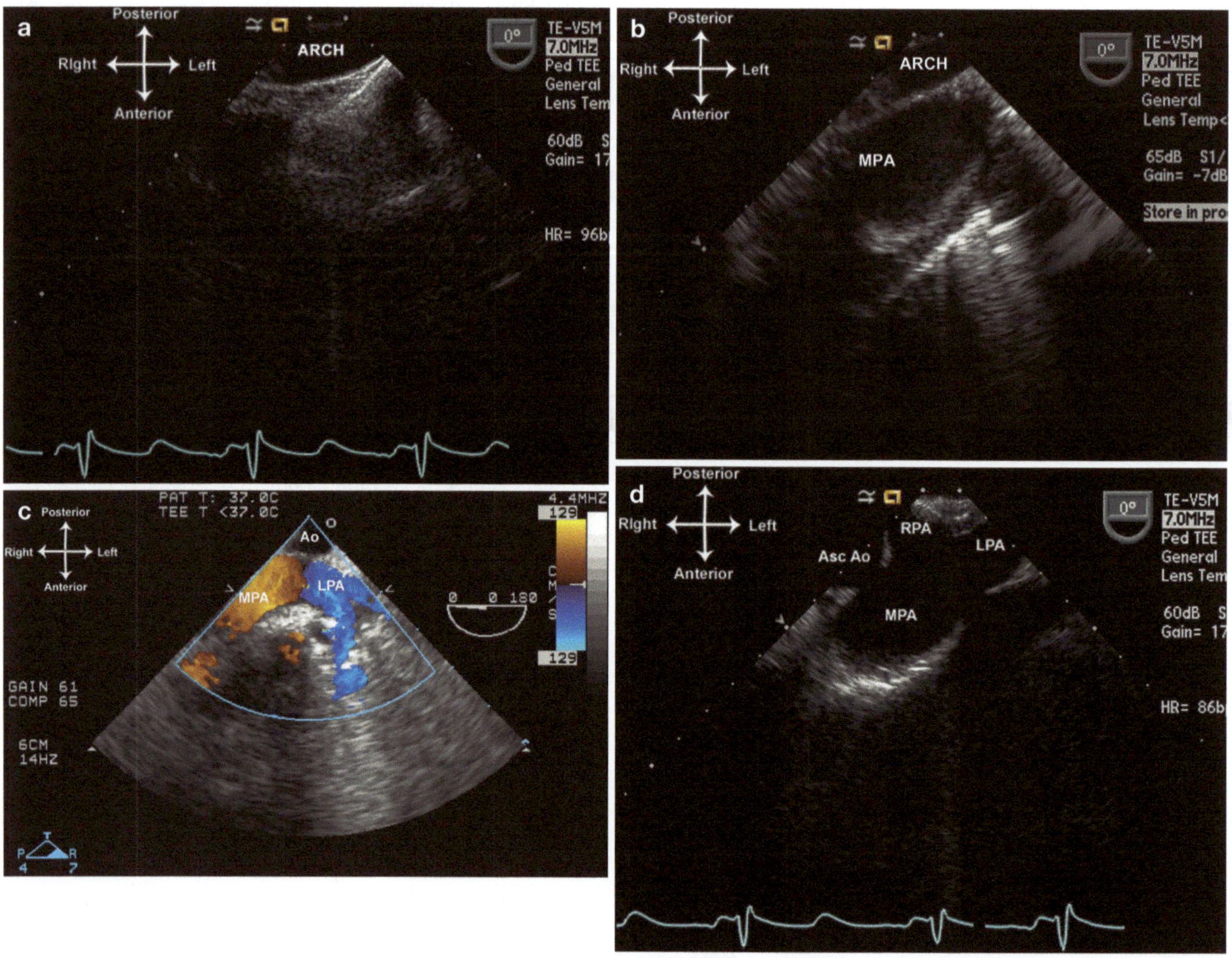

Fig. 4.42 Upper esophageal evaluation of the great arteries, multiplane angle 0°. When the probe is gradually withdrawn from a mid esophageal four chamber or the ascending aortic short axis view, the ascending aorta and transverse aortic arch (*ARCH*) are seen in an upper esophageal aortic arch long axis view (**a**). When the probe is rotated leftward (*counterclockwise*) and advanced slightly, both ARCH and main pulmonary artery (*MPA*), can be visualized (**b**). The left pulmonary artery (*LPA*) can be seen when the probe is then turned to the left and advanced slightly more to the upper esophageal pulmonary artery long axis view (**c**). The LPA is just inferior and anterior to the junction of transverse aortic arch and descending thoracic aorta (*Ao*). Turning the probe to the right (*clockwise*) and advancing further will provide a view of the MPA, right pulmonary artery (*RPA*), and sometimes the pulmonary artery bifurcation (**d**)

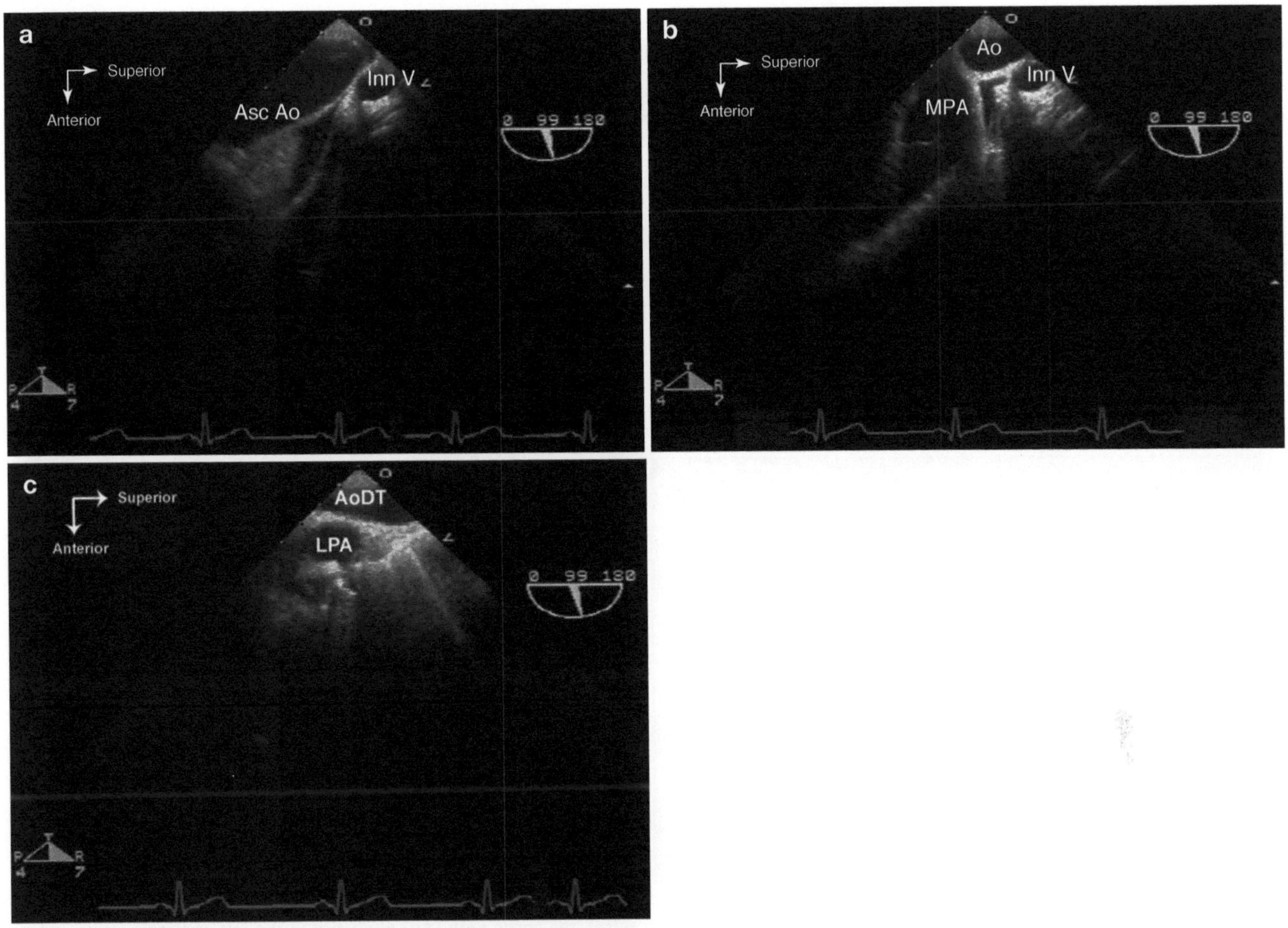

Fig. 4.43 Upper esophageal aortic arch short axis view (multiplane angle 90–100°). The probe is slowly turned from right to left (**a**, **b**) showing ascending aorta (*Asc Ao*), innominate vein (*Inn V*), aortic arch (*Ao*), and main pulmonary artery (*PA*). Note the position of the Inn V anterior and superior to the transverse aortic arch. Further leftward probe rotation and slight advancement displays the descending aorta (*AoDT*) and mid left pulmonary artery (*LPA*) (**c**)

well as slight withdrawal of the probe to produce the *upper esophageal aortic arch long axis view* (UE Ao Arch LAX, Figs. 4.5a and 4.42a), and the arch is followed with further leftward rotation as it becomes the descending aorta. At this point, if the probe is advanced slightly (Fig. 4.42b), a view will be obtained that we refer to in this textbook as the *upper esophageal pulmonary artery long axis view* (UE PA LAX, Figs. 4.5b and 4.42c, d) can be obtained, with the left pulmonary artery seen just below the level of the aortic arch, just as it becomes the descending aorta [51, 52]. It is at this level that color flow Doppler can demonstrate a patent ductus arteriosus, if present. With slight advancement of the probe and rightward rotation, the main and right pulmonary arteries (and sometimes the pulmonary artery bifurcation) again come into view (Figs. 4.5b and 4.42d). With further rightward rotation and probe advancement, the ME Asc Ao SAX view (Figs. 4.5l and 4.37) is once again obtained. An example of great artery evaluation (left aortic arch) is shown in Video 4.30. For a right aortic arch, the reverse process occurs: at the level of the UE Ao Arch LAX view, the TEE probe is rotated clockwise (rightward) and advanced/withdrawn to visualize the right sided aortic arch and descending aorta.

The same type of probe maneuvers can be performed at mid to upper esophageal level, using a multiplane angle of 90–120°, to visualize the great arteries from a more sagittal/longitudinal perspective. The ME Asc Ao LAX (Figs. 4.5m and 4.36a) provides a long axis view of the ascending aorta as it passes anterior to the right pulmonary artery, which can be seen in cross section. Further withdrawal of the probe, along with leftward probe rotation, produces the *upper esophageal aortic arch short axis view* (UE Ao Arch SAX, Fig. 4.5c), which displays the main pulmonary artery, along with a short axis view of the aortic arch and innominate vein (Fig. 4.43a, b). At this level, further leftward probe rotation and slight probe advancement will display the descending thoracic aorta and left pulmonary artery (sometimes with its lobar branch takeoffs) (Fig. 4.43c) [51]. Video 4.31 demonstrates this leftward sweep with the TEE probe in the UE Ao Arch SAX position, showing first the ascending aorta and main pulmonary artery, then the aortic arch, and finally the descending thoracic aorta and distal left pulmonary artery. Also in this UE Ao Arch SAX view, an LSVC (if present) can be visualized, as noted previously: leftward rotation of the probe will display a tubular (long axis)

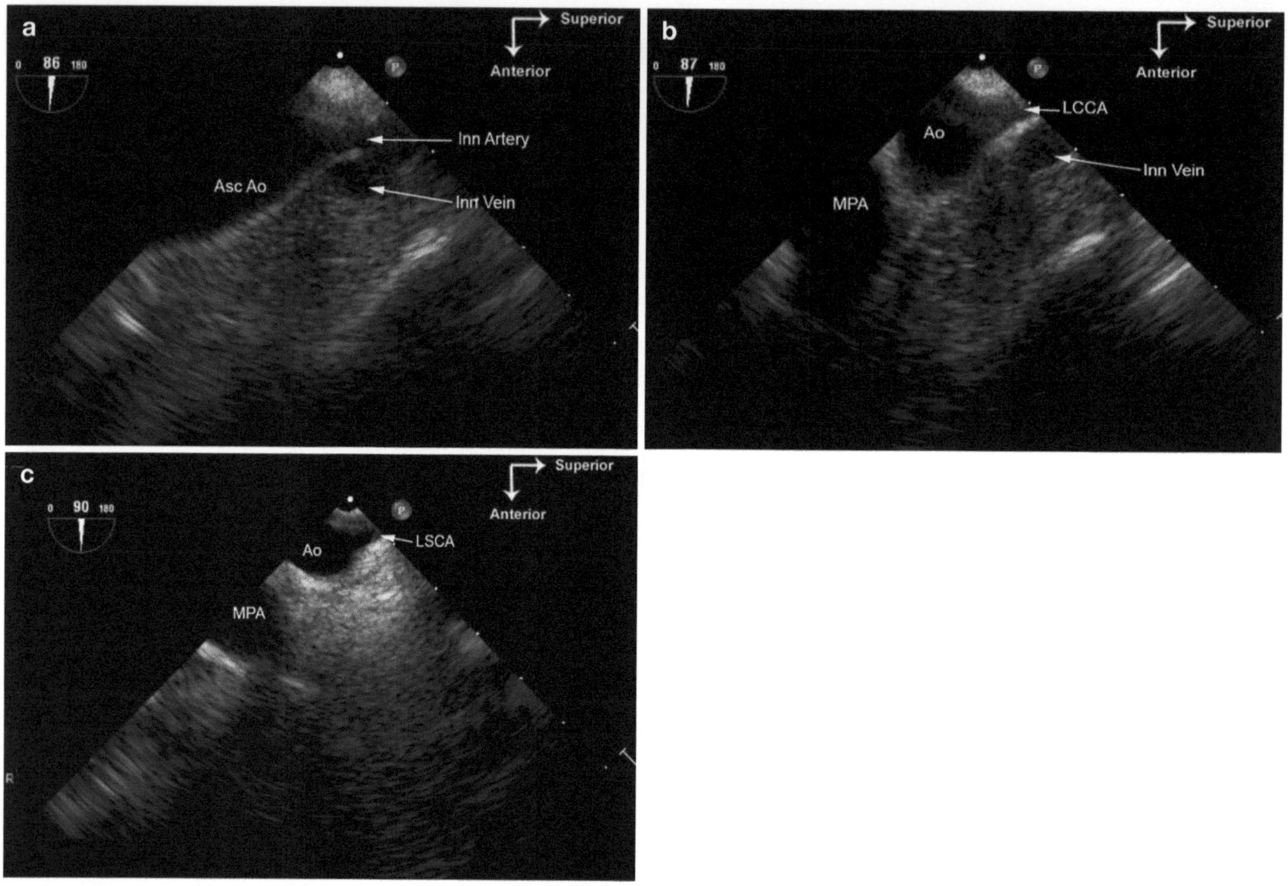

Fig. 4.44 Upper esophageal aortic arch short axis view (multiplane angle about 90°) used to display the aortic arch vessels, in a patient with a left aortic arch. (**a**) From an upper esophageal aortic arch short axis view, the transducer is first turned to the right to visualize the ascending aorta (*Asc Ao*); in this view the innominate artery (*Inn Artery*) is first seen. (**b**) As the transducer is rotated toward to the left (*counterclockwise*), the aortic arch (*Ao*) gives rise to the left common carotid artery (*LCCA*). (**c**) Further leftward rotation of the probe reveals the left subclavian artery (LSCA) origin. Note that the innominate vein (*Inn Vein*) is seen in cross section (short axis), anterior and superior to the aortic arch. *MPA* main pulmonary artery

view of the vessel as it descends anterior to the left pulmonary artery and drains to the heart (Fig. 4.12, Video 4.3).

The more superior vascular structures such as the individual aortic arch vessels (innominate/brachiocephalic, carotid, and subclavian arteries), as well as the innominate vein, are difficult to image by TEE but can sometimes be seen in the upper esophagus with the UE Ao Arch LAX and UE Ao Arch SAX views. Using the UE Ao Arch SAX view (multiplane angle about 90°), with right to left probe rotation, individual aortic arch vessels can be identified (Fig. 4.44, Video 4.32) [1, 53, 54]. The innominate vein can be visualized superior and anterior to the aortic arch, both by the UE Ao Arch LAX and SAX views. This view is sometimes useful for visualization of return of anomalous pulmonary venous return to the innominate vein or anomalies of innominate vein anatomy (Fig. 4.45, Video 4.33). However evaluation of these more superior vessels by TEE can be challenging, with visualization quite variable; thus TEE cannot be relied upon regularly for evaluation of pathology in these areas.

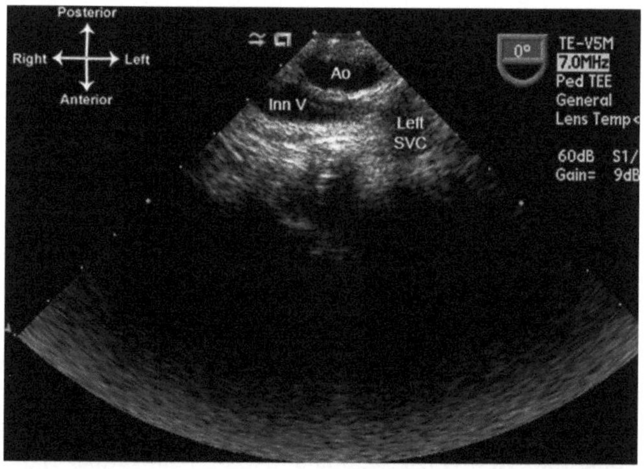

Fig. 4.45 Upper esophageal aortic arch long axis view in the patient from Fig. 4.12 with an absent right superior vena cava (*SVC*). The innominate vein (*Inn V*) is seen crossing anterior to the aortic arch (*Ao*) to connect with a left SVC, which then drains via a dilated coronary sinus into the right atrium (not shown). A catheter is faintly seen in the Inn V

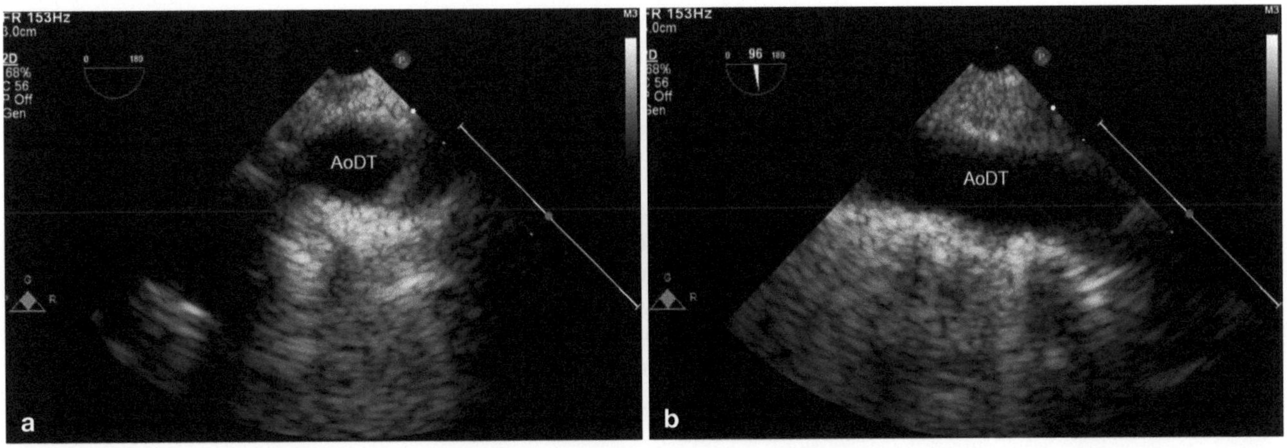

Fig. 4.46 Descending thoracic aorta views. In the mid esophageal window the probe is rotated to the left (*counterclockwise*) to visualize the aorta. A multiplane angle of 0° displays the descending thoracic aorta in cross section (**a**); changing the multiplane angle to 90–110° produces a long axis display of the descending aorta (**b**)

It should be noted that great artery evaluation is one of the more problematic aspects of TEE as discussed in Chap. 13. First, due to potential interference by right and left mainstem bronchi, visualization of the great arteries, particularly the branch pulmonary arteries, is more variable. Second, it can be very difficult to visualize the aortic arch in its entirety, particularly the aortic isthmus. Third, at these more superior levels the examiner must be careful not to withdraw the TEE probe completely out of the esophagus.

Descending Aorta

The descending thoracic aorta can be inspected by turning the shaft of the TEE probe (usually leftwards) such that it probe faces leftward and posteriorly toward the spine. With the multiplane angle at 0° the descending aorta can be viewed in cross section with the *descending aorta short axis* view (Desc Ao SAX, Figs. 4.5n and 4.46a, Video 4.34). At 90–110°, a portion of the aorta is visualized longitudinally using the *descending aorta long axis view* (Desc Ao LAX, Figs. 4.5o and 4.46b, Video 4.34). While these examples are shown at the level of mid esophagus, most of the descending thoracic aorta can be evaluated by maintaining the same view orientation, and alternately advancing and withdrawing the TEE probe to various levels within the esophagus.

Evaluation of Cardiac Malposition

The TEE evaluation of a patient with cardiac malposition can present even more significant challenges. With mesocardia and dextrocardia, many probe manipulations and imaging views will be the complete opposite of what is usually encountered in situs solitus and levocardia, and some images will be unlike any shown in this chapter (or any other reference). There is no standard way to evaluate these cardiac defects: each heart is different, many are unique, and no universal "template" applies. The best approach follows that used for all CHD diagnosis: a structure-based, systematic evaluation utilizing the segmental approach as outlined in this chapter. In fact, the segmental approach becomes even more important in this setting because of the high likelihood of visceroatrial situs abnormalities, such as heterotaxy, and more complex forms of CHD. In these instances a detailed and accurate assessment of all cardiac structures, including systemic and pulmonary venous drainage, becomes mandatory.

Nonetheless, in most patients with cardiac malposition, a good quality TEE study can generally be obtained because the esophagus remains in close proximity to the heart. There are a few instances, however, when the esophagus and stomach lie further away from the heart. In these cases, imaging can become more problematic.

Synopsis of the Segmental Approach by TEE

The segmental approach for the TEE evaluation of CHD—as outlined in this chapter—is summarized in Table 4.2. The individual cardiac segments and their corresponding cardiac structures are given in the first and second columns, and the accompanying TEE views that best visualize these structures are given in the third column. Table 4.2 serves as a useful cross reference linking the organized methodology outlined in this chapter, and the TEE views described in Table 4.1 and Fig. 4.5. It is important to remember that, while the views given in Table 4.2 apply to the majority of the congenital cardiac defects, the spectrum of the CHD is so vast and varied that exceptions will inevitably be encountered. Thus the

Table 4.2 Segmental approach by transesophageal echocardiography: recommended views

Segment	Structure(s)	Recommended TEE views
Cardiac position	Cardiac base to apex orientation	ME 4 Ch
Venous return	Systemic Venous Return	
	Hepatic vein/IVC	LE: Situs SAX, IVC LAX DTG: LAX, Sagittal
	Coronary sinus	LE: Situs SAX ME: 4 Ch, 2 Ch
	Right SVC	ME: 4 Ch, Asc Ao SAX, Bicaval TG: RV In (rightward rotation) DTG: LAX, Sagittal
	Left SVC	ME: 4 Ch, 2 Ch, Bicaval (leftward rotation) UE: PA LAX, Ao Arch SAX (leftward rotation)
	Innominate vein	UE: Ao Arch LAX, Ao Arch SAX
	Pulmonary Venous Return	ME: 4 Ch, Bicaval (both views with rightward and leftward rotation)
Atria	Right atrium/appendage	LE: Situs SAX, IVC LAX ME: 4 Ch, Bicaval DTG: LAX, Sagittal
	Left atrium/appendage	ME: 4 Ch (leftward rotation, anteflexion), 2 Ch DTG: LAX, Sagittal
	Interatrial septum	LE: Situs SAX, IVC LAX (lower part of atrial septum) ME: 4 Ch, Bicaval DTG: LAX, Sagittal
Atrioventricular junction, ventricles	Mitral valve/Left ventricle	ME: 4 Ch, 2 Ch, Mitral, LAX TG: Basal SAX, Mid SAX, 2 Ch, LAX DTG: LAX, Sagittal
	Tricuspid valve/Right ventricle	ME: 4 Ch, RV In-Out, Bicaval TG: RV In, Basal/Mid SAX (rightward rotation) DTG: LAX, Sagittal
	Interventricular septum	
	Inlet/membranous	ME: 4 Ch, RV In-Out, AV SAX, LAX, AV LAX DTG: LAX, Sagittal
	Trabecular/apical	ME: 4 Ch TG: Basal SAX, Mid SAX DTG: LAX, Sagittal
	Outlet/conal septum	ME: RV In-Out, AV SAX, LAX, AV LAX DTG: LAX, Sagittal
Ventriculo-arterial junction	Left ventricular outflow tract	ME: 4 Ch, LAX, AV LAX, AV SAX TG: LAX DTG: LAX, Sagittal
	Right ventricular outflow tract	ME: RV In-Out, 4 Ch (with anteflexion, slight probe withdrawal) TG: RV In (leftward rotation) DTG: Sagittal, LAX
	Aortic valve	ME: AV SAX, AV LAX, LAX TG: LAX DTG: LAX, Sagittal
	Pulmonary valve	ME: RV In-Out, AV SAX TG: RV In (leftward rotation) DTG: Sagittal, LAX
Great arteries	Main pulmonary artery	ME: Asc Ao SAX, Asc Ao LAX (leftward rotation) UE: PA LAX, Ao Arch LAX, Ao Arch SAX
	Right pulmonary artery	ME: Asc Ao SAX, Asc Ao LAX UE: PA LAX (rightward rotation)
	Left pulmonary artery	UE: PA LAX, Ao Arch SAX (leftward rotation)
	Ascending aorta	ME: Asc Ao SAX, Asc Ao LAX UE: Ao Arch LAX, Ao Arch SAX
	Aortic arch/head and neck vessels	UE: Ao Arch LAX, PA LAX, Ao Arch SAX
	Descending aorta	Desc Ao: SAX, LAX (both views from upper to lower esophagus)

Table 4.2 (continued)

Segment	Structure(s)	Recommended TEE views
Coronary arteries	Proximal coronary arteries	ME: AV LAX, AV SAX
	Mid to distal right, posterior descending	ME: 4 Ch (retroflexion)
	Circumflex, left anterior descending	ME: AV SAX, 2 Ch (with leftward rotation)

Ao aorta, *Ao Arch* aortic arch, *Asc Ao* ascending aortic, *AV* aortic valve, *Ch* chamber, *Desc* descending, *DTG* Deep transgastric, *In* inflow, *IVC* inferior vena cava, *LAX* long axis, *LE* lower esophageal, *ME* mid esophageal, *Out* outflow, *PA* pulmonary artery, *RV* right ventricular, SAX short axis, *SVC* superior vena cava, *TG* transgastric, *UE* upper esophageal. See Table 4.1 and Fig. 4.5 for a detailed description of the individual views

reader should not view this table as absolute and definitive, but rather a starting point, or handy guide, to assist in the evaluation of a patient with known or suspected CHD.

Summary

In this chapter we reviewed the basics of TEE probe manipulation and the standardized nomenclature for the different TEE windows and views. We outlined modified planes applicable to the patient with CHD that complement the views suggested in published guidelines for a comprehensive TEE examination We also presented a segmental, structure-based methodology to perform a complete TEE study in any patient with simple or complex CHD. The information from this chapter should serve as a framework that enables the reader to understand the information presented in subsequent chapters, and also to perform the TEE evaluation of the various congenital cardiac lesions as described. The approach outlined in this chapter presents an idealized, comprehensive TEE assessment applicable to most congenital cardiac lesions. However, it should be emphasized that that main goal of any examination—regardless of sequence or style—is the acquisition of anatomic, hemodynamic, and functional information in as much detail as possible. Thus, each TEE examination, including views and sequence, should be tailored to the individual patient and clinical situation. In some cases, additional TEE views might be obtained that complement or serve as alternates to those outlined in this chapter.

References

1. Shanewise JS, Cheung AT, Aronson S, et al. ASE/SCA guidelines for performing a comprehensive intraoperative multiplane transesophageal echocardiography examination: recommendations of the American Society of Echocardiography Council for Intraoperative Echocardiography and the Society of Cardiovascular Anesthesiologists Task Force for Certification in Perioperative Transesophageal Echocardiography. J Am Soc Echocardiogr. 1999;12:884–900.
2. VanPraagh R, Ongley PA, Swan HJ. Anatomic types of single or common ventricle in man. Morphologic and geometric aspects of 60 necropsied cases. Am J Cardiol. 1964;13:367–86.
3. Van Praagh R, Van Praagh S, Vlad P, Keith JD. Anatomic types of congenital dextrocardia: diagnostic and embryologic implications. Am J Cardiol. 1964;13:510–31.
4. Van Praagh R. The segmental approach to diagnosis in congenital heart disaease. In: Bergsma D, editor. Birth defects: original article series. Baltimore: Williams and Wilkins; 1972. p. 4–23.
5. Anderson RH, Becker AE, Freedom RM, et al. Sequential segmental analysis of congenital heart disease. Pediatr Cardiol. 1984;5:281–7.
6. Snider AR, Ritter SB, Serwer GA. Echocardiography in pediatric heart disease. 2nd ed. St Louis: Mosby; 1997.
7. O'Leary PW. The segmental approach to congenital heart disease. Pediatr Ultrasound Today. 1997;2:82–104.
8. Anderson RH. Terminology. In: Anderson RH, Baker EJ, Redington A, Rigby ML, Penny D, Wernovsky G, editors. Paediatric cardiology. 3rd ed. Philadelphia: Churchill Livingstone/Elsevier; 2009. p. 3–16.
9. Geva T. Nomenclature and segmental approach to congenital heart disease. In: Lai W, Mertens L, Cohen MS, Geva T, editors. Echocardiography in pediatric and congenital heart disease: from fetus to adult. illustrated ed. Chichester/Hoboken: Wiley; 2009. p. 22–33.
10. Gillis E, Springer R, O'Leary PW. Practical issues related to the examination, anatomic image orientation, and segmental cardiovascular analysis. In: Eidem BW, Ceteta F, O'Leary PW, editors. Echocardiography in pediatric and adult congenital heart disease. Philadelphia: Lippincott Williams & Wilkins; 2010.
11. Kimball TR, Michelfelder EC. Echocardiography. In: Allen HD, Driscoll DJ, Shaddy RE, Feltes TF, editors. Moss and Adams' heart disease in infants, children, and adolescents: including the fetus and young adult. 7th ed. Philadelphia: Lippincott Williams & Wilkins; 2008. p. 95–163.
12. Van Praagh R. The importance of segmental situs in the diagnosis of congenital heart disease. Semin Roentgenol. 1985;20:254–71.
13. Huhta JC, Hagler DJ, Seward JB, Tajik AJ, Julsrud PR, Ritter DG. Two-dimensional echocardiographic assessment of dextrocardia: a segmental approach. Am J Cardiol. 1982;50:1351–60.
14. Lai WW, Geva T, Shirali GS, et al. Guidelines and standards for performance of a pediatric echocardiogram: a report from the Task Force of the Pediatric Council of the American Society of Echocardiography. J Am Soc Echocardiogr. 2006;19:1413–30.
15. Transesophageal echocardiography in congenital heart disease. In: Stümper O, Sutherland GR, editors. London: Edward Arnold; 1994.
16. Weintraub R, Shiota T, Elkadi T, et al. Transesophageal echocardiography in infants and children with congenital heart disease. Circulation. 1992;86:711–22.
17. Bengur AR, Li JS, Herlong JR, Jaggers J, Sanders SP, Ungerleider RM. Intraoperative transesophageal echocardiography in congenital heart disease. Semin Thorac Cardiovasc Surg. 1998;10:255–64.
18. Muhiudeen Russell IA, Miller-Hance WC, Silverman NH. Intraoperative transesophageal echocardiography for pediatric patients with congenital heart disease. Anesth Analg. 1998;87:1058–76.
19. Shanewise JS, Shin JJ, Vezina DP, Cahalan MK. Comprehensive and abbreviated intraoperative TEE examination. In: Savage RM, Aronson S, Shernan SK, editors. Comprehensive textbook of perioperative transesophageal echocardiography. 2nd ed. Philadelphia: Lippincott Williams & Wilkins; 2010. p. 84–97.
20. Ayres NA, Miller-Hance W, Fyfe DA, et al. Indications and guidelines for performance of transesophageal echocardiography in the

patient with pediatric acquired or congenital heart disease: a report from the Task Force of the Pediatric Council of the American Society of Echocardiography. J Am Soc Echocardiogr. 2005;18:91–8.
21. Sundar S, DiNardo JA. Transesophageal echocardiography in pediatric surgery. Int Anesthesiol Clin. 2008;46:137–55.
22. Kamra K, Russell I, Miller-Hance WC. Role of transesophageal echocardiography in the management of pediatric patients with congenital heart disease. Paediatr Anaesth. 2011;21:479–93.
23. Muhiudeen IA, Silverman NH, Anderson RH. Transesophageal transgastric echocardiography in infants and children: the subcostal view equivalent. J Am Soc Echocardiogr. 1995;8:231–44.
24. Miller-Hance WC, Silverman NH. Transesophageal echocardiography (TEE) in congenital heart disease with focus on the adult. Cardiol Clin. 2000;18(4):861–92.
25. Stümper OF, Sreeram N, Elzenga NJ, Sutherland GR. Diagnosis of atrial situs by transesophageal echocardiography. J Am Coll Cardiol. 1990;16:442–6.
26. Van Praagh R, Weinberg PM, Smith SD, Foran RB, Van Praagh S. Malpositions of the heart. In: Adams FH, Emmanouilides GC, Riemenschneider TA, editors. Moss' heart disease in infants, children and adolescents. 4th ed. Baltimore: Williams & Wilkins; 1989. p. 530–80.
27. Van Praagh R, Van Praagh S. Morphologic anatomy. In: Keane JF, Lock JE, Fyler DC, editors. Nadas' pediatric cardiology. 2nd ed. Philadelphia: Saunders Elsevier; 2006. p. 27–37.
28. Pinheiro L, Nanda NC, Jain H, Sanyal R. Transesophageal echocardiographic imaging of the pulmonary veins. Echocardiography. 1991;8:741–8.
29. Stümper OF, Vargas-Barron J, Rijlaarsdam M, et al. Assessment of anomalous systemic and pulmonary venous connections by transoesophageal echocardiography in infants and children. Br Heart J. 1991;66:411–8.
30. Seiler C. How should we assess patent foramen ovale? Heart. 2004;90:1245–7.
31. Soliman OII, Geleijnse ML, Meijboom FJ, et al. The use of contrast echocardiography for the detection of cardiac shunts. Eur J Echocardiogr. 2007;8:S2–12.
32. Van Hare GF, Silverman NH. Contrast two-dimensional echocardiography in congenital heart disease: techniques, indications and clinical utility. J Am Coll Cardiol. 1989;13:673–86.
33. Schneider B, Zienkiewicz T, Jansen V, Hofmann T, Noltenius H, Meinertz T. Diagnosis of patent foramen ovale by transesophageal echocardiography and correlation with autopsy findings. Am J Cardiol. 1996;77:1202–9.
34. Woods TD, Patel A. A critical review of patent foramen ovale detection using saline contrast echocardiography: when bubbles lie. J Am Soc Echocardiogr. 2006;19:215–22.
35. Stoddard MF, Keedy DL, Dawkins PR. The cough test is superior to the Valsalva maneuver in the delineation of right-to-left shunting through a patent foramen ovale during contrast transesophageal echocardiography. Am Heart J. 1993;125:185–9.
36. Verghese ST, Nath A, Zenger D, Patel RI, Kaplan RF, Patel KM. The effects of the simulated Valsalva maneuver, liver compression, and/or Trendelenburg position on the cross-sectional area of the internal jugular vein in infants and young children. Anesth Analg. 2002;94:250–4.
37. Van Praagh R. Diagnosis of complex congenital heart disease: morphologic-anatomic method and terminology. Cardiovasc Intervent Radiol. 1984;7:115–20.
38. Van Praagh R. Normally and abnormally related great arteries: what have we learned? World J Pediatr Congenit Heart Surg. 2010;1:364–85.
39. Kumar N, Kumar M, Duran CM. A revised terminology for recording surgical findings of the mitral valve. J Heart Valve Dis. 1995;4:70–5.
40. Gillinov AM, Beyer EA, Gonzalez-Stawinski G, Mihaljevic T. Surgical considerations in mitral and tricuspid valve surgery. In: Savage RM, Aronson S, Shernan SK, editors. Comprehensive textbook of perioperative transesophageal echocardiography. 2nd ed. Philadelphia: Lippincott Williams & Wilkins; 2010. p. 474–86.
41. Shook DC, Essandoh M, Savage RM, Stewart WJ. Surgical considerations and assessment in nonischemic mitral valve surgery. In: Savage RM, Aronson S, Shernan SK, editors. Comprehensive textbook of perioperative transesophageal echocardiography. 2nd ed. Philadelphia: Lippincott Williams & Wilkins; 2010. p. 487–565.
42. Martinez RM, O'Leary PW, Anderson RH. Anatomy and echocardiography of the normal and abnormal tricuspid valve. Cardiol Young. 2006;16 Suppl 3:4–11.
43. Anderson RH. Anatomy. In: Anderson RH, Baker EJ, Redington A, Rigby ML, Penny D, Wernovsky G, editors. Paediatric cardiology. 3rd ed. Philadelphia: Churchill Livingstone/Elsevier; 2009. p. 17–55.
44. Rehfeldt KH. Two-dimensional transesophageal echocardiographic imaging of the tricuspid valve. Anesth Analg. 2012;114:547–50.
45. Maxted W, Nanda NC, Kim K, Roychoudhury D, Pinherio L. Transesophageal echocardiography identification and validation of individual tricuspid valve leaflets. Echocardiography. 1994;11:585–96.
46. Sanders SP. Echocardiography and related techniques in the diagnosis of congenital heart defects. Part II: atrioventricular valves and ventricles. Echocardiography. 1984;1:333–91.
47. Van Praagh S, LaCorte M, Fellows KE, et al. Supero-inferior ventricles: anatomic and angiographic findings in ten postmortem cases. In: Van Praagh R, Takao A, editors. Etiology and morphogenesis of congenital heart disease. Mt. Kisco: Futura; 1980. p. 317–78.
48. Van Praagh R. Segmental approach to diagnosis. In: Keane JF, Lock JE, Fyler DC, editors. Nadas' pediatric cardiology. 2nd ed. Philadelphia: Saunders Elsevier; 2006. p. 39–46.
49. Tynan MJ, Becker AE, Macartney FJ, Jimenez MQ, Shinebourne EA, Anderson RH. Nomenclature and classification of congenital heart disease. Br Heart J. 1979;41:544.
50. Hoffman P, Stümper O, Rydelwska-Sadowska W, Sutherland GR. Transgastric imaging: a valuable addition to the assessment of congenital heart disease by transverse plane transesophageal echocardiography. J Am Soc Echocardiogr. 1993;6:35–44.
51. Phoon CK, Rutkowski M. Transesophageal imaging of the mid to distal left pulmonary artery in congenital heart disease. J Am Soc Echocardiogr. 1999;12:663–8.
52. Tsai SK, Chang CI, Wang MJ, et al. The assessment of the proximal left pulmonary artery by transesophageal echocardiography and computed tomography in neonates and infants: a case series. Anesth Analg. 2001;93:594–7.
53. Nanda NC, Domanski MJ. Aortic valve, aorta, and aortic branches. In: Atlas of transesophageal echocardiography. 2nd ed. Philadelphia: Lippincott Williams & Wilkins; 2007. p. 112–90.
54. Honos GN, Dürrleman N, Denault AY, Buithieu J. Normal anatomy and flow. In: Denault AY, Couture P, Vegas A, Buithieu J, Tardif JC, editors. Transesophageal echocardiography multimedia manual: a perioperative transdisciplinary approach. 2nd ed. New York/London: Informa Healthcare; 2011. p. 65–95.

Functional Evaluation of the Heart by Transesophageal Echocardiography

5

Benjamin W. Eidem

Abstract
The noninvasive echocardiographic evaluation of ventricular performance is an essential tool in the clinician's assessment and management of children and adults with congenital heart disease (CHD). However the unique anatomic and physiologic features in these patients, which include nonstandard ventricular geometries as well as variable loading conditions, can make the quantitative assessment of ventricular function challenging, particularly by transesophageal echocardiography (TEE). Newer echocardiographic methods are enabling more accurate and quantitative evaluation of ventricular performance, both by the transthoracic as well as the transesophageal approach. This chapter discusses the current applications of TEE in the evaluation of ventricular function in patients with CHD.

Keywords
Transesophageal echocardiography • Congenital heart disease • Pediatric acquired heart disease • Ventricular function • Myocardial performance • Systolic function • Diastolic function

Introduction

The noninvasive echocardiographic evaluation of ventricular performance is an essential tool in the clinician's assessment and management of children and adults with congenital heart disease (CHD). As noninvasive methods have continued to evolve, the importance of global and regional ventricular function has become better appreciated. Alterations in both ventricular geometry and loading conditions are the hallmarks of many congenital heart lesions and can make the quantitative assessment of ventricular function challenging. While transesophageal echocardiography (TEE) has often historically been limited to a subjective assessment of ventricular function, newer echocardiographic methods allow more accurate and quantitative evaluation of ventricular performance by the transesophageal approach. This chapter focuses on the current applications of TEE in the evaluation of ventricular function in patients with CHD. Many of these concepts are also relevant to the assessment of ventricular function in children with acquired cardiovascular pathologies.

Transesophageal Echocardiographic Evaluation of Ventricular Function in Congenital Heart Disease

Indications

The majority of patients with CHD have excellent transthoracic echocardiographic (TTE) windows. However, TEE imaging is particularly helpful in those with challenging surface images, such as adults with CHD or postoperative

B.W. Eidem, MD, FACC, FAAP, FASE
Division of Pediatric Cardiology and Cardiovascular Diseases, Departments of Pediatrics and Medicine, Mayo Clinic, 200 First Street SW, Rochester, MN 55905, USA
e-mail: eidem.benjamin@mayo.edu

The online version of this chapter (doi:10.1007/978-1-84800-064-3_5) contains supplementary material, which is available to authorized users.

P.C. Wong, W.C. Miller-Hance (eds.), *Transesophageal Echocardiography for Congenital Heart Disease*, DOI 10.1007/978-1-84800-064-3_5, © Springer-Verlag London 2014

patients (Table 5.1). In addition, evaluation of ventricular function in the operating room [1–9] or during interventional cardiac catheterization procedures [10–13], is often best facilitated with TEE imaging.

Imaging Planes

Optimal imaging of the left ventricle (LV) is best achieved with a combination of the transgastric mid left ventricular short axis (TG Mid SAX), transgastric long axis (TG LAX), mid esophageal four chamber (ME 4 Ch), and mid esophageal two chamber (ME 2 Ch) views [14, 15]. The miniaturization of multiplane TEE probes allows for additional imaging planes that are also quite helpful in facilitating better endocardial border definition and optimizing Doppler alignment, particularly in patients with CHD-associated with altered ventricular anatomy and geometry.

Table 5.1 Specific indications for TEE assessment of ventricular function

Limited transthoracic image quality
Intra-operative assessment of ventricular function
Pre and postoperative assessment of ventricular performance
Identification of regional wall motion abnormalities suggesting ischemia
Ongoing postoperative assessment of response to medical or surgical or intervention
Evaluation of ventricular function in the critical care setting
Evaluation of unstable hemodynamics
Assessment of the integrity of the cardiac repair and its impact on ventricular function
Weaning from mechanical circulatory support
Evaluation of ventricular function during interventional cardiac catheterization procedures
Impact of procedure on ventricular performance

The TG Mid SAX, obtained at the mid papillary level, is the TTE equivalent of the parasternal short axis scan plane and readily facilitates the evaluation of radial ventricular function including LV shortening fraction (Fig. 5.1). This view is also optimal to evaluate regional wall motion abnormalities as all major coronary artery distributions are represented in this view.

The TG LAX view best visualizes the apex of the LV and is also helpful to assess regional wall motion. This plane, in addition to the deep transgastric long axis (DTG LAX) and sagittal (DTG Sagittal) views, allow for optimal spectral Doppler alignment with the left ventricular outflow tract, making quantitative assessment of LV cardiac output feasible.

The ME 4 Ch and ME 2 Ch views are easily obtained from the mid esophageal window. The ME 4 Ch view is most commonly used for simultaneous qualitative assessment of right ventricular (RV) and LV performance (Fig. 5.2a, b). In addition, longitudinal ventricular function is best evaluated in this view due to the optimal alignment with both lateral RV and LV walls. Overall assessment of volume status is also readily appreciated in this four chamber orientation. The ME 2 Ch view provides for biplane measurement of ventricular volume and LV ejection fraction (Fig. 5.2c, d, e).

Echocardiographic Assessment of Global Left Ventricular Systolic Function

Echocardiographic measures of LV systolic function include M-mode, two-dimensional (2D), three-dimensional (3D), and Doppler-derived indices of ventricular performance. Each of these measures can be readily obtained with TEE [17–42]. The majority of echocardiographic measures of LV systolic function represent ejection phase indices that rely

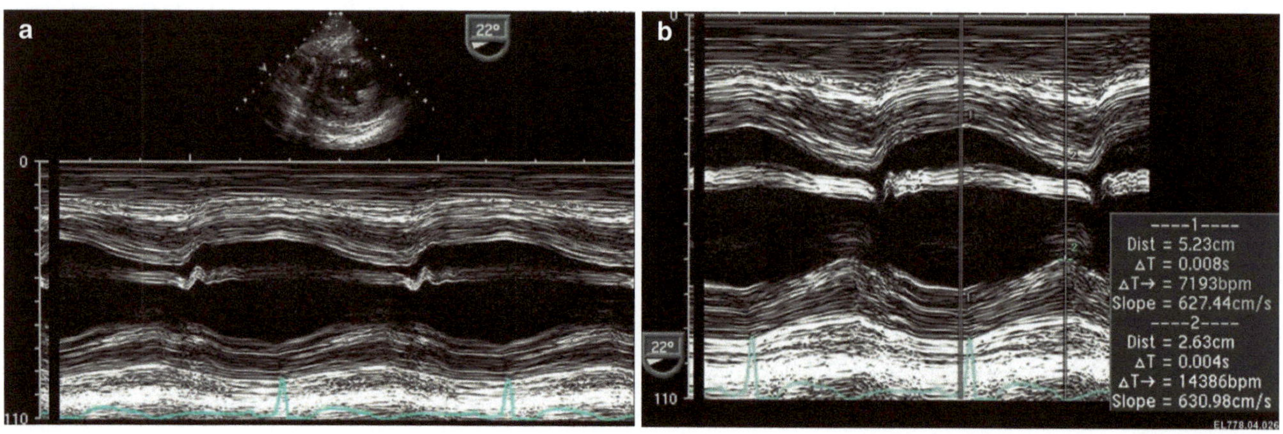

Fig. 5.1 Left ventricular shortening fraction. Transgastric mid short axis image at level of papillary muscles of the left ventricle (LV). (**a**) M-mode demonstrating left ventricular shortening. (**b**) M-mode derived shortening fraction (SF) of the LV:

$$SF\ \% = [LVEDD - LVESD]/LVEDD = [52\ mm - 26\ mm]/53\ mm = 50\%$$

LVEDD LV end-diastolic dimension, *LVESD* LV end-systolic dimension

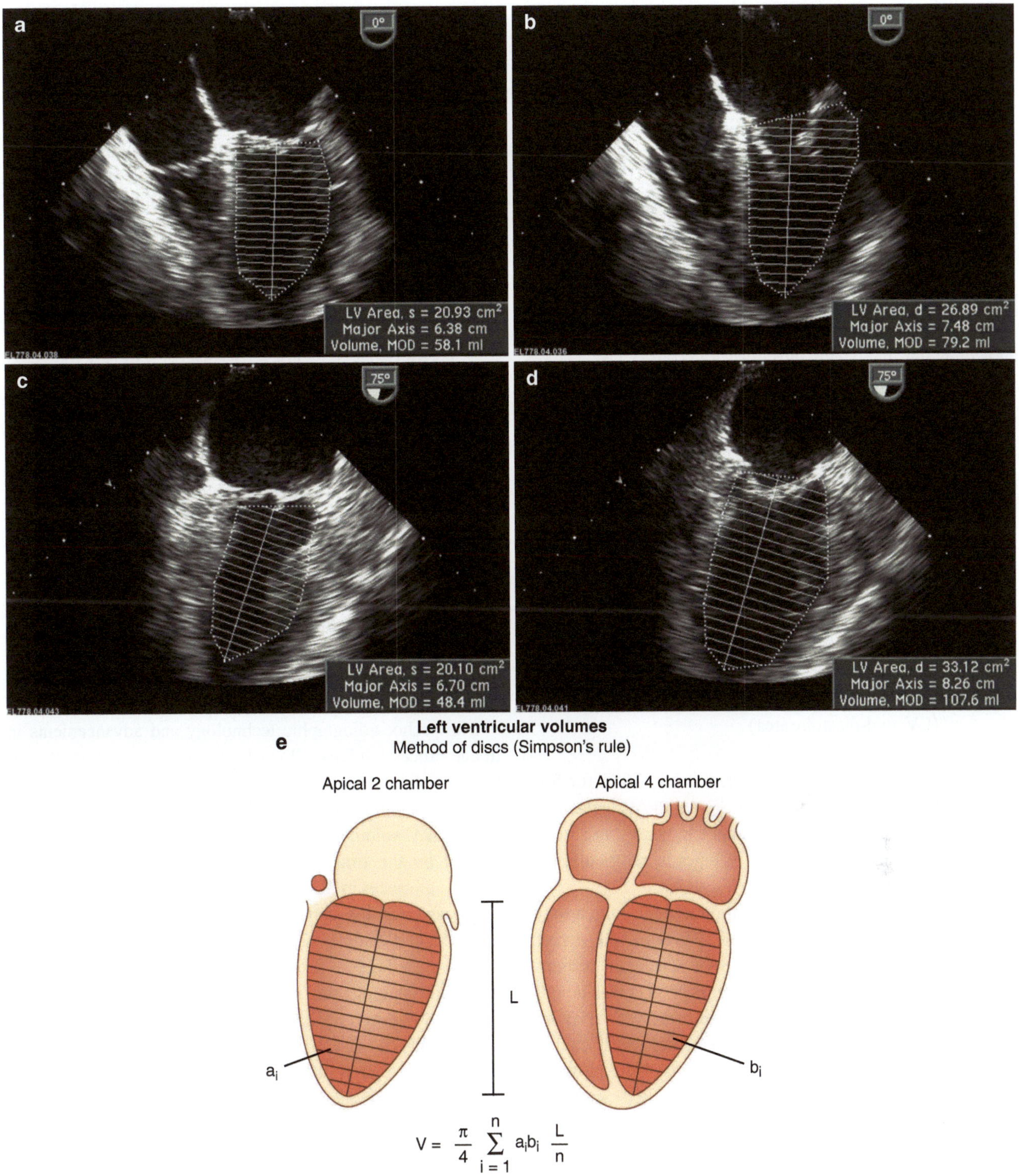

Fig. 5.2 Left ventricular ejection fraction. Four chamber (**a**, **b**) and two chamber (**c**, **d**) views at the level of the mid esophagus in systole (**a**, **c**) and diastole (**b**, **d**). These imaging planes allow quantitative assessment of left ventricular (*LV*) systolic function. Simpson's biplane methodology to calculate LV ejection fraction (**e**), figure adapted from Schiller et al. [16], with permission)

upon geometric assumptions inherent in the elliptical shape of the LV. More importantly, these measurements are significantly influenced by a variety of hemodynamic factors including altered ventricular preload and afterload, heart rate, LV mass, and myocardial contractility. The emergence of Doppler-derived measures of ventricular function has circumvented many of the geometric challenges inherent in this global assessment of ventricular performance. This is especially the case in the evaluation of RV performance as well as quantitative assessment of systolic function in patients with complex ventricular morphologies. Many of these techniques have been applied using TEE [43–51].

Left Ventricular Shortening Fraction and Fractional Area Change

One-dimensional wall motion analysis, or M-mode echocardiography, has traditionally been one of the most commonly utilized methods to measure the extent of LV shortening. Shortening fraction (SF) represents the change in LV short axis diameter that occurs during systole (Fig. 5.1):

$$\text{LVSF}(\%) = [\text{LVEDD} - \text{LVESD}] / \text{LVEDD} \times 100$$

LVEDD=LV end-diastolic dimension; LVESD=LV end-systolic dimension

Normal values for shortening fraction range between 28 and 44 %. The LV TG Mid SAX plane is the TEE view most frequently used to make these measurements. Similar to fractional shortening, fractional area change (FAC) can also be measured in this view by determining the change in LV area that occurs during the cardiac cycle:

$$\text{FAC} = [(\text{LV end-diastolic area}) - (\text{LV end-systolic area})] / (\text{LV end-diastolic area})$$

Normal values have been reported to be >36 % for fractional area change in adults. LVSF and FAC have been reported to be independent of changes in heart rate and age but are significantly impacted by changes in ventricular preload and afterload [52–56].

A concern regarding this evaluation was raised in a retrospective blinded analysis comparing TTE from TEE-derived FAC measured from LV TG Mid SAX images in pediatric patients with CHD [57]. Potential errors in this measurement were reported as well as significant interobserver variability. In spite of these findings the authors were not able to exclude echocardiographic experience and training of the investigators as potential factors accounting for the variability observed. In this study, TEE-derived FAC measurement was not possible in a significant number of patients due to inability to trace endocardial borders at end-systole. Technological advances since the publication of this work may facilitate this assessment in the current era.

Left Ventricular Ejection Fraction

Left ventricular ejection fraction (LVEF) is the most commonly measured parameter of ventricular systolic function. Global estimation of LVEF is often determined in a qualitative fashion; however, utilizing TTE or TEE, 2D imaging allows quantitative measurement of LVEF by assessing changes in ventricular volume during the cardiac cycle. The geometric model most commonly used for this measurement is the modified Simpson's biplane method (Fig. 5.2e) [16, 58–60]. By utilizing orthogonal four chamber and two chamber views of the LV (from an apical window during TTE), this geometric model calculates LV end-diastolic volume (LVEDV) and LV end-systolic volume (LVESV) by summing equal sequential slices of LV area from each of these scan planes. LVEF can then be calculated as:

$$\text{LVEF}(\%) = [\text{LVEDV} - \text{LVESV}] / \text{LVEDV} \times 100$$

Normal values for LVEF range between 56 and 78 %. Similar to LVSF, LVEF has been shown to be dependent on changes in ventricular loading conditions [52, 54–56, 61].

Accurate calculation of LV volume by TEE can be challenging due to foreshortening of the LV cavity. To circumvent this limitation, an area-length method to derive LVEF can also be used [24]. This method utilizes the short axis area of the LV and the long axis LV length and can be obtained by imaging the LV in the TG mid SAX and ME 4 Ch views. Determination of ventricular volume and EF by these TEE methods has been shown to correlate reasonably well with invasively measured parameters of ventricular function.

New echocardiographic technology and advancements in image processing have allowed improved acquisition of ventricular volumes. Studies have validated the ability of 3D echocardiography to obtain accurate and reproducible estimates of LV and RV volumes and EF [32–35, 62–64]. While initially limited by the time-consuming reconstruction of acquired images, advances in 3D TEE now allow for real time data display, significantly enhancing the quantitative assessment of ventricular volume and function (Chap. 19) [63, 65, 66].

Automated border detection (ABD) is another approach in imaging technology that utilizes acoustic quantification to differentiate the myocardium from the blood pool and thereby allows enhanced visualization of the endocardial border. End-diastolic and end-systolic LV area can be continuously displayed with this modality enabling determination of ventricular volume, FAC, and even pressure-volume or pressure-area loops. Excellent correlation of ABD with other noninvasive and invasive measurements of ventricular function has been reported in a few adult studies but data is lacking in patients with CHD and altered ventricular geometry [44, 46, 67–73].

Velocity of Circumferential Fiber Shortening and the Stress–Velocity Index

The rate of LV fiber shortening can be noninvasively assessed by M-mode echocardiography (a graphic display of distance over time). This measurement, termed the mean velocity of circumferential fiber shortening (V_{cf}), is normalized for LV end-diastolic dimension and can be obtained from the following equation:

$$V_{cf} = [\text{LVEDD} - \text{LVESD}] / [\text{LVEDD} \times \text{LVET}]$$

LVET = LV ejection time.

Reported normal values for mean V_{cf} are 1.5 ± 0.04 circumferences (circ)/sec (s) for neonates and 1.3 ± 0.03 circ/s for children between 2 and 10 years of age [54, 74, 75]. This index not only assesses the degree of fractional shortening but the rate at which this shortening occurs. To normalize V_{cf} for variation in heart rate, LVET is divided by the square root of the R-R interval to derive a rate-corrected mean velocity of circumferential fiber shortening (V_{cfc}). Normal V_{cfc} has been reported to be 1.28 ± 0.22 and 1.08 ± 0.14 circ/s in neonates and children, respectively [54, 74–79]. Because V_{cfc} values are corrected for heart rate, a significant decrease in V_{cfc} between the neonatal and childhood age groups has been attributed to increased systemic afterload with advancing age. V_{cf} is sensitive to changes in contractility and afterload but relatively insensitive to changes in preload. Similar to fractional shortening, this parameter relies on the elliptical shape of the LV and is invalid with altered LV geometry.

Because the majority of ejection phase indices, including SF, EF, and V_{cfc} are dependent upon the underlying loading state of the LV, measures of wall tension, namely circumferential and meridional end-systolic wall stress, have been proposed to assess myocardial systolic performance in a relatively load-independent fashion [80]. Colan and colleagues have previously described a stress-velocity index that is an inverse linear relationship between V_{cfc} and end-systolic wall stress (Fig. 5.3). This stress-velocity index is independent of preload, normalized for heart rate, and incorporates afterload resulting in a noninvasive measure of LV contractility that is independent of ventricular loading conditions [81]. This index can therefore provide a more accurate characterization of LV myocardial systolic performance, by differentiating states of increased ventricular afterload from decreased myocardial contractility. While both conditions can affect cardiac output, the former represents increased resistance to myocardial output despite normal myocardial contractility, while the latter represents a true impairment of myocardial contractile performance. While the stress-velocity index is appealing, the clinical application of this index has been limited by its cumbersome acquisition and the need for time-consuming offline processing which are often not suitable for rapid assessment of ventricular performance such as is typically required during TEE. This index is also limited in patients with altered ventricular geometry and wall thickness, features that are hallmarks of CHD.

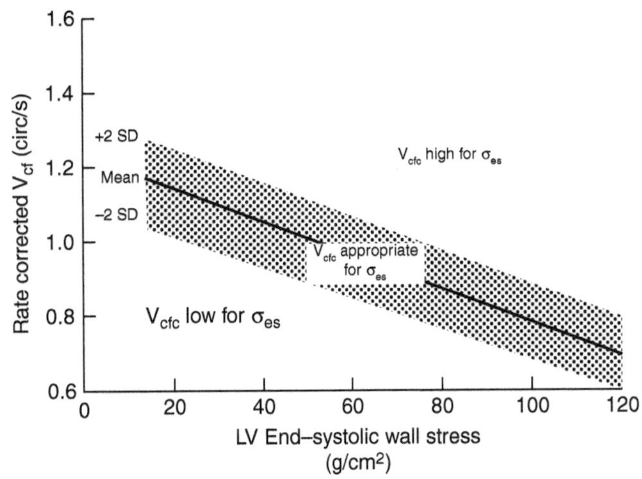

Fig. 5.3 Stress–velocity index for assessment of left ventricular systolic function. Graphic representation of the relationship between the mean rate-corrected velocity of circumferential left ventricular (*LV*) fiber shortening (V_{cfc}) and the LV end-systolic wall stress (σ_{es}). To normalize V_{cf} for variation in heart rate, it is divided by the square root of the R–R interval to derive a rate-corrected mean velocity of circumferential LV fiber shortening (V_{cfc}). Values above the upper limit of the mean relationship imply an increased inotropic state while values below the mean imply depressed contractility (From Colan et al. [81], with permission)

Doppler Parameters of Global Left Ventricular Systolic Function

Echocardiographic evaluation of systolic function has primarily relied upon one-dimensional measures of LV shortening or on 2D measures of LV volume changes that are often difficult to assess in patients with distorted ventricular geometry. Doppler measures of global ventricular function have been reported to be a potentially more reproducible and sensitive measure of ventricular function overcoming the limitations of other approaches.

Left Ventricular dP/dt

Doppler echocardiography can be utilized in the quantitative evaluation of LV systolic function. If mitral regurgitation (MR) is present, the peak and mean rate of change in LV systolic pressure (dP/dt) can be derived from the ascending portion of the continuous wave MR Doppler signal. This rate of change of ventricular pressure is determined during the isovolumic phase of the cardiac cycle before opening of the aortic valve. Utilizing the simplified Bernoulli equation, two velocity points along the MR Doppler envelope are selected from which a corresponding LV pressure change can be derived (Fig. 5.4). This change in LV pressure can then be divided by the change in time between the two Doppler velocities to derive the LV dP/dt. Normal values for mean dP/dt have been reported to be >1,200 mmHg/s for the LV. While more time consuming to perform, peak dP/dt

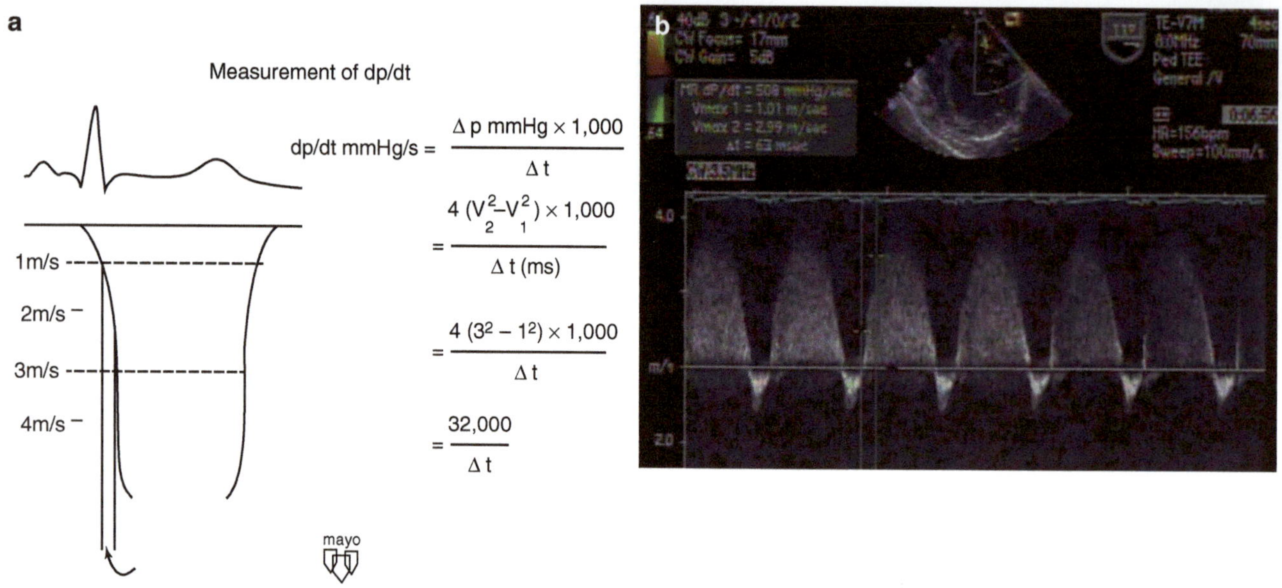

Fig. 5.4 Left ventricular dP/dt. (**a**) Measurement of dP/dt. (**b**) Calculation of left ventricular (LV) dP/dt from the mitral regurgitation (MR) jet. This still frame demonstrates the Doppler velocity curve of the MR jet obtained during TEE in a child with dilated cardiomyopathy and severe LV dysfunction. Utilizing the simplified Bernoulli equation, the LV dP/dt is the change in LV pressure measured from 1.0 to 3.0 m/s divided by the change in time between these two LV pressure points: LV dP/dt = (36 mmHg − 4 mmHg)/63 ms = 508 mmHg/s (normal >1,200 mmHg/s). Figure 5.4a used with permission from Mayo Clinic

correlates more accurately with invasive cardiac catheterization measurements. To ascertain peak LV dP/dt noninvasively, the MR signal is digitized to obtain the first derivative of the pressure gradient curve from which peak positive LV dP/dt can be calculated. While reflective of myocardial contractility, peak positive LV dP/dt is significantly affected by changes in preload and afterload [43, 82]. Peak negative LV dP/dt and the time constant of relaxation (Tau) can also be calculated from the MR signal, serving as indices of diastolic function.

Myocardial Performance Index

The myocardial performance index (MPI), also referred to as Tei index, is a Doppler-derived quantitative measure of global ventricular function that incorporates both systolic and diastolic time intervals [83–87]. The MPI is defined as the sum of isovolumic contraction time (ICT) and isovolumic relaxation time (IRT) divided by ejection time (ET) (Fig. 5.5):

$$\text{MPI} = (\text{ICT} + \text{IRT}) / \text{ET}$$

The components of this index are measured from routine pulsed wave Doppler signals at the atrioventricular valve and ventricular outflow tract of either the LV or RV (as an alternative, the comparable signals from tissue Doppler imaging, as described below, can be used). To derive the sum of ICT and IRT, the Doppler derived ejection time for either ventricle is subtracted from the Doppler interval between cessation and onset of the respective atrioventricular valve inflow signal (from the end of the Doppler A wave to the beginning of the Doppler E wave of the next cardiac cycle). Increasing values of the MPI correlate with increasing degrees of global ventricular functional impairment.

Both adult and pediatric studies have established normal values for the MPI [84, 86, 88]. In adults, normal LV and RV MPI values are 0.39 ± 0.05 and 0.28 ± 0.04, respectively. In children, similar values for the LV and RV are reported to be 0.35 ± 0.03 and 0.32 ± 0.03, respectively. The MPI has been shown to be a sensitive predictor of outcome in adult and pediatric patients with acquired and CHD [85, 86, 89–94]. One of the advantages of the MPI is the ease in which it can be obtained, both by TTE as well as TEE. Because the MPI incorporates measures of both systolic and diastolic performance, this index may be a more sensitive early measure of ventricular dysfunction in the absence of other overt changes in isolated systolic or diastolic echocardiographic indices. In addition, because the MPI is a Doppler-derived index, it has been reported to be easily applied to the assessment of both LV and RV function as well as complex ventricular geometries in patients with CHD [89, 90, 92, 93]. The MPI, however, does have major limitations. It is significantly affected by changes in loading conditions, particularly preload, and has a paradoxical change with high filling pressures or severe semilunar valve regurgitation ("pseudo-normalization"). In addition, the combined nature of this index fails to readily discriminate between abnormalities of systolic or diastolic performance.

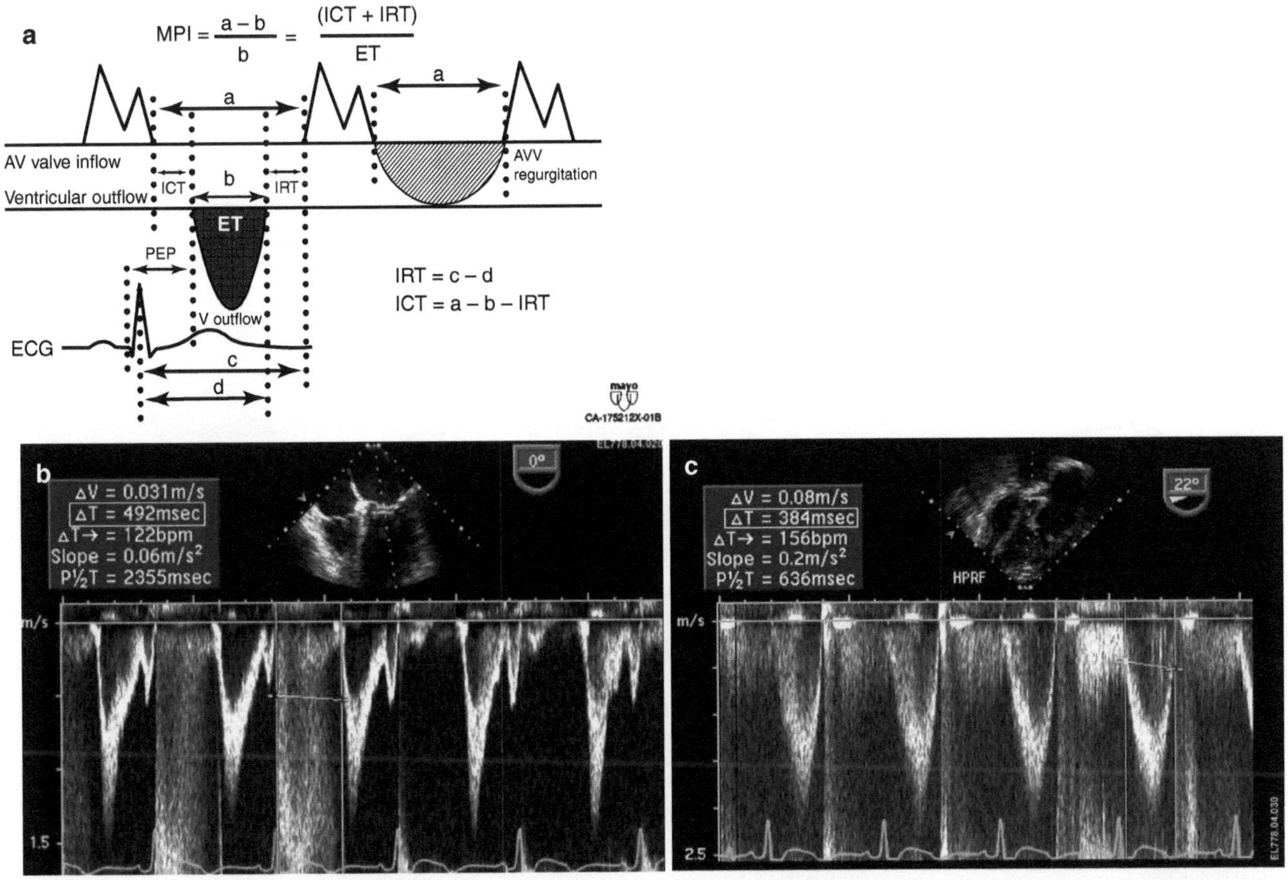

Fig. 5.5 Myocardial performance index (*MPI*) for assessment of left ventricular global function. *AV* atrioventricular, *AVV* atrioventricular valve, *ECG* electrocardiogram, *PEP* pre ejection period, *V* ventricular. (**a**) MPI represents the ratio of isovolumic contraction time (*ICT*) and isovolumic relaxation time (*IRT*) to ventricular ejection time (*ET*):

$$MPI = (ICT + IRT) / ET$$

(**b**) Mid esophageal four chamber view. The duration of ICT+IRT is measured from the cessation of mitral valve inflow to the onset of atrioventricular valve inflow of the next cardiac cycle (interval a). (**c**) Deep transgastric view with pulsed wave Doppler within the left ventricular outflow tract. Ventricular ejection time is measured from the onset to cessation of LV ejection (interval b)

$$LV\ MPI = (492 - 384) / 384 = 0.28$$

(Figure a from Eidem et al. [88], with permission)

Echocardiographic Assessment of Regional Left Ventricular Systolic Function

Two-Dimensional Imaging

Regional ventricular function can be assessed by examining wall motion and systolic wall thickening. TEE, particularly in the intraoperative setting, is ideally suited for this purpose. Changes in ventricular wall motion typically occur during periods of decreased coronary perfusion, as can be the case during surgical interventions. These wall motion alterations are characterized by reduced systolic thickening and decreased inward endocardial excursion.

In order to facilitate regional wall function assessment several schemes have been proposed that include specific nomenclature, a variable number of LV segmental divisions, and different methods of wall motion analysis. Two models of LV segmental division have been favored as follows: (1) the 16-segment LV model and (2) the 17-segment LV model. The former, established in 1989 [16], represents an effort by the American Society of Echocardiography Committee on Standards and forms the basis for the recommendations in the original guidelines for performing a comprehensive intraoperative multiplane TEE examination established by the American Society of Echocardiography and the Society of Cardiovascular Anesthesiologists [95]. The latter, proposed by the American Heart Association in 2002, aimed to standardize myocardial segmentation and nomenclature for all types of cardiac imaging modalities [96]. These two models as applicable to TEE imaging are illustrated in Figs. 5.6 and 5.7.

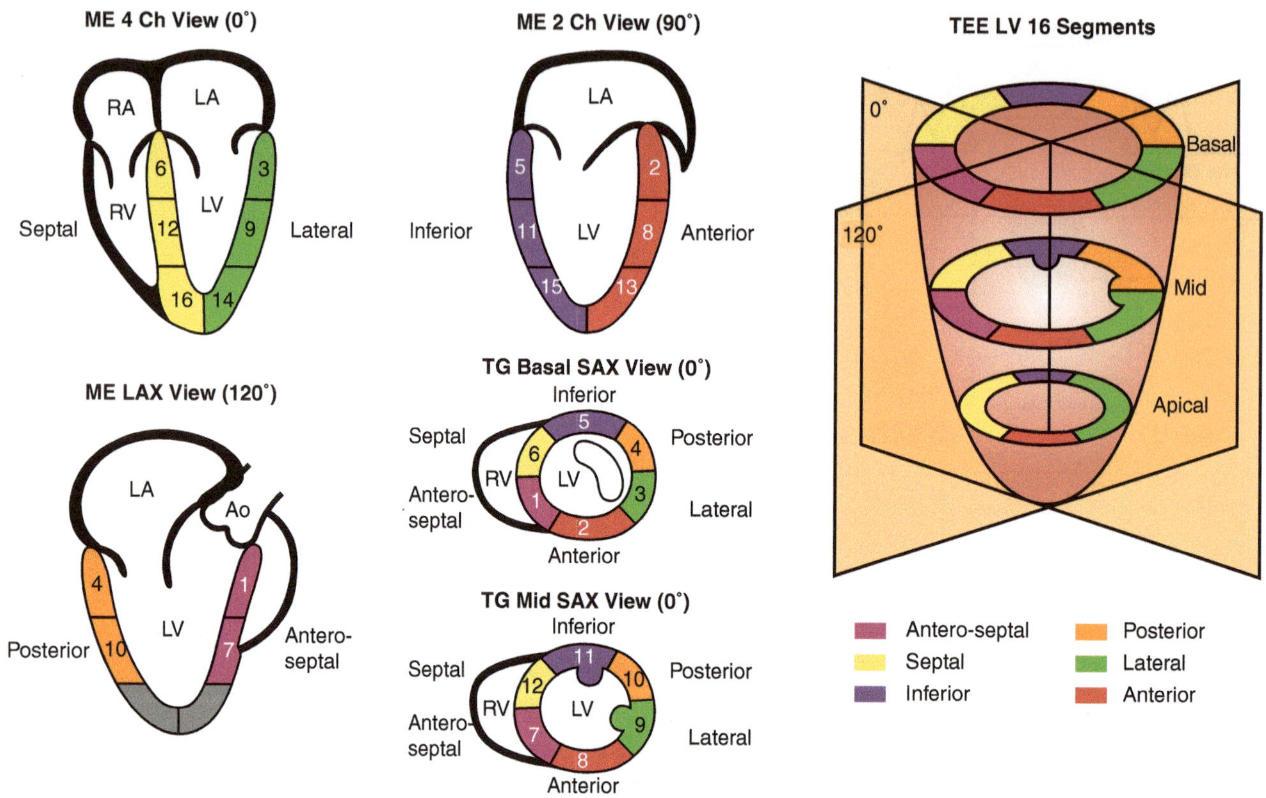

Fig. 5.6 SCA/ASE 16-segment model of the left ventricle

Basal segments	Mid segments	Apical segments
1. Basal antero-septal	7. Mid antero-septal	13. Apical anterior
2. Basal anterior	8. Mid anterior	14. Apical lateral
3. Basal lateral	9. Mid lateral	15. Apical inferior
4. Basal posterior	10. Mid posterior	16. Apical septal
5. Basal inferior	11. Mid inferior	
6. Basal septal	12. Mid septal	

Modified from Vegas [97], with permission from Springer

The 16-segment model divides the LV into three levels from base to apex: basal, mid, and apical. The basal and mid levels are each divided circumferentially into six segments, and the apical level into four. The 17-segment model added the apical cap or myocardial apex at the extreme tip of the LV beyond the chamber cavity. It was also suggested that the term 'inferior' might be more suitable than 'posterior' in reference to the ventricular walls. In the most recent recommendations for chamber quantification it is pointed out that the 16-segment model is more suitable for assessing wall motion abnormalities (as the apical segment does not move), while the 17-segment model is more appropriate for myocardial perfusion evaluation and comparison among various imaging modalities [97].

The TG Mid SAX view at the level of the papillary muscles is the suggested starting point to facilitate the qualitative evaluation of regional ventricular systolic function. Although there is significant variability in the myocardial blood supply by the coronary arteries, this cross-section allows for a prompt assessment of segmental wall function since all coronary artery territories are represented in this view (Fig. 5.8). Additional TEE cross-sections are needed to evaluate all myocardial segments as allowed by multiplanar imaging, including the ME 4 Ch, ME 2 Ch, and ME LAX views (Fig. 5.8). The visual assessment of wall motion should be graded as normal/hyperkinetic, hypokinetic (reduced systolic thickening), akinetic (absent systolic thickening), dyskinetic (paradoxical systolic motion), or aneurysmal (diastolic deformation).

The feasibility of this segmental functional analysis and its utility has been reported in infants with CHD. In a prospective study of neonates undergoing an arterial switch operation for transposition of the great arteries, segmental wall motion was examined in the TG Mid SAX and ME 4 Ch views [98]. The presence of severe wall motion abnormalities that persisted at the completion of surgery and were present in multiple segments was found to correlate with myocardial ischemia in this cohort. This highlights the importance of regional functional analysis in patients undergoing interventions that involve the coronary arteries, aortic root or any other procedures that can potentially impact coronary perfusion.

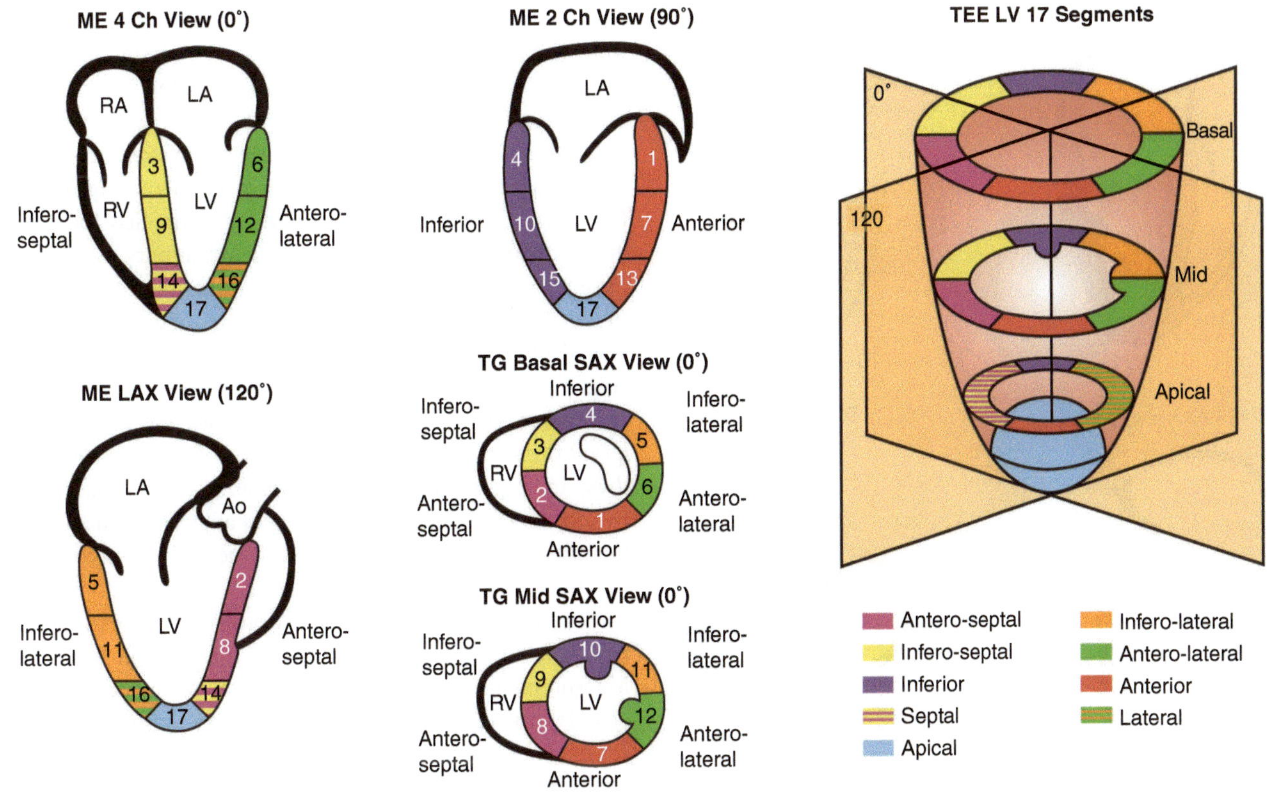

Fig. 5.7 AHA 17-segment model of the left ventricle

Basal segments	Mid segments	Apical segments
1. Basal anterior	7. Mid anterior	13. Apical anterior
2. Basal antero-septal	8. Mid antero-septal	14. Apical septal
3. Basal infero-septal	9. Mid infero-septal	15. Apical inferior
4. Basal inferior	10. Mid inferior	16. Apical lateral
5. Basal infero-lateral	11. Mid infero-lateral	17. Apex
6. Basal antero-lateral	12. Mid antero-lateral	

Modified from Vegas [97], with permission from Springer

Obviously, the two segmental models discussed apply principally to the LV in an anatomically "normal" heart—one with situs solitus, normal segments, and atrioventricular and ventriculoarterial connections (Chap. 4). As such, there will be limited direct application of these models for a number of congenital heart defects. Nonetheless the principles embodied in this segmental wall motion analysis—in particular, the evaluation of segmental wall kinetic motion—can be more generally applied to all forms of CHD. It facilitates a semi-quantitative, analytic assessment of wall motion and function even in hearts with very abnormal ventricular shape and morphology.

Tissue Doppler Imaging and Strain Rate Imaging

The assessment of regional systolic LV function, as detailed above, has centered upon the evaluation of segmental endocardial excursion and LV wall thickening. These semi-quantitative methods often fail to discriminate between active and passive myocardial motion. Newer echocardiographic modalities, including tissue Doppler imaging and strain rate imaging, offer a potentially more quantitative and accurate approach to the assessment of regional myocardial contraction and relaxation.

Tissue Doppler imaging (TDI, also known as Doppler tissue imaging or DTI) has been an addition to the armamentarium of the echocardiographer in recent years. By incorporating a high pass filter, tissue Doppler allows the display and quantitation of the low velocity high amplitude Doppler shifts present within the myocardium as opposed to the higher velocity lower amplitude Doppler signals more commonly measured within the blood pool (Fig. 5.9). Tissue Doppler echocardiography is less load-dependent than corresponding Doppler velocities from the blood pool and has systolic and diastolic components. These systolic velocities are heterogenous depending on ventricular wall and position.

Measurement of myocardial wall velocities by TDI has been shown to be a promising modality for assessment of longitudinal systolic performance [49, 51, 100]. Recent

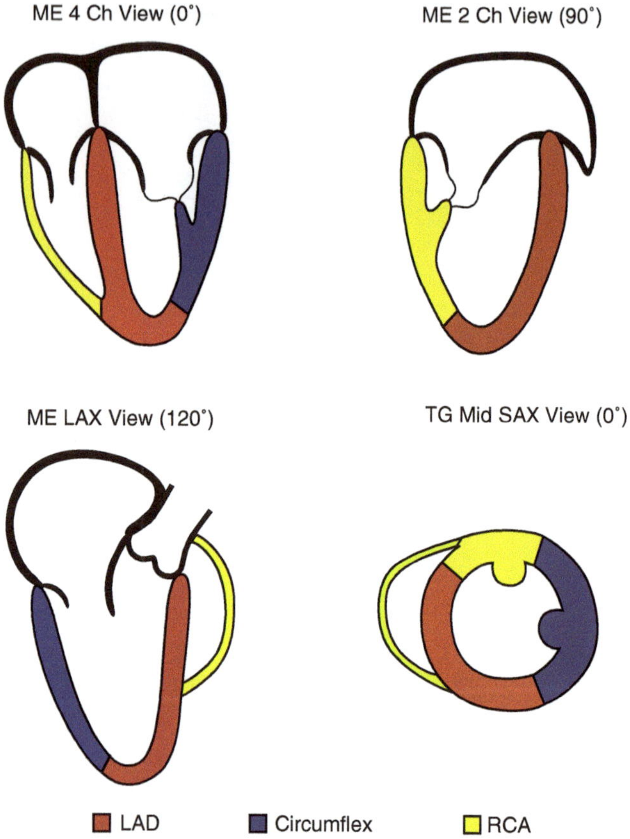

Fig. 5.8 Myocardial regions perfused by the major coronary arteries. The figure displays the typical myocardial territories perfused by the major coronary arteries

Left coronary circulation	Right coronary circulation
Left anterior descending (LAD) artery: (anterior, antero/infero septal walls)	Right coronary artery (RCA): (inferior wall, RV, SA and AV nodes)
Septal perforators	Posterior interventricular
Diagonal branches	Posterior Lateral
Posterior interventricular	Acute marginal
Circumflex (Cx) artery: (posterior, lateral walls)	Papillary muscles blood supply:
Obtuse marginal branches	AL by two arteries (obtuse + diagonal)
Posterior interventricular	PM by one artery (RCA or obtuse)

Dominance depends on which vessel (RCA or Cx) supplies the posterior interventricular branch. The majority of hearts (85 %) are right dominant. *AL* anterolateral, *AV* atrioventricular, *RV* right ventricle, *SA* sinotrial, *PM* posteromedial

Modified from Vegas [97], with permission from Springer

studies have demonstrated significant changes in mitral annular systolic TDI velocities in adult patients with LV dysfunction and elevated filling pressures [101, 102]. These indices have also been used to identify subclinical systolic ventricular dysfunction in pediatric patients [103]. Data in children following cardiac transplantation have also been found to correlate with hemodynamic parameters [104].

Tissue Doppler velocities, however, cannot differentiate between active contraction and passive motion, representing a major limitation when assessing regional myocardial function. Regional strain rate corresponds to the rate of regional myocardial deformation and can be calculated from the spatial gradient in myocardial velocity between two neighbouring points within the myocardium. Regional strain represents the amount of deformation (expressed as a percentage) or the fractional change in length caused by an applied force and is calculated by integrating the strain rate curve over time during the cardiac cycle. Strain measures the total amount of deformation in either the radial or longitudinal direction while strain rate calculates the velocity of shortening (Fig. 5.10). These two measurements reflect different aspects of myocardial function and therefore provide complementary information. In contrast to tissue Doppler velocities, these indices of myocardial deformation are not influenced by global heart motion or tethering of adjacent segments and therefore represent better indices of true regional myocardial function.

Studies have demonstrated regional differences in strain rate in adult patients after myocardial infarction [50, 105]. Measurements of radial and longitudinal strain rate have also been reported in normal children [106]. In addition, quantification of regional RV and LV function by strain rate and strain indexes after surgical repair of tetralogy of Fallot in children demonstrated that RV deformation abnormalities are associated with electrical depolarization abnormalities or chronic pulmonary regurgitation [107–110]. Further studies are needed to identify potential applications of strain rate imaging and related newer modalities (speckle-tracking and vector velocity imaging) in the evaluation of ventricular mechanics and regional assessment of myocardial function of both right and left ventricles in children [111]. It is hoped that future investigations can address the suitability of these approaches in the perioperative setting.

Echocardiographic Assessment of Diastolic Ventricular Function

2D and particularly Doppler echocardiography, have historically been essential noninvasive tools in the quantitative assessment of LV diastolic function. Abnormalities of ventricular compliance and relaxation can be demonstrated by characteristic changes in mitral inflow and pulmonary venous Doppler patterns [112]. Newer methodologies including tissue Doppler echocardiography and flow propagation velocities enhance the ability of echocardiography to define and quantitate these adverse changes in diastolic performance. Because diastolic dysfunction often precedes systolic dysfunction, careful assessment of diastolic function is mandatory in the noninvasive characterization and serial evaluation of patients with CHD.

Noninvasive evaluation of diastolic function in normal infants and children is influenced by a variety of factors

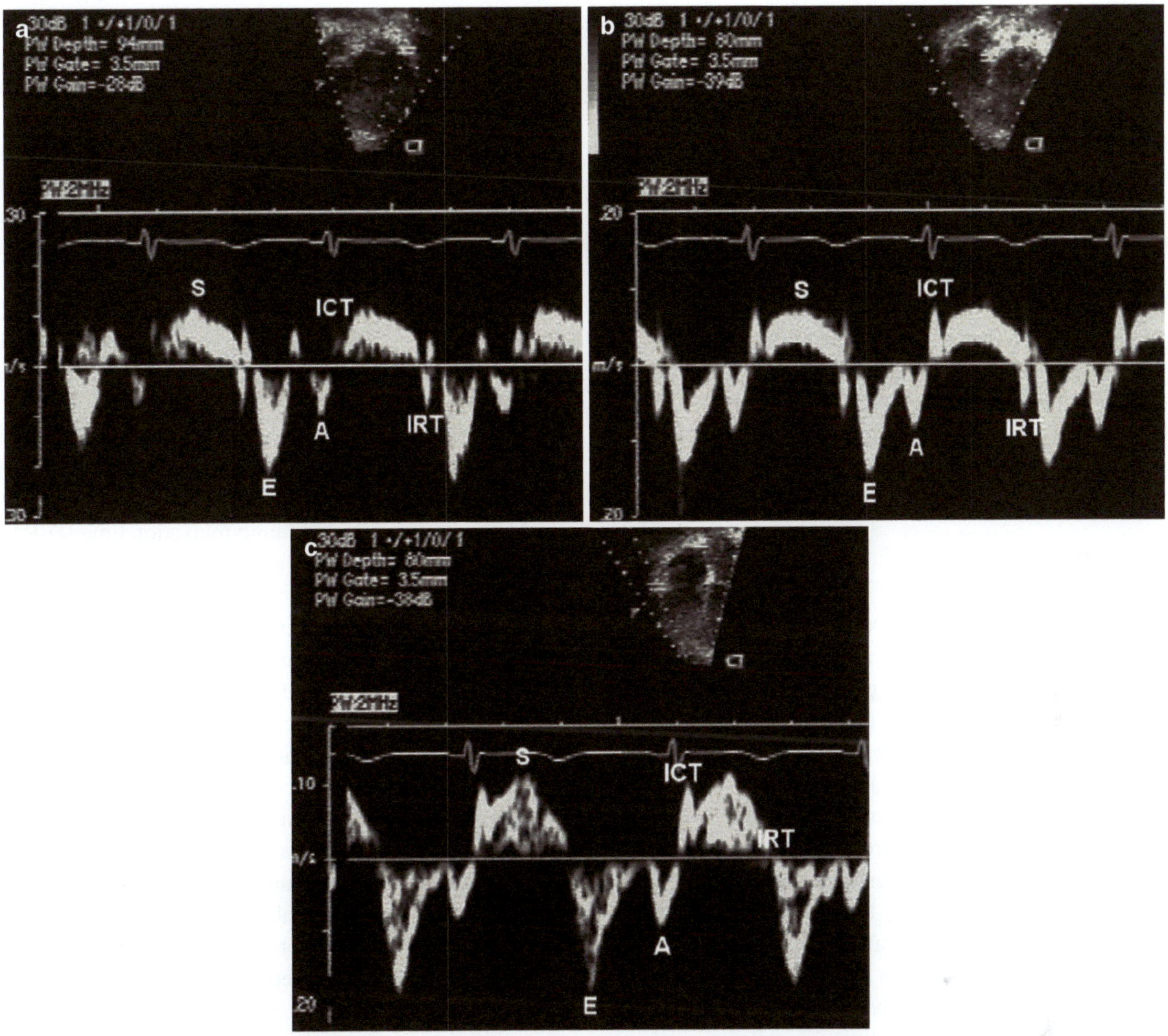

Fig. 5.9 Tissue Doppler imaging. Normal mitral annular (panel a), septal (panel b), and tricuspid annular (panel c) pulsed wave longitudinal Doppler tissue velocities. Note the characteristic normal pattern of a larger early diastolic velocity (E-wave) compared to late diastolic velocity (A-wave). The S-wave is the systolic wave. ICT, isovolumic contraction time; IRT, isovolumic relaxation time (From Eidem et al. [99], with permission)

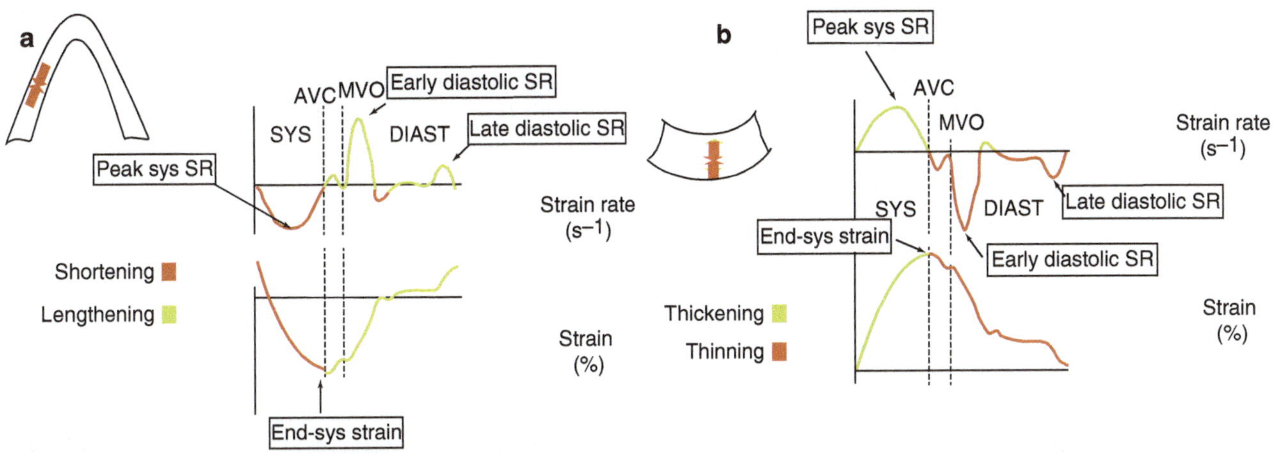

Fig. 5.10 Strain and strain rate imaging. Schematic representation of longitudinal (**a**) and radial (**b**) strain and strain rate imaging. In the longitudinal direction, strain represents myocardial shortening (systole) and lengthening (diastole) while strain rate represents the rate at which shortening or lengthening occurs. Similarly, radial strain represents myocardial thickening (systole) and thinning (diastole) while strain rate represents the rate at which thickening or thinning occurs. *AVC* aortic valve closure, *diast* diastole, *MVO* mitral valve opening, *SR* strain rate, *sys* systole/systolic (Figures used with permission from Luc Mertens, MD)

including age, heart rate, and the respiratory cycle. Reference values detailing both mitral and pulmonary venous Doppler velocities in a large cohort of normal children have been established using transthoracic imaging [113]. Similar to many echocardiographic parameters, these Doppler velocities are also significantly impacted by loading conditions making determination of diastolic dysfunction by using these parameters alone very challenging in patients with CHD.

Although the evaluation of diastolic function using TEE has been reported in adult patients in the perioperative setting, there are no formal studies addressing this application in the pediatric age group. The discussion that follows reviews general concepts of diastolic evaluation in children with the use of echocardiography and potential applications using the transesophageal modality.

Mitral Inflow Doppler

Mitral inflow Doppler is readily obtained from the ME 4 Ch view and represents the diastolic pressure gradient between the left atrium (LA) and LV (Fig. 5.11). The early diastolic filling wave, or E-wave, is the dominant diastolic wave in children and young adults and represents the peak LA to LV pressure gradient at the onset of diastole. The deceleration time of the mitral E-wave reflects the time period needed for equalization of LA and LV pressures. The late diastolic filling wave, or A-wave, represents the peak pressure gradient between the LA and LV in late diastole at the onset of atrial contraction. Normal mitral inflow Doppler is characterized by a dominant E-wave, a smaller A-wave, and a ratio of E- and A-waves (E:A ratio) between 1.0 and 3.0. Normal duration of mitral deceleration time as well as isovolumic relaxation time vary with age and have been reported in both

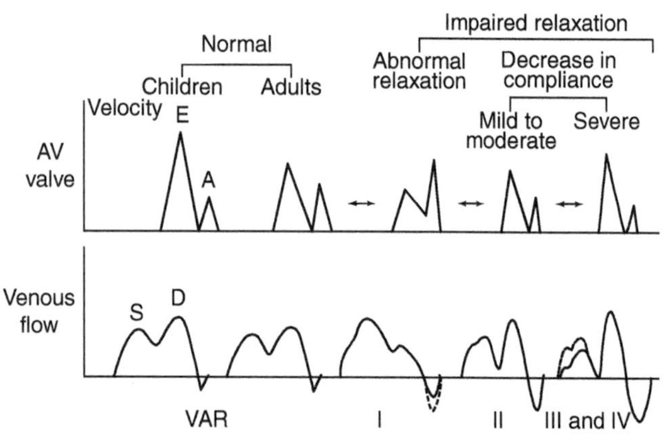

Fig. 5.11 Doppler patterns in diastolic dysfunction. Graphic representation of spectrum of changes in mitral and pulmonary venous inflow patterns associated with diastolic dysfunction in children. *A* atrial filling wave, *AV* atrioventricular, *D* pulmonary vein diastolic flow wave, *E* early filling wave, *S* pulmonary vein systolic flow wave, *VAR* vein atrial reversal wave (Modified from: Olivier et al. [114], with permission)

pediatric and adult populations [113, 115–118]. Mitral inflow Doppler velocities are not only impacted by changes in LV diastolic function but also by a variety of additional hemodynamic factors including age, altered loading conditions, heart rate, and changes in atrial and ventricular compliance. Interpretation of characteristic patterns of mitral inflow must be carefully evaluated with particular attention paid to the potential impact of each of these hemodynamic factors on the Doppler velocities.

The earliest stage of LV diastolic dysfunction demonstrated by mitral inflow Doppler is abnormal relaxation (Fig. 5.11). This Doppler pattern is characteristic of normal aging in adults and represents a mild decrease in the rate of LV relaxation with continued normal LA pressure. It is characterized by a reduced E-wave velocity, increased A-wave velocity, decreased E:A ratio <1.0, and a prolonged mitral deceleration time and isovolumic relaxation time (IVRT).

As diastolic dysfunction progresses, further changes in ventricular relaxation and compliance occur leading to an increase in LA pressure. Increased LA pressure normalizes the initial transmitral gradient between the LA and LV producing a "pseudo-normalized" mitral inflow Doppler pattern with increased E-wave velocity and E:A ratio, and normalized mitral deceleration and isovolumic relaxation time intervals (Fig. 5.11). This pseudo-normal Doppler pattern may be difficult to distinguish from normal mitral inflow Doppler; however, maneuvers that decrease ventricular preload, like the Valsalva maneuver, will uncover the underlying abnormalities of mitral inflow Doppler. In addition, evaluation of pulmonary venous inflow Doppler can help unmask this advanced degree of LV diastolic dysfunction (see below).

Further deterioration of LV diastolic function results in restrictive ventricular filling with an additional increase in LA pressure and a concomitant decrease in ventricular compliance. The Doppler pattern of restrictive LV filling is characterized by additional increases in E-wave velocity, reduction in A-wave velocity, an increased E:A ratio >3.0, and significant shortening of both mitral deceleration time and IVRT (Fig. 5.11) [115]. This pattern is typically seen in patients with restrictive cardiomyopathy and may also be seen in other conditions associated with restrictive physiology (i.e., acute post-transplant setting).

Pulmonary Venous Doppler

Pulmonary venous Doppler, combined with mitral inflow Doppler, provides a more comprehensive assessment of LA and LV filling pressures (Fig. 5.11) [119–121]. TEE is ideally suited to the acquisition and quantitation of pulmonary venous flows, particularly in patients with poor transthoracic windows [19, 20, 27, 122]. Pulmonary venous inflow consists of three distinct Doppler waves: a systolic wave (S-wave), a diastolic wave (D-wave), and a reversal wave that occurs with atrial contraction (Ar-wave). In normal adolescents and adults, the characteristic pattern of pulmonary venous inflow consists of a dominant S-wave, a smaller D-wave, and a small Ar-wave of low velocity and brief duration. In neonates and younger children, a dominant D-wave is often present with a similar brief low velocity, or even absent, Ar-wave.

With worsening LV diastolic dysfunction, LA pressure increases leading to diminished systolic forward flow into the LA from the pulmonary veins with relatively increased diastolic forward flow resulting in a diastolic dominance of pulmonary venous inflow (Fig. 5.11). More importantly, both the velocity and duration of the pulmonary venous atrial reversal wave are increased. Pediatric and adult studies have demonstrated that an Ar-wave duration >30 ms longer than the corresponding mitral A-wave duration or a ratio of pulmonary venous Ar-wave to mitral A-wave duration >1.2 is predictive of elevated LV filling pressure (Fig. 5.12) [113, 120]. Pulmonary venous flow variables as measured by TEE have been correlated with estimations of mean LA pressure in adults undergoing cardiovascular surgery [19].

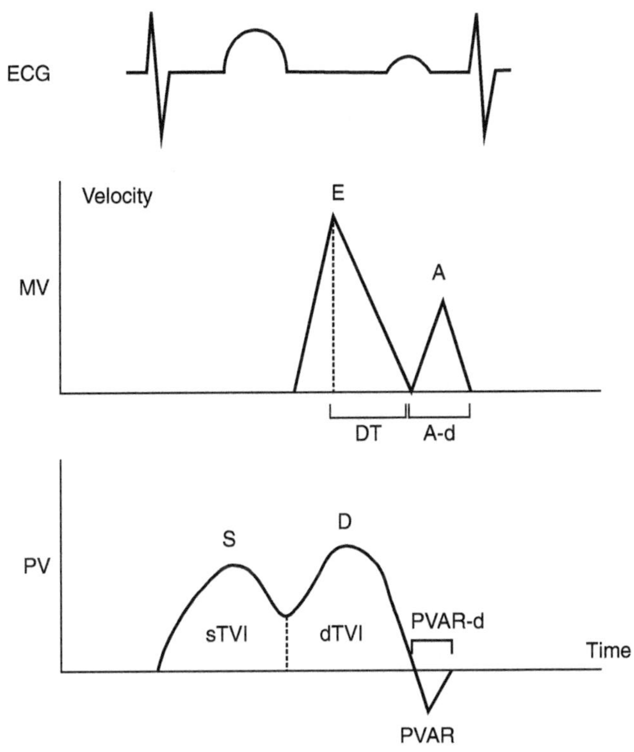

Fig. 5.12 Mitral valve and pulmonary venous Doppler tracings. Diagram depicting mitral valve (*MV*) and pulmonary vein (*PV*) Doppler flow tracings. *A* atrial filling wave, *A-d* duration of atrial filling wave, *D* pulmonary vein diastolic flow wave, *DT* mitral deceleration time, *dTVI* time velocity integral of pulmonary vein diastolic flow wave, *E* early filling wave, *ECG* electrocardiogram, *PVAR* pulmonary vein atrial reversal wave, *PVAR-d* duration of pulmonary vein atrial reversal flow, *S* pulmonary vein systolic flow wave, *sTVI* time velocity integral of pulmonary vein systolic flow wave (From O'Leary et al. [113], with permission)

Tissue Doppler Imaging

Tissue Doppler imaging is particularly well suited to the quantitative evaluation of LV diastolic function and can be easily obtained by either a transthoracic or transesophageal approach. Both early (Ea) and late (Aa) annular diastolic velocities can be readily obtained by tissue Doppler echocardiography (Fig. 5.9). Similar to systolic tissue Doppler velocities, differences in diastolic velocities exist between (1) the subendocardium and subepicardium, (2) from cardiac base to apex, and (3) between various myocardial wall segments. Previous studies have reported an excellent correlation between the early annular diastolic mitral velocity and simultaneous invasive measures of diastolic function at cardiac catheterization [123]. Early annular diastolic velocities also appear to be less sensitive to changes in ventricular preload compared to the corresponding early transmitral Doppler inflow velocity [101, 123, 124]. These diastolic tissue Doppler velocities, however, are impacted by significant alterations in preload. The influence of afterload on tissue Doppler velocities is less controversial with many studies documenting significant changes in systolic and diastolic annular velocities with changes in ventricular afterload [125–127]. Therefore, the clinical use of tissue Doppler velocities in patients with valvar stenoses or other etiologies of altered ventricular afterload need to be interpreted carefully in light of this limitation.

Tissue Doppler velocities have been shown to be clinically helpful in the discrimination between normal and abnormal transmitral Doppler filling patterns [101, 128–130]. In addition to changes incurred by loading conditions, alterations in LA pressure as well as LV end-diastolic pressure also affect the early transmitral diastolic velocity. However, the corresponding tissue Doppler velocity is characteristically decreased in patients with pseudo-normal filling allowing differentiation of this abnormal filling pattern from one of normal transmitral Doppler inflow. Clinical reports have suggested a ratio of the early transmitral inflow Doppler signal to the lateral mitral annular early diastolic velocity (mitral E/Ea) as a noninvasive measure of LV filling pressure. Nagueh and colleagues demonstrated a significant correlation of mitral E/Ea with invasively measured mean pulmonary capillary wedge pressure [101], and subsequent studies have further validated this ratio and reported its applicability in a variety of hemodynamic settings mostly in adult populations. Additional novel indices of LV diastolic function utilizing tissue Doppler echocardiography have been reported that may further expand the role of this modality in the clinical evaluation of LV filling pressures [130, 131].

Tissue Doppler has also been shown to be of considerable clinical value in the differentiation of constrictive from restrictive LV filling [132–135]. Evaluation of patients with constrictive pericarditis and restrictive cardiomyopathy with 2D echocardiography and even invasive cardiac catheterization may fail to confidently distinguish these two disease states. Because the myocardium in patients with constrictive pericarditis is most commonly normal, the corresponding tissue Doppler velocities are also normal. However, patients with restrictive cardiomyopathy have been shown to have significantly decreased early diastolic as well as systolic tissue Doppler velocities. Therefore evaluation of tissue Doppler velocities allows separation of these two distinct clinical entities.

Tissue Doppler Studies in Normal Children

A number of TTE studies have been performed in children to establish normal reference values of tissue Doppler velocities in this cohort [99, 136–141]. Similar to previously published adult reports, pediatric tissue Doppler velocities vary with age, heart rate, wall location, and myocardial layer. In addition, pulsed wave tissue Doppler velocities are also highly correlated with parameters of cardiac growth, most notably LVEDD and LV mass with the most significant changes in these velocities occurring during the first year of life (Fig. 5.13) [99]. In a published large series of infants and children, tissue Doppler velocities did not correlate significantly with other more commonly utilized measures of systolic and diastolic ventricular performance including LV fractional shortening, LV and RV MPI, and transmitral inflow Doppler [99]. This lack of correlation in part is likely due to pulsed wave tissue Doppler assessing longitudinal ventricular function while other more traditional 2D and Doppler methods assess radial and global measures of ventricular performance.

Similar to previously published adult normative data, normal values for the E/Ea ratio in children have also been

a

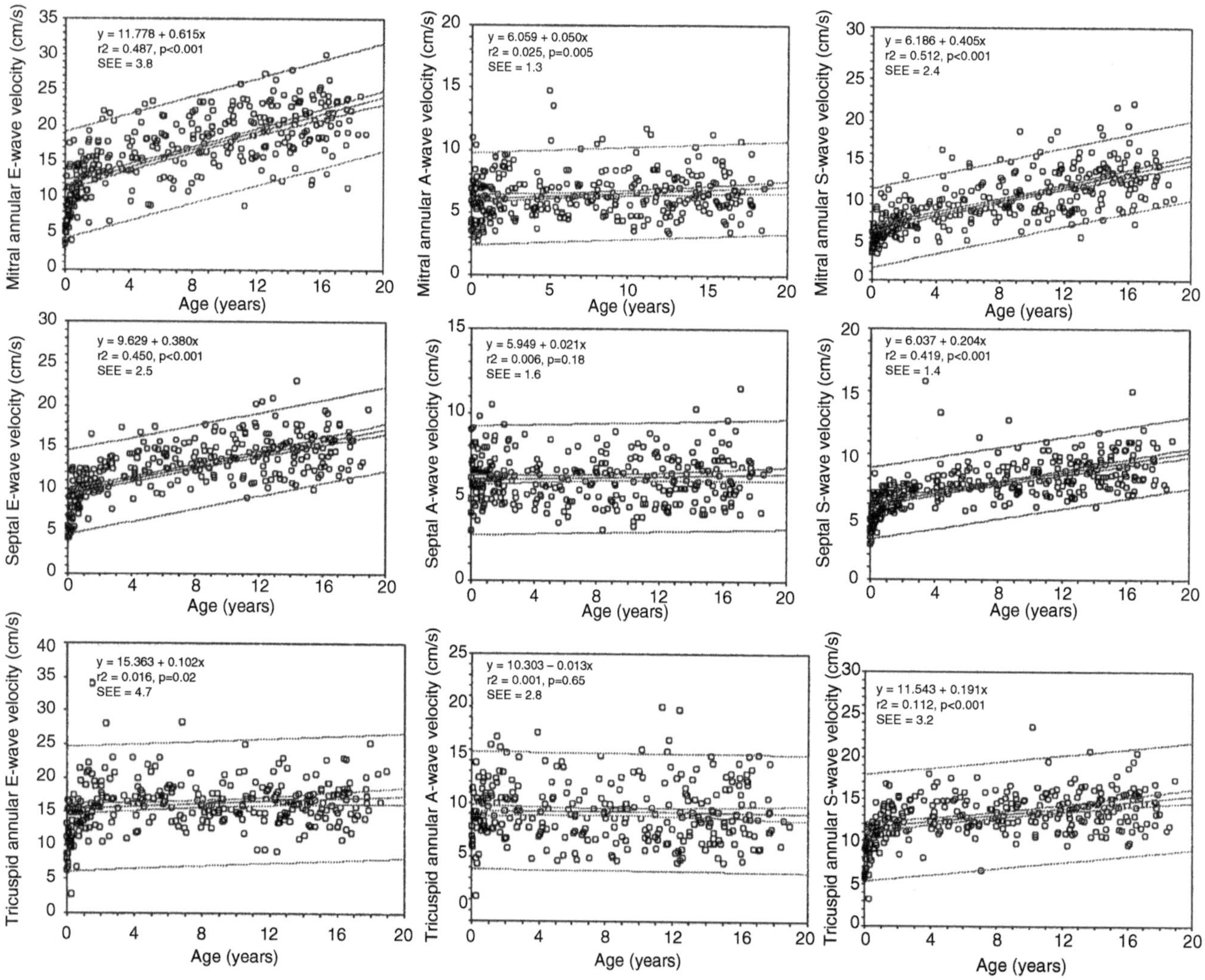

Fig. 5.13 Tissue Doppler velocities in children. Influence of age (**a**) and left ventricular end-diastolic dimension (**b**) on longitudinal systolic (S) and diastolic (E and A) pulsed wave tissue Doppler velocities in children (From: Eidem et al. [99], with permission)

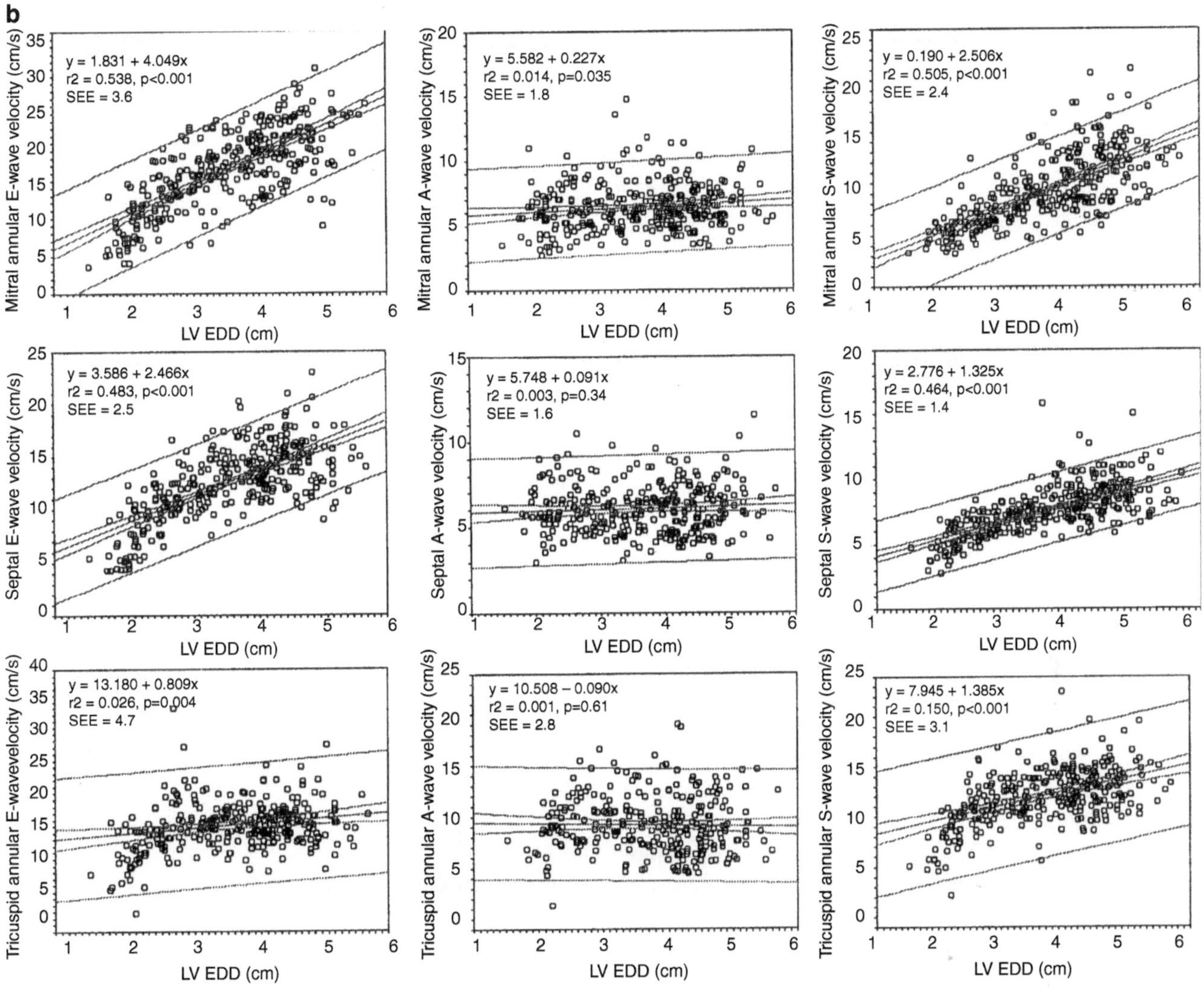

Fig. 5.13 (continued)

reported [99]. These values are also impacted by age, heart rate, ventricular wall location, LV dimension, and LV mass. Values for E/Ea are highest in neonates and decrease with advancing age primarily due to an increased Ea velocity over this time period. Data regarding simultaneous catheterization—echocardiographic measurements correlating the E/Ea ratio in children with invasive measures of LV filling pressure are limited to date. Two recent studies in children following cardiac transplantation demonstrate a poor correlation between these parameters. One study found E:E′ to be a poor predictor of simultaneously obtained, catheter-derived hemodynamic parameters in post-transplant children [142]. Another recent study reported that E/Ea does not correlate well with filling pressures observed after pediatric heart transplantation [104]. However, a septal E/Ea > 12 was associated with elevated pulmonary capillary wedge pressure and high-grade cellular rejection. In addition, a lateral tricuspid E/Ea > 10 was associated with elevated mean right atrial pressure. In a small cohort of children, invasive cardiac catheterization measures of LV function were compared to simultaneously obtained color M-mode and Doppler parameters of LV performance [139]. The ratio of early diastolic mitral annular tissue Doppler velocity to flow propagation velocity (Ea/Vp) correlated closely with invasive LV end-diastolic pressure while the septal Ea velocity correlated with the time constant of relaxation (Tau). Additional studies utilizing tissue Doppler to establish normal atrioventricular electromechanical coupling intervals have also been reported [141]. The applications and clinical value of tissue Doppler echocardiography obtained by transesophageal imaging deserve further evaluation.

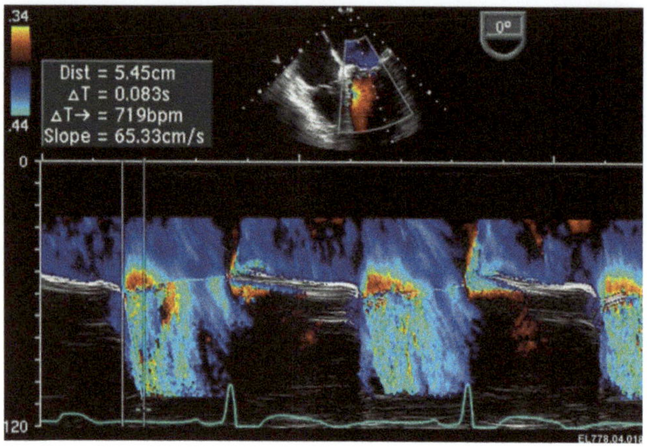

Fig. 5.14 Color M-mode Doppler flow propagation velocity. Measurement of flow propagation velocity (Vp) from color M-mode Doppler in the assessment of LV diastolic function. Vp is determined by the slope of the first clearly demarcated aliasing velocity (*white line*) during early left ventricular filling. In this 28 year old patient with aortic regurgitation, color M-mode during the intraoperative TEE examination demonstrated a normal Vp of 65 cm/s

Color M-Mode Flow Propagation Velocity

Flow propagation of early diastolic filling from the mitral annulus to the cardiac apex can be quantitated by color M-mode (Fig. 5.14). As opposed to mitral inflow Doppler, this propagation velocity has been shown to be significantly less affected by changes in heart rate, LA pressure, and loading conditions, and may therefore more accurately reflect changes in myocardial relaxation. Numerous studies have demonstrated a significant decrease in flow propagation velocity in patients with diastolic dysfunction of varying etiology [102, 143–145]. In addition, the ratio of the mitral annular Doppler tissue E-wave velocity to flow propagation velocity has also been shown to be a significant predictor of congestive heart failure and outcome in patients after myocardial infarction. This ratio of flow propagation and Doppler tissue imaging velocity may also be helpful in distinguishing a normal mitral inflow pattern from one of pseudo-normalized mitral inflow. In a small cohort of children undergoing simultaneous cardiac catheterization and TTE, Border and colleagues demonstrated a significant positive correlation between invasively measured LV end-diastolic pressure and the ratio of peak early transmitral Doppler flow velocity to flow propagation velocity (E/Vp) [146].

Echocardiographic Assessment of Right Ventricular Function

Echocardiographic assessment of RV function, either by transthoracic or transesophageal methods, has been limited due to the geometric shape of the RV. Doppler echocardiography has historically been useful in the noninvasive prediction of RV systolic and pulmonary artery pressures [147, 148]. However, quantification of RV systolic function by M-mode or 2D echocardiography has relied on the visual assessment of relative RV wall motion or semi-quantitative measurements of FAC in RV dimension or volume. Newer echocardiographic modalities that have shown promise in quantifying RV function include Doppler measures of RV performance (myocardial performance index, RV dP/dt, and Doppler tissue imaging) as well as acoustic quantification and 3D echocardiography.

Right Ventricular Myocardial Performance Index

As described previously, the MPI is a Doppler-derived measure of global ventricular function that can be applied to any ventricular geometry. Studies have validated the ability of the MPI to quantitatively assess RV function in adults and patients with CHD [88, 92]. In addition, the MPI has demonstrated prognostic power in discriminating outcome in patients with either RV or LV failure [89–91]. Care, however, must be exercised in using this index in patients with CHD with altered RV preload or afterload [55, 56, 149, 150]. The RV MPI has been shown to be relatively independent of changes in chronic loading conditions but the impact of acute changes in physiologic loading are significant and need further definition.

Right Ventricular dP/dt

Similar to the LV, the rate of pressure change over time can also be used as a measure of RV systolic function in patients with tricuspid regurgitation. RV dP/dt has been shown to correlate with invasive measures of RV performance [151–154]. RV dP/dt has also been demonstrated to be helpful in the serial assessment of RV function in children with hypoplastic left heart syndrome [153]. Similar to LV limitations with this parameter, RV dP/dt is impacted by changes in loading conditions.

Right Ventricular Tissue Doppler Imaging

Tissue Doppler imaging represents one of the most recent modalities applied to the quantitative evaluation of RV function. Tricuspid annular motion has been shown to correlate with RV function in previous studies [99, 137, 138, 140]. TDI has been reported to be a reproducible noninvasive method of assessing systolic and diastolic annular motion and RV function. While impacted by both afterload and preload, data in adults and children with TDI have demonstrated these velocities to be less influenced by altered preload than corresponding mitral or tricuspid inflow Doppler. Limited data is available regarding the applications of RV TDI in CHD [155].

Acoustic Quantification and Right Ventricular Function

Acoustic quantification utilizes automated border detection techniques to measure the absolute change and rate of change in RV volume. This modality has been shown to correlate with other invasive methods of RV functional assessment in adults with abnormalities of global RV function. Automated border methods have also shown good correlation with magnetic resonance imaging in assessing changes in RV volume and systolic function. Feasibility of acoustic quantification in the noninvasive transthoracic evaluation of RV function in normal children has also been reported [156, 157]. Ongoing investigation is needed to establish the potential of this technique for the identification and serial evaluation of RV dysfunction in children with the use of TEE.

Three-Dimensional Echocardiography and Right Ventricular Function

3D echocardiography has enabled the noninvasive evaluation of RV volume and function [158–160]. The ability of 3D echocardiography to evaluate RV geometry in multiple spatial planes allows for accurate assessment of changes in RV volume during the cardiac cycle. Application of live 3D TEE to the assessment of RV volume and systolic function in adults and children appears promising [161–164].

Echocardiographic Assessment of Single Ventricular Function in Patients with Complex Congenital Heart Disease

Quantitative measurement of ventricular function in patients with functional single ventricles can be challenging. In most cases, a visual estimate of systolic function from 2D images is used. Quantitative echocardiographic assessment is limited by complex ventricular geometry often with associated abnormalities of wall motion [165–167].

Similar to novel techniques used to assess RV function; Doppler echocardiography holds promise in the potential evaluation of global single ventricle function [114, 168–170]. However, only limited studies to date have addressed either dP/dt or the MPI in patients with functional single ventricles [93, 153, 171]. Data is lacking on the ability of these new Doppler indices to predict outcome in patients with complex single ventricle anatomy. Finally, 3D echocardiography also holds promise in the nongeometric assessment of ventricular volume and function but has yet to be comprehensively evaluated in patients with CHD with transesophageal imaging.

Summary

The assessment of ventricular performance in congenital pathology has been hindered by the fact that most cardiovascular anomalies are associated with abnormal ventricular geometry and altered loading conditions. Thus the application of classic parameters developed and widely utilized in the functional assessment of the structurally normal heart may not be suitable in the setting of CHD. The recently developed echocardiographic techniques discussed throughout this chapter have provided new insight into the functional abnormalities that may be present in this patient group. These modalities, initially investigated and applied during transthoracic imaging, should now allow for the functional assessment during TEE to evolve further from a qualitative to a more quantitative approach. The techniques described in this chapter, as well as promising techniques and technologies of the future such as 3D imaging, give hope towards being able to provide more detailed insights into the systolic and diastolic function in CHD patients with even the most complex cardiac anatomy and geometry.

Case Examples

Editor's Note: Several of the TEE images in this section (Videos 5.1b, 5.1d, 5.1e, 5.2b, 5.3d; Figs. 5.15a, b, 5.16a, 5.17) are displayed in a vertically inverted orientation with respect to equivalent views presented in Chap. 4 – Structural Evaluation and throughout the textbook. This represents a preference by some institutions to display TEE images in an orientation that mimics the equivalent transthoracic cross-sections.

Case 1

11 year old child referred for surgical closure of moderate-sized secundum atrial septal defect

Preoperative (Videos 5.1a, 5.1b) and postoperative TEE images (Videos 5.1c, 5.1d, 5.1e) from multiple views allow for qualitative assessment of ventricular size and function in this patient. The transgastric mid LV view as shown is Fig. 5.15 (Video 5.1e) provides for M-mode interrogation and determination of LV shortening fraction.

Case 2

22 year old patient with long QT syndrome referred for surgical excision of intracardiac right ventricular lead

Qualitative assessment of right and left ventricular systolic function by TEE in this case is displayed in Videos 5.2a and 5.2b. Representative M-mode images for determination of LV shortening fraction are shown in Figs. 5.16a and 5.16b; Doppler tracings obtained for calculation of LV MPI are illustrated in Figs. 5.16c and 5.16d.

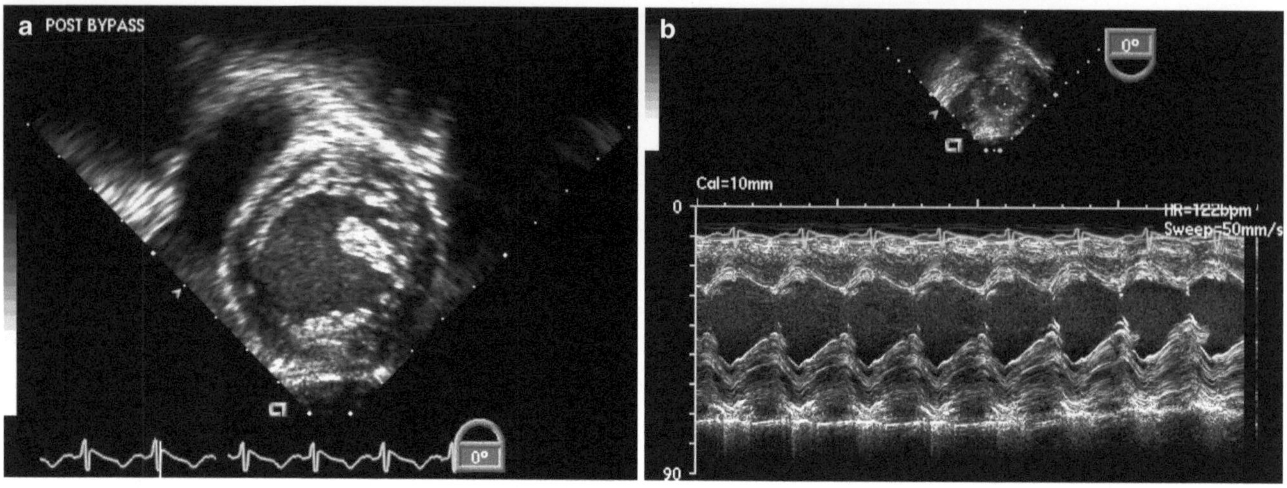

Fig. 5.15 (**a**) Still frame demonstrating the *elliptical shape* of the left ventricle in a transgastric view as shown in Video 5.1e. (**b**) Representative M-mode obtained during the TEE examination. The LV shortening fraction was 36 %. Note that the orientation of the M-mode beam with respect to the left ventricle during transesophageal/transgastric imaging may not correlate with that obtained during a transthoracic study

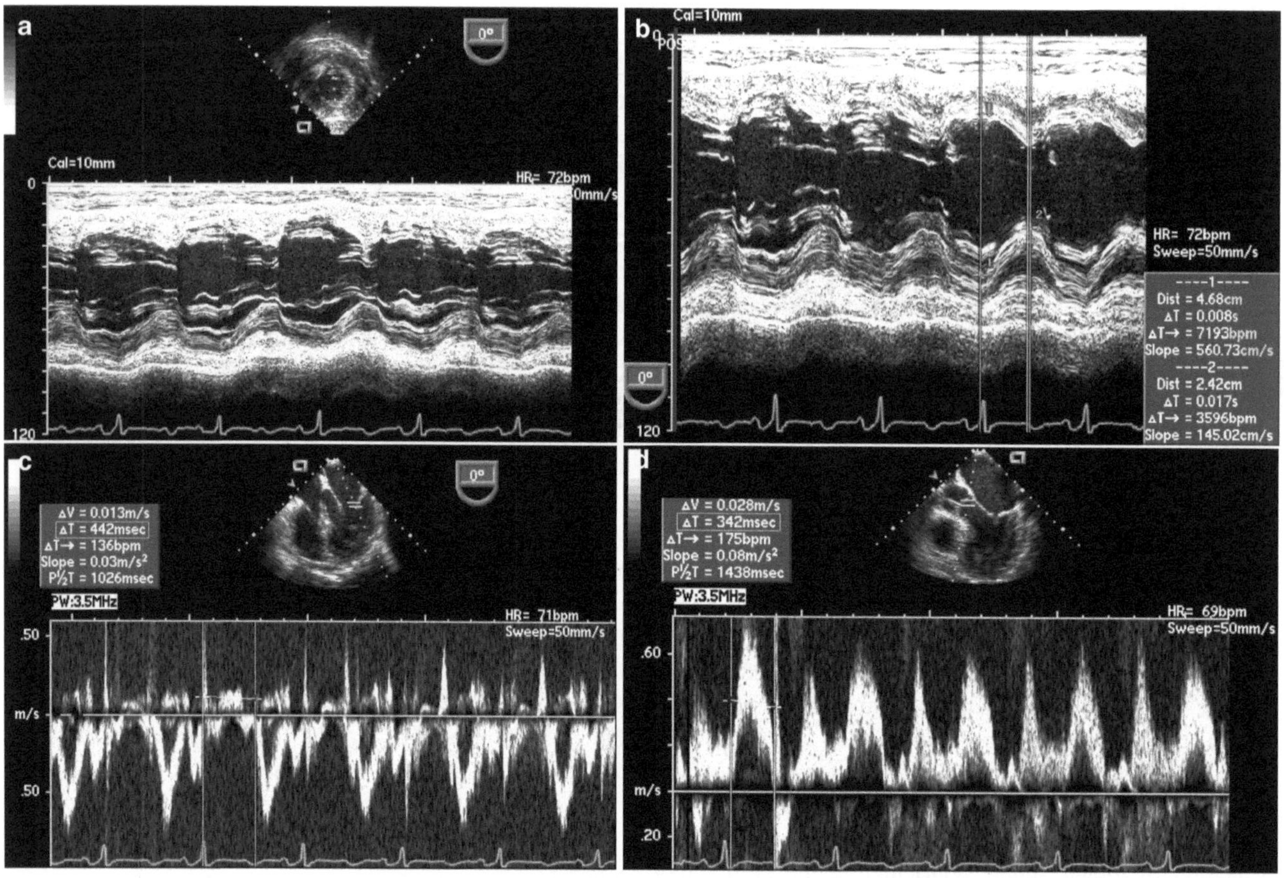

Fig. 5.16 (**a, b**) Representative M-mode images obtained during the TEE examination. The LV shortening fraction is = [(LVEDD) − (LVESD)]/(LVEDD) = [(47 mm) − (24 mm)]/(47 mm) = 49 %. (**c, d**) Measurement of the left ventricular myocardial performance index. (**c**) A pulsed wave Doppler signal is placed within the mitral valve inflow to obtain the mitral closure to opening interval (MV C-O, 442 ms). (**d**) A pulsed wave Doppler signal is placed within the left ventricular outflow tract to derive the ejection time (LVET, 342 ms). LV MPI = [(MV C-O) − (LVET)]/LVET = [(442 ms) − (342 ms)]/342 ms = 0.29

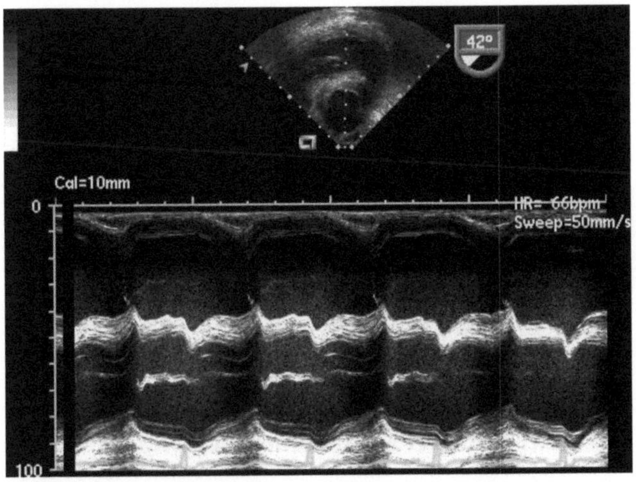

Fig. 5.17 M-mode echocardiogram obtained by transgastric imaging as shown in Video 5.3d. The paradoxical septal wall motion secondary to the right ventricular volume overload limits this method of quantitative assessment of ventricular function in this setting

Case 3

20 year old patient with history of tetralogy of Fallot and long-standing severe pulmonary regurgitation

Preoperative and postoperative TEE images are depicted in Videos 5.3a, 5.3b, 5.3c, 5.3d, and 5.3e. These views represent suitable imaging planes for qualitative interrogation of the ventricular functional abnormalities in this patient. The transgastric mid ventricular short axis view (Video 5.3d) is well suited for M-mode interrogation although, as shown in this case (Fig. 5.17), paradoxical septal motion may limit quantitative determination of LV systolic function.

References

1. Cyran SE, Kimball TR, Meyer RA, et al. Efficacy of intraoperative transesophageal echocardiography in children with congenital heart disease. Am J Cardiol. 1989;63:594–8.
2. Ritter SB. Transesophageal echocardiography in children: new peephole to the heart [comment]. J Am Coll Cardiol. 1990;16:447–50.
3. Stumper OF, Elzenga NJ, Hess J, Sutherland GR. Transesophageal echocardiography in children with congenital heart disease: an initial experience. J Am Coll Cardiol. 1990;16:433–41.
4. Ungerleider RM, Greeley WJ, Sheikh KH, et al. Routine use of intraoperative epicardial echocardiography and Doppler color flow imaging to guide and evaluate repair of congenital heart lesions. A prospective study. J Thorac Cardiovasc Surg. 1990; 100:297–309.
5. Fyfe DA, Kline CH, Sade RM, Greene CA, Gillette PC. The utility of transesophageal echocardiography during and after Fontan operations in small children. Am Heart J. 1991;122:1403–15.
6. Stevenson JG, Sorensen GK, Gartman DM, Hall DG, Rittenhouse EA. Transesophageal echocardiography during repair of congenital cardiac defects: identification of residual problems necessitating reoperation. J Am Soc Echocardiogr. 1993;6:356–65.
7. Stevenson JG. Role of intraoperative transesophageal echocardiography during repair of congenital cardiac defects. Acta Paediatr Suppl. 1995;410:23–33.
8. Ninomiya J, Yamauchi H, Hosaka H, et al. Continuous transoesophageal echocardiography monitoring during weaning from cardiopulmonary bypass in children. Cardiovasc Surg. 1997;5: 129–33.
9. Rice MJ, McDonald RW, Li X, Shen I, Ungerleider RM, Sahn DJ. New technology and methodologies for intraoperative, perioperative, and intraprocedural monitoring of surgical and catheter interventions for congenital heart disease. Echocardiography. 2002;19:725–34.
10. Stumper O, Witsenburg M, Sutherland GR, Cromme-Dijkhuis A, Godman MJ, Hess J. Transesophageal echocardiographic monitoring of interventional cardiac catheterization in children. J Am Coll Cardiol. 1991;18:1506–14.
11. Ludomirsky A. The use of echocardiography in pediatric interventional cardiac catheterization procedures. J Interv Cardiol. 1995;8:569–78.
12. Tumbarello R, Sanna A, Cardu G, Bande A, Napoleone A, Bini RM. Usefulness of transesophageal echocardiography in the pediatric catheterization laboratory. Am J Cardiol. 1993;71:1321–5.
13. Rigby ML. Transoesophageal echocardiography during interventional cardiac catheterisation in congenital heart disease. Heart. 2001;86 Suppl 2:II23–9.
14. Simon P, Mohl W. Intraoperative echocardiographic assessment of global and regional myocardial function. Echocardiography. 1990; 7:333–41.
15. Skiles JA, Griffin BP. Transesophageal echocardiographic (TEE) evaluation of ventricular function. Cardiol Clin. 2000;18:681–97, vii.
16. Schiller NB, Shah PM, Crawford M, et al. Recommendations for quantitation of the left ventricle by two-dimensional echocardiography. American Society of Echocardiography Committee on Standards, Subcommittee on Quantitation of Two-Dimensional Echocardiograms. J Am Soc Echocardiogr. 1989;2:358–67.
17. Abel MD, Nishimura RA, Callahan MJ, Rehder K, Ilstrup DM, Tajik AJ. Evaluation of intraoperative transesophageal two-dimensional echocardiography. Anesthesiology. 1987;66:64–8.
18. Nishimura RA, Abel MD, Housmans PR, Warnes CA, Tajik AJ. Mitral flow velocity curves as a function of different loading conditions: evaluation by intraoperative transesophageal Doppler echocardiography. J Am Soc Echocardiogr. 1989;2:79–87.
19. Kuecherer HF, Muhiudeen IA, Kusumoto FM, et al. Estimation of mean left atrial pressure from transesophageal pulsed Doppler echocardiography of pulmonary venous flow. Circulation. 1990;82: 1127–39.
20. Kuecherer HF, Kusumoto F, Muhiudeen IA, Cahalan MK, Schiller NB. Pulmonary venous flow patterns by transesophageal pulsed Doppler echocardiography: relation to parameters of left ventricular systolic and diastolic function. Am Heart J. 1991;122: 1683–93.
21. Muhiudeen IA, Kuecherer HF, Lee E, Cahalan MK, Schiller NB. Intraoperative estimation of cardiac output by transesophageal pulsed Doppler echocardiography. Anesthesiology. 1991;74:9–14.
22. Savino JS, Troianos CA, Aukburg S, Weiss R, Reichek N. Measurement of pulmonary blood flow with transesophageal two-dimensional and Doppler echocardiography. Anesthesiology. 1991;75:445–51.
23. Gorcsan 3rd J, Diana P, Ball BA, Hattler BG. Intraoperative determination of cardiac output by transesophageal continuous wave Doppler. Am Heart J. 1992;123:171–6.

24. Smith MD, MacPhail B, Harrison MR, Lenhoff SJ, DeMaria AN. Value and limitations of transesophageal echocardiography in determination of left ventricular volumes and ejection fraction. J Am Coll Cardiol. 1992;19:1213–22.
25. Stoddard MF, Dillon S, Peters G, Kupersmith J. Left ventricular ejection fraction is increased during transesophageal echocardiography in patients with impaired ventricular function. Am Heart J. 1992;123:1005–10.
26. Doerr HK, Quinones MA, Zoghbi WA. Accurate determination of left ventricular ejection fraction by transesophageal echocardiography with a nonvolumetric method. J Am Soc Echocardiogr. 1993;6:476–81.
27. Kuecherer HF, Foster E. Hemodynamics by transesophageal echocardiography. Cardiol Clin. 1993;11:475–87.
28. Rafferty T, Durkin M, Harris S, et al. Transesophageal two-dimensional echocardiographic analysis of right ventricular systolic performance indices during coronary artery bypass grafting. J Cardiothorac Vasc Anesth. 1993;7:160–6.
29. Sutton DC, Cahalan MK. Intraoperative assessment of left ventricular function with transesophageal echocardiography. Cardiol Clin. 1993;11:389–98.
30. Darmon PL, Hillel Z, Mogtader A, Mindich B, Thys D. Cardiac output by transesophageal echocardiography using continuous-wave Doppler across the aortic valve. Anesthesiology. 1994;80:796–805, discussion 25A.
31. Pu M, Griffin BP, Vandervoort PM, Leung DY, Cosgrove 3rd DM, Thomas JD. Intraoperative validation of mitral inflow determination by transesophageal echocardiography: comparison of single-plane, biplane and thermodilution techniques. J Am Coll Cardiol. 1995;26:1047–53.
32. Hozumi T, Yoshikawa J, Yoshida K, Akasaka T, Takagi T, Yamamuro A. Three-dimensional echocardiographic measurement of left ventricular volumes and ejection fraction using a multiplane transesophageal probe in patients. Am J Cardiol. 1996;78: 1077–80.
33. Troianos CA, Porembka DT. Assessment of left ventricular function and hemodynamics with transesophageal echocardiography. Crit Care Clin. 1996;12:253–72.
34. Kuhl HP, Franke A, Frielingsdorf J, et al. Determination of left ventricular mass and circumferential wall thickness by three-dimensional reconstruction: in vitro validation of a new method that uses a multiplane transesophageal transducer. J Am Soc Echocardiogr. 1997;10:107–19.
35. Kuhl HP, Franke A, Janssens U, et al. Three-dimensional echocardiographic determination of left ventricular volumes and function by multiplane transesophageal transducer: dynamic in vitro validation and in vivo comparison with angiography and thermodilution. J Am Soc Echocardiogr. 1998;11:1113–24.
36. Ochiai Y, Morita S, Tanoue Y, Kawachi Y, Tominaga R, Yasui H. Use of transesophageal echocardiography for postoperative evaluation of right ventricular function. Ann Thorac Surg. 1999;67:146–52, discussion 153.
37. Poelaert J, Schmidt C, Van Aken H, Hinder F, Mollhoff T, Loick HM. A comparison of transoesophageal echocardiographic Doppler across the aortic valve and the thermodilution technique for estimating cardiac output. Anaesthesia. 1999;54:128–36.
38. Kubota H, Furuse A, Kotsuka Y, et al. Cardiac function evaluated by transesophageal echocardiography during cardiopulmonary bypass. Jpn J Thorac Cardiovasc Surg. 2000;48:261–6.
39. Schiller NB. Hemodynamics derived from transesophageal echocardiography (TEE). Cardiol Clin. 2000;18:699–709.
40. Simmons LA, Weidemann F, Sutherland GR, et al. Doppler tissue velocity, strain, and strain rate imaging with transesophageal echocardiography in the operating room: a feasibility study. J Am Soc Echocardiogr. 2002;15:768–76.
41. Swaminathan M, Phillips-Bute BG, Mathew JP. An assessment of two different methods of left ventricular ejection time measurement by transesophageal echocardiography. Anesth Analg. 2003;97:642–7.
42. Poelaert JI, Schupfer G. Hemodynamic monitoring utilizing transesophageal echocardiography: the relationships among pressure, flow, and function. Chest. 2005;127:379–90.
43. Chen C, Rodriguez L, Guerrero JL, et al. Noninvasive estimation of the instantaneous first derivative of left ventricular pressure using continuous-wave Doppler echocardiography. Circulation. 1991;83:2101–10.
44. Greim CA, Roewer N, Laux G, Schulte am Esch J. On-line estimation of left ventricular stroke volume using transoesophageal echocardiography and acoustic quantification. Br J Anaesth. 1996;77:365–9.
45. Rhodes J, Marx GR, Tardif JC, et al. Evaluation of ventricular dP/dt before and after open heart surgery using transesophageal echocardiography. Echocardiography. 1997;14:15–22.
46. Declerck C, Hillel Z, Shih H, Kuroda M, Connery CP, Thys DM. A comparison of left ventricular performance indices measured by transesophageal echocardiography with automated border detection. Anesthesiology. 1998;89:341–9.
47. Kotoh K, Watanabe G, Ueyama K, et al. On-line assessment of regional ventricular wall motion by transesophageal echocardiography with color kinesis during minimally invasive coronary artery bypass grafting. J Thorac Cardiovasc Surg. 1999;117:912–7.
48. Vermes E, Houel R, Simon M, Le Besnerais P, Loisance D. Doppler tissue imaging to predict myocardial recovery during mechanical circulatory support. Ann Thorac Surg. 2000;70: 2149–51.
49. Skarvan K, Filipovic M, Wang J, Brett W, Seeberger M. Use of myocardial tissue Doppler imaging for intraoperative monitoring of left ventricular function. Br J Anaesth. 2003;91:473–80.
50. Skulstad H, Andersen K, Edvardsen T, et al. Detection of ischemia and new insight into left ventricular physiology by strain Doppler and tissue velocity imaging: assessment during coronary bypass operation of the beating heart. J Am Soc Echocardiogr. 2004;17: 1225–33.
51. David JS, Tousignant CP, Bowry R. Tricuspid annular velocity in patients undergoing cardiac operation using transesophageal echocardiography. J Am Soc Echocardiogr. 2006;19:329–34.
52. Borow KM, Neumann A, Marcus RH, Sareli P, Lang RM. Effects of simultaneous alterations in preload and afterload on measurements of left ventricular contractility in patients with dilated cardiomyopathy: comparisons of ejection phase, isovolumetric and end-systolic force-velocity indexes. J Am Coll Cardiol. 1992;20: 787–95.
53. Kimball TR, Daniels SR, Loggie JM, Khoury P, Meyer RA. Relation of left ventricular mass, preload, afterload and contractility in pediatric patients with essential hypertension. J Am Coll Cardiol. 1993;21:997–1001.
54. Rowland DG, Gutgesell HP. Noninvasive assessment of myocardial contractility, preload, and afterload in healthy newborn infants. Am J Cardiol. 1995;75:818–21.
55. Kjaergaard J, Snyder EM, Hassager C, Oh JK, Johnson BD. Impact of preload and afterload on global and regional right ventricular function and pressure: a quantitative echocardiography study. J Am Soc Echocardiogr. 2006;19:515–21.
56. Ozdemir K, Balci S, Duzenli MA, et al. Effect of preload and heart rate on the Doppler and tissue Doppler-derived myocardial performance index. Clin Cardiol. 2007;30:342–8.
57. Bailey JM, Shanewise JS, Kikura M, Sharma S. A comparison of transesophageal and transthoracic echocardiographic assessment of left ventricular function in pediatric patients with congenital heart disease. J Cardiothorac Vasc Anesth. 1995;9:665–9.
58. Silverman NH, Ports TA, Snider AR, Schiller NB, Carlsson E, Heilbron DC. Determination of left ventricular volume in children: echocardiographic and angiographic comparisons. Circulation. 1980;62:548–57.

59. Quinones MA, Waggoner AD, Reduto LA, et al. A new, simplified and accurate method for determining ejection fraction with two-dimensional echocardiography. Circulation. 1981;64:744–53.
60. Mercier JC, DiSessa TG, Jarmakani JM, et al. Two-dimensional echocardiographic assessment of left ventricular volumes and ejection fraction in children. Circulation. 1982;65:962–9.
61. Harrison MR, Clifton GD, Berk MR, DeMaria AN. Effect of blood pressure and afterload on Doppler echocardiographic measurements of left ventricular systolic function in normal subjects. Am J Cardiol. 1989;64:905–8.
62. Bashein G, Sheehan FH, Nessly ML, Detmer PR, Martin RW. Three-dimensional transesophageal echocardiography for depiction of regional left-ventricular performance: initial results and future directions. Int J Card Imaging. 1993;9:121–31.
63. Hozumi T, Yoshikawa J. Three-dimensional echocardiography using a multiplane transesophageal probe: the clinical applications. Echocardiography. 2000;17:757–64.
64. Mizelle KM, Rice MJ, Sahn DJ. Clinical use of real-time three-dimensional echocardiography in pediatric cardiology. Echocardiography. 2000;17:787–90.
65. Keller AM. Positional localization: three-dimensional transthoracic echocardiographic techniques for the measurement of cardiac mass, volume, and function. Echocardiography. 2000;17:745–8.
66. Azran MS, Kwong R, Chen FY, Shernan SK. A potential use for intraoperative three-dimensional transesophageal echocardiography in predicting left ventricular chamber dimensions and ejection fraction after aneurysm resection. Anesth Analg. 2010;111:1362–5.
67. Perez JE, Waggoner AD, Barzilai B, Melton HEJ, Miller JG, Sobel BE. On-line assessment of ventricular function by automatic boundary detection and ultrasonic backscatter imaging. J Am Coll Cardiol. 1992;19:313–20.
68. Gorcsan 3rd J, Romand JA, Mandarino WA, Deneault LG, Pinsky MR. Assessment of left ventricular performance by on-line pressure-area relations using echocardiographic automated border detection. J Am Coll Cardiol. 1994;23:242–52.
69. Gorcsan 3rd J, Denault A, Mandarino WA, Pinsky MR. Left ventricular pressure-volume relations with transesophageal echocardiographic automated border detection: comparison with conductance-catheter technique. Am Heart J. 1996;131:544–52.
70. Liu N, Darmon PL, Saada M, et al. Comparison between radionuclide ejection fraction and fractional area changes derived from transesophageal echocardiography using automated border detection. Anesthesiology. 1996;85:468–74.
71. Chandra S, Bahl VK, Reddy SC, Bhargava B, Malhotra A, Wasir HS. Comparison of echocardiographic acoustic quantification system and radionuclide ventriculography for estimating left ventricular ejection fraction: validation in patients without regional wall motion abnormalities. Am Heart J. 1997;133:359–63.
72. Denault AY, Gorcsan 3rd J, Mandarino WA, Kancel MJ, Pinsky MR. Left ventricular performance assessed by echocardiographic automated border detection and arterial pressure. Am J Physiol. 1997;272:H138–47.
73. Schmidlin D, Aschkenasy S, Vogt PR, Schmidli J, Jenni R, Schmid ER. Left ventricular pressure-area relations as assessed by transoesophageal echocardiographic automated border detection: comparison with conductance catheter technique in cardiac surgical patients. Br J Anaesth. 2000;85:379–88.
74. Tynan M, Reid DS, Hunter S, et al. Ejection phase indices of left ventricular performance in infants, children, and adults. Br Heart J. 1975;37:196–202.
75. Igarashi H, Shiraishi H, Endoh H, Yanagisawa M. Left ventricular contractile state in preterm infants: relation between wall stress and velocity of circumferential fiber shortening. Am Heart J. 1994;127:1336–40.
76. Fisher EA, DuBrow IW, Hastreiter AR. Comparison of ejection phase indices of left ventricular performance in infants and children. Circulation. 1975;52:916–25.
77. Gutgesell HP, Paquet M, Duff DF, McNamara DG. Evaluation of left ventricular size and function by echocardiography. Results in normal children. Circulation. 1977;56:457–62.
78. Henry WL, Ware J, Gardin JM, Hepner SI, McKay J, Weiner M. Echocardiographic measurements in normal subjects. Growth-related changes that occur between infancy and early adulthood. Circulation. 1978;57:278–85.
79. Ruschhaupt DG, Sodt PC, Hutcheon NA, Arcilla RA. Estimation of circumferential fiber shortening velocity by echocardiography. J Am Coll Cardiol. 1983;2:77–84.
80. Greim CA, Roewer N, Schulte am Esch J. Assessment of changes in left ventricular wall stress from the end-systolic pressure-area product. Br J Anaesth. 1995;75:583–7.
81. Colan SD, Borow KM, Neumann A. Left ventricular end-systolic wall stress-velocity of fiber shortening relation: a load-independent index of myocardial contractility. J Am Coll Cardiol. 1984;4:715–24.
82. Royse CF, Connelly KA, MacLaren G, Royse AG. Evaluation of echocardiography indices of systolic function: a comparative study using pressure-volume loops in patients undergoing coronary artery bypass surgery. Anaesthesia. 2007;62:109–16.
83. Tei C. New non-invasive index for combined systolic and diastolic ventricular function. J Cardiol. 1995;26:135–6.
84. Tei C, Ling LH, Hodge DO, et al. New index of combined systolic and diastolic myocardial performance: a simple and reproducible measure of cardiac function—a study in normals and dilated cardiomyopathy. J Cardiol. 1995;26:357–66.
85. Tei C, Dujardin KS, Hodge DO, Kyle RA, Tajik AJ, Seward JB. Doppler index combining systolic and diastolic myocardial performance: clinical value in cardiac amyloidosis. J Am Coll Cardiol. 1996;28:658–64.
86. Tei C, Nishimura RA, Seward JB, Tajik AJ. Noninvasive Doppler-derived myocardial performance index: correlation with simultaneous measurements of cardiac catheterization measurements. J Am Soc Echocardiogr. 1997;10:169–78.
87. Broberg CS, Pantely GA, Barber BJ, et al. Validation of the myocardial performance index by echocardiography in mice: a noninvasive measure of left ventricular function. J Am Soc Echocardiogr. 2003;16:814–23.
88. Eidem BW, Tei C, O'Leary PW, Cetta F, Seward JB. Nongeometric quantitative assessment of right and left ventricular function: myocardial performance index in normal children and patients with Ebstein anomaly. J Am Soc Echocardiogr. 1998;11:849–56.
89. Tei C, Dujardin KS, Hodge DO, et al. Doppler echocardiographic index for assessment of global right ventricular function. J Am Soc Echocardiogr. 1996;9:838–47.
90. Dujardin KS, Tei C, Yeo TC, Hodge DO, Rossi A, Seward JB. Prognostic value of a Doppler index combining systolic and diastolic performance in idiopathic-dilated cardiomyopathy. Am J Cardiol. 1998;82:1071–6.
91. Yeo TC, Dujardin KS, Tei C, Mahoney DW, McGoon MD, Seward JB. Value of a Doppler-derived index combining systolic and diastolic time intervals in predicting outcome in primary pulmonary hypertension. Am J Cardiol. 1998;81:1157–61.
92. Eidem BW, O'Leary PW, Tei C, Seward JB. Usefulness of the myocardial performance index for assessing right ventricular function in congenital heart disease. Am J Cardiol. 2000;86:654–8.
93. Williams RV, Ritter S, Tani LY, Pagoto LT, Minich LL. Quantitative assessment of ventricular function in children with single ventricles using the Doppler myocardial performance index. Am J Cardiol. 2000;86:1106–10.
94. Yasuoka K, Harada K, Toyono M, Tamura M, Yamamoto F. Tei index determined by tissue Doppler imaging in patients with pulmonary regurgitation after repair of tetralogy of Fallot. Pediatr Cardiol. 2004;25:131–6.
95. Shanewise JS, Cheung AT, Aronson S, et al. ASE/SCA guidelines for performing a comprehensive intraoperative multiplane

transesophageal echocardiography examination: recommendations of the American Society of Echocardiography Council for Intraoperative Echocardiography and the Society of Cardiovascular Anesthesiologists Task Force for Certification in Perioperative Transesophageal Echocardiography. J Am Soc Echocardiogr. 1999;12:884–900.

96. Cerqueira MD, Weissman NJ, Dilsizian V, et al. Standardized myocardial segmentation and nomenclature for tomographic imaging of the heart: a statement for healthcare professionals from the Cardiac Imaging Committee of the Council on Clinical Cardiology of the American Heart Association. Circulation. 2002;105:539–42.
97. Lang RM, Bierig M, Devereux RB, et al. Recommendations for chamber quantification: a report from the American Society of Echocardiography's Guidelines and Standards Committee and the Chamber Quantification Writing Group, developed in conjunction with the European Association of Echocardiography, a branch of the European Society of Cardiology. J Am Soc Echocardiogr. 2005;18:1440–63.
98. Rouine-Rapp K, Rouillard KP, Miller-Hance W, et al. Segmental wall-motion abnormalities after an arterial switch operation indicate ischemia. Anesth Analg. 2006;103:1139–46.
99. Eidem BW, McMahon CJ, Cohen RR, et al. Impact of cardiac growth on Doppler tissue imaging velocities: a study in healthy children. J Am Soc Echocardiogr. 2004;17:212–21.
100. McMahon CJ, Nagueh SF, Pignatelli RH, et al. Characterization of left ventricular diastolic function by tissue Doppler imaging and clinical status in children with hypertrophic cardiomyopathy. Circulation. 2004;109:1756–62.
101. Nagueh SF, Middleton KJ, Kopelen HA, Zoghbi WA, Quinones MA. Doppler tissue imaging: a noninvasive technique for evaluation of left ventricular relaxation and estimation of filling pressures. J Am Coll Cardiol. 1997;30:1527–33.
102. Nagueh SF, Mikati I, Kopelen HA, Middleton KJ, Quinones MA, Zoghbi WA. Doppler estimation of left ventricular filling pressure in sinus tachycardia. A new application of tissue Doppler imaging. Circulation. 1998;98:1644–50.
103. Sasaki N, Garcia M, Lytrivi I, et al. Utility of Doppler tissue imaging-derived indices in identifying subclinical systolic ventricular dysfunction in children with restrictive cardiomyopathy. Pediatr Cardiol. 2011;32:646–51.
104. Goldberg DJ, Quartermain MD, Glatz AC, et al. Doppler tissue imaging in children following cardiac transplantation: a comparison to catheter derived hemodynamics. Pediatr Transplant. 2011;15:488–94.
105. Derumeaux G, Ovize M, Loufoua J, Pontier G, Andre-Fouet X, Cribier A. Assessment of nonuniformity of transmural myocardial velocities by color-coded tissue Doppler imaging: characterization of normal, ischemic, and stunned myocardium. Circulation. 2000;101:1390–5.
106. Weidemann F, Eyskens B, Jamal F, et al. Quantification of regional left and right ventricular radial and longitudinal function in healthy children using ultrasound-based strain rate and strain imaging. J Am Soc Echocardiogr. 2002;15:20–8.
107. Weidemann F, Eyskens B, Mertens L, et al. Quantification of regional right and left ventricular function by ultrasonic strain rate and strain indexes after surgical repair of tetralogy of Fallot. Am J Cardiol. 2002;90:133–8.
108. Harada K, Toyono M, Yamamoto F. Assessment of right ventricular function during exercise with quantitative Doppler tissue imaging in children late after repair of tetralogy of Fallot. J Am Soc Echocardiogr. 2004;17:863–9.
109. Toyono M, Harada K, Tamura M, Yamamoto F, Takada G. Myocardial acceleration during isovolumic contraction as a new index of right ventricular contractile function and its relation to pulmonary regurgitation in patients after repair of tetralogy of Fallot. J Am Soc Echocardiogr. 2004;17:332–7.
110. Eyskens B, Ganame J, Taylor AM, et al. Reduced right ventricular deformation in children with severe pulmonary regurgitation after tetralogy of Fallot correction is associated with reduced exercise capacity. Circulation. 2005;112:17.
111. Friedberg MK, Mertens L. Tissue velocities, strain, and strain rate for echocardiographic assessment of ventricular function in congenital heart disease. Eur J Echocardiogr. 2009;10:585–93.
112. Nagueh SF, Appleton CP, Gillebert TC, et al. Recommendations for the evaluation of left ventricular diastolic function by echocardiography. J Am Soc Echocardiogr. 2009;22:107–33.
113. O'Leary PW, Durongpisitkul K, Cordes TM, et al. Diastolic ventricular function in children: a Doppler echocardiographic study establishing normal values and predictors of increased ventricular end-diastolic pressure. Mayo Clin Proc. 1998;73:616–28.
114. Olivier M, O'leary PW, Pankratz VS, et al. Serial Doppler assessment of diastolic function before and after the Fontan operation. J Am Soc Echocardiogr. 2003;16:1136–43.
115. Appleton CP, Hatle LK, Popp RL. Relation of transmitral flow velocity patterns to left ventricular diastolic function: new insights from a combined hemodynamic and Doppler echocardiographic study. J Am Coll Cardiol. 1988;12:426–40.
116. Nishimura RA, Abel MD, Hatle LK, Tajik AJ. Assessment of diastolic function of the heart: background and current applications of Doppler echocardiography. Part II. Clinical studies. Mayo Clin Proc. 1989;64:181–204.
117. Bessen M, Gardin JM. Evaluation of left ventricular diastolic function. Cardiol Clin. 1990;8:315–32.
118. Myreng Y, Smiseth OA. Assessment of left ventricular relaxation by Doppler echocardiography. Comparison of isovolumic relaxation time and transmitral flow velocities with time constant of isovolumic relaxation. Circulation. 1990;81:260–6.
119. Klein AL, Tajik AJ. Doppler assessment of pulmonary venous flow in healthy subjects and in patients with heart disease. J Am Soc Echocardiogr. 1991;4:379–92.
120. Appleton CP, Galloway JM, Gonzalez MS, Gaballa M, Basnight MA. Estimation of left ventricular filling pressures using two-dimensional and Doppler echocardiography in adult patients with cardiac disease. Additional value of analyzing left atrial size, left atrial ejection fraction and the difference in duration of pulmonary venous and mitral flow velocity at atrial contraction. J Am Coll Cardiol. 1993;22:1972–82.
121. Cohen GI, Pietrolungo JF, Thomas JD, Klein AL. A practical guide to assessment of ventricular diastolic function using Doppler echocardiography. J Am Coll Cardiol. 1996;27:1753–60.
122. Hoit BD, Shao Y, Gabel M, Walsh RA. Influence of loading conditions and contractile state on pulmonary venous flow. Validation of Doppler velocimetry. Circulation. 1992;86:651–9.
123. Sohn DW, Chai IH, Lee DJ, et al. Assessment of mitral annulus velocity by Doppler tissue imaging in the evaluation of left ventricular diastolic function. J Am Coll Cardiol. 1997;30:474–80.
124. Aranda JMJ, Weston MW, Puleo JA, Fontanet HL. Effect of loading conditions on myocardial relaxation velocities determined by Doppler tissue imaging in heart transplant recipients. J Heart Lung Transplant. 1998;17:693–7.
125. Oki T, Fukuda K, Tabata T, et al. Effect of an acute increase in afterload on left ventricular regional wall motion velocity in healthy subjects. J Am Soc Echocardiogr. 1999;12:476–83.
126. Muller S, Bartel T, Koopman J, Pandian NG, Erbel R, Pachinger O. Tissue Doppler analysis is hindered in abnormal wall motion and changes in afterload. Int J Cardiol. 2003;90:81–90.
127. Jacques DC, Pinsky MR, Severyn D, Gorcsan 3rd J. Influence of alterations in loading on mitral annular velocity by tissue Doppler echocardiography and its associated ability to predict filling pressures. Chest. 2004;126:1910–8.
128. Farias CA, Rodriguez L, Garcia MJ, Sun JP, Klein AL, Thomas JD. Assessment of diastolic function by tissue Doppler echocar-

diography: comparison with standard transmitral and pulmonary venous flow. J Am Soc Echocardiogr. 1999;12:609–17.
129. Garcia MJ, Thomas JD. Tissue Doppler to assess diastolic left ventricular function. Echocardiography. 1999;16:501–8.
130. Rivas-Gotz C, Khoury DS, Manolios M, Rao L, Kopelen HA, Nagueh SF. Time interval between onset of mitral inflow and onset of early diastolic velocity by tissue Doppler: a novel index of left ventricular relaxation: experimental studies and clinical application. J Am Coll Cardiol. 2003;42:1463–70.
131. Ruan Q, Rao L, Middleton KJ, Khoury DS, Nagueh SF. Assessment of left ventricular diastolic function by early diastolic mitral annulus peak acceleration rate: experimental studies and clinical application. J Appl Physiol. 2006;100:679–84.
132. Garcia MJ, Rodriguez L, Ares M, Griffin BP, Thomas JD, Klein AL. Differentiation of constrictive pericarditis from restrictive cardiomyopathy: assessment of left ventricular diastolic velocities in longitudinal axis by Doppler tissue imaging. J Am Coll Cardiol. 1996;27:108–14.
133. Oki T, Tabata T, Yamada H, et al. Right and left ventricular wall motion velocities as diagnostic indicators of constrictive pericarditis. Am J Cardiol. 1998;81:465–70.
134. Ha JW, Oh JK, Ommen SR, Ling LH, Tajik AJ. Diagnostic value of mitral annular velocity for constrictive pericarditis in the absence of respiratory variation in mitral inflow velocity. J Am Soc Echocardiogr. 2002;15:1468–71.
135. Ha JW, Ommen SR, Tajik AJ, et al. Differentiation of constrictive pericarditis from restrictive cardiomyopathy using mitral annular velocity by tissue Doppler echocardiography. Am J Cardiol. 2004;94:316–9.
136. Rychik J, Tian ZY. Quantitative assessment of myocardial tissue velocities in normal children with Doppler tissue imaging. Am J Cardiol. 1996;77:1254–7.
137. Harada K, Orino T, Yasuoka K, Tamura M, Takada G. Tissue Doppler imaging of left and right ventricles in normal children. Tohoku J Exp Med. 2000;191:21–9.
138. Kapusta L, Thijssen JM, Cuypers MH, Peer PG, Daniels O. Assessment of myocardial velocities in healthy children using tissue Doppler imaging. Ultrasound Med Biol. 2000;26:229–37.
139. Mori K, Hayabuchi Y, Kuroda Y, Nii M, Manabe T. Left ventricular wall motion velocities in healthy children measured by pulsed wave Doppler tissue echocardiography: normal values and relation to age and heart rate. J Am Soc Echocardiogr. 2000;13:1002–11.
140. Frommelt PC, Ballweg JA, Whitstone BN, Frommelt MA. Usefulness of Doppler tissue imaging analysis of tricuspid annular motion for determination of right ventricular function in normal infants and children. Am J Cardiol. 2002;89:610–3.
141. Swaminathan S, Ferrer PL, Wolff GS, Gomez-Marin O, Rusconi PG. Usefulness of tissue Doppler echocardiography for evaluating ventricular function in children without heart disease. Am J Cardiol. 2003;91:570–4.
142. Savage A, Hlavacek A, Ringewald J, Shirali G. Evaluation of the myocardial performance index and tissue Doppler imaging by comparison to near-simultaneous catheter measurements in pediatric cardiac transplant patients. J Heart Lung Transplant. 2010;29:853–8.
143. Nagueh SF, Kopelen HA, Quinones MA. Assessment of left ventricular filling pressures by Doppler in the presence of atrial fibrillation. Circulation. 1996;94:2138–45.
144. Sundereswaran L, Nagueh SF, Vardan S, et al. Estimation of left and right ventricular filling pressures after heart transplantation by tissue Doppler imaging. Am J Cardiol. 1998;82:352–7.
145. Nagueh SF, Lakkis NM, Middleton KJ, Spencer 3rd WH, Zoghbi WA, Quinones MA. Doppler estimation of left ventricular filling pressures in patients with hypertrophic cardiomyopathy. Circulation. 1999;99:254–61.
146. Border WL, Michelfelder EC, Glascock BJ, et al. Color M-mode and Doppler tissue evaluation of diastolic function in children: simultaneous correlation with invasive indices. J Am Soc Echocardiogr. 2003;16:988–94.
147. Yock PG, Popp RL. Noninvasive estimation of right ventricular systolic pressure by Doppler ultrasound in patients with tricuspid regurgitation. Circulation. 1984;70:657–62.
148. Zoghbi WA, Habib GB, Quinones MA. Doppler assessment of right ventricular filling in a normal population. Comparison with left ventricular filling dynamics. Circulation. 1990;82:1316–24.
149. Moller JE, Poulsen SH, Egstrup K. Effect of preload alternations on a new Doppler echocardiographic index of combined systolic and diastolic performance. J Am Soc Echocardiogr. 1999;12:1065–72.
150. Poelaert J, Ruggero A. Myocardial performance index and tissue Doppler systolic wave velocity are preload dependent. Anesthesiology. 2005;103:210; author reply 210; author reply 211.
151. Anconina J, Danchin N, Selton-Suty C, et al. Noninvasive estimation of right ventricular dP/dt in patients with tricuspid valve regurgitation. Am J Cardiol. 1993;71:1495–7.
152. Pai RG, Bansal RC, Shah PM. Determinants of the rate of right ventricular pressure rise by Doppler echocardiography: potential value in the assessment of right ventricular function. J Heart Valve Dis. 1994;3:179–84.
153. Michelfelder EC, Vermilion RP, Ludomirsky A, Beekman RH, Lloyd TR. Comparison of simultaneous Doppler- and catheter-derived right ventricular dP/dt in hypoplastic left heart syndrome. Am J Cardiol. 1996;77:212–4.
154. Kanzaki H, Nakatani S, Kawada T, Yamagishi M, Sunagawa K, Miyatake K. Right ventricular dP/dt/P(max), not dP/dt(max), noninvasively derived from tricuspid regurgitation velocity is a useful index of right ventricular contractility. J Am Soc Echocardiogr. 2002;15:136–42.
155. Noori NM, Mehralizadeh S, Khaje A. Assessment of right ventricular function in children with congenital heart disease. Doppler tissue imaging. Saudi Med J. 2008;29:1168–72.
156. Helbing WA, Bosch HG, Maliepaard C, et al. On-line automated border detection for echocardiographic quantification of right ventricular size and function in children. Pediatr Cardiol. 1997;18:261–9.
157. Geva T, Powell AJ, Crawford EC, Chung T, Colan SD. Evaluation of regional differences in right ventricular systolic function by acoustic quantification echocardiography and cine magnetic resonance imaging. Circulation. 1998;98:339–45.
158. Jiang L, Siu SC, Handschumacher MD, et al. Three-dimensional echocardiography. In vivo validation for right ventricular volume and function. Circulation. 1994;89:2342–50.
159. Fujimoto S, Mizuno R, Nakagawa Y, Dohi K, Nakano H. Estimation of the right ventricular volume and ejection fraction by transthoracic three-dimensional echocardiography. A validation study using magnetic resonance imaging. Int J Card Imaging. 1998;14:385–90.
160. Ota T, Fleishman CE, Strub M, et al. Real-time, three-dimensional echocardiography: feasibility of dynamic right ventricular volume measurement with saline contrast. Am Heart J. 1999;137:958–66.
161. Grison A, Maschietto N, Reffo E, et al. Three-dimensional echocardiographic evaluation of right ventricular volume and function in pediatric patients: validation of the technique. J Am Soc Echocardiogr. 2007;20:921–9.
162. Tamborini G, Brusoni D, Torres Molina JE, et al. Feasibility of a new generation three-dimensional echocardiography for right ventricular volumetric and functional measurements. Am J Cardiol. 2008;102:499–505.
163. Tamborini G, Muratori M, Brusoni D, et al. Is right ventricular systolic function reduced after cardiac surgery? A two- and three-dimensional echocardiographic study. Eur J Echocardiogr. 2009;10:630–4.
164. Vegas A, Meineri M. Core review: three-dimensional transesophageal echocardiography is a major advance for intraoperative

clinical management of patients undergoing cardiac surgery: a core review. Anesth Analg. 2010;110:1548–73.
165. Cheung YF, Penny DJ, Redington AN. Serial assessment of left ventricular diastolic function after Fontan procedure. Heart. 2000;83:420–4.
166. Mahle WT, Coon PD, Wernovsky G, Rychik J. Quantitative echocardiographic assessment of the performance of the functionally single right ventricle after the Fontan operation. Cardiol Young. 2001;11:399–406.
167. Earing MG, Cetta F, Driscoll DJ, et al. Long-term results of the Fontan operation for double-inlet left ventricle. Am J Cardiol. 2005;96:291–8.
168. Frommelt PC, Snider AR, Meliones JN, Vermilion RP. Doppler assessment of pulmonary artery flow patterns and ventricular function after the Fontan operation. Am J Cardiol. 1991;68:1211–5.
169. Penny DJ, Rigby ML, Redington AN. Abnormal patterns of intraventricular flow and diastolic filling after the Fontan operation: evidence for incoordinate ventricular wall motion. Br Heart J. 1991;66:375–8.
170. Bassareo PP, Tumbarello R, Piras A, Mercuro G. Evaluation of regional myocardial function by Doppler tissue imaging in univentricular heart after successful Fontan repair. Echocardiography. 2010;27:702–8.
171. Ikemba CM, Su JT, Stayer SA, et al. Myocardial performance index with sevoflurane-pancuronium versus fentanyl-midazolam-pancuronium in infants with a functional single ventricle. Anesthesiology. 2004;101:1298–305.

Systemic and Pulmonary Venous Anomalies

6

Theresa Ann Tacy

Abstract

Assessment of systemic and pulmonary venous anatomy represents a vital part of the echocardiographic evaluation of any patient with suspected congenital heart disease (CHD). Systemic and pulmonary venous anomalies can occur as known associations with both simple and complex forms of CHD, and their presence (or absence) can have important clinical implications. Moreover, knowledge of systemic and pulmonary venous return is necessary for the accurate classification of some of the more complex forms of CHD, and for understanding the underlying physiology in such patients. Anyone performing echocardiographic evaluation of possible systemic/pulmonary venous anomalies should have a comprehensive understanding of the normal anatomy of both systems, as well as the more common abnormalities involving each system and associated hemodynamic alterations. Transesophageal echocardiography (TEE) is well suited for evaluation of both systemic and pulmonary venous anomalies, due to the proximity of the esophagus and transducer to the sites of venous return and to the atrial chambers. This chapter presents a thorough discussion of congenital systemic and pulmonary venous anomalies and their evaluation by TEE.

Keywords

Transesophageal echocardiography • Pulmonary venous anomalies • Total anomalous pulmonary venous connection • Partial anomalous pulmonary venous connection • Systemic venous anomalies • Intraoperative monitoring

Introduction

There is a wide spectrum of anomalies of either the systemic or pulmonary venous connections, both in their clinical presentation as well as in their morphology [1, 2]. In the general population, the incidence of systemic venous anomalies is only 0.3–0.4 %, yet in the population of patients requiring surgery for congenital heart defects, these anomalies are more prevalent, occurring in 2.8–4.8 % of operative cases [3]. In view of the important implications of these anomalies in the surgical approach, it is important to define them prior to and immediately after surgical intervention. Transesophageal echocardiography (TEE) is well suited for evaluation of both pulmonary and systemic venous structures due to the proximity of the transducer to the sites of venous return and atrial chambers [4]. While diagnostic modalities such as magnetic resonance imaging, contrast enhanced magnetic resonance angiography, and computed axial tomography have advantages over echocardiography when viewing these structures, echocardiography still remains an important tool in the diagnosis and management of these abnormalities due to its relatively low cost, safety, and portability. These alternate imaging modalities will not supplant the role of the TEE

T.A. Tacy, MD
Division of Pediatric Cardiology, Department of Pediatrics, Lucile Packard Children's Hospital, Stanford University School of Medicine, 725 Welch Road, Suite 120, Palo Alto, CA 94304, USA
e-mail: tatacy@stanford.edu

The online version of this chapter (doi:10.1007/978-1-84800-064-3_6) contains supplementary material, which is available to authorized users.

P.C. Wong, W.C. Miller-Hance (eds.), *Transesophageal Echocardiography for Congenital Heart Disease*,
DOI 10.1007/978-1-84800-064-3_6, © Springer-Verlag London 2014

in the operating room in the near future, thus we serve our patients best by maintaining expertise in imaging these structures, especially when intraoperative detection of a residual venous obstruction or related problems will allow immediate revision.

Normally, imaging of the systemic veins with TEE is relatively straightforward. Yet systemic venous anatomy is highly variable, thus abnormalities may be missed if a full evaluation of the systemic veins is not pursued on a routine basis. Identification of an anomalous venous connection also requires a higher index of suspicion of its presence, instilled by either: (1) knowledge of associations between a particular lesion and anomalous pulmonary or systemic venous connections, or (2) associating the patient's clinical scenario with possible anomalous venous connections.

Pulmonary and systemic venous abnormalities present a unique diagnostic challenge to the echocardiographer. When performing a TEE, one is usually looking anteriorly from a posterior window to view cardiac structures. Looking at systemic veins and pulmonary veins requires stepping away from the familiarity of imaging anteriorly. To view the structures draining into the heart, one must image laterally and posteriorly from the esophagus to view the pulmonary veins, superiorly to image the superior vena cava (SVC) and innominate veins, and inferiorly to examine the inferior vena cava (IVC)/hepatic veins (HVs). The loss of cardiac structures within the image can be disorienting. This issue may be ameliorated by the use of "anchors", or easily found normal structures (e.g., the SVC), to understand the anatomic relationship of the structure you desire to interrogate (e.g. the right upper pulmonary vein) to the known structure (rightwards and superior), and maneuver to image the structure of interest (rotate rightward from the SVC in the sagittal plane). Making one's way through the complexities of cardiac anatomy in space requires context. A suggestion is to think of the anatomy in relational terms, and make your way through the body thusly, like you would follow driving directions. Such an approach will likely lead to more exploration of extracardiac anatomy, and ultimately a more comprehensive examination.

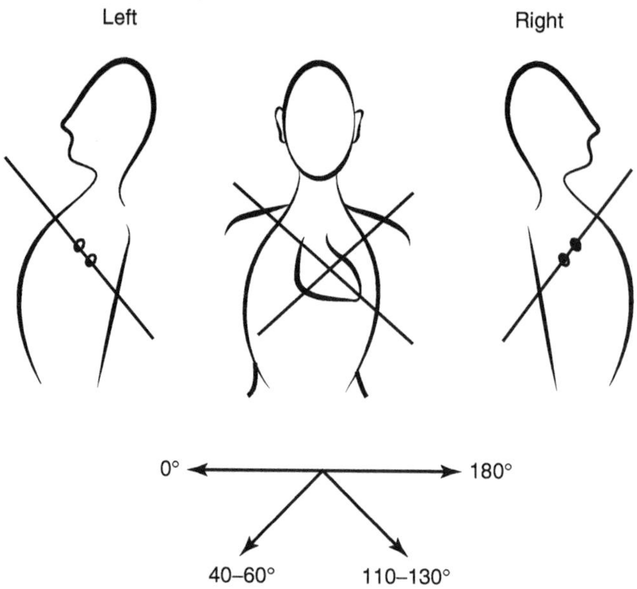

Fig. 6.1 Evaluation of pulmonary venous anatomy by TEE. In the center is a diagram of a person, facing front. The axis of 120° through the long axis of the left ventricle is drawn. When the person is viewed from the left side (*left image*), the anterior position of the left upper vein compared to the left lower vein is observed, as is the alignment of the 120° plane of imaging with both orifices. When the person is viewed from the right side (*right image*), the anterior position of the right upper vein compared to the right lower vein is observed, as is the alignment of the 60° plane of imaging with both orifices

Normal Systemic Venous Anatomy

The left innominate vein (LIV) is located anterior and superior to the ascending aorta, and travels in a horizontal plane. Its position is often helpful in locating the innominate artery, as the vein courses immediately anterior to the origin of the innominate artery from the aorta.

The SVC is a right sided structure (right SVC or RSVC) and courses anterior to the right pulmonary artery (RPA) in a relatively straight, cephalad to caudal fashion. The SVC courses parallel to and rightward of the ascending aorta. The SVC enters the right atrium (RA) adjacent to the interatrial septum. The IVC also courses relatively straight, through the liver, in a caudal to cephalad course. The HVs course into the IVC from an angle, to reflect their role in draining the respective lobes of the hepatic system.

Normal Pulmonary Venous Anatomy

In about 75–80 % of individuals there are four pulmonary veins with separate ostia into the left atrium (LA), however, accessory pulmonary veins can be present [5]. When there are four veins, the left pulmonary veins are located more superiorly than the right pulmonary veins. On each side, the superior veins join the LA in a more anterior position than the lower pulmonary veins (Fig. 6.1). The right middle and upper lobe veins join to form the right upper pulmonary vein (RUPV). The left upper pulmonary vein (LUPV) receives blood draining from the left upper lobe. The right and left lower pulmonary veins receive blood from the right and left lower lobes, respectively. A common vein—which occurs when upper and lower veins join proximal to the LA, resulting in a single orifice to the LA occurs more frequently on the left side [6]. The LUPV connects to the LA just superior to the orifice of the mouth of the left atrial appendage (LAA). The RUPV passes immediately behind the RSVC and inferior to the RPA.

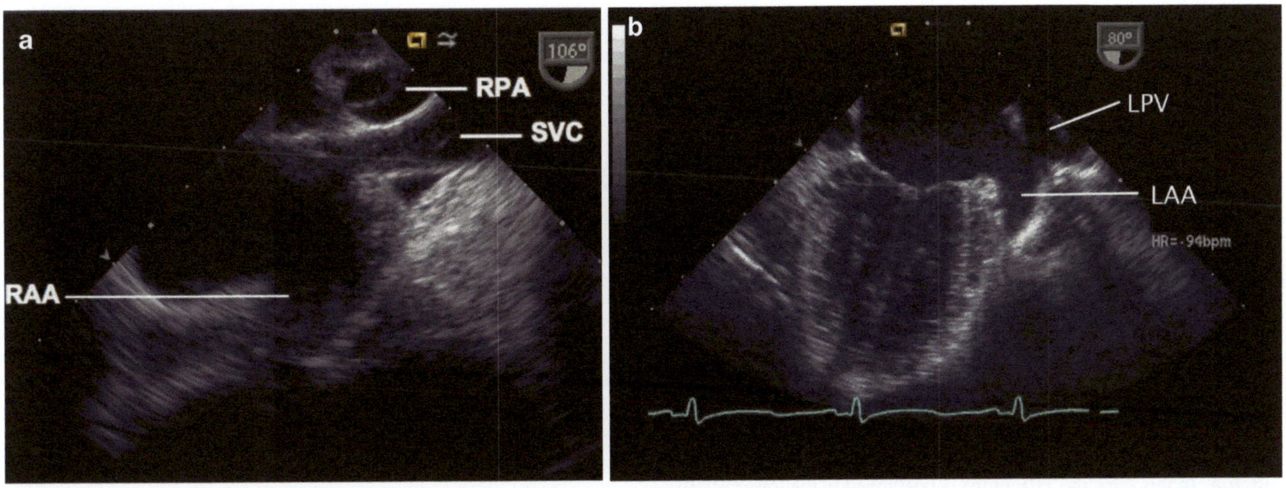

Fig. 6.2 (**a**) Transesophageal echocardiographic image of the right atrium viewed in the sagittal plane (mid esophageal bicaval view). The superior vena cava (*SVC*) is seen superiorly, and the right pulmonary artery (*RPA*) is seen in cross section as it courses behind the SVC. The broad-based right atrial appendage (*RAA*) is seen anteriorly. (**b**) Image of the left atrium in the mid esophageal two chamber view. The left upper pulmonary vein (*LPV*) is seen and directly anterior to this is the entrance of the narrow-based left atrial appendage (*LAA*) into the left atrial cavity

Transesophageal Imaging

Imaging of Normal Systemic Veins

Identification of the atrial appendages can assist in differentiating the atria. The broad-based, blunt appearance of the right atrial appendage (RAA) is best appreciated in the sagittal plane (90°) in the mid esophageal bicaval (ME Bicaval) view, where the base of the RAA is seen anterior to the entrance of the SVC (Fig. 6.2a, Video 6.1). The narrow finger-like LAA can be seen at 0° with flexion or withdrawal of the probe from the mid esophageal four chamber view (ME 4 Ch), or alternatively it can be displayed by rotating the plane to 90° to obtain the mid esophageal two chamber view (ME 2 Ch) (Fig. 6.2b, Video 6.2) [7]. Within the RA, the crista terminalis may be seen as a linear structure extending from the RA wall close to the IVC to the septum adjacent to the SVC. This may be mistaken for the atrial septum. However, if this were the case, then the IVC would drain into the LA. This potential error is easily avoided simply by recalling that the IVC normally drains to the RA.

A normal RSVC can be imaged by starting in a horizontal plane (0°) at the ME 4 Ch view, then withdrawing the probe to the SVC-RA junction. The SVC will be bisected by the imaging plane. Once seen at 0°, if the multiplane angle is then rotated to 90° and the probe withdrawn, the SVC may be imaged in its long axis in the ME Bicaval view. The SVC course anterior to the RPA will be obvious in this plane. If the ascending aorta is seen, then clockwise rotation will result in imaging of the SVC in the normal heart.

The course of the IVC and HVs can be imaged using the ME Bicaval view with probe advancement past the level of the diaphragm or a lower esophageal situs short axis (LE Situs SAX) or deep transgastric approach at 0°. The course of these structures can be visualized by manipulating the probe and advancing and withdrawing the transducer within the esophagus to visualize which atrium the IVC is entering, as well as to identify the HVs draining into the IVC (Fig. 6.3, Video 6.3). One must remember to observe all the poles of the HVs, as a separate entrance from a posterior lobe can be easily missed. Normally the IVC enters the RA very midline, just adjacent to the atrial septum. The long axis of the IVC, and its entrance to the atrium, can be seen using the lower esophageal IVC long axis (LE IVC LAX) view, with the imaging plane at 90°, however the left-right orientation of the image is lost in this view (Fig. 6.4, Video 6.4). Keeping the same image position while adjusting the multiplane angle to 0°, while imaging the IVC, produces the LE Situs SAX view below the level of the heart. The TEE probe can be rotated in a clockwise-counterclockwise direction to determine the relation of the infradiaphragmatic vessels to one another and to the spine.

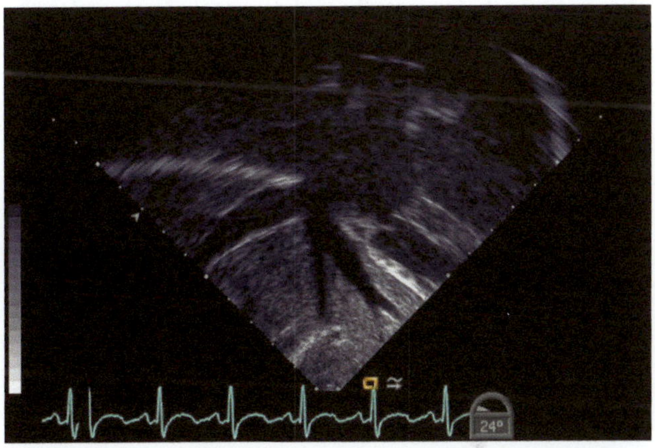

Fig. 6.3 The hepatic veins can be seen entering the right atrium in a nearly coronal plane from a deep transgastric window

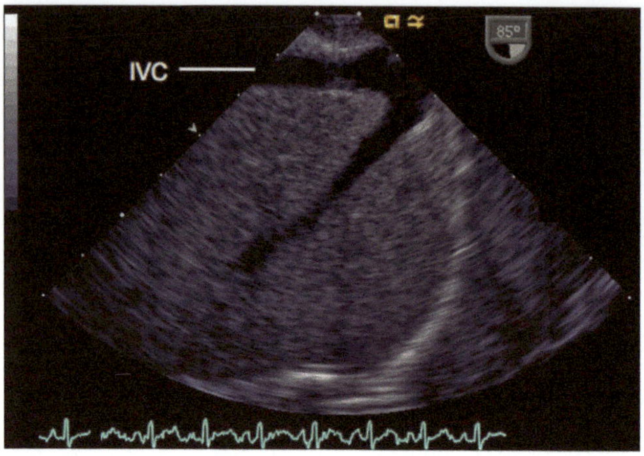

Fig. 6.4 In this view the TEE probe is positioned in the lower esophageal inferior vena cava long axis window (probe angle adjusted to a 90° plane) to demonstrate the inferior vena cava (*IVC*). This view can be obtained by advancing the imaging probe from the mid esophageal bicaval view further into the esophagus. A hepatic vein is joining the IVC anteriorly and superiorly

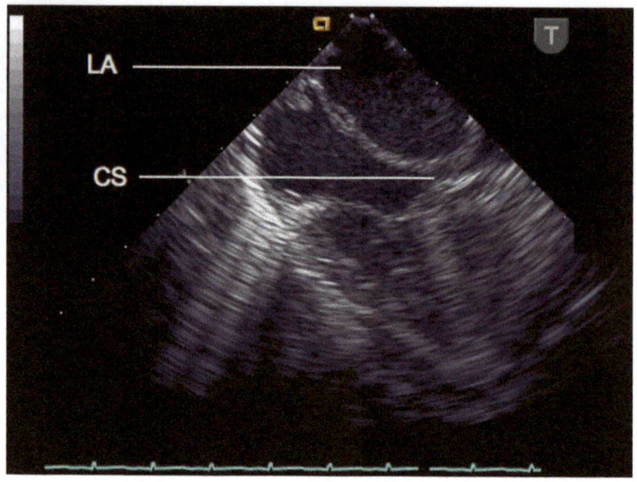

Fig. 6.5 In this mid esophageal four chamber view the probe has been retroflexed within the esophagus to demonstrate the coronary sinus (*CS*) and its relation to the left atrium (*LA*)

The probe is then gradually withdrawn to demonstrate the presence of a venous (Eustachian) valve within the RA, the roof of the RA, and the connection of the RA to the SVC.

The LIV can be imaged by starting from a ME 4 Ch view, rotating the transducer leftwards beyond the cardiac mass, towards the patient's spine, until the descending aorta is seen in its short axis (Desc Ao SAX view). Keeping this in the center of the image sector, the transducer orientation is changed to about 90°–120° (descending aorta long axis or Desc Ao LAX view), and the probe withdrawn to image the proximal descending aorta. With further withdrawal and slight rightward probe shaft rotation, the transverse arch can be more proximally imaged in the upper esophageal aortic arch short axis (UE Ao Arch SAX) view. In this view the innominate vein is seen in cross section (short axis), anterior and superior to the aortic arch. Multiplane angle rotation to about 90 ° displays the upper esophageal aortic arch long axis (UE Ao Arch LAX) view where the innominate vein may also be seen crossing anterior to the aortic arch [8]. Although these views are possible, the tracheal air column may preclude a complete examination of the vascular structures at this level.

The coronary sinus (CS) is seen in the ME 4 Ch view by retroflexing the probe, where it traverses the atrioventricular groove behind the LA before entering the RA (Fig. 6.5, Video 6.5). To depict the relation between the CS and an atrial septal defect (ASD), an oblique (130°) mid esophageal view is useful.

Imaging of Normal Pulmonary Veins

Several views can be used to evaluate the left and right pulmonary veins. Imaging begins with the transducer positioned behind the LA at 0°. From the ME 4 Ch view, the transducer is rotated leftwards (counterclockwise) to identify the left

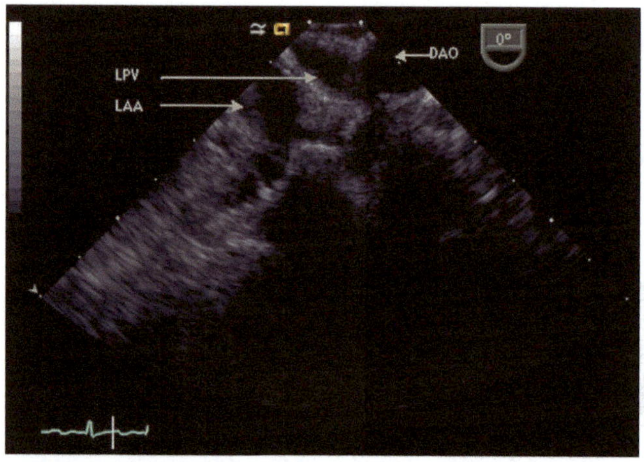

Fig. 6.6 In this image at 0°, the probe has been withdrawn and rotated leftwards (counterclockwise) from the mid esophageal four chamber view to demonstrate the relationship of the descending aorta (*DAO*), left upper pulmonary vein (*LPV*), and left atrial appendage (*LAA*) in a posterior to anterior position

pulmonary veins, which usually course between the LAA and descending aorta (Fig. 6.6, Video 6.6). The LUPV enters the LA just lateral to the LAA from an anterior to posterior pathway. The LUPV is identified by slightly withdrawing and turning the probe to the left (from the LAA). The LLPV is then displayed by turning slightly farther to the left and advancing the probe into the esophagus. The LLPV enters the LA just below the LUPV. Alternatively, the exam can start from the ME 2 Ch view. Once the LAA is identified, slight probe withdrawal and turning to the left will demonstrate the LUPV above the LAA. After centering the LUPV on the display and rotating the multiplane angle to ~100–120°, the LLPV can be seen. Because the LLPV courses in a more lateral to medial direction, it is less suitable than the LUPV for Doppler interrogation of pulmonary venous blood flow [9].

The horizontal or transverse plane (0°) is less suited to imaging the right pulmonary veins, but often the right pulmonary

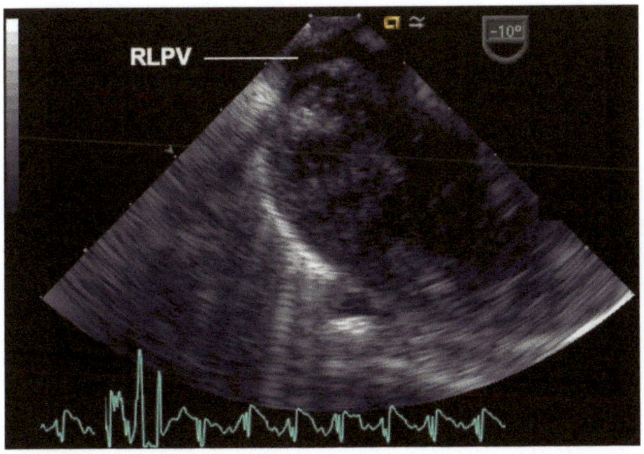

Fig. 6.7 In this image, the probe has been rotated rightwards (clockwise) in the mid esophageal four chamber view and advanced slightly within the esophagus to demonstrate the entrance of the right lower pulmonary vein (*RLPV*) into the left atrium

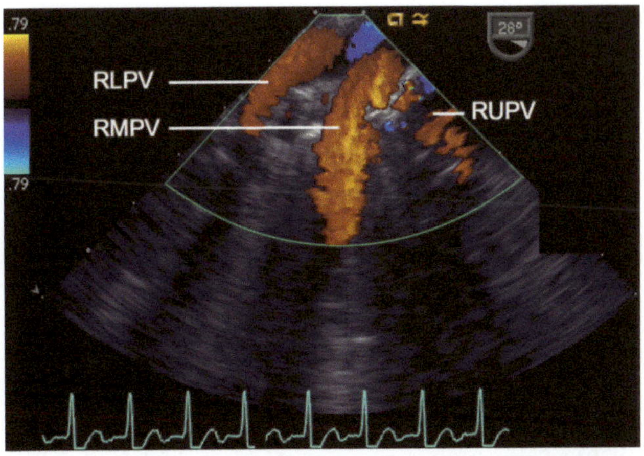

Fig. 6.9 View of the right pulmonary veins (*RLPV* right lower pulmonary vein, *RMPV* right middle pulmonary vein, *RUPV* right upper pulmonary vein) from a mid esophageal position, as they enter the left atrium. This view can be obtained with rightwards rotation of the probe, using an imaging plane of approximately 30–50°

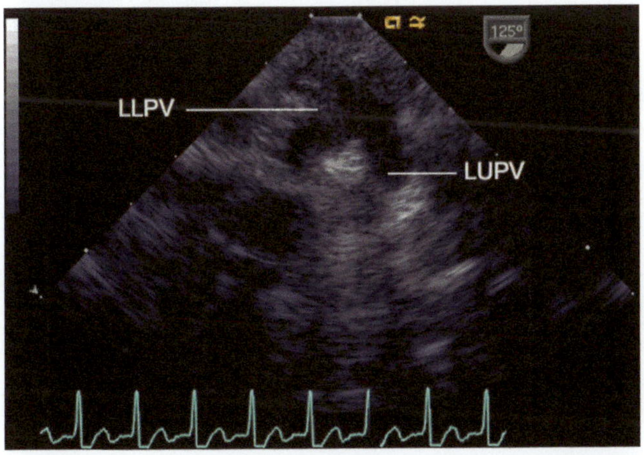

Fig. 6.8 View of the left pulmonary veins from a mid esophageal position (*LLPV* left lower pulmonary vein, *LUPV* left upper pulmonary vein) as they enter the left atrium, using an imaging plane of 125°. From the left atrium, the probe has been rotated leftwards to visualize the veins

veins can be viewed by first centering the RA in the image sector, then withdrawing the transducer until the RPA is encountered. The transducer is then rotated rightwards, and advanced slightly until RUPV flow is seen entering the LA from the right, and then the transducer advanced slightly further to image the RLPV (Fig. 6.7, Video 6.7).

Another approach is to image the pulmonary veins on each side, in their long axis, as they course towards the LA [8]. One way to approach this is to recall that on each side, the upper veins attach to the LA more anteriorly than the lower veins. To view the left pulmonary veins using a multiplane transducer, the angle should be at about 120° (Fig. 6.8, Video 6.8). One can start from the mid esophageal aortic valve long axis (ME AV LAX) view of the left ventricle (LV) and left ventricular outflow tract and rotate leftwards, withdraw the probe slightly and use color Doppler to assist in locating the pulmonary veins by detecting the flow as these enter the LA. If the descending aorta is encountered, the transducer has been rotated too far leftwards (imaging more posteriorly than necessary), and must return slightly anterior by rotating clockwise. Often, one or the other left pulmonary veins may be visualized first, and the transducer beam orientation can be adjusted ±20°–30° until both veins can be seen lengthwise as they approach the LA. On occasion secondary tributaries are also seen, as this view seems to image the pulmonary veins along a greater length.

For the right pulmonary veins, a similar approach may be taken, although at an almost perpendicular angle to the view for the left pulmonary veins. One can start at the mid esophageal right ventricular inflow-outflow (ME RV in-out) view, at about 30°–50°, and rotate rightwards (clockwise), to just past the SVC. Color Doppler may aid in initial identification and subsequent refinement of the imaging angle that will provide optimal views of the right pulmonary veins (Fig. 6.9, Video 6.9). When beginning to use this view, a helpful method of remembering which angle to use for the left and right pulmonary vein views is to recall that in the retrocardiac position, 120° provides imaging of the inflow and outflow of the LV, so it also provides imaging of the left veins when directed leftward and posteriorly. Similarly, in the retrocardiac position, 30°–50° provides imaging of the inflow and outflow of the right ventricle, and also provides imaging of the right veins when directed rightward and posteriorly.

Systemic Venous Abnormalities

Persistent Left Superior Vena Cava Draining to the Coronary Sinus

Over 90 % of cases of persistent left superior vena cava (LSVC) drain via a CS [10]. This condition is common, occurring in approximately 0.5 % of the general population [11–13] and in 3–10 % of patients with congenital heart defects [10, 14]. Although several reports cite total absence of the RSVC in 17 % of patients with a persistent LSVC [10, 14], this appears to be substantially less common in our experience.

Identification of an LSVC is important in a patient undergoing surgery, as it may alter the venous cannulation strategy. In addition, a LSVC to CS drainage pattern complicates atrial baffle procedures, because the CS is usually incorporated into the pulmonary venous atrium, which would not be wise given the increased volume of desaturated blood the CS would carry when an LSVC is connected to it [15].

The presence of bilateral SVCs has more significance in the execution of a bidirectional cavopulmonary anastomosis (BCPA). Some centers have reported increased risk for the bilateral BCPA in comparison to a single BCPA [16]. Central pulmonary artery (PA) hypoplasia may develop in this population after a bilateral BCPA, which may be ameliorated by the preservation of low grade antegrade pulmonary flow [17].

Bilateral SVCs may also impact heart transplantation, in that more LIV may need to be harvested with the donor heart, especially if the intended recipient has undergone a bilateral BCPA. In these patients, both the RSVC and LSVC can then be anastomosed to the donor LIV without need for additional reconstruction [15].

Other clinically important features of the presence of a LSVC may relate to the administration of retrograde cardioplegia and placement of catheters such as central venous lines and PA catheters as these may take an unusual course.

Transesophageal Echocardiography

A dilated CS may be identified as an echo-free region between the posterior mitral leaflet and the LA. To image the CS in its long axis, the examination is initiated in the ME 4 Ch view and the probe is slightly advanced within the esophagus (see Fig. 6.5). A short axis image of the CS can be seen anywhere from 90° to 120° in the ME 2 Ch and mid esophageal long axis (ME LAX) views (Fig. 6.10, Video 6.10). A dilated CS should initiate a search for a persistent LSVC. If this is not identified, other potential causes of a dilated CS should be investigated, such as anomalous pulmonary venous return or HVs draining to the CS, partial unroofing of the CS septum, CS orifice atresia or stenosis, elevated right atrial pressure, tricuspid regurgitation directed into the CS or coronary artery fistula to CS.

The LSVC courses anterior to the left pulmonary artery (LPA), between the left pulmonary veins and the LAA. This vessel can be visualized lengthwise from mid to upper esophageal positions at about 60°–80° (Fig. 6.11, Video 6.11), descending to the left of the aortic arch and in front of the LPA towards the atrioventricular groove, where it continues into the CS. Pulsed and color Doppler confirm the direction of LSVC flow as being towards the heart. Vessels that resemble an LSVC, and have the same embryologic origin from the left cardinal vein system, but have venous flow away from the heart include a left vertical vein in patients with anomalous pulmonary venous drainage to the LIV, and a levoatrial cardinal vein in patients with mitral atresia and intact atrial septum [18, 19]. If the LSVC cannot be adequately imaged, injection of agitated saline into a left arm vein or left jugular vein, which results in opacification of the CS, will confirm the diagnosis [20, 21]. Sagittal views at 90° (ME Bicaval view) are useful for determining if an RSVC is present. When bilateral superior cavae are present, the LIV is usually either hypoplastic or absent [22–25]. When absence of the RSVC occurs, it is usually in the presence of an LSVC draining to a CS or directly to the LA [26–28]. In these cases, the LIV is well-developed.

A dilated CS in association with a persistent LSVC has led to diagnostic errors as in some cases the opening of the CS in the RA has been misinterpreted for an ASD. This may be avoided by comprehensive anterior and posterior

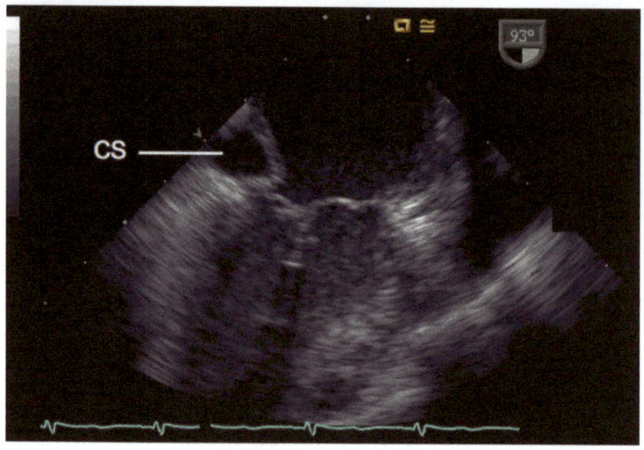

Fig. 6.10 In this mid esophageal two chamber view the left atrium and left ventricle are displayed. A dilated coronary sinus (*CS*) is demonstrated

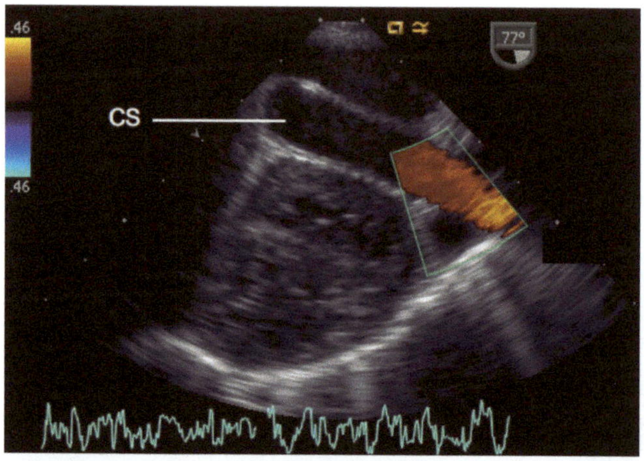

Fig. 6.11 View of the coronary sinus (*CS*) in its longitudinal plane. This receives a left superior vena cava as demonstrated by color flow mapping. This view can be obtained from initially obtaining the short axis view of the coronary sinus and rotating the transducer to 60°–80°

scanning from the ME 4 Ch view as the probe is anteflexed and retroflexed to display the anatomical details, color Doppler interrogation is applied, and structures of interest are examined in multiple planes.

Anomalous Subaortic Position of the Innominate Vein (Retroaortic Innominate Vein)

In approximately 1 % of patients with congenital heart disease (CHD), the LIV takes an anomalous course underneath the aortic arch [29–31]. This is seen more commonly in patients with tetralogy of Fallot or ventricular septal defect and pulmonary atresia. The incidence of a right aortic arch is higher in patients with this venous abnormality [29].

Its clinical significance lies in the potential for mistaking the LIV for a RPA, an error that may occur in the setting of branch PA hypoplasia [29]. The approach to venous cannulation during cardiac surgery may be affected by the presence of this anomaly.

Transesophageal Echocardiography

As the transesophageal windows may not allow for a comprehensive examination of the aortic arch and neighboring structures, this abnormality may not be easily assessed by TEE.

Persistent Left Superior Vena Cava Draining to the Left Atrium

In approximately 8 % of cases of a persistent LSVC, there is direct drainage of the LSVC into the roof of the LA. While this pattern may occur in right isomerism—a condition in which no CS is present [32], it is not diagnostic of this entity. Direct communication of the LSVC to the LA occurs rarely in isolation [33]. More commonly, this defect occurs in association with significant intracardiac anomalies such as ASD, common atrium, atrioventricular septal defect [14, 34–36], anomalous pulmonary venous return, coarctation of the aorta, tetralogy of Fallot, patent ductus arteriosus, transposition of the great arteries, and tricuspid atresia [35–37].

Transesophageal Echocardiography

The normal-sized CS is not easily visible on two-dimensional imaging. Due to the lack of dilation of the CS, this diagnosis can be missed unless the LSVC is visualized directly, or other very subtle clues are detected, such as a small or absent LIV and/or RSVC, which may lead to the search for an LSVC. Alternatively, if an LSVC has been noted (either by TEE or by the surgeon) but the CS is *not* dilated, one must have a strong suspicion that the LSVC drains directly into the LA. Contrast injection using agitated saline or albumin into a peripheral vein in the left arm or left head/neck vein will result in the appearance of "bubbles" in the LA.

Persistent LSVC Draining to a Coronary Sinus with a Coronary Sinus—Left Atrial Fenestration

This is similar to the entity described above (LSVC to CS), except a defect is present between the CS and the LA. This is also referred to as an unroofed CS. The CS orifice opens into the RA in its usual position. This condition may occur in isolation, or with associated heart malformations [38]. When atresia of one atrioventricular valve is present, the communication may represent the only egress of blood from the RA or LA in the absence of other communications at the atrial level [39–41]. Failure to recognize the defect in the CS septum may result in persistent interatrial shunting, and may cause postoperative cyanosis if the shunting is in the right to left direction.

Transesophageal Echocardiography

In the ME 4 Ch view, a dilated CS may present the first clue that an abnormality is present. The CS ostium may be dilated, and may be confused with a primum ASD—the mouth of the CS may be distinguished from a primum ASD on the basis of a normal-appearing mitral valve, and the CS orifice's location posterior to the MV annulus. This is observed as a defect that becomes more visible when the probe is advanced from the usual mitral valve/atrial septal junction to the CS view. In the ME 2 Ch view, the dilated CS is seen, as is the septum separating the CS from the LA. A defect in this septum can be clearly demonstrated using this imaging plane (Fig. 6.12, Video 6.12).

Contrast echocardiography is helpful, as injection into a left arm vein will result in sequential opacification of the LSVC, CS, LA (Fig. 6.13), and finally the RA via the CS orifice [38]. This sequence may be variable as it depends on regional pressure gradients. For example, if the shunt direction is predominantly left to right (that is, from the LA to the CS via the defect, to the RA), injection into the left arm will stream predominantly into the RA, with negative contrast seen from the LA into the CS.

Right Superior Vena Cava Connection to Left Atrium

Drainage of a RSVC predominately or entirely into the LA is a rare finding, and has been the subject of several case reports [42–50]. In two-thirds of cases, patients presented with cyanosis. In every patient presenting with cyanosis there was no LSVC. The second most common finding leading to the diagnosis of RSVC to LA is a brain abscess.

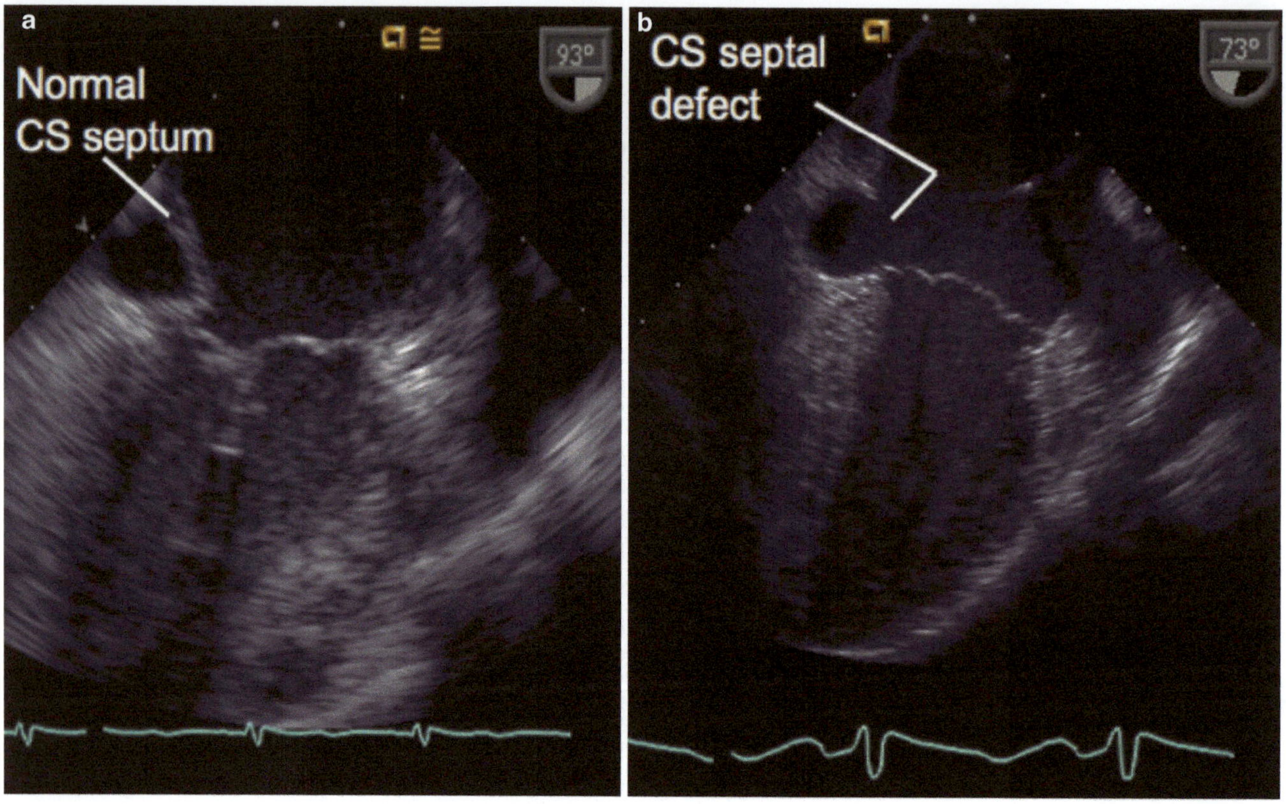

Fig. 6.12 (**a**) In the mid esophageal two chamber view, the normal coronary sinus (*CS*) septum is seen. In this patient the coronary sinus is dilated. (**b**) The absence of septum is evident in this patient with a coronary sinus septal defect

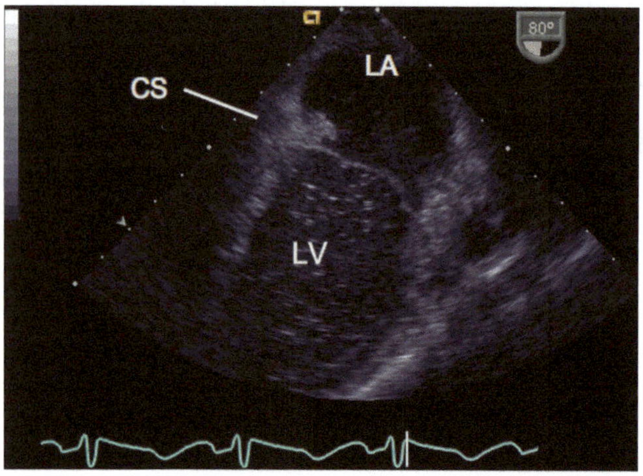

Fig. 6.13 In this image, which is the same orientation as demonstrated in Fig. 6.12, agitated saline was injected into the left arm. Opacification was seen first in the coronary sinus (*CS*), then a brief flash of contrast was seen entering the left atrium (*LA*), establishing the diagnosis of CS septal defect. This contrast was then washed back into the CS and into the right atrium, so that overall there was scant contrast seen in the left ventricle (*LV*) as shown

Transesophageal Echocardiography

The course and location of the RSVC is relatively normal until its entrance to the atrium. Thus, imaging along the long axis of the SVC in the ME Bicaval view will often demonstrate the course of the RSVC, including its entrance to the LA, and the prominent right sinoatrial fold can often be seen in this view (Fig. 6.14, Video 6.13).

Interrupted Inferior Vena Cava with Azygous Continuation

Interrupted IVC is a rare finding, occurring in only 0.6 % of patients with congenital heart defects [51]. In this entity, the portion of the IVC below the HVs is absent. The HVs drain directly into the RA, whereas the IVC connects to the azygous vein which drains to the SVC. Distal absence of the IVC is only rarely found as an isolated lesion. This anomaly is, however, common in patients with heterotaxy, and is the most pathognomonic finding in left isomerism [52].

Awareness of the caval-azygous abnormality is important: accidental ligation of the azygos vein has been reported to be fatal and venous cardiac catheterization can be troublesome in a patient with this condition [53]. The presence of IVC interruption has technical implications for venous cannulation at the time of cardiac surgery: the snare around the SVC cannula should be distal to the azygous or hemiazygous flow, if not the operative field will be flooded by the IVC flow [54].

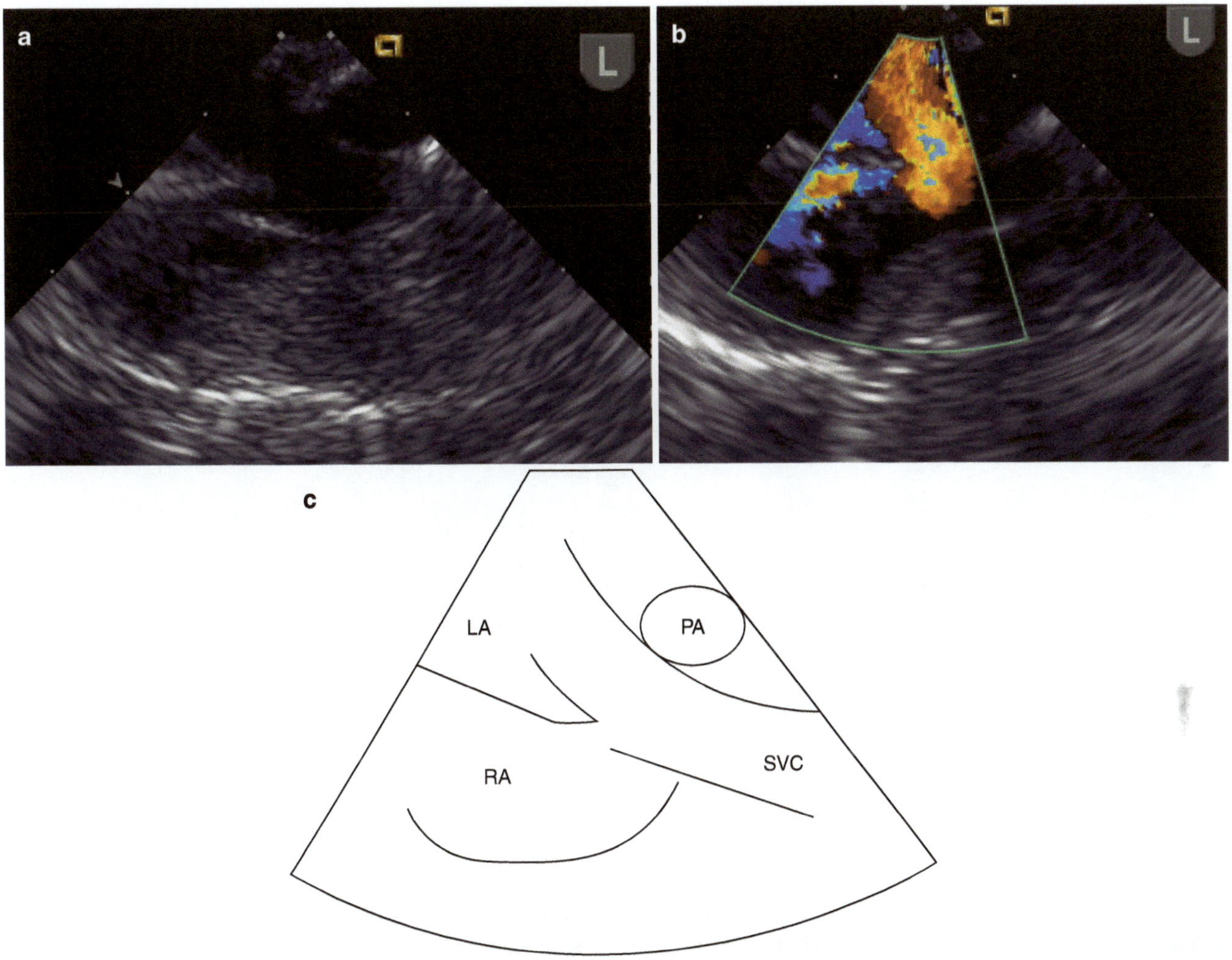

Fig. 6.14 This series of images in the longitudinal or sagittal plane in the mid esophageal bicaval view demonstrates the commitment of a right superior vena cava (*SVC*) to the left atrium (*LA*): (**a**) two-dimensional image; (**b**) Color Doppler demonstrates flow from the SVC entering both the LA (*red*) and right atrium (*RA*) (*blue*); (**c**) diagrammatic representation displaying the anatomy. The right pulmonary artery (*PA*) is depicted behind the SVC

In addition, cannulation of the hepatic veins as they enter the heart may be necessary.

It is important to diagnose this abnormality of venous anatomy in the patient with single ventricle physiology undergoing staged surgical palliation. The Kawashima operation, in which the flow from the SVC and the azygous continuation are routed to the pulmonary arteries via a bidirectional cavopulmonary anastomosis, results in diversion of 75 % of systemic venous return to the pulmonary arterial tree. The pulmonary vascular resistance must be able to accept this volume load at the time of surgery, and for this reason the cavopulmonary connection may be delayed in the patient with an interrupted IVC [15]. The exclusion of hepatic venous return from pulmonary blood flow may lead to development of diffuse pulmonary arteriovenous malformations (AVMs). Subsequent inclusion of HVs into pulmonary blood flow via an extracardiac conduit or lateral tunnel has resulted in resolution of the AVMs [55].

Transesophageal Echocardiography

Transesophageal imaging of this entity must be directed. When an attempt to view the IVC in its long axis as it enters the RA (Video 6.4) is not successful, search for the azygous vein should ensue (Fig. 6.15, Video 6.14). The azygous continuation can be visualized in the retrocardiac position thusly: one may begin by searching in the transverse or horizontal plane (0°) for a venous structure traveling in a paravertebral gutter. Alternately, a search for a vascular structure coursing in the longitudinal (90°) plane of the posterior chest (i.e., looking away from the heart, towards the spine) with cranially directed venous flow would suggest an azygous vein (Fig. 6.16, Video 6.15). Ideally the entrance of the azygous vein to the SVC should be visible and one might expect that the plane of imaging would be at 90° (ME Bicaval view). However, due to the orientation of the esophagus (parallel and to the left of the azygous course), and to the close proximity of the right mainstem bronchus, imaging of this

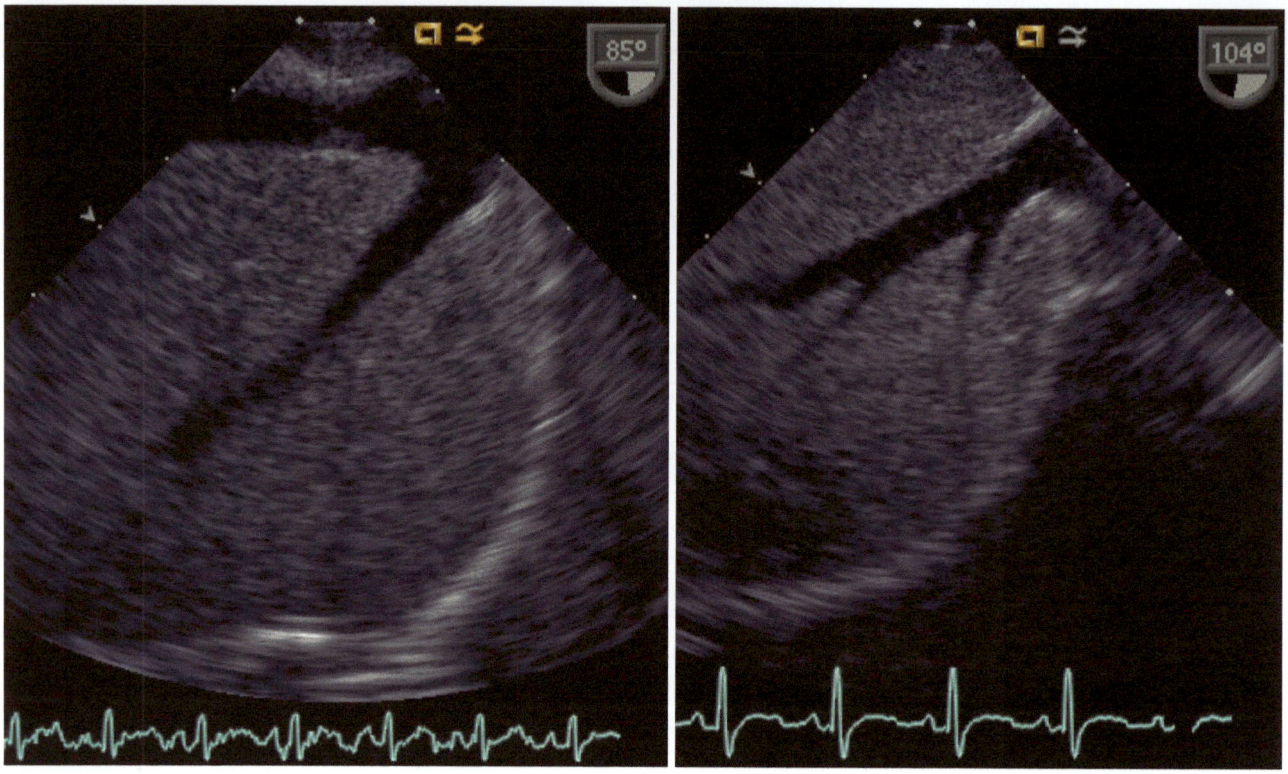

Fig. 6.15 This is a lower esophageal inferior vena cava long axis view in the sagittal plane displaying the findings in a patient with a normal inferior vena cava (*left image*) with hepatic veins joining this structure superiorly, in comparison to a corresponding image in a patient with an interrupted inferior vena cava (*right image*). In this view only hepatic veins are seen

structure may be less than rewarding. Figure 6.17 and Video 6.16 demonstrate a view of the azygous as it travels towards the SVC. At 90°, the distal azygous can be displayed coursing over the RPA seen in its short axis. This relationship between azygous and RPA also can also be appreciated from at the level of the mid esophageal ascending aortic short axis (ME Asc Ao SAX) view, with the multiplane angle at 0°, and with the probe withdrawn and turned clockwise. The RPA is first demonstrated, then the probe is slightly anteflexed to display venous flow directed away from the probe (i.e., anteriorly towards its entrance into the SVC).

Inferior Vena Cava Connection to Left Atrium

A left-sided IVC occurs with an incidence of 0.2–0.5 % [56]. Case reports include cases where the hepatic venous drainage is with the IVC to the LA [57], or is separate. In the latter situation, part or all of the abdominal portion of the right IVC is absent, but the intrathoracic segment which connects the common hepatic vein to the RA is present [58]. Blood from the lower part of the body drains to a left-sided IVC. At the level of about T12, the left sided IVC may:

- cross the aorta anteriorly to assume its normal right-sided course above the renal vessels (most common course) [59],
- drain to a hemiazygous vessel [60], or
- split into a vessel which communicates with the distal right IVC, and a second vessel as a hemiazygous continuation to a left-sided SVC [60, 61].

Transesophageal Echocardiography

Although it may not be feasible to fully characterize this anomaly by the transesophageal imaging approach, comprehensive scanning guided by color Doppler flow interrogation may assist in this assessment.

Pulmonary Venous Abnormalities

Partial Anomalous Pulmonary Venous Connection

Partial anomalous pulmonary venous connection (PAPVC) occurs infrequently, with an incidence of less than 0.4 % in autopsy series [62]. Most commonly, PAPVC is associated with an ASD, either secundum or sinus venosus type in >75 % of cases [63–65]. PAPVC is more common in the setting of a sinus venosus defect—occurring in up to 85 % of cases, compared to a 10–15 % incidence in patients with secundum ASDs [63, 65].

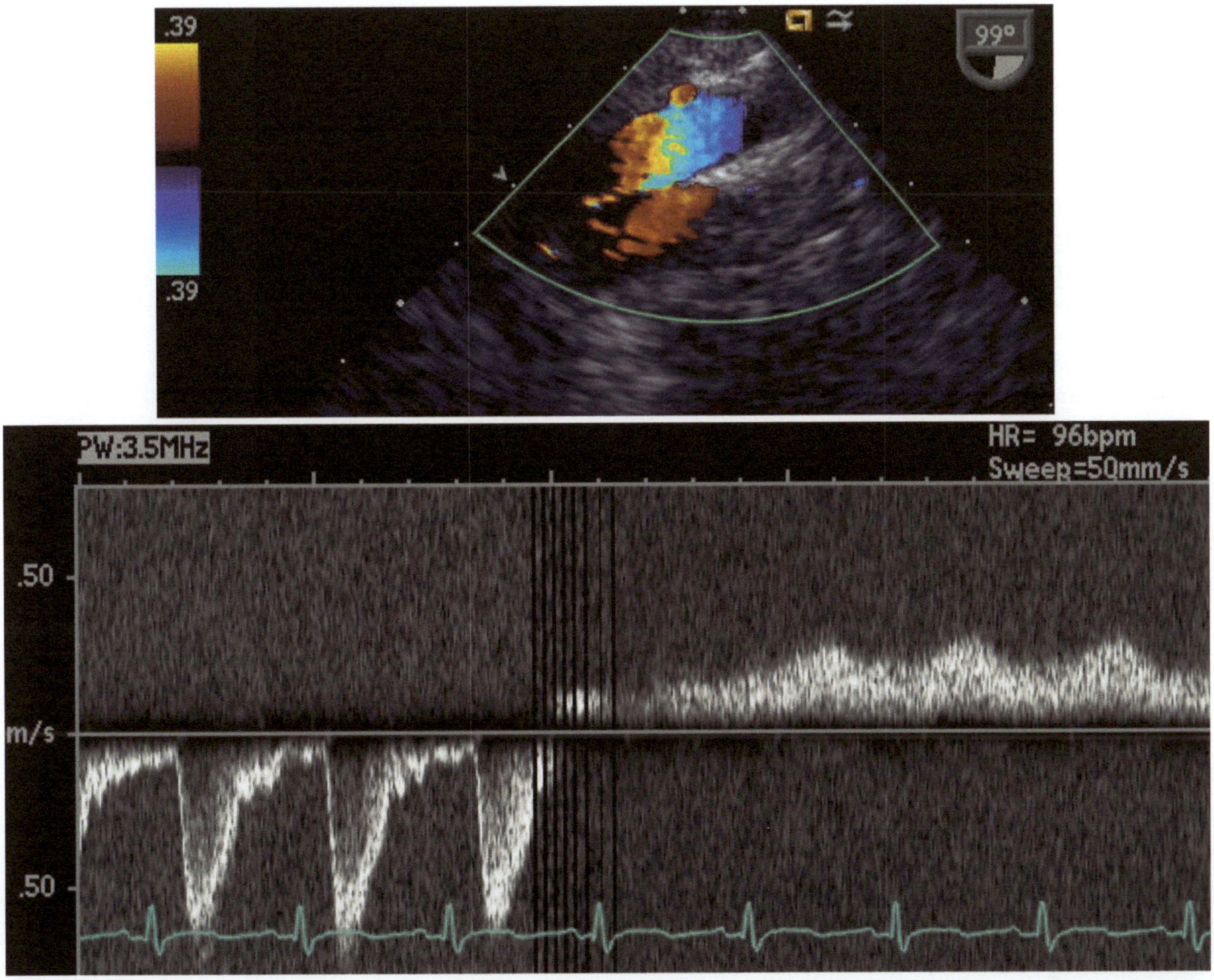

Fig. 6.16 In the top image, the TEE probe is in a low esophageal position, but has been rotated posteriorly; the transducer is oriented in the sagittal plane. Two vascular structures are seen coursing adjacent to each other. In the lower image, the pulsed Doppler sample has been moved from the descending aorta, which has pulsatile flow directed caudally, to the azygous vein that has venous flow traveling cranially

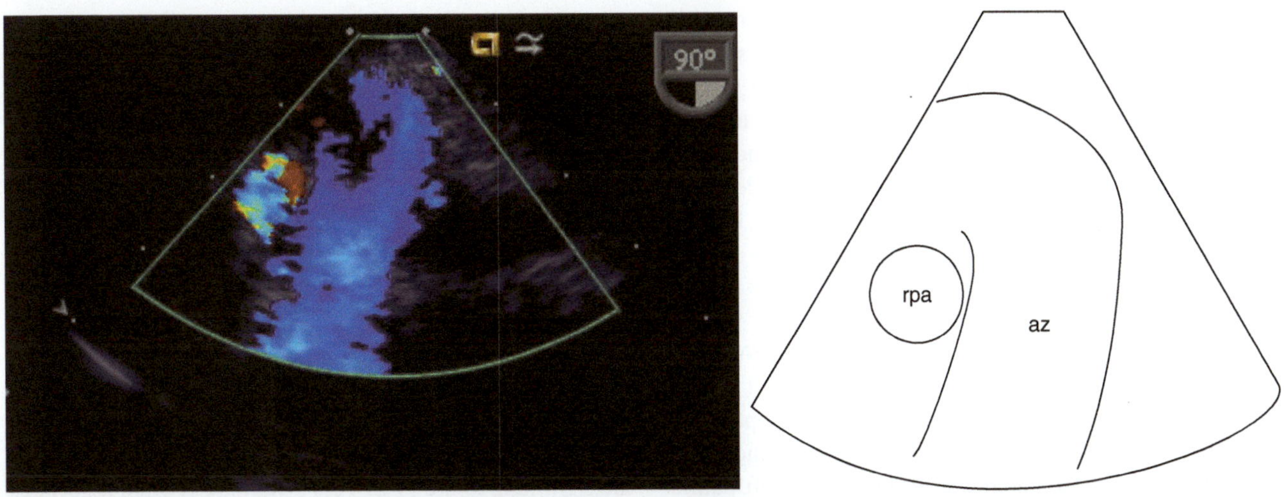

Fig. 6.17 View of the azygous (*az*) vein as it travels towards the superior vena cava. At 90°, the distal azygous vein can be seen coursing over the right pulmonary artery (*rpa*) seen in its short axis. This is a modified view obtained at the level of the mid esophagus

The physiologic disturbance caused by PAPVC depends on the number of anomalous pulmonary venous connections involved, site of the connection, status of the pulmonary venous bed, and the presence of an ASD or other CHD. When a pulmonary vein connects anomalously to the RA or SVC, blood is preferentially shunted to this anomalous vein because of the lower RA pressure, compared with LA pressure, and can produce significant right-sided volume overload.

By far the most common type of PAPVC is right-sided, occurring in up to 89 % in series reviews [8, 64, 65]. The most common sites for drainage of anomalous right pulmonary veins are the RSVC (36–52 %) and RA (12–52 %) [8, 66, 67]. Anomalous right pulmonary veins more commonly involve two or more lobes (75 %) than single lobes (25 %) [68]. When one or both left pulmonary veins drain anomalously, they may drain into the CS, or azygous vein, yet most commonly they drain to a left vertical vein before entering the left aspect of the LIV.

One anatomic factor that affects detection of this defect is the site of the anomalous pulmonary venous drainage; anomalous pulmonary veins draining into the RSVC and entering the SVC higher than 2 cm above its entrance to the RA may be difficult to detect [68].

Transesophageal Echocardiography

Detection rates for partial anomalous pulmonary venous drainage by TEE vary from 60 to 93 % [64]. The presence of four normally draining pulmonary veins into the LA does not exclude anomalous additional or accessory pulmonary veins [8]. With anomalous pulmonary venous drainage (either partial or total), color flow Doppler evaluation is an essential part of the examination, though Nyquist limits might need to be adjusted to highlight the anomalous venous drainage.

Anomalous right pulmonary veins draining to the SVC are often best visualized by imaging the SVC-RA junction at a multiplane angle of 0° (which transects the SVC in the horizontal plane), and withdrawing the imaging probe while observing the transition from high RA to the round shape of the SVC. This is performed by initially obtaining the ME Asc Ao SAX view. A change from this round shape to a teardrop appearance, suggests the point of entry of an anomalous right pulmonary vein into the SVC (Fig. 6.18, Video 6.17) [8]. Similarly, anomalous venous connections to the free wall of the RA can be assessed in this 0° plane by rotating rightwards and advancing the probe inferiorly towards the IVC.

The most common anomalous connection for PAPVC is for one or more left pulmonary veins to enter a left vertical vein draining superiorly into the LIV. The LIV empties into the SVC, which may be dilated if the shunt volume is significant. To assess the anomalous drainage, the left pulmonary veins are imaged longitudinally at about a multiplane angle of 120° as they course towards the LA from the lungs

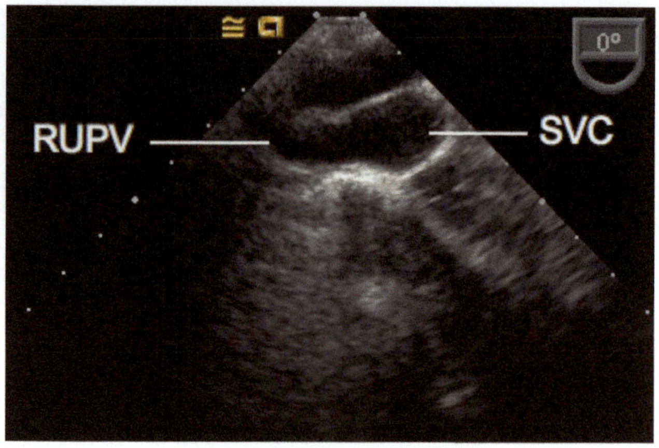

Fig. 6.18 From the mid esophageal ascending aortic short axis view with probe rotation to the right, multiplane angle 0°, the right upper pulmonary vein (*RUPV*) can be seen entering the superior vena cava (*SVC*). In real time imaging, the change in shape of the SVC from round to a teardrop shape is an indication that the patient has an anomalous connection of the RUPV to the SVC

[8]. In this case, instead of entering the LA, the anomalous pulmonary veins will enter a vessel lateral to the LA, which courses anteriorly to the LPA, and is headed in a cephalad direction.

Alternately, one can screen for entry of the left vertical vein into the LIV [8]. To image the LIV, as previously described, from the ME 4 Ch view, the transducer is rotated leftwards beyond the cardiac window, towards the patient's spine, until the Desc Ao SAX view is obtained. Maintaining the aorta in the center of the image sector, the transducer orientation is modified to display the Desc Ao LAX view at a multiplane angle of 90°-120°. With further probe withdrawal, the transverse arch can be more proximally imaged in the UE Ao Arch SAX view. The LIV will appear anterior to the upper thoracic aorta and transverse arch. At this point, at the level of the UE Ao Arch SAX, leftwards rotation of the transducer shaft should demonstrate any anomalous pulmonary veins and/or the vertical vein. Rightward rotation of the transducer will result in a long axis view of the SVC; with probe advancement, it becomes the ME Bicaval view. Anomalous right pulmonary veins entering the SVC can be seen with this latter view. Again, both imaging and color flow Doppler should be used for detection of anomalous pulmonary venous drainage.

Scimitar Syndrome

Scimitar syndrome is a rare condition consisting of either partial or total anomalous pulmonary venous drainage from the right lung to the IVC. This syndrome is often associated with a number of other abnormalities including a hypoplastic right lung and RPA, anomalous systemic arterial supply to the right lung from the abdominal aorta with or without pulmonary sequestration, abnormalities of the tracheobronchial architecture and of lung lobation, rightward displacement of the heart (meso- or dextrocardia), and pulmonary hypertension [69]. The anomalous vein resembles a Turkish sword, hence the combination of these findings is called "Scimitar Syndrome."

Affected patients present either in infancy or adulthood, depending on the clinical sequelae. In the adult form, it has been suggested that the syndrome has no serious clinical manifestations and that usually no therapy is indicated [70]. The infantile variant is marked by a higher incidence and severity of associated defects, heart failure, pulmonary hypertension, and significant mortality [71].

Surgery may involve occlusion of feeding arterial vessels alone, or baffling/anastomosis of the anomalous pulmonary veins to the LA.

A related entity, often termed "meandering left pulmonary vein" refers to cases in which right pulmonary venous drainage is via Scimitar vein to the LA. These cases often have other features of Scimitar syndrome, such as right pulmonary hypoplasia, but to a milder degree [72].

Transesophageal Echocardiography

Especially in the adult, the use of TEE or other diagnostic modalities is mandatory for confirmation of suspected Scimitar syndrome, especially to determine the exact site of the anomalous pulmonary venous connection to the IVC [73].

Imaging of the anomalous right pulmonary venous connection can begin at a multiplane angle of 0°, by placing the probe in a transgastric position. The probe is further advanced into the stomach to obtain the deep transgastric long axis (DTG LAX) view. From this plane, the multiplane angle is rotated to the deep transgastric sagittal (DTG sagittal) view (90°). Rightwards probe shaft rotation allows for the entire length of the IVC to be seen. The IVC can then be followed caudally by slightly advancing the probe, looking for turbulent flow of the anomalous Scimitar pulmonary vein as it enters the IVC, either below or above the level of the diaphragm (Fig. 6.19, Video 6.18) [73]. The multiplane angle can then be rotated back to 0° for further imaging of the Scimitar vein in an orthogonal plane. Alternatively, in the esophagus (while at 90°) in the ME Bicaval view, further probe advancement may allow for the anomalous vein to be visualized in the LE IVC LAX view as it drains into the IVC.

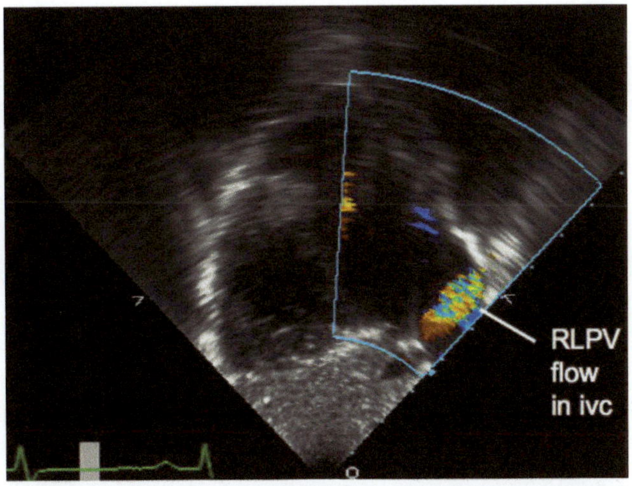

Fig. 6.19 This is a deep transgastric sagittal plane (about 110°) demonstrating by color Doppler turbulent flow from a right lower pulmonary vein (*RLPV*) draining into the posterior aspect of the inferior vena cava (*IVC*) above the diaphragm in this case

Partial Anomalous Pulmonary Venous Drainage Due to Malposition of Septum Primum

A variant in atrial septal morphology, leftward deviation of septum primum, can result in anomalous drainage of some of the pulmonary veins despite a normal attachment. Anomalous attachment of the superior portion of the septum primum has physiologic consequences [74]. When the septum deviates superiorly and anteriorly, flow through the foramen many be restricted, and this may lead to hypoplasia of the left atrioventricular valve. In one series of patients with left ventricular hypoplasia, leftward deviation of septum primum was observed by echocardiography in 37 % of patients with hypoplastic left heart syndrome [75]. When the septum deviates superiorly and posteriorly, normally connected right pulmonary veins can drain into the RA, yet the impact of this alteration in left atrioventricular valve size may be minimal [74].

Transesophageal Echocardiography

In these cases, the pulmonary veins connect normally, but due to the atrial septal deviation, the flow from several or all of the pulmonary veins may be directed to the RA (in the case of posterior and superior deviation of the septum) or may not be affected at all. Thus the TEE examination may be focused on imaging of the septal configuration, once normal pulmonary venous attachment has been recognized.

Beginning in the horizontal plane (0°) at mid esophageal level, one can start from a more inferior position within the esophagus, such as the level used to view the CS course through the posterior left atrial wall (ME 4 Ch view with probe retroflexion). As one withdraws the probe one can observe almost immediately, in the case of the posterior and leftward deviation, the abrupt turn of the septum primum toward the left lateral atrial wall. This will resemble a cor triatriatum, except for the fact that the septal wall of the superior chamber is absent. All pulmonary veins can be appreciated entering the LA normally, but by color flow Doppler, their flow is seen directed to the RA.

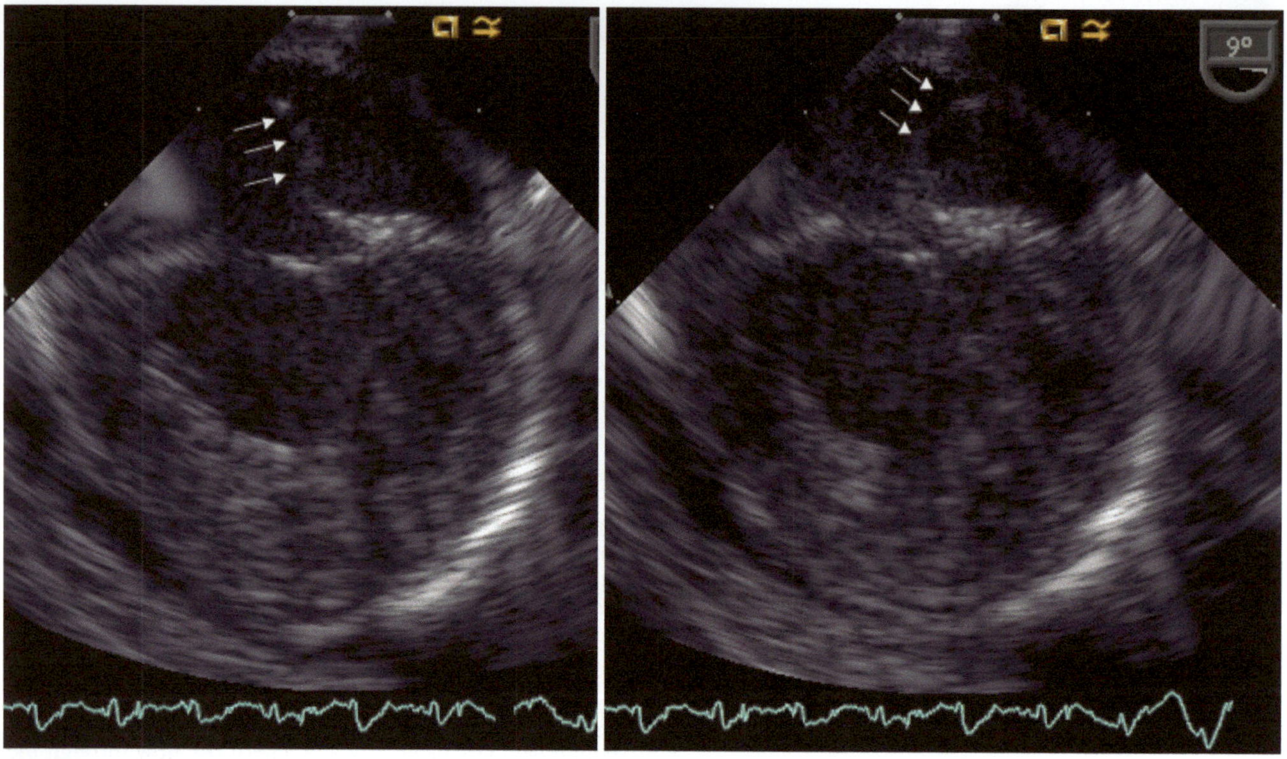

Fig. 6.20 Transesophageal echocardiogram from an infant with hypoplastic left heart syndrome. The *left image* is a mid esophageal four chamber view demonstrating a usual appearance for the septum primum. As one withdraws the probe within the esophagus, the septum is seen shifting to a more leftwards position (*right image*). The position of the interatrial septum is indicated by *arrows* in both images

In the case of anterior and leftward deviation of septum primum, one must withdraw the TEE probe almost to the level of the roof of the LA to observe the "curling" of the septum primum leftwards (Fig. 6.20, Video 6.19). The distance between this septum and the right pulmonary veins can be appreciated, as the entrance of the right pulmonary veins occurs more posteriorly than the affected septum. Often, the septal deviation does result in restricted flow across the foramen ovale. The color Doppler signal of the restricted atrial level shunt originates much further leftward and superiorly, and can be confused with left pulmonary venous flow if the echocardiographer is not aware of the position of the septum primum.

Total Anomalous Pulmonary Venous Connection

Total anomalous pulmonary venous connection (TAPVC) is defined as abnormal drainage of the pulmonary venous blood to the systemic venous system. This malformation represents about 2.2 % of all CHD [76].

TAPVC is usually classified by the location of the abnormal drainage as being supracardiac (45–55 %), cardiac (15–20 %), infracardiac (15–20 %), or mixed (5–10 %) [77]. Individual pulmonary vein size at diagnosis is a strong, independent predictor of survival in patients with TAPVC. An indexed pulmonary vein diameter sum of about 50 mm/m^2 (<25th percentile) or less has been associated with worse outcomes [78].

Transesophageal Echocardiography

Transesophageal imaging of TAPVC is well known to be associated with a risk of respiratory compromise related to compression of tracheobronchial structures [79], or hypotension by compressing the descending aorta [80] or the pulmonary venous confluence [81]. For these reasons the routine investigation of TAPVC using TEE in infants has been discouraged. In our institution the approach to TEE imaging in the TAPVC patient is to proceed with the study with extreme caution, carefully monitoring the arterial pressure tracing, as well as alerting the anesthesiologist to maneuvers more likely to cause compression anteriorly; namely anteflexion or withdrawal into a high esophageal position. Others have reported inserting the imaging probe after the sternotomy is performed, potentially increasing the margin of safety [82].

Complete evaluation of TAPVC prior to surgery includes: (1) identification of a venous confluence; (2) identification of individual veins joining the confluence; (3) identification of the site or sites of drainage; (4) evaluation of any obstruction to the pulmonary venous flow; and (5) evaluation of intracardiac anatomy and assessment for associated cardiac lesions [83].

Supracardiac TAPVC

In the case of TAPVC of the supracardiac type, the pulmonary venous confluence is usually located between the esophagus and the LA. The lengthwise orientation of the confluence is in a nearly horizontal plane, although this may be variable. The confluence is often located just posterior and inferior to the central pulmonary arteries, and the pulmonary veins travel almost parallel to the ipsilateral branch pulmonary arteries, in a posterior and inferior relationship (Fig. 6.21, Video 6.20). Often this relationship is helpful in locating either individual veins or the confluence.

Transesophageal Echocardiography

The very close proximity of the confluence to the probe often becomes a challenge in TEE imaging, as anatomic context may be lost. For supracardiac TAPVC, one technique is to begin at the ME 4 Ch view and identify the confluence (Video 6.21). Subsequently adjust the transducer beam angle to demonstrate the long axis of the pulmonary venous confluence. Once the pulmonary venous chamber has been identified, the next goal is to identify individual veins. The right veins can be searched for by keeping the confluence central in the image sector, adjusting the transducer multiplane angle to 30°–50°, and rotating the probe rightwards (clockwise), to just past the SVC. Color Doppler aids in initial identification. The left pulmonary veins can be searched for by going back to the view affording the long axis display of the confluence, from there adjusting the transducer angle to about 120°, and rotating the probe leftwards (counterclockwise), to just before encountering the descending aorta.

Drainage of supracardiac TAPVC is most commonly via a left vertical vein emptying to the left side of the LIV (Fig. 6.22). The imaging approach is similar to that previously described for partial anomalous pulmonary venous drainage into the LIV. To image the vertical vein, one can interrogate the left aspect of the LIV for any venous structures

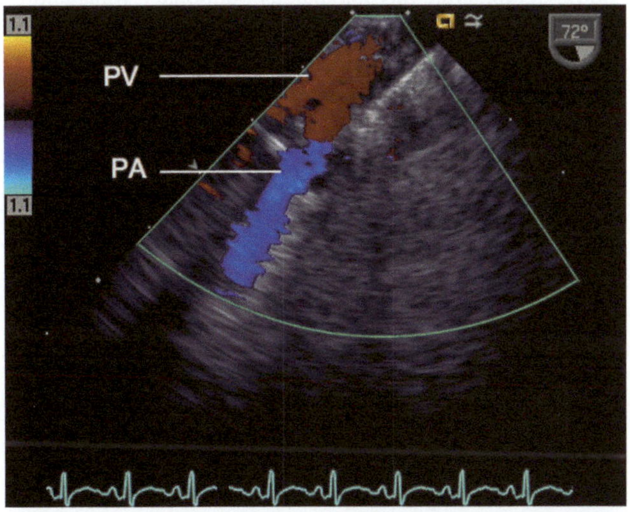

Fig. 6.21 This view is oriented to identify the right pulmonary veins (*PV*). Close relationship between pulmonary veins and pulmonary arteries is evident in this image—the pulmonary artery (*PA*) being directly anterior, and usually slightly superior to the pulmonary veins

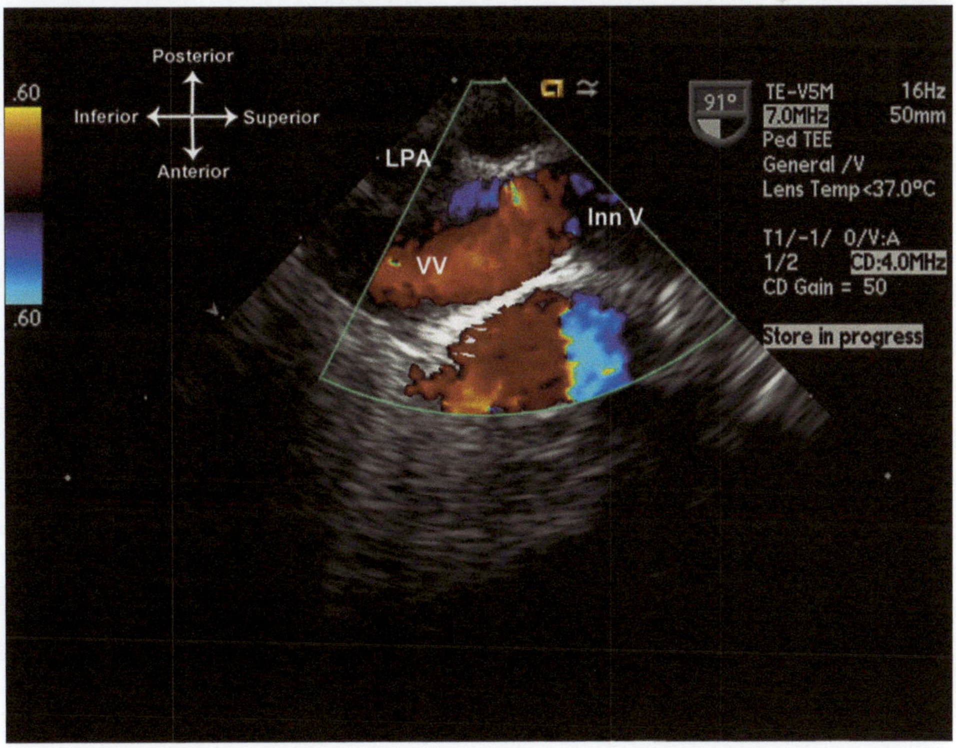

Fig. 6.22 Total anomalous pulmonary venous connection to the left innominate vein. This image is obtained from an upper esophageal aortic arch short axis view with leftward rotation of the probe. A large vertical vein (*VV*), arising from the *left side* of the pulmonary venous confluence, travels superiorly, coursing anterior to the left pulmonary artery (*LPA*) to insert into the leftward aspect of the left innominate vein (*Inn V*). The length of the vertical vein is best seen in this sagittal plane

draining into it: from a ME 4 Ch view, rotate transducer towards the spine until the Desc Ao SAX view is obtained. Changing transducer plane to about 90°–120° displays the Desc Ao LAX. With further probe withdrawal and maintaining the same imaging plane of approximately 90°, the transverse arch can be seen in the UE Ao Arch SAX view. In the case of TAPVC to a left vertical vein, the dilated LIV will appear in its short axis anterior to the upper thoracic aorta and transverse arch. Leftwards rotation of the transducer should demonstrate any anomalous pulmonary veins and/or the vertical vein, which travels anterior to the LPA course. Alternatively the examination can begin once the pulmonary confluence is identified behind the heart and this is followed to establish or confirm its course and site of drainage (Fig. 6.22, Video 6.21). In a supracardiac type of connection, obstruction can occur in the ascending vertical vein connecting the pulmonary venous confluence to the LIV. Passage of the vertical vein between the LPA and the left bronchus (hemodynamic vise) can cause compression of the vertical vein [84].

Infracardiac TAPVC

If a confluence is present in infracardiac TAPVC, it will be located in a more inferior location than in the supracardiac type (Fig. 6.23, Video 6.22). Often however there is no true pulmonary venous "confluence" per se, but a vertically oriented "Christmas tree" type of pattern, of individual pulmonary veins joining into one common vein in a staggered fashion [85]. In each case the vertical vein descends inferiorly through the diaphragm through the esophageal hiatus to connect with the portal vein or the ductus venosus. The vertical vein in this setting is also referred to as a descending vein (Video 6.23). With the infracardiac type of pathology, obstruction is commonly seen either at the ductus venosus or within the hepatic sinusoids, where the pulmonary venous flow must travel to connect to the IVC.

Transesophageal Echocardiography

The preoperative TEE assessment of infracardiac TAPVC can be challenging. The techniques described above (supracardiac TAPVC) can be used to visualize the individual right and left pulmonary veins as they return to the vertical vein. A cross-section of the vertical vein can be imaged behind the heart using the ME 4 Ch view, and by advancing the TEE probe slowly toward the stomach, the vertical vein can be followed below the diaphragm. Anteflexion and slight rightward rotation of the probe, producing the LE Situs SAX view, can demonstrate the entrance of the vertical vein into the liver and its anastomosis with the portal vein or ductus venosus. Color flow Doppler may show aliasing at the point of connection, indicating obstruction, and a mean gradient can sometimes be obtained by spectral Doppler. In some cases, imaging of this form of TAPVC may be difficult, and limited to evaluation of individual veins for focal stenosis.

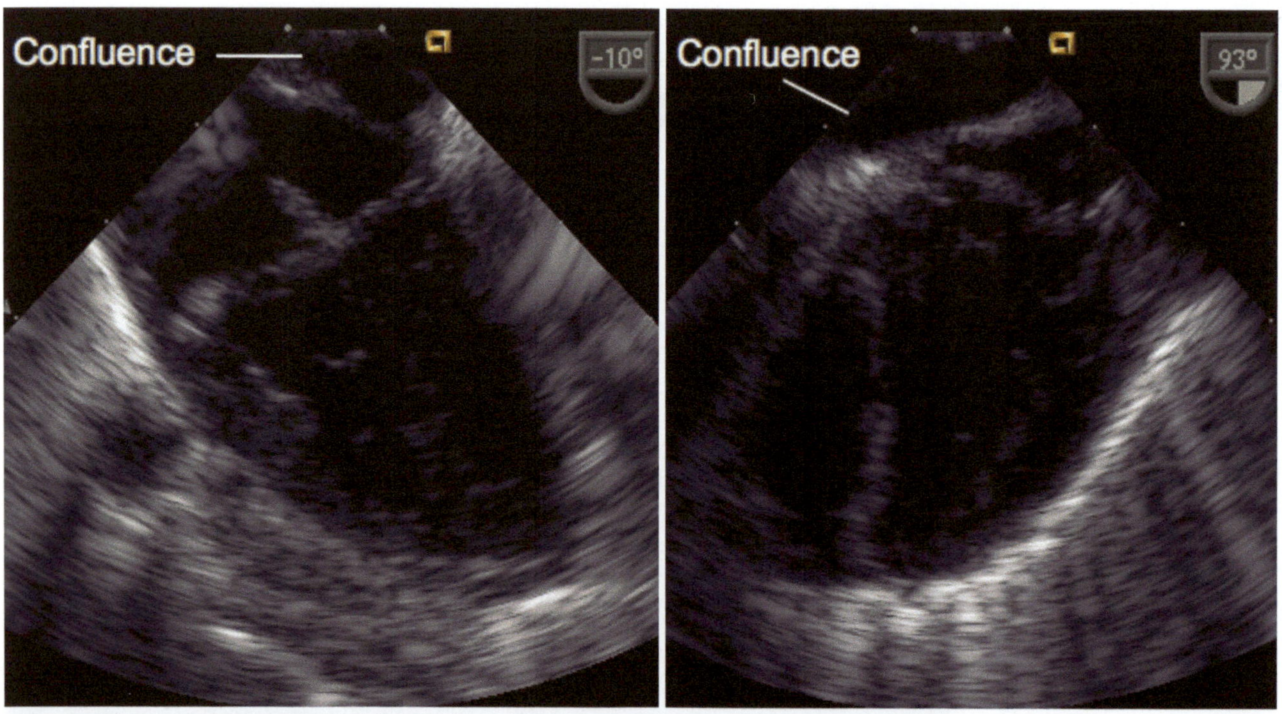

Fig. 6.23 In the *left image*, the pulmonary venous confluence is identified posteriorly in the mid esophageal four chamber view. The transducer beam is then adjusted to an orthogonal plane in order to image the confluence in a long axis orientation (*right image*)

Cardiac Type of TAPVC

Pulmonary veins in this setting drain either directly to the RA (Fig. 6.24, Video 6.24) or to the CS. In these cases there is no confluence, and imaging of the pulmonary venous pathway is often performed in the horizontal plane (ME 4 Ch view). When all or some of the pulmonary veins drain to the CS, this structure will be notably dilated due to the increase flow through it, and the CS can take an unusual, more vertical orientation.

Transesophageal Echocardiography

To image TAPVC to the CS, the biggest challenge is separating the CS from the LA, as the CS is so hugely dilated it is difficult to identify its margins. In the ME 4 Ch view, manipulating the probe up and down within the esophagus will facilitate the identification of which chamber is receiving the pulmonary venous drainage (Fig. 6.25, Video 6.25).

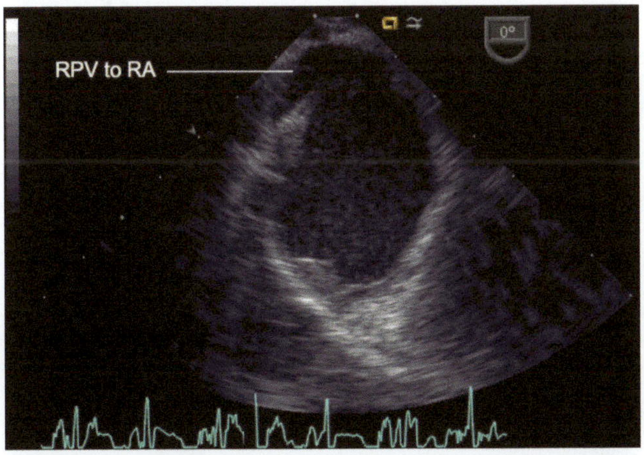

Fig. 6.24 Direct drainage of a right pulmonary vein (*RPV*), in this case, a right lower pulmonary vein, to the right atrium is demonstrated in mid esophageal four chamber view with clockwise transducer rotation

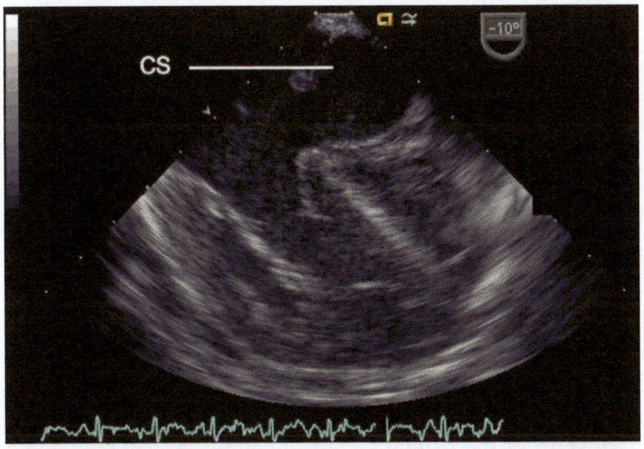

Fig. 6.25 In this mid esophageal four chamber view with the probe advanced and retroflexed, a dilated coronary sinus (*CS*) is shown

Mixed TAPVC

Patients may have a combination of the above drainage types, resulting in a mixed type of TAPVC, which presents a challenge in the assessment by TEE. As in most cases in children, this diagnosis is made by transthoracic echocardiography and preoperative TEE complements this evaluation.

Transesophageal Echocardiography

It is recommended to always explore usual additional sites of pulmonary venous drainage and assess for either flow disturbance or an abnormal venous signal indicating venous blood flow away from the heart. Usual sites of interrogation include: the left side of the LIV for anomalous LUPV drainage, the lateral wall of the RA and SVC for anomalous right pulmonary venous drainage, portal vein or ductus venosus (subdiaphragmatic) region, and the CS. All of the techniques described above can and should be applied to the evaluation of mixed TAPVC.

Surgical Considerations for TAPVC Repair

Conventional surgical repair of TAPVC has involved anastomosis of the pulmonary venous confluence directly to the LA in supracardiac types, and may have modifications—such as anastomosis between the pulmonary venous confluence and the descending vertical vein to the LA in cases of infracardiac TAPVC. These modifications are an attempt to minimize the potential for anastomotic stricture and pulmonary venous obstruction postoperatively. Mortality has decreased to 5 % in the current era, yet factors such as infracardiac venous connection, earlier age at operation, obstructed venous connection, and small pulmonary veins all confer higher operative risks [86].

There is a low (9 % in one longitudinal series) [86] but persistent incidence of post repair pulmonary vein stenosis after an uneventful repair of TAPVC. Recurrence typically occurs soon after the initial surgery and rapidly progresses with pulmonary venous thickening and fibrosis, often diffusely throughout the parenchyma [87]. Patients with bilateral pulmonary vein stenosis have a dismal prognosis; earlier postoperative pathology is more rapidly progressive.

The sutureless technique (Fig. 6.26) has evolved—initially developed to address the challenge of pulmonary vein stenosis, the application of this technique is broadening to include patients with risk factors for TAPVC surgery, such as early repair, small patient size, and small pulmonary vein dimensions [88]. The technique avoids a direct suture line into the pulmonary vein wall. As applied to pulmonary vein stenosis, the affected side is first exposed from the lateral aspect, and a longitudinal incision is made in the pulmonary

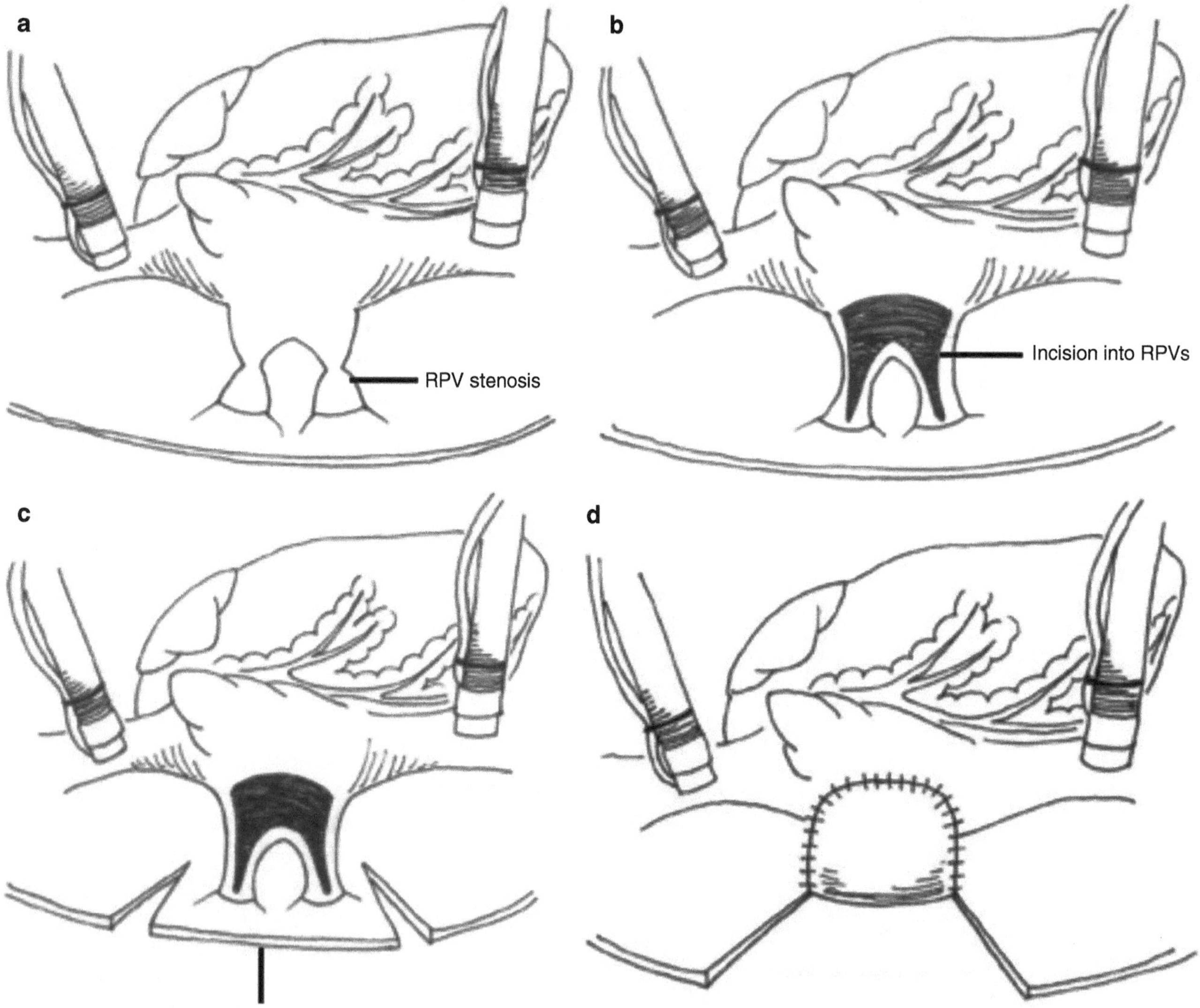

Fig. 6.26 The sutureless technique is demonstrated, as applied to a patient with right pulmonary vein (*RPV*) stenosis. In (**a**), the pericardium is opened and the RPV stenosis exposed. In (**b**), a longitudinal incision is made into each affected pulmonary vein, and extended laterally to the pericardial attachment to the heart. In (**c**), a tongue of pericardium is created around the pulmonary veins, and (**d**), folded anteriorly, with suturing of the pericardium to the LA, avoiding any suturing to pulmonary venous walls (Images courtesy Laura Brantman, NP)

vein to open the area of narrowing. A tongue of pericardium is taken from the site of pulmonary vein entrance into the pericardial space, and is then sutured around the pulmonary vein entrance to the LA, using the lateral walls of the LA. This is in an attempt to prevent distortion of the suture line, reduce local turbulence, and prevent a subsequent spiral of pulmonary venous intimal hypertrophy and progressive local obstruction.

Postoperative Echocardiography

The primary purpose of postoperative TEE is to thoroughly evaluate each pulmonary vein for stenosis. Even in the absence of preoperative evidence of individual pulmonary vein stenosis, unfavorable torsion on the pulmonary venous confluence may result in kinking of an individual vein (Figs. 6.27 and 6.28, Videos 6.26 and 6.27). In the case of direct anastomosis of the pulmonary venous confluence to the LA, interrogation of the anastomotic site is also indicated (Fig. 6.29, Video 6.28). It is difficult to assess the absolute dimension of the anastomotic site postoperatively, since the venoatrial connection is elliptical in shape. For this reason, measurements and assessment in several planes is warranted. In addition, it may be difficult to identify each of the pulmonary veins or the patient's clinical condition may preclude a comprehensive evaluation. Despite these challenges, the postoperative Doppler evaluation can provide important

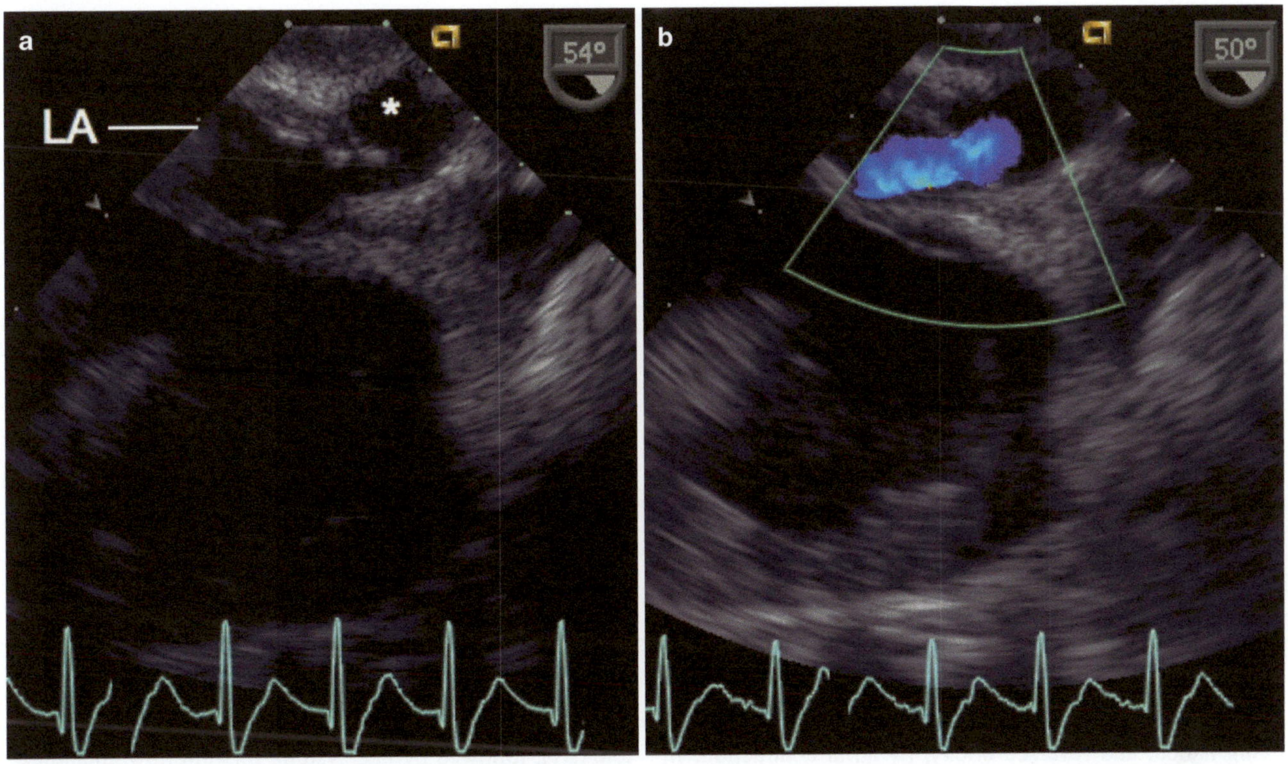

Fig. 6.27 (**a**) This is an image exclusively examining the right pulmonary veins after direct anastomosis of the pulmonary venous confluence to the left atrium (*LA*). There was torsion of the anastomosis, with localized narrowing of the right upper pulmonary vein entrance to the LA. The *asterisk* indicates dilation of the RUPV proximal to the site of obstruction. (**b**) Displays a single frame of the color Doppler interrogation

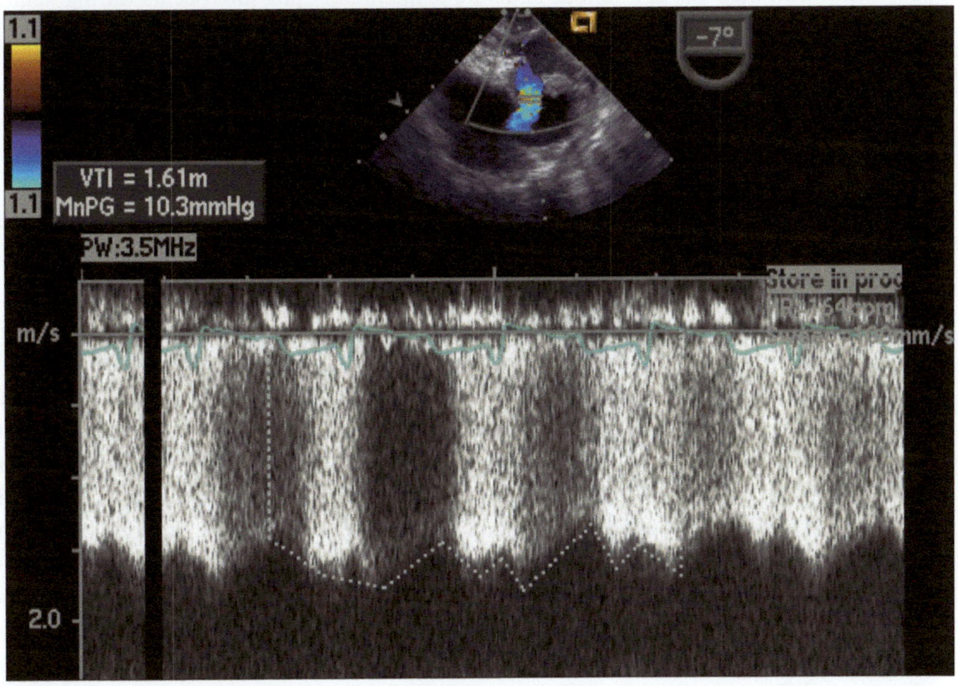

Fig. 6.28 Spectral Doppler interrogation in the same patient displayed in Fig. 6.27 demonstrates a significant mean gradient and loss of the normal phasic flow, related to the obstruction across the right upper pulmonary vein

information. Turbulent flow strongly suggests residual stenosis or inadequate repair of the anastomosis [89–91]. Spectral Doppler information is very helpful for both baseline and follow-up quantitative information, if performed after separation from cardiopulmonary bypass. If TEE is not feasible, epicardial imaging can be considered.

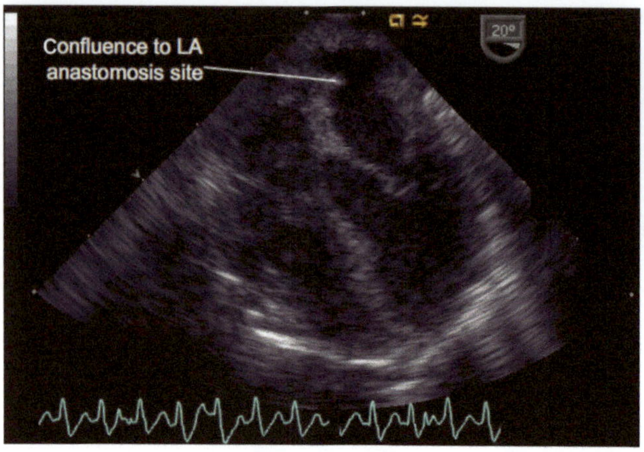

Fig. 6.29 In the mid esophageal four chamber view, the anastomotic site between the pulmonary venous confluence and left atrium is well seen

Systemic Venous Doppler: Normal and Abnormal Patterns

The normal flow in the SVC is characterized by a biphasic forward flow in systole and early diastole, with forward flow being halted, and reversed briefly, by atrial contraction. In children, the systolic flow is greater than the diastolic flow (assessed by either flow velocity or velocity time integral).

In the evaluation of systemic venous obstruction, the assessment of the pattern is often more important than the Doppler gradient. Stenosis in a venous structure is manifest primarily by loss of the phasic pattern of flow. The absolute gradient may vary depending on the preload status of the patient at the time, as well as the capacitance of the venous bed proximal to the obstruction. Systemic venous obstruction is most often caused by extrinsic compression by a mass, but can also be a postsurgical complication, especially after baffling of an anomalous RUPV to the SVC—RA junction (Fig. 6.30, Video 6.29). Other causes of SVC obstruction in the pediatric population include narrowing from multiple pacing leads in the patient with a transvenous pacing system, obstruction from indwelling catheters, or thrombus, always a consideration in the patient with a chronic illness requiring longstanding venous catheter placement. Imaging in the longitudinal or sagittal plane (90°) by interrogating the ME Bicaval view is most helpful to viewing the vessel and narrowing itself, whereas supplemental imaging in the horizontal plane (0°) at multiple levels may be critical to assessing the cause of the obstruction, if unknown. Deep transgastric views, when available, can provide excellent angles for color flow and spectral Doppler evaluation of SVC inflow.

The normal flow pattern in the HVs is toward the RA in systole and diastole, with a mildly dominant systolic flow signal, yet the forward flow waves are interrupted by a reverse flow signal. There is also flow reversal in atrial systole. Thus the normal hepatic venous signal has a to-and-fro appearance. Doppler evaluation of the hepatic veins can be performed from both the LE Situs SAX and LE IVC LAX views.

A study assessing venous flow patterns in children by Doppler echocardiography noted a significant decrease in peak velocities in all veins during expiration [92]. This decrease was found to be more prominent in the HVs as compared to the SVC.

Pulmonary Venous Doppler: Normal and Abnormal Patterns

The normal pulmonary venous Doppler signal in adults has been well-described. The standard of imaging is to use pulsed wave Doppler and place the sample volume within the pulmonary vein (2 cm from the left atrial entrance in the adult). The normal pulmonary venous pattern in animal models and humans without cardiovascular disease has been characterized by a triphasic forward flow pattern, with one brief period of flow reversal. Brief and low velocity reverse pulmonary vein flow can occur during LA contraction (A wave). After atrial contraction, there is atrial relaxation in early systole, so the LA pressure is lower than the pulmonary venous pressure, thus pulmonary vein forward flow occurs in early systole (S1), followed by late systolic forward flow, thought to reflect the forward flow through the pulmonary bed as a result of right ventricular contraction (S2). During ventricular relaxation and filling of the LV from the LA, pulmonary vein diastolic forward flow occurs (D wave) when the fall in LV pressure occurs during ventricular relaxation and the mitral valve opens (Fig. 6.31) [93]. In children, a biphasic forward flow pattern is more common, with S1 and S2 being indistinguishable in most patients. The usual pattern in infants is S wave dominance [92].

Pulmonary vein stenosis may occur as an isolated lesion or secondary to surgery or other interventions. The techniques described to image the pulmonary veins in the irrespectives longitudinal planes as they approach the LA are ideal for aligning the flow signal to be parallel with the Doppler beam. It is emphasized that as in the case of systemic venous obstruction, while assessing for venous flow abnormalities the evaluation of the pattern is often more important than assessment of the Doppler gradient (Fig. 6.32). Stenosis is primarily manifest by loss of phasic flow pattern [94]. The velocity does not necessarily reflect the severity of the obstruction, as flow may be redistributed away from the lung segment drained by the stenotic vein. In any case, in venous signals, the mean Doppler gradient assessed over 1–2 cardiac cycles provides more useful hemodynamic assessment than a measurement at an isolated point in the cardiac cycle. Magnetic resonance imaging studies have shown that unilateral pulmonary vein stenosis is associated with reduced systolic forward flow and diastolic flow reversal in the ipsilateral branch PA, whereas the controlateral PA showed increased systolic flow and continuous forward flow in diastole [95]. If a prominent A wave is observed in the pulmonary venous Doppler, that could indicate

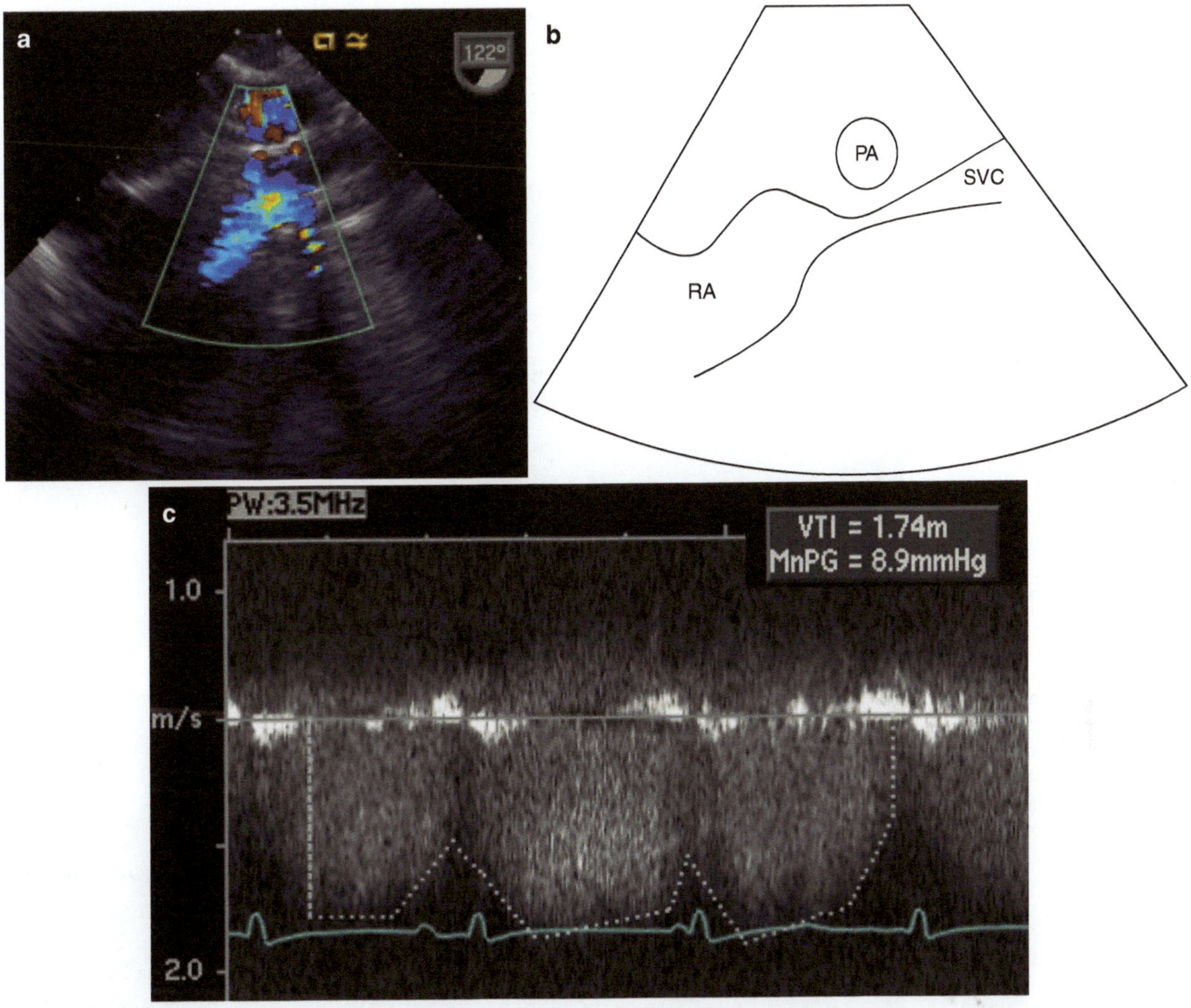

Fig. 6.30 (**a**) Immediate postoperative TEE performed following repair of sinus venosus atrial septal defect. Flow disturbance was seen in the lower aspect of the superior vena cava. (**b**) Diagrammatic representation of findings. (**c**) Significant obstruction was demonstrated by spectral Doppler with a mean gradient of almost 9 mmHg. The repair was revised with resolution of the venous obstruction

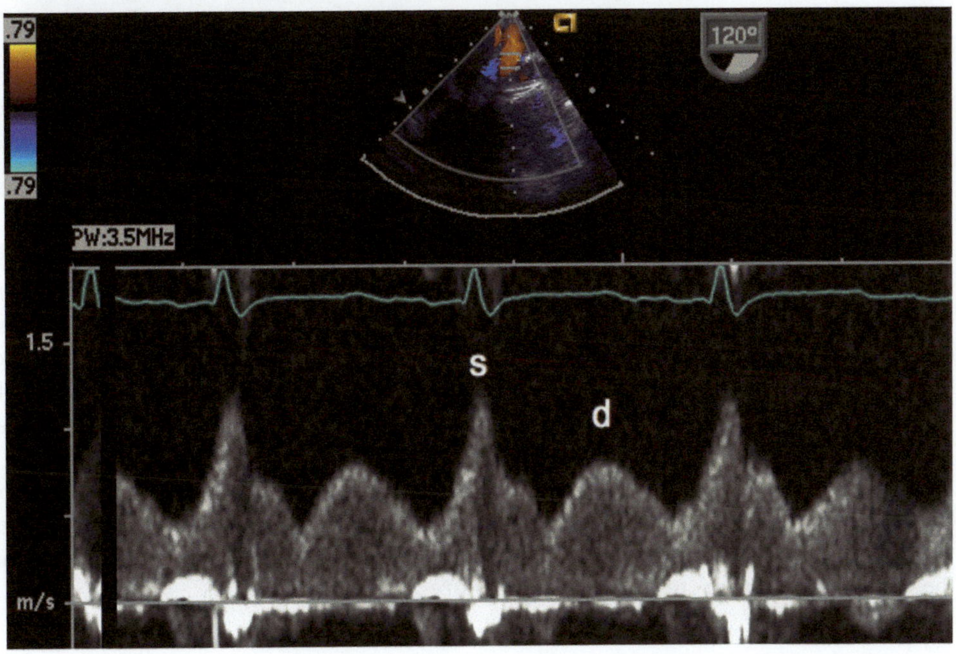

Fig. 6.31 A normal pulmonary venous Doppler tracing is demonstrated. See text for discussion

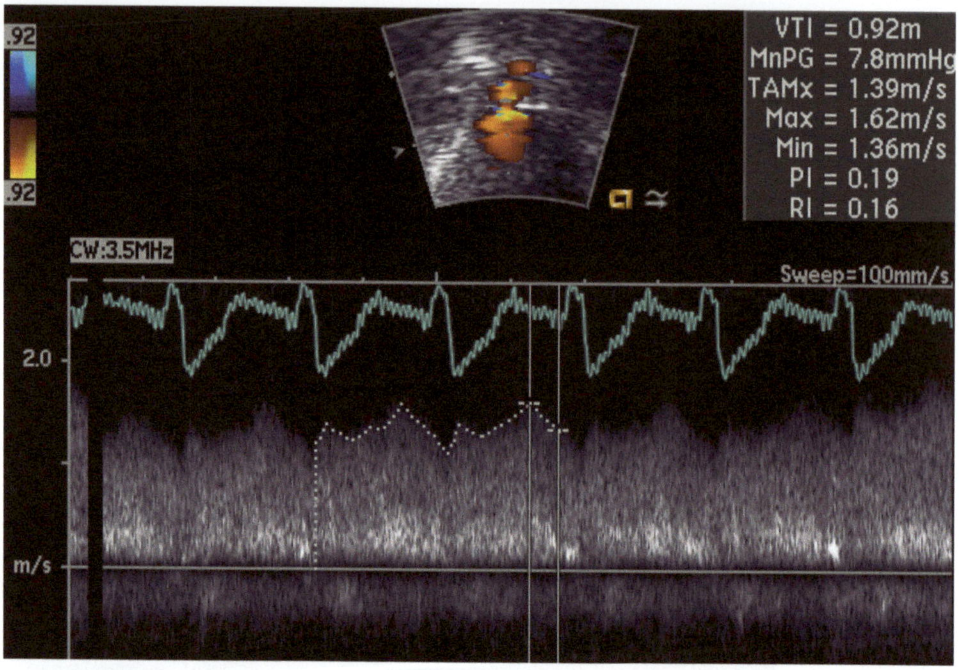

Fig. 6.32 This venous Doppler pattern has nearly complete loss of its phasic pattern, and a mean gradient of nearly 8 mmHg is measured over several cardiac cycles. This is consistent with venous obstruction

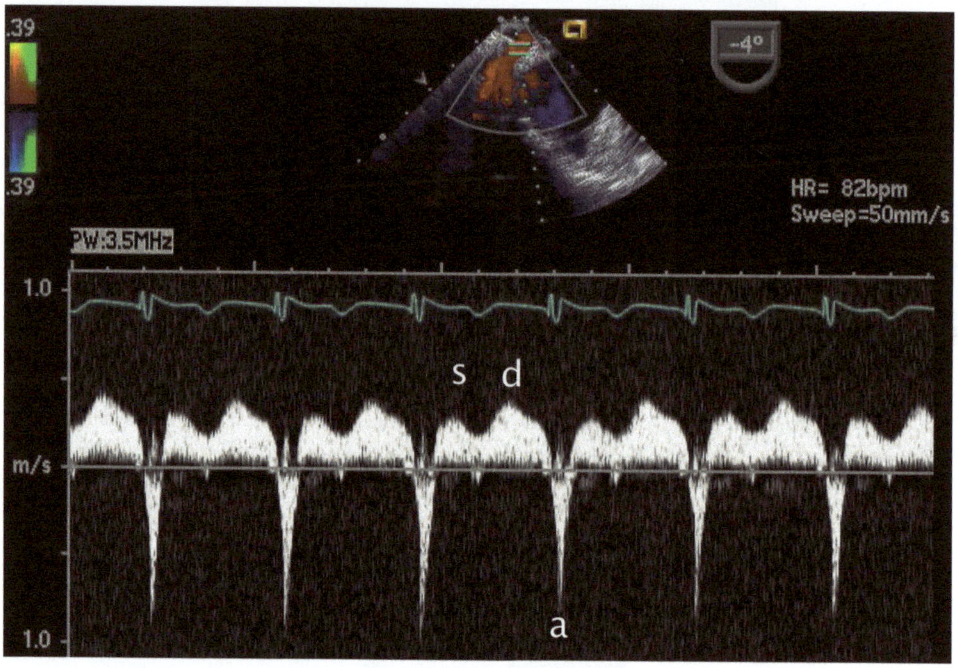

Fig. 6.33 This patient had the new appearance of pulmonary venous large A wave reversal in the postoperative period, consistent with the diagnosis of a junctional rhythm

either left atrial hypertension from diastolic dysfunction, or an abnormal rhythm, such as a junctional rhythm (Fig. 6.33).

Summary

The ability to image and correctly diagnose unusual venous abnormalities relies significantly on the skills of the echocardiographer to image and identify normal venous structures. Once accustomed to interrogating normal structures, diagnosis of subtle or even unexpected variations from normal anatomy are facilitated. The transesophageal approach is well known to contribute to the evaluation of variants and anomalies that affect the systemic and pulmonary veins. In the perioperative setting, TEE interrogation allows for assessment of the adequacy of the intervention for anomalies of venous structures and exclusion of hemodynamically significant residual pathology.

References

1. Geva T, Van Praagh S. Abnormal systemic venous connections. In: Allen HD, Driscoll DJ, Shaddy RE, Feltes TF, editors. Moss and Adams heart disease in infants, children, and adolescents. 7th ed. Philadelphia: Lippincott Williams & Wilkins; 2008. p. 792–817.
2. Geva T, Van Praagh S. Anomalies of the pulmonary veins. In: Allen HD, Driscoll DJ, Shaddy RE, Feltes TF, editors. Moss and Adams heart disease in infants, children, and adolescents. 7th ed. Philadelphia: Lippincott Williams & Wilkins; 2008. p. 781–92.
3. Loogen F, Rippert R. Anomalies of the large body and lung veins. Z Kreislaufforsch. 1958;47:677–90.
4. Stumper O, Vargas-Barron J, Rijlaarsdam M, et al. Assessment of anomalous systemic and pulmonary venous connections by transoesophageal echocardiography in infants and children. Br Heart J. 1991;66:411–8.
5. Ho SY. Pulmonary vein ablation in atrial fibrillation: does anatomy matter? J Cardiovasc Electrophysiol. 2003;14:156–7.
6. Stanford W, Breen JF. CT evaluation of left atrial pulmonary venous anatomy. Int J Cardiovasc Imaging. 2005;21:133–9.
7. Masani ND. Transoesophageal echocardiography in adult congenital heart disease. Heart. 2001;86 Suppl 2:II30–40.
8. Ammash NM, Seward JB, Warnes CA, et al. Partial anomalous pulmonary venous connection: diagnosis by transesophageal echocardiography. J Am Coll Cardiol. 1997;29:1351–8.
9. Shanewise JS, Cheung AT, Aronson S, et al. ASE/SCA guidelines for performing a comprehensive intraoperative multiplane transesophageal echocardiography examination: recommendations of the American Society of Echocardiography Council for Intraoperative Echocardiography and the Society of Cardiovascular Anesthesiologists Task Force for Certification in Perioperative Transesophageal Echocardiography. J Am Soc Echocardiogr. 1999; 12:884–900.
10. Meadows WR, Sharp JT. Persistent left superior vena cava draining into the left atrium without arterial unsaturation. Am J Cardiol. 1965;16:273–9.
11. Bunger PC, Neufeld DA, Moore JC, et al. Persistent left superior vena cava and associated structural and functional considerations. Angiology. 1981;32:601–8.
12. Cobb RJ, Mendelson DS, Norton KI. Persistent left superior vena cava: case report and review. Mt Sinai J Med. 1987;54: 171–3.
13. Campbell M, Deuchar DC. The left-sided superior vena cava. Br Heart J. 1954;16:423–39.
14. Cha EM, Khoury GH. Persistent left superior vena cava. Radiologic and clinical significance. Radiology. 1972;103:375–81.
15. Gandy K, Hanley F. Management of systemic venous anomalies in the pediatric cardiovascular surgical patient. Semin Thorac Cardiovasc Surg Pediatr Card Surg Annu. 2006;9:63–74.
16. Iyer GK, Van Arsdell GS, Dicke FP, et al. Are bilateral superior vena cavae a risk factor for single ventricle palliation? Ann Thorac Surg. 2000;70:711–6.
17. Reddy VM, McElhinney DB, Moore P, et al. Outcomes after bidirectional cavopulmonary shunt in infants less than 6 months old. J Am Coll Cardiol. 1997;29:1365–70.
18. Kaneda T, Onoe M, Matsuda M, et al. Patent levoatrial cardinal vein without left heart hypoplasia. Ann Thorac Surg. 2006; 81:740–2.
19. Bernstein HS, Moore P, Stanger P, et al. The levoatriocardinal vein: morphology and echocardiographic identification of the pulmonary-systemic connection. J Am Coll Cardiol. 1995; 26:995–1001.
20. Snider AR, Ports TA, Silverman NH. Venous anomalies of the coronary sinus: detection by M-mode, two-dimensional and contrast echocardiography. Circulation. 1979;60:721–7.
21. Stewart JA, Fraker TDJ, Slosky DA, et al. Detection of persistent left superior vena cava by two-dimensional contrast echocardiography. J Clin Ultrasound. 1979;7:357–60.
22. Winter FS. Persistent left superior vena cava; survey of world literature and report of thirty additional cases. Angiology. 1954; 5:90–132.
23. Utley JR, Mobin-Uddin K. Absent left innominate vein: sign of persistent left superior vena cava. Ann Thorac Surg. 1975; 19:101–2.
24. Jureidini SB, Hormann JW, Williams J, et al. Morphometric assessment of the innominate vein in the prediction of persistent left superior vena cava. J Am Soc Echocardiogr. 1998;11:372–6.
25. Huhta JC, Smallhorn JF, Macartney FJ, et al. Cross-sectional echocardiographic diagnosis of systemic venous return. Br Heart J. 1982;48:388–403.
26. Choi JY, Anderson RH, Macartney FJ. Absent right superior caval vein (vena cava) with normal atrial arrangement. Br Heart J. 1987;57:474–8.
27. Lenox CC, Zuberbuhler JR, Park SC, et al. Absent right superior vena cava with persistent left superior vena cava: implications and management. Am J Cardiol. 1980;45:117–22.
28. Marin-Garcia J, Sanmarti J, Moller JH. Congenital absence of the right superior vena cava: report of two cases. Eur J Cardiol. 1978;7:293–7.
29. Choi JY, Jung MJ, Kim YH, et al. Anomalous subaortic position of the brachiocephalic vein (innominate vein): an echocardiographic study. Br Heart J. 1990;64:385–7.
30. Gerlis LM, Ho SY. Anomalous subaortic position of the brachiocephalic (innominate) vein: a review of published reports and report of three new cases. Br Heart J. 1989;61:540–5.
31. Nii M, Matsuoka S, Mori K, et al. Digital subtraction angiography, magnetic resonance imaging and echocardiographic findings in patients with an anomalous subaortic left brachiocephalic vein. Cardiol Young. 1997;7:172–7.
32. Moller JH, Nakib A, Anderson RC, et al. Congenital cardiac disease associated with polysplenia. A developmental complex of bilateral "left-sidedness". Circulation. 1967;36:789–99.
33. Davis WH, Jordaan FR, Snyman HW. Persistent left superior vena cava draining into the left atrium, as an isolated anomaly. Am Heart J. 1959;57:616–22.
34. Raghib G, Ruttenberg H, Anderson R, et al. Termination of the left superior vena cava in left atrium, atrial septal defect and absence of the coronary sinus. A developmental complex. Circulation. 1965; 31:906–18.
35. Blank E, Zuberbuhler JR. Left to right shunt through a left atrial left superior vena cava. Am J Roentgenol Radium Ther Nucl Med. 1968;103:87–92.
36. Taybi H, Kurlander G, Lurie P, et al. Anomalous systemic venous connection to the left atrium or to a pulmonary vein. Am J Roentgenol Radium Ther Nucl Med. 1965;94:62–77.
37. Shumacker HBJ, King H, Waldhausen JA. The persistent left superior vena cava. Surgical implications, with special reference to caval drainage into the left atrium. Ann Surg. 1967;165:797–805.
38. Schmidt KG, Silverman NH. Cross-sectional and contrast echocardiography in the diagnosis of interatrial communications through the coronary sinus. Int J Cardiol. 1987;16:193–9.
39. Rose AG, Beckman CB, Edwards JE. Communication between coronary sinus and left atrium. Br Heart J. 1974;36:182–5.
40. Freedom RM, Culham JA, Rowe RD. Left atrial to coronary sinus fenestration (partially unroofed coronary sinus). Morphological and angiocardiographic observations. Br Heart J. 1981;46:63–8.
41. Beckman CB, Moller JH, Edwards JE. Alternate pathways to pulmonary venous flow in left-sided obstructive anomalies. Circulation. 1975;52:509–16.
42. Akalin H, Uysalel A, Ozyurda U, et al. The triad of persistent left superior vena cava connected to the coronary sinus, right superior

vena cava draining into the left atrium, and atrial septal defect: report of a successful operation for a rare anomaly. J Thorac Cardiovasc Surg. 1987;94:151–3.
43. Arora G, Carlson KM, Neish SR. Anomalies of systemic venous return: right superior vena cava draining to the left atrium. Pediatr Cardiol. 2005;26:115–6.
44. Leys D, Manouvrier J, Dupard T, et al. Right superior vena cava draining into the left atrium with left superior vena cava draining into the right atrium. Br Med J (Clin Res Ed). 1986;293:855.
45. Mukhopadhyay S, Mehta V, Yusuf J, et al. Anomalous drainage of the right superior vena cava into the left atrium. Indian Heart J. 2004;56:70–1.
46. Oppido G, Pace Napoleone C, Turci S, et al. Right superior vena cava draining in the left atrium: anatomical, embryological, and surgical considerations. Ann Thorac Surg. 2006;81:2313–5.
47. Recto MR, Sobczyk WL, Yeh TJ. Right superior vena cava draining predominantly into the left atrium causing cyanosis in a young child. Pediatr Cardiol. 2004;25:163–4.
48. Samir K, Fraisse A, Rauzier JM, et al. Anomalous drainage of the right superior vena cava to the left atrium. Eur J Cardiothorac Surg. 2003;23:1051.
49. Van Praagh S, Geva T, Lock JE, et al. Biatrial or left atrial drainage of the right superior vena cava: anatomic, morphogenetic, and surgical considerations—report of three new cases and literature review. Pediatr Cardiol. 2003;24:350–63.
50. Vassallo M, Pascotto M, Pisacane C, et al. Right superior vena cava draining into the left atrium: prenatal diagnosis and postnatal management. Ultrasound Obstet Gynecol. 2006;27:445–8.
51. Anderson RC, Adams PJ, Burke B. Anomalous inferior vena cava with azygos continuation (infrahepatic interruption of the inferior vena cava). Report of 15 new cases. J Pediatr. 1961;59:370–83.
52. Applegate KE, Goske MJ, Pierce G, et al. Situs revisited: imaging of the heterotaxy syndrome. Radiographics. 1999;19:837–52, discussion 853–4.
53. Beedie RJ, Yeo W, Morcos SK. Congenital absence of the intrahepatic segment of the inferior vena cava with azygos continuation presenting as a mediastinal mass. Postgrad Med J. 1989;65:253–5.
54. Manzer R, Sutton RG, Ploessl J, et al. Cardiopulmonary bypass venous cannulation challenges in a paediatric patient with complex congenital heart disease: a case report. Perfusion. 1997;12:203–6.
55. McElhinney DB, Kreutzer J, Lang P, et al. Incorporation of the hepatic veins into the cavopulmonary circulation in patients with heterotaxy and pulmonary arteriovenous malformations after a Kawashima procedure. Ann Thorac Surg. 2005;80:1597–603.
56. Baldridge EDJ, Canos AJ. Venous anomalies encountered in aortoiliac surgery. Arch Surg. 1987;122:1184–8.
57. Burri H, Vuille C, Sierra J, et al. Drainage of the inferior vena cava to the left atrium. Echocardiography. 2003;20:185–9.
58. Goor D, Lillehei C. Congenital malformations of the heart. New York: Grune and Stratton; 1975.
59. Mayo J, Gray R, St Louis E, et al. Anomalies of the inferior vena cava. AJR Am J Roentgenol. 1983;140:339–45.
60. Haswell DM, Berrigan TJJ. Anomalous inferior vena cava with accessory hemiazygos continuation. Radiology. 1976;119:51–4.
61. Hurwitt E, Escher D, Citrin L. Surgical correction of cyanosis due to entrance of left superior vena cava into left auricle. Surgery. 1955;38:903–14.
62. Healy JEJ. An anatomic survey of anomalous pulmonary veins: their clinical significance. J Thorac Surg. 1952;23:433–44.
63. Senocak F, Ozme S, Bilgic A, et al. Partial anomalous pulmonary venous return. Evaluation of 51 cases. Jpn Heart J. 1994; 35:43–50.
64. Wong ML, McCrindle BW, Mota C, et al. Echocardiographic evaluation of partial anomalous pulmonary venous drainage. J Am Coll Cardiol. 1995;26:503–7.
65. Gustafson RA, Warden HE, Murray GF, et al. Partial anomalous pulmonary venous connection to the right side of the heart. J Thorac Cardiovasc Surg. 1989;98:861–8.
66. Hijii T, Fukushige J, Hara T. Diagnosis and management of partial anomalous pulmonary venous connection. A review of 28 pediatric cases. Cardiology. 1998;89:148–51.
67. Kiseleva IP, Malsagov GU. Differential diagnosis of anomalous pulmonary venous return. A clinical-roentgenological study. Cor Vasa. 1984;26:140–6.
68. Ferrari VA, Scott CH, Holland GA, et al. Ultrafast three-dimensional contrast-enhanced magnetic resonance angiography and imaging in the diagnosis of partial anomalous pulmonary venous drainage. J Am Coll Cardiol. 2001;37:1120–8.
69. Brown JW, Ruzmetov M, Minnich DJ, et al. Surgical management of scimitar syndrome: an alternative approach. J Thorac Cardiovasc Surg. 2003;125:238–45.
70. Dupuis C, Charaf LA, Breviere GM, et al. The "adult" form of the scimitar syndrome. Am J Cardiol. 1992;70:502–7.
71. Dupuis C, Charaf LA, Breviere GM, et al. "Infantile" form of the scimitar syndrome with pulmonary hypertension. Am J Cardiol. 1993;71:1326–30.
72. Holt PD, Berdon WE, Marans Z, et al. Scimitar vein draining to the left atrium and a historical review of the scimitar syndrome. Pediatr Radiol. 2004;34:409–13.
73. Idris MT. Diagnostic aid of transesophageal echocardiography in an adult case of scimitar syndrome: confirmation of the findings at surgery and review of the literature. J Am Soc Echocardiogr. 1998;11:387–92.
74. Cohen MS, Weinberg P, Coon PD, et al. Deviation of atrial septum primum in association with normal left atrioventricular valve size. J Am Soc Echocardiogr. 2001;14:732–7.
75. Chin AJ, Weinberg PM, Barber G. Subcostal two-dimensional echocardiographic identification of anomalous attachment of septum primum in patients with left atrioventricular valve underdevelopment. J Am Coll Cardiol. 1990;15:678–81.
76. Ferencz C, Rubin JD, McCarter RJ, et al. Congenital heart disease: prevalence at livebirth. The Baltimore-Washington Infant Study. Am J Epidemiol. 1985;121:31–6.
77. Craig JM, Darling RC, Rothney WB. Total pulmonary venous drainage into the right side of the heart; report of 17 autopsied cases not associated with other major cardiovascular anomalies. Lab Invest. 1957;6:44–64.
78. Jenkins KJ, Sanders SP, Orav EJ, et al. Individual pulmonary vein size and survival in infants with totally anomalous pulmonary venous connection. J Am Coll Cardiol. 1993;22:201–6.
79. Gilbert TB, Panico FG, McGill WA, et al. Bronchial obstruction by transesophageal echocardiography probe in a pediatric cardiac patient. Anesth Analg. 1992;74:156–8.
80. Lunn RJ, Oliver WCJ, Hagler DJ, et al. Aortic compression by transesophageal echocardiographic probe in infants and children undergoing cardiac surgery. Anesthesiology. 1992;77:587–90.
81. Frommelt PC, Stuth EA. Transesophageal echocardiographic in total anomalous pulmonary venous drainage: hypotension caused by compression of the pulmonary venous confluence during probe passage. J Am Soc Echocardiogr. 1994;7:652–4.
82. Chang YY, Chang CI, Wang MJ, et al. The safe use of intraoperative transesophageal echocardiography in the management of total anomalous pulmonary venous connection in newborns and infants: a case series. Paediatr Anaesth. 2005;15:939–43.
83. Reddy SC, Chopra PS, Rao PS. Mixed-type total anomalous pulmonary venous connection: echocardiographic limitations and angiographic advantages. Am Heart J. 1995;129:1034–8.
84. Bennetts J, Caldarone C. Partial and total anomalous pulmonary venous connection: surgical perspective. eMedicine Specialties: Pediatrics, Cardiothoracic Surgery; 2006.

85. Kawashima Y, Matsuda H, Nakano S, et al. Tree-shaped pulmonary veins in infracardiac total anomalous pulmonary venous drainage. Ann Thorac Surg. 1977;23:436–41.
86. Karamlou T, Gurofsky R, Al Sukhni E, et al. Factors associated with mortality and reoperation in 377 children with total anomalous pulmonary venous connection. Circulation. 2007;115:1591–8.
87. Caldarone CA, Najm HK, Kadletz M, et al. Relentless pulmonary vein stenosis after repair of total anomalous pulmonary venous drainage. Ann Thorac Surg. 1998;66:1514–20.
88. Yun TJ, Coles JG, Konstantinov IE, et al. Conventional and sutureless techniques for management of the pulmonary veins: evolution of indications from postrepair pulmonary vein stenosis to primary pulmonary vein anomalies. J Thorac Cardiovasc Surg. 2005; 129:167–74.
89. Snider AR, Silverman NH, Turley K, et al. Evaluation of infradiaphragmatic total anomalous pulmonary venous connection with two-dimensional echocardiography. Circulation. 1982;66:1129–32.
90. Cooper MJ, Teitel DF, Silverman NH, et al. Study of the infradiaphragmatic total anomalous pulmonary venous connection with cross-sectional and pulsed Doppler echocardiography. Circulation. 1984;70:412–6.
91. Smallhorn JF, Freedom RM. Pulsed Doppler echocardiography in the preoperative evaluation of total anomalous pulmonary venous connection. J Am Coll Cardiol. 1986;8:1413–20.
92. Ayabakan C, Ozkutlu S. Normal patterns of flow in the superior caval, hepatic and pulmonary veins as measured using Doppler echocardiography during childhood. Cardiol Young. 2003;13:143–51.
93. Appleton CP. Hemodynamic determinants of Doppler pulmonary venous flow velocity components: new insights from studies in lightly sedated normal dogs. J Am Coll Cardiol. 1997;30: 1562–74.
94. Grosse-Wortmann L, Al-Otay A, Goo HW, et al. Anatomical and functional evaluation of pulmonary veins in children by magnetic resonance imaging. J Am Coll Cardiol. 2007;49:993–1002.
95. Roman KS, Kellenberger CJ, Macgowan CK, et al. How is pulmonary arterial blood flow affected by pulmonary venous obstruction in children? A phase-contrast magnetic resonance study. Pediatr Radiol. 2005;35:580–6.

Atrial Abnormalities and Atrial Septal Defects

7

Louis I. Bezold

Abstract

Transesophageal echocardiography (TEE) allows for a comprehensive assessment of atrial chamber and interatrial septal anatomy. Due to the posterior position of the probe and its proximity to atrial structures, high resolution imaging of the atria and atrial septum represent a particular strength of this modality. Combined with color flow mapping and spectral Doppler interrogation, TEE is able to characterize communications at the atrial level, anatomic variants of the atria, and pathologic conditions that may affect these structures. This chapter focuses on the role of TEE in the characterization of atrial septal defects and atrial abnormalities such as juxtaposition of the atrial appendages and cor triatriatum.

Keywords

Transesophageal echocardiography • Atrial septal defects • Atrial communications • Patent foramen ovale • Atrial abnormalities • Juxtaposition of the atrial appendages • Cor triatriatum

Introduction

Transesophageal echocardiography (TEE) provides for a comprehensive evaluation of atrial chamber and interatrial septal anatomy in essentially all patients in whom this modality is feasible. Due to the proximity of the interrogating probe to the posterior aspect of the heart, high resolution imaging of atrial structures is a particular strength of the technology. This imaging approach, combined with Doppler assessment, is able to define atrial anatomy and details of the interatrial septum including communications at this level, as well as provide information regarding variants and pathologies that may affect these structures. This chapter addresses the role of TEE in the characterization of atrial septal defects and conditions such as juxtaposition of the atrial appendages and cor triatriatum.

L.I. Bezold, MD
Department of Pediatrics, Kentucky Children's Hospital,
University of Kentucky College of Medicine, 800 Rose St., MN 150,
Lexington 40536, KY, USA
e-mail: louis.bezold@uky.edu

General Comments

Transthoracic echocardiographic (TTE) evaluation of the atria, including complete evaluation of the interatrial septum for the presence of shunting, can be challenging in older children, teenagers, and adults due to limited subcostal acoustic windows. TEE overcomes this limitation while providing for optimal visualization of both atria, including the atrial appendages and venous connections [1–4]. TEE is often utilized and demonstrated to be highly useful in the operating room and/or cardiac catheterization laboratory to define atrial anatomy, presence, size, and location of septal defects, to evaluate postoperative results in related interventions, and to assist in transcatheter interventions that involve the atrial septum. Although a number of centers do not routinely use intraoperative TEE for straightforward surgical closures of secundum atrial septal defects, this imaging approach can be extremely helpful in documenting adequate cardiac de-airing prior to separation from cardiopulmonary bypass, and for facilitating overall intraoperative care.

The online version of this chapter (doi:10.1007/978-1-84800-064-3_7) contains supplementary material, which is available to authorized users.

P.C. Wong, W.C. Miller-Hance (eds.), *Transesophageal Echocardiography for Congenital Heart Disease*,
DOI 10.1007/978-1-84800-064-3_7, © Springer-Verlag London 2014

Pulmonary and systemic venous connections can often be verified by TEE (Chap. 6). Evaluation for intracardiac thrombi, particularly to exclude an atrial thrombus prior to cardioversion in atrial fibrillation, or in potential "low-flow" states such as may be the case in the postoperative Fontan patient, can be more completely and accurately accomplished by TEE as compared to TTE (Chap. 16). This is particularly true in patients who have undergone previous modifications of the Fontan procedure such as direct atriopulmonary connections, which are generally seen in older patients with poor transthoracic acoustic windows.

In patients with neurologic findings suggestive of transient ischemic attacks or cerebral vascular accidents, the use of TEE, particularly in combination with agitated saline injection, increases the sensitivity in the detection of right-to-left flow through a patent foramen ovale.

The early experience regarding the applications of three-dimensional TEE in the evaluation of anomalies of the atria and atrial septum has already demonstrated unique benefits and in some cases superior morphologic assessment as compared to two-dimensional (2D) TEE (Chaps. 19 and 20) [5–10].

Atrial Septal Defects

Atrial septal defects (ASDs) are relatively common, accounting for approximately 7–8 % of congenital heart disease (CHD) [11]. These can occur in isolation, or may be associated with other congenital cardiac abnormalities. Communications that allow for interatrial shunting may be due to either morphologic defects involving the interatrial septum or in a location outside the confines of the septum as discussed below. The location of the defect generally reflects its underlying embryologic origin. The hemodynamic perturbations and clinical findings of a defect are largely related to its anatomic location and size, as modified by the presence or absence of potentially associated structural cardiac lesions and the relative pulmonary and systemic vascular resistances.

This chapter will focus on isolated defects, which are usually classified according to their location. Isolated ASDs include those involving the fossa ovalis (secundum ASD), defects either superior or inferior to the fossa ovalis and involving the connections of the vena cavae (superior or inferior sinus venosus type ASDs, for superior and inferior vena cava respectively), and coronary sinus defects. A patent foramen ovale (PFO) also represents a communication between the right and left atria. Although generally not considered a true ASD in the strictest sense because there is no true deficiency of atrial septal tissue [12], PFOs may become clinically significant in situations where an elevation in right atrial pressure causes right-to-left interatrial shunting through the foramen, thus representing a potential risk for paradoxical embolization. So-called primum ASDs (partial atrioventricular septal or canal defects) are considered under atrioventricular septal defects and they will be addressed only briefly in this chapter. These defects are discussed in depth in Chap. 8.

Secundum Atrial Septal Defect

Secundum ASDs, the most common type of ASD (~70 % of ASDs), are generally located within the area bordered by the limbus of the fossa ovalis. They generally result from a deficiency the in septum primum, of variable size and extent. These defects may constitute single communications, or so-called fenestrated defects with multiple orifices. They may be variably positioned, which can influence efforts at transcatheter closure. Fenestrated ASDs are often associated with an aneurysmal septum primum of the foramen. Care must be taken to identify the Eustachian valve of the right atrium (RA), which connects to the limbus of the fossa ovalis and may be mistaken for the lower edge of an ASD by echocardiography or at the time of surgery. If this error occurs during the echocardiographic evaluation, the size of the ASD could be overestimated. If it occurs during surgery, attachment of an ASD patch to this structure will have the unintended effect of diverting inferior vena cava flow directly into the left atrium (LA), resulting in significant cyanosis.

Secundum ASDs may occur in isolation or in association with many other congenital cardiac defects, including other types of ASDs [13–16]. Most secundum ASDs occur sporadically, however some occur in conjunction with defined syndromes (such as Holt-Oram or heart-hand syndrome) or gene defects [17–22].

Primum Atrial Septal Defect

Primum ASDs are the second most common type of ASD (~20 % of all ASDs). These defects are located in the most inferior and posterior portion of the atrial septum, involving the atrioventricular septum, and are invariably associated with a large "cleft" (or commissure) in the anterior leaflet of the mitral valve. They comprise one part of the spectrum of atrioventricular septal (endocardial cushion) defects, hence they are also called partial atrioventricular canal defects. These defects are discussed in full detail in Chap. 8.

Sinus Venosus Atrial Septal Defect

Sinus venosus ASDs (~10 % of ASDs) are characterized by a communication between the atrial chambers in juxtaposition to either the superior or inferior vena cava. Associated malposition of the insertion of either the superior or inferior vena cava results in these structures straddling the atrial septum with the interatrial communication generally located within the orifice of the overriding caval vein. Superior sinus venosus defects (also known as superior vena caval defects) are located immediately inferior or caudal to the orifice of the superior vena cava and above the superior limbus of the fossa ovalis. This is the most common type of defect. Anomalous drainage of the right upper as well as in some cases, the right middle pulmonary vein often accompanies this type of defect [23, 24].

The less common inferior sinus venosus defects (also known as inferior vena caval defects) are located immediately superior/cranial to the orifice of the inferior vena cava (posterior and inferior to the fossa ovalis, which may demonstrate hypoplasia or anterior displacement of the posterior limbus). These defects are also associated with partial anomalous right pulmonary venous drainage [25–28].

Sinus venosus defects result from a deficiency in the wall that normally separates the LA from the respective caval veins. Since they are located outside the confines of the atrial septum, it has been suggested that they do not represent 'true' septal defects.

Coronary Sinus Atrial Septal Defect

Coronary sinus ASDs are rare (<1 % of ASDs) and result from either a partial deficiency or complete absence (unroofed coronary sinus) of the superior aspect of the common wall between the coronary sinus and the LA. Interatrial shunting occurs through the defect in the coronary sinus wall on the left atrial side, which is continuous with the coronary sinus opening on the right atrial side of the septum. There may be additional deficiency of atrial septal tissue surrounding the coronary sinus orifice on the right side. A common association is a persistent left superior vena cava draining to the coronary sinus [29]. These defects may also be seen in complex CHD in association with heterotaxy syndrome, atrial situs abnormalities, and with other anomalies of systemic venous return [30–32].

Patent Foramen Ovale

A PFO is present in approximately 15–30 % of normal adult hearts. Inter-atrial shunting can potentially occur if right atrial pressure exceeds left atrial pressure (right-to-left) or with normal atrial pressures if the flap valve (septum primum) of the foramen ovale is incompetent (left-to-right shunt). Transient increases in right atrial pressure do occur normally during early ventricular systole and with inspiration and can be induced by the Valsalva maneuver. A persistent, large Eustachian valve can also direct inferior vena caval blood preferentially towards the fossa ovalis and potentially across a PFO throughout the cardiac cycle [33]. An important issue related to a PFO is its potential association with paradoxical embolism and stroke, rare complications in children. TEE is more sensitive than transthoracic imaging for detection of PFO shunting. The injection of agitated saline via a peripheral or central venous catheter enhances the sensitivity of detecting a PFO [34, 35]. The presence of an atrial septal aneurysm in association with a PFO has been implicated in an increased risk of paradoxical emboli and neurologic events [36–40].

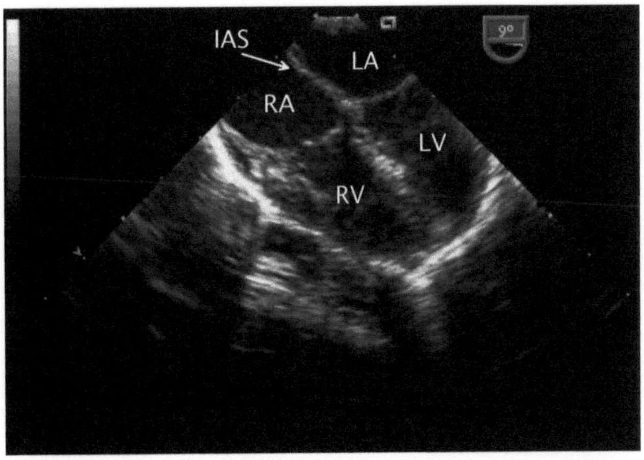

Fig. 7.1 The mid esophageal four chamber view represents a starting point in the evaluation of atrial septal defects as this cross-section displays both atria, the interatrial septum (*IAS*), atrioventricular valves, and ventricular inflows. *LA* left atrium, *LV* left ventricle, *RA* right atrium, *RV* right ventricle

Transesophageal Echocardiographic Evaluation

The interatrial septum is generally well oriented with respect to 2D imaging and Doppler interrogation with the probe at the mid esophageal four chamber (ME 4 Ch) view [41]. Probe rotation clockwise in an otherwise normal heart may enhance this view. Evaluation of the atrial septum thus begins in this view (plane ~0°–20°). This cross section demonstrates both atria and the interatrial septum (Fig. 7.1, Video 7.1). Slight probe retroflexion, if possible without losing contact with the anterior esophagus, optimizes imaging. Right and left probe shaft rotation enhances visualization of right-sided or left-sided structures respectively.

Secundum ASDs, in general, are adequately visualized in this view with slight clockwise probe shaft rotation (Fig. 7.2, Video 7.2). Color flow Doppler interrogation in this plane demonstrates the presence and direction of shunting across the interatrial septum that can be verified by pulsedwave Doppler. This assessment also assists in the characterization of the flow across an interatrial communication in terms of the presence or absence of restriction (Fig. 7.3, Video 7.3). Slight probe withdrawal may be required to visualize small superior secundum defects, or probe advancement for small inferior

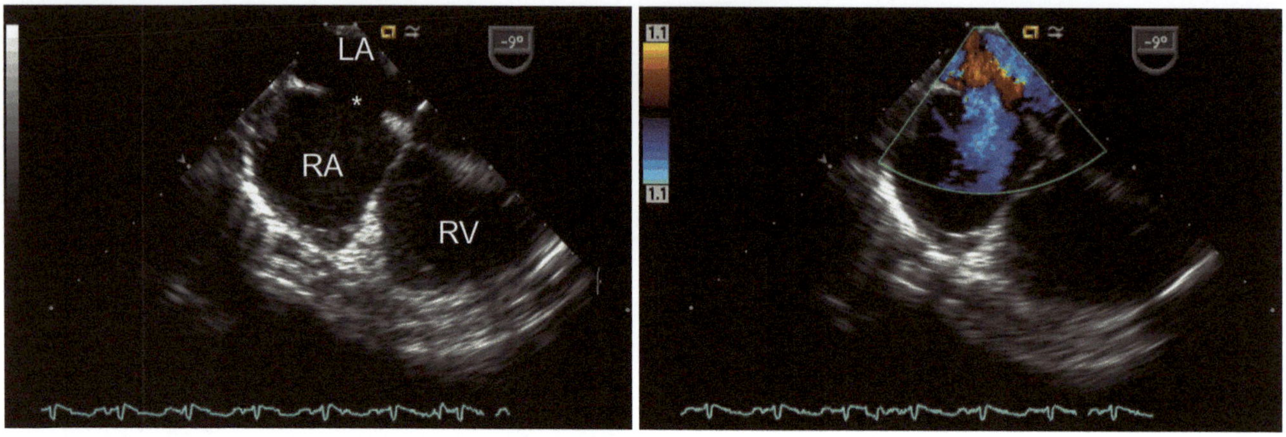

Fig. 7.2 *Left panel:* Centrally located secundum atrial septal defect (*asterisk*) shown as seen in the mid esophageal four chamber view. *Right panl:* Color flow Doppler interrogation demonstrates left-to-right shunting across the defect (*blue signal*). Note that the probe has been rotated rightwards in this view to focus on the atrial communication. *LA* left atrium, *RA* right atrium, *RV* right ventricle

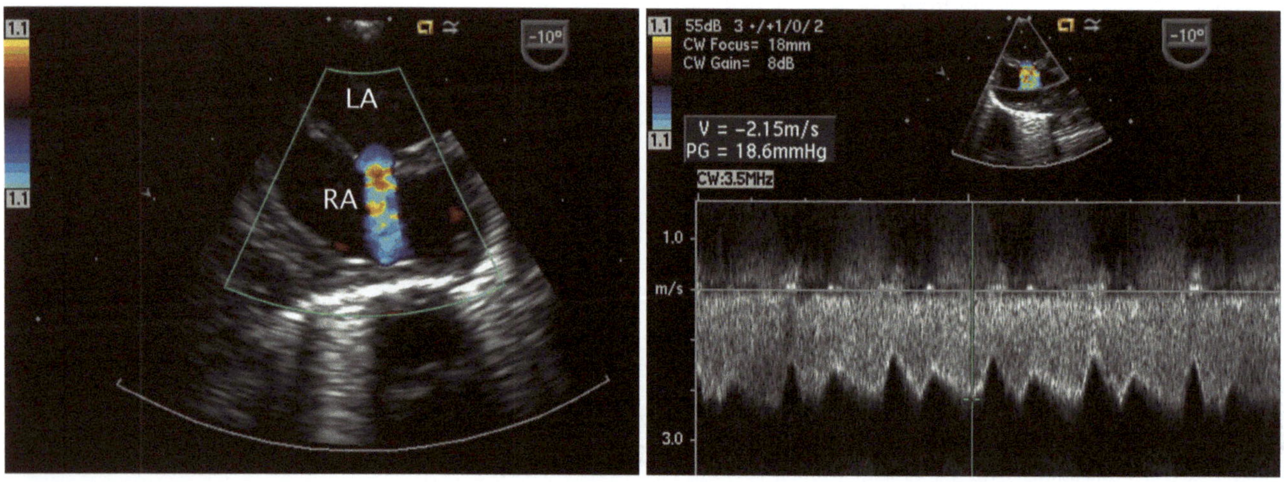

Fig. 7.3 *Left panel:* Image of the interatrial septum in the mid esophageal four chamber view with rightwards probe rotation. Note the aliased nature (mosaic of colors) of the jet across the atrial communication consistent with restriction across a small secundum atrial septal defect. The interatrial septum bulges in the rightwards direction suggesting elevated left atrial pressures. *Right panel:* Spectral Doppler interrogation confirms the restricted, high velocity flow across the defect with reduced phasic variation. *LA* left atrium, *RA* right atrium

secundum defects. Minimal probe shaft movements enhance the 2D evaluation allowing for examination of the defect in relation to adjacent structures as well as interrogation of the rims of the defect (Fig. 7.4). At times, smaller and/or more eccentric atrial defects will be detected in a standard TEE view (e.g. ME 4 Ch) *only* when a thorough sweep is performed of the septum. This emphasizes the importance of full sweeps when assessing communications at the atrial septum, as well as many other defects (Video 7.4).

Progressive withdrawal of the probe in the ME 4 Ch view to above the level of the fossa ovalis demonstrates the superior aspect of the interatrial septum—the location of superior sinus venosus defects (Fig. 7.5, Video 7.5)—as well as the superior vena cava in cross-section. Anomalous drainage of the pulmonary veins as they enter the vena cavae can be seen from these views and attempts to visualize all veins should be made. The ME 4 Ch view also allows for 2D assessment

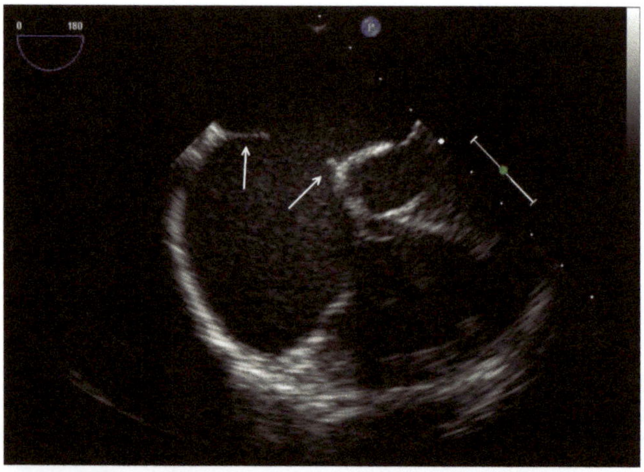

Fig. 7.4 Image displays the rims (*arrows*) of a secundum atrial septal defect in the mid esophageal four chamber view with slight rightwards probe rotation

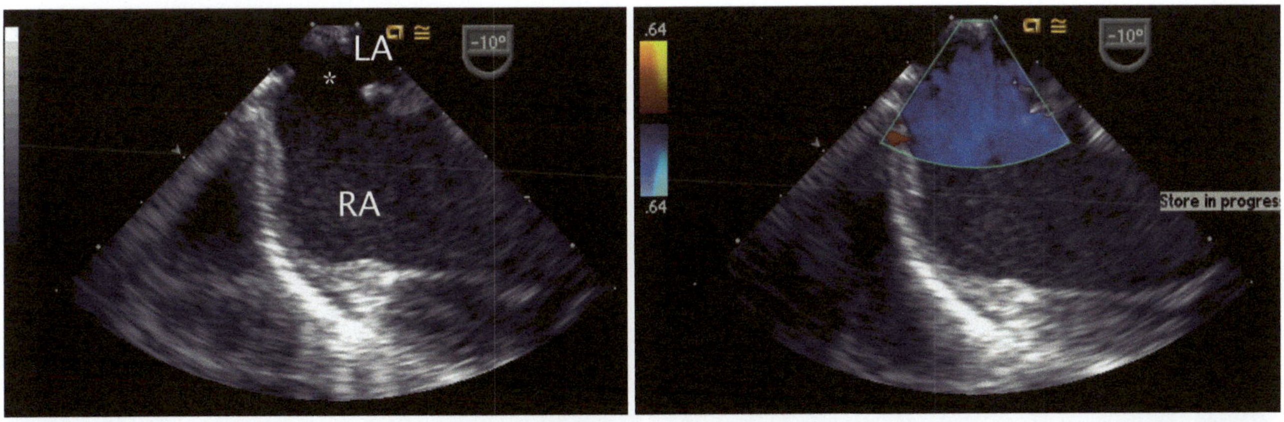

Fig. 7.5 *Left panel:* Superior sinus venosus atrial septal defect (*asterisk*) as seen by withdrawal of the imaging probe above the level of the fossa ovalis from a mid esophageal position. *Right panel:* Color Doppler imaging demonstrating flow across the defect. *LA* left atrium, *RA* right atrium

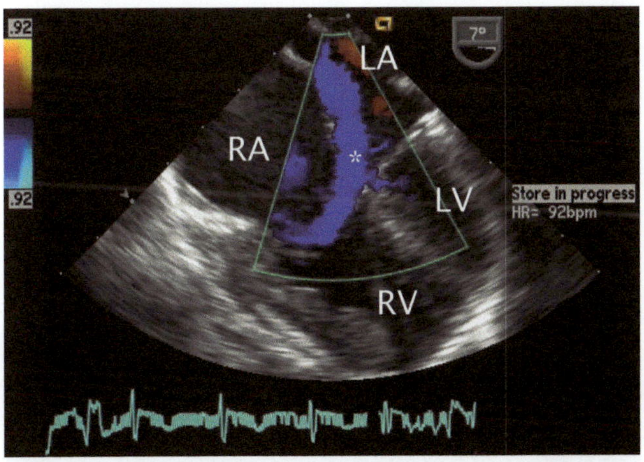

Fig. 7.6 Color Doppler image displaying left-to-right shunting across a primum atrial septal defect (*asterisk*) in the mid esophageal four chamber view. *LA* left atrium, *LV* left ventricle, *RA* right atrium, *RV* right ventricle

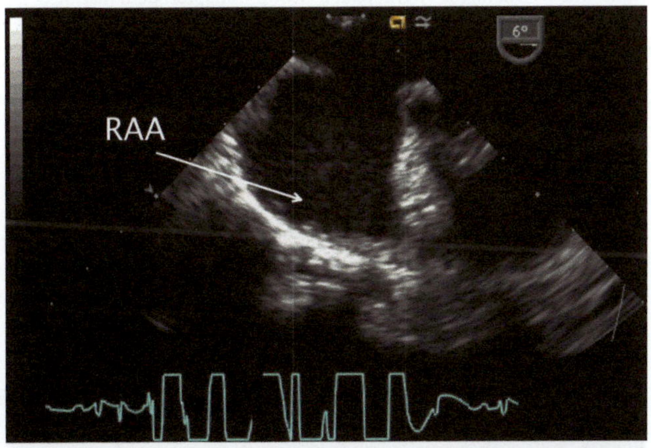

Fig. 7.7 Transesophageal image displaying the broad-based right atrial appendage (*RAA*). There is also a moderate to large secundum atrial septal defect present

of primum ASDs and Doppler interrogation of the atrioventricular valves (Fig. 7.6, Video 7.6; discussed in detail in Chap. 8).

Clockwise turning of the probe in the ME 4 Ch view visualizes the remainder of the RA. The proximal aspect of the right atrial appendage (RAA) can be seen with slight probe withdrawal (Fig. 7.7, Video 7.7), in addition to portions of the tricuspid valve and right ventricular inflow (Fig. 7.8, Video 7.8) with clockwise probe shaft rotation. Tricuspid valve inflow and the degree of tricuspid regurgitation can be assessed from this window as well as in the mid esophageal right ventricular inflow-outflow (ME RV In-Out) and transgastric right ventricular inflow (TG RV In) views. Determination of the Doppler peak velocity of tricuspid regurgitation can be used to estimate right ventricular and pulmonary artery systolic pressures. Pulmonary artery diastolic pressure may be predicted by measurement of theend-diastolic velocity of pulmonary regurgitation from the ME RV In-Out, mid esophageal aortic valve short axis (ME AV SAX), or deep transgastric sagittal (DTG Sagittal) views. Increased tricuspid valve inflow and pulmonary outflow Doppler velocities may be seen within the context of large ASDs with significantly increased pulmonary to systemic blood flow (Qp:Qs) ratios. Increased flow across these structures does not necessarily represent valvar stenosis and in most cases are regarded as 'flow-related gradients'. Pulmonary hypertension is quite rare, but may occur in patients with isolated ASDs over a period of many years.

Returning to the ME 4 Ch view, sometimes requiring slight further clockwise turning, as well as advancement or withdrawal of the probe, connection of the right pulmonary veins to the LA posteriorly can be demonstrated (Figs. 7.9 and 7.10, Videos 7.9 and 7.10; also refer to Chap. 6).

The sweep continues from the ME 4 Ch view with counterclockwise turning of the probe shaft to better visualize the LA (Fig. 7.11, Video 7.11). Probe advancement and retroflexion will enhance visualization of the coronary sinus and

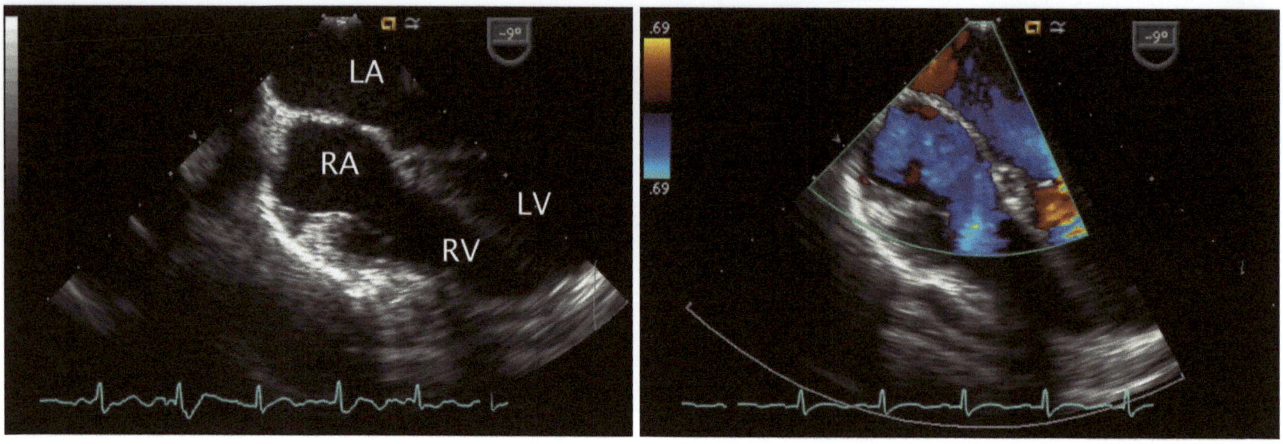

Fig. 7.8 *Left panel:* Image obtained by turning of the imaging probe from the mid esophageal four chamber view clockwise to visualize right-sided structures. *Right panel:* Color Doppler demonstrates an intact atrial septum and laminar tricuspid inflow in this example. *LA* left atrium, *LV* left ventricle, *RA* right atrium, *RV* right ventricle

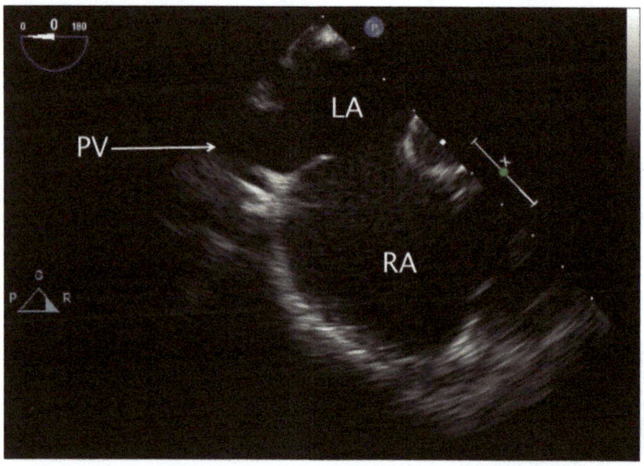

Fig. 7.9 Mid esophageal view with clockwise probe shaft rotation to examine the right pulmonary venous connections (*PV*) into the left atrium (*LA*). *RA* right atrium

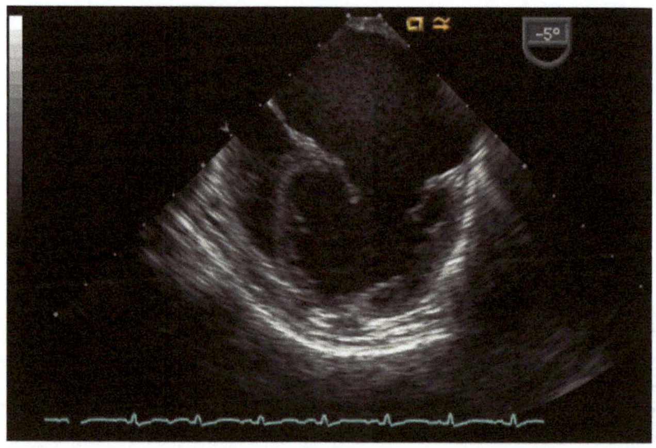

Fig. 7.11 Mid esophageal four chamber image obtained with counterclockwise rotation of the imaging probe demonstrates the left atrium (dilated due to mitral regurgitation in this example)

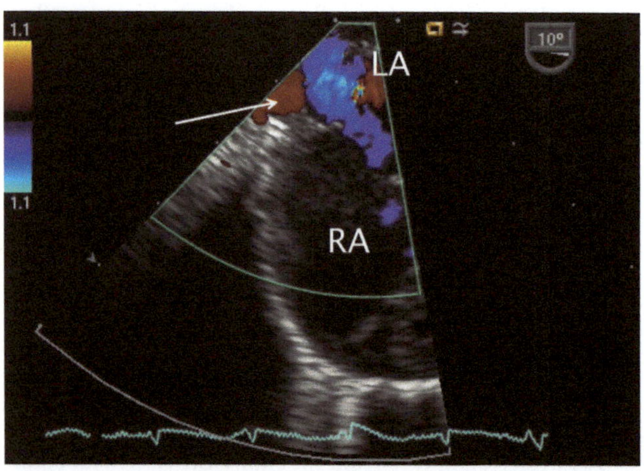

Fig. 7.10 Color flow Doppler in a similar plane as shown in Fig. 7.9 to assess drainage of the right upper pulmonary vein (*red color* flow shown by *arrow*) into the left atrium (*LA*). *RA* right atrium

identify areas of unroofing, if present. Continued further counterclockwise rotation of the probe in conjunction with advancement or withdrawal demonstrates the left pulmonary venous connections to the left atrial posterior-lateral wall (Fig. 7.12, Video 7.12). Color and pulsed wave Doppler can be applied to facilitate this assessment (Fig. 7.13, Video 7.13). Pulmonary vein stenosis, although rare in most uncomplicated ASDs, may be suggested by aliasing/turbulence by color Doppler (Fig. 7.14, Video 7.14). This finding should be confirmed by spectral Doppler interrogation. This view may demonstrate a dilated coronary sinus in cross section if a persistent left superior vena cava to coronary sinus connection is present (Fig. 7.15, Video 7.15). Anterior to the entry of the left pulmonary veins with slight probe withdrawal to nearly a ME AV SAX plane, the proximal portion of the left atrial appendage (LAA) can be seen from this window (Fig. 7.16, Video 7.16). Forward axial rotation of the

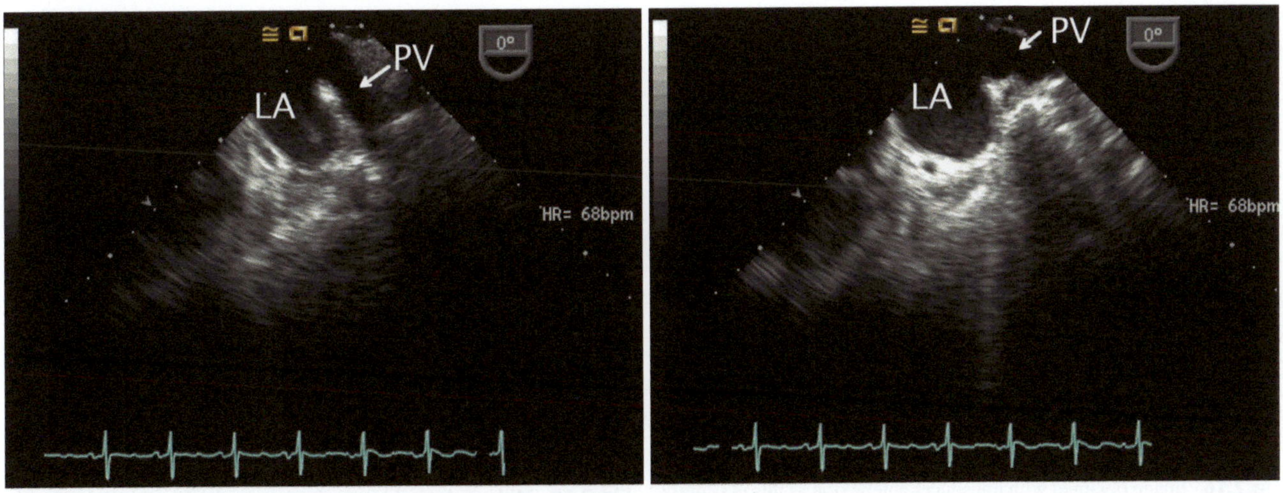

Fig. 7.12 The courses of two left sided pulmonary veins (*PV*) into the left atrium (*LA*) are demonstrated. *Left panel:* The left upper pulmonary vein is seen coursing in an anterior to posterior direction. *Right panel:* The more horizontal course of the left lower vein is demonstrated as it runs lateral to medial. Note the two different orientations of these veins as they enter the left atrium

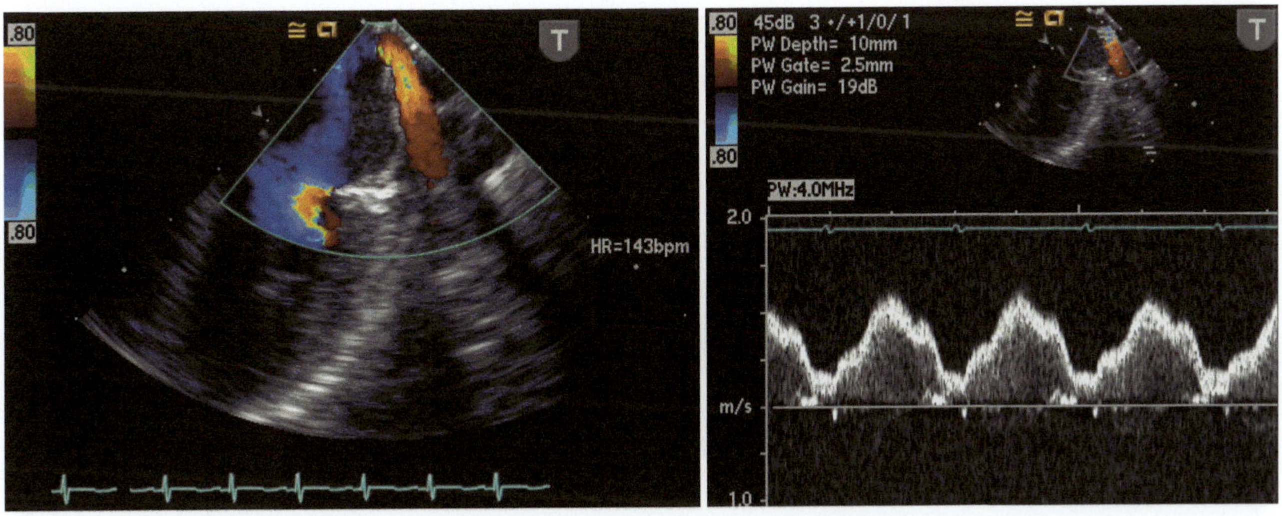

Fig. 7.13 Color flow Doppler imaging (*left panel*) and spectral tracing (*right panel*) complements the two-dimensional evaluation of the pulmonary veins. Note the characteristic normal systolic and diastolic nature of the pulmonary venous flow

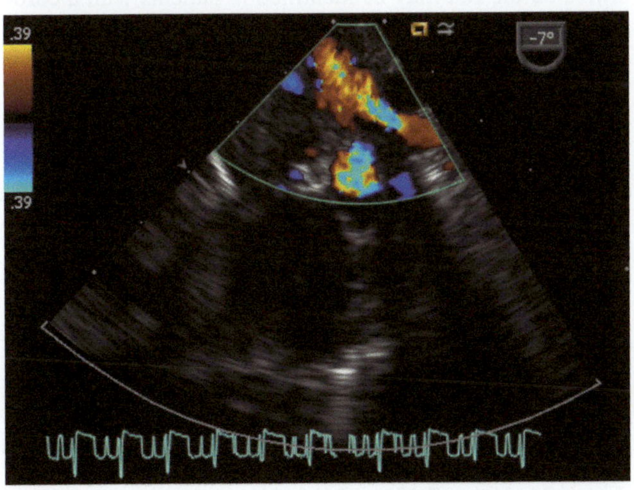

Fig. 7.14 Transesophageal color Doppler image of the left upper pulmonary vein as it courses towards the let atrium. Aliasing is seen by color flow interrogation that should prompt further investigation, including spectral Doppler interrogation

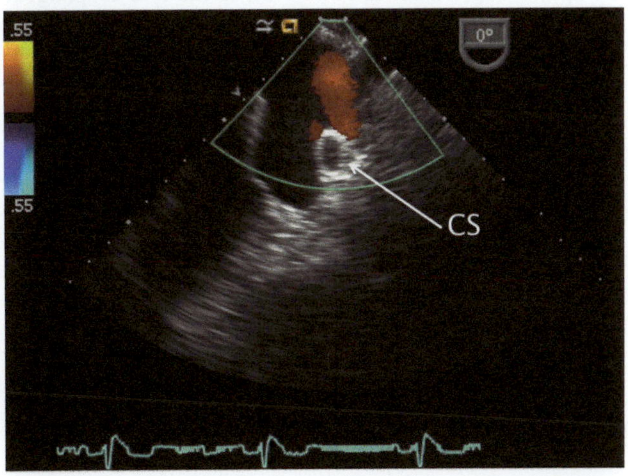

Fig. 7.15 Image displays a dilated coronary sinus (*CS, arrow*) as seen in cross-section (*arrow*) below the left pulmonary venous inflow. This may indicate the presence of a persistent left superior vena cava

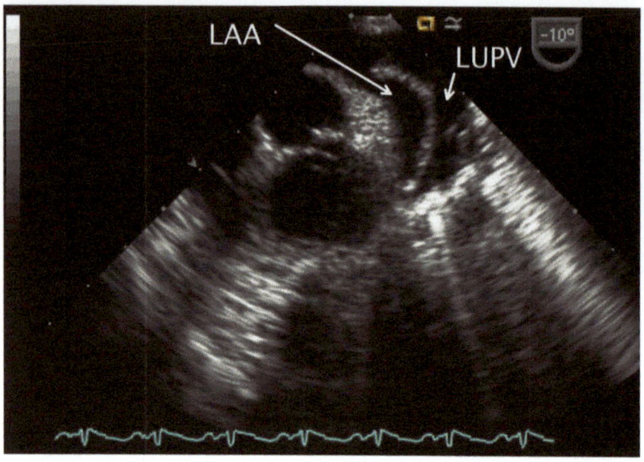

Fig. 7.16 Image obtained with transducer anteflexion as this is slightly withdrawn to a nearly mid esophageal aortic valve short axis plane. This cross-section displays the left atrial appendage (*LAA*) anteriorly located in relation to the left upper pulmonary vein (*LUPV*)

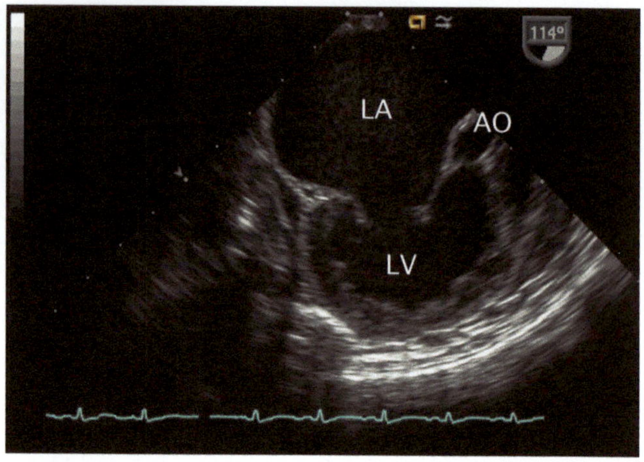

Fig. 7.18 Mid esophageal long axis view (multiplane angle 114°) corresponding to same patient displayed in Fig. 7.11. This image confirms the large dimensions of the left atrium (*LA*) and displays the left ventricle (*LV*) and aortic root (*AO*).

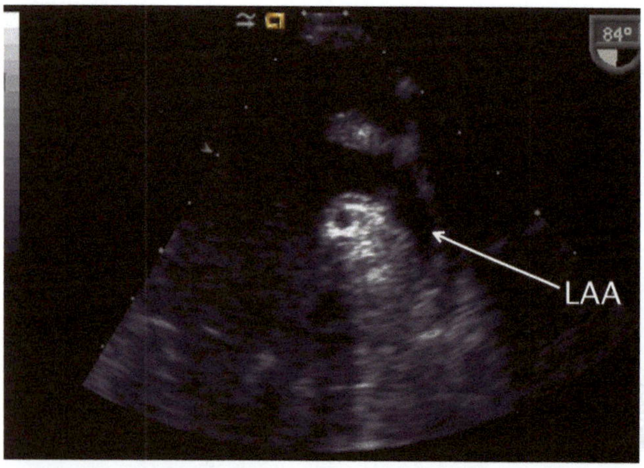

Fig. 7.17 Mid esophageal two chamber view demonstrating the anterior position (*arrow*) of the left atrial appendage (*LAA*)

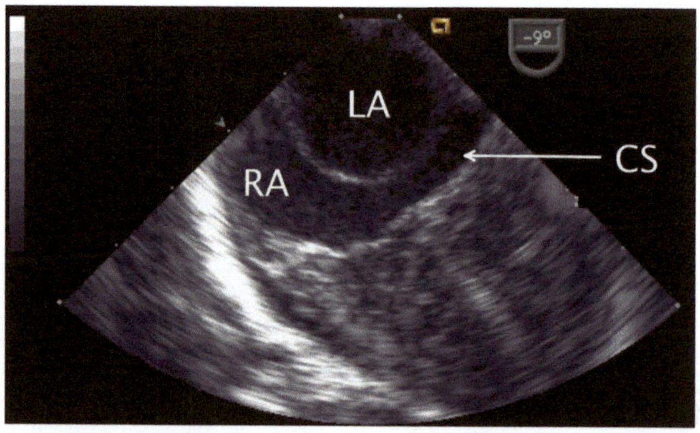

Fig. 7.19 Image obtained after slightly advancing the probe in the mid esophageal four chamber view. The coronary sinus (*CS*) in seen in long axis as it courses along the atrioventricular groove to drain into the right atrium (*RA*). *LA* left atrium

multiplane angle from the ME 4 Ch to the mid esophageal two chamber (ME 2 Ch) view (angle ~90°) displays the LA in an orthogonal plane and the LAA in long axis (Fig. 7.17, Video 7.17). Further counterclockwise turning of the TEE probe may visualize a left superior vena cava in long axis if one is present. From the ME 2 Ch plane forward transducer rotation displays a mid esophageal long axis (ME LAX) view (angle ~110°) and demonstrates the LA, mitral valve, and left ventricular outflow (Fig. 7.18, Video 7.18).

Slight advancement of the probe in the ME 4 Ch will allow for visualization successively of the coronary sinus as it courses longitudinally along the posterior atrioventricular groove (Fig. 7.19, Video 7.19), along with the coronary sinus orifice as it normally drains into the RA, and the lower portion of the interatrial septum. This is also the area where deficiency of atrial septal tissue surrounding the coronary sinus orifice on the RA may be identified in patients with a coronary sinus-type ASD. A dilated coronary sinus should not be confused for a primum ASD. Agitated saline injection into a left arm vein or left jugular vein will demonstrate contrast in the coronary sinus and drainage into the RA if a persistent left superior vena cava to coronary sinus connection is present (Fig. 7.20, Video 7.20) (Chap. 6).

From the ME 4 Ch view, clockwise turning of the probe and forward angle rotation displays the mid esophageal bicaval (ME Bicaval) view, angle ~90°–110°. This provides an excellent cross-section of the entire atrial septum (superior to inferior) (Figs. 7.21 and 7.22, Videos 7.21 and 7.22). The majority of the interatrial septum will be oriented optimally with respect to 2D and Doppler imaging from this view. This window is ideal for confirming the presence of superior (Fig. 7.23, Video 7.23) and inferior sinus venosus defects,

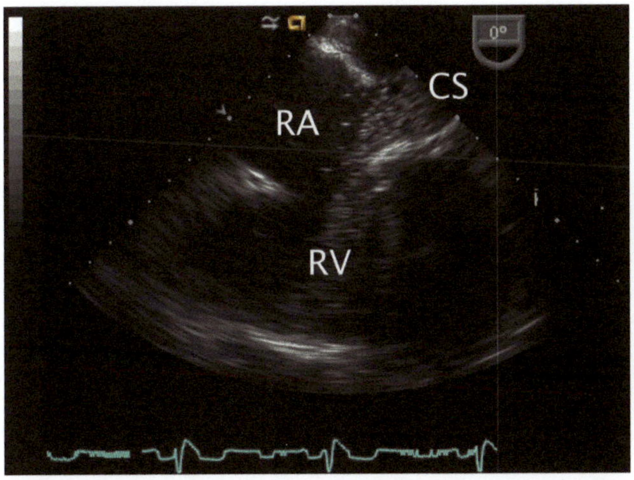

Fig. 7.20 Injection of agitated saline into a left arm vein in a patient with a persistent left superior vena cava demonstrating contrast in the coronary sinus (*CS*) thus confirming the connection. *RA* right atrium, *RV* right ventricle

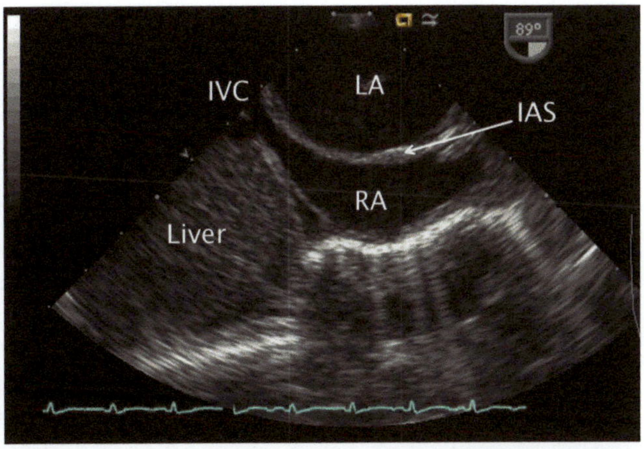

Fig. 7.22 Image of a mid esophageal bicaval view displaying a dilated left atrium (*LA*) with bulging of the interatrial septum (*IAS*) towards the right atrium (*RA*). The inferior vena cava (*IVC*) is also seen in this view it enters the RA

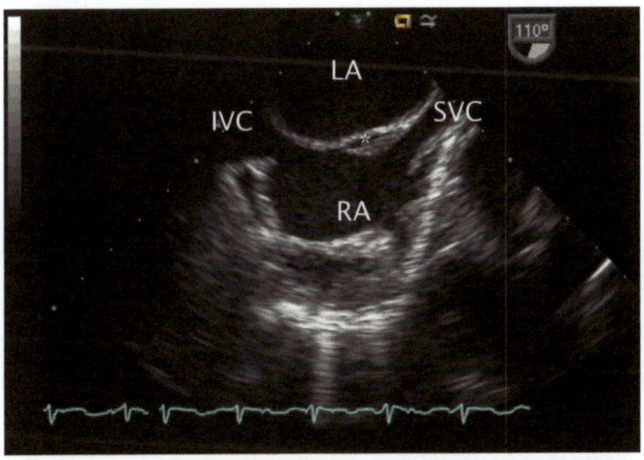

Fig. 7.21 Mid esophageal bicaval view displaying the entire atrial septum. The flap valve of the foramen is well seen (*asterisk*). *IVC* inferior vena cava, *LA* left atrium, *RA* right atrium, *SVC* superior vena cava

secundum defects (Figs. 7.24, 7.25, and 7.26, Videos 7.24, 7.25, and 7.26), and a PFO [42–44]. As mentioned, contrast echocardiography with a Valsalva (or simulated Valsalva maneuver during mechanical ventilation) may be required for the detection of shunting across a PFO.

Slight clockwise/counterclockwise probe turning from the ME Bicaval view may be necessary to optimally visualize an ASD depending upon its size and location. Withdrawal of the probe while in this view displays the superior vena cava in long axis. Probe advancement provides long axis imaging of the inferior vena cava (Fig. 7.22, Video 7.22). Anomalous pulmonary veins entering either vena cavae may be seen from these views with appropriate probe withdrawal and/or advancement (Fig. 7.27, Video 7.27)

While in the ME 4 Ch view, advancement of the probe displays the lower esophageal situs short axis (LE Situs SAX) view. The junction of the inferior vena cava into the RA and upper portion of the vena cava can be seen in this cross-section. Further clockwise turning of the probe may be necessary during this sweep. This view can also be useful in the assessment of inferior vena cava-type of sinus venosus defects and anomalous pulmonary veins entering the vena cava.

Forward axial rotation of the imaging probe through the ME RV In-Out view (angle ~60°), allows more complete anatomic assessment of the tricuspid valve, right atrial, and ventricular size, and right ventricular outflow tract and pulmonary valve. This view is particularly helpful to demonstrate right ventricular volume overload and systolic function (Fig. 7.28, Video 7.28) in the setting of communications at the atrial level. The transgastric mid short axis (TG Mid SAX) view also provides information regarding right ventricular size and magnitude of atrial level shunting in these lesions (Fig. 7.29, Video 7.29).

Further views of the interatrial septum can also be obtained from the deep transgastric window. Once the DTG Sagittal view is obtained (angle ~90°–100°) clockwise probe rotation as necessary allows for the entire interatrial septum to be displayed; the multiplane angle can be adjusted for optimal visualization of the atrial septum (Figs. 7.30, 7.31, and 7.32, Videos 7.30, 7.31, and 7.32). The deep transgastric windows complement the assessments of ASDs (Fig. 7.33, Video 7.33) and in some cases allow for details of the anatomy not visualized in other views to be demonstrated.

Evaluation of right atrial and right ventricular size, which generally reflect the relative volume of left-to-right shunting through an ASD, provides a qualitative assessment of the clinical significance of the defect. Pertinent TEE windows

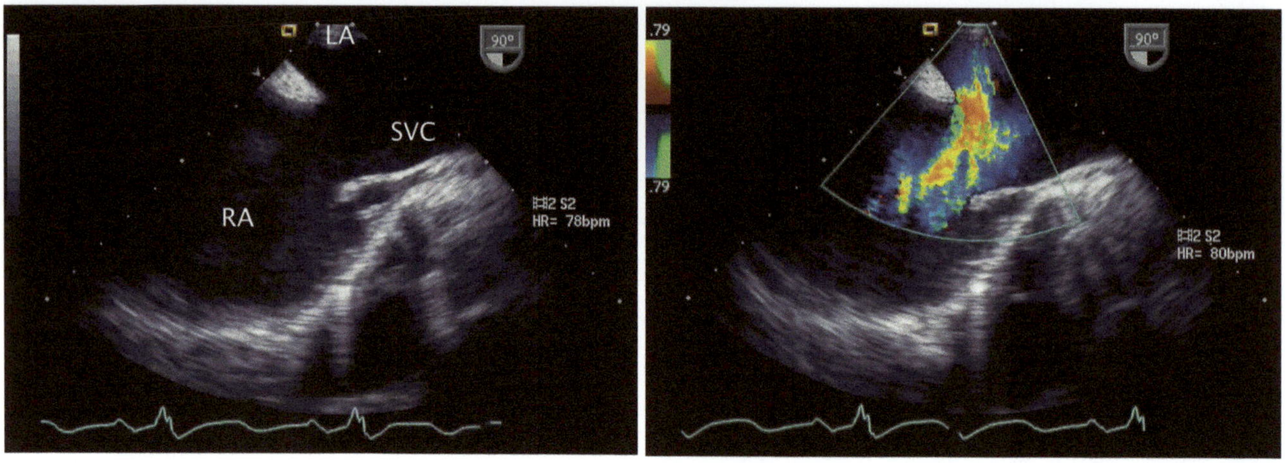

Fig. 7.23 *Left panel:* Two-dimensional image of a superior sinus venosus defect in the mid esophageal bicaval view. The superior vena cava (*SVC*) frequently straddles the interatrial septum in this defect. *Right panel:* Color flow Doppler confirms left-to-right shunting across the atrial communication. *LA* left atrium, *RA* right atrium

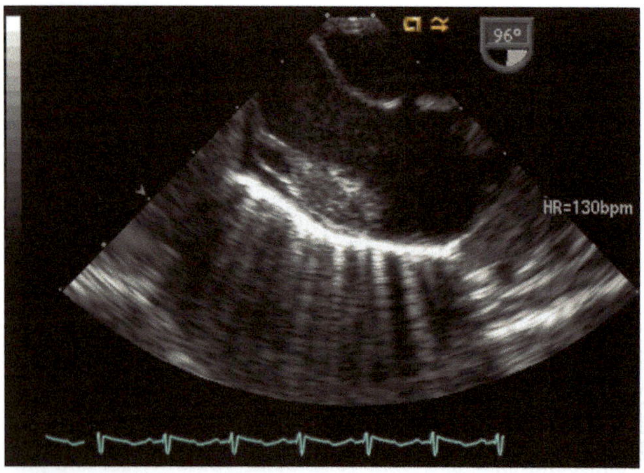

Fig. 7.24 Small secundum atrial septal defect as shown in the mid esophageal bicaval view

include: at the mid esophageal level the 4 Ch, RV In-Out and Bicaval views (Fig. 7.34, Video 7.34); at the transgastric level the RV In, Basal SAX, and Mid SAX views; and at the deep transgastric window the DTG Sagittal view and modified cross-sections. Qualitative assessment of right and left ventricular systolic function and color and spectral Doppler evaluation of associated lesions, as appropriate, are also indicated. Normal biventricular systolic function with flattening of the interventricular septum in diastole is a common finding in defects resulting in right ventricular volume overload.

The considerations in the echocardiographic assessment of atrial level communications are summarized in Table 7.1.

Surgical and Transcatheter Considerations

Preprocedure Assessment

Preoperative TEE evaluation focuses on confirming the size and location of the ASD, exclusion of additional congenital cardiac lesions, and assessment of atrial and ventricular chamber size and ventricular systolic function. Pulmonary venous anatomy should be evaluated, particularly in patients with sinus venosus ASDs. Care should be taken not to mistake a redundant Eustachian valve in the RA for the atrial septum and potentially misdiagnose an ASD that does not exist. Likewise, as discussed, a dilated coronary sinus should not be interpreted to represent a primum-type communication. Doppler evaluation of the atrial shunt and quantitation of the degree and peak velocity of tricuspid regurgitation should be performed.

In patients with a secundum ASD or PFO deemed suitable for transcatheter device closure, TEE evaluation includes size and location of the communication, evaluation of adequacy of atrial septal tissue rims (particularly the retroaortic rim), exclusion of additional septal defects, evaluation for atrial septal aneurysm (Fig. 7.35, Video 7.35), and assessment of ventricular chamber size and function [45–50]. The relationship of the defect to the vena cavae and atrioventricular valves and balloon sizing of the ASD or tunnel length of the PFO for suitable device selection are also important features to be evaluated. These considerations are discussed in detail Chap. 17.

For some severe forms of CHD, an ASD is actually necessary to maintain a physiology compatible with survival. In these types of patients, restrictive or non-existent atrial communications may require catheter-based interventions. These are aimed at either creating or enlarging an atrial communication allowing for either enhanced mixing of systemic and pulmonary venous blood (e.g. d-transposition of the great arteries) or decompression of venous return typically in cases of atrioventricular valve stenosis or atresia (Fig. 7.36, Video 7.36). These interventions might also benefit from TEE guidance, particularly in infants, as this patient group may be quite ill. TEE may limit radiation exposure and enhance the safety of these procedures.

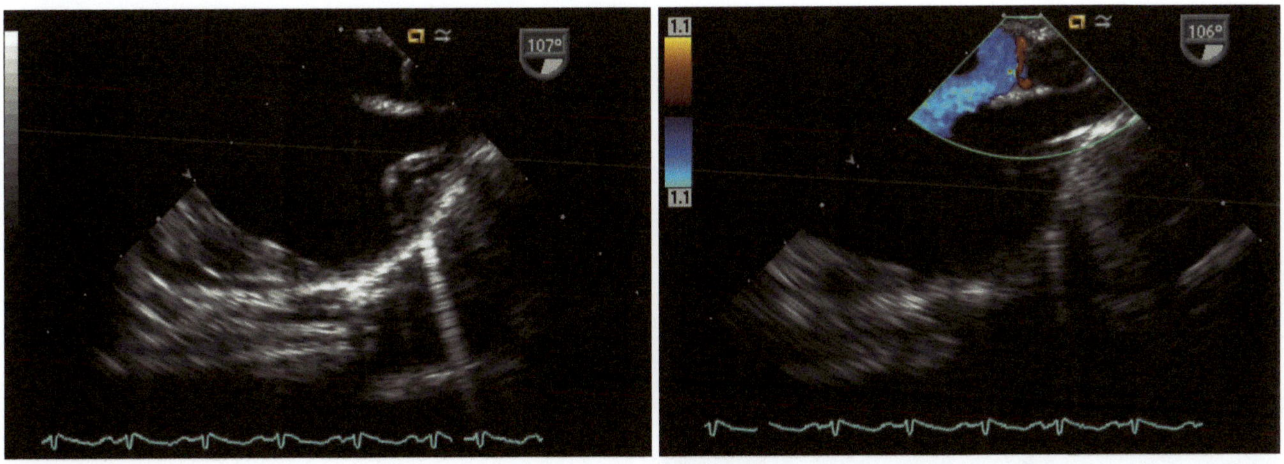

Fig. 7.25 Images demonstrate a high secundum atrial septal defect in the mid esophageal bicaval view (*left panel*) and corresponding color flow Doppler (*right panel*)

Fig. 7.26 Large secundum atrial septal defect (*left panel*) with associated left-to-right shunting (*right panel*). Note the slightly more inferior location of this defect as compared to the communication illustrated in a similar imaging plane in Fig. 7.25

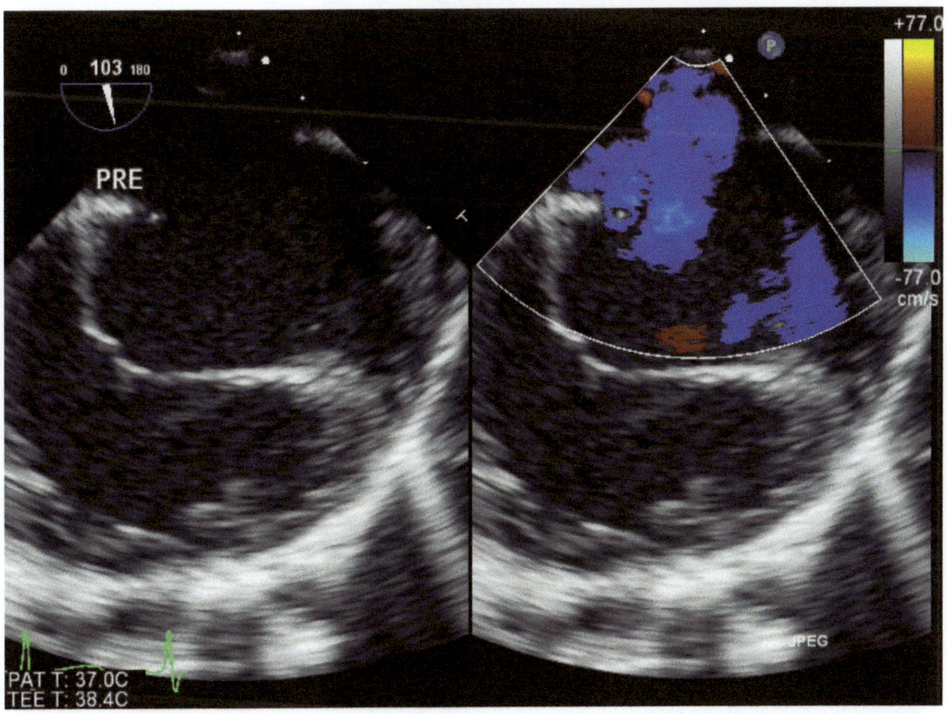

Postprocedure Assessment

Postoperative evaluation following surgical closure of an ASD begins with confirmation of adequate cardiac de-airing. Evaluation of the surgical repair involves exclusion of residual atrial level shunting (Figs. 7.37 and 7.38, Videos 7.37 and 7.38), quantification of atrioventricular valve regurgitation, and assessment of ventricular systolic function following weaning from cardiopulmonary bypass. In surgeries involving closure of sinus venosus ASDs with redirection of anomalous pulmonary veins it is very important to exclude vena caval or pulmonary venous obstruction post repair [51–53].

TEE is useful for ASD/PFO occlusion device positioning and during deployment confirms the adequacy of device position after release. Postdevice evaluation includes: (1) assessment of residual shunting, (2) evaluation of the vena cava and right pulmonary veins to exclude impingement of the device into these structures, and (3) Doppler assessment of atrioventricular valve inflow and regurgitation, and aortic valve regurgitation (particularly in cases with small retroaortic septal rims where the device arms straddle the aortic root). Ventricular systolic function should also be evaluated. Also refer to Chap. 17 for an in depth discussion of this subject.

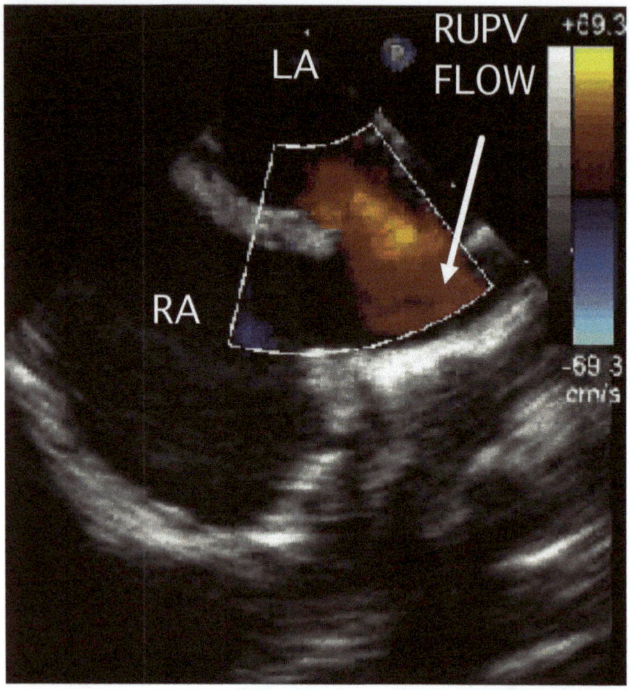

Fig. 7.27 Image demonstrates flow from the right upper pulmonary vein (*RUPV*) directed towards the superior vena cava-right atrial junction in a superior sinus venosus defect. *LA* left atrium, *RA* right atrium. Image courtesy of Thomas M. Burch, MD

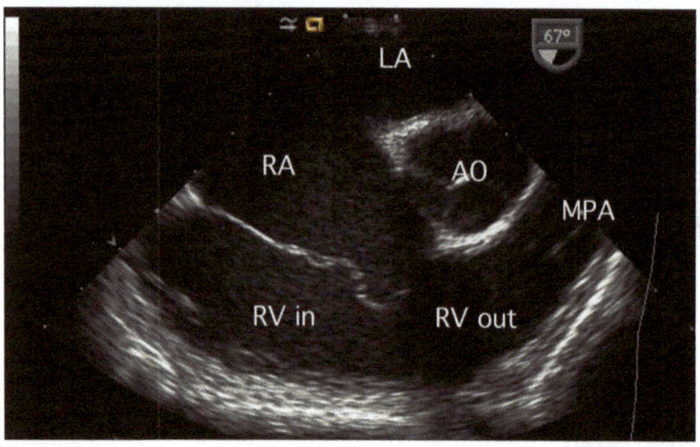

Fig. 7.28 Image of a mid esophageal right ventricular inflow-outflow view. This cross-section is useful in the comprehensive assessment of atrial septal defects as it displays the tricuspid valve, left atrium (*LA*), right atrial (*RA*) and right ventricular (*RV*) sizes, right ventricular inflow (*RV in*) and outflow (*RV out*) tract, pulmonary valve, and proximal main pulmonary artery (*MPA*). *AO* aorta

Juxtaposition of the Atrial Appendages

The atrial appendages normally lie on opposite sides of the roots of the great arteries. Juxtaposition of the atrial appendages, in which both appendages are oriented side by side on either the right ("right juxtaposition"), or much more commonly on the left ("left juxtaposition") was first described in 1954 [54]. This atrial anomaly is quite rare (found in ~0.8 % of congenital heart lesions). In most cases the atria are otherwise usually arranged (rarely, it is seen in left atrial isomerism) [55, 56]. Left juxtaposition is generally felt to be more

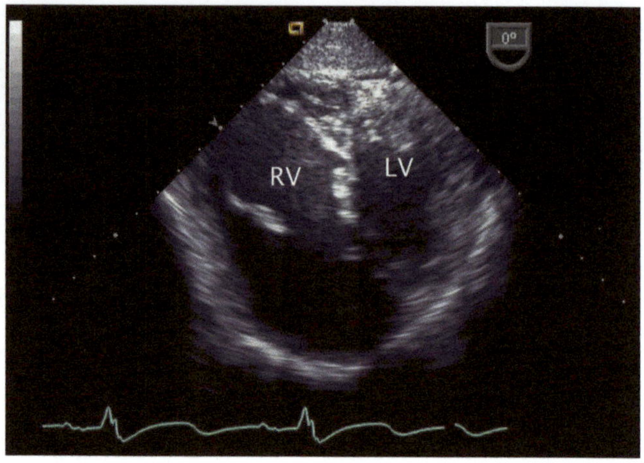

Fig. 7.29 Transgastric mid short-axis view demonstrating a large, volume loaded right ventricle (*RV*) in a patient with a large atrial septal defect. *LV left ventricle*

significant clinically [57, 58]. Juxtaposition of the atrial appendages is generally not seen in isolation, usually being found in conjunction with other complex congenital cardiac lesions, with left juxtaposition most commonly found in association with cyanotic conditions such as transposition of the great arteries, tricuspid atresia, and heterotaxy syndromes [55, 56, 59–61]. There is often some degree of hypoplasia of the right heart structures. Right juxtaposition has been described in conjunction with double outlet right ventricle and ventricular septal defect [61]. Although not hemodynamically significant *perse*, juxtaposition of the atrial appendages may have implications for catheter-based interventions as well as surgical procedures. Juxtaposed atrial appendages may be confused with an ASD if the abnormal septal configuration is not recognized [62–64].

Non invasive diagnosis of left juxtaposition of the atrial appendages is possible by TTE, however it represents a challenging diagnosis requiring a high level of suspicion [65]. Echocardiographic features include: (1) abnormalities of the plane of the atrial septum and (2) direct visualization of the abnormally oriented atrial appendage coursing anterior to the atria and posterior to the great arteries. TEE can provide further anatomic confirmation of this lesion in most cases [60].

Transesophageal Echocardiographic Evaluation

An important consideration in the TEE evaluation of this anomaly is recognition of the characteristic morphologic features of the atrial appendages and the normal orientation of the atrial septum [66]. Normally, the RAA is broad-based and displays a triangular shape (Fig. 7.7, Video 7.7), whereas the LAA is narrow-based relative to the remainder of the atrium and has an elongated shape (Fig. 7.16, Video 7.16). The abnormal orientation of the appendages in juxtaposition can be suspected/confirmed by recognizing these unique morphologies. In addition the abnormal orientation of the

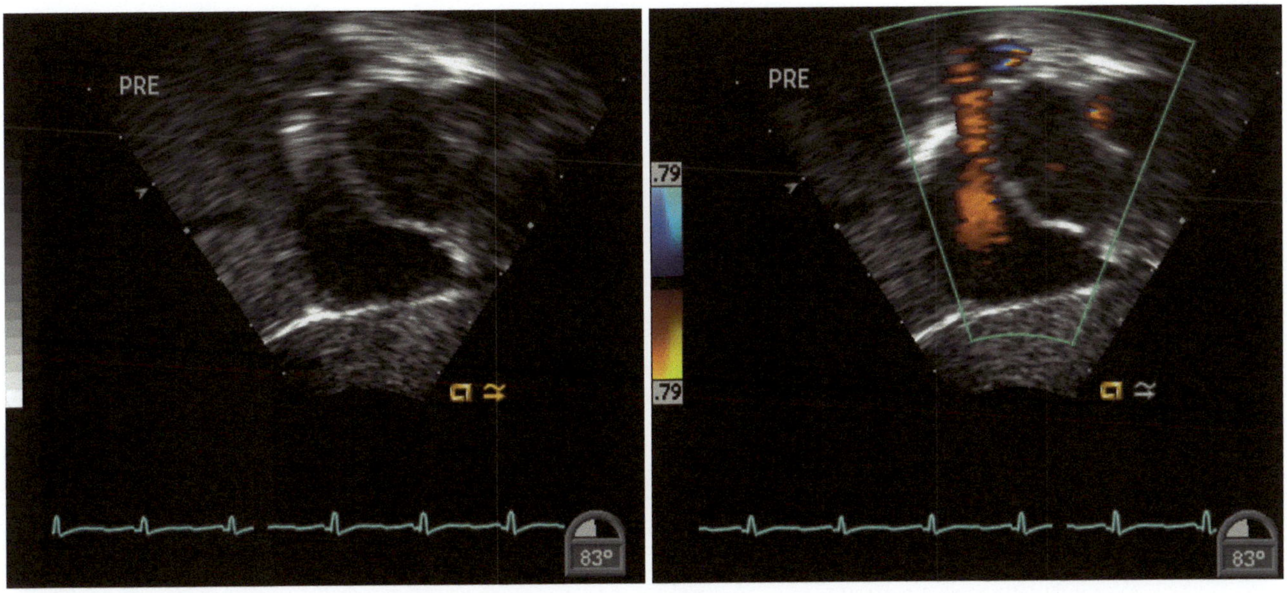

Fig. 7.30 Deep transgastric sagittal images of the atrial septum displaying two-dimensional (*left panel*) and color information (*right panel*). The interatrial septum appears intact by two-dimensional imaging

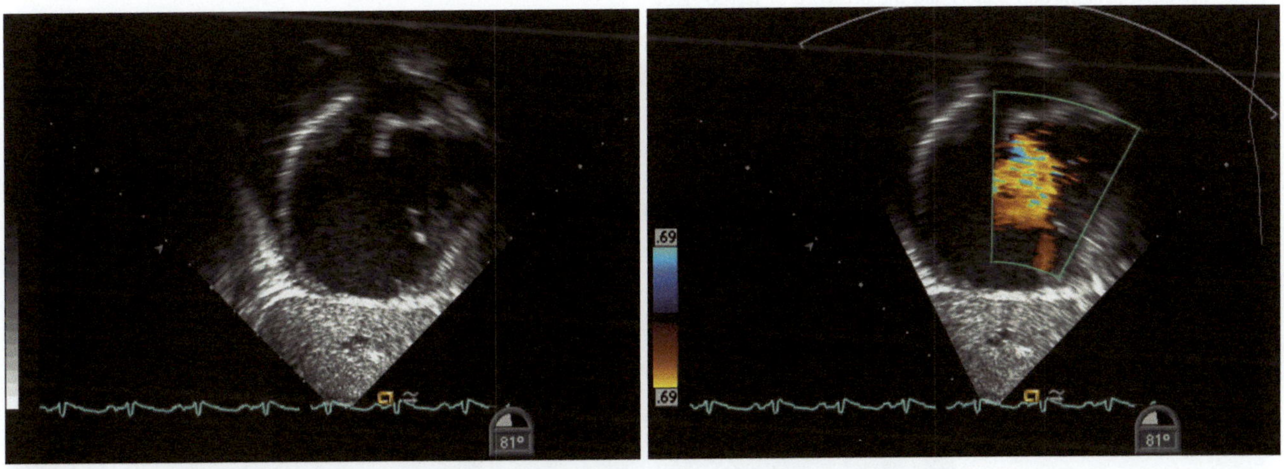

Fig. 7.31 Images obtained in the same cross-sections as shown in Fig. 7.30. In this example, the presence of a secundum atrial septal defect is demonstrated

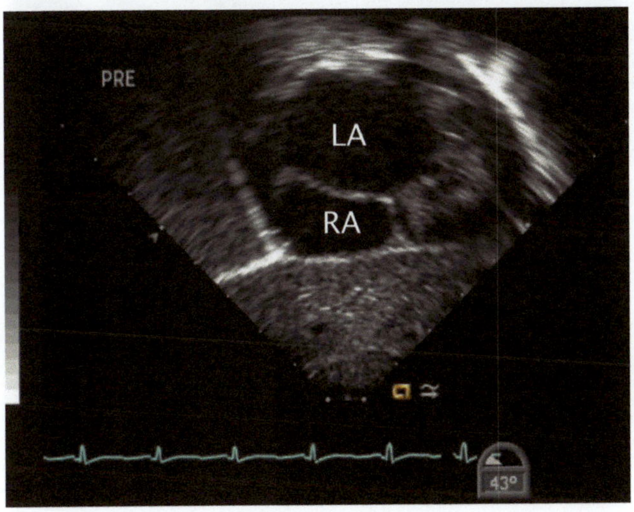

Fig. 7.32 The image displays a modified plane in the deep transgastric window that also allows for echocardiographic assessment of the interatrial septum. *LA* left atrium, *RA* right atrium

interatrial septum may provide a clue. The characteristic findings in left juxtaposition of the atrial appendages are lateral deviation of the posterior portion of the atrial septum (Fig. 7.39, Video 7.39) and a right to left horizontal (frontal) orientation of the antero-superior portion of the atrial septum that forms the posterior wall of the junction of the RAA with the atrial cavity [60]. These features are best demonstrated from several views.

The atrial septum is well seen from ME 4 Ch view, which in this anomaly would display the frontal deviation of the superior septum and opening of the left-deviated RAA behind the posterior great artery and anterior to the body of the LA (Fig. 7.40, Video 7.40). It should be emphasized that assessment of this anomaly in the ME 4 Ch view requires sweeps spanning multiple planes from the posterior to the anterior aspect of the heart. The characteristic echocardiographic features of juxtaposed appendages can also be seen

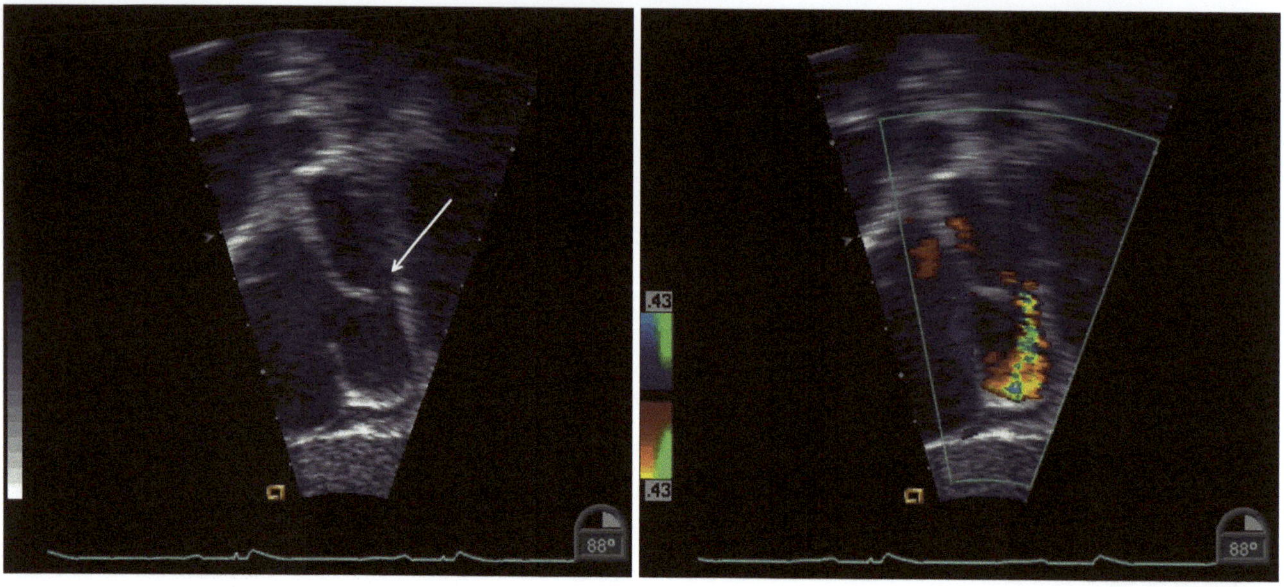

Fig. 7.33 Images of an inferior sinus venosus defect as obtained from a modified deep transgastric sagittal view (same view as shown in Figs. 7.30 and 7.31). Note the deficiency (*arrow*) in the inferior aspect of the interatrial septum (*left panel*) and the presence of left-to-right shunting across this region (*right panel*). The Eustachian valve is also seen. Additional planes in this window may provide information regarding associated anomalies of pulmonary venous drainage

Fig. 7.34 Mid esophageal images in orthogonal planes that assist in the determination of right ventricular (*RV*) size and function. Moderate right ventricular dilation is shown. (*LV*) left ventricle

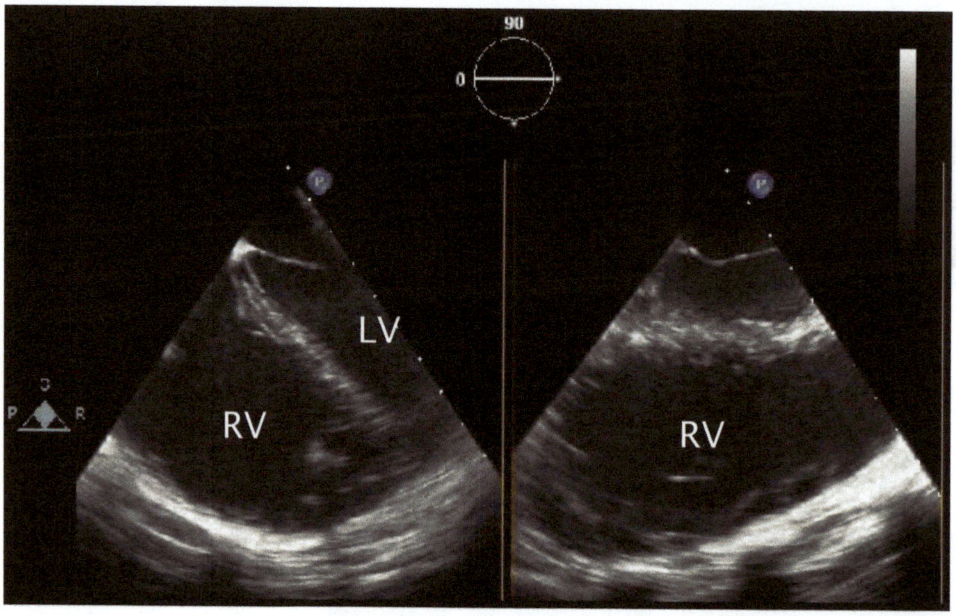

as the imaging probe is slowly withdrawn from the ME 4 Ch, multiplane angle axially rotated forward and adjusted between the ME AV SAX and mid esophageal ascending aortic short axis (ME Asc Ao SAX) views. Slight anteflexion of the probe may be helpful. In the ME RV In-Out view the RAA can also be demonstrated coursing behind the posterior great artery and anterior to the LA.

From the ME 4 Ch view, clockwise probe shaft rotation and forward axial rotation to an angle ~90°–95° displays the entire atrial septum as visualized in the ME Bicaval view. The characteristic septal malalignment, with posterior deviation of the superior portion and anterior deviation of the inferior portion can be also seen from this view. The ME LAX and mid esophageal ascending aorta long axis (ME Asc Ao LAX) views can also demonstrate the RAA behind the posterior great artery and anterior to the LA.

Probe withdrawal from a TG Basal SAX/LE Situs SAX planes with anteflexion may demonstrate the appendage crossing behind the great arteries. Further views of the interatrial septum displaying the septal malalignment and opening of the abnormally oriented atrial appendage can also be obtained from the deep transgastric views with clockwise/

Table 7.1 Atrial communications

Summary of important considerations for TEE assessment
Anatomy of the atrial septal defect or patent foramen ovale
Size and location of defect (single versus fenestrated)
Septal rims
Septal anatomy
Direction of atrial level shunt
Drainage of pulmonary veins
Atrial chamber size
Doppler assessment of atrioventricular valves (regurgitation); mitral valve anatomy (prolapse, cleft)
Assessment for possible pulmonary hypertension
Estimation of right ventricular systolic pressure by tricuspid regurgitation jet velocity
Estimation of right ventricular diastolic pressure by pulmonary regurgitation end-diastolic velocity
Identification and evaluation of other associated congenital cardiac lesions
Ventricular chamber size and systolic function

counterclockwise adjustments as necessary and anterior to posterior sweeping (Fig. 7.41, Video 7.41). Evaluation of associated defects (particularly transposition of the great arteries, tricuspid valve obstructive lesions, and ASDs) should also be undertaken as indicated.

Color and pulsed-wave Doppler can help to distinguish between flow across an ASD and flow in an atrial appendage in cases where 2D imaging is inconclusive. Tricuspid valve obstructive lesions other than atresia can co-exist with other complex congenital heart defects, particularly transposition of the great arteries thus careful Doppler evaluation of the tricuspid valve is warranted. Color flow Doppler can facilitate identification of an associated ASD, which may have a more anterior opening due to the abnormal septal configuration. Appropriate Doppler evaluation of any additional associated lesions and routine assessment of ventricular function are also indicated. Finally, thrombi can form in a juxtaposed appendage and should be assessed for [67].

Salient features of the echocardiographic evaluation of juxtaposed atrial appendages are summarized in Table 7.2.

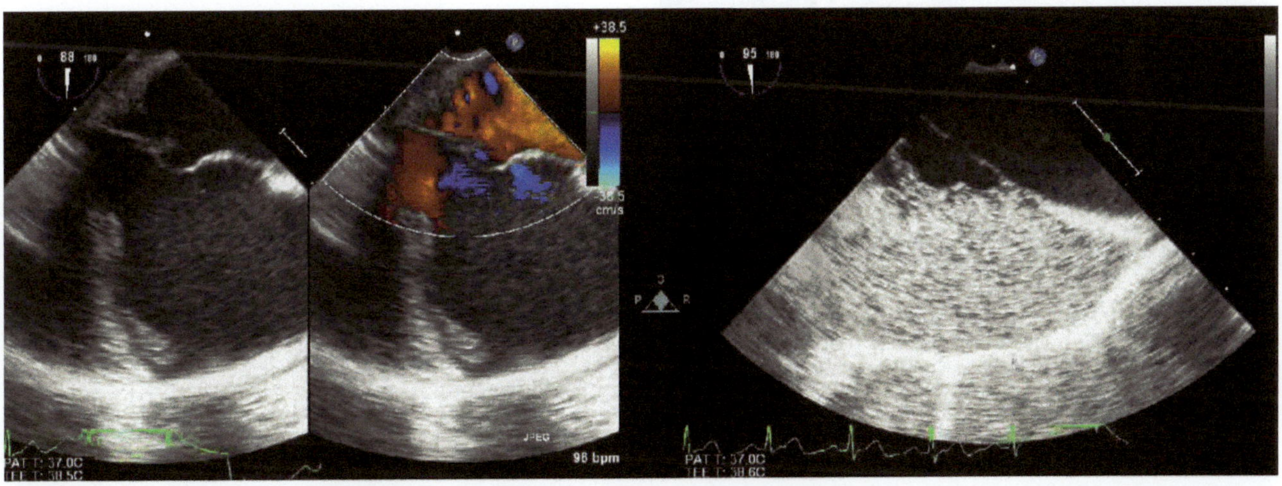

Fig. 7.35 Images demonstrate an aneurysm of the interatrial septum as shown by two-dimensional imaging (*left panel*), color flow mapping (*middle panel*), and contrast echocardiography (*right panel*). Injection of agitated saline into a lower extremity vein was performed to assess for the presence of a patent foramen ovale in a child with a history of multiple strokes

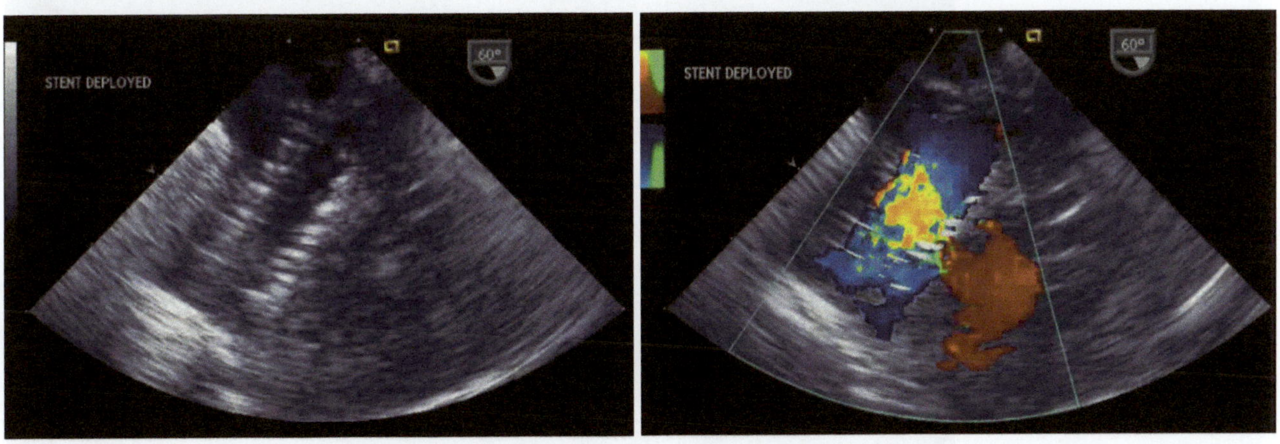

Fig. 7.36 *Left panel:* Two-dimensional image of an atrial septal stent placed following radiofrequency perforation of the interatrial septum in a critically ill infant with hypoplastic left heart syndrome and an intact atrial septum. *Right panel:* Color Doppler depicts flow across the central aspect of the stent

Surgical and Transcatheter Considerations

Juxtaposed atrial appendages may be found incidentally at the time of surgical intervention for other complex heart defects. This anomaly usually has little impact on outcome in the present surgical era. Atrial baffle procedures (Senning or Mustard), which are rarely performed today, could conceivably be complicated by this anomaly. On occasion this may influence a Fontan connection or atrial cannulation for cardiopulmonary bypass. However, the associated lesions generally have much greater surgical implications than the juxtaposed appendages [59].

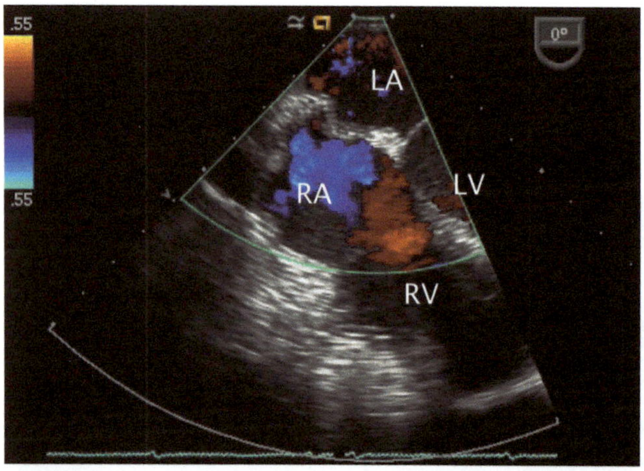

Fig. 7.37 Mid esophageal four chamber imaging with color flow interrogation to assess the results of the surgical intervention following patch closure of a secundum atrial septal defect. *LA* left atrium, *LV* left ventricle, *RA* right atrium, *RV* right ventricle

Although not usually a setting where TEE is routinely utilized, a more important consideration worth mentioning concerns performance of balloon atrial septostomy in patients with *d*-transposition of the great arteries and left juxtaposition of the atrial appendages. An increased risk of inadvertent placement of the balloon catheter tip into the abnormally oriented RAA has been reported that, if not recognized, can lead to complications during attempted septostomy. The combination of 2D imaging and Doppler interrogation may avoid mistaking the base or mouth of a juxtaposed RAA for an atrial communication in this instance. In addition, recognition of the abnormal atrial septal configuration and the often unusual placement/orientation of the ASD/PFO in this anomaly by TEE can assist in catheter manipulation, save valuable time, and potentially increase the margin of safety of the procedure. This may be important in clinically unstable, cyanotic neonates in whom time is of the essence.

Cor Triatriatum

Cor triatriatum consists of a congenital fibromuscular membrane dividing either the RA or LA into proximal (venous) and distal (atrial) chambers. The term "cor triatriatum", when used alone, usually refers to a left atrial membrane, also sometimes called "cor triatriatum sinister". Although by far the most common form of the defect, this is a rare cardiac anomaly, accounting for less than 2–4 % of all congenital heart disease. An even less common form of this lesion may affect the RA (cor triatriatum dexter) and will not be discussed in depth.

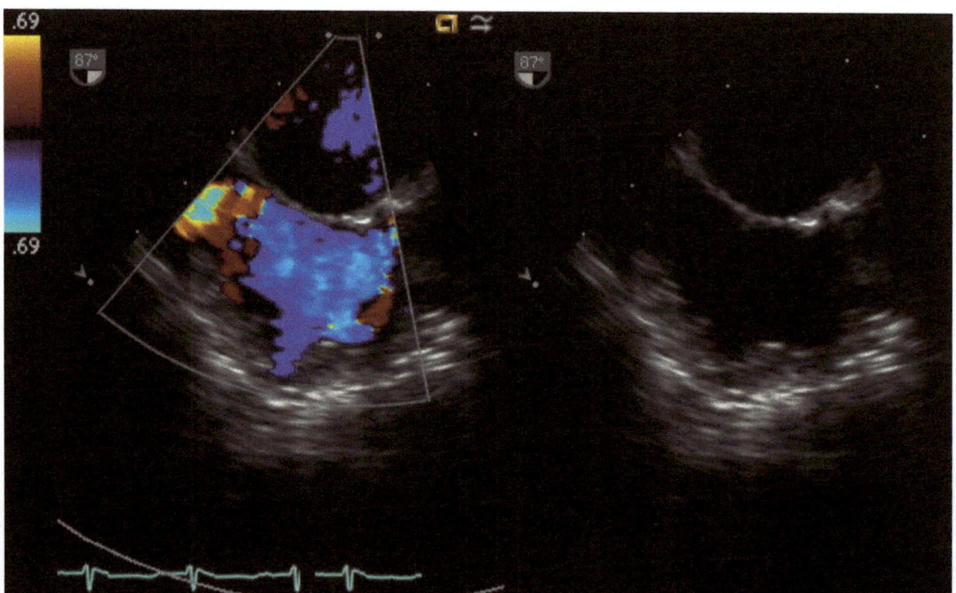

Fig. 7.38 Images display the post surgical evaluation of a secundum atrial septal defect in the mid esophageal bicaval plane. No residual shunting is detected across the patch

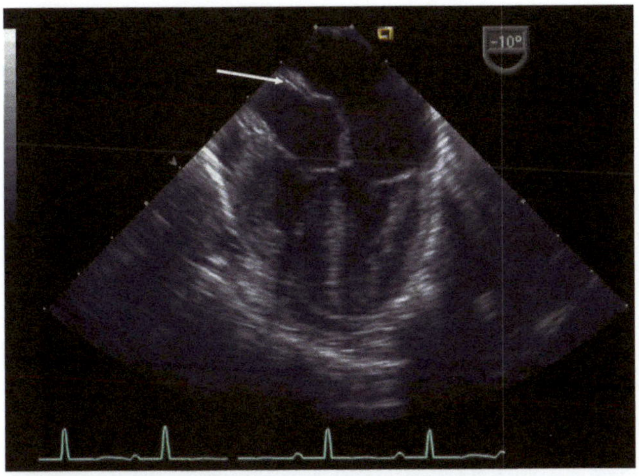

Fig. 7.39 Note the abnormal orientation (*arrow*) of the interatrial septum in a patient with juxtaposed left atrial appendages

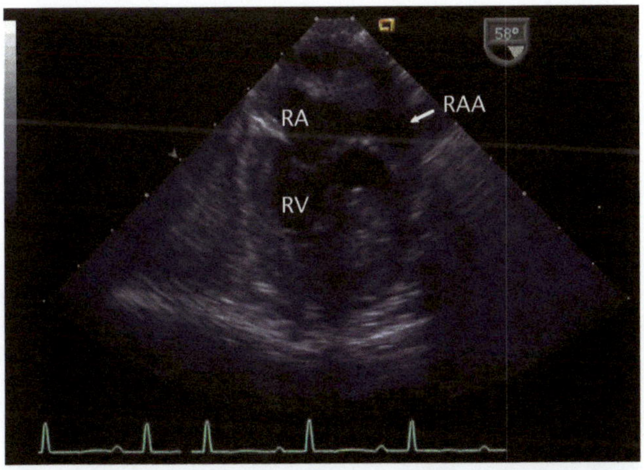

Fig. 7.40 Image displays the abnormal position of the right atrial appendage (*RAA*) as it extends from the right atrium (*RA*) to lie next to the left atrial appendage in left juxtaposition of the atrial appendages. The abnormal orientation of the interatrial septum is also appreciated in this view. *RV* right ventricle

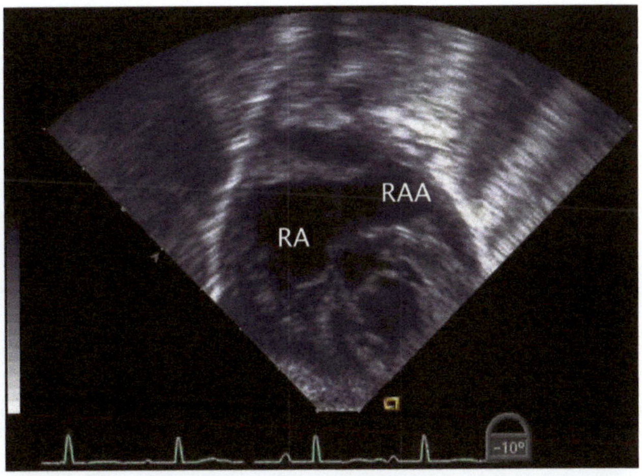

Fig. 7.41 This deep transgastric image further displays the anatomy/orientation of the atrial appendages in the infant shown in Figs. 7.39 and 7.40 with juxtaposition of the atrial appendages. Note the position of the right atrial appendage (*RAA*) on the *left side* (left juxtaposition). Associated defects in this patient included double outlet right ventricle/malposed great arteries (Taussig Bing Anomaly). *RA* right atrium

Table 7.2 Juxtaposition of atrial appendages

Summary of important considerations for TEE assessment
Anatomy of the juxtaposed atrial appendage
Right versus left juxtaposition
Identification and evaluation of other associated congenital cardiac lesions
Left juxtaposition
Transposition of the great arteries, tricuspid stenosis/atresia
Heterotaxy syndrome, left atrial isomerism
Right juxtaposition
Ventricular septal defects, double outlet right ventricle
Other
Atrial septal defects
Thrombi

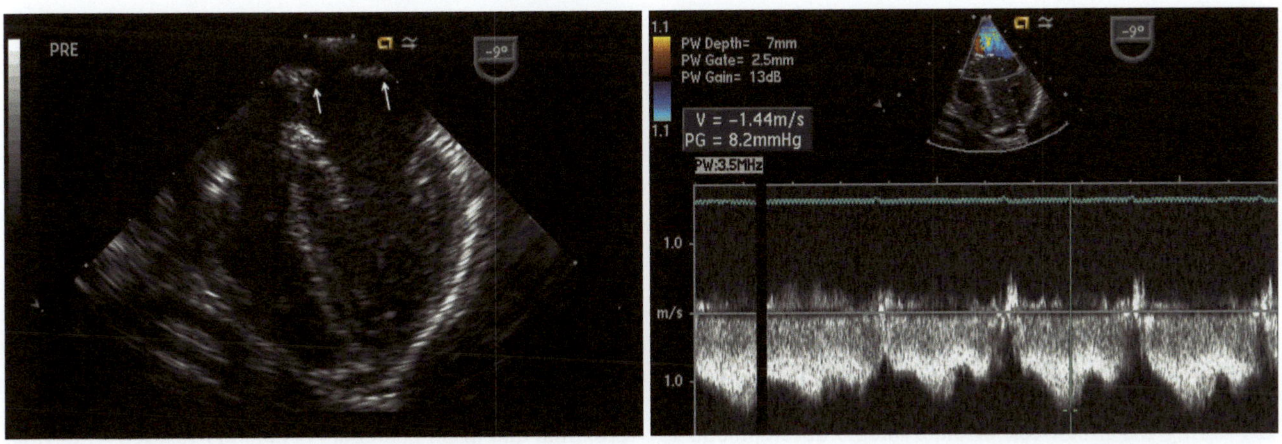

Fig. 7.42 *Left panel:* Mid esophageal view depicting a cor triatriatum membrane (*arrows*). *Right panel:* Spectral Doppler analysis across the orifice of the membrane is performed to determine the severity of obstruction. Although a peak velocity is measured in this tracing, parameters considered more representative of the degree of obstruction include the mean gradient across this region and characterization of the flow pattern. Phasic flow with velocities that return to the baseline suggests that there is not significant obstruction

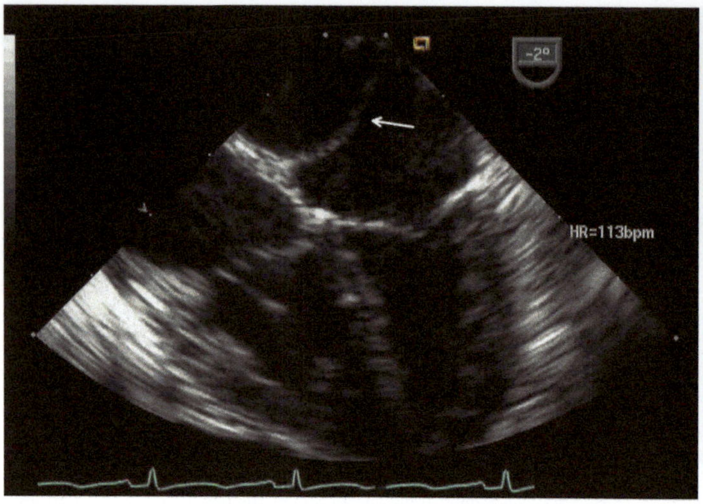

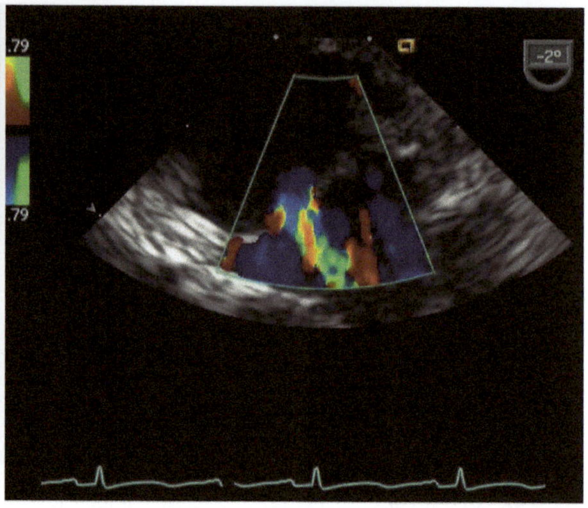

Fig. 7.43 In contrast to the images shown in Fig. 7.42, the cor triatriatum membrane (*arrow*) in this patient was of an obstructive nature. Note the division of the left atrium by the membrane into proximal and distal portions. Color Doppler displays aliased flow across the small central orifice that serves for the egress of blood across the membrane

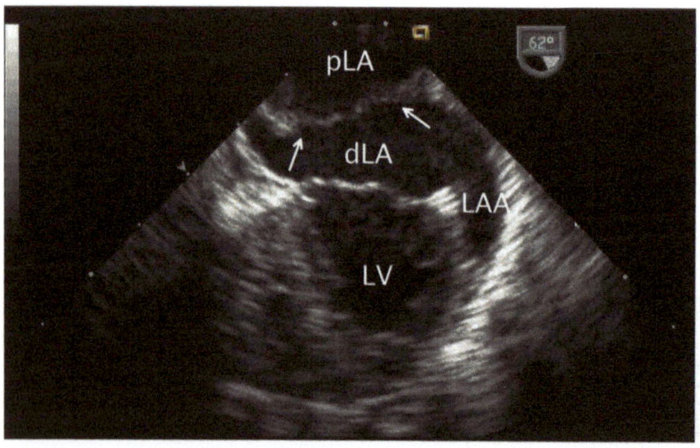

Fig. 7.44 In this mid esophageal view it is seen that the left atrial appendage (*LAA*) lies below the level of the membrane (*arrows*) in cor triatriatum. This is in contrast to a supravalvar mitral ring where the appendage lies above the membrane. *dLA* distal left atrium, *pLA* proximal left atrium, *dLA* distal left atrium, *LV* left ventricle

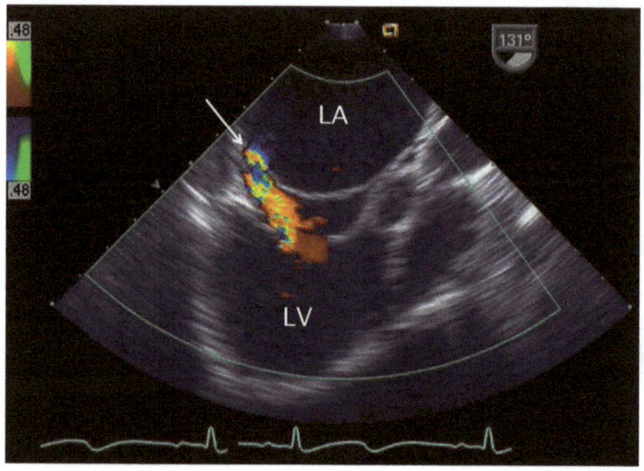

Fig. 7.45 Mid esophageal long-axis view demonstrates a cor triatriatum membrane with a small eccentric posteriorly located orifice. Note the aliased color flow (*arrow*) consistent with obstruction across this area. *LA* left atrium, *LV* left ventricle

Cor triatriatum is associated with other cardiac defects in up to 50 % of cases, most commonly secundum ASD, patent ductus arteriosus, left superior vena cava, and ventricular septal defect. Rare reported associations include tricuspid atresia, Ebstein anomaly of the tricuspid valve, tetralogy of Fallot, atrioventricular septal defect, Shone syndrome and coarctation of the aorta, sinus venosus ASD, and partial/total anomalous pulmonary venous return. Atrial septal communications, when present, typically but not invariably open into the distal (atrial) chamber [68–79].

Cor triatriatum is generally felt to be the result of inadequate incorporation of the common pulmonary vein into the LA during the fifth week of embryologic development. In the usual form, the LA is divided into proximal and distal chambers by a fibromuscular membrane usually with a single (less commonly multiple) restrictive orifice. The location of the LAA with respect to the obstructing membrane is the key anatomic feature that differentiates cor triatriatum from supravalvar mitral ring/stenosis. In cor triatriatum, the LAA is invariably found distal to the membrane in the same chamber with the mitral annulus (atrial chamber). The pulmonary veins drain into the proximal chamber, thus creating a form of pulmonary venous obstruction, which is often moderate to severe and accounts for the typical early clinical presentation of this lesion. However, if the connection between the proximal and distal chambers is not very restrictive, or if an ASD communicating with the pulmonary venous chamber is

Table 7.3 Cor triatriatum (sinister)

Summary of important considerations for TEE assessment
Anatomy of cor triatriatum membrane
Relationship of membrane to left atrial appendage
Exclude partial cor triatriatum
Degree of pulmonary venous obstruction by the cor triatriatum membrane
Anatomy of pulmonary venous return
Assessment of pulmonary hypertension
Presence/absence of atrial septal defect or patent foramen ovale
Determination of which left atrial chamber an existing atrial septal defect/patent foramen ovale communicates with
Evaluation of other associated congenital cardiac lesions
Right heart: tricuspid atresia, Ebstein anomaly, tetralogy of Fallot
Left heart: Shone syndrome, coarctation of the aorta
Miscellaneous: ventricular septal defect, patent ductus arteriosus, sinus venosus atrial septal defect
Ventricular chamber size and systolic function

present allowing a "pop-off" for pulmonary venous return, the hemodynamics may be less significantly affected and the diagnosis may be masked [80, 81]. Partial forms of cor triatriatum also occur, with only the right or left pulmonary veins draining into the proximal chamber.

In cor triatriatum dexter, as indicated, a membrane divides the RA. This is considered the result of a persistent right valve of the sinus venosus. The RA is partitioned (to a greater or lesser degree) into a proximal chamber that includes superior/inferior vena caval return, coronary sinus drainage and atrial septum, and a distal chamber that includes the RAA and tricuspid valve. Patients with cor triatriatum dexter are usually asymptomatic and this is most often reported as an incidental finding, however cases with associated ASDs, hypoplastic right sided structures, Ebstein anomaly, and coronary venous anomalies have been documented [82–84]. If the membrane is sufficiently obstructive, these patients can be cyanotic due to preferential streaming of systemic venous (deoxygenated) blood through an ASD and into the LA.

TTE can generally demonstrate the salient features of cor triatriatum, however TEE may provide optimal views and is useful in assessing the surgical repair [85].

Transesophageal Echocardiographic Evaluation

Anatomic evaluation of cor triatriatum involving the LA begins at the ME 4 Ch view (Fig. 7.42, Video 7.42). Slight retroflexion of the imaging probe maintaining adequate contact optimizes this view and may help prevent compression of the potentially hypertensive pulmonary venous chamber by the probe. Slight counterclockwise turning of the probe and/or rotation of the imaging plane optimally visualizes the LA and demonstrates the obstructing membrane crossing the atrium proximal to the orifice of the LAA. Probe advancement and withdrawal allows scanning of the entire membrane from inferior to superior in this plane. Color Doppler interrogation of a cor triatriatum membrane from the ME 4 Ch and 2 Ch views will most clearly identify the orifice(s) draining to the distal chamber, usually appearing as high velocity, turbulent flow with a lack of phasic variation in the presence of obstruction (Fig. 7.43, Video 7.43).

The connection of the left pulmonary veins proximal to the membrane can be demonstrated from this view (may require further counterclockwise turning and slight advancement or withdrawal of the probe to identify the upper and lower veins). The initial assessment of the left ventricular inflow also begins from this view. Completion of the anatomic evaluation of the LA, cor triatriatum membrane, LAA, and mitral valve/left ventricular inflow (including exclusion of a supravalve mitral ring and/or an abnormal subvalvar mitral apparatus) should be performed via progressive forward axial rotation of the multiplane angle through the following views: mid esophageal mitral commissural (ME Mitral, angle ~60°–70°), ME 2 Ch, and ME LAX (angle 100°–130°) views. Slight counterclockwise probe turning may be necessary. Through this sweep, the LAA will be seen primarily in long axis and the left atrial membrane will be seen attaching to the lateral atrial wall just above the appendage and below the left pulmonary veins (Fig. 7.44, Video 7.44).

Returning to the ME 4 Ch view, clockwise turning of the probe visualizes the mid portion of the interatrial septum to allow for evaluation of associated secundum ASD and/or PFO. Axial rotation of the multiplane angle to the ME Bicaval view, which provides further evaluation of the interatrial septum and systemic venous return, may be performed either at this point or later in the study, if desired. Specific determination of which left atrial chamber (venous or atrial) an interatrial communication enters should be sought in all cases.

In cases with eccentric orifices (Fig. 7.45, Video 7.45), interrogation in multiple planes is essential with forward/backward axial rotation and probe turning as needed to obtain a more ideal Doppler angle of interrogation. TEE windows for Doppler assessment of the membrane in these cases may include the ME Bicaval, ME LAX, ME Mitral, and the DTG views. Spectral Doppler interrogation of the jet across the orifice can be used to estimate the pressure gradient across the membrane to assist in characterizing the severity of pulmonary venous obstruction. Additional information to be obtained from a combination of views includes left ventricular inflow Doppler interrogation (mitral stenosis, regurgitation) and left ventricular diastolic assessment.

Color and pulsed Doppler evaluation of the interatrial septum to assess for associated secundum ASD and/or PFO should be performed as previously described. Spectral Doppler determination of the peak and mean velocity of left-to-right flow across an ASD communicating with the proximal (venous) chamber can be used to estimate pressure in that chamber. The degree of tricuspid regurgitation should be assessed as well as determination of the Doppler peak velocity of tricuspid regurgitation in order to estimate right ventricular and pulmonary artery systolic pressures. Pulmonary artery diastolic pressure should also be estimated as described in prior sections of this chapter.

Identification of the course and connection of the pulmonary veins may be facilitated by the use of color and spectral Doppler from the ME 4 Ch view with clockwise probe turning for right, and counterclockwise turning for left veins respectively. Color Doppler may also demonstrate the pulmonary veins from the ME Bicaval view, with turning of the probe shaft as described above.

Right ventricular size, wall thickness, and qualitative systolic function, in addition to right atrial size and interventricular septal configuration, may reflect the degree of pulmonary hypertension present and should be evaluated. Pertinent transesophageal and gastric windows include: ME 4 Ch, ME RV In-Out, TG RV In, TG Basal SAX, and TG Mid SAX views. Qualitative assessment of left ventricular systolic function and color/spectral Doppler evaluation of additional associated lesions, as appropriate, is indicated.

Anatomic evaluation of cor triatriatum dexter is similarly performed with a focus on TEE imaging of the systemic venous return, RA, and atrial septum from the LE Situs SAX and lower esophageal inferior vena cava long axis (LE IVC LAX), ME 4 Ch, ME RV In-Out, ME Bicaval, and TG RV In views.

Relevant aspects of the echocardiographic evaluation of this defect are summarized in Table 7.3.

Surgical Considerations

Preoperative Assessment

Important considerations in the preoperative assessment of cor triatriatum involve the following evaluations, as described above: (1) complete left heart examination including attempts to confirm pulmonary venous return (exclude partial anomalous pulmonary venous connections or partial cor triatriatum), (2) 2D imaging of the left atrial membrane, (3) Doppler evaluation of the degree of obstruction across the membrane and estimation of pulmonary venous chamber pressure, (4) exclusion of additional left heart obstructive lesions (supravalve mitral ring, mitral stenosis, left ventricular outflow tract and aortic valve abnormalities/stenosis), (5) Doppler determination of the degree of mitral regurgitation, and (6) evaluation of left ventricular size and qualitative systolic function. Appropriate preoperative evaluation of the right heart includes: (1) right atrial and right ventricular sizes and qualitative right ventricular systolic function, (2) assessment of tricuspid regurgitation severity, and (3) estimation of right ventricular systolic pressure. Presence and anatomic details of any ASD(s) must be determined. Additional associated cardiac structural lesions should be sought out and evaluated as well.

Postoperative Assessment

Surgical intervention for this anomaly typically involves resection of the membrane. Postoperative evaluation includes confirmation of adequate cardiac de-airing and evaluation of the adequacy of the repair. This involves: (1) exclusion of a residual membrane and left atrial obstruction, (2) evaluation of the atrial septum for shunting, because resection of the membrane might be performed through a right atriotomy and an incision in the atrial septum, (3) re-evaluation of tricuspid regurgitation severity and estimation of right ventricular systolic pressure, and (4) qualitative assessment of biventricular systolic function. If other procedures were performed for associated lesions, the adequacy of the surgical intervention for these procedures should be assessed as well.

Summary

TEE contributes to the diagnostic evaluation of interatrial communications and plays an important role in the management of patients affected by these defects in both the operating room and cardiac catheterization settings. Likewise, the transesophageal imaging approach facilitates the characterization of atrial variants and pathologies affecting atrial structures. Further advancements in imaging technologies are likely to further expand the benefits and applications of TEE in the assessment of these structures and corresponding anomalies.

References

1. Seward JB, Khandheria BK, Edwards WD, et al. Biplanar transesophageal echocardiography: anatomic correlations, image orientation, and clinical applications. Mayo Clin Proc. 1990;65:1193–213.
2. Tardif JC, Schwartz SL, Vannan MA, et al. Clinical usefulness of multiplane transesophageal echocardiography: comparison to biplanar imaging. Am Heart J. 1994;128:156–66.
3. Kronzon I, Tunick PA, Freedberg RS, et al. Transesophageal echocardiography is superior to transthoracic echocardiography in the diagnosis of sinus venosus atrial septal defect. J Am Coll Cardiol. 1991;17:537–42.
4. Lin SL, Ting CT, Hsu TL, et al. Transesophageal echocardiographic detection of atrial septal defect in adults. Am J Cardiol. 1992;69:280–2.
5. Hamdan R, Mirochnik N, Celermajer D, et al. Cor Triatriatum Sinister diagnosed in adult life with three dimensional transesophageal echocardiography. BMC Cardiovasc Disord. 2010;10:54.

6. Saric M, Perk G, Purgess JR, et al. Imaging atrial septal defects by real-time three-dimensional transesophageal echocardiography: step-by-step approach. J Am Soc Echocardiogr. 2010;23:1128–35.
7. Faletra FF, Nucifora G, Ho SY. Imaging the atrial septum using real-time three-dimensional transesophageal echocardiography: technical tips, normal anatomy, and its role in transseptal puncture. J Am Soc Echocardiogr. 2011;24:593–9.
8. Johri AM, Witzke C, Solis J, et al. Real-time three-dimensional transesophageal echocardiography in patients with secundum atrial septal defects: outcomes following transcatheter closure. J Am Soc Echocardiogr. 2011;24:431–7.
9. Perez L, Razzouk A, Bansal RC. Real time three-dimensional transesophageal echocardiographic evaluation of a sinus venosus atrial septal defect. Echocardiography. 2011;28:E82–4.
10. Roberson DA, Cui W, Patel D, et al. Three-dimensional transesophageal echocardiography of atrial septal defect: a qualitative and quantitative anatomic study. J Am Soc Echocardiogr. 2011; 24:600–10.
11. Feldt RH, Avasthey P, Yoshimasu F, et al. Incidence of congenital heart disease in children born to residents of Olmsted County, Minnesota, 1950–1969. Mayo Clin Proc. 1971;46:794–9.
12. Anderson RH, Brown NA, Webb S. Development and structure of the atrial septum. Heart. 2002;88:104–10.
13. Ferreira SM, Ho SY, Anderson RH. Morphological study of defects of the atrial septum within the oval fossa: implications for transcatheter closure of left-to-right shunt. Br Heart J. 1992;67:316–20.
14. Brassard M, Fouron JC, van Doesburg NH, et al. Outcome of children with atrial septal defect considered too small for surgical closure. Am J Cardiol. 1999;83:1552–5.
15. Riggs T, Sharp SE, Batton D, et al. Spontaneous closure of atrial septal defects in premature vs. full-term neonates. Pediatr Cardiol. 2000;21:129–34.
16. McMahon CJ, Feltes TF, Fraley JK, et al. Natural history of growth of secundum atrial septal defects and implications for transcatheter closure. Heart. 2002;87:256–9.
17. Basson CT, Cowley GS, Solomon SD, et al. The clinical and genetic spectrum of the Holt-Oram syndrome (heart-hand syndrome). N Engl J Med. 1994;330:885–91.
18. Basson CT, Bachinsky DR, Lin RC, et al. Mutations in human TBX5 [corrected] cause limb and cardiac malformation in Holt-Oram syndrome. Nat Genet. 1997;15:30–5.
19. Schott JJ, Benson DW, Basson CT, et al. Congenital heart disease caused by mutations in the transcription factor NKX2–5. Science. 1998;281:108–11.
20. Vaughan CJ, Basson CT. Molecular determinants of atrial and ventricular septal defects and patent ductus arteriosus. Am J Med Genet. 2000;97:304–9.
21. Garg V, Kathiriya IS, Barnes R, et al. GATA4 mutations cause human congenital heart defects and reveal an interaction with TBX5. Nature. 2003;424:443–7.
22. Ching YH, Ghosh TK, Cross SJ, et al. Mutation in myosin heavy chain 6 causes atrial septal defect. Nat Genet. 2005;37:423–8.
23. Van Praagh S, Carrera ME, Sanders SP, et al. Sinus venosus defects: unroofing of the right pulmonary veins—anatomic and echocardiographic findings and surgical treatment. Am Heart J. 1994;128: 365–79.
24. Jean D, Girard F, Couture P, et al. Transesophageal echocardiographic diagnosis of sinus venosus-type atrial septal defect associated with partial anomalous venous connections during cardiac surgery in adults. J Cardiothorac Vasc Anesth. 1995;9:438–41.
25. Davia JE, Cheitlin MD, Bedynek JL. Sinus venosus atrial septal defect: analysis of fifty cases. Am Heart J. 1973;85:177–85.
26. al Zaghal AM, Li J, Anderson RH, et al. Anatomical criteria for the diagnosis of sinus venosus defects. Heart. 1997;78:298–304.
27. Li J, Al Zaghal AM, Anderson RH. The nature of the superior sinus venosus defect. Clin Anat. 1998;11:349–52.
28. Van Praagh S, Geva T, Lock JE, et al. Biatrial or left atrial drainage of the right superior vena cava: anatomic, morphogenetic, and surgical considerations—report of three new cases and literature review. Pediatr Cardiol. 2003;24:350–63.
29. Sunaga Y, Hayashi K, Okubo N, et al. Transesophageal echocardiographic diagnosis of coronary sinus type atrial septal defect. Am Heart J. 1992;124:1657–9.
30. Quaegebeur J, Kirklin JW, Pacifico AD, et al. Surgical experience with unroofed coronary sinus. Ann Thorac Surg. 1979;27:418–25.
31. Freedom RM, Culham JA, Rowe RD. Left atrial to coronary sinus fenestration (partially unroofed coronary sinus). Morphological and angiocardiographic observations. Br Heart J. 1981;46:63–8.
32. Franz C, Mennicken U, Dalichau H, et al. Abnormal communication between the left atrium and the coronary sinus. Presentation of 2 cases and review of the literature. Thorac Cardiovasc Surg. 1985;33:113–7.
33. Schneider B, Zienkiewicz T, Jansen V, et al. Diagnosis of patent foramen ovale by transesophageal echocardiography and correlation with autopsy findings. Am J Cardiol. 1996;77:1202–9.
34. Waggoner AD, Davila-Roman VG, Hopkins WE, et al. Comparison of color flow imaging and peripheral venous saline contrast during transesophageal echocardiography to evaluate right-to-left shunt at the atrial level. Echocardiography. 1993;10:59–66.
35. Belkin RN, Pollack BD, Ruggiero ML, et al. Comparison of transesophageal and transthoracic echocardiography with contrast and color flow Doppler in the detection of patent foramen ovale. Am Heart J. 1994;128:520–5.
36. Hagen PT, Scholz DG, Edwards WD. Incidence and size of patent foramen ovale during the first 10 decades of life: an autopsy study of 965 normal hearts. Mayo Clin Proc. 1984;59:17–20.
37. Fisher DC, Fisher EA, Budd JH, et al. The incidence of patent foramen ovale in 1,000 consecutive patients. A contrast transesophageal echocardiography study. Chest. 1995;107:1504–9.
38. Agnetti A, Carano N, Sani E, et al. Cryptogenic stroke in children: possible role of patent foramen ovale. Neuropediatrics. 2006;37:53–6.
39. Bartz PJ, Cetta F, Cabalka AK, et al. Paradoxical emboli in children and young adults: role of atrial septal defect and patent foramen ovale device closure. Mayo Clin Proc. 2006;81:615–8.
40. Meissner I, Khandheria BK, Heit JA, et al. Patent foramen ovale: innocent or guilty? Evidence from a prospective population-based study. J Am Coll Cardiol. 2006;47:440–5.
41. Hausmann D, Daniel WG, Mugge A, et al. Value of transesophageal color Doppler echocardiography for detection of different types of atrial septal defect in adults. J Am Soc Echocardiogr. 1992; 5:481–8.
42. Oh JK, Seward JB, Khandheria BK, et al. Visualization of sinus venosus atrial septal defect by transesophageal echocardiography. J Am Soc Echocardiogr. 1988;1:275–7.
43. Watanabe F, Takenaka K, Suzuki J, et al. Visualization of sinus venosus-type atrial septal defect by biplane transesophageal echocardiography. J Am Soc Echocardiogr. 1994;7:179–81.
44. Pascoe RD, Oh JK, Warnes CA, et al. Diagnosis of sinus venosus atrial septal defect with transesophageal echocardiography. Circulation. 1996;94:1049–55.
45. Hellenbrand WE, Fahey JT, McGowan FX, et al. Transesophageal echocardiographic guidance of transcatheter closure of atrial septal defect. Am J Cardiol. 1990;66:207–13.
46. Ishii M, Kato H, Inoue O, et al. Biplane transesophageal echo-Doppler studies of atrial septal defects: quantitative evaluation and monitoring for transcatheter closure. Am Heart J. 1993;125:1363–8.
47. Hijazi ZM, Cao Q, Patel HT, et al. Transesophageal echocardiographic results of catheter closure of atrial septal defect in children and adults using the Amplatzer device. Am J Cardiol. 2000;85:1387–90.
48. Latiff HA, Samion H, Kandhavel G, et al. The value of transesophageal echocardiography in transcatheter closure of atrial septal defects in the oval fossa using the Amplatzer septal occluder. Cardiol Young. 2001;11:201–4.

49. Figueroa MI, Balaguru D, McClure C, et al. Experience with use of multiplane transesophageal echocardiography to guide closure of atrial septal defects using the Amplatzer device. Pediatr Cardiol. 2002;23:430–6.
50. Kleinman CS. Echocardiographic guidance of catheter-based treatments of atrial septal defect: transesophageal echocardiography remains the gold standard. Pediatr Cardiol. 2005;26:128–34.
51. Stevenson JG. Role of intraoperative transesophageal echocardiography during repair of congenital cardiac defects. Acta Paediatr Suppl. 1995;410:23–33.
52. Rosenfeld HM, Gentles TL, Wernovsky G, et al. Utility of intraoperative transesophageal echocardiography in the assessment of residual cardiac defects. Pediatr Cardiol. 1998;19:346–51.
53. Tempe DK, Sharma S, Banerjee A, et al. The utility of transesophageal echocardiography for detecting residual shunt in a patient undergoing atrial septal defect repair. Anesth Analg. 2007;104: 777–8.
54. Dixon AS. Juxtaposition of the atrial appendages; two cases of an unusual congenital cardiac deformity. Br Heart J. 1954;16:153–64.
55. Frescura C, Thiene G. Juxtaposition of the atrial appendages. Cardiovasc Pathol. 2012;21(3):169–79.
56. Van Praagh S, O'Sullivan J, Brili S, et al. Juxtaposition of the morphologically left atrial appendage in solitus and inversus atria: a study of 18 postmortem cases. Am Heart J. 1996;132: 391–402.
57. Van Praagh S, O'Sullivan J, Brili S, et al. Juxtaposition of the morphologically right atrial appendage in solitus and inversus atria: a study of 35 postmortem cases. Am Heart J. 1996;132:382–90.
58. Lai WW, Ravishankar C, Gross RP, et al. Juxtaposition of the atrial appendages: a clinical series of 22 patients. Pediatr Cardiol. 2001;22:121–7.
59. Anjos RT, Ho SY, Anderson RH. Surgical implications of juxtaposition of the atrial appendages. A review of forty-nine autopsied hearts. J Thorac Cardiovasc Surg. 1990;99:897–904.
60. Stumper O, Rijlaarsdam M, Vargas-Barron J, et al. The assessment of juxtaposed atrial appendages by transoesophageal echocardiography. Int J Cardiol. 1990;29:365–71.
61. Zhang YQ, Yu ZQ, Zhong SW, et al. Echocardiographic assessment of juxtaposition of the right atrial appendage in children with congenital heart disease. Echocardiography. 2010;27:878–84.
62. Tyrrell MJ, Moes CA. Congenital levoposition of the right atrial appendage. Its relevance to balloon septostomy. Am J Dis Child. 1971;121:508–10.
63. Rice MJ, Seward JB, Hagler DJ, et al. Left juxtaposed atrial appendages: diagnostic two-dimensional echocardiographic features. J Am Coll Cardiol. 1983;1:1330–6.
64. Lee ML, Wu MH, Wang JK, et al. Echocardiographic features of left juxtaposed atrial appendages associated with dextro-transposition of the great arteries. Pediatr Cardiol. 1996;17:63–6.
65. Chin AJ, Bierman FZ, Williams RG, et al. 2-dimensional echocardiographic appearance of complete left-sided juxtaposition of the atrial appendages. Am J Cardiol. 1983;52:346–8.
66. Tuccillo B, Stumper O, Hess J, et al. Transoesophageal echocardiographic evaluation of atrial morphology in children with congenital heart disease. Eur Heart J. 1992;13:223–31.
67. Viswanathan S, Vaidyanathan B, Kumar RK. Thrombus in a juxtaposed right atrial appendage. Cardiol Young. 2007;17:574.
68. Van Praagh R, Corsini I. Cor triatriatum: pathologic anatomy and a consideration of morphogenesis based on 13 postmortem cases and a study of normal development of the pulmonary vein and atrial septum in 83 human embryos. Am Heart J. 1969;78:379–405.
69. Marin-Garcia J, Tandon R, Lucas RVJ, et al. Cor triatriatum: study of 20 cases. Am J Cardiol. 1975;35:59–66.
70. Roper PC, Wright JS, McCredie RM, et al. Cor triatriatum associated with unilateral anomalous pulmonary venous drainage in an infant. Aust Paediatr J. 1981;17:122–4.
71. Hess J, Brenken U, Eygelaar A, et al. Successful management of cor triatriatum associated with anomalous pulmonary/systemic venous connection in an infant. Pediatr Cardiol. 1982;2:319–22.
72. Ostman-Smith I, Silverman NH, Oldershaw P, et al. Cor triatriatum sinistrum. Diagnostic features on cross sectional echocardiography. Br Heart J. 1984;51:211–9.
73. Grifka RG, Vincent JA. Abnormalities of the left atrium and mitral valve, including mitral valve prolapse. In: Garson AT, Bricker JT, Fisher DJ, et al., editors. The science and practice of pediatric cardiology. 2nd ed. Baltimore: Williams and Wilkins; 1998.
74. Binotto MA, Aiello VD, Ebaid M. Coexistence of divided left atrium (cor triatriatum) and tetralogy of Fallot. Int J Cardiol. 1991;31:97–9.
75. Kerensky RA, Bertolet BD, Epstein M. Late discovery of cor triatriatum as a result of unilateral pulmonary venous obstruction. Am Heart J. 1995;130:624–7.
76. Eidem BW, Cetta F. Unusual finding of cor triatriatum in a newborn with hypoplastic left heart syndrome. J Am Soc Echocardiogr. 2001;14:850–2.
77. Ito M, Kikuchi S, Hachiro Y, et al. Congenital pulmonary vein stenosis associated with cor triatriatum. Ann Thorac Surg. 2001;71: 722–3.
78. Hiramatsu T, Komori S, Okamura Y, et al. Surgical case of partial anomalous pulmonary venous connection to superior vena cava with cor triatriatum: Williams' modification and excision of diaphragm. Heart Vessels. 2008;23:433–5.
79. Tachibana K, Takagi N, Osawa H, et al. Cor triatriatum and total anomalous pulmonary venous connection to the coronary sinus. J Thorac Cardiovasc Surg. 2007;134:1067–9.
80. Jacobstein MD, Hirschfeld SS. Concealed left atrial membrane: pitfalls in the diagnosis of cor triatriatum and supravalve mitral ring. Am J Cardiol. 1982;49:780–6.
81. Krasemann Z, Scheld HH, Tjan TD, et al. Cor triatriatum: short review of the literature upon ten new cases. Herz. 2007; 32:506–10.
82. Fiorilli R, Argento G, Tomasco B, et al. Cor triatriatum dexter diagnosed by transesophageal echocardiography. J Clin Ultrasound. 1995;23:502–4.
83. Inoue Y, Tomomasa T, Okada Y, et al. Divided right atrium associated with extensive coronary vein abnormalities. Pediatr Cardiol. 2002;23:68–70.
84. Eroglu ST, Yildirir A, Simsek V, et al. Cor triatriatum dexter, atrial septal defect, and Ebstein's anomaly in an adult given a diagnosis by transthoracic and transesophageal echocardiography: a case report. J Am Soc Echocardiogr. 2004;17:780–2.
85. Shuler CO, Fyfe DA, Sade R, et al. Transesophageal echocardiographic evaluation of cor triatriatum in children. Am Heart J. 1995;129:507–10.

Atrioventricular Septal Defects and Atrioventricular Valve Anomalies

8

Mark K. Friedberg and Norman H. Silverman

Abstract

Transesophageal echocardiography plays a major role during the surgical intervention of congenital pathologies that affect the atrioventricular junction and atrioventricular valves. The prebypass examination can refine the planned surgical procedure, while the postbypass assessment can detect clinically significant residual findings that otherwise would not have been identified, thereby prompting a return to cardiopulmonary bypass and subsequent reintervention. This chapter focuses on the morphologic features and corresponding echocardiographic findings, as displayed by transesophageal imaging, of the most common congenital anomalies that involve the atrioventricular junction. Particular emphasis is placed on atrioventricular septal defects and malformations affecting the atrioventricular valves.

Keywords

Transesophageal echocardiography • Atrioventricular septal defects • Atrioventricular canal defects • Endocardial cushion defects • Atrioventricular valves • Atrioventricular valve anomalies • Congenital mitral valve anomalies • Congenital tricuspid valve anomalies • Ebstein anomaly • Prosthetic mitral valve • Mitral valve prolapse • Infectious endocarditis

Introduction

Transesophageal echocardiography (TEE) has had a major impact on surgery of the atrioventricular (AV) valves in children [1]. Prebypass information obtained by TEE may alter the planned surgical procedure, while postbypass TEE can detect clinically significant residual findings that would otherwise not have been identified, thereby prompting a return to cardiopulmonary bypass and subsequent reintervention [2, 3]. TEE has also expanded the anatomic and hemodynamic assessment in patients with congenital heart disease (CHD), particularly in those with challenging or limited transthoracic echocardiographic examinations (TTE) such as adults, patients with surgical dressings, or poorly characterized studies [4]. In view of excellent transthoracic imaging in children, the principal use of TEE at most institutions largely centers around the intraoperative evaluation.

This chapter reviews the pertinent anatomic and TEE features of the most common congenital lesions affecting the AV junction, with particular emphasis on AV septal defects and pathology of the AV valves. The reader is encouraged to refer to Chap. 4 for a detailed discussion regarding TEE evaluation of AV valves and related structures in the normal heart.

M.K. Friedberg, MD (✉)
Division of Cardiology, Department of Pediatrics,
The Labatt Family Heart Center, The Hospital for Sick Children,
University of Toronto, 555 University Avenue,
Toronto, ON, M5G 1X8, Canada
e-mail: mark.friedberg@sickkids.ca

N.H. Silverman, MD, DSc (Med), FACC, FASE, FAHA, FCP(SA)
Division of Pediatric Cardiology, Department of Pediatrics,
Lucile Packard Children's Hospital,
Stanford University School of Medicine, Palo Alto, CA, USA

The online version of this chapter (doi:10.1007/978-1-84800-064-3_8) contains supplementary material, which is available to authorized users.

P.C. Wong, W.C. Miller-Hance (eds.), *Transesophageal Echocardiography for Congenital Heart Disease*,
DOI 10.1007/978-1-84800-064-3_8, © Springer-Verlag London 2014

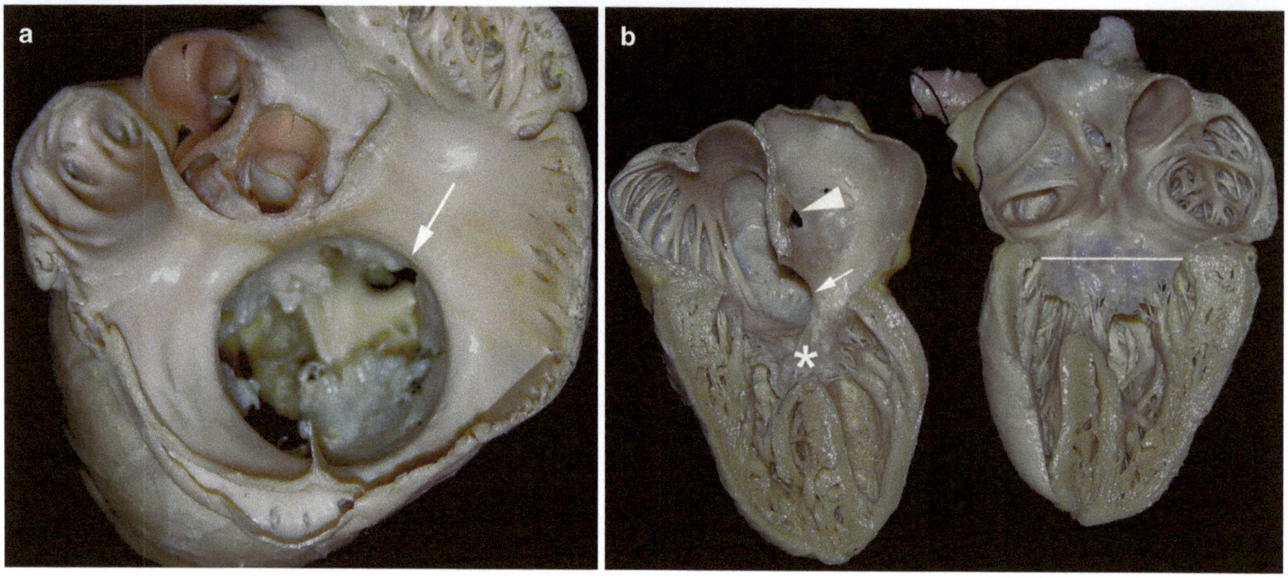

Fig. 8.1 (**a**) Pathologic specimen displaying a common atrioventricular valve *en face* as viewed from the atrial perspective. An *arrow* marks the common atrioventricular junction. The superior and inferior bridging leaflets are seen extending along the crest of the interventricular septum below. (**b**) Pathologic specimen of a heart with an atrioventricular septal defect sectioned in the equivalent of the echocardiographic four chamber view. *Arrowhead* region of the fossa ovalis, *arrow* interatrial communication (primum atrial septal defect), *asterisk* ventricular communication (inlet ventricular septal defect). The *horizontal line* represents the plane of the common atrioventricular valve annulus (Images by courtesy of Dianne Spicer)

Atrioventricular Septal Defects

Atrioventricular septal defects (AVSDs), also termed AV canal or endocardial cushion defects, result from abnormal development of the embryologic endocardial cushions. They occur in 0.19 per 1,000 live births, constituting 4–5%of all congenital heart lesions. The endocardial cushions play an integral role in the formation of the atrial and ventricular septa as well as both AV valves. Thus an abnormality of endocardial cushion development can be expected to affect a number of intracardiac structures.

Morphology

In AVSD, atrial and ventricular septation are deficient, and rather than separating into distinct mitral and tricuspid orifices, the AV junction remains common (Fig. 8.1). This lesion represents a spectrum of anomalies that can be further divided into *complete* and *incomplete* (*partial*) forms of AVSD. In *complete* AVSD, the inferior portion of the atrial septum and the posterior portion of the ventricular septum are absent, resulting in a "scooped out" appearance to the ventricular inlet, with large contiguous atrial (ASD) and ventricular septal defects (VSD) that allow shunting to occur at both levels. In addition, one large common AV valve is present. This is the most common form of AVSD in children. In the case of *incomplete* AVSDs, there is partial fusion between the superior and inferior bridging leaflets to form two separate AV orifices. When the AV valvar leaflets adhere to the ventricular septum and completely prevent any ventricular communication, an *ostium primum ASD* results. If on the other hand the leaflets attach to the ventricular septum but do not completely obstruct communication between the ventricles, then a small VSD can be present. Rarely, a form of incomplete AVSD is produced when the AV valve leaflets adhere completely to the inferior portion of the interatrial septum, preventing any atrial shunting but allowing ventricular shunting to occur. This is known as a *VSD of the AV canal type*. Regardless of whether an AVSD is complete or incomplete, there is a common anatomic feature shared by both: a large defect in the AV septum, extending above and below the crux of the heart. What differentiates the complete and incomplete forms is the degree of septation of the AV valves, in addition to the manner and extent to which the AV valve(s) attaches to the crest of the ventricular (or atrial) septum, thereby determining whether atrial or ventricular shunting (or both) can occur. Other forms of incomplete AV canal defects include a common atrium (in which no atrial septum is present), and isolated cleft left AV valve (LAVV or mitral valve), in which no atrial or ventricular communication is present.

The terminology used in the classification of AVSDs has been the subject of confusion and even controversy [5]. This is related to the fact that nomenclature such as *intermediate* and *transitional* has also been applied to describe variant forms of the complete and partial defects. To complicate matters further, in many cases these terms have been used interchangeably. When considered as different entities, an

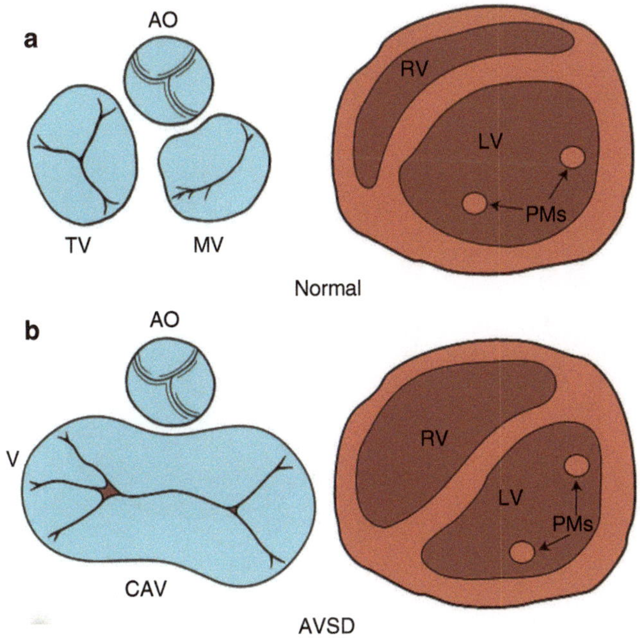

Fig. 8.2 Diagrammatic representation of the atrioventricular (*AV*) junction (on the left in blue) and the papillary muscles within the ventricle (on the right in pink), as seen from a caudal view. The normal heart is shown in *panel a* and an atrioventricular septal defect (AVSD) is shown in *panel b*. In contrast to the normal heart, in an AVSD the aortic valve is sprung anteriorly and superiorly (*panel b, left*); the papillary muscles are closely spaced and rotated (*panel b, right*). *AO* aortic valve, *CAV* common atrioventricular valve, *LV* left ventricle, *MV* mitral valve, *PMs* papillary muscles, *RV* right ventricle, *TV* tricuspid valve. Modifed from Silverman NH, The Secundum Atrial Septal Defect and Atrioventricular Septal Defects. In: Freedom R and Braunwald E, Atlas of Heart Diseases. St. Louis, Current Medicine LLC, 1996, with permission from Springer

intermediate AVSD refers to a variant of the complete form of the defect in the setting of a common AV valve annulus and two distinct AV valvar orifices separated by a tongue of tissue. These types of defects are characterized by a primum ASD and a nonrestrictive VSD. From a physiologic perspective, these defects are no different than the common type of complete AVSD. A *transitional* defect has been regarded a variant of the partial form of AVSD. This is the defect characterized by two distinct AV valve annuli, a primum ASD, a cleft LAVV, and a small inlet VSD, frequently restrictive in nature, due to partial obliteration of the ventricular communication by valvar tissue. The physiology of this defect mimics that of the typical partial AVSD (ostium primum ASD and cleft LAVV). It has been argued, however, that categorization of defects into these variants is unnecessary and only two main forms of the defect, complete and partial should be recognized [5, 6]. The main distinction should then relate to two aspects of the anatomy: (1) arrangement of the valvar leaflets relative to the AV orifices and (2) relationship of the bridging leaflets of the common valve and the septal structures. For the purpose of this chapter the classification scheme of complete and partial defects will be used.

In AVSD, there is always a common AV valve annulus (Fig. 8.1) [7]. In the complete defect, the common AV valve resembles its embryonic form and has five leaflets (Fig. 8.2). The superior bridging leaflet, a derivative of the embryonic superior endocardial cushion, and the inferior bridging leaflet, a derivative of the embryonic inferior cushion, straddle the atrial and ventricular septa and cross the area normally occupied by the AV septum. A mural (lateral) leaflet in the left side of the AV valve orifice completes the left component of the common AV valve. The right side of the common AV valve consists of the two components of the bridging leaflets as well as the anterior and posterior (mural) leaflets. The meeting point or zone of apposition between the left components of the bridging leaflets is the so-called '*cleft*'. This has also been considered to represent a commissure and alternatively may be referred to as such [8].

The *Rastelli classification* of complete AVSDs, based on the morphology of the superior bridging leaflet, degree of bridging, and its chordal attachments, was originally considered to have prognostic implications. Although now less important surgically, this scheme is still widely used (Fig. 8.3) [9]. In our previously published experience of *Rastelli type A* AVSD, which accounted for 89 % of the complete form of AVSD, the superior bridging leaflet attaches to the ventricular septum. In that report Down syndrome was present in 58 % of the patients with this type of lesion but not with the other complete forms of AVSD [10]. In *Rastelli type B*, which accounted for 2 % of cases, the superior bridging leaflet attaches to a septal papillary muscle on the right side of the ventricular septum. However, it is often difficult to differentiate between the Rastelli types A and B. In *Rastelli type C*, which accounted for 9 %, the least developed or most primitive form of AVSD, the superior bridging leaflet extends to the anterior papillary muscle within the right ventricle. In this arrangement there are no chordal attachments to the septum and the freestanding right ventricular papillary muscle supports the right component of the superior bridging leaflet [11].

A number of other morphologic characteristics are present in AVSD. The positions of the left ventricular papillary muscles are rotated counter-clockwise (when viewed from the apex) due to counter-clockwise rotation of the LAVV commissures. The anterolateral papillary muscle is situated more medially at 'three o'clock', and the posteromedial papillary muscle is situated more laterally at 'five o'clock', compared with their normal positions at 'four o'clock' and 'seven o'clock', respectively as viewed from the parasternal left ventricular short axis view by TTE (Fig. 8.2) [10]. Papillary muscle rotation and approximation may cause a functionally parachute LAVV. Therefore, recognition of both papillary muscles within the left ventricle is important because repair of the LAVV may create an acquired parachute mitral valve deformity. In the normal heart the aortic valve is wedged

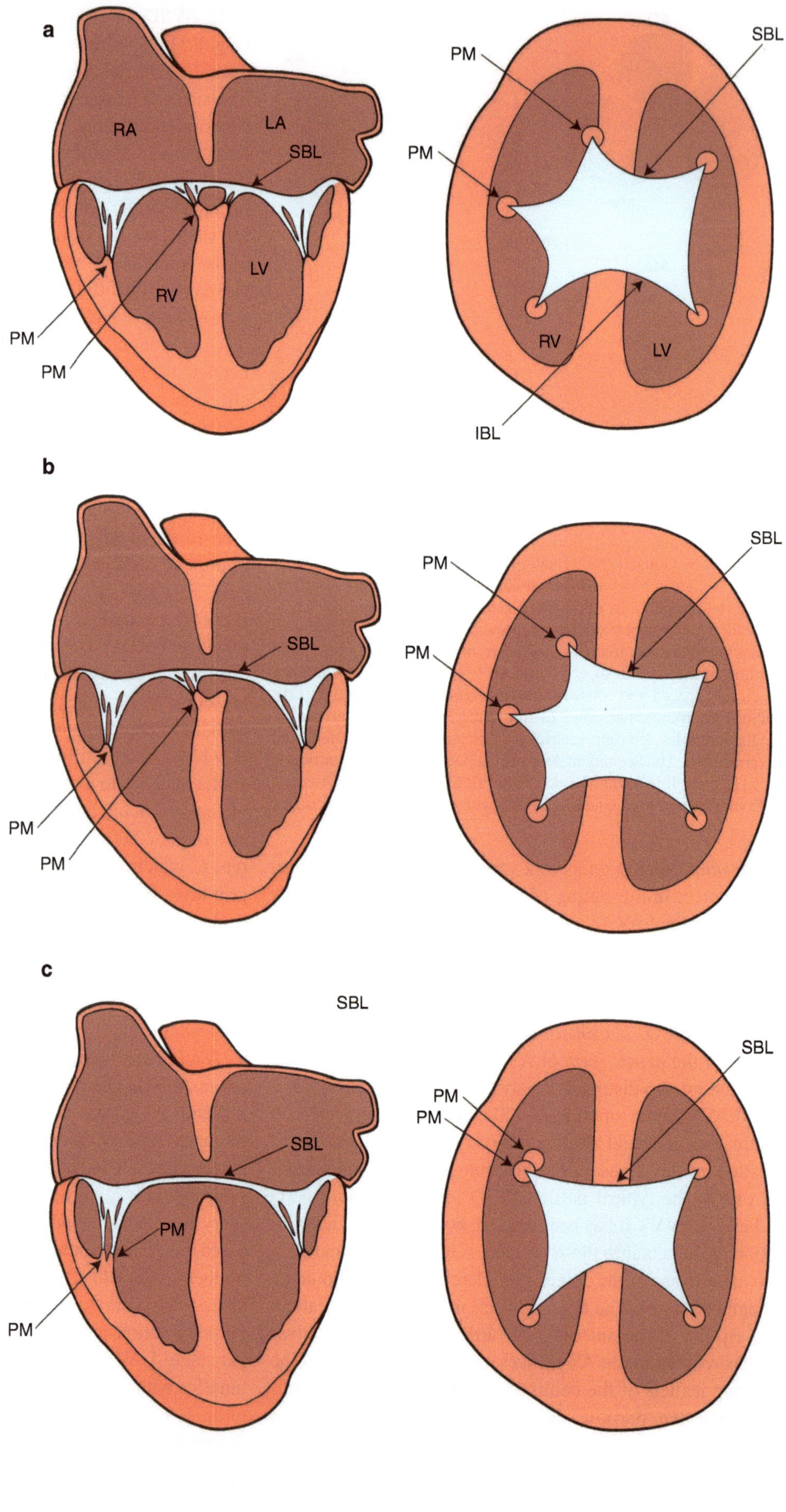

Fig. 8.3 Diagrammatic representation of the Rastelli classification of atrioventricular septal defects as assessed by transesophageal echocardiography in the mid esophageal four chamber (*on the left*) and deep transgastric sagittal views (*on the right*). In *type A* (*panel a*), the superior bridging leaflet attaches to the crest of the interventricular septum. In *type B* (*panel b*), the superior bridging leaflet attaches to a septal papillary muscle on the right aspect of the ventricular septum. In *type C* (*panel c*), the superior bridging leaflet is large and undivided. It extends to the anterior papillary muscle within the right ventricle. *IBL* inferior bridging leaflet, *LA* left atrium, *LV* left ventricle, *PM* papillary muscle, *RA* right atrium, *RV* right ventricle, *SBL* superior bridging leaflet. Modifed from Silverman NH, The Secundum Atrial Septal Defect and Atrioventricular Septal Defects. In: Freedom R and Braunwald E, Atlas of Heart Diseases. St. Louis, Current Medicine LLC, 1996, with permission from Springer

between the mitral and tricuspid valves. In contrast, in AVSD, the aorta is "sprung" anteriorly and superiorly due to the lack of two separate AV orifices between which the aortic valve is normally situated (Fig. 8.2) [12]. These morphologic features, along with a discrepancy in the length of the left ventricular inlet and outlet (Fig. 8.4), create elongation and narrowing of the left ventricular outflow tract (LVOT), producing the so-called '*goose-neck*' deformity characteristic of AVSDs initially described by its angiographic appearance.

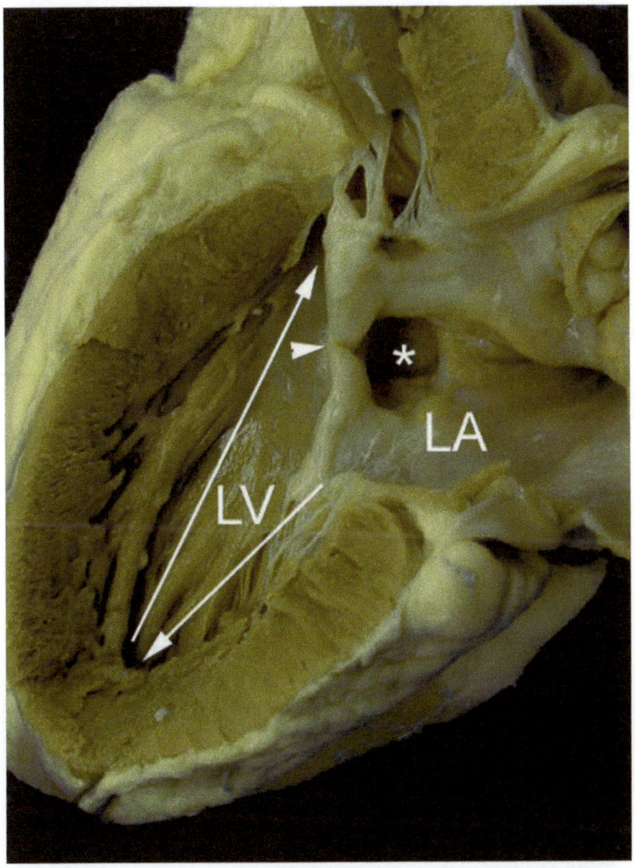

Fig. 8.4 Specimen of an ostium primum atrial septal defect demonstrating length disproportion between the inlet (*arrow* pointing down) and the outlet portions of the left ventricle (LV) from the apex (*arrow* pointing up). The *asterisk* is seen within the ostium primum atrial defect and the ventricular margins of this defect are the so-called 'cleft' (*arrowhead*) representing the fused origin of the superior and inferior bridging leaflets. *LA* left atrium

Shunting of blood in AVSD depends upon the attachment of the AV valve(s) to the septum and the direction of regurgitant valve jets. In diastole shunting is largely atrial, whereas in systole it is largely between the ventricles. If the valve leaflets adhere to the crest of the ventricular septum, as they do in ostium primum ASD, then the shunting is interatrial, whereas if the leaflets adhere to the interatrial septum as they do in isolated VSDs, the shunting is interventricular (Fig. 8.5). A left ventricular to right atrial shunt can be present, and less frequently in some cases, depending on the hemodynamics, right ventricular to left atrial shunts can be seen. These shunts are compounded by additional left ventricular to left atrial and right ventricular to right atrial regurgitant jets.

In most cases, atrial level shunting is holodiastolic in nature and occurs in the left-to-right direction, however, flow reversal (e.g., right-to-left shunting) may occur briefly during the cardiac cycle related to associated pathology and hemodynamic status. The magnitude of shunting at the ventricular level is primarily determined by the size of the defect and the pulmonary vascular resistance. In regards to flow direction, left-to-right ventricular level shunting typically occurs during systole and is enhanced by a low pulmonary vascular resistance. Bidirectional shunting with right-to-left shunting in diastole, or predominant right-to-left shunting are seen in the setting of increased pulmonary vascular tone. Right ventricular to left atrial shunting in systole, although uncommonly seen, may contribute to arterial desaturation.

Pathophysiology

AVSDs represent a group of lesions that result in a volume load to the heart. The presence of an intracardiac communication(s) in these defects typically leads to left-to-right shunting and

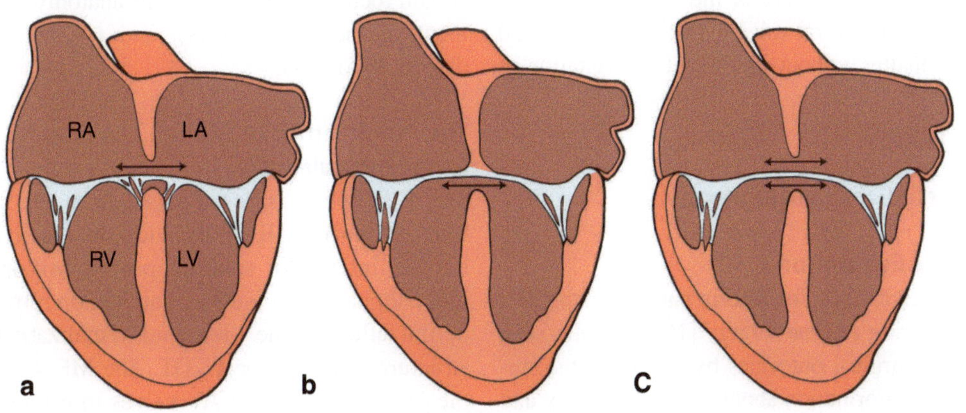

Fig. 8.5 Graphics depict atrial level shunting through an ostium primum atrial septal defect in *panel a*, ventricular level shunting in *panel b*, and combined atrial and ventricular shunting in *panel c*. Refer to text for details. *LA* left atrium, *LV* left ventricle, *RA* right atrium, *RV* right ventricle. Modifed from Silverman NH, The Secundum Atrial Septal Defect and Atrioventricular Septal Defects. In: Freedom R and Braunwald E, Atlas of Heart Diseases. St. Louis, Current Medicine LLC, 1996, with permission from Springer

increased pulmonary blood flow. The concomitant presence of AV valve regurgitation further exacerbates the ventricular volume overload. In the case of complete defects, the symptomatology is magnified due to shunts both at atrial and ventricular levels, frequent ventriculo-atrial shunts, and the presence of pulmonary hypertension. The elevated pulmonary artery pressure also imposes a pressure load on the right ventricle. Due to these factors, patients with complete AVSDs are generally in significant congestive heart failure; these symptoms account for the fact that complete AVSDs require corrective surgery during infancy. In some cases, elevated pulmonary vascular resistance limits left-to-right shunting and in fact, as mentioned, may even lead to predominant right-to-left shunting resulting in cyanosis. In the case of partial defects with a VSD, interventricular pressure restriction across the small defect limits the degree of ventricular left-to-right shunting, thereby minimizing pulmonary overcirculation and volume overload. Nonetheless these patients can still present with congestive symptoms if there is hemodynamically significant LAVV regurgitation. In partial defects without significant LAVV regurgitation, the physiology mimics that of any other atrial level communication, and clinical symptoms might be minimal or absent. In this case, left-to-right atrial level shunting is determined by the relative compliances of the ventricular chambers.

Management Considerations

A number of surgical techniques have been applied to the surgical correction of AVSDs. In complete defects, the goal of the intervention is reconstruction of the common AV valve to achieve two separate and competent AV valves, along with closure of the LAVV cleft, closure of the intracardiac communications, and repair of associated defects. This can be accomplished by a variety of approaches (i.e., single patch, double-patch, and modified techniques) [13–15]. The objectives of the surgical repair in partial AVSDs are to eliminate shunting, in the majority of cases by patch closure of the primum septal defect, and closure of the cleft to create the equivalent of an anterior mitral valve leaflet that coapts well with the posterior leaflet without significant regurgitation or stenosis.

Transesophageal Echocardiography

Preoperative TEE Evaluation

The most common indication for TEE in patients with CHD is for assessment during cardiac surgery [16]. Intraoperative TEE has improved surgical outcomes by providing the surgeon with real-time information about cardiac anatomy and valvular function [3, 17]. TEE can confirm or exclude preoperative transthoracic information and assess the immediate preoperative hemodynamics and ventricular function. In addition, important findings and key anatomic and hemodynamic features can be directly demonstrated to the perioperative providers for immediate review just prior to commencement of the operation. Preoperative TEE may also facilitate the placement of central venous catheters, selection of anesthetic agents, and use of preoperative inotropic support by demonstrating ventricular systolic function and size (refer to Chaps. 3 and 15) [18, 19]. However, in keeping with the recommendations of the Task Force of the Pediatric Council of the American Society of Echocardiography on pediatric TEE, as in the case of all congenital cardiac defects, an AVSD and its anatomical features should be defined completely preoperatively by transthoracic imaging [16]. The prebypass TEE should then confirm the TTE findings. Pertinent points to be addressed by the prebypass TEE include:

- The atrial communication(s)
- The type and extent of the ventricular communication(s)
- Atrioventricular valve morphology and function
- Shunting patterns and AV valve regurgitation
- Commitment of the AV junction to the underlying ventricular mass and the size of the ventricles (balance)
- Associated cardiac anomalies, including patent ductus arteriosus, left superior vena cava to coronary sinus, and coexistent lesions of moderate complexity such as tetralogy of Fallot

In addition, on the prebypass TEE, the operator should search for additional VSDs that might require surgical intervention as these may be easily missed in previous TTE imaging. The echocardiographer should also document the degree of AV valve regurgitation to facilitate comparison with any residual regurgitation after repair.

Intraoperative Imaging

Two-Dimensional Imaging of Complete Defects

As previously mentioned, the preoperative examination should focus on the details of the anatomy, functional assessment of the AV valves(s), and evaluation of associated defects as follows:

The Atrioventricular Septum and Common Atrioventricular Valve

The AV septum is best imaged from the mid esophageal four chamber (ME 4 Ch) view in the axial orientation. Further inferior or superior probe positioning within the mid esophagus, as well as anteflexion/retroflexion, allows optimization of the view and visualization of additional structures such as the LVOT. The ME 4 Ch demonstrates the relationship of the AV valves to each other and to the

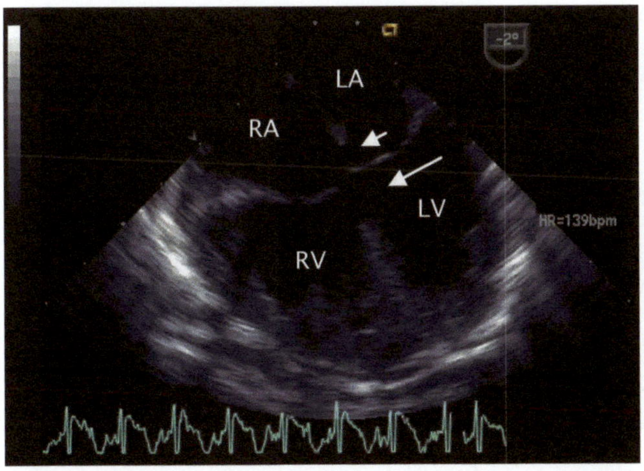

Fig. 8.6 Mid esophageal four chamber view demonstrating a complete atrioventricular septal defect. The primum atrial septal defect (*short arrow*) and inlet ventricular septal defect (*long arrow*) that characterize this malformation are shown. *LA* left atrium, *LV* left ventricle, *RA* right atrium, *RV* right ventricle

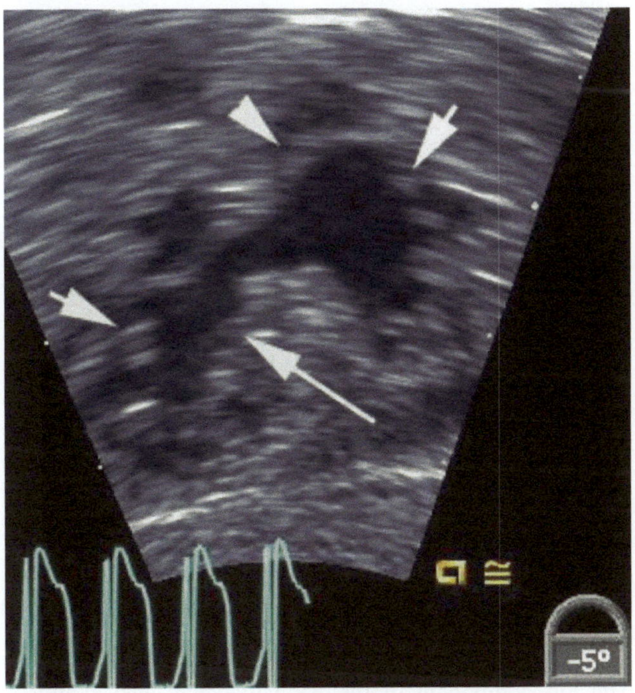

Fig. 8.7 Deep transgastric view showing the open common atrioventricular valve *en face*. The valve morphology is well seen in this view including the superior bridging leaflet (*arrowhead*), inferior bridging leaflet (*long arrow*) and the right and left mural leaflets (*short arrows*)

septa. In this defect, the AV valves insert onto the interventricular septum at the same level (Fig. 8.6, Video 8.1). Septal attachments of the chordae tendineae and papillary muscle apparatus of the LAVV define the 'cleft' or commissure between the superior and inferior bridging leaflets. The echocardiographer should assess the anatomical boundaries of the atrial and septal components of the defect. Scanning posteriorly (probe retroflexion) from the ME 4 Ch view defines the posterior limits of the atrial and ventricular components of the septal defect. Locating the crux of the heart (coronary sinus) with retroflexion of the transducer followed by slight anteflexion defines the position of the inferior components of the AV valve as it crosses the septum. The superior component is correspondingly defined in this plane by anteflexing the probe so that the bridging leaflet is observed crossing the anterior aspect of the defect. Anterior angulation of the transducer by cephalad retraction of the probe and further anteflexion from the ME 4 Ch view to a 'five chamber view' defines the anterior extent of the septal defects, the relationship of the chordae tendineae to the underlying ventricular septum and the LVOT, and the aortic root.

The morphology of the common AV valve and chordal attachments should be assessed in multiple planes including those displayed by the ME 4 Ch, mid esophageal long axis (ME LAX), TG basal short axis (TG Basal SAX), transgastric two chamber (TG 2 Ch), deep transgastric long axis (DTG LAX), and deep transgastric sagittal (DTG Sagittal) views. The ME 4 Ch view is particularly useful for defining the Rastelli type, although the operator must be cognizant of the scan plane passing through the superior leaflet (Fig. 8.3). This is achieved by pulling the transducer cephalad from this view into the upper esophagus, applying anteflexion and then directing the scan plane slightly posterior by advancing the transducer to the level of the mid esophagus until the superior bridging leaflet is identified. Transgastric and deep transgastric short axis views of the ventricles that display the common AV valve *en face*, much like a transthoracic subcostal view, also assist in the determination of Rastelli type as well as degree of balance of the AV valve over the ventricles, and attachments of the valve to the left and right ventricular papillary muscles (Figs. 8.3 and 8.7, Video 8.2). Because the plane of the AV junction is oriented more vertically in patients with an AVSD, the true short axis view in this anomaly is obtained using a more sagittal plane, which may require further angulation of the probe, by rotation and anteflexion [10, 20]. It is usually helpful to advance the probe into the stomach, apply anteflexion and then further advance the probe while it is flexed to increase its anterior curvature. The probe may then be gently withdrawn while maintaining anteflexion towards the esophago-gastric junction, until the optimal image comes into view. This "in between" deep transgastric view with multiplane angle between 0° (DTG LAX view) and 90° (DTG Sagittal view) is optimal to display the common AV valve *en face* (Fig. 8.8, Video 8.3).

There is considerable morphologic and functional variation in the AV valves and their support apparatus. Short axis

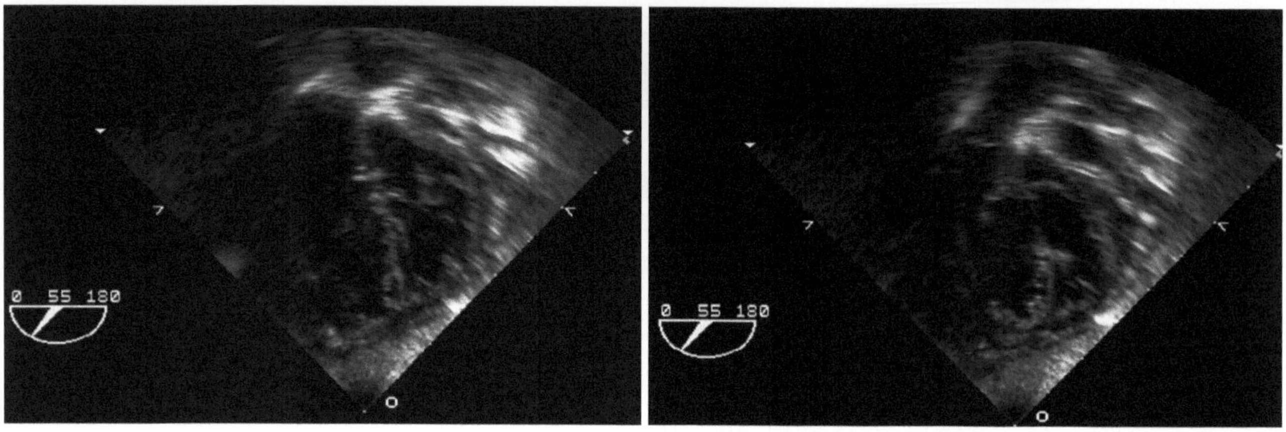

Fig. 8.8 Deep transgastric views at 55° display common atrioventricular valve *en face* in infant with complete atrioventricular septal defect. *Left panel* depicts closed valve in systolic frame and *right panel* opened valve in diastolic frame

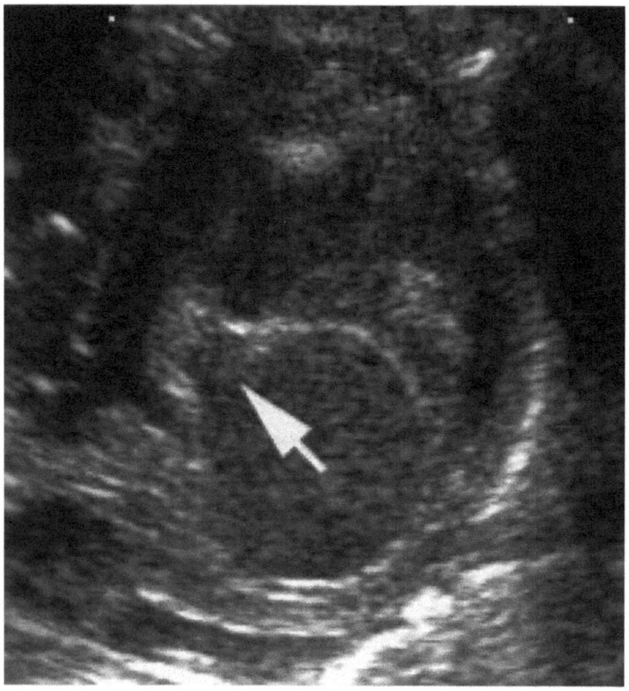

Fig. 8.9 Transthoracic parasternal short axis image demonstrating a cleft in left atrioventricular valve (*arrow*) pointing toward the inlet septum in an atrioventricular septal defect

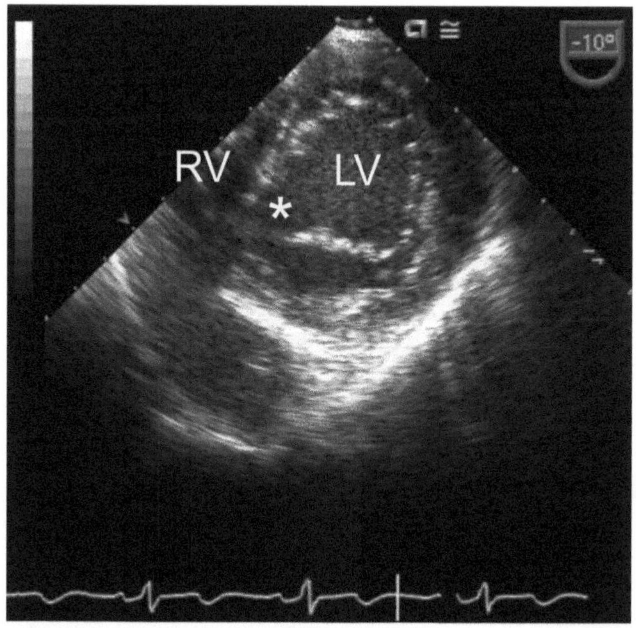

Fig. 8.10 Transgastric basal short axis view displaying cleft in the left atrioventricular valve (*asterisk*) in a patient with an atrioventricular septal defect. *LV* left ventricle, *RV* right ventricle

scanning of the entire AV orifice from a transgastric or deep transgastric plane displays the five leaflets of the common AV valve and the cleft between the left-sided components of the bridging leaflets (Fig. 8.7, Video 8.2). In AVSD, the cleft always points toward the inlet septum (Figs. 8.9 and 8.10, Videos 8.4 and 8.5), while an isolated cleft that is not part of an AVSD points to the LVOT [20–22]. The morphology of the left component of the AV valve should also be examined by imaging in the ME LAX view with the transducer plane at approximately 120^0 (Fig. 8.11, Video 8.6). The left component of the AV valve may also exhibit a double orifice, which can be identified in the *en face* view (Fig. 8.12, Video 8.7) [23, 24].

The Interatrial Communication

An ostium primum type atrial septal communication is found in most AVSDs. In a study examining the cross-sectional echocardiographic findings in AVSDs, a primum ASD was identified in nearly all patients (170 out of 171) [10]. Among the entire cohort, 74 % had a complete AVSD and 25 % a partial defect. A single patient had only a VSD component and cleft mitral valve.

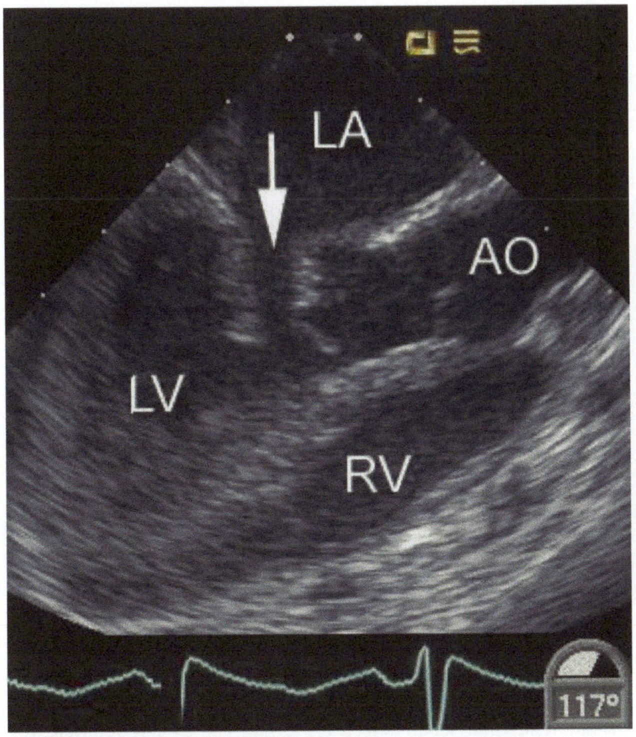

Fig. 8.11 Mid esophageal long axis view displaying a cleft in the left-sided component of a common atrioventricular valve (*arrow*). This is associated with abnormal motion of this region of the valve as shown. In this defect the cleft points towards the septum. *AO* aorta, *LA* left atrium, *LV* left ventricle, *RV* right ventricle

The ostium primum ASD can be defined from a number of views, but is best outlined when the atrial septum is perpendicular to the transducer. This can be accomplished in the ME 4 Ch view (approximately 0^0) by rotating the shaft of the transducer slightly clockwise to focus on the interatrial septum (Fig. 8.13, Video 8.8). The size of the ostium primum defect may vary from very large to extremely small. When the interatrial septum is well formed, it can be defined in the ME 4 Ch view as extending from the interatrial groove down to the lower edge of the inferior rim of the oval fossa. The ostium primum defect extends from the lower edge of the true atrial septum to the conjoined AV valve bridging leaflets inferiorly [10].The junction of the lower end of the atrial septum and an enlarged coronary sinus due to the connection of a left superior vena cava should not be confused with an ostium primum defect, particularly because the two structures are adjacent to each other. The coronary sinus is situated just anterior to the crux of the heart, and an ostium primum defect is located anterior to the coronary sinus. The ostium primum defect can also be identified from the mid esophageal bicaval (ME Bicaval) view with the plane at approximately 90^0. Shunting across the ostium primum defect occurs during diastole and in most cases flow is laminar and low velocity. Aliasing and higher than expected flow velocities can be seen depending on the size of the defect and relative amount of blood flow across it.

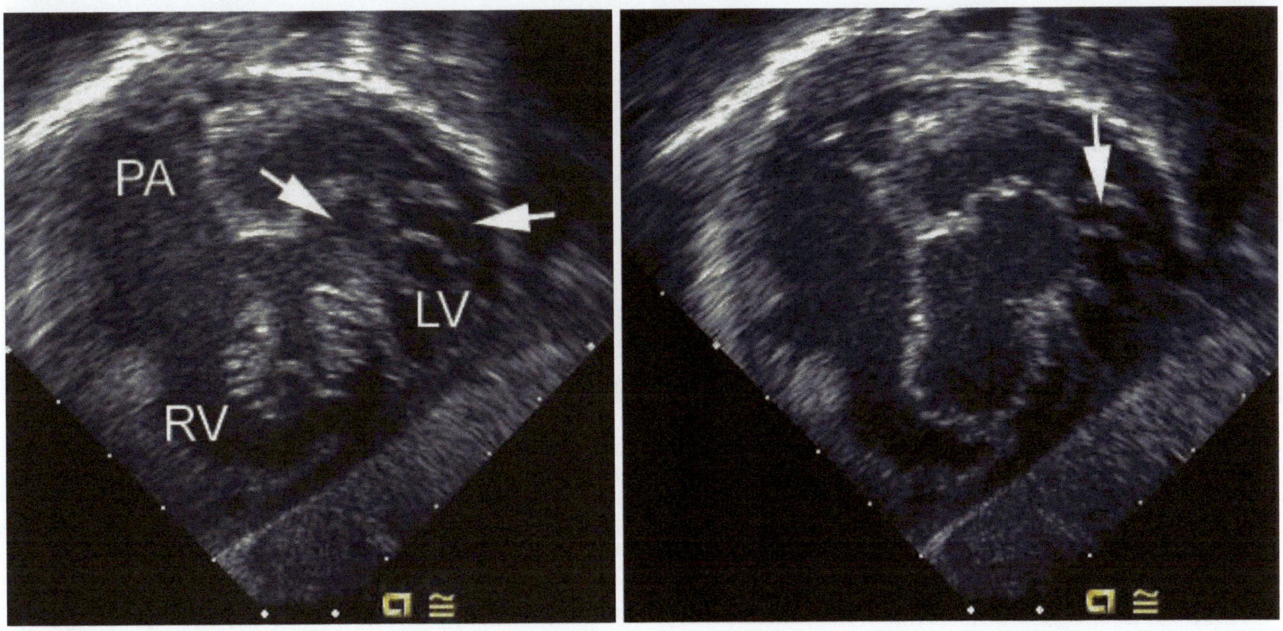

Fig. 8.12 *Left panel*, deep transgastric sagittal transesophageal echocardiographic image of a child with an atrioventricular septal defect and double-orifice of the left component of the atrioventricular valve. The left component is marked by the *arrows* during systole. *Right panel*, corresponding diastolic frame demonstrating the common atrioventricular valve orifice *en face* with its right and left components. An *arrow* notes the area of double orifice. *LV* left ventricle, *PA* pulmonary artery, *RV* right ventricle

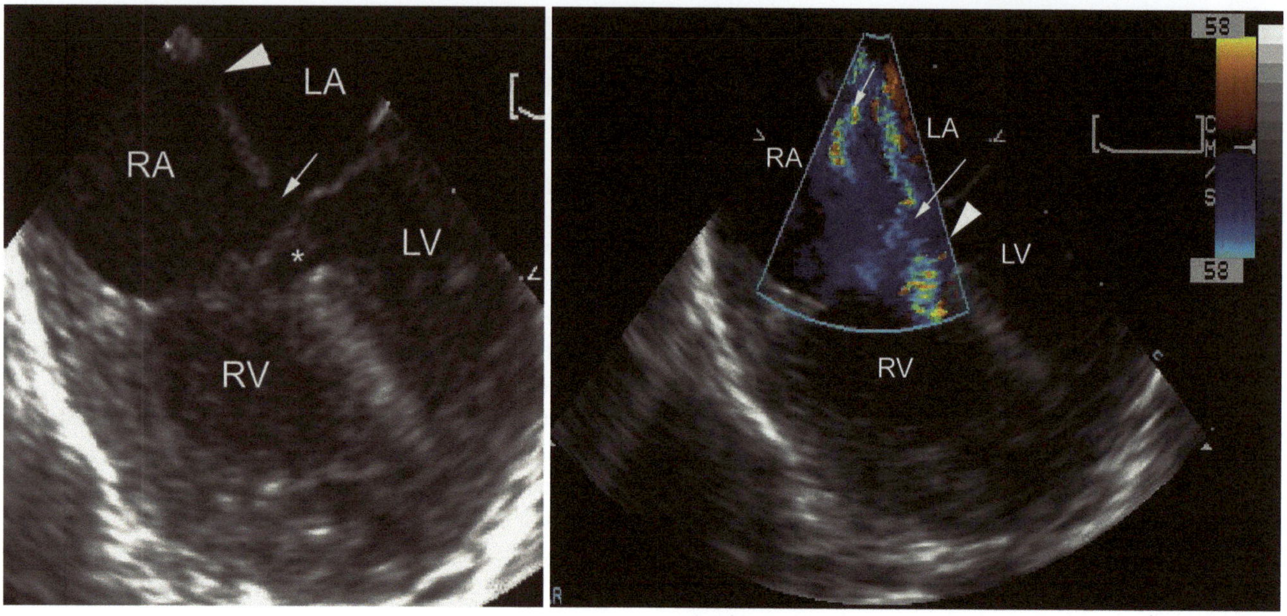

Fig. 8.13 *Left panel*, mid esophageal four chamber view depicting an atrioventricular septal defect. There is dual atrial level shunting at both the level of the ostium primum (*arrow*) and ostium secundum defect (*arrowhead*). The *asterisk* within the ventricular mass shows the ventricular septal defect surrounded by aneurysmal tissue, or so-called '*tricuspid pouch*'. *Right panel*, the color flow information is superimposed upon the morphologic image showing the left-to-right atrial shunting across both atrial communications (*arrows*). The accelerative flow in the region of the tricuspid pouch (*arrowhead*) indicates the presence of a small ventricular septal defect. *LA* left atrium, *LV* left ventricle, *RA* right atrium, *RV* right ventricle

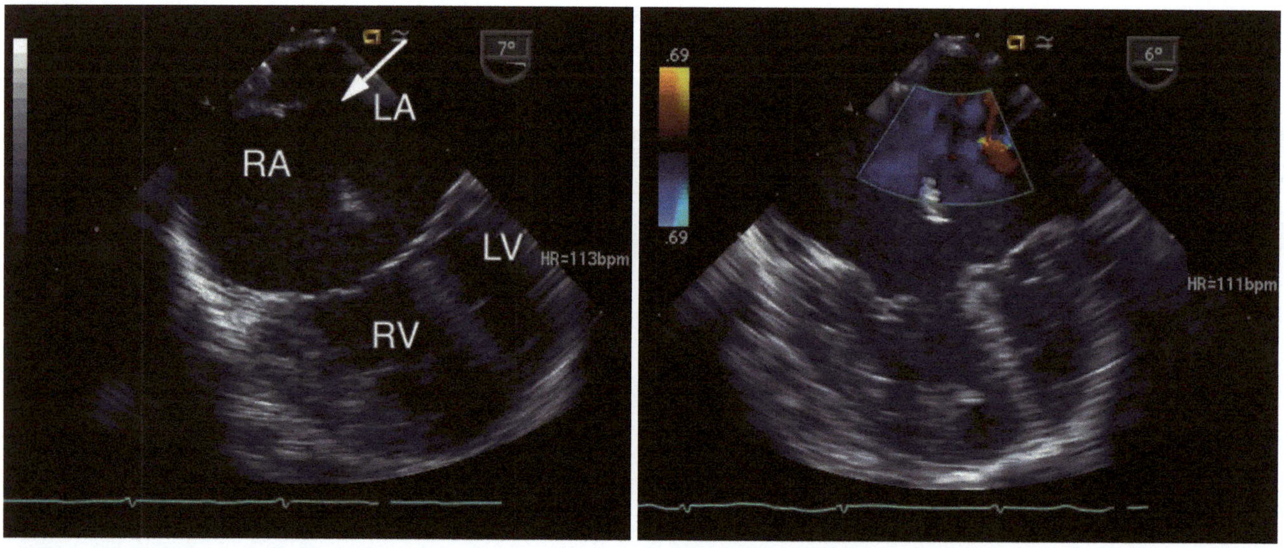

Fig. 8.14 *Left panel*, a large secundum atrial septal defect is seen (*arrow*) in association with an atrioventricular septal defect. *Right panel*, color interrogation demonstrates atrial level left-to-right shunting (*blue flow*). *LA* left atrium, *LV* left ventricle, *RA* right atrium, *RV* right ventricle

Ostium secundum ASDs are also frequently present (Figs. 8.13 and 8.14, Videos 8.8 and 8.9). In isomerism of the atrial appendages, the atrial septum can be almost completely absent with only a strand of atrial tissue remaining.

The Ventricular Component of the Defect

The ventricular component of the AVSD is displayed best in the ME 4 Ch view where its central portion below the bridging AV leaflets is seen (Fig. 8.15, Video 8.10). Other planes such as the ME LAX, TG Basal SAX, transgastric mid short axis (TG Mid SAX) and the deep transgastric views should also be used (Fig. 8.16, Video 8.11) to assess the ventricular communication(s). Isolated ventricular defects are rare (1 out of 171 patients with AVSDs in series described previously) and have been classified as 'VSDs of the AV canal type' (Fig. 8.17, Video 8.12). These differ from

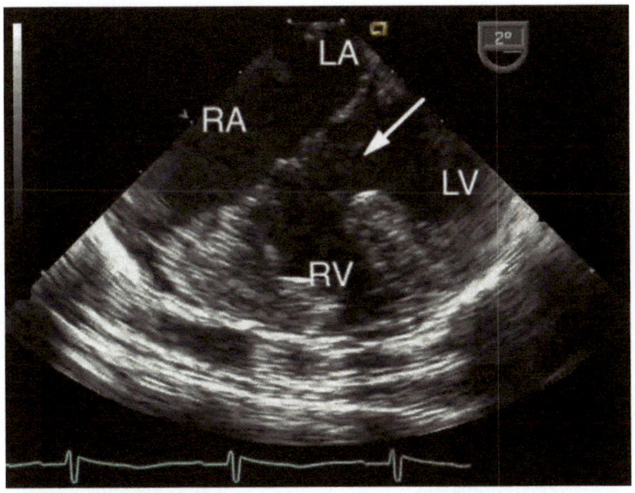

Fig. 8.15 The large ventricular component of a complete atrioventricular septal defect is shown (*arrow*). The right ventricular hypertrophy reflects the elevated pulmonary artery pressure that characterizes the lesion. *LA* left atrium, *LV* left ventricle, *RA* right atrium, *RV* right ventricle

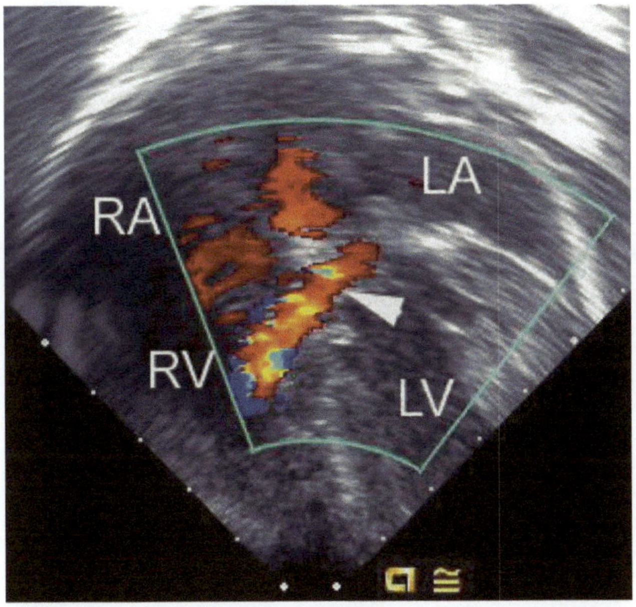

Fig. 8.16 Deep transgastric image obtained as a four chamber equivalent view showing a shunt jet (*arrowhead*) originating within the left ventricle (*LV*) associated with a flow convergence signal before it passes through the ventricular component of an atrioventricular septal defect into the right ventricle (*RV*). *LA* left atrium, *RA* right atrium

true isolated VSDs in the inlet septum (discussed in Chap. 9) in that they are located more posteriorly and have typical associations such as rotated papillary muscles and a cleft in the left component of the AV valve [25]. They can also have chordae from the left AV valve attaching to the crest of the ventricular septum.

The proximity of the VSD to the AV valves and their chordal apparatus may obscure the defect in diastole.

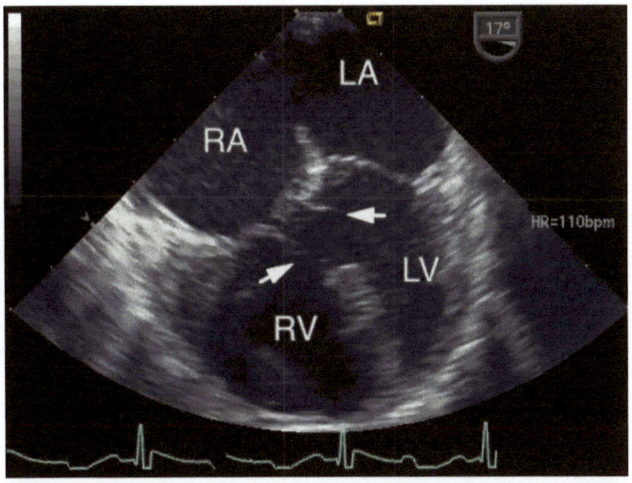

Fig. 8.17 Mid esophageal four chamber view depicting a ventricular septal defect of the 'atrioventricular canal-type'. In this defect separate atrioventricular valve orifices were present and the atrial communication was of the secundum-type. Several chordal attachments (*arrows*) are seen from the atrioventricular valves to the crest of the ventricular septum. Note the lack of normal offsetting of the atrioventricular valves. *LA* left atrium, *LV* left ventricle, *RA* right atrium, *RV* right ventricle

Therefore, the ventricular component of the defect is best defined during systole when the AV valve leaflets are closed and the chordal apparatus tensed. During systole, the valve leaflets move away from the ventricular component of the defect exposing the VSD and its relationship to the underlying papillary muscles and/or the ventricular septum. In those situations when the defect is not easily visualized because of dense chordal attachments to the crest of the interventricular septum, flow may still be detected by Doppler color flow imaging (Fig. 8.13, Video 8.8). The atrial component of the defect can be difficult to define when the common AV valve is open, especially if small, as there is complete communication between the atria and ventricles. This may be better appreciated when the valve is closed. Thus, definition of the components of the defect should be performed during the full cardiac cycle.

AVSDs intrinsically have elongation of the LVOT and shortening of the left ventricular inflow, creating inlet–outlet disproportion (Fig. 8.4) as mentioned. This is in contrast to the left ventricle in the normal heart where the inlet and outlet are of equal length. Anterior angulation of the transducer from the deep transgastric window and a multiplane angle of 90^0 to visualize the aortic root (DTG Sagittal view) demonstrates the 'gooseneck deformity' of the LVOT (Fig. 8.18, Video 8.13) [10]. The outflow tract can also be imaged from the ME LAX and ME 4 Ch view with anteflexion of the imaging probe. Chordal attachments of the AV valve leaflets, and in some instances accessory left AV valve tissue can also contribute to LVOT obstruction (Fig. 8.19, Video 8.14).

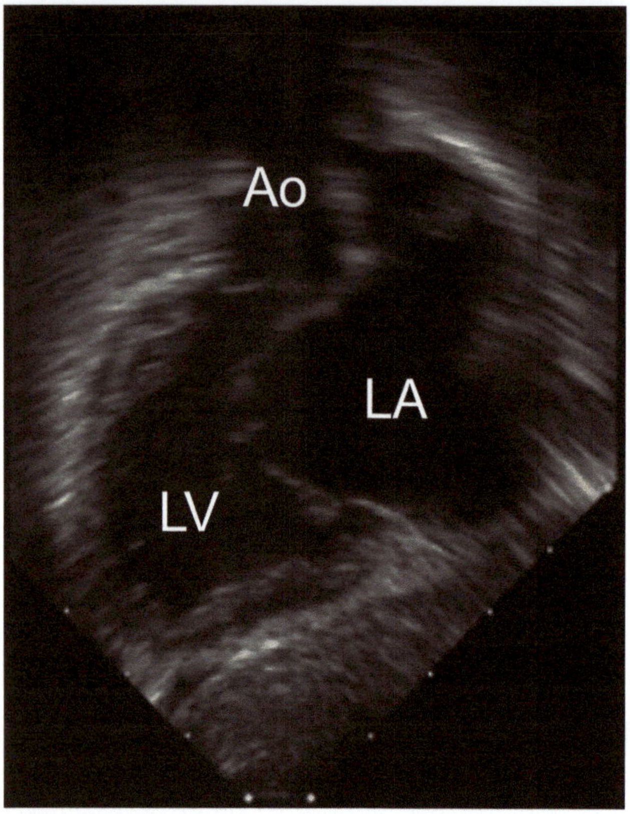

Fig. 8.18 The 'goose neck' deformity of the left ventricular outflow tract that characterizes an atrioventricular septal defect is shown in this deep transgastric sagittal view. *Ao* aorta, *LA* left atrium, *LV* left ventricle

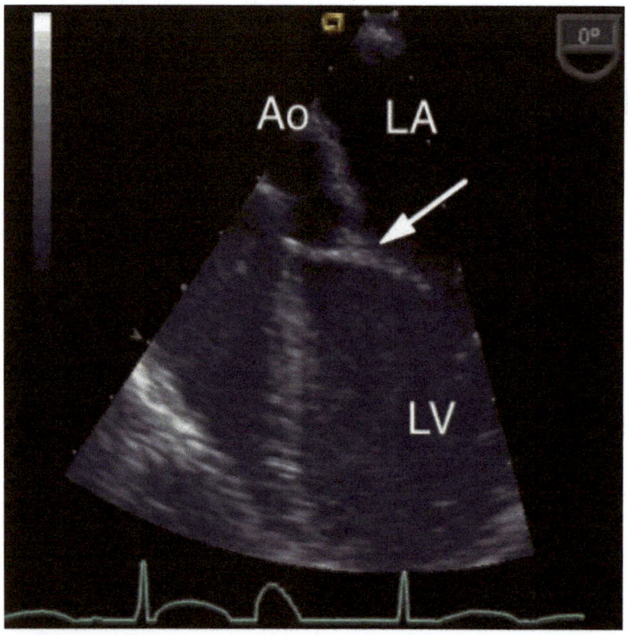

Fig. 8.19 Modified mid esophageal four chamber view with anterior transducer angulation displaying chordal attachments of the left atrioventricular valve across the left ventricular outflow tract onto the interventricular septum (*arrow*). This can result in outflow tract obstruction. *Ao* aorta, *LA* left atrium, *LV* left ventricle

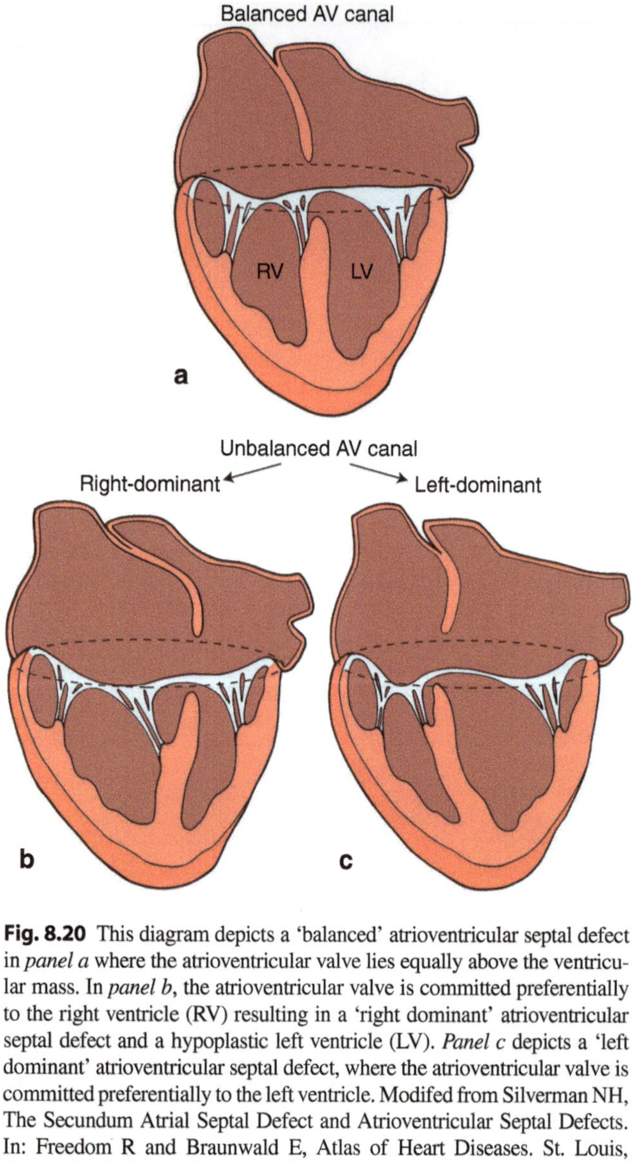

Fig. 8.20 This diagram depicts a 'balanced' atrioventricular septal defect in *panel a* where the atrioventricular valve lies equally above the ventricular mass. In *panel b*, the atrioventricular valve is committed preferentially to the right ventricle (RV) resulting in a 'right dominant' atrioventricular septal defect and a hypoplastic left ventricle (LV). *Panel c* depicts a 'left dominant' atrioventricular septal defect, where the atrioventricular valve is committed preferentially to the left ventricle. Modifed from Silverman NH, The Secundum Atrial Septal Defect and Atrioventricular Septal Defects. In: Freedom R and Braunwald E, Atlas of Heart Diseases. St. Louis, Current Medicine LLC, 1996, with permission from Springer.

Commitment of the Atrioventricular Junction to the Ventricles

Usually the right and left portions of the AV junction are equally committed to their respective ventricles, however, preferential commitment to either ventricle can occur in approximately 5–10 % of cases, resulting in left, or more commonly right ventricular dominance (Fig. 8.20) [10, 26]. This is also known as an *unbalanced* AVSD.

The commitment of the AV orifice to the underlying ventricles by TEE can be defined from the ME 4 Ch view (Fig. 8.21, Video 8.15), but additional views (including the TG Basal SAX and deep transgastric views) provide further comprehensive assessment. Unbalance of AV tissue over the ventricles, ventricular hypoplasia or the presence of a single left ventricular papillary muscle may preclude a biventricular repair. Unbalanced AVSDs are commonly associated

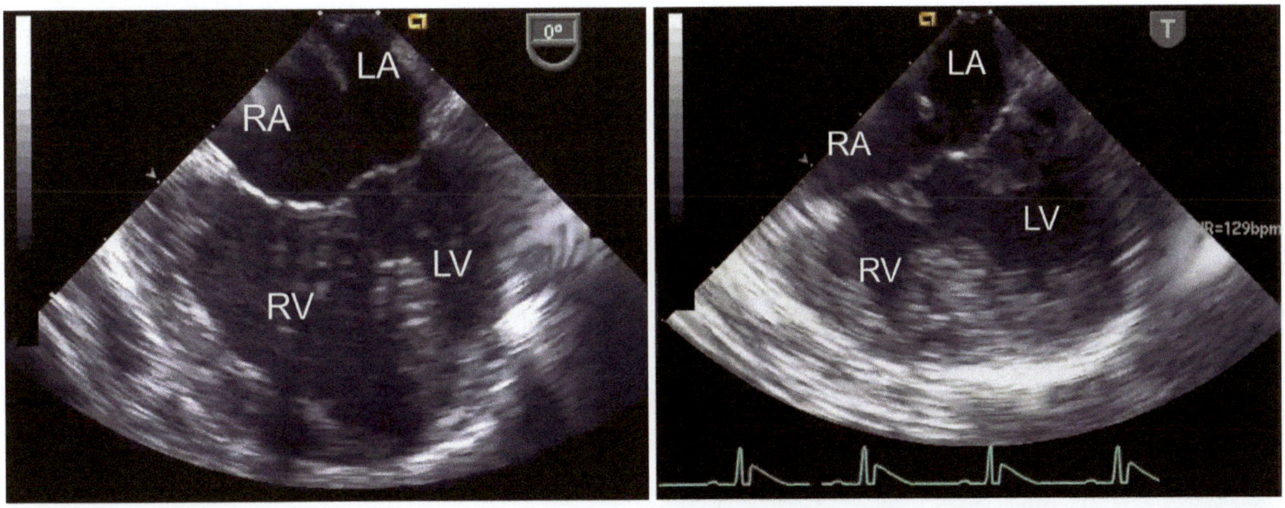

Fig. 8.21 The figure displays unbalanced atrioventricular septal defects in the mid esophageal four chamber view (*left panel*, right dominant defect; *right panel*, left dominant defect). *LA* left atrium; *LV* left ventricle; *RA* right atrium; *RV* right ventricle

with heterotaxy syndromes, particularly right atrial isomerism (asplenia). This is further discussed in Chap. 10.

As this represents an important issue for surgical planning, echocardiographic criteria have been investigated to determine the extent of unbalance in order to discriminate between balanced and unbalanced forms of the defect. This is particularly relevant to settings where the degree of unbalance is not extreme, being readily determined by qualitative assessment. A parameter studied by TTE has been referred to as 'atrioventricular valve index' (AVVI) [27].This is obtained from a subcostal left anterior oblique cross section (*en face* view), where the relationship between the common AV valve and ventricular septum are visualized. The orifice of the common AV valve is traced in diastole and after a line in drawn corresponding to the plane of the interventricular septum, the respective areas of the left and right components are determined. In its initial description, the AVVI was expressed as the ratio of the area of the smaller AV valve component to the larger component. Most recently, a modified AVVI has been used to correlate anatomic type of AVSD and surgical decision-making [28]. For this purpose the index was simplified, being derived by dividing the LAVV area by the total AV valve area. An AVVI of <0.4 was considered to define right dominance and >0.6, left dominance. Although, not formally studied by transesophageal imaging, this index can also be derived from deep transgastric interrogation using the equivalent *en face* view, allowing for evaluation of balance versus unbalance at the time of surgical intervention.

Two-Dimensional Imaging of Incomplete (Partial) Defects

As indicated, in all forms of AVSD the AV junction consists of a single annulus, but there may be a single valve orifice (the complete form), or two separate orifices (the partial form), formed by a tongue of tissue connecting the two bridging leaflets and dividing the common orifice. Functionally separated AV orifices also occur when only an atrial or ventricular component of the defect is present. An isolated ventricular component of an AVSD occurs only rarely, as previously noted. An isolated atrial component (ostium primum ASD) occurs much more frequently and results from fusion of the bridging leaflets with the ventricular septum. A cleft in the mitral valve, best seen in views that display the valve in its short axis, can be associated with variable degrees of regurgitation.

Partial AVSDs may exhibit redundant tissue prolapsing through the interventricular communication into the right ventricle, also known as *tricuspid pouch*. This is comprised by connecting tissue between the bridging leaflets and tissue from the superior bridging leaflet and its tensor apparatus [10, 29]. This structure can be seen in the ME 4 Ch view (Fig. 8.22, Video 8.16) and short axis images of the common AV valve from the transgastric and deep transgastric windows, and has an identical appearance to that of tricuspid tissue tags or membranous ventricular septum aneurysm found with perimembranous VSDs. The size of the tricuspid pouch can be quite prominent.

Doppler Evaluation of Defects

The detection of shunting patterns by color flow Doppler is important for the surgical repair as well for prognosis [10, 30, 31]. This applies to both the evaluation of intracardiac communications and valve regurgitation. Color flow mapping facilitates the assessment of intracardiac shunting (Figs. 8.14, 8.16, and 8.23, Videos 8.9 and 8.11) and is particularly helpful in the assessment of flow when there is limited potential for interventricular shunting under the superior bridging leaflet (restrictive VSD) in the setting of a partial AVSD (Fig. 8.13, Video 8.8). The peak velocity of the jet across the ventricular level shunt, as obtained from spectral Doppler interrogation, represents the pressure gradient between the ventricles in the absence of right ventricular outflow tract obstruction (RVOTO). This can be used to estimate right ventricular and pulmonary artery pressures by applying the simplified Bernoulli equation as follows:

Right Ventricular Systolic Pressure = Systemic Systolic Pressure—Peak Gradient Across Ventricles

Peak Gradient Across Ventricles = 4 (Peak VSD Velocity)^2

Valves with similar morphology can display quite different degrees of regurgitation and functional impairment. Color Doppler interrogation requires an assessment in multiple views of all defects (Fig. 8.24, Video 8.17). Particularly in patients with a partial form of AVSD, the site where regurgitation occurs is important for surgical repair. AV valve regurgitation through the left-sided cleft is frequently directed centrally and may be part of a left ventricular to right atrial shunt. (Fig. 8.25, Video 8.18) The jet may also be directed leftwards and becomes a left ventricular to left atrial shunt. This may be related to mural leaflet hypoplasia of the left component of the AV valve [30]. Right ventricular to right atrial regurgitation may also be substantial (Fig. 8.26, Video 8.19). Often, multiple jets are present (Figs. 8.25 and 8.26, Videos 8.18 and 8.19).

Precise definition of the regurgitant jet is important for accurate interpretation of a pressure gradient in patients with partial defects. A left ventricular to right atrial regurgitant velocity will yield a high estimated gradient due to the large pressure difference between the two chambers, and if this is misinterpreted as a tricuspid regurgitant velocity, the true

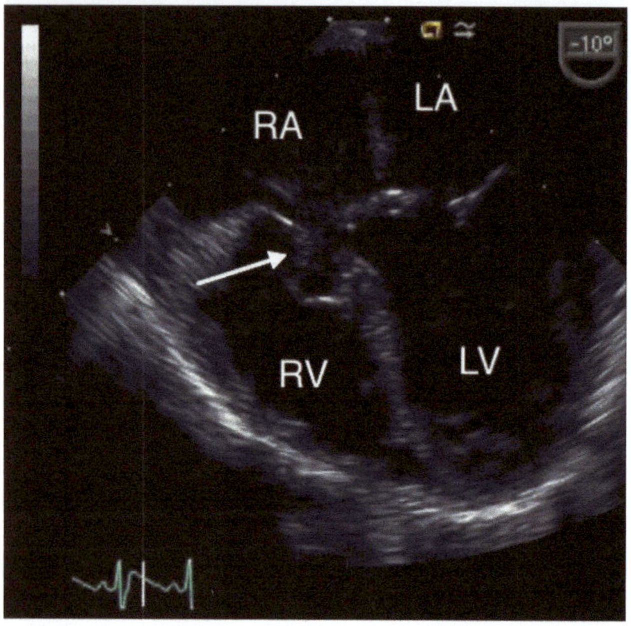

Fig. 8.22 Mid esophageal four chamber view displays a tricuspid pouch lesion (*arrow*) in a patient with a partial atrioventricular septal defect. *LA* left atrium, *LV* left ventricle, *RA* right atrium, *RV* right ventricle

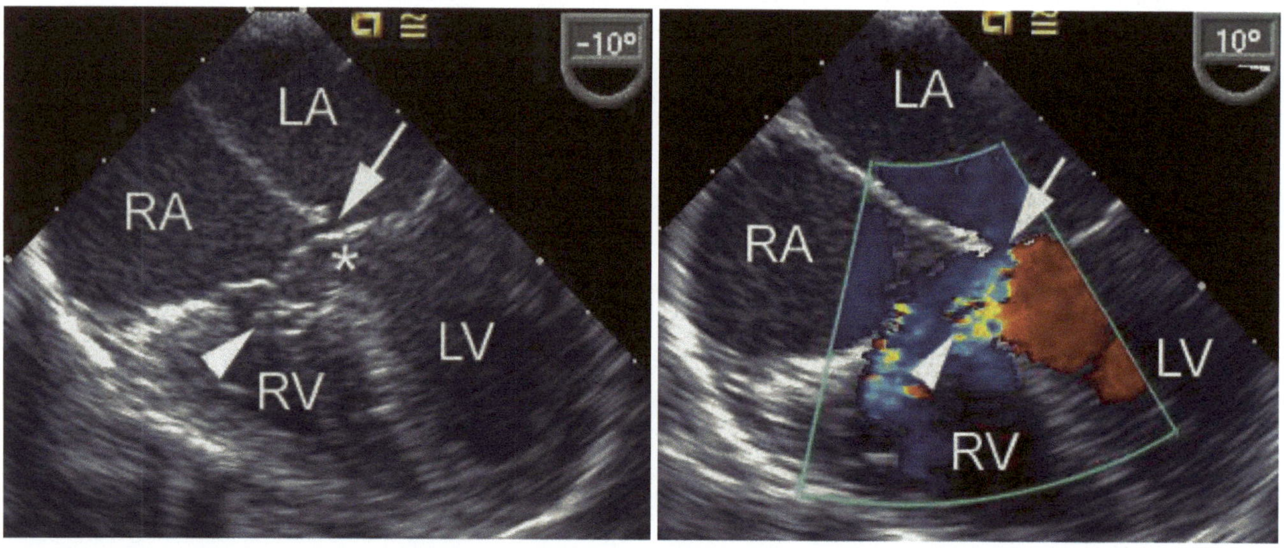

Fig. 8.23 The figure demonstrates an atrioventricular septal defect in a two-dimensional mid esophageal four chamber view in the *left panel* and corresponding color flow mapping demonstrating left-to-right shunting in the *right panel*. The *arrow* points to a small primum atrial septal defect. The *arrowhead* points to a tricuspid pouch and the *asterisk* indicates the ventricular septal defect. *LA* left atrium, *LV* left ventricle, *RA* right atrium, *RV* right ventricle

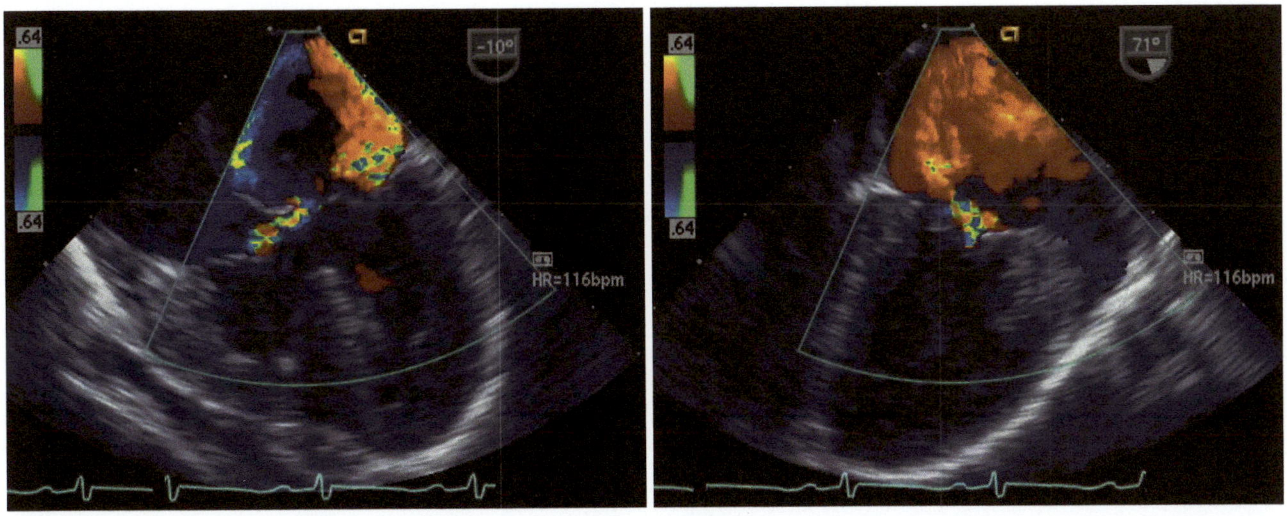

Fig. 8.24 The figure displays a complete atrioventricular septal defect in different transesophageal echocardiographic cross-sections. Color flow mapping demonstrates intracardiac shunting in addition to a significant regurgitant jet across the left component of the common atrioventricular valve. The characteristics of the regurgitant jet are further defined by multiplane imaging, highlighting the importance of color Doppler interrogation in multiple views

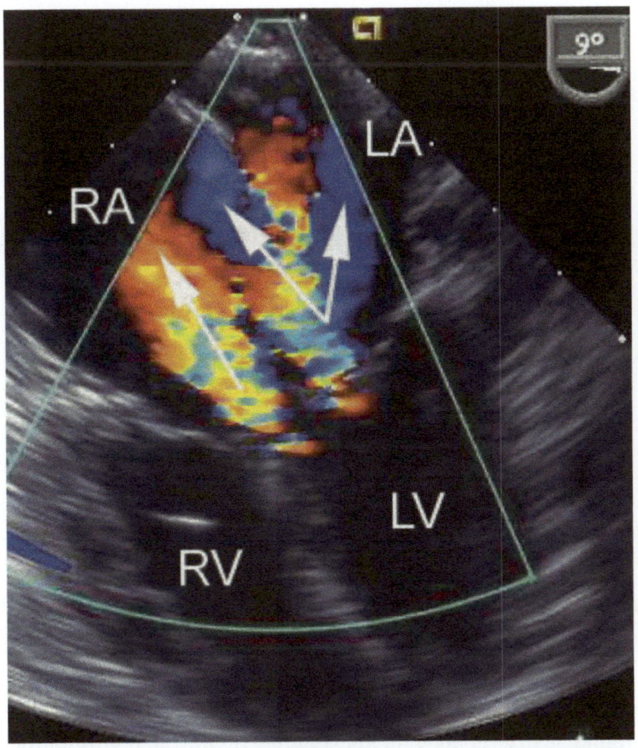

Fig. 8.25 Preoperative mid esophageal four chamber view displaying an atrioventricular septal defect. Color flow mapping depicts multiple regurgitant jets. The *arrows* point to regurgitation from the left ventricle (*LV*) into both the left atrium (*LA*) and right atrium (*RA*), split by the atrial septum, as well as a separate jet from the left-sided component of the atrioventricular septal defect directed into the RA (left ventricular to right atrial shunt). *RV* right ventricle

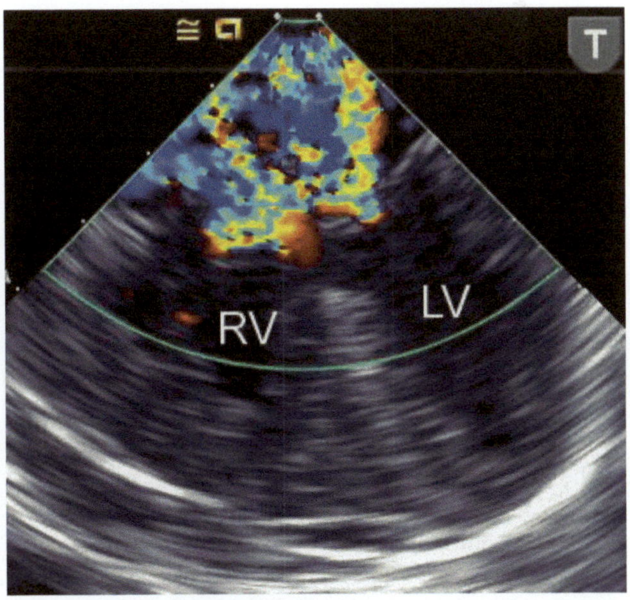

Fig. 8.26 The image shows preoperative color flow information obtained in a mid esophageal four chamber view using a pediatric biplane transesophageal probe in a small infant with a complete atrioventricular septal defect. Significant regurgitation is depicted from both the left and right atrioventricular valvar components, during systole. *LV* left ventricle, *RV* right ventricle

right ventricular pressure could mistakenly be overestimated. If, under the circumstances described here, an accurate right ventricular to right atrial jet can be identified and interrogated by spectral Doppler, a much lower velocity might be recorded.

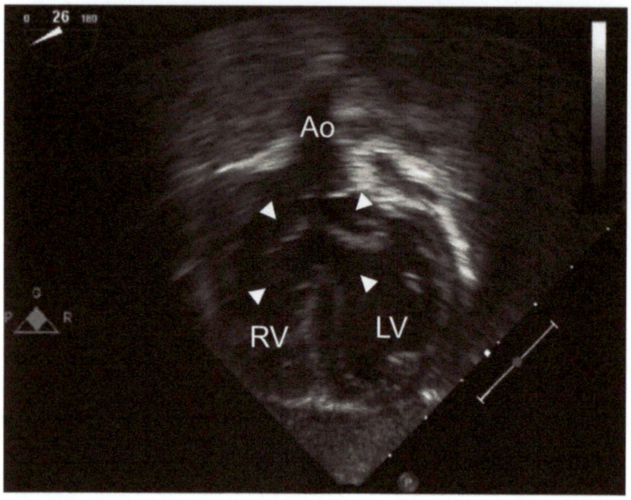

Fig. 8.27 Deep transgastric long axis view in infant with Down syndrome and 'tet-canal defect'. Note the relationship of the aorta (*Ao*) to the common atrioventricular valve (*arrowheads*). The characteristic aortic override in tetralogy of Fallot is well seen. *LV* left ventricle, *RV* right ventricle

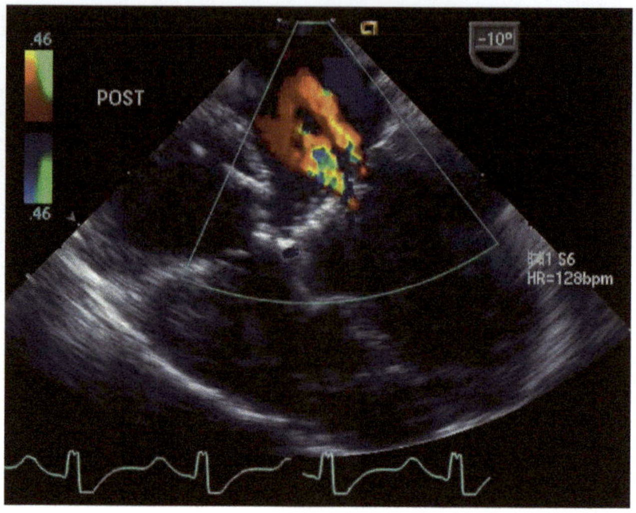

Fig. 8.28 Postoperative transesophageal echocardiogram following repair of a complete atrioventricular septal defect. Color Doppler interrogation demonstrates two small jets of left atrioventricular valve regurgitation. The jet closest to the interatrial septum represents regurgitation across a residual cleft

Associated Cardiac Lesions

Additional muscular VSDs can be found in 10 % of patients with AVSDs [10]. Color Doppler flow mapping facilitates demonstration of these defects but when pulmonary hypertension is present these lesions may be missed. Decreasing the color flow Doppler scale can increase the sensitivity for low velocity color flow signals and sometimes uncover associated muscular VSDs. Tetralogy of Fallot is an important conotruncal malformation that can be seen in combination with an AVSD. This lesion is colloquially referred to as a 'tet-canal' defect. In this setting, the Rastelli type C defect is most commonly found (Fig. 8.27, Video 8.20). Down syndrome is present in the majority of these patients. The echocardiographic findings in this lesion are those previously mentioned for AVSDs, in addition to the features that characterize tetralogy as discussed in Chap. 12 (i.e., RVOT obstruction, aortic override). Other lesions less frequently encountered include valvar pulmonary stenosis, double outlet right ventricle, transposition of the great arteries, and truncus arteriosus. Subaortic stenosis may contribute to LVOTO and may be associated with aortic coarctation [32]. Patent ductus arteriosus is also common, particularly in patients with Down syndrome. Other chromosomal and genetic abnormalities can also be associated with AVSDs [33]. A high percentage of heterotaxy patients will have AVSDs (refer to Chap. 10). In this setting, double outlet right ventricle is a common association. The comprehensive preoperative TEE evaluation in the patient with an AVSD should also include an assessment of associated lesions as described throughout this textbook for each of the respective defects.

Postoperative TEE Evaluation

The most important goal of the postbypass TEE study is to identify significant hemodynamic abnormalities that should be addressed at the time of surgery. Important lesions requiring revision/reintervention include: residual LAVV valve regurgitation or stenosis, residual or additional VSDs, and LVOT obstruction (LVOTO) [34]. These problems, along with the need for permanent pacemaker insertion/revision, are the major indications for reoperation in patients with AVSDs, and a major cause of morbidity and mortality.

TEE has been shown to identify and estimate the severity of valvar regurgitation [35, 36].This imaging modality has been used to accurately localize mitral regurgitant lesions in adults and found to improve the assessment of patients with significant mitral regurgitation [37, 38]. Likewise, intraoperative TEE is also used to assess LAVV function after surgery in children with AVSDs (Fig. 8.28, Video 8.21) [39, 40]. Severe LAVV regurgitation was found by TEE post AVSD surgery in 5 % of patients in one study [17]. Further repair was undertaken so that no patient left the operating room with severe regurgitation. It is of interest that this study found a discrepancy in the degree of mitral regurgitation identified by intraoperative TEE versus predischarge TTE in 45 % of patients. In most cases (81 %), the degree of mitral regurgitation on the predischarge TTE was worse than that found by TEE in the operating room. This may be due to lower systemic blood pressures and higher heart rates at the time of surgery, underestimating the true severity of AV valve regurgitation. It was concluded that the grade of mitral regurgitation by intraoperative TEE does not predict the severity of regurgitation at follow-up as imaged by TTE and it was suggested that TEE findings should be interpreted in

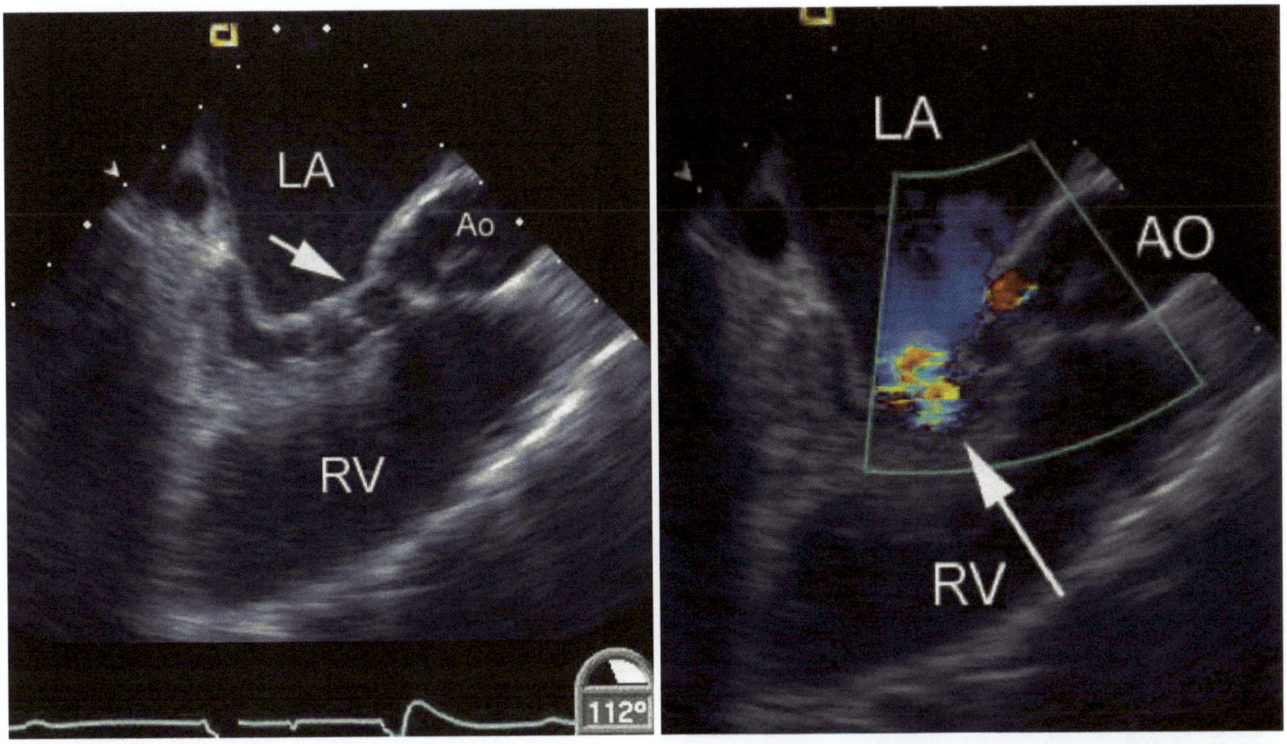

Fig. 8.29 *Left panel*, diastolic frame in a mid esophageal long axis view displaying mitral valve stenosis resulting from cleft closure (*arrow*) following repair of an atrioventricular septal defect. The left atrium (*LA*) appears dilated. Narrowing of the left ventricular outflow tract is also noted in association with multiple chordal attachments across the subaortic region onto the ventricular septum. *Right panel*, color flow information superimposed on the morphologic data shows a turbulent jet across the left ventricular inflow corresponding to mitral stenosis (*arrow*). The coronary sinus appears mildly dilated. *Ao*/*AO* aorta, *RV* right ventricle

the light of the hemodynamic status. Others have also found discrepancies in the severity of mitral valve regurgitation by intraoperative TEE and subsequent TTE [41, 42]. However, these discrepancies were generally not large enough to necessitate reoperation in early to mid-term follow up, leading the authors to conclude that intraoperative TEE may be used as a tool to predict durability of surgical results and to decrease the incidence of reoperation in complete AVSDs. In other studies, an excellent correlation has been identified between intraoperative color flow assessment of LAVV regurgitation and immediate postoperative evaluation [43]. The need for reoperation was found to correlate significantly with the severity of LAVV regurgitation ($r=0.68$) and intraoperative imaging was found to accurately predict the development of early postoperative heart failure and subsequent reoperation for AVSD [43].

We believe that it may not be possible to reliably assess the real degree of regurgitation because of loading conditions as well as changes in myocardial contractility, blood pressure, systemic vascular resistance, and wear and tear as the repair settles into the postoperative functional status. One of the significant errors that can be made is a too rapid report to the surgeon that the regurgitation is minimal immediately after separation from cardiopulmonary bypass. Therefore the initial post-repair TEE assessment should be followed by a later evaluation made prior to removal of the imaging probe.

The difficulties in the echocardiographic assessment of mitral valve regurgitation in children after repair of AVSD were underscored in a recent study [44]. The cohort in this report included children enrolled in a multicenter drug study (enalapril) 6 months following repair of AVSD. The evaluation of the severity of mitral regurgitation by TTE was based in the following criteria: (1) qualitative assessment; (2) measurement of vena contracta width with respect to body size; (3) calculation of vena contracta area; and (4) determination of mitral regurgitant volume and fraction. Among the quantitative parameters evaluated, the methods used in the assessment of the vena contracta were found to be minimally superior to qualitative mitral regurgitation grading. Values for regurgitant volume and fraction were frequently negative. This, in addition to poor interobserver agreement in these parameters, limited their utility.

Stenosis of the left component of the AV valve occurs most commonly after closure of the cleft in the setting of a parachute valve, and in some cases, a double-orifice LAVV. Doppler interrogation during postbypass TEE imaging in the ME 4 Ch view should recognize obstruction to left ventricular inflow so that the surgeon can relieve some of the sutures closing the cleft, or adjust an annuloplasty, if this was undertaken. This assessment can also be performed in the mid esophageal two chamber (ME 2 Ch) and ME LAX views (Fig. 8.29, Video 8.22). In this situation, the best possible balance between hemodynamically tolerable LAVV stenosis and regurgitation needs to be achieved. In rare instances, implantation of a mitral prosthesis becomes necessary; however, this is problematic in smaller patients due to the small size of the LAVV annulus.

An important aspect of the postoperative evaluation in AVSDs is interrogation for the presence of residual intracardiac shunts. Color Doppler is essential in this evaluation and when subsequent reoperation is required to address residual/recurrent hemodynamically significant shunts (Fig. 8.30, Video 8.23).

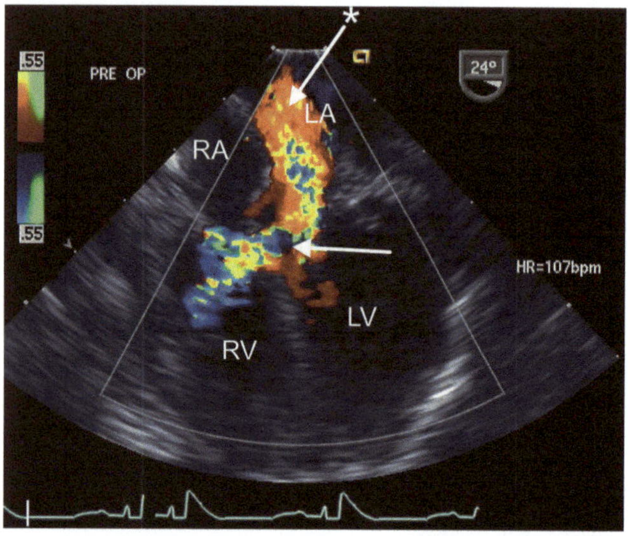

Fig. 8.30 Preoperative transesophageal echocardiogram in an infant requiring reoperation to address a residual inlet ventricular septal defect (*arrow*) as well as significant regurgitation across a large left atrioventricular valve cleft related to suture dehiscence (*arrow with asterisk*). Both lesions are well characterized by color flow imaging in the mid esophageal four chamber view. *LA* left atrium, *LV* left ventricle, *RA* right atrium, *RV* right ventricle

AVSDs, as previously stated, can be associated with LVOTO (Fig. 8.29, Video 8.22) [32]. Potential mechanisms of residual or new onset LVOTO include discrete subaortic fibrous stenosis, tunnel stenosis, accessory LAVV tissue and chordae, redundant LAVV tissue and apparatus, aneurysm of the mitral valve, abnormal papillary muscles, anteroseptal twist, malaligned aorta over the septum, hypertrophic muscle, and mitral valve prosthesis [45–47]. Although LVOTO usually becomes significant only in the period following surgery, the echocardiographer should investigate for LVOTO at the time of intraoperative TEE, especially in the postbypass evaluation (Fig. 8.31, Video 8.24), as any obstruction to flow may need to be addressed at time of surgery.

TEE is also of significant benefit in the recognition of other less common but important complications resulting from the repair of these defects. These problems include unusual intracardiac shunts (Fig. 8.32, Video 8.25) and the rare instance when inferior vena caval flow may be inadvertently directed into the left atrium. The use of contrast echocardiography can be particularly useful in the evaluation of these issues (Fig. 8.33, Video 8.26).

Three-Dimensional Echocardiographic Imaging

Three-dimensional (3D) TTE has been used to define the anatomy of the primum ASD in AVSDs and found to provide important information regarding the spatial orientation and alignment of the endocardial cushion region relative to the ventricles. The ability to determine this alignment and to predict the corresponding size and orientation of the AV valve has important clinical implications and would be essential for considering ASD or VSD

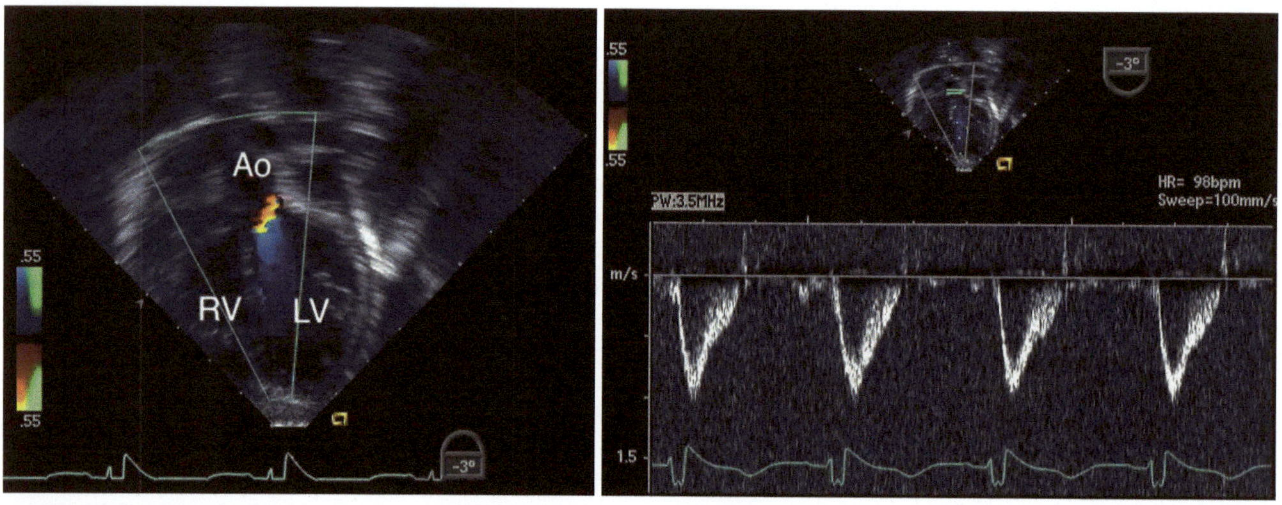

Fig. 8.31 Deep transgastric long axis view obtained following repair of an atrioventricular septal defect. The image displays interrogation of the left ventricular outflow tract using a combination of Doppler modalities (color flow mapping on the *left panel* and spectral Doppler on the *right panel*). No evidence of obstruction was demonstrated in this case. Note the favorable angle for pulsed wave Doppler interrogation of the outflow tract in this view. *Ao* aorta, *LV* left ventricle, *RV* right ventricle

closure (i.e., a biventricular repair), as opposed to consideration of surgical management along the single ventricle pathway [48]. This type of information, when available at the time of intraoperative TEE, would enhance the options for surgical intervention.

3D imaging has also been used to facilitate the preoperative anatomic definition of AVSDs and to predict AV valve regurgitation in children after repair by evaluating the morphology of the valve leaflets [49]. The early experience found that most often two jets of LAVV regurgitation were present in these patients after repair. One jet emanated medially from a residual 'cleft'. The second jet originated laterally from the region of the mural leaflet. These locations were related to the relative sizes of the individual leaflets. When the origin of the jet was directed medially, this was most often associated with a smaller inferior leaflet component. When the regurgitant jet originated laterally, near the coaptation site of the superior and inferior leaflet, this was associated with a smaller mural leaflet. As 3D technology has evolved, subsequent studies have also documented the applications of this approach in regards to anatomic and functional information prior to surgical intervention in these patients [50, 51]. A recent quantitative study of real-time 3D echocardiography in children following repair of AVSD demonstrated that significant mitral valve regurgitation was associated with leaflet prolapse, larger annular area, and papillary muscle displacement in this patient group [52]. A particular strength of this technology, in addition to the diagnostic applications already mentioned, is considered its ability to define complex AV valve and LVOT abnormalities [53].

Transesophageal 3D imaging has also been applied in the assessment of these lesions. An early experience in a small number of patients reported acquisition of 3D data sets to define LAVV morphology and function in patients with AVSDs undergoing patch augmentation of the LAVV for either regurgitation or LVOTO [54]. This reconstructive 3D TEE approach, using a rotational device built into a multiplane two-dimensional (2D) TEE probe, provided clear intracardiac images as there was no interposition of ribs or

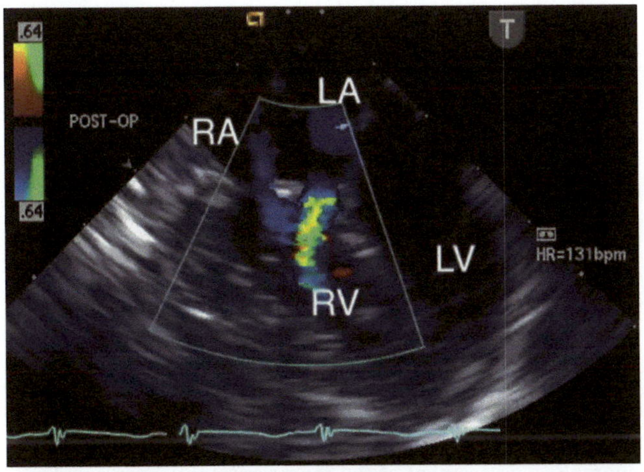

Fig. 8.32 Postbypass transesophageal echocardiogram obtained in the mid esophageal four chamber view demonstrates flow by color Doppler from the left atrium (*LA*) into the right ventricle (*RV*; *blue jet*). This communication, representing a left-to-right shunt, was inadvertently created during repair of the defect. The echocardiographic findings led to revision of the repair. *LV* left ventricle, *RA* right atrium

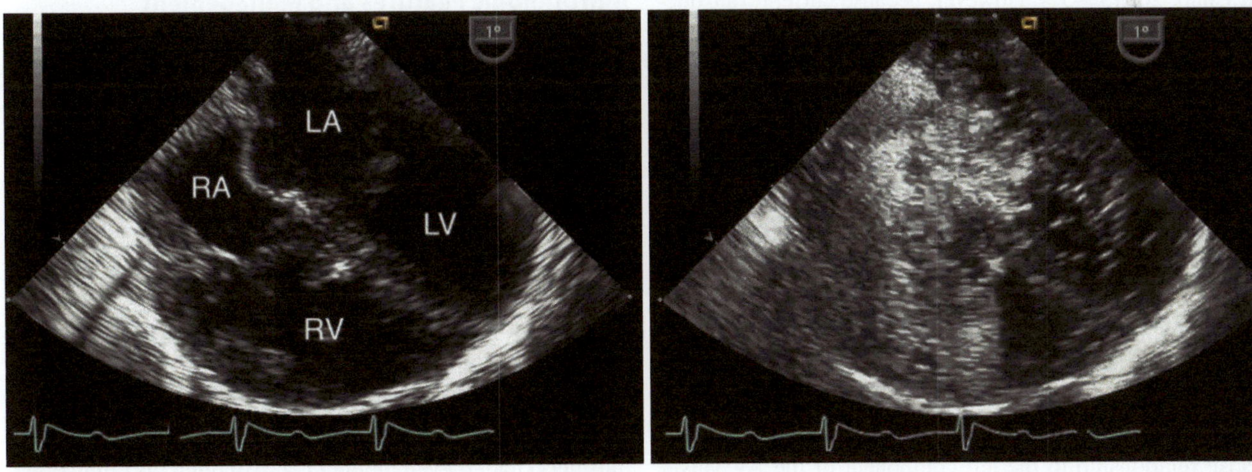

Fig. 8.33 *Left panel*, mid esophageal four chamber view obtained immediately after separation from bypass following repair of a complete atrioventricular septal defect. Both atrial and ventricular septal patches are seen. *Right panel*, contrast study performed to evaluate a small color Doppler signal suggestive of residual ventricular level shunting (not shown). Agitated saline injected through a femoral venous catheter demonstrated opacification of the right atrium with unexpected almost immediate appearance of contrast in the superior aspect of the left atrium. The concern for mistaken partial incorporation of inferior vena cava flow into the LA (right-to-left shunt) was raised. This was confirmed upon return to bypass. After revision of the repair a repeat contrast study demonstrated a normal flow pattern and no residual shunts. *LA* left atrium, *LV* left ventricle, *RA* right atrium, *RV* right ventricle

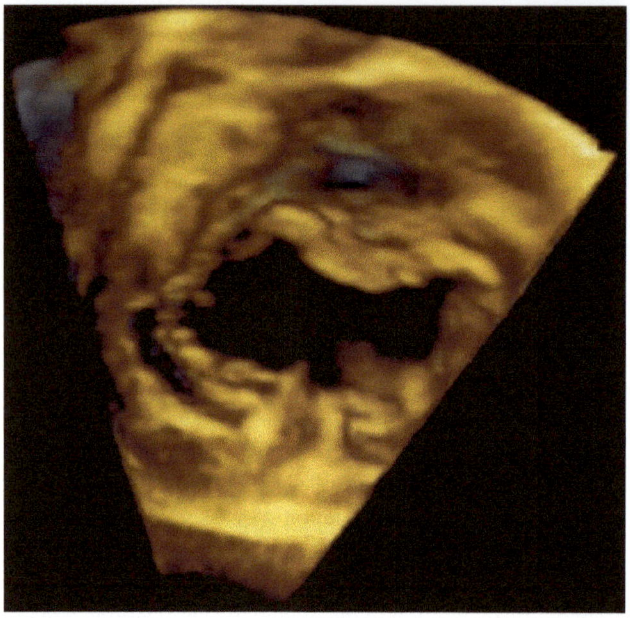

Fig. 8.34 Three-dimensional image obtained by transesophageal echocardiography in an older child displaying *en face* view of a complete atrioventricular septal defect. Note the detailed definition of the common atrioventricular valve components (Image by courtesy of David A. Roberson, M.D.)

lungs and the use of a high-frequency TEE transducer optimized image quality in children. Heart rate and respiratory gating were necessary, but when kept relatively constant under moderate/deep sedation, excellent data were acquired.

The availability of real-time 3D TEE represents a major advancement for the evaluation of AVSDs and has already been shown to facilitate this assessment (refer to Chap. 19 and Chap. 20) [55–57]. However, because current transducers are designed for adults, the experience in the pediatric age group has been limited to older children. Real-time 3D TEE allows for further definition of the morphological features of these defects. *En face* views can be reconstructed from the atrial and ventricular aspects to determine the precise anatomy of the valve leaflets (Fig. 8.34, Video 8.27). This approach enables the sites and mechanisms of valve regurgitation to be defined, and then displayed in a surgical view. In addition, during 3D imaging of these defects color flow Doppler interrogation can be adjusted so that the proximal isovelocity surface acceleration (PISA), the vena contracta (representing the regurgitant jet as it traverses the defect in the valve), and the aliased jets above can be identified in a precise relationship to the left component of the AV valve. The valve image can then be removed or retained allowing visualization of the exact appearance and size of the vena contracta. These techniques in early studies have been found to aid in the surgical planning of either primary or secondary repair of AVSDs and associated residual lesions. Similar benefits are also expected to be applicable to real-time 3D TEE.

Availability of 3D TEE using miniaturized probes in the future should allow for improved intraoperative morphologic definition of the repaired AV valve, potentially providing the surgeon with information that would allow appropriate manipulation of the valve leaflets at the time of surgery, thereby reducing the incidence of postoperative AV valve problems.

Congenital Mitral Valve Anomalies

Congenital mitral valve anomalies are rare in children but can have serious implications. These malformations include: (1) mitral stenosis, (2) parachute deformity, (3) supravalve mitral ring, (4) double-orifice mitral valve, (5) isolated cleft in the mitral valve, (6) mitral arcade, (7) straddling mitral valve, and (8) congenital valvar regurgitation.

The discussion that follows reviews the morphologic features that characterize each of these lesions and addresses relevant aspects of management, focusing on surgical approaches. A brief overview of the pathophysiology of mitral valve disease is presented. The role of TEE in the evaluation of these lesions is discussed, including goals of the preoperative examination, aspects of interest in the TEE study for each of the anomalies, assessment of the most commonly associated valvar functional abnormalities, and the postoperative interrogation. The experience to date regarding the applications of 3D imaging in congenital mitral valve anomalies is summarized.

Specific Anomalies

Morphologic Features and Management

Congenital Mitral Stenosis

Morphology—Congenital mitral stenosis was detected in 1.2 % of autopsied patients with CHD and in 0.42 % of all cardiac patients [58]. As an isolated entity this lesion occurs very rarely. Most commonly it is found within the context of mitral valve hypoplasia associated with Shone's complex (discussed below) or in combination with other congenital pathology such as aortic coarctation [59]. Congenital mitral stenosis is usually characterized by abnormalities of all valve components and as such is defined by dysplasia of the entire mitral valve apparatus, i.e., thickened valve leaflets with rolled edges, short tendinous chords, and obliterated interchordal spaces. The lesion can also occur with papillary muscle(s) underdevelopment [12]. Although the clinical features are most notably those associated with obstruction to left ventricular inflow, valvar regurgitation also represents a manifestation of the disease.

Management Considerations—Congenital mitral stenosis is a difficult lesion to manage in infancy, accounting for significant morbidity and mortality. Interventions are necessary when obstruction is significant enough to cause symptoms. Since the pathology is complex in nature, aggressive medical management is always attempted first consisting primarily of diuretic therapy. Catheter-based procedures have been used in an effort to decrease the transvalvar mitral gradient and achieve symptomatic improvement [60]. Depending on the nature of the pathology, various surgical techniques have been applied in an effort to alleviate the obstruction [61]. These include valvotomy, commissurotomy, splitting of chordal structures and/or papillary muscles. In contrast to acquired mitral stenosis resulting from rheumatic heart disease, in most cases of congenital mitral stenosis commissurotomy is not adequate as the sole approach. Alternate strategies to valve repair include: (1) mitral valve replacement, in some cases requiring suturing the prosthesis in supra-annular position or annular enlargement; (2) placement of conduits between the left atrium and left ventricle, including replacement of the mitral valve with a pulmonary autograft (Ross II procedure); (3) single ventricle palliation, particularly in the presence of concomitant left-sided obstructive lesions; and (4) cardiac transplantation.

Parachute Mitral Valve

Morphology—A single papillary muscle in the left ventricle is the hallmark of a parachute mitral valve. Tendinous chords from the mitral valve leaflets insert onto this papillary muscle, or closely associated groups of papillary muscles, leading to the formation of the parachute deformity. A parachute mitral valve is commonly associated with other left-sided obstructive heart lesions. The constellation of lesions that include a parachute mitral valve, supravalvar mitral ring, subaortic stenosis, and coarctation of the aorta is referred to as Shone's complex [62]. An incomplete (partial) form or variant implies the presence of fewer than these four components. A concomitant supravalvar mitral ring was recognized in 71 % of the patients with a parachute mitral valve deformity in one series, making it the most frequently detected left heart obstructive lesion in the presence of a parachute mitral valve [63]. The association of a parachute mitral valve with LVOTO is well established; however, mitral stenosis may also be associated with RVOTO, e.g. tetralogy of Fallot [64, 65].

Management Considerations—The surgical repair of a parachute mitral valve creating stenosis is challenging as full visualization of the mitral support apparatus, particularly in young patients can be extremely difficult, even more so in the case of concomitant left-sided obstructed lesions. In a case series of 12 patients with congenital mitral stenosis (9 of a parachute-type) the pathology was approached through an apical left ventriculotomy [66]. The management of this lesion may involve splitting of chordal structures and division of the single or closely spaced papillary muscle(s) enhancing the egress of left atrial blood into the left ventricle. The success rate of these types of interventions in alleviating the obstruction may be variable and likely significantly influenced by the associated lesions.

Supravalvar Mitral Ring

Morphology—A supravalvar mitral ring is a membrane lying in the funnel of the mitral valve leaflets, constricting left ventricular inflow. This anomaly almost always exists as part of a complete or partial Shone's complex, and is rarely an isolated lesion. Therefore, a supravalvar mitral ring should be strongly suspected when typical lesions comprising the Shone's complex are present and when the annulus of the mitral valve is hypoplastic. Conversely, identification of a supravalvar mitral ring should prompt a search for the other cardiac defects associated with Shone's complex.

Management Considerations—Resection of a mitral valve ring is accomplished by peeling away the obstructive web from the surface of the leaflets on the left atrial aspect of the valve. In the majority of cases this is successful in relieving the inflow obstruction and allowing for the valve leaflets to move freely during diastole. At the time of surgery other lesions are addressed as indicated. This lesion, if the main cause of mitral inflow obstruction, is associated with a better prognosis as compared to other mitral valve pathology, thus identification of this particular entity is important when a patient presents with mitral stenosis.

Double-Orifice Mitral Valve

Morphology—Double-orifice mitral valve, an uncommon mitral valve lesion found in 1 % of autopsied cases of CHD, may lead to mitral stenosis, mitral regurgitation or both [67]. Various nomenclature (classic form, double parachute mitral valve) and classification schemes (complete bridge type, incomplete type, and hole type) have been proposed for this lesion based on the size and location of the two mitral valve orifices [23, 24, 67]. For practical purposes two morphological subtypes can be considered: one subtype is caused by a fibrous tissue 'bridge' across the left-sided orifice and is associated with AVSDs (Fig. 8.12, Video 8.7) [68]. The second subtype is caused by duplication of the mitral orifice, with each sub-orifice supported by its own tensor apparatus (Fig. 8.35) [12, 24]. These two forms cannot be easily distinguished from each other by echocardiography. Double-orifice mitral valve can also be found in the setting of a primum ASD, truncus arteriosus, left heart obstructive lesions, the CHARGE association (coloboma of the eye, heart defects, choanal atresia, growth retardation, genital and/or urinary abnormalities, ear abnormalities, and deafness), and other lesions [67, 69].

Management Considerations—In a series of 46 patients that included children and adolescents with a double-orifice mitral valve, surgical intervention specifically to address the valve was required in the minority of patients who underwent repair of associated cardiac pathologies [67].

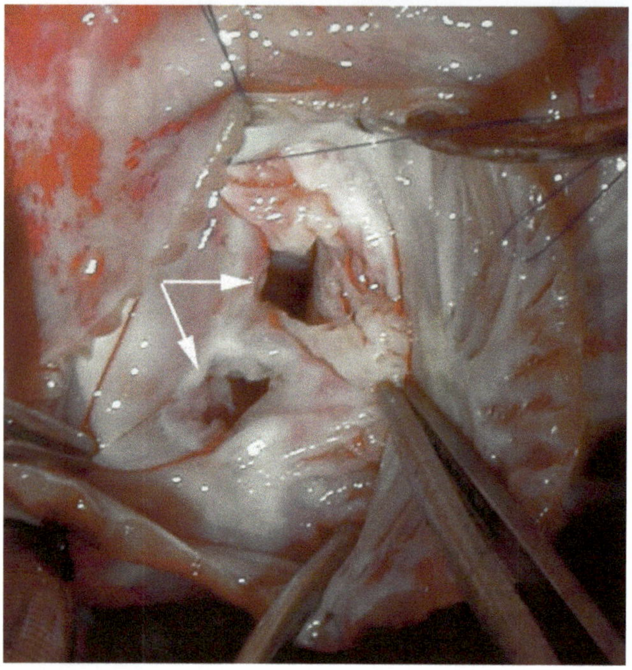

Fig. 8.35 Intraoperative photograph taken from a patient with duplication of the mitral valve (double-orifice mitral valve) showing the two distinct valve orifices (*arrows*)

It was reported that the long-term morbidity related to the valve pathology was low. Surgical repair of double-orifice mitral valve, most often in the setting of AVSDs, has been reasonably successful, usually by partial closure of the cleft in the anterior bridging leaflet [70–72]. In general, mitral stenosis does not occur after closure of the cleft.

Isolated Cleft of the Mitral Valve

Morphology—An isolated cleft in the anterior leaflet of the mitral valve can exist unassociated with an AVSD. In fact it has been proposed that this represents a distinct morphologic entity from the cleft of the left-sided valve of an AVSD [73]. The pathology is usually restricted to the leaflet. Findings may include leaflet dysplasia characterized by thickened and rolled edges.

Management Considerations—The most frequent indication for surgical intervention in this lesion is the presence of mitral regurgitation. The repair of an isolated mitral valve cleft usually consists of approximation of the edges of the anterior leaflet by direct suture closure. In some cases, particularly beyond childhood, more extensive valve reconstruction may be required using autologous pericardium [74]. A concomitant valve annuloplasty may be necessary.

Mitral Arcade

Morphology—An arcade represents a rare mitral valve lesion. First described in pathology specimens and subsequently by echocardiography, it consists of a bridge of fibrous tissue running along the free aspect of the anterior mitral leaflet connecting the two papillary muscles, forming an arch-like structure that obstructs the mitral orifice [75, 76]. The papillary muscle heads may be hypertrophied and closely approximated, compounding the problem at the mitral orifice [59, 77]. In these patients, mitral stenosis is the predominant presenting clinical abnormality. However, the tendinous chords are thickened and short, restricting the movement of the anterior leaflet and preventing complete closure of the mitral valve orifice, frequently also leading to mitral regurgitation. Although mitral arcade most commonly manifests in childhood, there are cases of presentation later in life due to mitral regurgitation [78, 79].

Management Considerations—Among mitral valve malformations, a mitral arcade represents a difficult lesion to successfully address surgically due to the complexity of the pathology and usually severe nature of the valve abnormalities that result in stenosis and/or regurgitation. The lack of supporting chordal structures in most cases requires extensive valve reconstruction that may include removal of fibrous tissue, creation of artificial supporting structures, splitting of papillary muscles, commissurotomy, and annuloplasty. Alternative strategies applied to the management of congenital mitral valve disease, mentioned previously, may also be required in this lesion.

Straddling Mitral Valve

Morphology—The straddling mitral valve also represents a rare defect. The term "straddling" in general implies anomalous attachments of valvar support structures (chordae, papillary muscles or both) into both ventricles, thus by definition this requires the presence of a communication at the ventricular level [80]. In this anomaly, the mitral valve straddles the septum through an anterior VSD, considered of the malalignment type. The leaflet that straddles the ventricular septum typically has an associated cleft [81], however, it is unusual for it to exhibit regurgitation. Frequently there are associated abnormal ventriculoarterial connections such as double outlet right ventricle and transposition of the great arteries [82]. Other more complex defects can be present, including those characterized by ventricular hypoplasia. In some cases, straddling valves also demonstrate 'override', meaning that the annulus is connected to ventricles on both sides of the interventricular septum.

Management Considerations—The straddling mitral valve frequently presents a significant surgical challenge. In most cases the options for surgical intervention involve sacrificing chordal structures, without creating a flail valve or risking the potential for mitral regurgitation, chordal transfer, or valve replacement. The single ventricle pathway may be favored in some patients.

Congenital Mitral Valve Regurgitation

Morphology—In the pediatric age group, mitral valve regurgitation is usually secondary in nature. It may result from conditions associated with left ventricular dysfunction (i.e., cardiomyopathy, myocarditis, anomalous origin of coronary artery), endocarditis, rheumatic heart disease, and systemic degenerative diseases. Additional causes include congenital pathology of the types discussed earlier in this chapter, such as AVSD, cleft mitral valve, and anomalies of the valve itself in association with other left heart malformations. This reflects the fact that mitral valve competence relies upon normal function and integrity of the entire valvular unit (annulus, leaflets, chordae tendineae, papillary muscles, adjacent left ventricular myocardium). Thus abnormalities in any of these components can result in mitral valve dysfunction.

Although rare, the entity of primary (isolated) congenital mitral regurgitation is well recognized. In many cases dysplasia and thickening of the valve leaflets is seen in association with tethering and shortening of chordal structures leading to a regurgitant valvar orifice. An element of mitral stenosis can also be found in primary regurgitant lesions.

The Carpentier nomenclature of mitral valve regurgitation, proposed in the late 1970s, continues to be used and deserves mention [83]. This classification is based on mitral leaflet motion as follows: *type I* has normal leaflet motion; *type II* has increased leaflet motion, and *type III* has restricted motion. This functional classification of mitral regurgitation is detailed in Table 8.1.

Management Considerations—A number of techniques have been utilized in the surgical treatment of mitral regurgitation depending on the nature of the anomaly/anomalies. The objective in all cases is reconstruction and retention of native tissue if feasible. Approaches include reduction in annular size, leaflet reduction, and chordal shortening among others. Mitral valve replacement is considered a last resort, particularly in infants and young children.

Table 8.1 Carpentier functional classification of mitral regurgitation

Type I lesions
Characterized by normal leaflet motion
Caused by:
Deformation and dilation of valvar annulus
Clefts in the leaflets
Partial agenesis of the tissue of the leaflets
Mitral regurgitant jet directed centrally
Type II lesions
Result from increased leaflet motion
Caused by:
Absence of tendinous chords
Elongation of tendinous chords
Elongation of papillary muscles
Mitral regurgitant jet directed away from pathological leaflet
Type III lesions
Result from restricted leaflet motion
Subdivided into types IIIa and IIIB:
Type IIIa: leaflet motion restricted during systole and diastole
Usually associated with mitral stenosis
Caused by commissural fusion or shortening of chords
Eccentric mitral regurgitant jet more likely in the direction of pathological restricted leaflet or central jet of both leaflets involved
Type IIIb: leaflet motion restricted during systole
Posterior leaflet typically involved
Caused by displacement of papillary muscle(s) or segment of ventricular wall
Mitral regurgitant jet directed towards restricted leaflet

Pathophysiology

It is important to consider that although the main physiologic impact of congenital anomalies that affect the mitral valve may result from isolated stenosis or regurgitation, in many cases both functional abnormalities are present. The inflow obstruction that characterizes congenital mitral stenosis, whether due primarily to valvar pathology or supporting structures, is associated with a progressive increase in left atrial pressure and elevation of pulmonary venous pressure. This results in reflex pulmonary arteriolar vasoconstriction and right ventricular hypertension. The malformations that produce mitral stenosis can have a variable clinical presentation depending upon the severity of the obstruction. In cases of mild stenosis, patients can remain free of symptoms. However, severe mitral valve stenosis is likely to be associated with poor growth and manifestations of congestive heart failure, particularly in infants. Associated obstruction of left-sided structures complicates the clinical course.

With mitral valve regurgitation, there is progressive left atrial dilation as the chamber expands to accommodate the regurgitant volume. With mild to moderate degrees of dilation, left atrial compliance is such that the chamber is able to maintain a relatively low pressure as dilation occurs. However with increasing amounts of left atrial dilation, eventually compliance decreases, leading to significant elevation of left atrial and pulmonary venous pressures, and resulting in pulmonary hypertension. The regurgitant volume, in addition, represents a load on the heart, potentially impairing myocardial performance. Although initially well compensated, long-standing mitral regurgitation can result in significant morbidity.

Transesophageal Echocardiography

Preoperative TEE Evaluation

The main objectives of the preoperative TEE examination in mitral valve anomalies are to:

- Define morphology and function of the mitral valve and of its support apparatus
- Obtain measurements of the mitral valve annulus, preferably from several different planes
- Determine whether the primary pathology is stenosis or regurgitation (or both)

- If stenosis is present, define the nature of the obstruction, and any additional level(s) of obstruction
- If regurgitation is present, assess the mechanism of regurgitation
- Evaluate the hemodynamic severity of stenosis/regurgitation and secondary effects on cardiac structures
- Estimate right ventricular/pulmonary artery pressures
- Characterize associated lesions as indicated
- Assess left atrial and ventricular size, and ventricular function

Intraoperative Imaging

It is important to recognize that the mitral valve apparatus consists of multiple structures that include the leaflets, annulus, chordae papillary muscles, and the left ventricle. As such, it is imperative to carefully examine each of these components and to methodically characterize the involved pathology. TEE imaging of the left atrium, mitral valve, and left ventricle can be achieved from a combination of views that include the ME 4 Ch, ME 2 Ch, mid esophageal aortic valve long axis (ME AV LAX), ME LAX, TG Basal SAX, TG Mid SAX, TG 2 Ch, transgastric long axis (TG LAX), and deep transgastric views.

Congenital Mitral Stenosis

Most of the characteristic features of congenital mitral stenosis can be demonstrated in cross-sections displayed in the views noted above, including thick and dysplastic mitral valve leaflets, restricted funnel-shaped opening, and stiff movement of the leaflets due to short tendinous chords (Fig. 8.36). In congenital mitral stenosis the leaflets typically are more echoreflective than normal; there is often poor leaflet motion, and the valve domes during ventricular diastole (Figs. 8.37 and 8.38, Videos 8.28 and 8.29). Mitral valve leaflet thickening frequently extends onto the tendinous chords resulting in obliteration of interchordal spaces and lending the subvalvar mitral apparatus an echodense, crowded appearance.

The severity of mitral stenosis is sometimes difficult to determine in children by assessment of the transmitral gradient, because a high-pressure gradient may not be generated even in the presence of severe mitral stenosis. This is due to the frequent association of an atrial communication and/or multiple levels of left-sided obstruction (see discussion below) [59, 64]. The original description of Shone and colleagues noted that in the presence of coarctation, mitral stenosis was not readily apparent until the coarctation was resected [62].

Color flow Doppler is invaluable for morphological definition of the lesion: determining the level(s) of obstruction, assessing severity of stenosis, and defining the direction of the jets across the stenotic mitral valve (Fig. 8.37, Video 8.28) [84]. Pulsed and continuous wave Doppler can then be

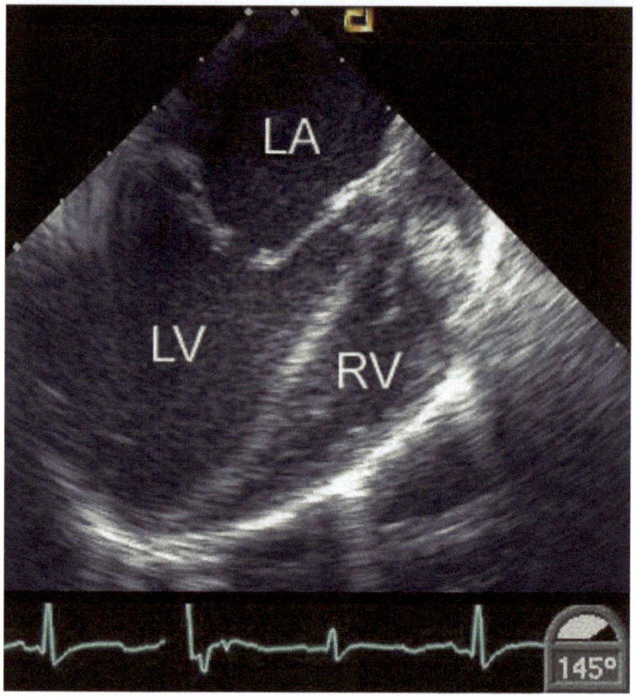

Fig. 8.36 Mid esophageal long axis view demonstrates mitral stenosis. There is reduced leaflet excursion in diastole and substantial stenosis (thickened and rolled edges at the tips of the valvar leaflets). *LA* left atrium, *LV* left ventricle, *RV* right ventricle

aligned appropriately (Fig. 8.39). Both spectral modalities are frequently applied, in particular continuous wave Doppler when velocities exceed the Nyquist limit of pulsed wave Doppler interrogation resulting in aliasing (refer to Chap. 1). As previously stated, in children with mitral valve stenosis the peak diastolic velocity is often less than 2 meters per second (m/s) because of associated atrial communications. The pressure half-time (PHT, or time for the mitral gradient to fall to half its peak value) may also be less than in the adult with acquired mitral stenosis [63, 84]. In fact, because of faster heart rates, there may be no E-F slope to measure the PHT, and the flow velocity of atrial contraction (A wave in the spectral Doppler tracing) may be higher than the velocity of early filling (E wave). Clinically significant mitral valve obstruction is suggested when peak velocities exceed 2 m/s.

Parachute Mitral Valve

The single papillary muscle can be identified at the mid esophageal level in the ME 4 Ch and ME 2 Ch views where the mitral valve leaflets appear echogenic and have restricted motion in most affected patients (Fig. 8.40). However, the anatomy is best seen in short axis views particularly those obtained by transgastric imaging (TG Mid SAX and TG 2 Ch views), where the single papillary muscle is usually detected in a posteromedial position within the left ventricle (Fig. 8.41, Video 8.30).

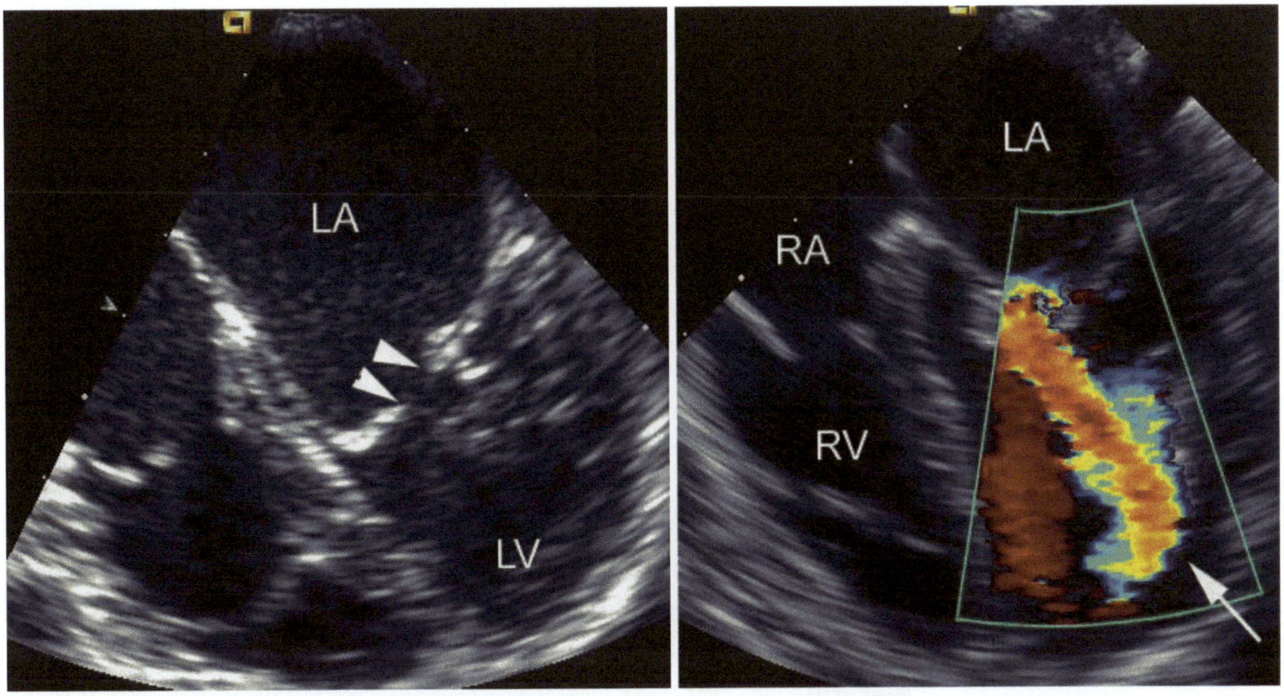

Fig. 8.37 *Left panel*, mid esophageal four chamber image in diastole displaying an abnormal mitral valve. The mitral valve exhibits grossly abnormal leaflets and small ridges could be construed as a supravalvar mitral ring (*arrowheads*). *Right panel* frame demonstrates a turbulent color jet and region of flow convergence at the mitral valve. The degree of flow velocity acceleration is significant and reaches the left ventricular apex (*arrow*) before it turns round, while maintaining its dimensions until distorted by the apical wall, indicating the severity of the obstruction. *LA* left atrium, *LV* left ventricle, *RA* right atrium, *RV* right ventricle

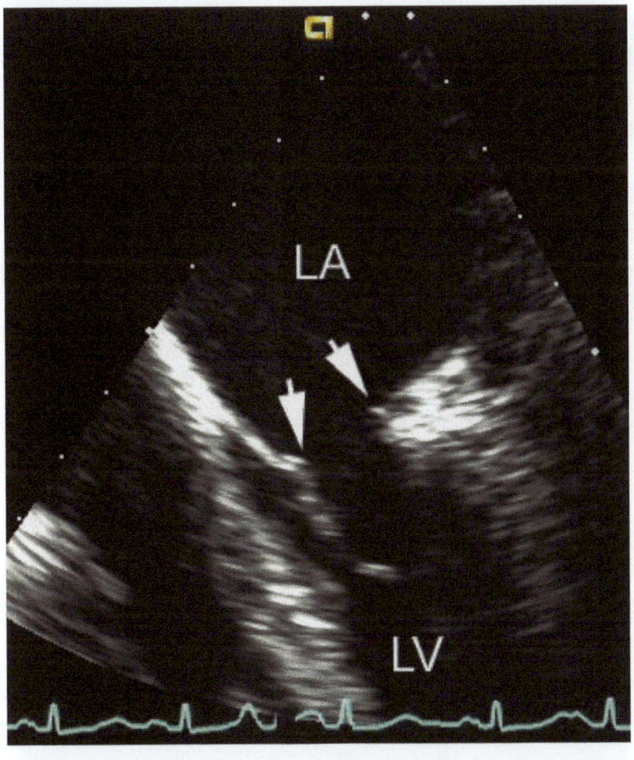

Fig. 8.38 Mid esophageal four chamber view demonstrates a distorted, funnel-shaped mitral inflow. The *arrows* indicate a small supravalvar mitral ring. The left atrium appears substantially enlarged. *LA* left atrium, *LV* left ventricle

Supravalvar Mitral Ring

The abnormalities of the area of the ring and mitral valve are best recognized from the ME 4 Ch and ME 2 Ch views (Figs. 8.38 and 8.42, Videos 8.29 and 8.31) [85]. Alternate cross sections of the mitral valve as provided by the mid esophageal mitral valve commissural (ME Mitral; Fig. 8.43, Video 8.32) and ME LAX views (Fig. 8.44, Video 8.33) can also adequately display the pathology [86]. The supravalvar ring may be difficult to detect because it lies within the atrial surface of the valve leaflets, usually within 1–3 mm of the mitral valve annulus. The membrane of the supravalvar mitral ring may prolapse into the mitral valve orifice during diastole. During systole, it may adhere to the atrial surface of the mitral valve leaflets, but appears to dissociate slightly from them during diastole. When the left atrial appendage is visualized, it is always seen proximal to the supramitral ring, in contrast to cor triatriatum, in which the appendage is distal to the membrane (refer to Chap. 7).

In only about 10 % of patients with a supramitral ring will this pathology itself cause significant obstruction. In the remainder, associated lesions (such as a parachute mitral valve) are the cause of mitral stenosis. The lack of clinically detectable stenosis can be explained by the frequent presence of an atrial communication and/or a large, non-obstructive opening in the supravalvar mitral ring [77, 87]. Color Doppler imaging shows evidence of flow convergence toward the

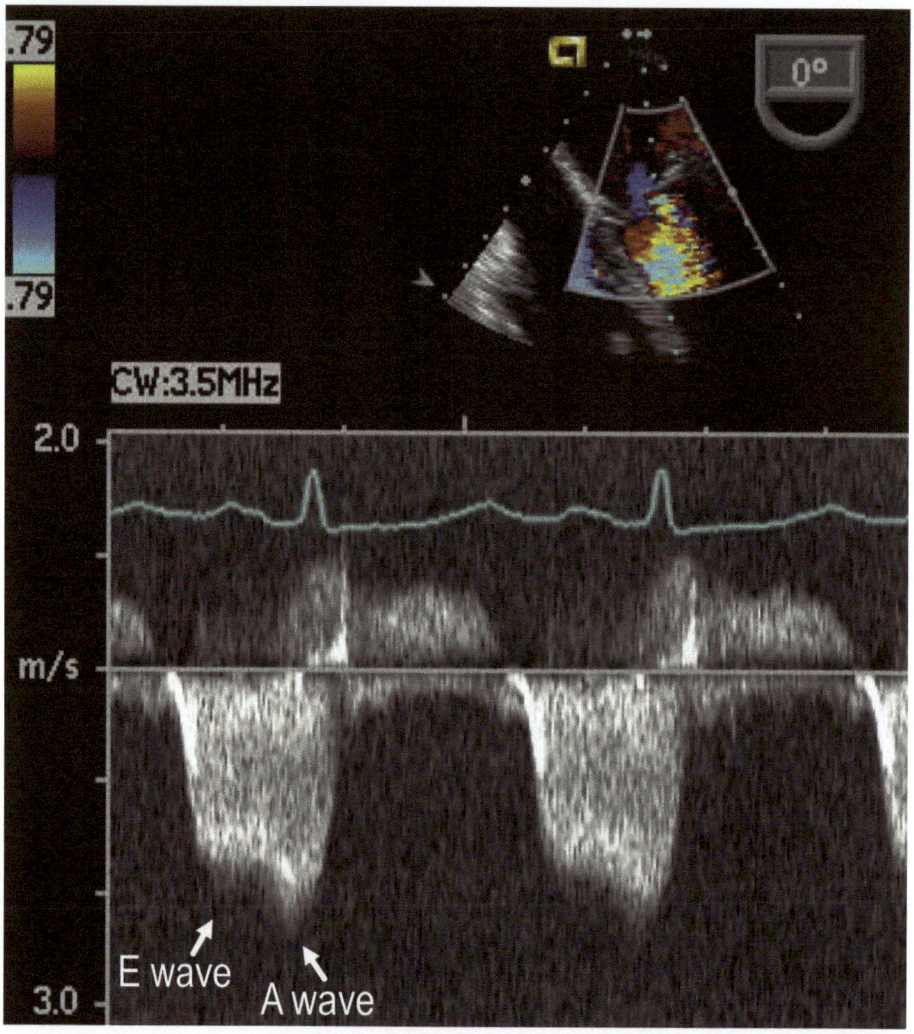

Fig. 8.39 Continuous wave Doppler recording sampled across the mitral valve leaflets, from the standard mid esophageal four chamber reference image, in a child with congenital mitral stenosis. The mitral inflow velocities are increased with the A wave near 2.4 m/s and an abnormal flow pattern with E wave and A wave reversal

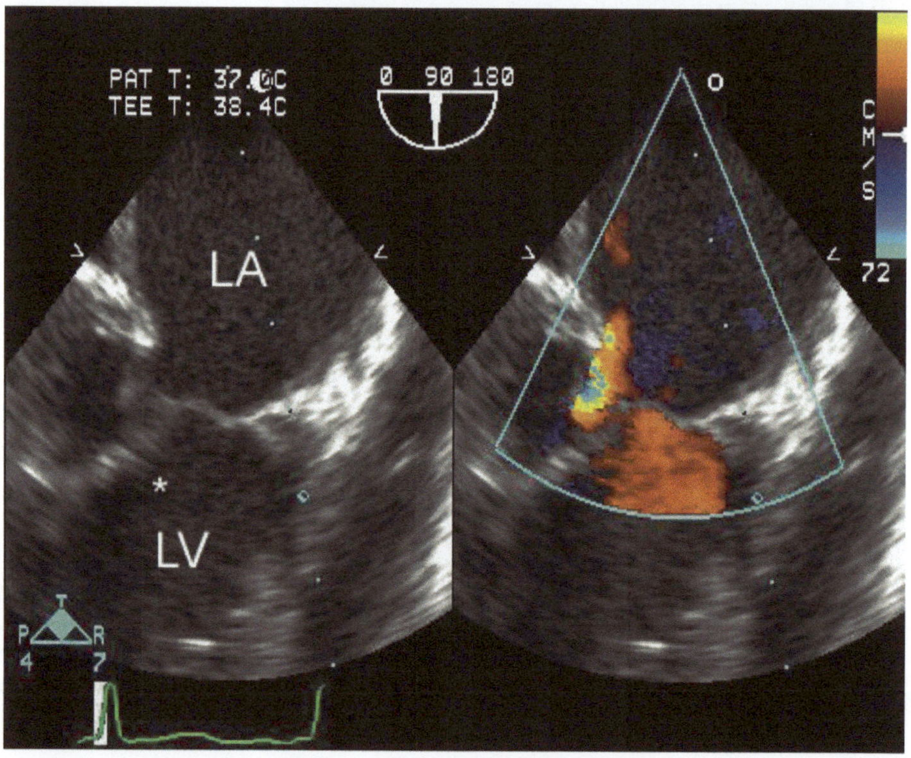

Fig. 8.40 Mid esophageal two chamber view shows a dilated left atrium (*LA*) and a single left ventricular (*LV*) papillary muscle (*asterisk*). There is flow acceleration across the mitral valve at end diastole (aliased flow)

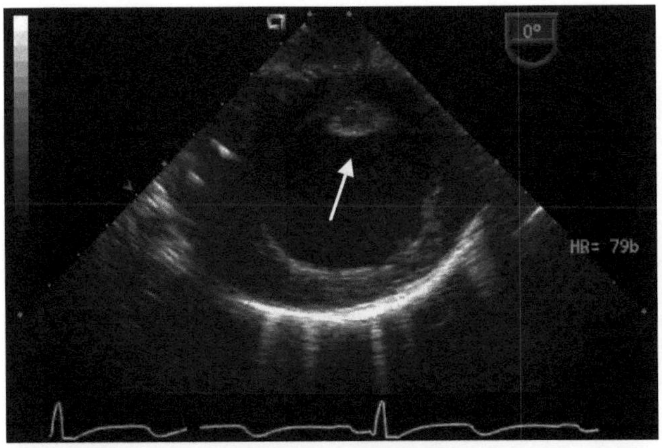

Fig. 8.41 Transgastric imaging in the mid left ventricular short axis view demonstrates a single posteromedial papillary muscle (*arrow*) in a child with a parachute mitral valve deformity

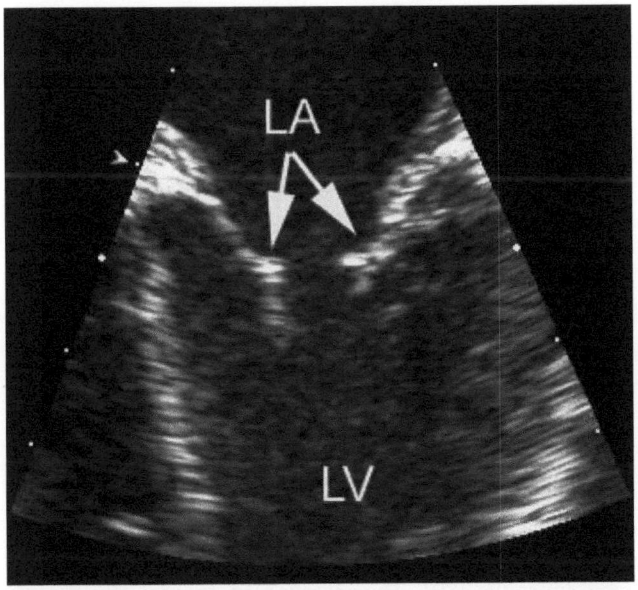

Fig. 8.42 Still frame obtained in a mid esophageal four chamber view in a child with a parachute mitral valve and a prominent supravalvar mitral ring (*arrows*) within the funnel of the open valvar leaflets. *LA* left atrium, *LV* left ventricle

center of the supravalvar ring and valve (Figs. 8.44 and 8.45, Videos 8.33 and 8.34), as well as a smaller flow area through the mitral annulus than would be expected. Spectral Doppler interrogation in the absence of an interatrial communication assists in the determination of the severity of obstruction across the mitral valve (Fig. 8.46). However, when an atrial defect is present, the Doppler flow across the valve can provide less information about this lesion than for many other conditions. This is because the volume of flow through the valve is less than expected due to left-to-right atrial shunting. In addition, in the presence of associated lesions that cause mitral stenosis, the separate contribution of the supravalvar

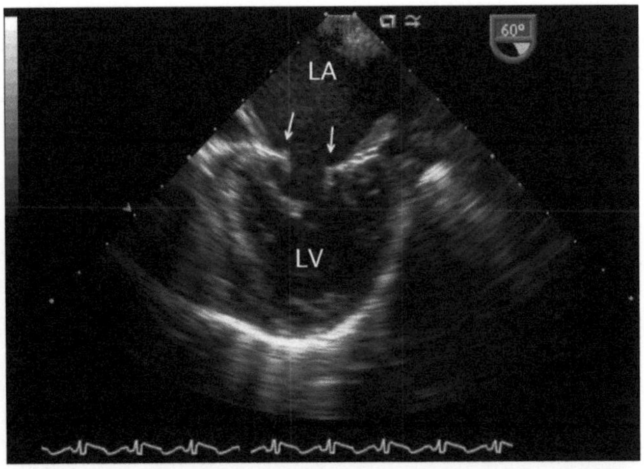

Fig. 8.43 Mitral valve commissural view, obtained at 60°, demonstrates the supravalvar ridges (*arrows*) that characterize a mitral ring. *LA* left atrium, *LV* left ventricle (Figure by courtesy of Louis I. Bezold, M.D.)

ring itself to the total inflow obstruction might be difficult, if not impossible, to quantitate.

Double-Orifice Mitral Valve

The typical echocardiographic finding in this lesion is that of two separate valvar orifices opening into the left ventricle. Although both orifices may be of equal size, more commonly they are unequal, the smaller orifice usually located in the anterolateral aspect of the left ventricle. The short axis echocardiographic plane at the level of the valve orifice, achievable by imaging in the TG Basal SAX view, equivalent to the transthoracic parasternal left ventricular short axis (Fig. 8.47, Video 8.35), is best for detecting this lesion. This anomaly may also be seen from the ME 4 Ch and ME 2 Ch views (Fig. 8.48, Video 8.36), as well as with deep transgastric imaging (Fig. 8.49) [88]. Color flow Doppler demonstrates the relative velocities through the orifices, and can depict the division of flow into two streams, each entering a separate orifice. The spectral Doppler flow characteristics are normal unless stenosis is present. It is important to recognize the fact that in double-orifice mitral valve other anomalies of the tensor apparatus can be found and should be defined [24].

Isolated Cleft of the Mitral Valve

Sweeps between a transgastric short axis view at the level of the mitral valve leaflets (TG Basal SAX) and deep transgastric views, which also display the LVOT (DTG LAX or DTG Sagittal), effectively identify the cleft pointing in the direction of the LVOT (Fig. 8.50, Video 8.37) [22, 63]. As previously indicated, this is in contrast to the cleft in AVSDs which points toward the inlet ventricular septum. There may be attachment of tendinous chords arising from the margins of the cleft to the ventricular septum, which in turn may

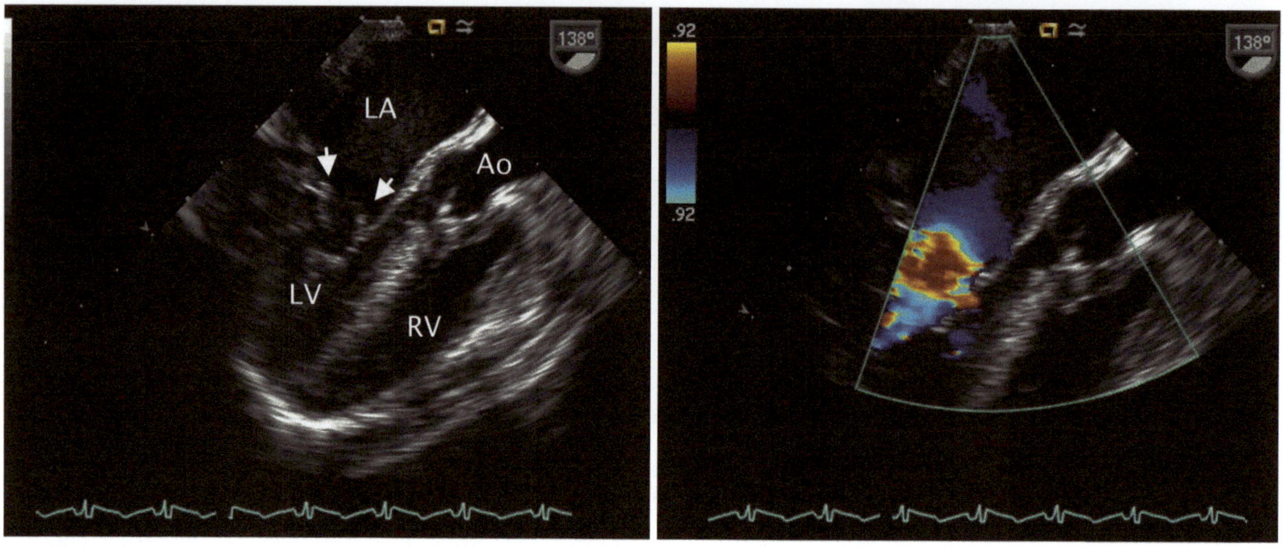

Fig. 8.44 Mid esophageal long axis views recorded from the same infant depicted in Fig. 8.43. *Left panel*, the supravalvar mitral membrane is well seen (*arrows*). There is associated narrowing of the left ventricular outflow tract and mild hypoplasia of the aortic annulus. *Right panel*, superimposed color Doppler depicts aliasing of flow at the level of the mitral annulus consistent with the inflow obstruction. *Ao* aorta, *LA* left atrium, *LV* left ventricle, *RV* right ventricle (Figure by courtesy of Louis I. Bezold, M.D.)

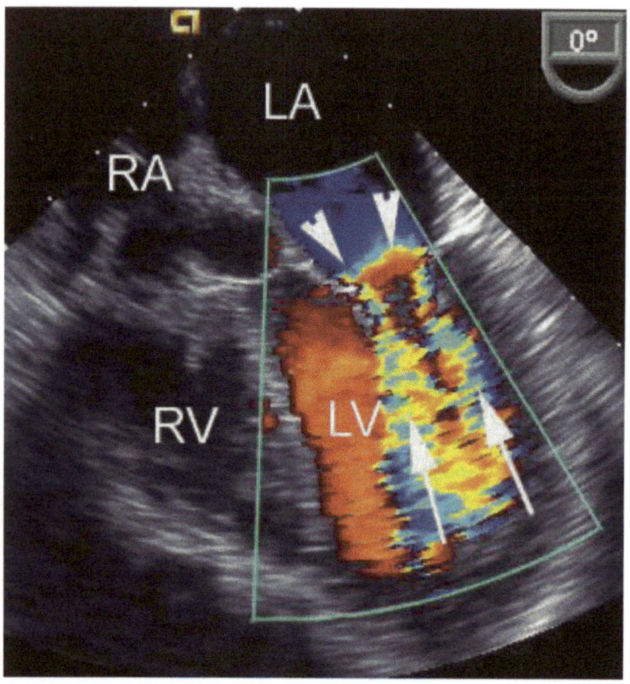

Fig. 8.45 This mid esophageal four chamber view shows the area of flow convergence (*arrowheads*) between the left atrium (*LA*) and left ventricle (*LV*) due to a supravalvar mitral ring. Additionally, two jets of mitral inflow are seen during diastole (*two arrows*), reflecting two areas of stenosis in this abnormal mitral valve. *RA* right atrium, *RV* right ventricle

cause LVOTO detectable by Doppler echocardiography. This is best evaluated in the ME 4 Ch, ME LAX, TG LAX, and deep transgastric views. Color flow mapping facilitates the assessment of regurgitation through the cleft.

Mitral Arcade

TEE is useful in the diagnostic evaluation of these cases [78]. Characteristically the mitral valve apparatus appears abnormal with thick and shortened chordal attachments and obliterated chordal spaces (Fig. 8.51, Video 8.38). Color Doppler imaging demonstrates flow aliasing at the level of the mitral valve inflow and in some cases multiple small jets can be observed across the valvar openings between the fused chordal structures.

Straddling Mitral Valve

The main goal in the evaluation of the straddling mitral valve is to characterize in detail the supporting structures and tension apparatus [89]. The insertion of chordal attachments may be onto a papillary muscle well within the apex of the right ventricle, to the right aspect of the interventricular septum or to the crest of the ventricular septum. Suggested views for evaluating the extent of straddling and the cleft include those where the mitral valve supporting structures are optimally seen as well as their relationships to the interventricular septum (ME 4Ch, ME LAX, TG Basal SAX). The deep transgastric views are particularly helpful in this evaluation. Sweeps that provide cross-sections of the ventricular chambers, interventricular septum, and outflow tracts from a posterior to anterior orientation are extremely valuable. This assessment is primarily done by 2D imaging (Fig. 8.52, Video 8.39). Doppler can then be applied to evaluate the mitral valve in views that provide for functional assessment as described below. Other important aspects of the anatomy should be defined, particularly the VSD, ventriculoarterial connections, and associated lesions.

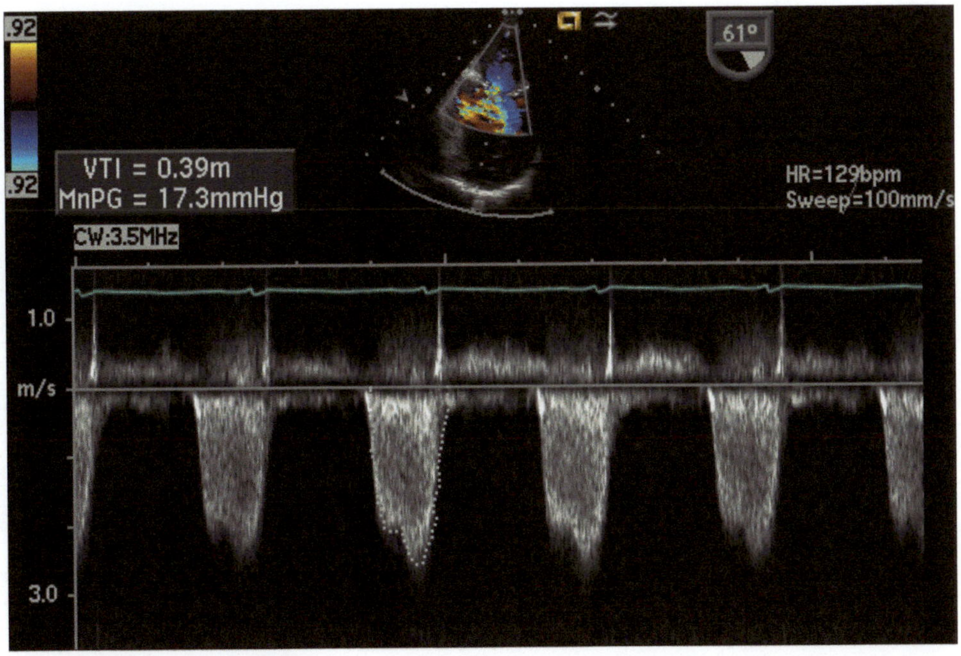

Fig. 8.46 Spectral Doppler tracing across left ventricular inflow obtained in the mid esophageal mitral commissural view in same infant depicted in Figs. 8.43 and 8.44. A transvalvar mean gradient of approximately 17 mmHg was recorded consistent with severe mitral inflow obstruction (Figure by courtesy of Louis I. Bezold, M.D.)

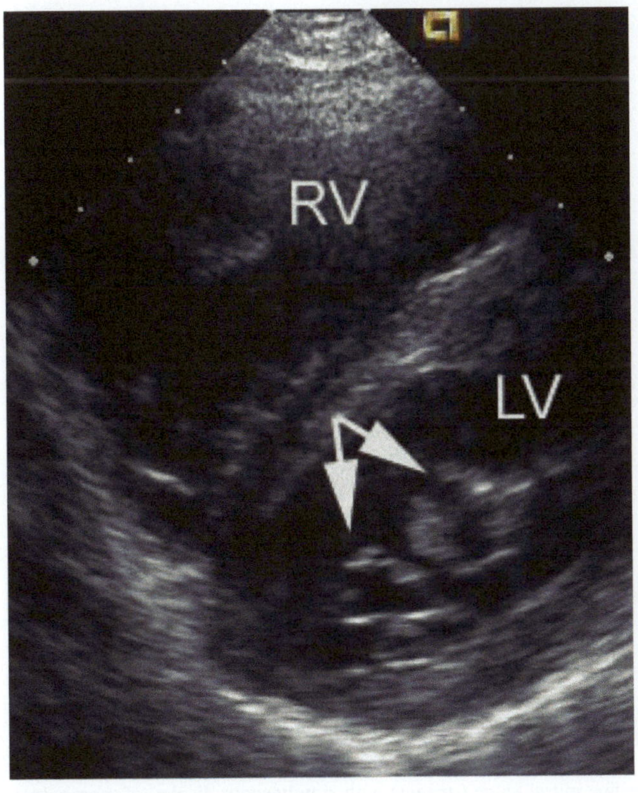

Fig. 8.47 Transthoracic left ventricular parasternal short axis image depicting a double-orifice mitral valve (*arrows*). *LV* left ventricle, *RV* right ventricle

Congenital Mitral Valve Regurgitation

In the evaluation of congenital mitral regurgitation suitable TEE views are those that display the left ventricular inflow as detailed previously (Fig. 8.53, Video 8.40). Specific aspects of the anatomy that should be examined include annular dimensions measured in multiple views, morphology and motion of the leaflets, and support apparatus. The exam should allow the evaluation of secondary changes of cardiac structures associated with volume overload.

Assessment of Mitral Valve Stenosis and Regurgitation

The intraoperative assessment of the severity of mitral stenosis in children relies mostly upon qualitative and semiquantitative data. In this evaluation, the main consideration is the 2D appearance of the valve leaflets and supporting structures (i.e., leaflet thickening, valve excursion in diastole, valve opening), annular dimensions, color flow pattern across the valve (i.e., presence and location of turbulence, flow convergence), and spectral Doppler assessment. Additional echocardiographic parameters evaluate the hemodynamic repercussions of the inflow obstruction, such as the magnitude of left atrial dilation and degree of pulmonary/right ventricular hypertension, as derived by the peak velocity of tricuspid or pulmonary regurgitant jet (if present) or inferred from other criteria (i.e., position of interventricular septum, right ventricular dilation/hypertrophy/function). Pulmonary venous flow patterns have also been investigated in the intraoperative setting to estimate mean left atrial pressure. As mean left atrial pressure increases, a shift in the normal pattern of predominant systolic pulmonary venous flow to one of predominant early diastolic flow has been observed [90]. However, there are limitations in this assessment that include factors such as those leading to left atrial hypertension, effects of acute versus chronic elevations, influence of

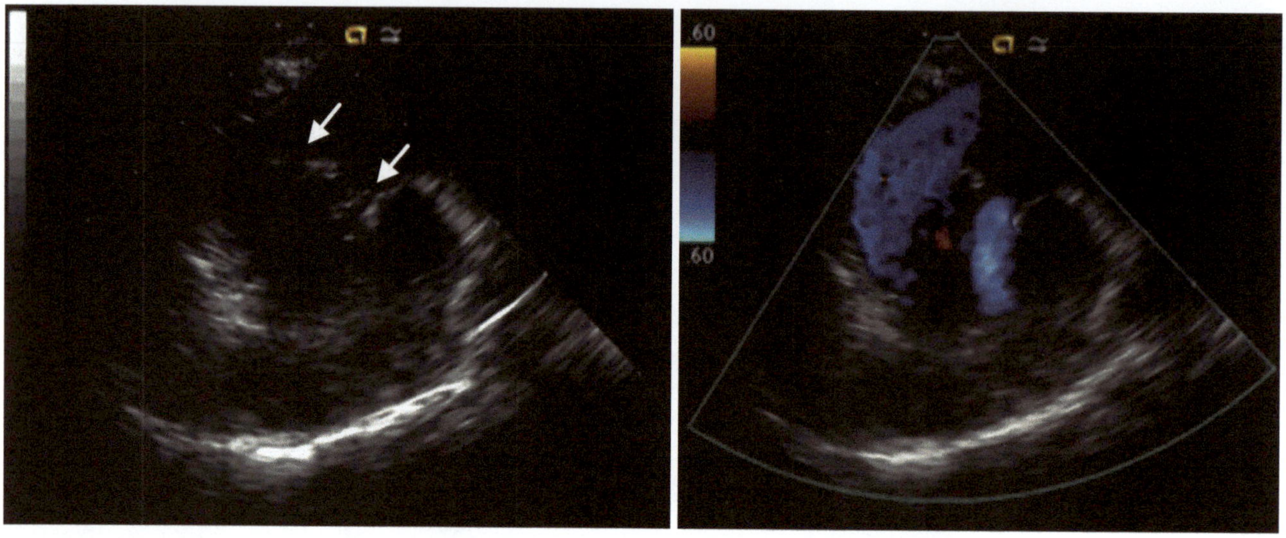

Fig. 8.48 Mid esophageal two chamber view depicting a double-orifice mitral valve. Two-dimensional imaging (*left panel*) shows two distinct valvar orifices during diastole (*arrows*). Color flow (*right panel*) appears more prominent across the more posterior valvar opening

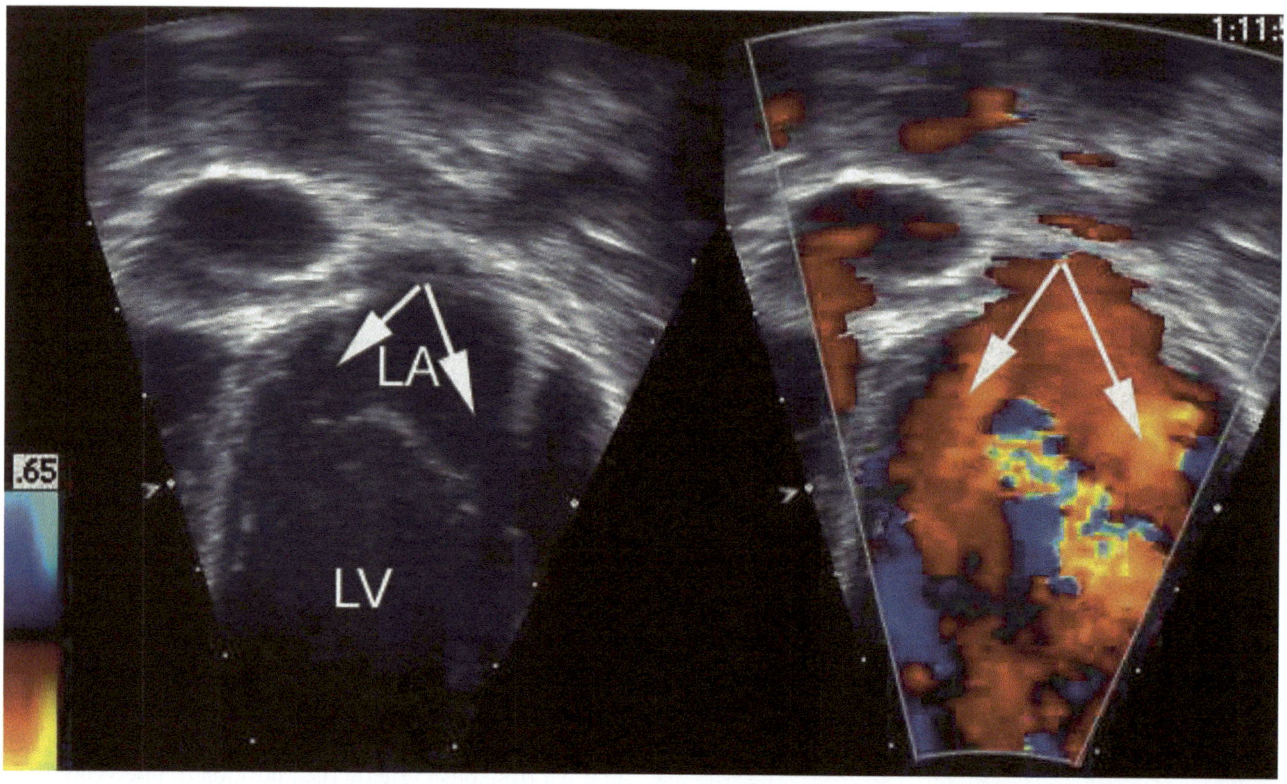

Fig. 8.49 Deep transgastric diastolic image in a patient with a double-orifice mitral valve (*arrows*) with simultaneous display of morphology (*left panel*) and flow information (*right panel*). *LA* left atrium, *LV* left ventricle

associated defects, and importantly, the lack of validation of this echocardiographic parameter in the pediatric age group.

Several indices have been applied in the evaluation of mitral valve stenosis including estimation of the diastolic pressure gradient as derived from the flow-velocity curve across the valve and mitral valve area derivation (from PHT, 2D planimetry, continuity equation, and PISA) [91]. Among these indices, calculation of the transmitral mean gradient continues to be favored as it is relatively easy to obtain in the intraoperative setting. However, it is important to

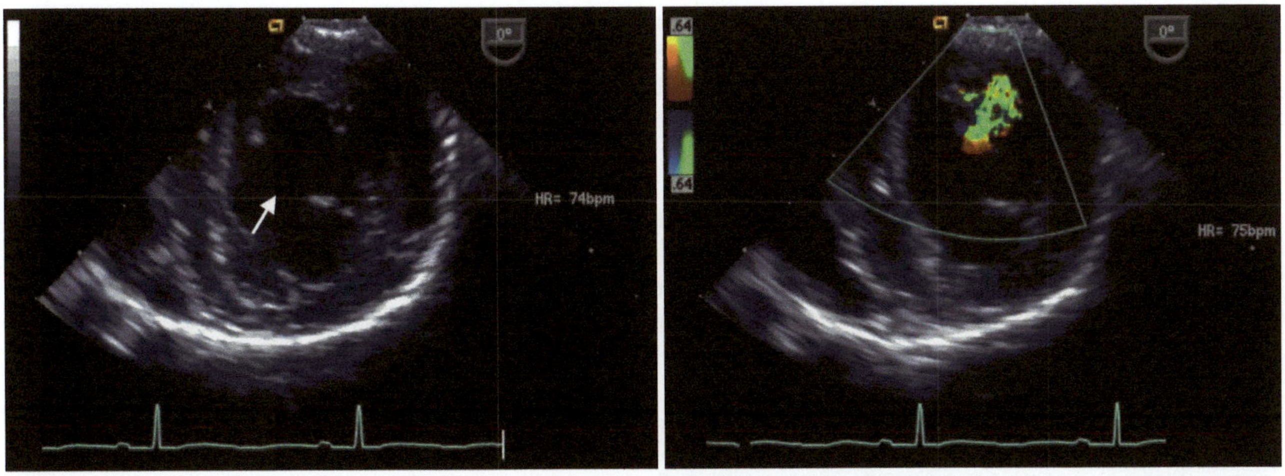

Fig. 8.50 Transgastric basal short axis views displaying the mitral valve *en face*. In the two-dimensional image (*left panel*) the mitral cleft is indicated by the *arrow*; corresponding color Doppler interrogation (*right panel*) depicts an associated jet of mitral regurgitation across the valvar cleft

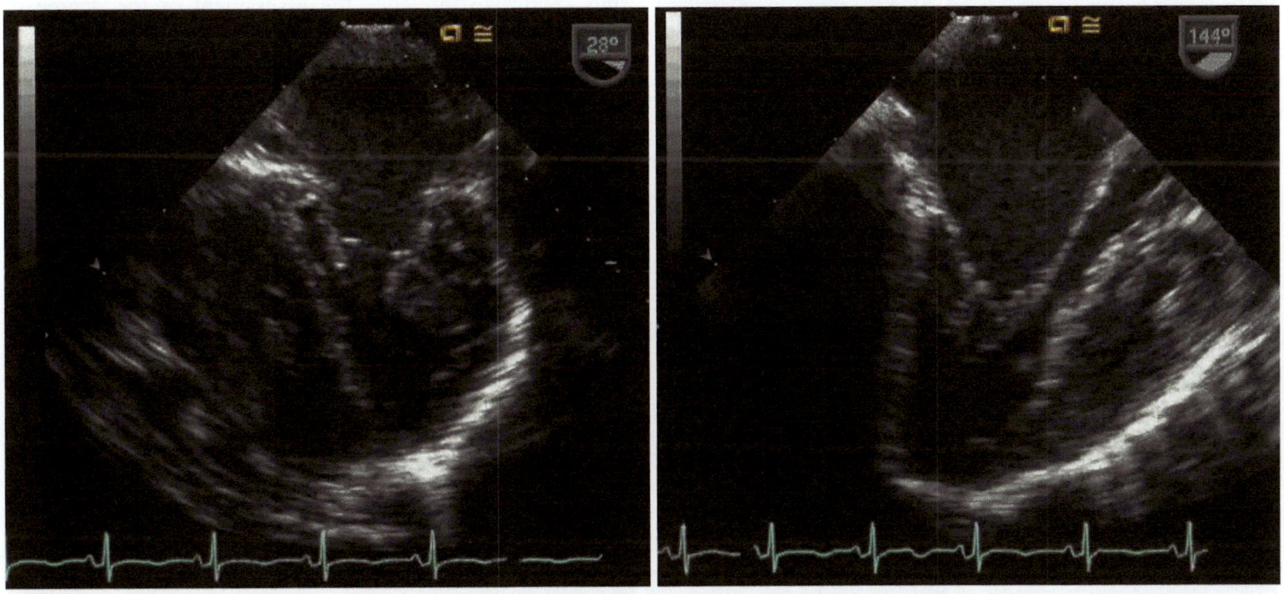

Fig. 8.51 Multiplane imaging of the mitral valve demonstrating restricted diastolic opening and marked thickening of the leaflets and support apparatus. The leaflets appear to insert directly into bulky subvalvar structures without definitive chordae, suggesting the presence of a mitral arcade (confirmed at surgery)

acknowledge a number of caveats/limitations regarding the use of this parameter: 1) an optimal angle of interrogation is critical in obtaining an accurate mitral inflow velocity, and 2) values for mean gradients are impacted by changes in cardiac output (flow and heart rate) and the presence of shunts (either intracardiac or great artery level). Related to this, as previously noted, is the fact that in the presence of multiple levels of obstruction, the severity of mitral valve inflow obstruction can be underestimated. Conversely, the presence of large left-to-right shunts (such as a large VSD) and mitral valvar regurgitation can increase the transmitral flow velocity, thereby overestimating the degree of obstruction. Mean gradients therefore should be evaluated within this context and considered as supporting evidence in severity assessment. In general, mean gradients under 5 mmHg are consistent with mild obstruction, between 5 and 10 mmHg moderate, and exceeding 10 mmHg suggest severe stenosis. The parameters to derive mitral valve area, although well validated in adult patients, in general are less applicable to children. In addition, from a practical standpoint, these measurements can be very difficult to obtain in an operating room environment.

In regards to the evaluation of mitral regurgitation, an even greater number of echocardiographic parameters have been considered [92]. In general, the assessment of disease severity relies upon: (1) morphologic features, such as the appearance of the leaflets (malcoaptation, prolapse, flail) and degree of annular dilation, (2) color and spectral Doppler parameters, and (3) degree of dilation of related cardiac structures (i.e., left atrium, left ventricle).

Doppler color flow mapping represents an essential modality in the assessment of the severity of mitral regurgitation. To a significant extent this evaluation relies upon visualization of the turbulent systolic regurgitant flow from the left ventricle into the left atrium, and qualitative assessment of the area of the regurgitant jet relative to that of the left atrium. Other parameters that should also be examined include the direction of the regurgitant jet(s), number of jets, density of regurgitant signal in the continuous wave Doppler tracing (dense signal consistent with more severe disease), presence/extent of pulmonary vein systolic flow reversal (assisted by spectral Doppler), and mitral inflow profile (higher velocities obtained with increasing severity of regurgitation in addition to a dominant E wave pattern). Although these types of assessments are performed on a routine basis, a number of important caveats should be recognized in regards to color flow mapping of regurgitant jets. The evaluation is significantly influenced by a number of technical and hemodynamic variables other than regurgitant flow and volume; equipment settings (e.g., gain) can impact image display and under/overestimate disease severity. In addition, factors such as inotropic state, volume status, vascular resistance—all of which can change in the postbypass setting—can also influence the assessment of the degree of regurgitation. Other factors such as wall impingement and fluid entrainment of the regurgitant jet, left atrial dimension, differences between left atrial and left ventricular pressures, can impact the size of the mitral regurgitant jet by color flow imaging. Another important aspect is the fact that the color Doppler image display represents velocities of moving blood elements and is not volumetric in nature as discussed in Chap. 1.

A number of echocardiographic indices provide a quantitative volumetric assessment of the regurgitant flow. These include calculations of regurgitant volume, regurgitant area, and effective regurgitant orifice area. The techniques required to derive these indices, however, have a number of limitations and are not of practical value in the intraoperative setting. The measurement of the vena contracta by color

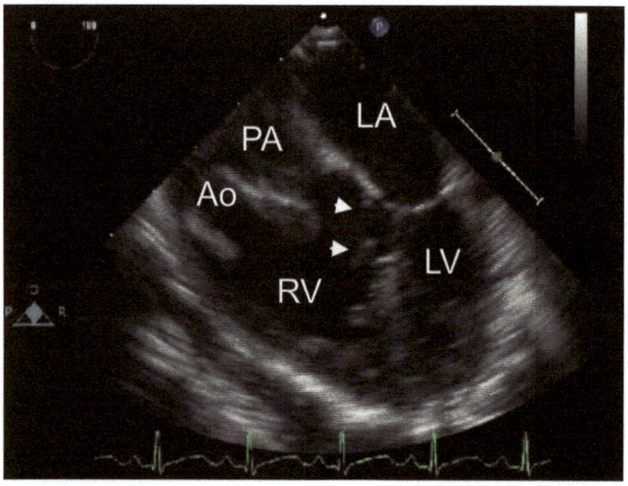

Fig. 8.52 Transesophageal echocardiogram depicting a straddling mitral valve in a child with double outlet right ventricle. The image is obtained by transducer anteflexion after the mid esophageal four chamber view is obtained. Chordal attachments from the mitral valve are seen to straddle the ventricular septum and insert on the right ventricular aspect near the crest of the ventricular septum (*arrowheads*). The abnormal, side-by-side spatial orientation of the great arteries is shown. *Ao* aorta; *LA* left atrium; *LV* left ventricle; *PA* pulmonary artery; *RV* right ventricle

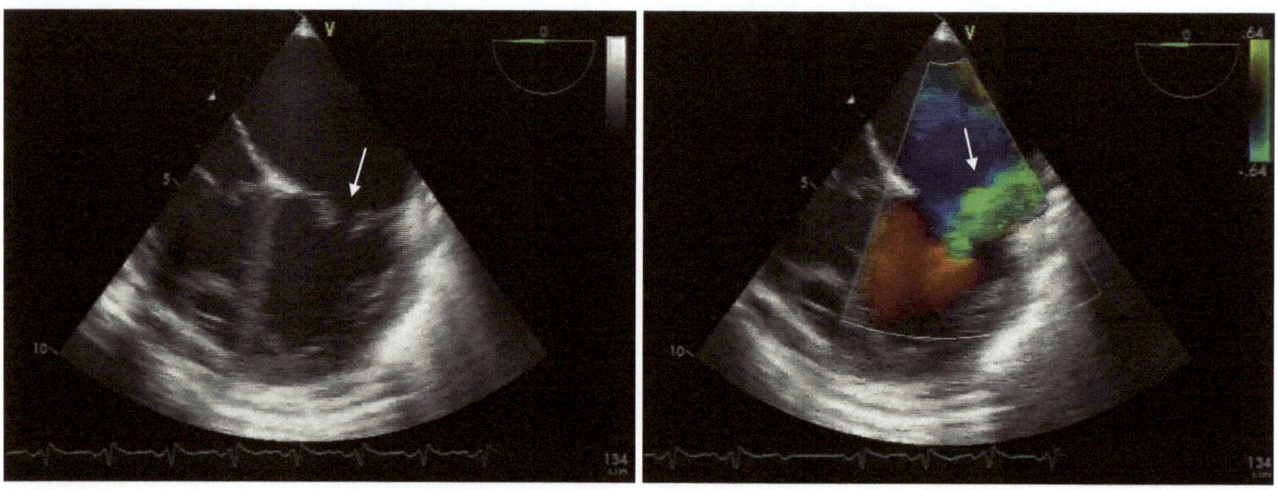

Fig. 8.53 *Left panel*, mid esophageal four chamber view depicting a thickened mitral valve with lack of systolic coaptation (*arrow*) in infant with congenital mitral regurgitation. *Right panel*, color flow Doppler identifies the broad regurgitant, aliased jet across the mitral orifice (*arrow*)

Doppler (narrowest cross-sectional area of jet width as it emerges regurgitant orifice) represents a semiquantitative parameter that has been used as a surrogate for regurgitant orifice area, a reliable index of the severity of mitral regurgitation. This measurement is helpful in the evaluation of eccentric jets but not in the presence of multiple jets (which is often the case when mitral regurgitation is seen following repair of a congenital mitral valve abnormality). Another concern is the fact that the accuracy of this method requires mapping in multiple planes to overcome limitations related to an asymmetric orifice, also presenting a challenge for immediate postbypass evaluation. In this regard, 3D imaging offers a significant advantage.

Postoperative TEE Evaluation

As discussed previously for AVSDs, an important role of postbypass TEE is to detect residual lesions that require further surgical attention [3, 93]. In congenital lesions affecting the mitral valve, an important concern is the balance between residual stenosis versus residual regurgitation. Postbypass TEE can aid in making this determination by examining the parameters previously discussed [94].

Three-Dimensional Echocardiographic Imaging

A number of publications have reported on the role of 3D echocardiography in CHD, including the assessment of congenital anomalies that affect the mitral valve [95–102]. Many of the applications of 3D imaging have already been explored for several of the malformations discussed in preceeding sections of this chapter [103–107]. The 3D TTE experience is congenital mitral valve disease is increasing as the benefits of the technology are being widely recognized. In regards to 3D TEE imaging, the reports, although limited mostly to adults due to the lack of suitable probes for children, already demonstrate clear benefits and incremental value over conventional 2D imaging [108]. The collective data thus far indicates: (1) enhanced characterization of morphologic abnormalities (spatial orientation/relationships, extent of deformities); (2) increased understanding of complex anatomic relationships; (3) better appreciation of disease severity and mechanisms of valve disease; and (4) contributions to clinical decision-making, in particular, guiding surgical management. As 3D technology continues to evolve it is anticipated that additional benefits will be derived.

Congenital Tricuspid Valve Anomalies

Isolated anomalies of a congenital nature that affect the tricuspid valve are relatively rare. In most cases, these malformations coexist in the presence of associated defects. Congenital tricuspid valve anomalies include Ebstein malformation, dysplasia, straddling, and other very unusual defects (i.e., double orifice tricuspid valve, parachute tricuspid valve). These lesions for the most part represent a spectrum of disease involving both the leaflets and subvalvar structures. The primary functional consequences of these abnormalities are tricuspid regurgitation and/or stenosis. The discussion that follows focuses on the two most common congenital tricuspid valve malformations, namely, Ebstein anomaly and tricuspid valve dysplasia. The morphologic features and management strategies are reviewed as well as relevant aspects of the pathophysiology of tricuspid valve disease. The goals of preoperative transesophageal imaging in these lesions, salient features of the exam, and postoperative evaluation are discussed. Atresia of the tricuspid valve is addressed in Chap. 10 along with other lesions that comprise the single ventricle category.

Specific Anomalies

Morphologic Features and Management

Ebstein Anomaly

Morphology—Ebstein anomaly represents a spectrum of congenital abnormalities of the tricuspid valve [109–111]. In this lesion there is displacement of the proximal attachments of the tricuspid valve leaflets, dysplasia of the leaflets, abnormalities in their distal attachments, and frequently associated tricuspid regurgitation. It is considered that the underlying right ventricular myocardium is also affected in this malformation [112].

In the more common forms of Ebstein anomaly, leftward and inferior displacement of the proximal attachments involves the septal and posterior (inferior or mural) leaflets, while the anterior (also referred as anterosuperior) leaflet is usually normally attached to the annulus, but enlarged and 'sail-like' [113]. The displacement of the septal and posterior leaflets is caused by partial or complete adherence to the underlying myocardium, due to lack of apoptosis-induced delamination during early valvar development. Because of the inferior displacement of these leaflets, a portion of the anatomic right ventricle becomes contiguous with the right atrium; this portion of the right ventricle is termed "atrialized" right ventricle. The remainder of the right ventricle (distal to the attachment of the displaced leaflets) is known as the "functional" right ventricle, and there can be considerable variation in size and function of this ventricular chamber. Depending upon tricuspid leaflet development and mobility, there is also a variable degree of tricuspid regurgitation, which can range from mild to very severe.

Management Considerations—The most common indications for surgical intervention in Ebstein anomaly are the presence of cyanosis and heart failure. The neonate with concomitant RVOTO may require surgical palliation by means of a systemic to pulmonary artery shunt, frequently, in the form of a modified Blalock-Taussig shunt. A number of different strategies have been applied to the critically ill neonate with intractable heart failure resulting from severe tricuspid valve regurgitation [114]. One palliative approach consists of creating functional tricuspid atresia by placing a fenestrated tricuspid valve patch in the annular position that obstructs virtually all right ventricular inflow, effectively converting the patient to a form of tricuspid valve atresia (Starnes right ventricular exclusion procedure) [115, 116]. Performed in combination with a reduction right atrioplasty, atrial septectomy, and placement of a systemic to pulmonary artery shunt, this operation assumes the eventual goal of Fontan completion. Cardiac transplantation represents an alternate option in these infants. In the older patient, valve repair/reconstruction can be attempted. Several strategies have been reported that include creation of a monocusp valve, leaflet augmentation, sliding leaflet valvuloplasties, cone repairs, plication of atrialized right ventricle, annular reduction, and a variety of other approaches with variable results [117–120]. In some cases a 'one and a half' ventricle management is utilized that usually combines some form of tricuspid valvuloplasty and creation of a bidirectional cavopulmonary anastomosis (Glenn shunt) [121].The goal is to effectively unload the right heart and limit the regurgitant volume. The 'one and a half' ventricle approach is discussed in further detail in Chap. 10.

Dysplastic Tricuspid Valve

Morphology—Isolated congenital tricuspid regurgitation may arise from abnormalities of the tricuspid architecture other than Ebstein malformation [122]. These rare causes of congenital isolated tricuspid regurgitation include tricuspid valve dysplasia, defined primarily by thickened and malformed tricuspid leaflets and short tendinous chords [123]. The tricuspid leaflets may adhere to the underlying myocardium [110].The dysplastic valve in this setting typically has normal proximal attachments to the AV groove.

Management Considerations—The clinical presentation of severe forms of tricuspid valve dysplasia associated with tricuspid regurgitation mimics that of Ebstein malformation. However, the underlying myocardium in this lesion is usually normal, thus ventricular performance is less likely to be compromised, leading to a more favorable overall prognosis. The pathology may be amenable to surgical intervention [124] and include similar strategies to those applied in Ebstein anomaly, namely, valve repair, replacement, creation of tricuspid atresia and cardiac transplantation.

Pathophysiology

Related to the anatomic spectrum of tricuspid valve malformations (Ebstein anomaly and the dysplastic valve), there are also a wide range of functional abnormalities that determine the pathophysiology of these lesions [125, 126]. The main factors that influence the clinical manifestations are the severity of the tricuspid regurgitation, magnitude of the right-to-left shunt at atrial level, and the degree of right ventricular dysfunction. Mild forms of Ebstein anomaly or valvar dysplasia can present as an incidental finding and the patient may remain completely asymptomatic. At the other end of the spectrum, patients can have significant symptomatology associated with functional limitations, cyanosis, and/or arrhythmias that mandate interventions. The severely symptomatic infant represents a major challenge in terms of clinical management and overall poor prognosis.

Additional anomalies are common in these lesions. A large patent ductus in the neonate with Ebstein anomaly affects clinical management because it maintains elevated pulmonary arterial pressure and can prevent antegrade flow through the pulmonary valve. This 'functional pulmonary atresia' may be difficult to distinguish from true stenosis or atresia of the pulmonary valve. The presence of pulmonary regurgitation by Doppler flow or contrast echocardiography excludes true pulmonary atresia [127]. ASDs are present in almost all patients with Ebstein anomaly and can be considered part of the lesion; right-to-left shunting is generally seen through these defects. In some cases, RVOTO can be present related to the anterior leaflet of the tricuspid valve. Rhythm disturbances can occur due to (a) AV bypass tracts (Wolff-Parkinson-White syndrome) causing supraventricular tachycardia, and (b) atrial dilation leading to atrial fibrillation/flutter. A thinned right ventricular musculature may worsen right ventricular function. Other less frequent associations include VSDs, tetralogy of Fallot, and mitral valve anomalies.

Transesophageal Echocardiography

Preoperative TEE Evaluation

Prebypass TEE has had a major impact in the surgical management of patients with tricuspid valve pathology, particularly in Ebstein anomaly. An important aspect of the TEE examination is to define the morphologic features of the tricuspid valve and supporting structures in order to determine suitability for valve repair. More precise delineation of valve anatomy and function allows refinement of the surgical plan, enhancing the likelihood of a successful intervention [1]. The main objectives of the intraoperative evaluation for this or any other tricuspid valve malformation are to:

- Provide anatomical details of the tricuspid valvar apparatus
- Determine the presence and severity of functional abnormalities related to the malformation
- Assess right and left ventricular systolic performance
- Evaluate associated cardiovascular defects

Intraoperative Imaging

Comprehensive evaluation of the tricuspid valve is feasible by TEE (refer to Chap. 4) [128].The right atrium, tricuspid valve, inflow and trabecular portions of the right ventricle are adequately demonstrated in the ME 4 Ch, mid esophageal right ventricular inflow-outflow (ME RV In-Out), transgastric right ventricular inflow (TG RV In), and deep transgastric views. These views are essential in the examination of tricuspid valve disease. Additional views complement the evaluation.

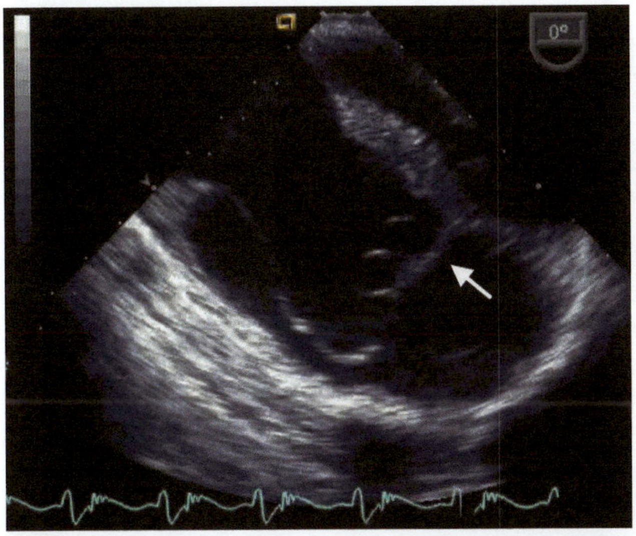

Fig. 8.54 The characteristic features of Ebstein anomaly are displayed in this mid esophageal four chamber view including: apical septal leaflet displacement (*arrow*), redundancy of the anterior leaflet, and atrialization of the right ventricle

Ebstein Anomaly

The characteristic anatomic features of Ebstein anomaly can be well defined by TEE. In the normal heart the septal tricuspid leaflet inserts only slightly towards the apex in comparison with the mitral valve insertion to the ventricular septum. The exaggerated degree of displacement of the septal tricuspid leaflet in Ebstein anomaly (Fig. 8.54, Video 8.41) can be determined by measuring the distances between mitral and tricuspid septal insertion and the apex (ratio between these two distances of >1.5) or the distance between the two points of insertion (>8 mm/m^2 of body surface area) in the ME 4 Ch view [129]. Reduced mobility of the septal leaflet may also be seen. The ME 4 Ch view also allows for definition of the AV junction and the extent of the atrialized right ventricle (Fig. 8.55, Video 8.42). The arrangement of the valve attachments forms an oblique plane that has its largest distance from the right AV groove on the septal surface of the right ventricle as best seen in the ME 4 Ch view (Figs. 8.56 and 8.57) [129].The displacement of the posterior leaflet can be demonstrated in the deep transgastric views in coronal (DTG LAX) and sagittal (DTG Sagittal) planes (Fig. 8.58) [130]. The degree of displacement can be judged from the position of the AV groove. If this is not well seen, the Eustachian valve within the right atrium, which lies close to the AV groove and is often prominent in Ebstein anomaly, can be displayed by the ME 4 Ch view (with retroflexion of the TEE probe) and may aid in defining the distance of displacement of the tethered septal and posterior leaflet(s). The TG RV In, TG Basal SAX (rightward probe rotation) and ME RV In-Out views are also excellent for demonstrating tethering of the posterior leaflet to the underlying myocardium.

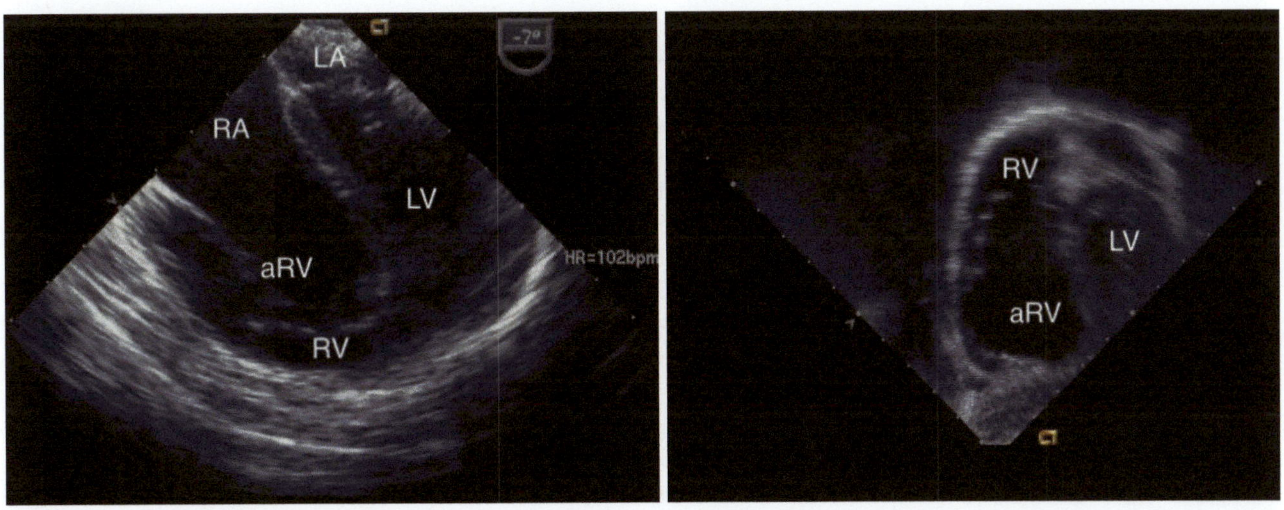

Fig. 8.55 *Left panel*, mid esophageal four chamber view of severe form of Ebstein anomaly displaying adherence of the tricuspid septal leaflet to the underlying myocardium and displacement of the valvar coaptation point well into the apex of the right ventricle (*RV*). *Right panel*, deep transgastric sagittal view depicts the degree of atrialization of the RV (*aRV*). Note the small size of the 'true' or 'functional' *RV*. *LA* left atrium, *LV* left ventricle, *RA* right atrium

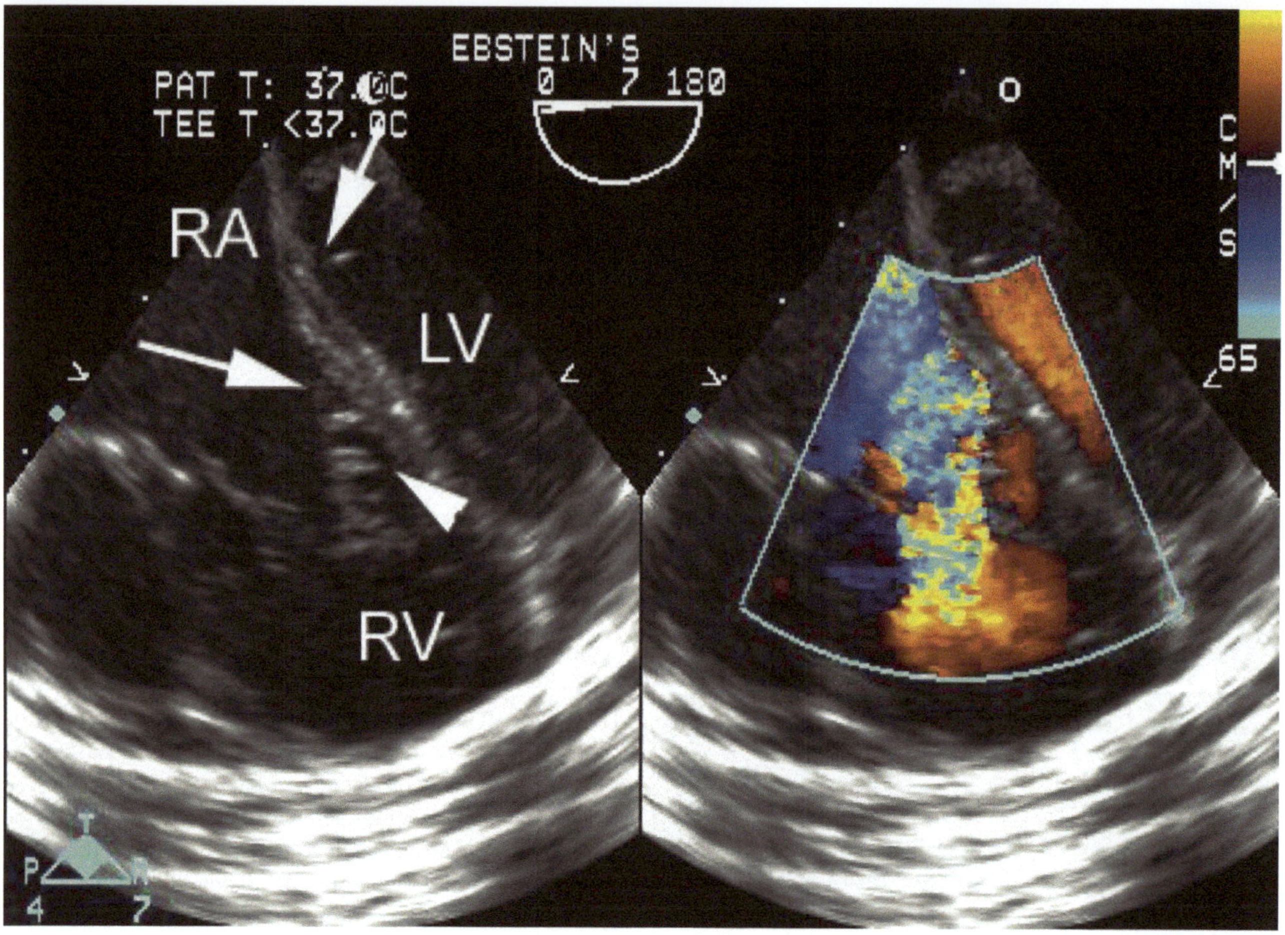

Fig. 8.56 Figure shows a simultaneous mid esophageal four chamber display of morphology (*left panel*) and color flow information (*right panel*) in a patient with Ebstein malformation. The *arrows* indicate the septal attachment of the mitral valve annulus in the left ventricle (*LV*) and the attachment of the apically displaced septal leaflet of the tricuspid valve in the right ventricle (*RV*). An *arrowhead* defines the tips of the tendinous chords arising from the papillary muscles. The color Doppler signal shows aliasing of flow into the *RV* from the right atrium (*RA*)

The anterior leaflet can be interrogated in several planes. The proximal anterior leaflet is attached to the annulus normally, as can be seen in the ME 4 Ch view. Motion of the anterior and septal leaflets can also be appreciated in this view. These features can also be displayed in the TG RV In and deep transgastric views (DTG LAX, DTG Sagittal, and modified views; Fig. 8.59). Using a combination of these cross-sections allows for better assessment of the severity of displacement and the size of the 'atrialized' right ventricle (Fig. 8.55, Video 8.42), while observations and measurements in just one reference plane may fail to predict the degree of severity and the need for extensive surgical intervention [131].

Planning the appropriate surgical approach is based not only on the degree of displacement of the leaflets, but also on the mode of distal attachment of the anterior leaflet [130–132]. As indicated, the valve may be tethered by a number of chordal attachments or may be attached by a band of muscle to the underlying ventricular myocardium. The former is known as a hyphenated attachment [130, 133]. The degree of this attachment can be assessed by echocardiography, although the more severe forms cannot be differentiated. Echocardiographic recognition of tethering, when severe, is important because it allows the surgeon to differentiate those cases where an annuloplasty can be performed from those where the severe tethering will not allow "liberation" of the leaflet. 3D TEE has been shown to enhance the 2D visualization of leaflet tethering [134].

Presence of linear attachments and tethering to the right ventricular free wall, especially of the large anterior leaflet, may result in obstruction between the inlet and outlet portions of the right ventricle and preclude reconstructive-types of operation [133].While linear attachments and tethering of the anterior leaflet are usually noted in the views described above, the degree of obstruction may be difficult to assess because blood flow may occur only through commissures of an immobile valve or through the interstices of the leaflets.

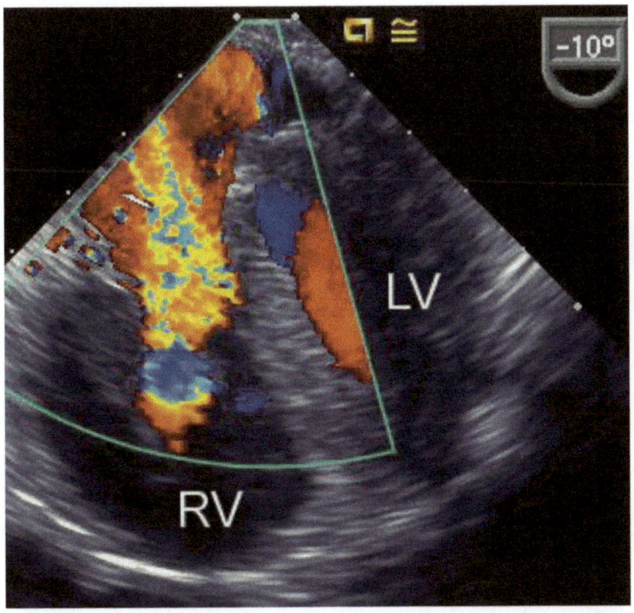

Fig. 8.57 Mid esophageal four chamber view in a patient with Ebstein anomaly demonstrating the origin of the tricuspid regurgitant jet towards the apex of the right ventricle (*RV*) and area of flow convergence (proximal isovelocity surface area or PISA) proximal to the apposed valvar leaflets. The tricuspid leaflets are remarkably displaced inferiorly relative to the hinge point of the mitral leaflets in the left ventricle (*LV*). From the size of the PISA the degree of tricuspid regurgitation appears significant

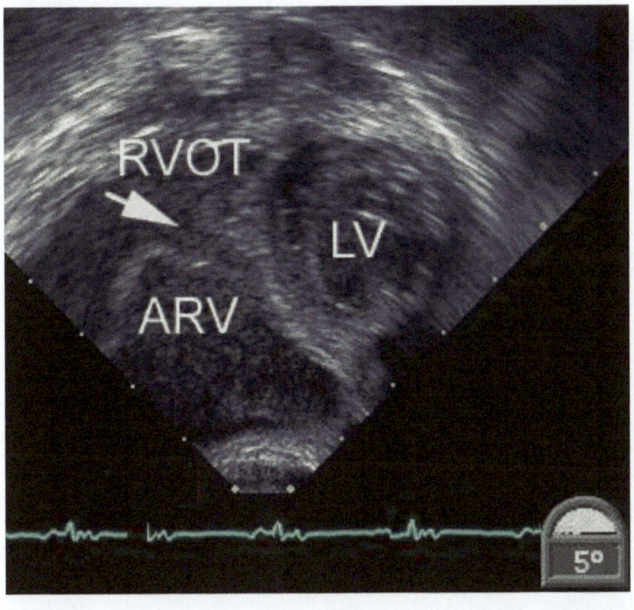

Fig. 8.58 This deep transgastric with posterior transducer angulation demonstrates the displacement of the opposed edges of the septal and posterior (mural) leaflets within the right ventricular outflow tract (*arrow*) and the area of the atrialized right ventricle (*ARV*) lying close to the diaphragm. *LV* left ventricle, *RVOT* right ventricular outflow tract

The use of contrast echocardiography using agitated saline injected into a systemic vein has been suggested in evaluating such obstruction. Rapid filling of the left heart with contrast indicating a large right-to-left shunt may suggest severe obstruction to right ventricular inflow. Conversely, rapid appearance of contrast within the RVOT and a small amount of right-to-left shunting is more likely to represent minimal to no inflow obstruction [135].

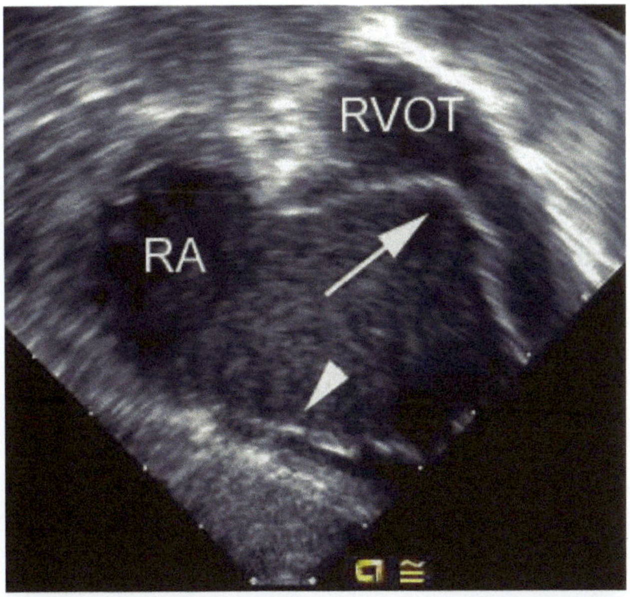

Fig. 8.59 Deep transgastric modified view demonstrating the redundant anterior tricuspid valve leaflet (*large arrow*) and the posterior leaflet (*arrowhead*) adherent to the underlying ventricular myocardium in a patient with Ebstein malformation. *RA* right atrium, *RVOT* right ventricular outflow tract

The echocardiographic features of leaflet dysplasia in this malformation include dense echo reflection and leaflet thickening, which may be observed in almost all planes. In addition to the morphologic abnormalities of the tricuspid valve, the right atrium is typically dilated in Ebstein anomaly, in a significant number of cases to a marked extent. In the neonate this may reflect long-standing tricuspid valve regurgitation throughout fetal life.

Doppler ultrasound effectively demonstrates the tricuspid regurgitation that is present in almost all patients with this anomaly although the severity is variable, reflecting the spectrum of disease. Spectral Doppler interrogation is essential in the TEE evaluation as it provides information on diastolic inflow velocities across the tricuspid valve, facilitates the evaluation of the systolic RVOT velocities, and allows for estimation of pulmonary artery pressures. A relevant application of spectral Doppler in this setting also consists of the assessment of left ventricular outflow tract velocities to exclude obstruction resulting from septal shifting. In some cases the left ventricle can be compressed exhibiting a "pancaked" appearance (Fig. 8.60, Video 8.43).

An important aspect of the preoperative evaluation is an assessment of the functional state of the right ventricle in terms of chamber volume and systolic performance.

A common finding in this lesion is a reduction in the size of the functional right ventricle, particularly in cases when there is obstruction to right ventricular output. This assessment as well as the qualitative evaluation of right ventricular function should be accomplished in multiple views, including those suggested above for the evaluation of the tricuspid valve apparatus. It is relevant to also consider surveillance of left ventricular performance, as functional impairment may co-exist resulting from altered geometry and detrimental ventricular-ventricular interactions.

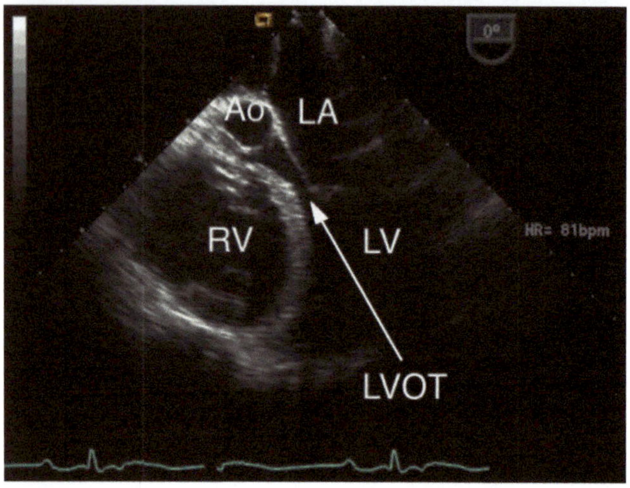

Fig. 8.60 Mid esophageal four chamber view demonstrating bulging of the interventricular septum towards the left ventricle (septal shift), resulting in narrowing of the left ventricular outflow tract (LVOT) and a "pancaked" appearance of the left ventricle (*LV*). *Ao* aorta, *LA* left atrium, *RV* right ventricle

Patients with congenitally corrected transposition of the great arteries (refer to Chap. 12) may display tricuspid (left-sided) valve abnormalities similar to Ebstein anomaly, thus the term "Ebstenoid" appearance (Fig. 8.61).

Tricuspid Valve Dysplasia

Intraoperative TEE plays an important role in defining the anatomy in tricuspid valve dysplasia. The same TEE views described in the evaluation of Ebstein anomaly can be utilized to assess the morphologic and functional abnormalities in this lesion. In some cases it might be difficult to distinguish clearly between primary tricuspid valve dysplasia and Ebstein malformation. This discrimination relies to a significant extent on the echocardiographic assessment of the insertion of the septal leaflet of the tricuspid valve and degree of displacement—normal in tricuspid valve dysplasia versus significant in Ebstein anomaly (Fig. 8.62, Video 8.44).

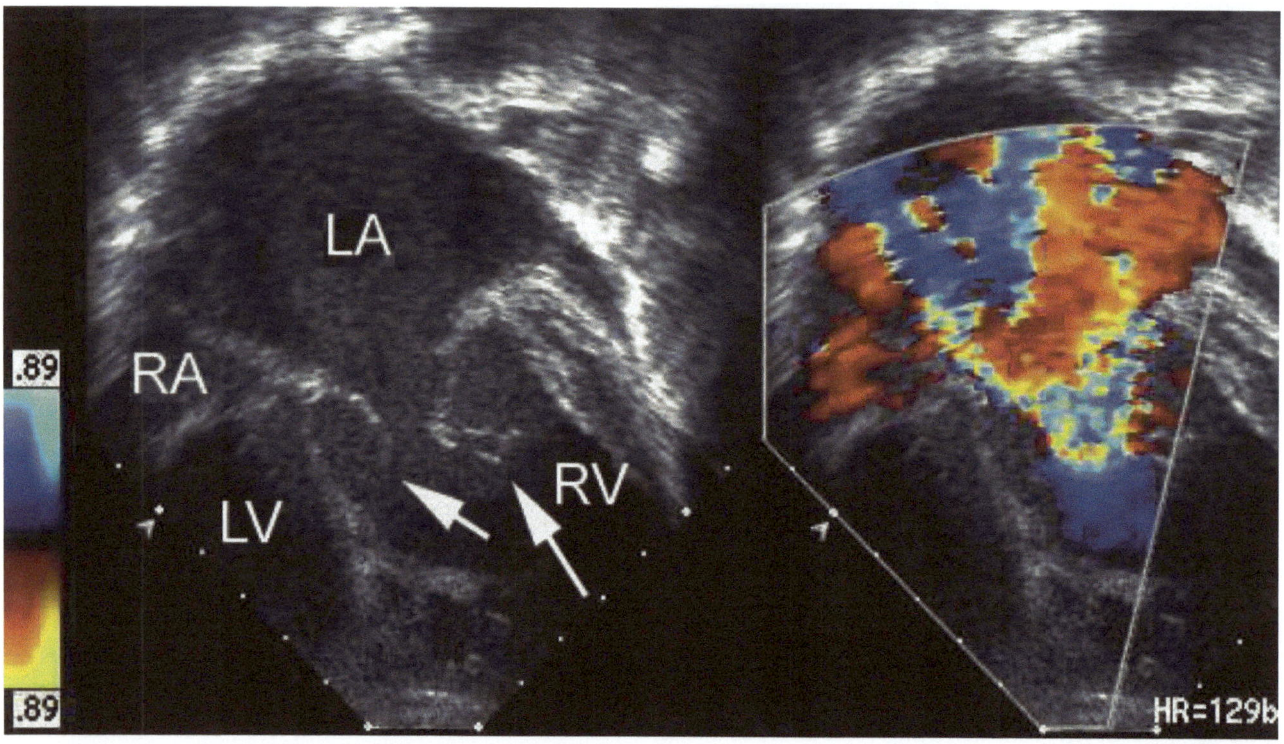

Fig. 8.61 Deep transgastric systolic frame (*left panel*) displays the anatomical features in a patient with congenitally corrected transposition (*l*-TGA). Dysplasia and lack of coaptation of the tricuspid leaflets (left atrioventricular or systemic atrioventricular valve; *arrows*) is shown. Note the significant degree of annular dilation. There is an associated large jet of tricuspid regurgitation as depicted by color flow mapping (*right panel*). *LA* left atrium, *LV* left ventricle, *RA* right atrium, *RV* right ventricle

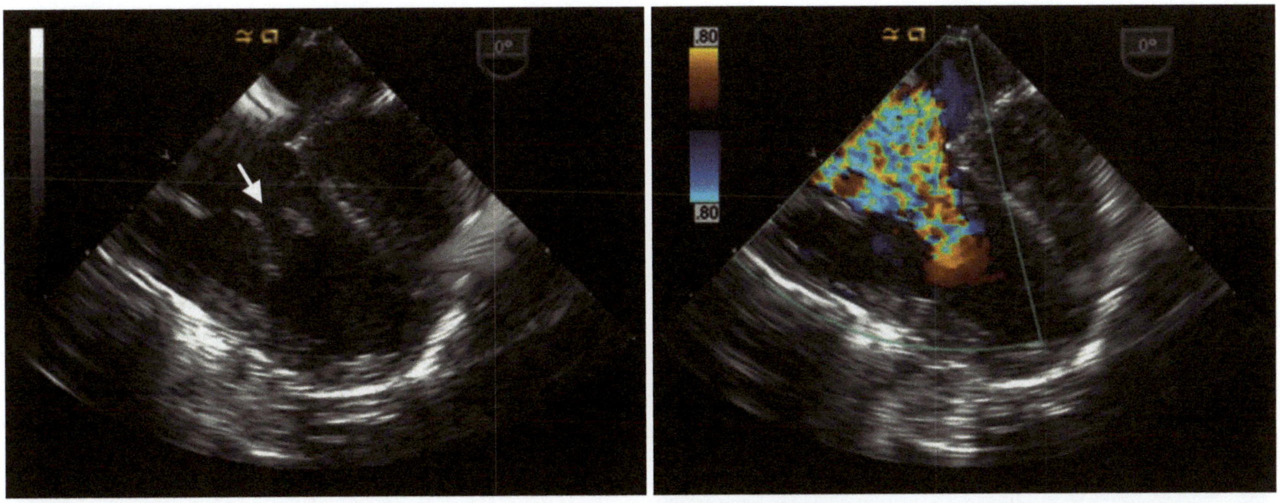

Fig. 8.62 Mid esophageal four chamber view (*left panel*) displaying an abnormal tricuspid valve with thickened and dysplastic leaflets that coapt poorly during systole (*arrow*). Associated severe regurgitation is present (*right panel*). There is an exaggerated degree of normal offset of the atrioventricular valves onto the septum suggesting a more likely diagnosis of Ebstein anomaly over that of tricuspid valvar dysplasia, where normally hinged leaflets are present

Assessment of Tricuspid Regurgitation

An important goal in tricuspid valve repair surgery is the detection and severity grading of valvar regurgitation [136]. Color Doppler interrogation, however, can be challenging due to factors such as distorted anatomy secondary to dilated cardiac chambers and unusual orientation of regurgitant jets. In Ebstein anomaly the examination should consider that the regurgitant jet frequently originates distal to the true valvar annulus, near or at the region where the displaced valvar leaflets are attached to the right ventricular endocardial surface. Thus sweeps that display the right ventricular inlet from an anterior to a posterior aspect are essential in this evaluation. This is important in both, the preoperative and postoperative evaluation.

Several parameters have been applied in the quantitative evaluation of tricuspid regurgitation by echocardiography including jet area by color Doppler, calculation of regurgitant orifice area, and measurement of the width of the vena contracta by color flow imaging [137]. These parameters, however, have not been fully validated in children or may not be applicable to congenital tricuspid valve pathology. Thus, for practical purposes in the intraoperative setting, the evaluation of tricuspid regurgitation is semi-quantitative, derived from the visual assessment that grades the degree of regurgitation from trivial to severe. Supporting criteria for severity grading may include the extent of right atrial and inferior vena cava dilation and the presence of systolic flow reversal in the vena cava and hepatic veins.

Postoperative TEE Evaluation

The focus of the postrepair TEE assessment is the determination of residual tricuspid regurgitation, exclusion of hemodynamically significant tricuspid stenosis, as well as the evaluation of myocardial function and adequacy of the repair of associated defects (Fig. 8.63). In the setting of valve replacement, a comprehensive evaluation should be performed that focuses on prosthetic valve function (refer to Chap. 16) [138, 139].

Three-Dimensional Echocardiograpic Imaging

The 3D imaging modality has been applied to the pre and postoperative evaluation of valve repair in Ebstein anomaly and allows for additional morphologic and functional evaluation than that provided by 2D imaging (refer to Chap. 19 and Chap. 20). As such, real-time 3D TEE is likely to significantly expand the contributions of intraoperative imaging in this malformation [140].

Additional Applications of TEE in Pathologies Affecting the Atrioventricular Valves

Prosthetic Mitral Valve

In adult patients, TEE has been shown to be an excellent modality for imaging prosthetic valves in the mitral position with an overall sensitivity of 96 % for detection of abnormalities [141, 142]. TEE has also been useful to investigate mitral valve prosthetic function in children (refer to Chap. 16) [143].The most common prosthetic valve abnormalities that may require TEE interrogation include abnormal motion of the leaflets, resulting in prosthetic valve stenosis or regurgitation, and infective

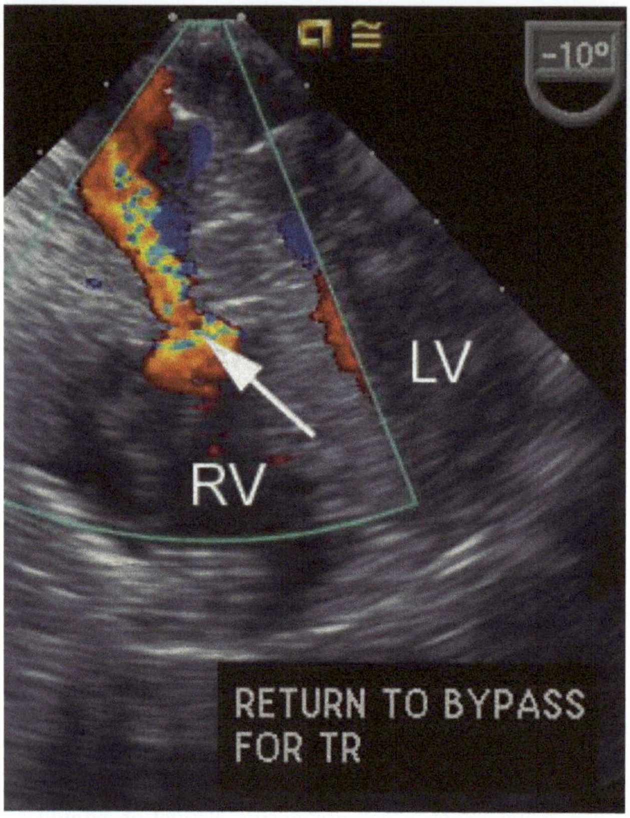

Fig. 8.63 Mid esophageal four chamber view demonstrating the residual degree of tricuspid regurgitation following annuloplasty for Ebstein malformation. This image, taken after a second return to cardiopulmonary bypass, still demonstrates tricuspid regurgitation through a very narrow tricuspid orifice (*arrow*), but without hemodynamic evidence of stenosis. This degree of regurgitation was considered acceptable for weaning from cardiopulmonary bypass. *LV* left ventricle, *RV* right ventricle

endocarditis. Seating puffs that occur inside the sewing ring should be differentiated from paravalvar leaks which occur outside the sewing ring (Fig. 8.64). Leaflet motion analysis is feasible by TEE in most patients with a prosthetic mitral valve and this modality has a higher rate of success than TTE for single-disk and bileaflet prostheses (Fig. 8.65) [144]. TEE has also been shown to be valuable in the detection of prosthetic valve infective endocarditis (discussed in detail in Chap. 16) [145].

Mitral Valve Prolapse

Mitral valve prolapse can occur as an isolated phenomenon in an otherwise healthy individual or in those with connective tissue disorders such as Marfan syndrome [146]. As discussed in Chap. 4, the posterior leaflet of the mitral valve can be divided into three scallops namely, P1, P2 and P3. The most common site of prolapse is the middle scallop, or P2, and the adjacent segment of the anterior leaflet (referred to as A2). However, multiple scallops can be involved. The affected regions typically display a floppy appearance, thickening, and myxomatous changes. The prolapse can cause mitral regurgitation representing a potential risk factor for infectious endocarditis. TEE is indicated if imaging is not adequate by TTE to define the presence of prolapse, its mechanism, or the extent of mitral regurgitation. TEE represents an important tool to guide the repair and examine the operative results. The concerns of infectious endocarditis and chordal rupture represent additional main indications for TEE interrogation in mitral valve prolapse.

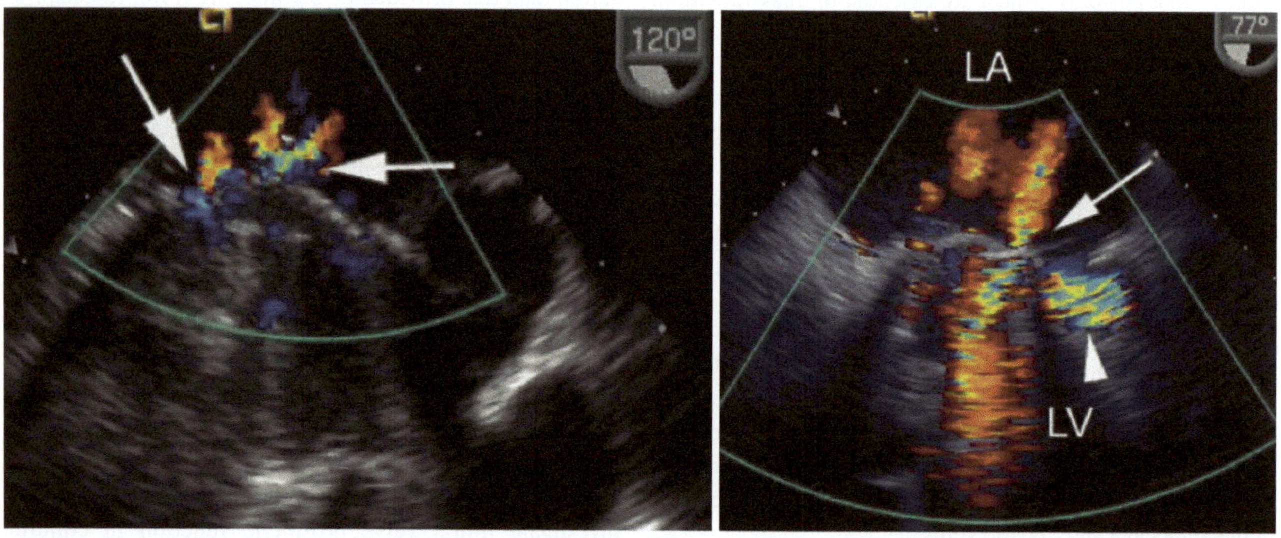

Fig. 8.64 *Left panel*, mid esophageal long axis view focusing on a St. Jude® mitral valve prosthesis in annular position. The image depicts the characteristic seating puffs in systole, present at the circumference of the metal leaflet opposing the ring and also at the junction of the two linear portions of the valvar leaflet in the center. The *arrows* indicate that these regurgitant jets are lying within the metal annulus clearly identified in this image and these are therefore not paravalvar leaks. *Right panel*, both a seating puff (*arrow*) and a paravalvar leak (*arrowhead*) are displayed in this mid esophageal mitral commissural equivalent view at 77°. The paravalvar leak is directed into a large pouch in the sub mitral area. *LA* left atrium, *LV* left ventricle

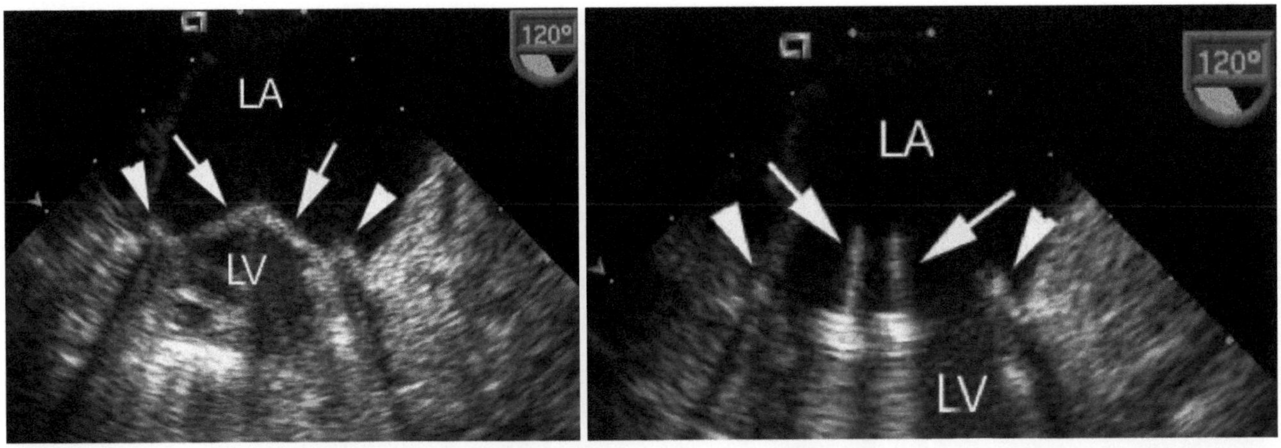

Fig. 8.65 In the two figures, obtained in a mid esophageal long axis view, the St. Jude® mitral prosthesis is seen positioned between the left atrium (*LA*) and left ventricle (*LV*). *Left panel*, the two leaflets of the prosthetic valve are depicted in the apposed position during systole (*arrows*) and the annulus is well seen (*arrowheads*). *Right panel*, the prosthetic valvar leaflets are seen in the open position (*arrows*) during diastole and demonstrate a marked degree of reverberation at the hinge points. The annular ring is more clearly identified with the valvar leaflets open (*arrowheads*)

The TEE evaluation of the mitral valve in this pathology consists of imaging in multiple planes. A comprehensive examination is important because in some cases, only certain portions of the valve/tension apparatus can be affected. A systematic, methodical approach allows for accurate localization of the pathology that accounts for mitral regurgitation [37, 38]. By rotating the transducer through several planes each segment/scallop can be evaluated to define the origin of the regurgitant jet(s). In most cases the exam starts at the ME 4 Ch and navigates the entire valve annulus while moving across the ME mitral commissural, ME 2 Ch, ME LAX, and transgastric basal short axis views (Refer to Chap. 4). At each of these views the transducer can be manipulated to display anterior and posterior valvar components as well as rotated to interrogate rightward or leftward valvar regions, relative to the position of the probe. Additional long axis views of the valve at the transgastric level (TG LAX and TG 2 Ch) can offer complementary information.

Mitral prolapse represents a pathology where 3D TEE has played a significant role. In contrast to 2D TEE where evaluation of the valve requires rotation of the scanning plane in multiple views as described, 3D TEE provides a detailed structural display of the valve without the need for collecting serial 2D images and mentally reconstructing the 3D anatomy. Superimposed color information provides for localization of regurgitant jets. Importantly, the technique also allows for the valvar structures to be displayed from a surgical perspective, facilitating the repair. The benefit of 3D TEE technology in mitral valve disease continues to be documented in the literature, mostly in the adult population and in those patients suitable for imaging with currently available 3D TEE probes [147, 148].

Ruptured Tendinous Chords

Rupture of the mitral chordae is rare in children, even in those with Marfan syndrome and complications of mitral valve involvement usually only manifest towards the end of the second decade [146, 149]. In this setting, rupture of mitral chords is usually asymptomatic and only rarely causes acute hemodynamic deterioration [150, 151]. TEE in this case will demonstrate the ruptured chords appearing as mobile echogenic structures that may prolapse into the left atrium in systole and can be associated with significant mitral regurgitation. Rupture of tendinous chords can also result from bacterial endocarditis (see below). In this situation, chordal rupture can lead to acute and massive mitral regurgitation and severe hemodynamic compromise (Figs. 8.66 and 8.67).

Infectious Endocarditis

Echocardiography is a central diagnostic modality for infectious endocarditis (IE) and its potential complications and should be performed in most cases when this diagnosis is suspected and transthoracic imaging is not diagnostic (also refer to Chap. 16). In adult patients, TEE is more sensitive than TTE for detection of intracardiac vegetations and for complications such as annular abscesses, but it may be overused as a screening test. Therefore debate exists to whether TTE or TEE should be performed as the initial echocardiographic modality for IE [152, 153]. As noted throughout this textbook, children generally have better TTE windows than adults, thus smaller vegetations can be more easily detected. The decision then whether to perform TTE

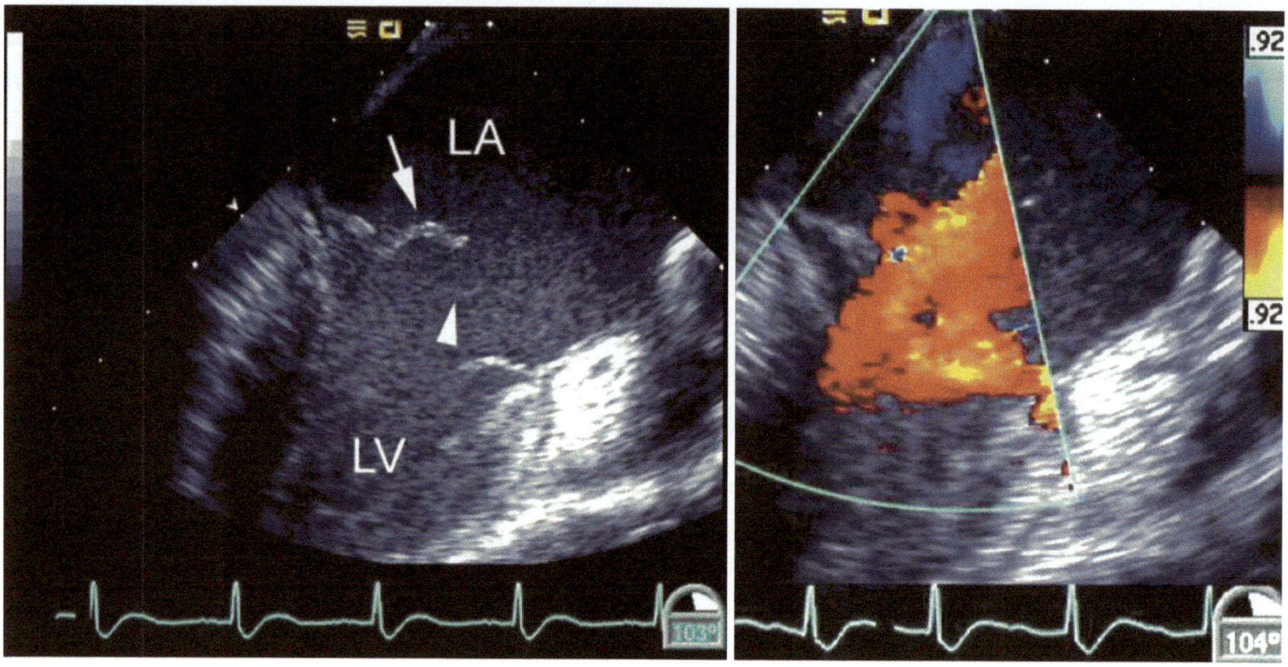

Fig. 8.66 *Left panel*, mid esophageal long axis view in a young patient with Marfan syndrome and a ruptured mitral chord due to acute infectious endocarditis. The flail mitral leaflet is seen (*arrow*) as well as the ruptured chords (*arrowhead*). *Right panel*, the associated massive degree of mitral regurgitation is demonstrated. *LA* left atrium, *LV* left ventricle

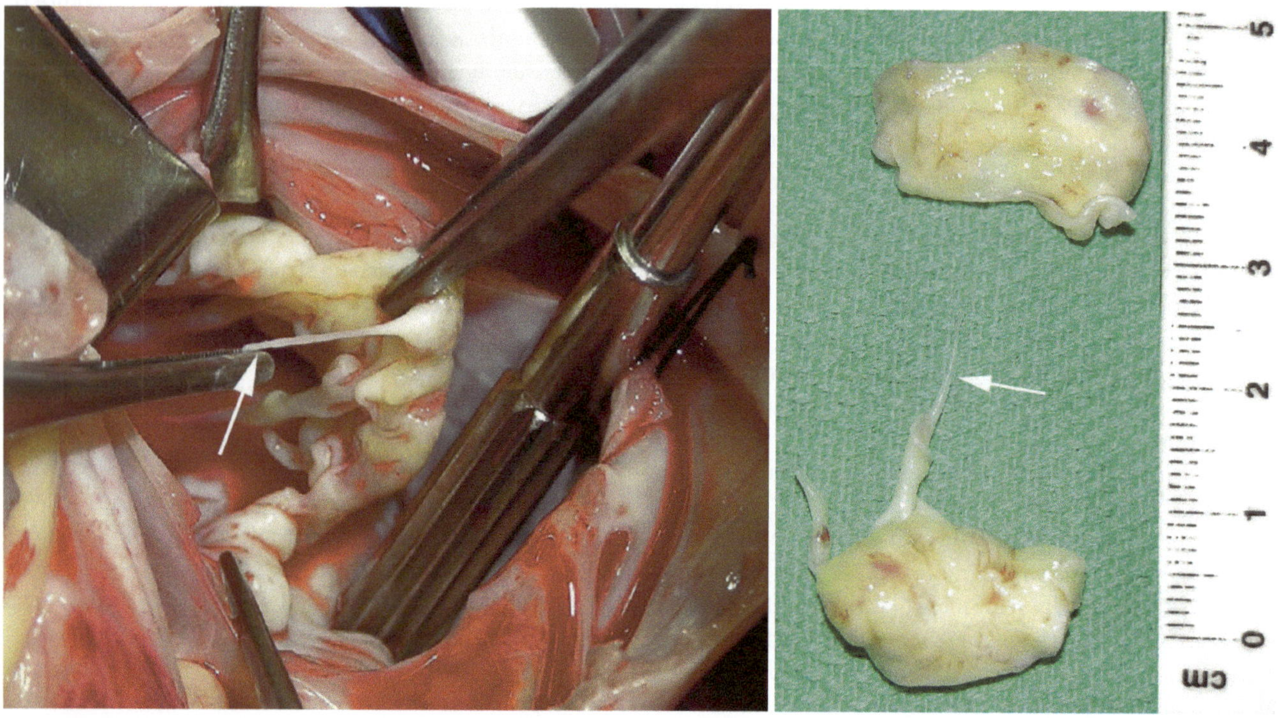

Fig. 8.67 Intraoperative photographs from patient shown in Fig. 8.66 demonstrating in the *left panel* a ruptured chord as is held by the forceps (*arrow*). Note the thickened, redundant mitral leaflets. The valve was excised as shown in the *right panel* and a mitral valve prosthesis was placed. An *arrow* indicates the ruptured chord

or TEE in children with suspected IE depends on the clinical situation [154, 155]. If the clinical suspicion for IE is low or transthoracic imaging is likely to be of good quality, then TTE is a reasonable first choice [156]. On the other hand, when transthoracic imaging produces poor images, TEE should be performed. However, before proceeding to TEE, the modified Duke criteria should be fulfilled as discussed in Chap. 16. If TTE provides negative results and the clinical suspicion for IE remains low, then other clinical entities should be considered and TEE is probably unnecessary. Also, if TTE identifies vegetations but the likelihood of complications is low, then subsequent TEE is unlikely to affect management of the patient. On the other hand, if clinical suspicion of IE or its complications is high, such as in the presence of a prosthetic valve, staphylococcal bacteremia, or new onset AV block, then a negative TTE study will not definitively exclude IE or resultant complications and TEE should be undertaken. Also, if the TTE is negative but the diagnosis of IE continues to be considered due to clinical or bacteriological suspicion, then TEE should be performed. Sometimes repeat examination after 7–10 days can be useful, as vegetations initially too small to have been visualized by TTE may have sufficiently increased in size to be detected by TEE. Extension of the infectious process or development of complications can also be detected on repeat examination. TEE should also be performed in cases where there is an initial positive TTE for IE and a high risk for cardiac complications such as perivalvular infection [154]. Multiplane TEE may be useful in identifying vegetations, which may appear as echogenic, mobile masses on the valve leaflets. The most common site in children is the mitral valve (Fig. 8.68), followed by the aortic valve. Valvular regurgitation may be present (Fig. 8.69). Surgery is indicated for complications including heart failure, recurrent embolic events, and annular abscess. In some cases the potentially aggressive nature of the microorganism might dictate the need for surgical intervention. After completion of medical and/or surgical treatment, repeat echocardiography should be undertaken to establish a baseline for follow-up that documents valvular morphology, presence of vegetations, valvular regurgitation, and ventricular function. This can be done by TTE, but as with the pretreatment study, TEE should be performed in the event of poor or difficult transthoracic imaging [154].

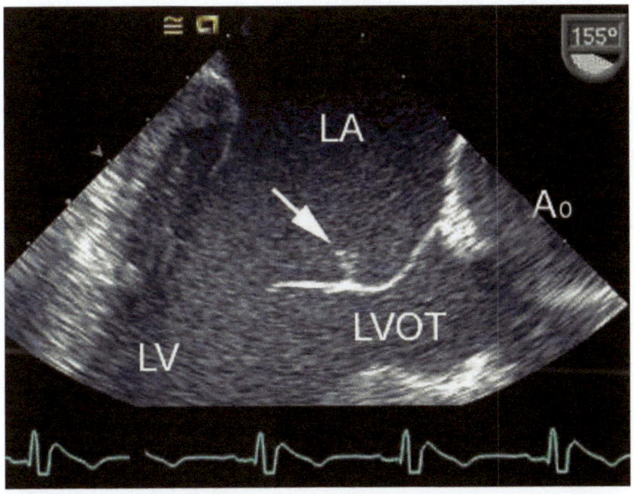

Fig. 8.68 Mid esophageal long axis view demonstrates a vegetation (*arrow*) on the anterior mitral leaflet in a patient with a repaired Taussig-Bing malformation, in whom an arterial switch operation was performed. *Ao* aorta, *LA* left atrium, *LV* left ventricle, *LVOT* left ventricular outflow tract

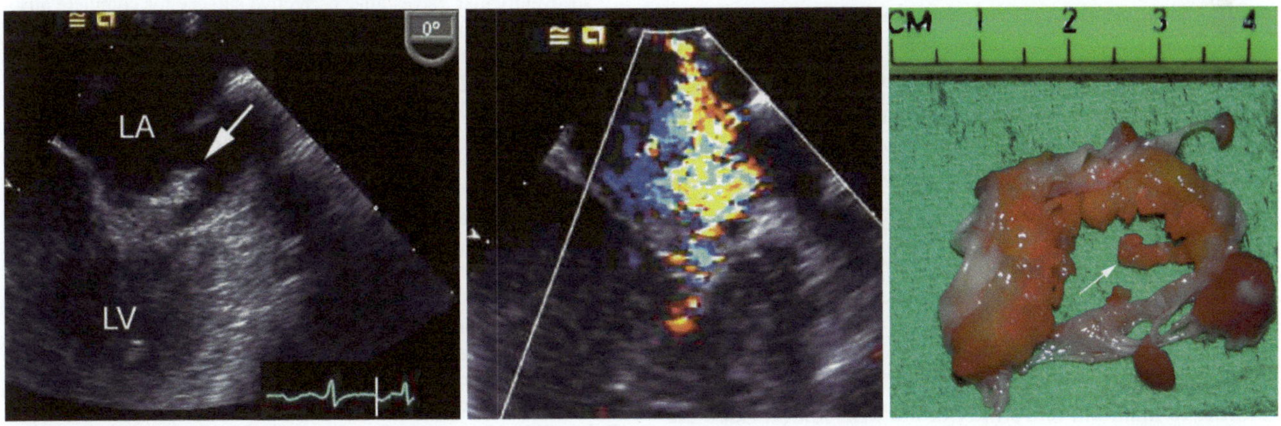

Fig. 8.69 *Left panel*, mid esophageal four chamber view depicting a vegetation on the atrial surface of the mitral valve (*arrow*). *Middle panel*, color flow mapping demonstrates valvar regurgitation associated with this vegetation. *Right panel*, the excised mitral valve and papillary muscle heads are shown taken shortly after the transesophageal echocardiogram. A vegetation is seen arising from the posterior leaflet (*arrow*) and the valve is extremely deformed by pan-endocarditis. *LA* left atrium, *LV* left ventricle

Summary

TEE plays an important role in the evaluation of malformations that affect the AV junction and in the assessment of congenital anomalies of the AV valves. In fact, among all the potential applications of TEE, AV valve evaluation represents one of the most important, most well recognized, and most useful. It was one of the first applications to be studied extensively following the introduction of the technology. In addition to being the subject of a significant clinical experience, AV valve evaluation has been the focus of many publications on TEE. There are clear and very compelling reasons why TEE assumes such importance in AV valve evaluation. Defects involving the AV septum and AV valves are frequently complex in nature, requiring comprehensive imaging assessment in order to develop appropriate management plans. TEE has been shown to provide detailed and highly accurate morphologic characterization of these pathologies, along with assessment of associated functional and hemodynamic abnormalities, and evaluation of coexistent cardiovascular defects. The significant intraoperative benefits of this modality have been well documented—for guiding and refining the surgical plan and, more importantly, for evaluating the adequacy of the surgical intervention. Recent experience with real-time 3D TEE imaging, although limited thus far to older children and adults, demonstrates superior benefits compared to 2D in pathology affecting the AV septum and AV valves. These include improved morphologic characterization of defects, enhanced appreciation of mechanisms of valve disease and assessment of disease severity, and better ability to guide surgical management.

Surgery for AVSDs and the AV valves continues to represent one of the most common indications for the use of the TEE in CHD. Even centers that do not routinely incorporate TEE in their standard of care during congenital heart surgery consider the assessment of these lesions a clear indication for the use of the modality. Future advances in imaging technology, particularly as these relate to the miniaturization of probes with real-time 3D capabilities, are expected to further enhance the benefits of TEE imaging in the evaluation of these defects.

Editor's Note

In order to maintain uniformity of the TEE image/video display throughout this textbook, selected figures (Figures 8.11, 8.29, 8.36, and 8.66) and videos (Videos 8.6 and 8.22) in this chapter have been inverted vertically relative to their orientation when originally acquired. The original image/video display format submitted by the authors followed their preference to present TEE images in an anatomic orientation equivalent to that of transthoracic echocardiography.

References

1. Randolph GR, Hagler DJ, Connolly HM, et al. Intraoperative transesophageal echocardiography during surgery for congenital heart defects. J Thorac Cardiovasc Surg. 2002;124:1176–82.
2. Cyran SE, Kimball TR, Meyer RA, et al. Efficacy of intraoperative transesophageal echocardiography in children with congenital heart disease. Am J Cardiol. 1989;63:594–8.
3. Stevenson JG, Sorensen GK, Gartman DM, Hall DG, Rittenhouse EA. Transesophageal echocardiography during repair of congenital cardiac defects: identification of residual problems necessitating reoperation. J Am Soc Echocardiogr. 1993;6:356–65.
4. Miller-Hance WC, Silverman NH. Transesophageal echocardiography (TEE) in congenital heart disease with focus on the adult. Cardiol Clin. 2000;18:861–92.
5. Mahle WT, Shirali GS, Anderson RH. Echo-morphological correlates in patients with atrioventricular septal defect and common atrioventricular junction. Cardiol Young. 2006;16 Suppl 3:43–51.
6. Ebels T, Elzenga N, Anderson RH. Atrioventricular septal defects. In: Anderson RH, Baker EJ, Penny DJ, Redington AN, Rigby ML, Wernovsky G, editors. Paediatric cardiology: expert consult—online and print. 3rd ed. Philadelphia: Churchill Livingstone; 2009. p. 553–89.
7. Becker AE, Anderson RH. Atrioventricular septal defects: What's in a name? J Thorac Cardiovasc Surg. 1982;83:461–9.
8. Anderson RH, Zuberbuhler JR, Penkoske PA, Neches WH. Of clefts, commissures, and things. J Thorac Cardiovasc Surg. 1985; 90:605–10.
9. Rastelli G, Kirklin JW, Titus JL. Anatomic observations on complete form of persistent common atrioventricular canal with special reference to atrioventricular valves. Mayo Clin Proc. 1966;41:296–308.
10. Silverman NH, Zuberbuhler JR, Anderson RH. Atrioventricular septal defects: cross-sectional echocardiographic and morphologic comparisons. Int J Cardiol. 1986;13:309–31.
11. Silverman NH. The secundum atrial septal defect and atrioventricular canal defects. In: Braunwald E, Freedom RM, editors. Atlas of heart diseases: congenital heart disease. New York: Mosby; 1996.
12. Becker AE, Anderson RH. Pathology of congenital heart disease. London: Butterworth Heinemann; 1981. p. 140.
13. Krasemann T, Debus V, Rellensmann G, et al. Regurgitation of the atrioventricular valves after corrective surgery for complete atrioventricular septal defects—comparison of different surgical techniques. Thorac Cardiovasc Surg. 2007;55:229–32.
14. Hoohenkerk GJ, Bruggemans EF, Rijlaarsdam M, Schoof PH, Koolbergen DR, Hazekamp MG. More than 30 years' experience with surgical correction of atrioventricular septal defects. Ann Thorac Surg. 2010;90:1554–61.
15. Karl TR, Provenzano SC, Nunn GR, Anderson RH. The current surgical perspective to repair of atrioventricular septal defect with common atrioventricular junction. Cardiol Young. 2010;20 Suppl 3:120–7.
16. Ayres NA, Miller-Hance W, Fyfe DA, et al. Indications and guidelines for performance of transesophageal echocardiography in the patient with pediatric acquired or congenital heart disease: report from the task force of the Pediatric Council of the American Society of Echocardiography. J Am Soc Echocardiogr. 2005;18:91–8.
17. Lee HR, Montenegro LM, Nicolson SC, Gaynor JW, Spray TL, Rychik J. Usefulness of intraoperative transesophageal echocardiography in predicting the degree of mitral regurgitation secondary to atrioventricular defect in children. Am J Cardiol. 1999;83:750–3.
18. Andropoulos DB. Transesophageal echocardiography as a guide to central venous catheter placement in pediatric patients undergoing cardiac surgery. J Cardiothorac Vasc Anesth. 1999;13:320–1.
19. Fyfe DA, Ritter SB, Snider AR, et al. Guidelines for transesophageal echocardiography in children. J Am Soc Echocardiogr. 1992;5:640–4.

20. Beppu S, Nimura Y, Sakakibara H, et al. Mitral cleft in ostium primum atrial septal defect assessed by cross-sectional echocardiography. Circulation. 1980;62:1099–107.
21. Anderson RH, Ebels T, Zuberbuhler JR, Silverman NH. The left valve in atrioventricular septal defect-anatomic and echocardiographic features. In: Anderson RH, Neches WH, Park SC, Zuberbuhler JR, editors. Perspectives in paediatric cardiology. New York: Futura, Mount Kisco; 1988. p. 299–310.
22. Smallhorn JF, de Leval M, Stark J, et al. Isolated anterior mitral cleft. Two dimensional echocardiographic assessment and differentiation from "clefts" associated with atrioventricular septal defect. Br Heart J. 1982;48:109–16.
23. Trowitzsch E, Baño-Rodrigo A, Burger BM, Colan SD, Sanders SP. Two-dimensional echocardiographic findings in double orifice mitral valve. J Am Coll Cardiol. 1985;6:383–7.
24. Baño-Rodrigo A, Van Praagh S, Trowitzsch E, Van Praagh R. Double-orifice mitral valve: a study of 27 postmortem cases with developmental, diagnostic and surgical considerations. Am J Cardiol. 1988;61:152–60.
25. Chin AJ, Bierman FZ, Sanders SP, Williams RG, Norwood WI, Castaneda AR. Subxyphoid 2-dimensional echocardiographic identification of left ventricular papillary muscle anomalies in complete common atrioventricular canal. Am J Cardiol. 1983;51:1695–9.
26. Bharati S, Lev M. The spectrum of common atrioventricular orifice (canal). Am Heart J. 1973;86:553–61.
27. Cohen MS, Jacobs ML, Weinberg PM, Rychik J. Morphometric analysis of unbalanced common atrioventricular canal using two-dimensional echocardiography. J Am Coll Cardiol. 1996;28:1017–23.
28. Jegatheeswaran A, Pizarro C, Caldarone CA, et al. Echocardiographic definition and surgical decision-making in unbalanced atrioventricular septal defect: a Congenital Heart Surgeons' Society multiinstitutional study. Circulation. 2010;122:S209–15.
29. Kudo T, Yokoyama M, Imai Y, Konno S, Sakakibara S. The tricuspid pouch in endocardial cushion defect. Am Heart J. 1974;87:544–9.
30. Ebels T, Becker AE. Surgery for left ventricular outflow tract stenosis in atrioventricular septal defect [letter]. J Thorac Cardiovasc Surg. 1988;96(2):344.
31. Meijboom EJ, Wyse RK, Ebels T, et al. Doppler mapping of postoperative left atrioventricular valve regurgitation. Circulation. 1988;77:311–5.
32. Freedom RM, Dische MR, Rowe RD. Pathologic anatomy of subaortic stenosis and atresia in the first year of life. Am J Cardiol. 1977;39:1035–44.
33. Digilio MC, Marino B, Toscano A, Giannotti A, Dallapiccola B. Atrioventricular canal defect without Down syndrome: a heterogeneous malformation. Am J Med Genet. 1999;85:140–6.
34. Bando K, Turrentine MW, Sun K, et al. Surgical management of complete atrioventricular septal defects. A twenty-year experience. J Thorac Cardiovasc Surg. 1995;110:1543–52; discussion 1552–4.
35. Castello R, Lenzen P, Aguirre F, Labovitz AJ. Quantitation of mitral regurgitation by transesophageal echocardiography with Doppler color flow mapping: correlation with cardiac catheterization. J Am Coll Cardiol. 1992;19:1516–21.
36. Sadoshima J, Koyanagi S, Sugimachi M, Hirooka Y, Takeshita A. Evaluation of the severity of mitral regurgitation by transesophageal Doppler flow echocardiography. Am Heart J. 1992;123:1245–51.
37. Foster GP, Isselbacher EM, Rose GA, Torchiana DF, Akins CW, Picard MH. Accurate localization of mitral regurgitant defects using multiplane transesophageal echocardiography. Ann Thorac Surg. 1998;65:1025–31.
38. Lambert AS, Miller JP, Merrick SH, et al. Improved evaluation of the location and mechanism of mitral valve regurgitation with a systematic transesophageal echocardiography examination. Anesth Analg. 1999;88:1205–12.
39. Dahm M, Iversen S, Schmid FX, Drexler M, Erbel R, Oelert H. Intraoperative evaluation of reconstruction of the atrioventricular valves by transesophageal echocardiography. Thorac Cardiovasc Surg. 1987;35(2):140–2.
40. Drexler M, Erbel R, Dahm M, Mohr-Kahaly S, Oelert H, Meyer J. Assessment of successful valve reconstruction by intraoperative transesophageal echocardiography (TEE). Int J Card Imaging. 1986;2:21–30.
41. Kim HK, Kim WH, Hwang SW, et al. Predictive value of intraoperative transesophageal echocardiography in complete atrioventricular septal defect. Ann Thorac Surg. 2005;80:56–9.
42. Sreeram N, Kaulitz R, Stumper OF, Hess J, Quaegebeur JM, Sutherland GR. Comparative roles of intraoperative epicardial and early postoperative transthoracic echocardiography in the assessment of surgical repair of congenital heart defects. J Am Coll Cardiol. 1990;16:913–20 [see comments].
43. Canter CE, Sekarski DC, Martin TC, Guitierrez FR, Spray TL. Intraoperative evaluation of atrioventricular septal defect repair by color flow mapping echocardiography. Ann Thorac Surg. 1989;48:544–50.
44. Prakash A, Lacro RV, Sleeper LA, et al. Challenges in echocardiographic assessment of mitral regurgitation in children after repair of atrioventricular septal defect. Pediatr Cardiol. 2012;33:205–14.
45. Piccoli GP, Ho SY, Wilkinson JL, Macartney FJ, Gerlis LM, Anderson RH. Left-sided obstructive lesions in atrioventricular septal defects: an anatomic study. J Thorac Cardiovasc Surg. 1982;83:453–60.
46. Silverman NH, Gerlis LM, Ho SY, Anderson RH. Fibrous obstruction within the left ventricular outflow tract associated with ventricular septal defect: a pathologic study. J Am Coll Cardiol. 1995;25:475–81.
47. Van Arsdell GS, Williams WG, Boutin C, et al. Subaortic stenosis in the spectrum of atrioventricular septal defects. Solutions may be complex and palliative. J Thorac Cardiovasc Surg. 1995;110:1534–41. discussion 1541–2.
48. Marx GR, Fulton DR, Pandian NG, et al. Delineation of site, relative size and dynamic geometry of atrial septal defects by real-time three-dimensional echocardiography. J Am Coll Cardiol. 1995;25:482–90.
49. Acar P, Laskari C, Rhodes J, Pandian N, Warner K, Marx G. Three-dimensional echocardiographic analysis of valve anatomy as a determinant of mitral regurgitation after surgery for atrioventricular septal defects. Am J Cardiol. 1999;83:745–9.
50. Lange A, Mankad P, Walayat M, Palka P, Burns JE, Godman MJ. Transthoracic three-dimensional echocardiography in the preoperative assessment of atrioventricular septal defect morphology. Am J Cardiol. 2000;85:630–5.
51. Singh A, Romp RL, Nanda NC, et al. Usefulness of live/real time three-dimensional transthoracic echocardiography in the assessment of atrioventricular septal defects. Echocardiography. 2006;23:598–608.
52. Takahashi K, Mackie AS, Thompson R, et al. Quantitative real-time three-dimensional echocardiography provides new insight into the mechanisms of mitral valve regurgitation post-repair of atrioventricular septal defect. J Am Soc Echocardiogr. 2012;25(11):1231–44.
53. Kutty S, Smallhorn JF. Evaluation of atrioventricular septal defects by three-dimensional echocardiography: benefits of navigating the third dimension. J Am Soc Echocardiogr. 2012;25:932–44.
54. Barrea C, Levasseur S, Roman K, et al. Three-dimensional echocardiography improves the understanding of left atrioventricular valve morphology and function in atrioventricular septal defects undergoing patch augmentation. J Thorac Cardiovasc Surg. 2005;129:746–53.
55. Piatkowski R, Budaj-Fidecka A, Scislo P, Kochanowski J, Spiewak M, Opolski G. Transesophageal real time three-dimensional echocardiography in assessment of partial atrioventricular septal defect. Echocardiography. 2009;26:1092–4.

56. Faletra FF, Nucifora G, Ho SY. Real-time 3-dimensional transesophageal echocardiography of the atrioventricular septal defect. Circ Cardiovasc Imaging. 2011;4:e7–9.
57. Cheng HL, Huang CH, Tsai HE, Chen MY, Fan SZ, Hsiao PN. Intraoperative assessment of partial atrioventricular septal defect with a cleft mitral valve by real-time three-dimensional transesophageal echocardiography. Anesth Analg. 2012;114:731–4.
58. Nadas AS, Fyler DC. Pediatric cardiology. Philadelphia: W.B. Saunders Co; 1972. p. 683.
59. Rosenquist GC. Congenital mitral valve disease associated with coarctation of the aorta: a spectrum that includes parachute deformity of the mitral valve. Circulation. 1974;49:985–93.
60. Moore P, Adatia I, Spevak PJ, et al. Severe congenital mitral stenosis in infants. Circulation. 1994;89:2099–106.
61. Serraf A, Zoghbi J, Belli E, et al. Congenital mitral stenosis with or without associated defects: an evolving surgical strategy. Circulation. 2000;102:III166–71.
62. Shone JD, Sellers RD, Anderson RC, Adams PJ, Lillihei CW, Edwards JE. The developmental complex of "parachute mitral valve," supravalvular ring of left atrium, subaortic stenosis, and coarctation of aorta. Am J Cardiol. 1963;11:714–25.
63. Banerjee A, Kohl T, Silverman NH. Echocardiographic evaluation of congenital mitral valve anomalies in children. Am J Cardiol. 1995;76:1284–91.
64. Collins-Nakai RL, Rosenthal A, Castaneda AR, Bernhard WF, Nadas AS. Congenital mitral stenosis. A review of 20 years' experience. Circulation. 1977;56:1039–47.
65. Benry J, Leachman RD, Cooley DA, Klima T, Lufschanowski R. Supravalvular mitral stenosis associated with tetralogy of Fallot. Am J Cardiol. 1976;37:111–4.
66. Barbero-Marcial M, Riso A, De Albuquerque AT, Atik E, Jatene A. Left ventricular apical approach for the surgical treatment of congenital mitral stenosis. J Thorac Cardiovasc Surg. 1993;106: 105–10.
67. Zalzstein E, Hamilton R, Zucker N, Levitas A, Gross GJ. Presentation, natural history, and outcome in children and adolescents with double orifice mitral valve. Am J Cardiol. 2004;93:1067–9.
68. Warnes C, Somerville J. Double mitral valve orifice in atrioventricular defects. Br Heart J. 1983;49:59–64.
69. Das BB, Pauliks LB, Knudson OA, et al. Double-orifice mitral valve with intact atrioventricular septum: an echocardiographic study with anatomic and functional considerations. J Am Soc Echocardiogr. 2005;18:231–6.
70. Lee CN, Danielson GK, Schaff HV, Puga FJ, Mair DD. Surgical treatment of double-orifice mitral valve in atrioventricular canal defects. Experience in 25 patients. J Thorac Cardiovasc Surg. 1985; 90:700–5.
71. Ohta N, Sakamoto K, Kado M, et al. Surgical repair of double-orifice of the mitral valve in cases with an atrioventricular canal defects. Jpn J Thorac Cardiovasc Surg. 2001;49:656–9.
72. Sharma V, Burkhart HM, Schaff HV, Cabalka AK, Grogan MA, Dearani JA. Double-orifice left atrioventricular valve in patients with atrioventricular septal defects: surgical strategies and outcome. Ann Thorac Surg. 2012;93:2017–20. discussion 2020–1.
73. Abadir S, Fouilloux V, Metras D, Ghez O, Kreitmann B, Fraisse A. Isolated cleft of the mitral valve: distinctive features and surgical management. Ann Thorac Surg. 2009;88:839–43.
74. Perier P, Clausnizer B. Isolated cleft mitral valve: valve reconstruction techniques. Ann Thorac Surg. 1995;59:56–9.
75. Castaneda AR, Anderson RC, Edwards JE. Congenital mitral stenosis resulting from anomalous arcade and obstructing papillary muscles. Report of correction by use of ball valve prosthesis. Am J Cardiol. 1969;24:237–40.
76. Grenadier E, Sahn DJ, Valdes-Cruz LM, Allen HD, Oliveira Lima C, Goldberg SJ. Two-dimensional echo Doppler study of congenital disorders of the mitral valve. Am Heart J. 1984;107:319–25.
77. Ruckman RN, Van Praagh R. Anatomic types of congenital mitral stenosis: report of 49 autopsy cases with consideration of diagnosis and surgical implications. Am J Cardiol. 1978;42:592–601.
78. Kim SJ, Shin ES, Park MK, Choi SH, Lee SG. Congenital mitral insufficiency caused by anomalous mitral arcade in an elderly patient: use of echocardiography and multidetector computed tomography for diagnosis. Circ J. 2005;69:1560–3.
79. Perez JA, Herzberg AJ, Reimer KA, Bashore TM. Congenital mitral insufficiency secondary to anomalous mitral arcade in an adult. Am Heart J. 1987;114:894–5.
80. Milo S, Ho SY, Macartney FJ, et al. Straddling and overriding atrioventricular valves: morphology and classification. Am J Cardiol. 1979;44:1122–34.
81. Soto B, Ceballos R, Nath PH, Bini RM, Pacifico AD, Bargeron LMJ. Overriding atrioventricular valves. An angiographic-anatomical correlate. Int J Cardiol. 1985;9:323–39.
82. Freedom RM, Bini R, Dische R, Rowe RD. The straddling mitral valve: morphological observations and clinical implications. Eur J Cardiol. 1978;8:27–50.
83. Carpentier A, Branchini B, Cour JC, et al. Congenital malformations of the mitral valve in children. Pathology and surgical treatment. J Thorac Cardiovasc Surg. 1976;72:854–66.
84. Hatle L, Brubakk A, Tromsdal A, Angelsen B. Noninvasive assessment of pressure drop in mitral stenosis by Doppler ultrasound. Br Heart J. 1978;40:131–40.
85. Ascione L, Caso P, De Leva F, et al. Transesophageal color flow echocardiographic evaluation of supravalve mitral ring in an adult patient. Echocardiography. 1994;11:231–5.
86. Snider AR, Roge CL, Schiller NB, Silverman NH. Congenital left ventricular inflow obstruction evaluated by two-dimensional echocardiography. Circulation. 1980;61:848–55.
87. Jacobstein MD, Hirschfeld SS. Concealed left atrial membrane: pitfalls in the diagnosis of cor triatriatum and supravalve mitral ring. Am J Cardiol. 1982;49:780–6.
88. Hoffman P, Stumper O, Groundstroem K, Sutherland G. The transesophageal echocardiographic features of double-orifice left atrioventricular valve. J Am Soc Echocardiogr. 1993;6:94–100.
89. Fraisse A, del Nido PJ, Gaudart J, Geva T. Echocardiographic characteristics and outcome of straddling mitral valve. J Am Coll Cardiol. 2001;38:819–26.
90. Kuecherer HF, Muhiudeen IA, Kusumoto FM, et al. Estimation of mean left atrial pressure from transesophageal pulsed Doppler echocardiography of pulmonary venous flow. Circulation. 1990;82:1127–39.
91. Baumgartner H, Hung J, Bermejo J, et al. Echocardiographic assessment of valve stenosis: EAE/ASE recommendations for clinical practice. J Am Soc Echocardiogr. 2009;22:1–23. quiz 101–2.
92. Zoghbi WA, Enriquez-Sarano M, Foster E, et al. Recommendations for evaluation of the severity of native valvular regurgitation with two-dimensional and Doppler echocardiography. J Am Soc Echocardiogr. 2003;16:777–802.
93. Bettex DA, Schmidlin D, Bernath MA, et al. Intraoperative transesophageal echocardiography in pediatric congenital cardiac surgery: a two-center observational study. Anesth Analg. 2003;97: 1275–82.
94. Rosenfeld HM, Gentles TL, Wernovsky G, et al. Utility of intraoperative transesophageal echocardiography in the assessment of residual cardiac defects. Pediatr Cardiol. 1998;19:346–51.
95. Salustri A, Spitaels S, McGhie J, Vletter W, Roelandt JR. Transthoracic three-dimensional echocardiography in adult patients with congenital heart disease. J Am Coll Cardiol. 1995;26: 759–67.
96. Espinola-Zavaleta N, Vargas-Barron J, Keirns C, et al. Three-dimensional echocardiography in congenital malformations of the mitral valve. J Am Soc Echocardiogr. 2002;15:468–72.

97. Baker GH, Shirali G, Ringewald JM, Hsia TY, Bandisode V. Usefulness of live three-dimensional transesophageal echocardiography in a congenital heart disease center. Am J Cardiol. 2009;103:1025–8.
98. Simpson JM, Miller O. Three-dimensional echocardiography in congenital heart disease. Arch Cardiovasc Dis. 2011;104:45–56.
99. Badano LP, Boccalini F, Muraru D, et al. Current clinical applications of transthoracic three-dimensional echocardiography. J Cardiovasc Ultrasound. 2012;20:1–22.
100. Shirali GS. Three-dimensional echocardiography in congenital heart disease. Echocardiography. 2012;29:242–8.
101. Vettukattil JJ. Three dimensional echocardiography in congenital heart disease. Heart. 2012;98:79–88.
102. Zhang L, Xie M, Balluz R, Ge S. Real time three-dimensional echocardiography for evaluation of congenital heart defects: state of the art. Echocardiography. 2012;29:232–41.
103. Baird CW, Bengur AR, Bensky A, Watts LT. Congenital absence of posteromedial papillary muscle and anterior mitral leaflet chordae: the use of three-dimensional echocardiography and approach in complex pediatric mitral valve disease. J Thorac Cardiovasc Surg. 2010;139:e75–7.
104. Pawelec-Wojtalik M, Iorio FS, Anwar AM, El Midany AA. Importance of accurate diagnosis using real-time three-dimensional echocardiography in the surgical treatment of congenital intramitral ring in infants. Interact Cardiovasc Thorac Surg. 2011;13:669–71.
105. Seguela PE, Dulac Y, Acar P. Double-orifice mitral valve assessed by two- and three-dimensional echocardiography in a newborn. Arch Cardiovasc Dis. 2011;104:361–2.
106. Bhattacharyya S, West C, Chinasamy D, Senior R, Li W. Utility of three-dimensional echocardiography for assessment of double-orifice mitral valve. Eur Heart J Cardiovasc Imaging. 2012;13:672.
107. Valverde I, Rawlins D, Austin C, Simpson JM. Three-dimensional echocardiography in the management of parachute mitral valve. Eur Heart J Cardiovasc Imaging. 2012;13:446.
108. Tani T, Kim K, Fujii Y, et al. Mitral valve repair for double-orifice mitral valve with flail leaflet: the usefulness of real-time three-dimensional transesophageal echocardiography. Ann Thorac Surg. 2012;93:e97–8.
109. Anderson KR, Zuberbuhler JR, Anderson RH, Becker AE, Lie JT. Morphologic spectrum of Ebstein's anomaly of the heart: a review. Mayo Clin Proc. 1979;54:174–80.
110. Becker AE, Becker MJ, Edwards JE. Pathologic spectrum of dysplasia of the tricuspid valve. Features in common with Ebstein's malformation. Arch Pathol. 1971;91:167–78.
111. Martinez RM, O'Leary PW, Anderson RH. Anatomy and echocardiography of the normal and abnormal tricuspid valve. Cardiol Young. 2006;16 Suppl 3:4–11.
112. Seward JB. Ebstein's anomaly: ultrasound imaging and hemodynamic evaluation. Echocardiography. 1993;10:641–64.
113. Nihoyannopoulos P, McKenna WJ, Smith G, Foale R. Echocardiographic assessment of the right ventricle in Ebstein's anomaly: relation to clinical outcome. J Am Coll Cardiol. 1986;8:627–35.
114. Knott-Craig CJ, Overholt ED, Ward KE, Ringewald JM, Baker SS, Razook JD. Repair of Ebstein's anomaly in the symptomatic neonate: an evolution of technique with 7-year follow-up. Ann Thorac Surg. 2002;73:1786–92.
115. Starnes VA, Pitlick PT, Bernstein D, Griffin ML, Choy M, Shumway NE. Ebstein's anomaly appearing in the neonate. A new surgical approach. J Thorac Cardiovasc Surg. 1991;101:1082–7.
116. Reemtsen BL, Fagan BT, Wells WJ, Starnes VA. Current surgical therapy for Ebstein anomaly in neonates. J Thorac Cardiovasc Surg. 2006;132:1285–90.
117. Dearani JA, Oleary PW, Danielson GK. Surgical treatment of Ebstein's malformation: state of the art in 2006. Cardiol Young. 2006;16 Suppl 3:12–20.
118. Stulak JM, Dearani JA, Danielson GK. Surgical management of Ebstein's anomaly. Semin Thorac Cardiovasc Surg Pediatr Card Surg Annu. 2007;10:105–11.
119. Van Arsdell G. Can we modify late functional outcome in Ebstein anomaly by altering surgical strategy? J Am Coll Cardiol. 2008; 52:467–9.
120. Brown ML, Dearani JA. Ebstein malformation of the tricuspid valve: current concepts in management and outcomes. Curr Treat Options Cardiovasc Med. 2009;11:396–402.
121. Quinonez LG, Dearani JA, Puga FJ, et al. Results of the 1.5-ventricle repair for Ebstein anomaly and the failing right ventricle. J Thorac Cardiovasc Surg. 2007;133:1303–10.
122. Hornberger LK, Sahn DJ, Kleinman CS, Copel JA, Reed KL. Tricuspid valve disease with significant tricuspid insufficiency in the fetus: diagnosis and outcome. J Am Coll Cardiol. 1991;17: 167–73.
123. McElhinney DB, Silverman NH, Brook MM, Hanley FL, Stanger P. Asymmetrically short tendinous cords causing congenital tricuspid regurgitation: improved understanding of tricuspid valvar dysplasia in the era of color flow echocardiography. Cardiol Young. 1999;9:300–4.
124. Reddy VM, McElhinney DB, Brook MM, Silverman NH, Stanger P, Hanley FL. Repair of congenital tricuspid valve abnormalities with artificial chordae tendineae. Ann Thorac Surg. 1998;66:172–6.
125. Attenhofer Jost CH, Connolly HM, Dearani JA, Edwards WD, Danielson GK. Ebstein's anomaly. Circulation. 2007;115:277–85.
126. Paranon S, Acar P. Ebstein's anomaly of the tricuspid valve: from fetus to adult: congenital heart disease. Heart. 2008;94:237–43.
127. Smallhorn JF, Izukawa T, Benson L, Freedom RM. Noninvasive recognition of functional pulmonary atresia by echocardiography. Am J Cardiol. 1984;54:925–6.
128. Rehfeldt KH. Two-dimensional transesophageal echocardiographic imaging of the tricuspid valve. Anesth Analg. 2012;114: 547–50.
129. Ports TA, Silverman NH, Schiller NB. Two-dimensional echocardiographic assessment of Ebstein's anomaly. Circulation. 1978;58: 336–43.
130. Roberson DA, Silverman NH. Ebstein's anomaly: echocardiographic and clinical features in the fetus and neonate. J Am Coll Cardiol. 1989;14:1300–7.
131. Shiina A, Seward JB, Tajik AJ, Hagler DJ, Danielson GK. Two-dimensional echocardiographic—surgical correlation in Ebstein's anomaly: preoperative determination of patients requiring tricuspid valve plication vs replacement. Circulation. 1983;68:534–44.
132. Shiina A, Seward JB, Edwards WD, Hagler DJ, Tajik AJ. Two-dimensional echocardiographic spectrum of Ebstein's anomaly: detailed anatomic assessment. J Am Coll Cardiol. 1984;3:356–70.
133. Zuberbuhler JR, Allwork SP, Anderson RH. The spectrum of Ebstein's anomaly of the tricuspid valve. J Thorac Cardiovasc Surg. 1979;77:202–11.
134. Ahmed S, Nanda NC, Nekkanti R, Pacifico AD. Transesophageal three-dimensional echocardiographic demonstration of Ebstein's anomaly. Echocardiography. 2003;20:305–7.
135. Silverman NH, Birk E. Ebstein's malformation of the tricuspid valve: cross-sectional echocardiography and Doppler. In: Anderson RH, Park SC, Zuberbuhler JR, editors. Perspectives in pediatric cardiology. New York: Futura Publishing, Mount Kisco; 1988. p. 113–25.
136. Fram DB, Missri J, Therrien ML, Chawla S. Assessment of Ebstein's anomaly and its surgical repair using transesophageal echocardiography and color flow mapping. Echocardiography. 1991;8:367.
137. Tribouilloy CM, Enriquez-Sarano M, Bailey KR, Tajik AJ, Seward JB. Quantification of tricuspid regurgitation by measuring the width of the vena contracta with Doppler color flow imaging: a clinical study. J Am Coll Cardiol. 2000;36:472–8.

138. Pibarot P, Dumesnil JG. Doppler echocardiographic evaluation of prosthetic valve function. Heart. 2012;98:69–78.
139. Zoghbi WA, Chambers JB, Dumesnil JG, et al. Recommendations for evaluation of prosthetic valves with echocardiography and doppler ultrasound: a report From the American Society of Echocardiography's Guidelines and Standards Committee and the Task Force on Prosthetic Valves, developed in conjunction with the American College of Cardiology Cardiovascular Imaging Committee, Cardiac Imaging Committee of the American Heart Association, the European Association of Echocardiography, a registered branch of the European Society of Cardiology, the Japanese Society of Echocardiography and the Canadian Society of Echocardiography, endorsed by the American College of Cardiology Foundation, American Heart Association, European Association of Echocardiography, a registered branch of the European Society of Cardiology, the Japanese Society of Echocardiography, and Canadian Society of Echocardiography. J Am Soc Echocardiogr. 2009;22:975–1014. quiz 1082–4.
140. van Noord PT, Scohy TV, McGhie J, Bogers AJ. Three-dimensional transesophageal echocardiography in Ebstein's anomaly. Interact Cardiovasc Thorac Surg. 2010;10:836–7.
141. Khandheria BK, Seward JB, Oh JK, et al. Value and limitations of transesophageal echocardiography in assessment of mitral valve prostheses. Circulation. 1991;83:1956–68.
142. Nellessen U, Schnittger I, Appleton CP, et al. Transesophageal two-dimensional echocardiography and color Doppler flow velocity mapping in the evaluation of cardiac valve prostheses. Circulation. 1988;78:848–55.
143. Scott PJ, Blackburn ME, Wharton GA, Wilson N, Dickinson DF, Gibbs JL. Transoesophageal echocardiography in neonates, infants and children: applicability and diagnostic value in everyday practice of a cardiothoracic unit. Br Heart J. 1992;68:488–92.
144. Muratori M, Montorsi P, Teruzzi G, et al. Feasibility and diagnostic accuracy of quantitative assessment of mechanical prostheses leaflet motion by transthoracic and transesophageal echocardiography in suspected prosthetic valve dysfunction. Am J Cardiol. 2006;97:94–100.
145. Pedersen WR, Walker M, Olson JD, et al. Value of transesophageal echocardiography as an adjunct to transthoracic echocardiography in evaluation of native and prosthetic valve endocarditis. Chest. 1991;100:351–6.
146. Pyeritz RE, Wappel MA. Mitral valve dysfunction in the Marfan syndrome. Clinical and echocardiographic study of prevalence and natural history. Am J Med. 1983;74:797–807.
147. Biaggi P, Gruner C, Jedrzkiewicz S, et al. Assessment of mitral valve prolapse by 3D TEE angled views are key. JACC Cardiovasc Imaging. 2011;4:94–7.
148. Hien MD, Rauch H, Lichtenberg A, et al. Real-time three-dimensional transesophageal echocardiography: improvements in intraoperative mitral valve imaging. Anesth Analg. 2012;116(2):287–95.
149. van Karnebeek CD, Naeff MS, Mulder BJ, Hennekam RC, Offringa M. Natural history of cardiovascular manifestations in Marfan syndrome. Arch Dis Child. 2001;84:129–37.
150. Grenadier E, Keidar S, Sahn DJ, et al. Ruptured mitral chordae tendineae may be a frequent and insignificant complication in the mitral valve prolapse syndrome. Eur Heart J. 1985;6:1006–15.
151. Grenadier E, Alpan G, Keidar S, Palant A. The prevalence of ruptured chordae tendineae in the mitral valve prolapse syndrome. Am Heart J. 1983;105:603–10.
152. Reynolds HR, Jagen MA, Tunick PA, Kronzon I. Sensitivity of transthoracic versus transesophageal echocardiography for the detection of native valve vegetations in the modern era. J Am Soc Echocardiogr. 2003;16:67–70.
153. Thangaroopan M, Choy JB. Is transesophageal echocardiography overused in the diagnosis of infective endocarditis? Am J Cardiol. 2005;95:295–7.
154. Baddour LM, Wilson WR, Bayer AS, et al. Infective endocarditis: diagnosis, antimicrobial therapy, and management of complications: a statement for healthcare professionals from the Committee on Rheumatic Fever, Endocarditis, and Kawasaki Disease, Council on Cardiovascular Disease in the Young, and the Councils on Clinical Cardiology, Stroke, and Cardiovascular Surgery and Anesthesia, American Heart Association: endorsed by the Infectious Diseases Society of America. Circulation. 2005;111:e394–434.
155. Penk JS, Webb CL, Shulman ST, Anderson EJ. Echocardiography in pediatric infective endocarditis. Pediatr Infect Dis J. 2011;30:1109–11.
156. Humpl T, McCrindle BW, Smallhorn JF. The relative roles of transthoracic compared with transesophageal echocardiography in children with suspected infective endocarditis. J Am Coll Cardiol. 2003;41:2068–71.

Ventricular Septal Defects

9

Grace C. Kung and Pierre C. Wong

Abstract

The term "ventricular septal defect" (VSD) denotes a gap or opening in the ventricular septum. There are several anatomically distinct types of VSDs, differing both in morphology as well as location within the ventricular septum. Transesophageal echocardiography (TEE) plays a very important role in the evaluation of VSDs, primarily in the intraoperative setting, as a method of monitoring surgical VSD closure. In addition, TEE also provides essential information and guidance during device closure of certain types of VSDs, either in the cardiac catheterization laboratory or via the perventricular approach. This chapter discusses the anatomy and morphology of the different types of VSDs, along with their echocardiographic evaluation by TEE.

Keywords

Heart defects • Congenital • Heart septal defects • Ventricular septal defect • Echocardiography • Transesophageal echocardiography • Pediatric cardiac surgery

The term "ventricular septal defect" (VSD) denotes a gap or opening in the ventricular septum [1]. This group of defects comprises several anatomically distinct types, differing both in morphology as well as location within the ventricular septum. Collectively, VSDs constitute one of the most common, if not the most common, forms of congenital heart disease [1, 2]. Transesophageal echocardiography (TEE) has proven a particularly useful tool in the preoperative and postoperative evaluation of a ventricular septal defect. The utility and accuracy of TEE for congenital heart disease, and particularly for VSD assessment, have been well reported [3–8]. However, VSD evaluation is not always straightforward: the different types of VSDs vary in location, shape and size, and given the curved, three-dimensional nature of the ventricular septum, not all will be optimally visualized with a single TEE view. Thus, a more thorough and systematic evaluation of the ventricular septum—using a combination of different TEE views—is often necessary to evaluate fully the ventricular septum. This chapter discusses the detailed TEE evaluation of VSDs, in accordance with principles previously detailed in this book (see Chap. 4) as well as the American Society of Echocardiography guidelines for the use of TEE in the pediatric population [9].

G.C. Kung, MD (✉) • P.C. Wong
Division of Cardiology, Children's Hospital Los Angeles, Department of Pediatrics, Keck School of Medicine, University of Southern California, 4650 Sunset Blvd, MS #34, Los Angeles, CA 90027, USA
e-mail: gkung@chla.usc.edu; pwong@chla.usc.edu

The online version of this chapter (doi:10.1007/978-1-84800-064-3_9) contains supplementary material, which is available to authorized users.

P.C. Wong, W.C. Miller-Hance (eds.), *Transesophageal Echocardiography for Congenital Heart Disease*,
DOI 10.1007/978-1-84800-064-3_9, © Springer-Verlag London 2014

Morphologic Classification of Ventricular Septal Defect

The classification of a VSD has traditionally been based on its location (Fig. 9.1). The portion of the ventricular septum just adjacent to the atrioventricular (AV) valves by the crux of the heart is the inlet (AV canal) septum and these types of defects have been variously called inlet or AV canal type VSDs. Defects in this area will also be discussed in a separate chapter about AV septal (AV canal) defects (Chap. 8). The outlet septum consists of the muscular septum, also know as conal (or infundibular) septum, the muscle that sits between the two great arteries and separates the outflow tracts. One must remember that in a morphologic right ventricle (RV), a cuff of muscle lies beneath the pulmonary valve and pulmonary artery, known as the conus or infundibulum (Fig. 9.2). Deficiency or absence of conal septum results in a VSD adjacent to the semilunar valves; such a defect has been variously termed an outlet septal, subarterial, subpulmonary, doubly committed, supracristal or conal septal VSD. Straightforward, isolated defects in this region are usually small in size but may involve distortion of the right aortic valve cusp due to the proximity of the lesion to the cusp. This distortion may result in prolapse of the cusp through the VSD, and associated aortic regurgitation.

When there is malalignment or displacement of the conus and conal septum from the remainder of the plane of muscular trabecular septum, specifically the portion of ventricular septum comprised by the two limbs (the 'Y') of septal band (or *trabecula septomarginalis*), the resultant defect is oftentimes referred to as a *malalignment* VSD. This type of defect is usually characterized by anterior or posterior malalignment of the conal septum. Such defects can have a more complex three-dimensional nature, with the surrounding margins not completely oriented in the same plane. In these defects the borders of the VSD can variously comprise muscular (trabecular

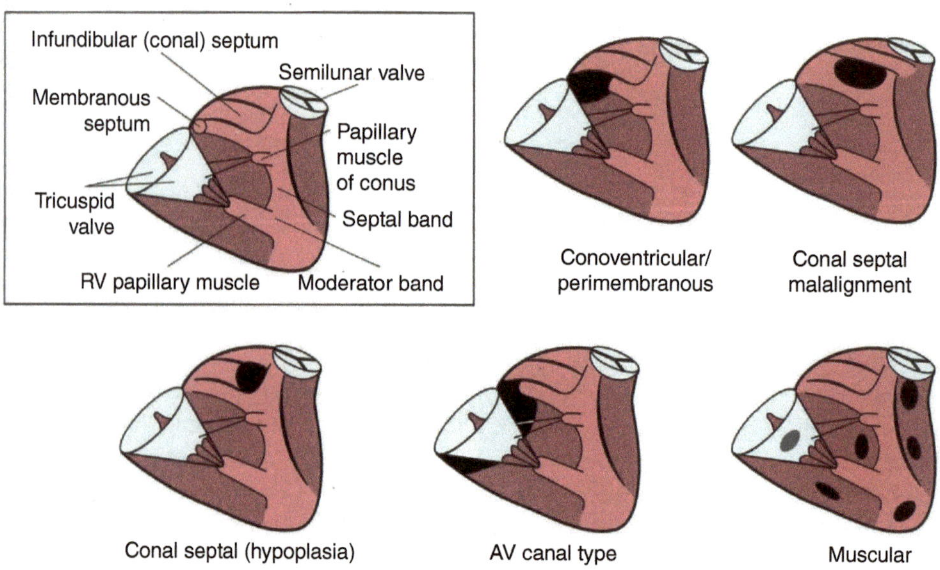

Fig. 9.1 Location of various types of ventricular septal defects (By permission of Weinburg [47])

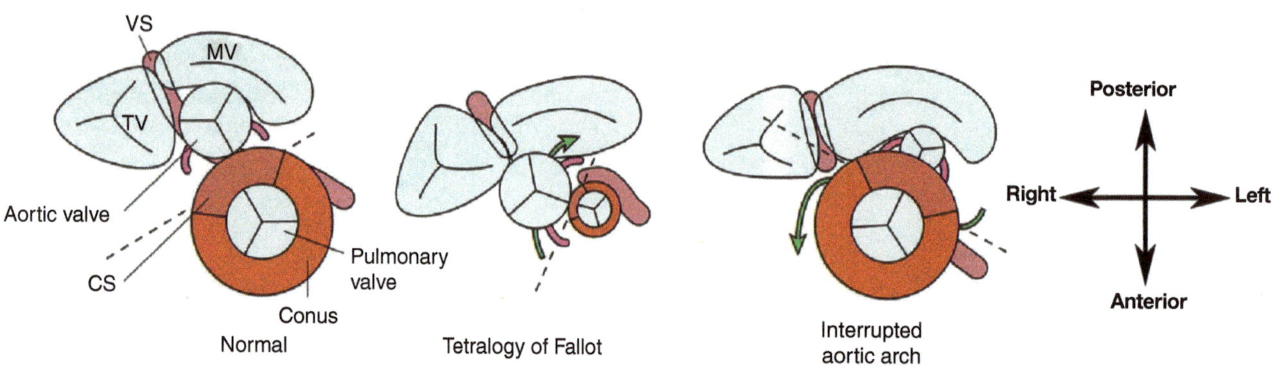

Fig. 9.2 Relationship of conus muscle to outflow tracts and ventricular septum in normal anatomy, anterior malalignment in tetralogy of Fallot, and posterior malalignment in interrupted aortic arch. *CS* conal septum, *MV* mitral valve, *TV* tricuspid valve, *VS* ventricular septum (By permission of: Weinburg [47])

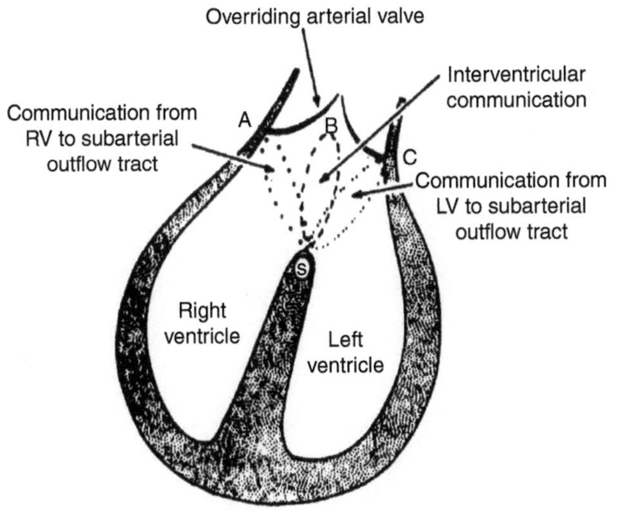

Fig. 9.3 Diagram showing three communications (A–S, B–S, C–S) potentially termed the "ventricular septal defect" in a patient with an overriding semilunar valve. (**A**) Infundibular septum; (**B**) Coapted leaflets of overriding semilunar valve; (**C**) Ventriculoinfundibular fold or area of arterial-atrioventricular valve fibrous continuity. *S* septal crest (By permission of: Macartney et al. [10])

septum), conal septum, a semilunar valve (or valves), ventriculo-infundibular fold, or intervalvular fibrosa (Fig. 9.3). Since the surgical repair of such defects can involve a complex re-routing of blood flow to the appropriate semilunar valve, closure of a ventricular communication in such instances often occurs by attachment of the patch to muscular rims that differ from those that comprise the actual borders of the VSD [10]. Thus, the "true" VSD can differ from the "surgical" VSD. Moreover, in this type of VSD the malaligned conal septum can impinge upon the outflow tract beneath a semilunar valve, resulting in obstruction of the affected outflow tract and hypoplasia of the associated semilunar valve and great artery. With in tetralogy of Fallot and some cases of double outlet right ventricle, the conal septum is malaligned anteriorly and superiorly resulting in narrowing of the right ventricular outflow tract (RVOT) and possibly hypoplasia of the pulmonary valve. This malalignment also results in the aorta overriding the remaining plane of the interventricular septum, hence the aortic valve forms the "roof" of the VSD. Conversely, posterior malalignment of the conal septum results in narrowing of the left ventricular outflow tract (LVOT) and possible accompanying hypoplasia of the aortic valve. This type of defect has a high association with aortic arch obstruction, including coarctation or interruption of the aorta.

Perimembranous (also known as conoventricular, membranous, infracristal, or paramembranous) VSDs involve the membranous portion of ventricular septum. The membranous septum is a specific region seen best by pathology as a thin region of the ventricular septum adjacent to the tricuspid valve and aortic valve. There is no muscle in this region and the superior portion is bordered by the aortic valve. As its name suggests, in pathologic specimens, this region is thin and almost transparent, easily transilluminated when held up to light. The term *peri*-membranous implies that such VSDs often represent not only a deficiency of membranous septum, but also extension to areas surrounding the membranous septum. Defects in this region can extend to the right and left aortic valve cusps as well, due to their proximity to the membranous septum. There can also be redundant, aneurysmal tricuspid valve tissue, which sometimes partially (or even completely) occludes the underlying defect. At times, the true defect in the septum may be large but the effective orifice quite small secondary to the tricuspid valve tissue. Thus, the tricuspid valve should be assessed for any incompetence. In some instances, VSD flow travels through the perimembranous VSD directly into the right atrium, or alternatively it is deflected via tricuspid valve tissue into the right atrium. This condition results in a left ventricle (LV) to right atrial shunt, also known as a "Gerbode" defect.

The remainder of the trabecular septum is considered just that—the trabecular or muscular septum. Defects in this portion of the septum are known as muscular VSDs, and can occur anywhere along the muscular septum—mid, anterior, apical, and posterior. Both posterior muscular and inlet/AV canal defects are situated close to the posterior border of ventricular septum, but the posterior muscular VSDs are located more inferiorly. Muscular VSDs can be of any size and shape; they can be single or multiple. When there are numerous separate muscular VSDs of varying size, the ventricular septum is popularly referred to as the so-called "Swiss cheese" septum. Upon surgical inspection, these multiple defects may in fact be a single large defect that has flow seen through multiple trabeculations on the right ventricular side by color flow Doppler. Indeed, due to the heavy trabeculations and oftentimes associated right ventricular hypertrophy from a large and longstanding shunt, the individual defects can be very difficult to assess surgically or challenging to address if they are located deep in the right ventricular (RV) apex as the surgeon is inspecting from the RV side.

There are two additional considerations regarding VSDs. First, combinations of different types of VSDs can occur together, such as a large perimembranous VSD coexisting with one or more muscular VSDs. Second, despite the specific locations of each type of VSD, in some instances a large enough defect will extend and overlap into various regions, such as a large perimembranous VSD extending into the inlet septum. The TEE examiner should be aware of both of these possibilities.

Evaluation of Ventricular Septal Defects by TEE

The ventricular septum can be well imaged by TEE [11]. Starting from the standard transverse plane at 0° or so in the mid esophageal four chamber (ME 4 Ch) view, the crux of the

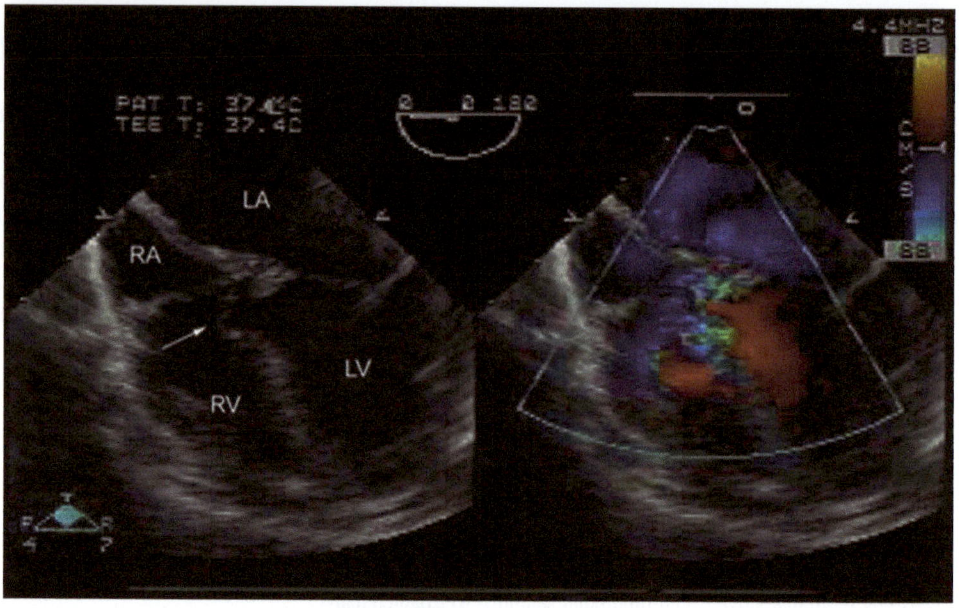

Fig. 9.4 *Left sided* image from mid esophageal four chamber view (multiplane angle 0°) shows a perimembranous ventricular septal defect (VSD) with tricuspid valve aneurysmal tissue as noted by the *arrow*. *Right sided* image demonstrates left to right shunting by color flow Doppler across the VSD. *LA* left atrium, *LV* left ventricle, *RA* right atrium, *RV* right ventricle

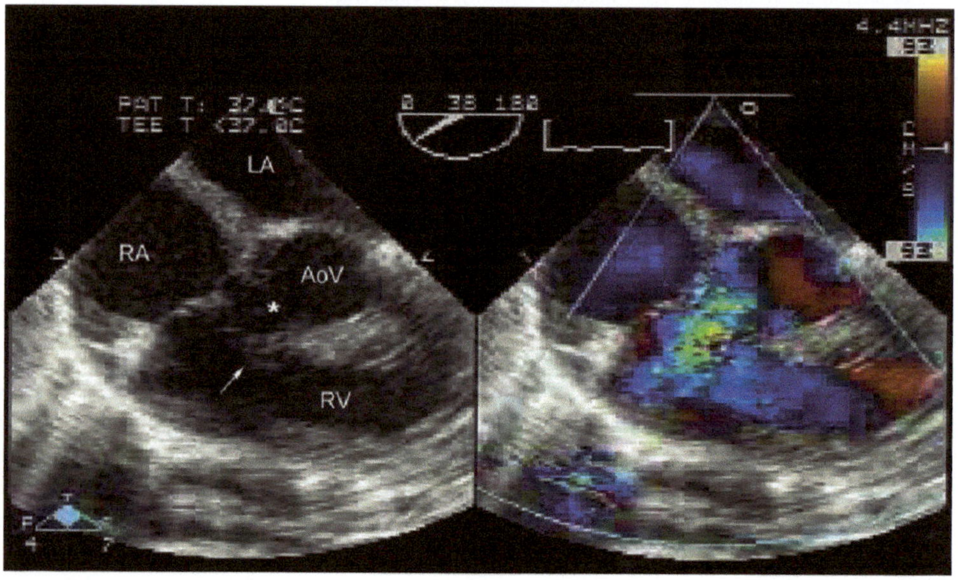

Fig. 9.5 Modified mid esophageal right ventricular inflow-outflow view with multiplane angle ~40° shows a perimembranous VSD *(asterisk)* with aneurysmal tricuspid valve tissue shown by *arrow*. This view is comparable to a parasternal short axis view of the aortic valve. *AoV* aortic valve, *LA* left atrium, *RA* right atrium, *RV* right ventricle

heart, the inlet septum, and most of the muscular trabecular septum can be well seen from the AV valves down to the apex as previously described. By withdrawing the probe and flexing anteriorly (anteflexing) from the crux, we pass through the perimembranous region adjacent to the tricuspid valve when the LVOT is in view. From here, a perimembranous defect can be seen by two-dimensional (2D) imaging and any involvement of tricuspid valve aneurysmal tissue can be detected (Fig. 9.4, Video 9.1). Color flow Doppler demonstrates the shunting through a perimembranous VSD well, and there is usually a favorable angle of interrogation for spectral Doppler (pulsed and continuous wave). If there is any LV to right atrial shunting through the perimembranous VSD, it can be adequately seen in the ME 4 Ch view (multiplane angle 0°).

It is also important to assess for any prolapse of tissue into the LVOT or for any other evidence of sub-aortic obstruction such as a discrete membrane or ridge. Another important consideration is that the size of the defect in the septum as noted by imaging, and the effective orifice as shown by color flow Doppler, can be quite different if aneurysmal tricuspid valve tissue causes partial obstruction of the defect. If anteflexion is continued with slight withdrawal of the probe, the image can be brought to that of a mid esophageal right ventricular inflow-outflow (ME RV In-Out) view (multiplane angle 60–90°). This view (Chap. 4) is comparable to an inverted transthoracic parasternal short axis view, and images perimembranous as well as outlet septal (supracristal) defects quite nicely (Fig. 9.5, Video 9.2).

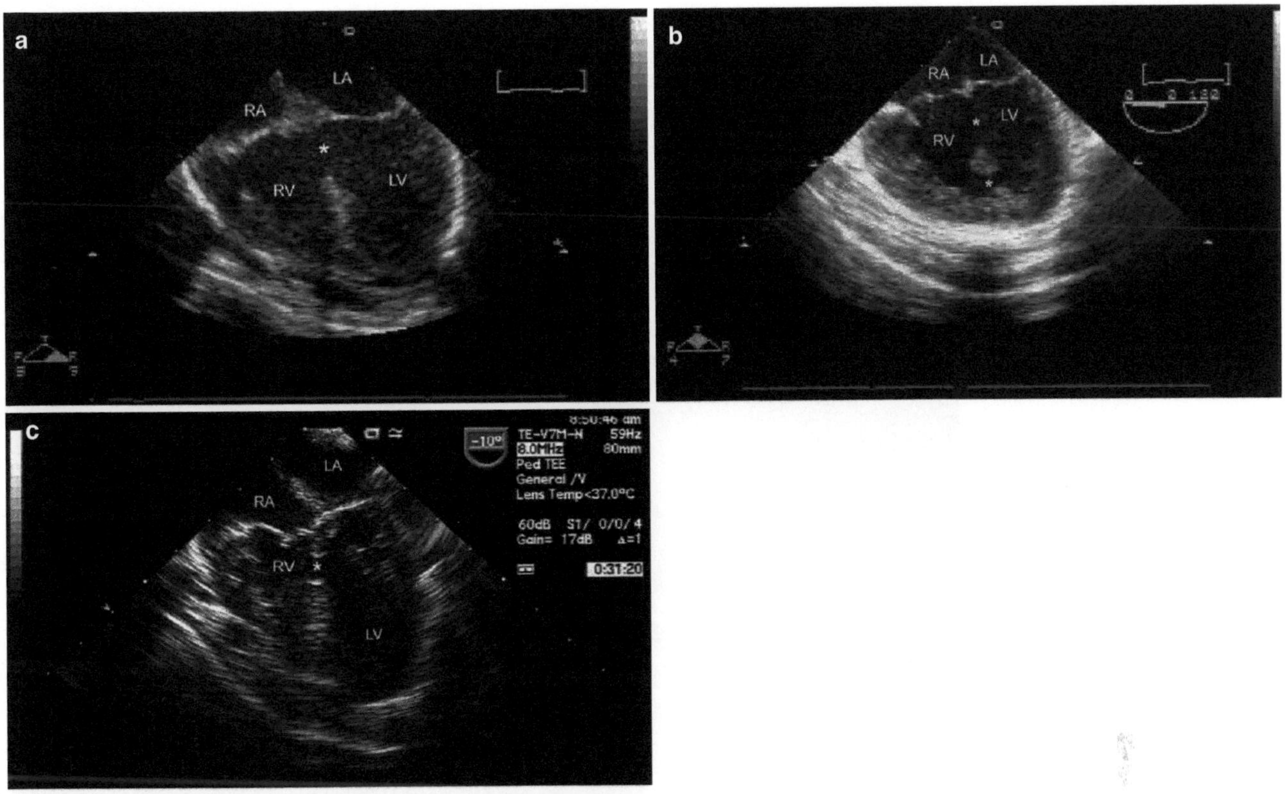

Fig. 9.6 Examples of muscular ventricular septal defect (VSD), shown from mid esophageal four chamber view. (**a**) Shows a large inlet VSD (*) at the level of the crux of the heart. (**b**) Shows large inlet and apical muscular VSDs (*). (**c**) shows right ventricular hypoplasia with small posterior muscular VSD (*). For all figures, multiplane angle is approximately 0°. *LA* left atrium, *LV* left ventricle, *RA* right atrium, *RV* right ventricle

Evaluation of the muscular (trabecular) septum can be performed effectively from the ME 4 Ch view, multiplane angle 0°. Retroflexion of the probe allows evaluation of inlet and muscular VSDs. With probe anteflexion, the mid and anterior muscular VSD can be visualized. Imaging should be used in conjunction with color flow Doppler mapping, as many muscular VSDs (particularly smaller defects) might not be well seen solely with 2D imaging. It is important to maintain an adequate size color flow Doppler sector, and carefully evaluate all portions of the muscular ventricular septum. This is particularly important with apical muscular VSDs, which are generally farther from the TEE probe and can be easily missed if the color flow sector is not extended completely to the apex (Fig. 9.6). Representative muscular VSDs are displayed in Videos 9.3 through 9.7 as follows: Video 9.3-large inlet defect; Video 9.4a-moderate size mid-muscular defect; Video 9.4b-a mid-muscular VSD in a patient with D-transposition of the great arteries and RV to LV shunting; Video 9.5-a small apical muscular VSD seen more readily with color flow Doppler; Videos 9.6 and 9.7-several defects in different locations of the muscular septum. Additional visualization of the mid and apical portions of muscular septum can also be provided by advancing the TEE probe into the stomach (transgastric position) while maintaining probe anteflexion, to obtain the transgastric basal short axis (TG Basal SAX) and mid short axis (TG Mid SAX) views (Video 9.4a). These views can be useful for visualizing postero-inferior and apical muscular VSDs that are sometimes difficult to image from other TEE windows.

As with any type of imaging, all anatomy should be evaluated from more than one plane. With modern multiplane TEE transducers, there is the luxury of being able to sweep from a transverse (0°) plane to the sagittal (90°) plane and beyond (even to 180°), while evaluating all planes in between. It should be remembered that every heart is different and, as often seen with congenital heart disease, the heart might not occupy its usual position. Therefore the multiplane angles given in this text are not absolute, and might need to be adjusted to obtain an optimal visualization of the VSD. Some patients have a better sagittal view at 80° or 110° rather than directly at 90°. Each patient must be assessed individually.

With the transducer oriented in a long axis plane (multiplane angle 100–130°), the mid esophageal long axis (ME LAX) view is obtained, providing excellent visualization of the LVOT. With slight rightward (counterclockwise) rotation, the RVOT can be visualized, and more anterior superior VSDs, as well as defects in the outlet septum (see below), can be well seen. This particular view, in association with the complementary mid esophageal RV inflow-outflow (ME RV In-Out) view (multiplane angle 60–90°),

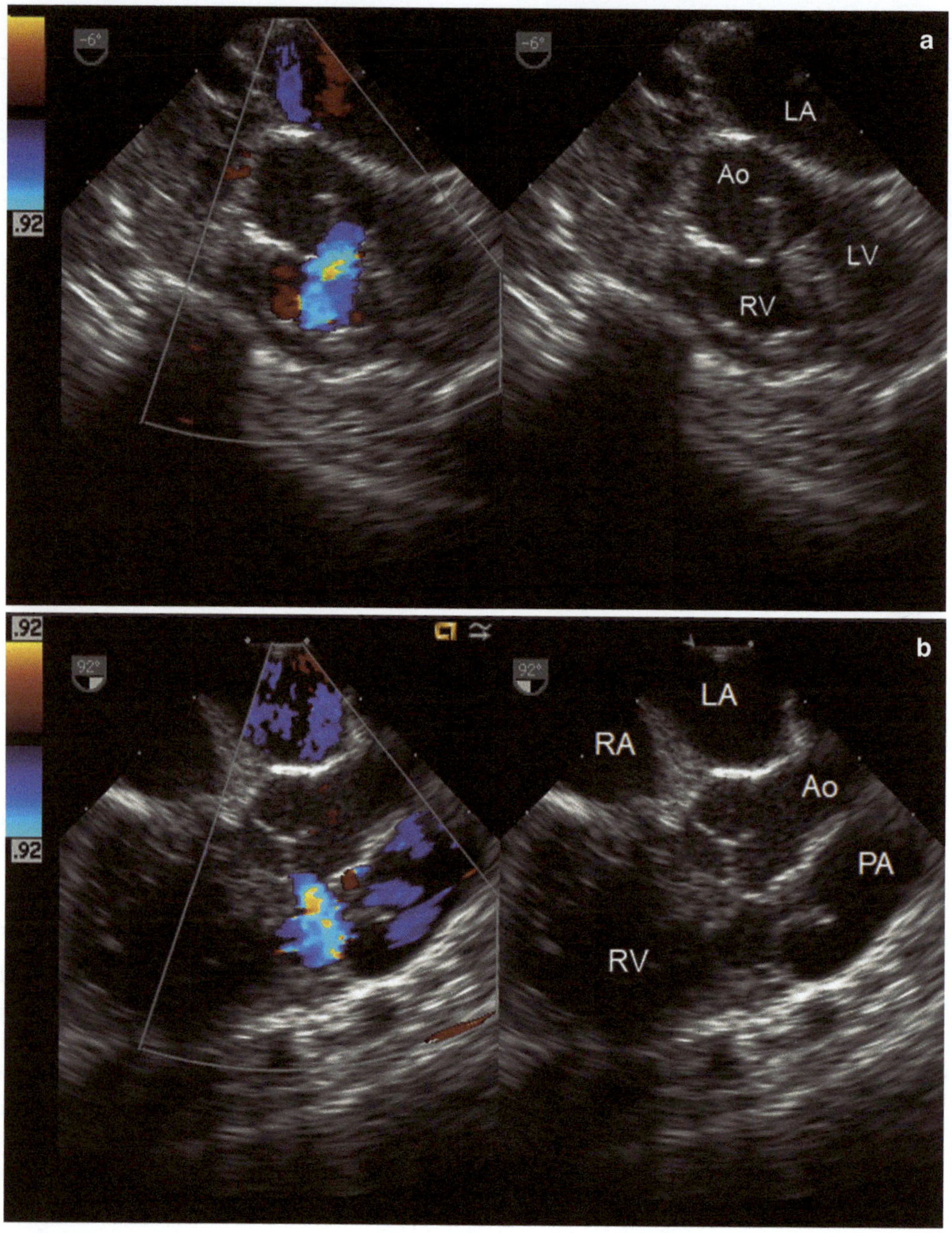

Fig. 9.7 Supracristal ventricular septal defect visualized from mid esophageal position, with a multiplane angle of 0° (**a**) and 90° (**b**). Note the right coronary cusp of aortic valve partly protruding through the defect. *Ao* aorta, *LA* left atrium, *LV* left ventricle, *PA* main pulmonary artery, *RA* right atrium, *RV* right ventricle

provides excellent visualization of any LV or RV outflow tract obstruction, either valvar or subvalvar (Video 9.8). In the case of the RV outflow tract, subpulmonary obstruction due to a superiorly displaced moderator band and/or anomalous muscles bundles, also known as double chambered RV, becomes much more visible when utilizing these TEE views. Double chambered RV carries a well-known association with perimembranous VSDs [12].

Supracristal VSDs can be visualized in several planes. Using the ME (Chap. 4) view and with the multiplane angle at 0° the defect can be seen although probe anteflexion is often necessary because of the more anterior and superior location of the defect (Fig. 9.7a). As noted previously, the standard ME RV In-Out view can also be helpful for distinguishing perimembranous from supracristal defects; when viewed as a clock face, perimembranous defects are seen between 7 and 10 o'clock, and supracristal defects from 3 to 6 o'clock, analogous to the views obtained with an inverted transthoracic parasternal short axis view. The supracristal defect is often seen very well seen from a near sagittal plane in the mid esophageal window, using the ME RV In-Out view, with a multiplane angle between 80 and 90°. With this view, the deficient conal septum becomes readily apparent, along with the location of the VSD directly adjacent to both semilunar valves. The semilunar valves can sometimes be seen in fibrous continuity with each other. If an aortic cusp prolapses through the defect, the protruding cusp is readily seen by both imaging and

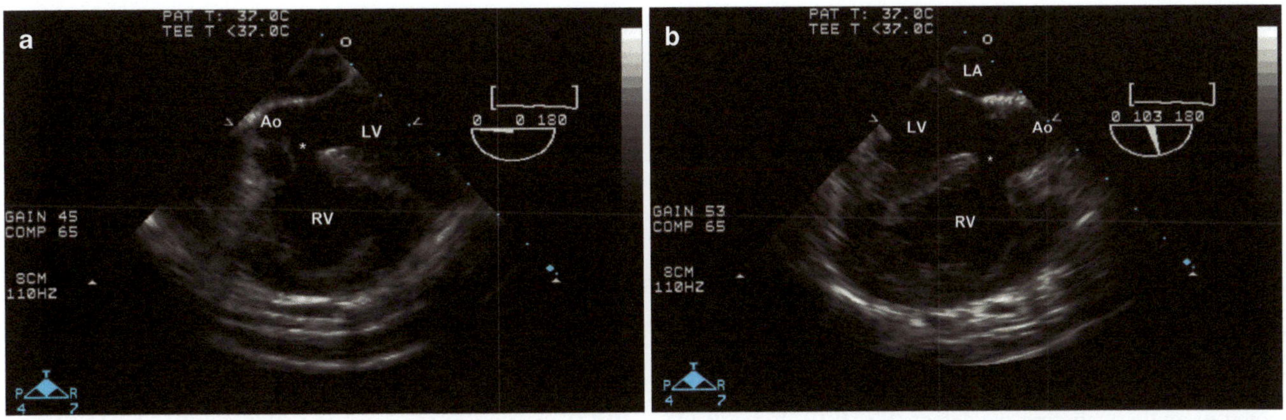

Fig. 9.8 Modified mid esophageal aortic valve short axis view at 0° (**a**) and modified mid esophageal long axis view at a multiplane angle of 100° (**b**). These views show the overriding aorta with anteriorly malaligned conal septum and large malalignment ventricular septal defect (*) in a patient with tetralogy of Fallot. *Ao* aorta, *LA* left atrium, *LV* left ventricle, *RV* right ventricle

color flow Doppler (Fig. 9.7b, Video 9.9). During the evaluation of supracristal VSDs, the LVOT and aortic valve should also be evaluated, with special attention paid to any possible aortic valve distortion and/or aortic valve insufficiency. For this type of VSD, the ME RV In-Out view provides a good angle of interrogation for spectral Doppler quantification of the VSD jet.

The ME LAX view (multiplane angle 100–130°) is also excellent for assessing malalignment VSDs. As mentioned previously, these defects may be categorized as being anteriorly or posteriorly malaligned depending on the positioning of the conal septum. *Posterior* malalignment of the conal septum will result in protrusion of the conal septum into the LVOT resulting in varying degrees of sub-aortic narrowing and obstruction; this type of defect is often associated with aortic arch hypoplasia, coarctation, or interruption. *Anterior* malalignment of the conal septum often results in an aorta that overrides the VSD, with varying degrees of subpulmonary and pulmonary valve narrowing and obstruction due to to the conal septum protruding into the RVOT—namely, tetralogy of Fallot (Fig. 9.8, Video 9.10). With a posterior malalignment VSD, a significant degree of LVOT obstruction might not be fully recognized since some blood can flow left to right through the VSD into the low resistance pulmonary vascular bed, and a significant gradient might not be seen across the LVOT by Doppler assessment. In such cases, evaluation by 2D imaging of the LVOT and aortic valve, including linear measurements of LVOT structures such as aortic valve annulus, plays an important role [13]. It is imperative to recognize and understand this anatomy and physiology at the time of the preoperative study so that these issues may be discussed with the surgeon prior to initiating the surgery.

Certain TEE views produce images that closely resemble their transthoracic counterparts (e.g. parasternal short axis view, noted above). Thus, keeping the probe in an anteflexed

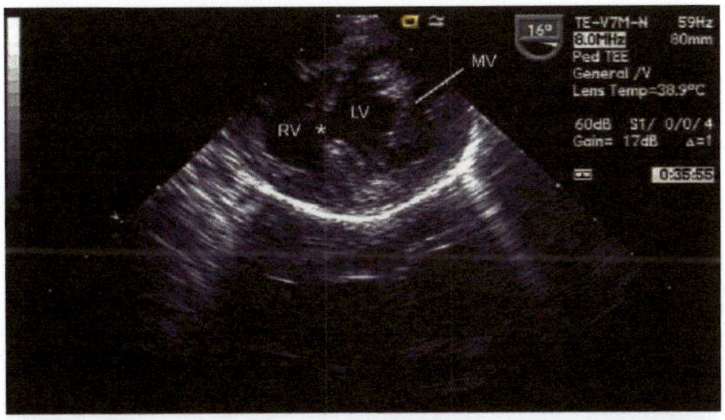

Fig. 9.9 Transgastric mid short axis view of the ventricles with *en-face* visualization of the mitral valve and small mid-muscular ventricular septal defect (*). *LV* left ventricle, *MV* mitral valve, *RV* right ventricle

position (multiplane angle 0°) and advancing into the lower esophageal and transgastric positions will produce the TG Basal SAX and TG Mid SAX views, which are analogous to the parasternal short axis views of the mid and apical portions of the ventricles. As noted above, these views can be useful for visualizing mid and apical muscular VSDs, both by imaging and color flow Doppler (Video 9.4a). In addition, the LV can be quantitatively assessed for function and septal wall motion. Thus the muscular septum can be thoroughly interrogated as the evaluation extends towards the apex (Fig. 9.9) and then superiorly towards the lower and mid esophagus. These views can be obtained with a combination of withdrawing and advancing the probe while retro or anteflexing.

With further advancement and anteflexion of the TEE probe, the deep transgastric views can produce excellent images comparable to the subcostal (subxiphoid) views in transthoracic imaging [14–16]. As with much of pediatric subcostal imaging, the image should be inverted on the screen. In the deep transgastric position with multiplane angle at 0–10°, the deep transgastric long axis (DTG LAX) view produces images comparable to that of a subcostal coronal plane. The crux of the heart and inlet septum can be visualized as well as most of the muscular septum, including lower muscular and apical septum. With further advancement and anteflexion of the probe, the imaging plane steers more posteriorly to visualize the LVOT and the membranous septum. Perimembranous VSDs can be well seen from the coronal sections produced by the DTG LAX view as well as the deep transgastric sagittal (DTG Sagittal) view (multiplane angle 80–110°), the latter with clockwise rotation of the probe to angle slightly away from the RVOT. Often, redundant aneurysmal tissue can be noted partially occluding the defect (Fig. 9.10, Video 9.11). Again, the LVOT should be assessed for associated subaortic stenosis or aortic regurgitation. When available, the deep transgastric position provides an excellent viewpoint from which to assess the LVOT in cases of sub-aortic or aortic valve obstruction. These views afford the best angle to obtain spectral Doppler interrogation since the LVOT is directly in line with the cursor. When using the DTG LAX view, further withdrawal of the probe will bring the RVOT into view but oftentimes optimal contact with the stomach can be lost at this point since the RVOT is fairly anterior. Transitioning to a DTG Sagittal view with a multiplane angle of 80–110° is comparable to the transthoracic subcostal sagittal plane, and this view can sometimes provide better imaging of the anterior RVOT. The short axis plane of the ventricles can be seen, and this view usually provides the best planes to image the RVOT in cases of tetralogy of Fallot and double chambered RV since the malaligned conal septum and anomalous muscle bundles can be clearly seen (Fig. 9.11, Video 9.12). This TEE view also provides an excellent angle for spectral Doppler assessment of RVOT obstruction. When increased velocities are obtained in the RVOT, a detailed 2D evaluation should also be performed for anatomic correlation, because in addition to RVOT obstruction, increased velocities in the outflow tract can occur for other reasons: (a) flow-related increases in velocity due to the presence of a significant left to right shunt, and (b) a high velocity flow transmitted from the adjacent VSD.

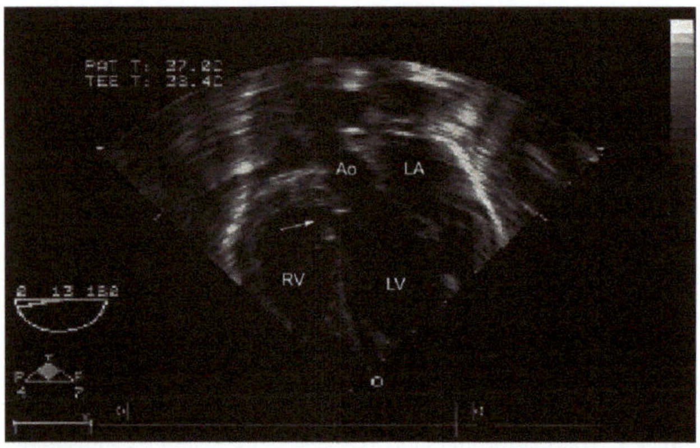

Fig. 9.10 Deep transgastric long axis view (multiplane angle 0–20°) with the *arrow* showing a perimembranous ventricular septal defect and also demonstrating an optimal angle of interrogation for assessing the left ventricular outflow tract by Doppler. *LA* left atrium, *LV* left ventricle, *RV* right ventricle

It should be noted that deep transgastric views are not always available. For example, in some instances of dextrocardia where the stomach and the heart are not on the same side of the body, this view might be difficult or impossible to obtain.

When evaluating the ventricular septum by TEE, color flow Doppler is an essential component of the examination. With color Doppler, a small VSD not visible by 2D imaging becomes apparent. Also, the magnitude and direction of a shunt can be assessed. It is important to remember that, given the range of congenital heart lesions and physiology that can

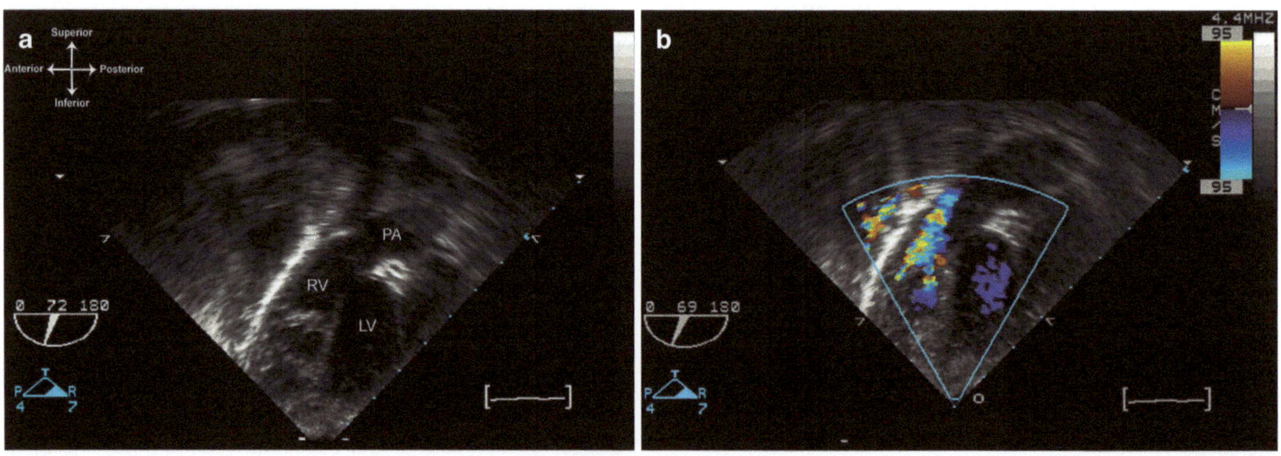

Fig. 9.11 Double chambered right ventricle (*RV*) as seen from the modified deep transgastric sagittal view (multiplane angle about 70°). (**a**) Shows the prominent mid-cavitary muscle bundles in the right ventricle. (**b**) Shows turbulent color flow Doppler across these muscle bundles. Note that this view provides an excellent angle for spectral Doppler evaluation of the RV outflow tract. *LV* left ventricle, *PA* pulmonary artery

be encountered, a defect in the ventricular septum might not always shunt from left to right. If a patient has pulmonary hypertension and a defect is seen by 2D imaging, once color is added, the characteristic appearance of aliasing seen with high velocity flow might not be present. Instead there may only be a low velocity non-aliased left to right shunt or even a right to left shunt. Thus the direction of flow by color Doppler is important to facilitate the physiologic assessment. In addition to color flow Doppler, spectral Doppler can help assess the direction and gradient of the flow through a defect (although an optimal spectral Doppler angle might not be available).

It is also important to remember that in the presence of a large defect, there may be additional smaller muscular defects not readily seen since the ventricular pressures are similar and the majority of the blood flow is through the larger defect. To aid in the detection of these defects, the color flow Doppler Nyquist limit can be decreased to identify lower velocity shunts However in some cases the smaller defects might not be detected until the postoperative evaluation; after the larger defect is closed and there is now a larger pressure differential between the two chambers, the smaller defects become more readily apparent. Moreover in some instances an apparently large, single muscular VSD reveals upon closer inspection that it is actually comprised of two smaller defects separated by a muscle bridge or bundle. Identification of this type of defect has important surgical implications. The potential for multiple VSDs underscores the importance of performing a complete and thorough TEE evaluation of all portions of the ventricular septum, using both 2D imaging and color flow Doppler.

As a general rule, it is recommended that the echocardiographer perform as much 2D imaging as possible to define the cardiac anatomy before turning on color flow Doppler. Excessive use of color flow Doppler is a common occurrence, particularly when the examiner has limited experience with TEE and/or unfamiliarity with the displayed anatomy. However, there will always be instances when this balance might not be possible due to time constraints or instability of the patient. In such cases, rapid collection of important physiologic information (for example, a residual VSD as noted by color flow Doppler) becomes the most important priority.

Intraoperative Evaluation of VSDs

Transesophageal imaging has become an important tool in the operative assessment of a patient with congenital heart disease. TEE can be performed after the induction of anesthesia, and prior to surgery, to confirm the anatomic findings. At times, the findings from the TEE study may alter the surgical approach. More importantly, the TEE can be performed immediately postoperatively to assess the surgical result and determine if any residual disease is present that might need to be addressed. Thus, in many instances TEE plays an integral role during VSD surgery, helping to guide the surgeon before and immediately after cardiopulmonary bypass [11, 17–26].

Preoperative Assessment

Preoperative VSD evaluation by TEE includes a complete assessment of number, size, and morphology of the VSD(s), using 2D imaging as well as color flow/spectral Doppler, as detailed above. However, as previously noted, it is important not only to assess the VSD, but associated lesions as well. These commonly include associated obstructions of the outflow tracts and semilunar valve involvement. In more complex cases of congenital heart disease, it is essential not only to note the size of the VSD, but sometimes more importantly how the defect is related to the outflow tracts and semilunar valves, for example in the instance of double outlet right ventricle with malposed great vessels. If the VSD is closely related to one of the great vessels, it can usually be addressed surgically and just patch-closed. However, if the aorta is far removed from the defect and an arterial switch operation cannot be performed, then closing (baffling) this VSD to the aorta becomes a much larger and more complicated undertaking—one that could result in significant LVOT obstruction. One must take into account the depth of the defect and how much of the RV would be interfered with by the VSD patch/baffle. All these anatomic considerations affect the surgical decision as to whether the VSD can be closed and if so, how to close the defect. In addition, the relationship of the AV valves to the defect is important. If there is straddling or override of one of the AV valves over the VSD, surgical closure of the defect might not be feasible.

Postoperative Assessment

If the VSD is the only surgical issue to be addressed, then that should be the focus of the postoperative study, although other factors such as ventricular function and valve function should be a standard part of the study as well. Depending upon the location of the defect, the area should be interrogated by 2D imaging as well as color flow Doppler to assess for any residual shunts (Fig. 9.12). If indeed a shunt is found, it should be interrogated by spectral Doppler to assess the pressure difference between ventricles as an indication of pulmonary arterial pressures (in the absence of RVOT obstruction). The AV valve function should be assessed, especially if there was manipulation of AV valve tissue during the surgery. Semilunar valve function, particularly the aortic valve, should be carefully evaluated for any leaflet prolapse or regurgitation, even if it was normal on the

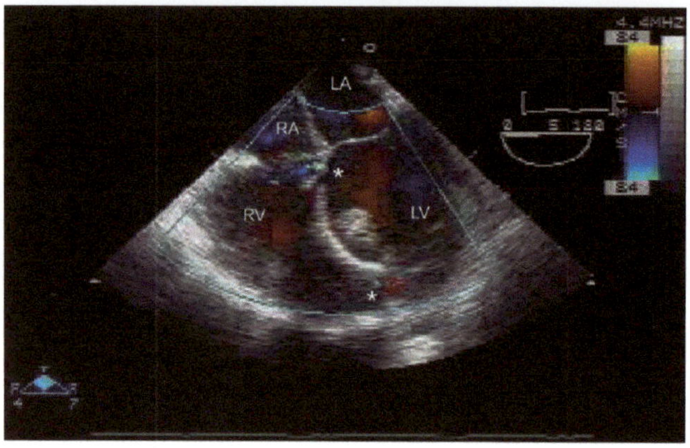

Fig. 9.12 Postoperative evaluation of patient 6, note the large patch and two small residual VSDs noted by color Doppler (*). *LA* left atrium, *LV* left ventricle, *RA* right atrium, *RV* right ventricle

preoperative evaluation. Any new incidence of significant aortic valve regurgitation, especially if eccentric and not central, should raise the possibility of leaflet entrapment/perforation if the VSD was in the vicinity of the outlet or membranous septum. A potential difficulty arises when a residual shunt is identified and deciding whether or not it is hemodynamically significant enough to re-address, as this means reinstitution of cardiopulmonary bypass to revise the repair. Important data that can assist surgical decision-making include the number and size (by color flow Doppler imaging) of residual VSD(s). Yang et al. noted that a residual VSD color jet diameter (measured by TEE) ≥ 4 mm predicted the need for immediate reoperation, while a 3 mm defect could be significant and required additional intraoperative hemodynamic evaluation [26]. Dodge-Khatami et al. found that residual defects less 2 mm were not hemodynamically significant, and likely to close spontaneously [27]. In equivocal cases, direct surgical measurement of right sided oxygen saturations (superior vena cava and pulmonary artery) can be used to estimate the degree of left to right shunting. If a ratio of pulmonary to systemic blood flow [Qp:Qs] exceeds 1.5:1, several investigators recommend a return to cardiopulmonary bypass to close the residual shunt [26, 27]. The location of a residual VSD can also play a role in determining whether to reoperate. For example, a small residual defect close to the aortic valve, in which a high velocity jet could potentially damage the valve, might require revision. In most cases, the decision whether to reintervene depends upon collection and assimilation of all available information, including the TEE study, as well as communication among the surgeon, cardiologist, and anesthesiologist. This decision should also be guided by the knowledge that residual shunts following VSD closure are commonly seen, but most are hemodynamically insignificant and with time; a large percentage of these shunts spontaneously resolve, particularly those with a diameter <3 mm [26–29].

With other complex lesions, outflow tracts and semilunar valve function must be evaluated thoroughly since these outflow tracts can often involve the areas where the VSD has been closed. As noted above, in the case of a posteriorly malaligned VSD, the subaortic area might appear narrow on the preoperative evaluation but demonstrate no gradient since blood is allowed to flow left to right through the VSD. However, once the VSD has been closed, the entire cardiac output must flow through the LVOT and at that time significant obstruction can become apparent. This physiology, however, must be anticipated preoperatively and brought to the attention of the surgeon, who can then inspect and address the LVOT intraoperatively.

TEE in the Cardiac Catheterization Lab

Newer innovations in technology have made possible the intervention of cardiac defects in the cardiac catheterization laboratory, and TEE has proven to play a very important role for several of these procedures. One of the first procedures to use TEE guidance was device closure of atrial septal defects [30–32]. Now, muscular VSDs can be closed by device as well [33–36]. Perimembranous VSDs can also be device-closed via interventional catheterization techniques [37], but at the time of this writing, the principal membranous VSD device under investigation has not been approved in the United States. However, this device continues to be used internationally [38, 39]. The primary utility of TEE in this role is to assist the interventional cardiologist in placing the catheter appropriately across the VSD for device deployment and then positioning of the device during and after deployment. More recently, three-dimensional TEE has shown considerable promise in guiding percutaneous closure of both muscular and perimembranous VSDs [40, 41]. See Chap. 17 for a more complete description of the use of TEE for congenital heart disease treatment in the cardiac catheterization laboratory.

Recently, a hybrid catheterization/surgical approach has gained increasing interest for closure of both muscular and perimembranous VSDs. Also known as *perventricular* closure of VSDs, this technique employs a limited surgical sternotomy, followed by placement of a guide wire and delivery sheath directly through the right ventricular free wall, then across the VSD. The VSD device is delivered via the sheath through the defect, then deployed utilizing continuous TEE monitoring and guidance for proper device positioning [36, 42–44]. Perventricular VSD device closure relies almost completely upon TEE or epicardial echocardiography to guide all phases of the procedure; little (if any) fluoroscopy is generally used [45].

Enlargement of a small, restrictive VSD is occasionally necessary in some patients in whom a large VSD is desirable, e.g. double outlet right ventricle requiring single ventricle palliation. In such instances, perventricular or cardiac catheterization techniques can be used for creation, enlargement, and/or stenting of the restrictive VSD [46]. Such procedures also benefit greatly from the use of TEE for continuous monitoring and guidance during the procedure. A number of factors—stent placement, VSD size, Doppler flow profile across the defect, and cardiac function—can be evaluated both before and after the procedure.

Summary

It is a well known fact that VSDs represent one of the most recognized and frequently encountered forms of CHD. However the term "ventricular septal defect" is itself a broad categorization, comprising several distinct anatomic subtypes that differ in terms of defect morphology, location, size, and clinical presentation/ importance. While VSDs can occur in isolation, they can also be seen in association with more complex congenital heart defects such as tetralogy of Fallot, double outlet right ventricle, truncus arteriosus, and other lesions. Therefore, VSDs will often be one of cardiac lesions that require evaluation whenever TEE is performed for congenital heart surgery or interventional cardiology procedures. It is important for the practitioner to have a solid understanding of the use and utility of TEE for VSD evaluation, particularly in regard to the anatomy and physiology of the different defects, and the surgical/interventional procedures performed specifically to correct them.

References

1. Keane JF, Fyler DC. Ventricular septal defect. In: Keane JF, Lock JE, Fyler DC, Nadas AS, editors. Nadas' pediatric cardiology. 2nd ed. Philadelphia: Saunders; 2006. p. 527–47.
2. McDaniel NL, Gutgesell HP. Ventricular septal defects. In: Moss AJ, Allen HD, editors. Moss and Adams' heart disease in infants, children, and adolescents: including the fetus and young adult. 7th ed. Philadelphia: Lippincott Williams & Wilkins; 2008. p. 667–82.
3. Benheim A, Karr SS, Sell JE, Midgley FM, Holley D, Martin GR. Routine use of transesophageal echocardiography and color flow imaging in the evaluation and treatment of children with congenital heart disease. Echocardiography. 1993;10:583–93.
4. Fyfe DA, Kline CH. Transesophageal echocardiography for congenital heart disease. Echocardiography. 1991;8:573–86.
5. Ritter SB. Pediatric transesophageal color flow imaging 1990: the long and short of it. Echocardiography. 1990;7:713–25.
6. Ritter SB. Transesophageal real-time echocardiography in infants and children with congenital heart disease. J Am Coll Cardiol. 1991; 18:569–80.
7. Stümper O, Kaulitz R, Elzenga NJ, et al. The value of transesophageal echocardiography in children with congenital heart disease. J Am Soc Echocardiogr. 1991;4:164–76.
8. Weintraub R, Shiota T, Elkadi T, et al. Transesophageal echocardiography in infants and children with congenital heart disease. Circulation. 1992;86:711–22.
9. Ayres NA, Miller-Hance W, Fyfe DA, et al. Indications and guidelines for performance of transesophageal echocardiography in the patient with pediatric acquired or congenital heart disease: a report from the Task Force of the Pediatric Council of the American Society of Echocardiography. J Am Soc Echocardiogr. 2005;18: 91–8.
10. Macartney FJ, Rigby ML, Anderson RH, Stark J, Silverman NH. Double outlet right ventricle. Cross sectional echocardiographic findings, their anatomical explanation, and surgical relevance. Br Heart J. 1984;52:164–77.
11. Tee SD, Shiota T, Weintraub R, et al. Evaluation of ventricular septal defect by transesophageal echocardiography: intraoperative assessment. Am Heart J. 1994;127:585–92.
12. Wong PC, Sanders SP, Jonas RA, et al. Pulmonary valve-moderator band distance and association with development of double-chambered right ventricle. Am J Cardiol. 1991;68:1681–6.
13. Salem MM, Starnes VA, Wells WJ, et al. Predictors of left ventricular outflow obstruction following single-stage repair of interrupted aortic arch and ventricular septal defect. Am J Cardiol. 2000;86: 1044–7.
14. Hoffman P, Stümper O, Rydelwska-Sadowska W, Sutherland GR. Transgastric imaging: a valuable addition to the assessment of congenital heart disease by transverse plane transesophageal echocardiography. J Am Soc Echocardiogr. 1993;6:35–44.
15. Muhiudeen IA, Silverman NH, Anderson RH. Transesophageal transgastric echocardiography in infants and children: the subcostal view equivalent. J Am Soc Echocardiogr. 1995;8:231–44.
16. Miller-Hance WC, Silverman NH. Transesophageal echocardiography (TEE) in congenital heart disease with focus on the adult. Cardiol Clin. 2000;18(4):861–92.
17. Bengur AR, Li JS, Herlong JR, Jaggers J, Sanders SP, Ungerleider RM. Intraoperative transesophageal echocardiography in congenital heart disease. Semin Thorac Cardiovasc Surg. 1998;10:255–64.
18. Cyran SE, Kimball TR, Meyer RA, et al. Efficacy of intraoperative transesophageal echocardiography in children with congenital heart disease. Am J Cardiol. 1989;63:594–8.
19. Cyran SE, Myers JL, Gleason MM, Weber HS, Baylen BG, Waldhausen JA. Application of intraoperative transesophageal echocardiography in infants and small children. J Cardiovasc Surg (Torino). 1991;32:318–21.
20. Muhiudeen I, Silverman N. Intraoperative transesophageal echocardiography using high resolution imaging in infants and children with congenital heart disease. Echocardiography. 1993;10: 599–608.
21. Randolph GR, Hagler DJ, Connolly HM, et al. Intraoperative transesophageal echocardiography during surgery for congenital heart defects. J Thorac Cardiovasc Surg. 2002;124:1176–82.
22. Rosenfeld HM, Gentles TL, Wernovsky G, et al. Utility of intraoperative transesophageal echocardiography in the assessment of residual cardiac defects. Pediatr Cardiol. 1998;19:346–51.
23. Smallhorn JF. Intraoperative transesophageal echocardiography in congenital heart disease. Echocardiography. 2002;19:709–23.
24. Stevenson JG, Sorensen GK, Gartman DM, Hall DG, Rittenhouse EA. Transesophageal echocardiography during repair of congenital cardiac defects: identification of residual problems necessitating reoperation. J Am Soc Echocardiogr. 1993;6:356–65.
25. Stevenson JG. Utilization of intraoperative transesophageal echocardiography during repair of congenital cardiac defects: a survey of North American centers. Clin Cardiol. 2003;26:132–4.
26. Yang SG, Novello R, Nicolson S, et al. Evaluation of ventricular septal defect repair using intraoperative transesophageal echocardiography: frequency and significance of residual defects in infants and children. Echocardiography. 2000;17:681–4.
27. Dodge-Khatami A, Knirsch W, Tomaske M, et al. Spontaneous closure of small residual ventricular septal defects after surgical repair. Ann Thorac Surg. 2007;83:902–5.

28. Kurokawa S, Honma T, Taneoka M, Imai H, Baba H, Nomura M. Can intraoperative TEE correctly measure residual shunt after surgical repair of ventricular septal defects? J Anesth. 2010;24:343–50.
29. Hanna BM, El-Hewala AA, Gruber PJ, Gaynor JW, Spray TL, Seliem MA. Predictive value of intraoperative diagnosis of residual ventricular septal defects by transesophageal echocardiography. Ann Thorac Surg. 2010;89:1233–7.
30. Hijazi ZM, Cao Q, Patel HT, Rhodes J, Hanlon KM. Transesophageal echocardiographic results of catheter closure of atrial septal defect in children and adults using the Amplatzer device. Am J Cardiol. 2000;85:1387–90.
31. Mazic U, Gavora P, Masura J. The role of transesophageal echocardiography in transcatheter closure of secundum atrial septal defects by the Amplatzer septal occluder. Am Heart J. 2001;142:482–8.
32. Vaidyanathan B, Simpson JM, Kumar RK. Transesophageal echocardiography for device closure of atrial septal defects: case selection, planning, and procedural guidance. JACC Cardiovasc Imaging. 2009;2:1238–42.
33. Holzer R, Balzer D, Cao QL, Lock K, Hijazi ZM, Amplatzer Muscular Ventricular Septal Defect Investigators. Device closure of muscular ventricular septal defects using the Amplatzer muscular ventricular septal defect occluder: immediate and mid-term results of a U.S. registry. J Am Coll Cardiol. 2004;43:1257–63.
34. Van der Velde ME, Sanders SP, Keane JF, Perry SB, Lock JE. Transesophageal echocardiographic guidance of transcatheter ventricular septal defect closure. J Am Coll Cardiol. 1994;23:1660–5.
35. Van der Velde ME, Perry SB. Transesophageal echocardiography during interventional catheterization in congenital heart disease. Echocardiography. 1997;14:513–28.
36. Bacha EA, Cao QL, Galantowicz ME, et al. Multicenter experience with perventricular device closure of muscular ventricular septal defects. Pediatr Cardiol. 2005;26:169–75.
37. Fu YC, Bass J, Amin Z, et al. Transcatheter closure of perimembranous ventricular septal defects using the new Amplatzer membranous VSD occluder: results of the U.S. phase I trial. J Am Coll Cardiol. 2006;47:319–25.
38. Hu HB, Jiang SL, Xu ZY, Huang LJ, Zhao SH, Zhen H. Transcatheter closure of perimembranous ventricular septal defects by a new Amplatzer membranous ventricular septal defect occluder: a single center study in Beijing. Chin Med J (Engl). 2008;121:573–6.
39. Zheng Q, Zhao Z, Zuo J, et al. A comparative study: early results and complications of percutaneous and surgical closure of ventricular septal defect. Cardiology. 2009;114:238–43.
40. Acar P, Abadir S, Aggoun Y. Transcatheter closure of perimembranous ventricular septal defects with Amplatzer occluder assessed by real-time three-dimensional echocardiography. Eur J Echocardiogr. 2007;8:110–5.
41. Perk G, Lang RM, Garcia-Fernandez MA, et al. Use of real time three-dimensional transesophageal echocardiography in intracardiac catheter based interventions. J Am Soc Echocardiogr. 2009;22:865–82.
42. Pedra CA, Pedra SR, Chaccur P, et al. Perventricular device closure of congenital muscular ventricular septal defects. Expert Rev Cardiovasc Ther. 2010;8:663–74.
43. Xing Q, Pan S, An Q, et al. Minimally invasive perventricular device closure of perimembranous ventricular septal defect without cardiopulmonary bypass: multicenter experience and mid-term follow-up. J Thorac Cardiovasc Surg. 2010;139:1409–15.
44. Bendaly EA, Hoyer MH, Breinholt JP. Mid-term follow up of perventricular device closure of muscular ventricular septal defects. Catheter Cardiovasc Interv. 2011;78(4):577–82.
45. Gan C, An Q, Lin K, et al. Perventricular device closure of ventricular septal defects: six months results in 30 young children. Ann Thorac Surg. 2008;86:142–6.
46. Meadows J, Pigula F, Lock J, Marshall A. Transcatheter creation and enlargement of ventricular septal defects for relief of ventricular hypertension. J Thorac Cardiovasc Surg. 2007;133:912–8.
47. Weinburg PM. Morphology of congenital heart disease. In: Freedom RM, Braunwald E, editors. Atlas of heart disease: congenital heart disease, vol. XII. Philadelphia: Current Medicine; 1997. p. 412.

Evaluation of the Single Ventricle

10

Pierre C. Wong

Abstract

The terms "single ventricle" and "functional single ventricle" apply to a broad group of congenital cardiac lesions that, despite their marked anatomic heterogeneity, share a common, unifying characteristic: a biventricular intracardiac repair cannot be performed to separate the systemic and pulmonary circulations. In essence, a single functional ventricular pumping chamber supplies both the systemic and pulmonary vascular beds; oxygenated and deoxygenated blood blend together, and all patients exhibit some degree of systemic arterial desaturation. In the management of these patients, the ultimate goal is to separate the systemic and pulmonary circulations such that deoxygenated systemic venous blood returns passively to the pulmonary arteries without the assistance of a separate pumping chamber. The resultant physiology, known as Fontan physiology, forms the basis for the current management of the single ventricle patient. Transesophageal echocardiography (TEE) can play an important role in the diagnostic evaluation of single ventricle patients. The most common application of TEE is in the intraoperative setting—preoperatively, to verify anatomy and physiology, and postoperatively, to evaluate the results of cardiac surgery. However, there are other non-operative settings in which TEE can be utilized to evaluate the detailed anatomy of the single ventricle patient, and to examine some of the possible problems and complications in operated patients. This chapter explores the use of TEE in the single ventricle patient.

Keywords

Single ventricle • Univentricular heart • Congenital heart disease • Echocardiography • Transesophageal echocardiography • Fontan operation • Pediatric cardiac surgery • Palliative surgery • Hypoplastic left heart syndrome • Tricuspid atresia • Heterotaxy

Introduction

The term "single ventricle", as used by specialists in congenital heart disease (CHD), is recognizably broad and nonspecific, encompassing a wide spectrum of cardiac lesions with differing pathologic anatomy and embryologic derivations. In its strictest sense, the term single ventricle refers to the class of lesions known as univentricular heart, in which one ventricular chamber is rudimentary or absent, and therefore unable to function as an independent, separate chamber [1, 2]. However from a surgical (and more utilitarian) sense, the use of the term "single ventricle" has been expanded to include all manner of cardiac lesions in which a biventricular

P.C. Wong, MD
Division of Cardiology, Children's Hospital Los Angeles, Department of Pediatrics, Keck School of Medicine, University of Southern California, 4650 Sunset Blvd, Mailstop #34, Los Angeles, CA 90027, USA
e-mail: pwong@chla.usc.edu

The online version of this chapter (doi:10.1007/978-1-84800-064-3_10) contains supplementary material, which is available to authorized users.

P.C. Wong, W.C. Miller-Hance (eds.), *Transesophageal Echocardiography for Congenital Heart Disease*,
DOI 10.1007/978-1-84800-064-3_10, © Springer-Verlag London 2014

intracardiac repair cannot be performed or may not be considered the optimal approach to separate the systemic and pulmonary circulations, and therefore only one functional ventricular pumping chamber supplies the systemic circulation [3, 4]. Systemic and pulmonary venous blood must, of necessity, commingle, producing mixing physiology and obligate systemic arterial hypoxemia. Because of the wide anatomic diversity of cardiac defects that can produce this physiology, the more generic term "functional single ventricle" is also used to describe such patients.

The most common application of transesophageal echocardiography (TEE) for single ventricle evaluation is in the intraoperative setting—preoperatively, to verify anatomy and physiology, and postoperatively, to evaluate the results of cardiac surgery. However, there are other non-operative settings in which TEE can be utilized to evaluate the detailed anatomy of the single ventricle patient. For example, in the adolescent or adult patient with complex single ventricle anatomy, TEE can serve as a supplemental (or even initial) tool for diagnostic evaluation. Postoperative Fontan patients are notorious for having marginal to poor transthoracic echocardiographic windows, and in this setting TEE can be used for improved evaluation.

This chapter discusses the TEE evaluation of the single ventricle patient. The focus will be upon those patients who, from an anatomic standpoint, have only one truly functional ventricle. As will be evident, there is great diversity among this group of patients, with each class of defect having its own distinctive anatomic and physiologic characteristics. Knowledge of these distinguishing features greatly facilitates their TEE assessment.

Author's note: As previously mentioned in Chap. 4, some of the standardized TEE terminology defined in that chapter might seem confusing when applied to the abnormal and unusual anatomy found in many single ventricle defects—for example, using the mid esophageal *four* chamber view for a double inlet ventricle with only *three* principal chambers. Nonetheless, for consistency's sake we will continue to utilize the standardized views and nomenclature defined in Chap. 4, and will denote modifications to those views when applicable. It is recommended that the reader have a reasonable degree of familiarity with the TEE views, probe positions and probe manipulations described in that chapter.

General Considerations for TEE Evaluation

As mentioned above, the term "single ventricle" comprises a heterogeneous group of lesions, and the TEE evaluation must be tailored to the anatomic considerations specifically associated with each cardiac lesion. Moreover, as is true with all CHD, considerable anatomic variation exists within any single group of cardiac defects, and the examiner must anticipate and prepare for this. The TEE study will rarely be the first diagnostic examination performed on a single ventricle patient; prior imaging and diagnostic information will usually be available, and the examiner should be thoroughly familiar with this information. Nonetheless the examiner should approach the TEE examination with a fresh perspective, because the TEE study will occasionally reveal new findings and/or modify previous ones. Moreover, in some instances the study provides important additional information that is considered vital in the formulation of a surgical plan or other therapeutic strategy. Whenever possible, a complete and systematic examination should be performed (see Chap. 4); the more complex the anatomy, the more meticulous and complete the TEE examination needs to be. In the sections that follow, the different types of single ventricle defects will be discussed, along with their most common anatomic features. Certain anatomic variations and abnormalities (such as a left superior vena cava to coronary sinus, pulmonary venous anomalies, patent ductus arteriosus) are common to a number of different pathologies, and these will not be repeated with each type of cardiac defect. However they again underline the importance of performing as complete a study as possible.

Single Ventricle: Anatomic Types

Hypoplastic Left Heart Syndrome

Hypoplastic left heart syndrome (HLHS) comprises a spectrum of lesions characterized by varying degrees of left sided hypoplasia [5, 6]. The classic constellation of associated cardiac defects includes mitral stenosis/mitral atresia, aortic valve atresia, a diminutive left ventricle (LV), a markedly hypoplastic ascending aorta, and hypoplastic aortic arch and aortic isthmus with a posterior aortic shelf (coarctation). However, the spectrum of HLHS can vary from mitral and aortic valve atresia, a tiny ascending aorta, and virtually no LV cavity, to mild mitral and aortic valve hypoplasia, antegrade flow across the aortic valve, and mild ascending aortic and LV hypoplasia. Nonetheless despite the anatomic variability, all cases of HLHS share a defining characteristic: an inability of the left sided structures to independently support the systemic circulation. Thus the right ventricle (RV) assumes the primary role as the systemic pumping chamber, providing blood to the systemic circulation via forward flow through the main pulmonary artery and patent ductus arteriosus (in the unoperated patient) or, if surgically palliated, via a Norwood-type procedure (see below).

The TEE evaluation of HLHS patients is relatively straightforward, focusing on the key features relevant for the patient's physiology and anatomy. Most of these features can be evaluated from the level of the mid esophagus; the most

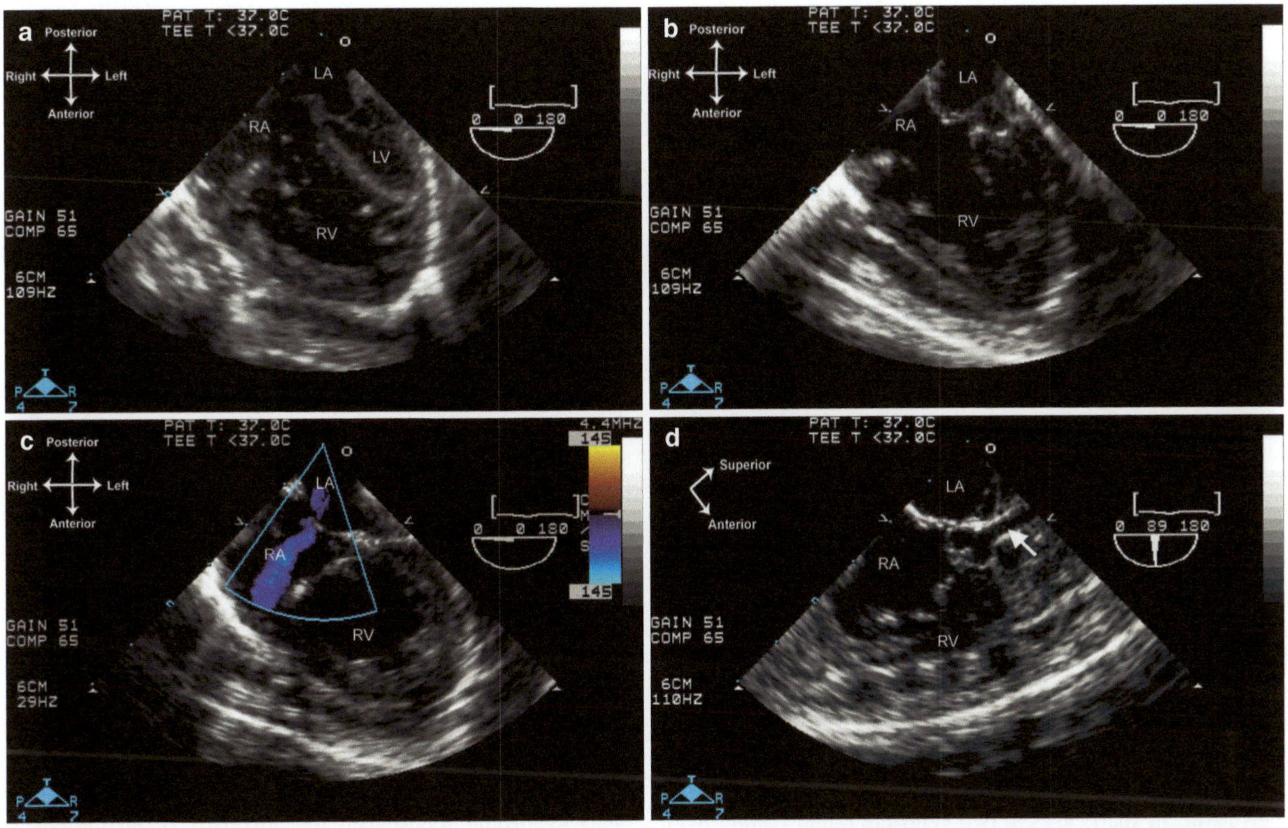

Fig. 10.1 Hypoplastic left heart syndrome, as viewed from the mid esophageal four chamber view. There can be significant anatomic variation ranging from mitral stenosis and left ventricle hypoplasia (**a**) to virtual absence of these structures (**b**). The atrial septum can be adequately visualized and interrogated by color Doppler also in this plane (**c**). The mid esophageal long axis view (**d**) allows for visualization of the aortic valve and diminutive proximal ascending aorta (*arrow*). *LA* left atrium, *LV* left ventricle, *RA* right atrium, *RV* right ventricle

useful initial view is the mid esophageal four chamber (ME 4 Ch) view, multiplane angle 0°. From here, the multiplane angle can be varied as needed for optimal visualization of the different cardiac structures. Specific TEE evaluation should include systemic and pulmonary venous return, atrial septal patency, tricuspid valve anatomy and regurgitation (if present), RV morphology, function, and wall motion abnormalities (if present), and pulmonary valve function (Fig. 10.1, Video 10.1). If mitral and/or aortic valve are patent, flow across these valves can also be evaluated. Coronary artery origins can be viewed from a modified mid esophageal aortic valve short axis (ME AV SAX) view, with probe anteflexion and multiplane angles between 0 and 45°. Other intracardiac anomalies associated with HLHS, such as anomalous pulmonary venous return and left superior vena cava (SVC) to a dilated coronary sinus can also be seen by TEE using the mid esophageal views. The hypoplastic ascending aorta can best be visualized in the mid esophageal aortic valve long axis (ME AV LAX) view with a multiplane angle approximately 80–90° (Fig. 10.1c); an accurate ascending aortic diameter can also be measured. Ductal patency can be evaluated by imaging and color flow Doppler in the upper esophageal aortic arch short axis (UE Ao Arch SAX) and upper esophageal pulmonary artery long axis (UE PA LAX) views; there will usually be low velocity right to left shunting in systole, and left to right shunting in diastole. However the hypoplastic transverse aortic arch and proximal descending thoracic aorta are generally difficult to visualize fully by TEE; evaluation of these structures is better accomplished by other modalities such as transthoracic echocardiography. When HLHS is associated with a very small or absent atrial communication, a small decompressing vein can sometimes be present, connecting the left atrium/pulmonary veins to the innominate vein. Known as a *levoatrial cardinal vein*, it serves as an alternate pathway to re-route pulmonary venous blood back to the right heart [7]. If present, it can sometimes be visualized with an UE Ao Arch SAX and UE PA LAX views, using leftward rotation to demonstrate the vein as it returns to the innominate vein.

Hypoplastic Right Heart Syndrome

Hypoplastic right heart syndrome encompasses a spectrum of cardiac lesions characterized by pulmonary atresia (either a formed but imperforate pulmonary valve, also known as membranous atresia, or long-segment muscular atresia), varying degrees of RV hypoplasia, and an intact ventricular septum. This class of cardiac defects is often referred to as pulmonary atresia/intact ventricular septum. The tricuspid valve is patent but hypoplastic, with the degree of tricuspid hypoplasia generally correlating with the extent of RV hypoplasia. In moderate hypoplasia, only two major portions of the RV (inflow and outflow) are present; the apical (trabecular) portion is either truncated or absent. This is termed a "bipartite" RV. In the most severe cases, only a tiny RV (usually the inflow portion) is present and this is termed a "unipartite" RV. Such patients have an obligate right to left shunt across the atrial septum, and a good-sized LV and aortic valve. Given the absence of antegrade flow from RV to pulmonary artery, patients require an alternate source of pulmonary blood flow, usually from a patent ductus arteriosus (PDA). As RV hypoplasia becomes more severe, there is an increasing likelihood of persistent embryonic sinusoidal connections (also known as ventriculo-coronary arterial communications) between the RV and the epicardial coronary arteries [8]. Some of these sinusoidal connections can contain stenoses that result in portions of the myocardium being perfused primarily or exclusively by the hypertensive RV; this situation is termed RV dependent coronary artery perfusion. In such cases, a two ventricle repair cannot even be considered, as the RV cannot be decompressed [9].

In the absence of RV-dependent coronary circulation, a determination must be made whether a hypoplastic right heart syndrome patient is a candidate for a two ventricle repair, or whether the patient should undergo single ventricle palliation. This determination is largely based upon an assessment of the degree of RV hypoplasia, which in turn is based primarily upon an evaluation of tricuspid valve annulus and RV size. The minimum tricuspid and RV dimensions that dictate the choice of one vs. two ventricle strategy vary among different institutions, and the published criteria continue to be evolve with time and increasing experience. Some centers use a tricuspid valve annulus z score anywhere between <−3 to −10 as a cutoff [10–13], some use the RV morphology (unipartite vs. bi/tripartite) [14], some use an estimation of RV diastolic volume [15], and some use a combination of these criteria. Whatever the method, if the tricuspid valve and RV are deemed too hypoplastic for a two ventricle circulation, then initial surgery is undertaken with the intention of single ventricle palliation—specifically, planned future bidirectional Glenn and Fontan procedures (discussed below). In this case, a systemic-pulmonary artery shunt (Blalock-Taussig shunt) is initially performed, often in conjunction with an atrial septectomy to assure unobstructed mixing of right and left atrial blood. In patients with milder forms of tricuspid valve and RV hypoplasia, a two ventricle (vs. "one and a half") approach can be considered. In these instances antegrade flow across the RV outflow tract is established in the newborn period, with the expectation that the increased blood flow through the RV will stimulate growth of this chamber. This can be accomplished surgically by reconstruction of the RV outflow tract, usually performed in combination with a systemic-pulmonary shunt (such as a Blalock-Taussig shunt) [16]. An alternative strategy utilizes interventional catheterization techniques to establish antegrade flow across the RV outflow tract, including catheter perforation of the pulmonary valve (using balloon, laser, or radiofrequency methods), along with transcatheter stenting of the ductus arteriosus [14, 17]. With either surgical or transcatheter approach, some patients experience enough growth of their RV that they can function effectively with two ventricle physiology [14, 18]. Eventually, these patients can undergo closure of the systemic-pulmonary shunt and, if an atrial defect is still present, it can also be closed. In other patients, the RV continues to be moderately hypoplastic and a "one and a half repair" is subsequently undertaken. In this type of operation, a bidirectional Glenn procedure (discussed below) is performed to allow SVC blood to drain directly to the pulmonary arteries, while leaving inferior vena cava (IVC) blood to return to the RV and then be ejected directly into the main and branch pulmonary arteries. At the time of the Glenn operation, the atrial septal defect, if present, is often closed [19].

The TEE evaluation of the patient with hypoplastic right heart syndrome focuses on the adequacy of an interatrial communication, as well as the degree of tricuspid valve and RV hypoplasia. The atrial septum can be assessed from the ME 4 Ch and mid esophageal bicaval (ME Bicaval) views. The tricuspid valve and hypoplastic RV are best seen using a combination of MV 4 Ch (Fig. 10.2a, Video 10.2) and mid esophageal right ventricle inflow-outflow (ME RV In-Out) views (Fig. 10.2b, c, Video 10.2). Tricuspid and pulmonary valve annular diameters can also be measured using these views; as mentioned above, the tricuspid valve annulus diameter plays a very important role in determining whether intervention should be undertaken for a one or two ventricle strategy [15, 19, 20]. Coronary artery sinusoidal flow can sometimes be seen with color flow Doppler, but coronary artery stenoses cannot be diagnosed by echocardiography and therefore must be evaluated by angiography. Left ventricular and mitral valve function should be evaluated carefully, also from the midesophageal views, specifically the ME 4 Ch, mid esophageal two chamber (ME 2 Ch), mitral commissural (ME Mitral), and long axis (ME LAX) views. Additional information regarding LV and mitral valve function can be provided by the transgastric views: the transgastric basal and mid short axis (TG Basal SAX, TG Mid SAX) and transgastric two-chamber (TG 2 Ch) and transgastric long axis (TG LAX) views. Some patients can have significant LV outflow tract obstruction due to bowing of the ventricular septum that produces mid-cavitary obstruction, and this should also be evaluated carefully with a combination of mid esophageal (ME 4 Ch, ME LAX), transgastric (TG LAX), and deep transgastric long axis (DTG LAX) and deep

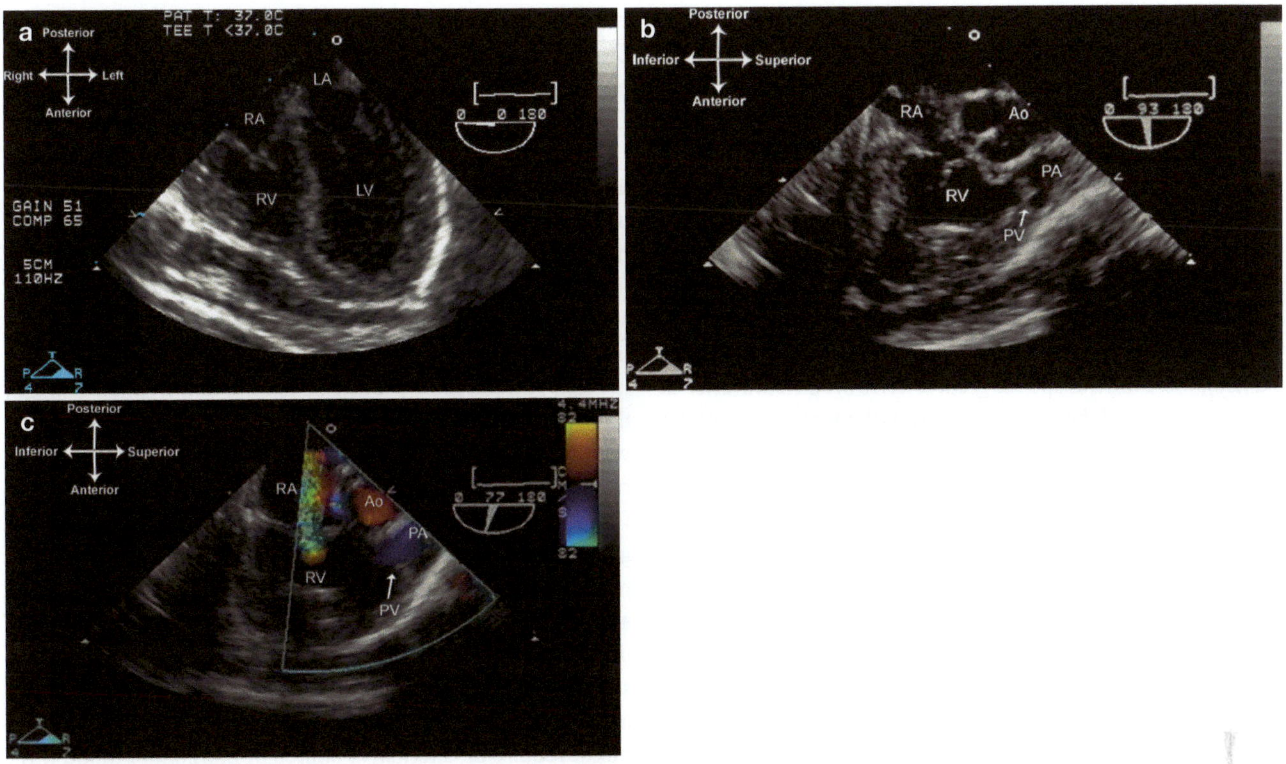

Fig. 10.2 Pulmonary atresia/intact ventricular septum, also known as hypoplastic right heart. The right ventricular cavity is small, muscular, and non-apex forming as displayed in the mid esophageal four chamber view (**a**). The trabecular portion of the right ventricle is typically underdeveloped, as shown in the mid esophageal right ventricular inflow-outflow views (**b**, **c**). Note the presence of an imperforate pulmonary valve without antegrade flow. There is significant tricuspid insufficiency. *Ao* ascending aorta, *LA* left atrium, *LV* left ventricle, *PA* main pulmonary artery, *PV* pulmonary valve, *RA* right atrium, *RV* right ventricle

transgastric sagittal (DTG Sagittal) views. The pulmonary valve, if present, can be evaluated and its annulus measured in the ME RV In-Out view, using a multiplane angle of 60–90° (Fig. 10.2b). The branch pulmonary arteries and ductus arteriosus are not always well seen, but ductal left to right flow can often be detected by color flow Doppler in the UE PA LAX and UE Ao Arch SAX views, using leftward probe rotation (when there is a left aortic arch).

Tricuspid Atresia

Patients with tricuspid atresia have no functional tricuspid valve. Often, there is complete absence of the tricuspid valve, with only a muscular shelf seen in the tricuspid position. In some instances the tricuspid valve is formed and present but imperforate (so-called "membranous" tricuspid atresia). In either case, there is obligate right to left shunting across the atrial septum, and complete mixing of deoxygenated and oxygenated blood at atrial level. There is generally a small RV cavity, with marked hypoplasia of the inflow portion but variable trabecular and infundibular portions, and usually (but not always) a communication between the LV and the hypoplastic RV. This communication has variously been termed a ventricular septal defect (VSD), or alternatively a *bulboventricular foramen* (BVF) [21, 22]—it generally is located between the LV and RV inflow portion, but can also be seen closer to the apex or infundibulum of the small RV. In the majority of cases, this defect will be the site of obstruction to LV to RV shunting, though obstruction can occur at the outlet valve itself (the valve arising from the RV) or in the subvalvar infundibulum [21]. The ventriculo-arterial connection can vary, and one of the most recognized classification systems for tricuspid atresia is based upon the relationship of the great arteries [23]. A summary of this classification system is given in Table 10.1. In general, this system's nomenclature is not widely used when clinicians describe and discuss tricuspid atresia, but it still serves to underline the most important anatomic features relevant to this anomaly, namely (a) great artery origin/relationship, (b) VSD/BVF size, and (c) whether aortic or pulmonary outflow obstruction is present. In Type I, seen in 70–80 % of patients with tricuspid atresia [24], the aorta arises in normal position from the LV, there is ventriculo-arterial concordance, and the aortic valve is of normal size and function. The pulmonary artery arises from the small RV chamber, and the amount of pulmonary blood flow depends upon the size of the VSD/BVF and the degree of subpulmonary stenosis (if present). Type I can be further classified into three subtypes, based upon the size of the VSD and degree of pulmonary outflow obstruction: Type Ia (no VSD, pulmonary atresia), Type Ib (small VSD, pulmonary stenosis); Type Ic (large VSD, no pulmonary stenosis). If the ventricular defect is large and there is no subpulmonary stenosis, the patient can have excessive pulmonary blood flow leading to pulmonary overcirculation and congestion. If there is obstruction at the ventricular defect or subpulmonary level, there can be reduced antegrade flow leading to systemic arterial hypoxemia (Fig. 10.3, Video 10.3). The patient is then dependent upon an alternative source of pulmonary blood flow such as a patent ductus arteriosus or surgically created shunt. With Type II, seen in 12–25 % of patients with tricuspid atresia [24], there are transposed great arteries (ventriculo-arterial discordance), and the aorta arises from the small RV outflow chamber, generally to the right of the pulmonary artery, or D-transposed. Type II is also classified into three subgroups, based on the degree of pulmonary outflow obstruction: Type IIa (pulmonary atresia), Type IIb (pulmonary stenosis), Type IIc (no pulmonary stenosis). In general, with Type II tricuspid atresia there is either subaortic stenosis or subpulmonary stenosis, depending on the size of the VSD/BVF (through which blood must pass from LV to RV to aorta) and position of the infundibular septum. Type IIc is the most common form: in such cases the pulmonary valve (which arises from the LV) is usually of normal size and function. The ventricular defect is often surrounded by a muscular rim, and if small enough, there can be marked subaortic stenosis, often in association with hypoplasia of the aorta and aortic coarctation or interruption (in many cases requiring a patent ductus arteriosus for systemic perfusion). Such patients invariably require surgery to alleviate or bypass the subaortic stenosis, as well as repair the aortic arch. Conversely, Types IIa and IIb (which are much less common) have pulmonary outflow obstruction, usually due to posterior malalignment of infundibular septum that can produce significant subpulmonary stenosis and decreased pulmonary blood flow [25]. Such patients might require an alternative source of pulmonary blood flow, such as a ductus arteriosus or surgically created shunt. In these instances the VSD/BVF and aorta are generally of good size, and there is no obstruction to systemic blood flow. Types I and II are by far the most common forms of tricuspid atresia.

Table 10.1 Classification of tricuspid atresia

Type I	**Normally related great arteries**
Ia	Intact ventricular septum and pulmonary atresia
Ib	Small ventricular septal defect and pulmonary stenosis
Ic	Large ventricular septal defect, no pulmonary stenosis
Type II	**Transposed great arteries**
IIa	Ventricular septal defect with pulmonary atresia
IIb	Ventricular septal defect with pulmonary stenosis
IIc	Ventricular septal defect, no pulmonary stenosis
Type III	**Transposition or malposition of the great arteries**
	Associated complex lesions, including L-transposition of the great arteries, double outlet right ventricle, double outlet left ventricle, truncus arteriosus

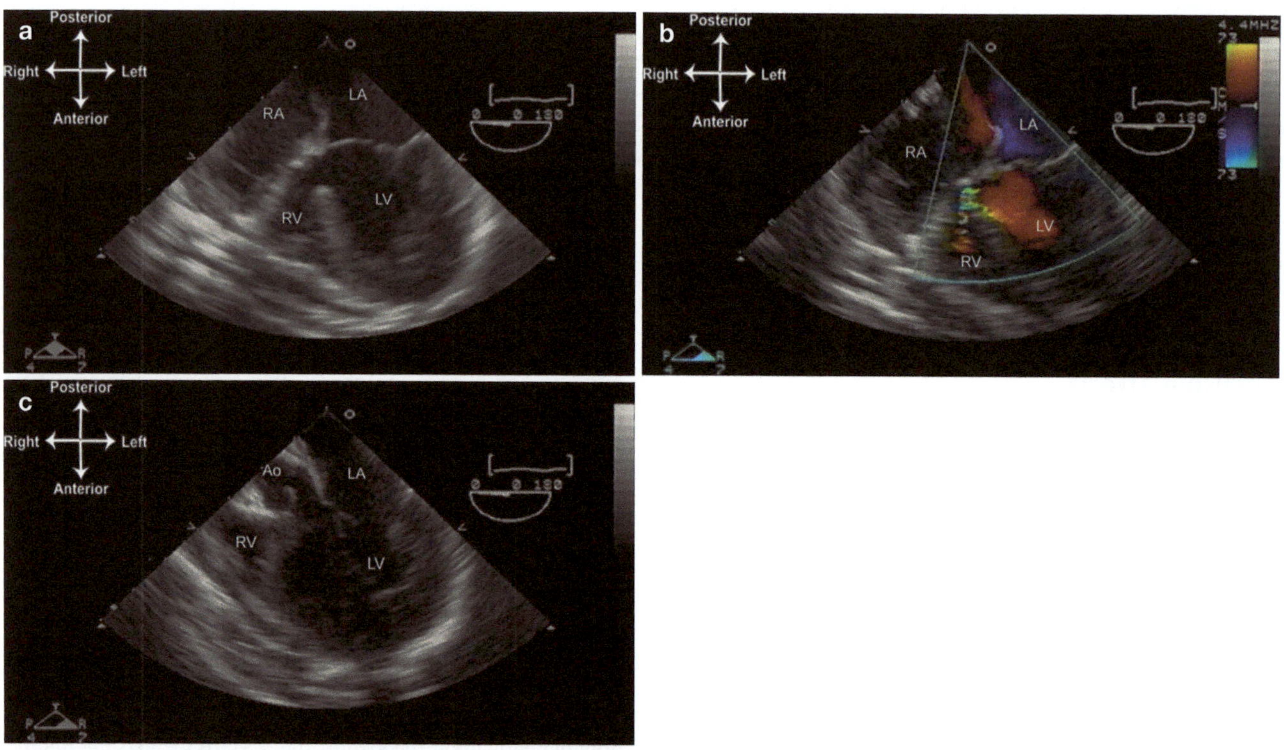

Fig. 10.3 Tricuspid atresia, normally related great arteries. (**a**) The mid esophageal four chamber view demonstrating lack of visible tricuspid valve; only a muscular shelf is seen, as well as a hypoplastic right ventricular chamber. (**b**) There is a small ventricular septal defect or bulboventricular foramen with turbulent left to right shunting. (**c**) Withdrawal and slight anteflexion of the TEE probe demonstrates the aortic valve (*Ao*) arising from the left ventricle. *LA* left atrium, *LV* left ventricle, *RA* right atrium, *RV* right ventricle.

Type III is much more rare, seen in about 3–6 % of patients with tricuspid atresia, and it is a less specific category that includes a number of other defects such as L-transposition of the great arteries, truncus arteriosus, etc. [24].

The TEE evaluation of tricuspid atresia focuses upon atrial septal patency and shunting, mitral valve and LV function, the position of the great arteries and ventriculo-arterial relationship, and outflow tract patency including the size of the VSD/BVF. Much of this evaluation can be performed from the level of the mid esophagus, particularly the ME 4 Ch view for evaluation of atrial septum, mitral valve, LV and great arteries as well as VSD/BVF. Supplemental evaluation of these structures can also be provided by other mid esophageal views: ME Bicaval (systemic venous return, atrial septum), ME LAX (mitral valve, semilunar valves, VSD/BVF), ME RV In-Out (VSD/BVF). The deep transgastric views (DTG LAX, DTG Sagittal) can also provide good visualization of the mitral valve and VSD/BVF, as well as the aortic and pulmonary outflow tracts. The DTG views are also useful for spectral Doppler evaluation of the outflow tracts. In patients with transposed great arteries, the size of the ventricular defect, and potential for subaortic stenosis, should be evaluated carefully (Fig. 10.4, Video 10.4). If the VSD/BVF and/or the subaortic area are felt to be potentially obstructive, the pulmonary valve should be evaluated with the anticipation of a possible Damus-Kaye-Stansel (DKS) operation. The evaluation of the VSD/BVF and the DKS operation are discussed below. In tricuspid atresia patients with transposed great arteries, left juxtaposition of the atrial appendages can sometimes be encountered [26, 27]. Care should be taken to recognize this entity and not confuse it with a large atrial septal defect; in fact, the orientation of the true atrial septal defect is often different from what is normally encountered [28]. This entity is best evaluated from a modified ME AV SAX view first retroflexed, then slowly anteflexed to demonstrate the right atrial appendage just anterior to the left atrial appendage. An example of left juxtaposition of the atrial appendages is given in Chap. 12—Conotruncal Malformations.

In tricuspid atresia patients with normally related great arteries, the size of the interventricular communication and determination of the presence and degree of pulmonary outflow tract obstruction are essential. If pulmonary blood flow is unobstructed, limitation by means of pulmonary artery banding is usually undertaken; if blood flow is reduced, interventions to increase pulmonary blood flow will need to be considered. Some patients have just enough restriction to pulmonary blood flow that they are neither overcirculated nor excessively cyanotic—in other words, they are well balanced.

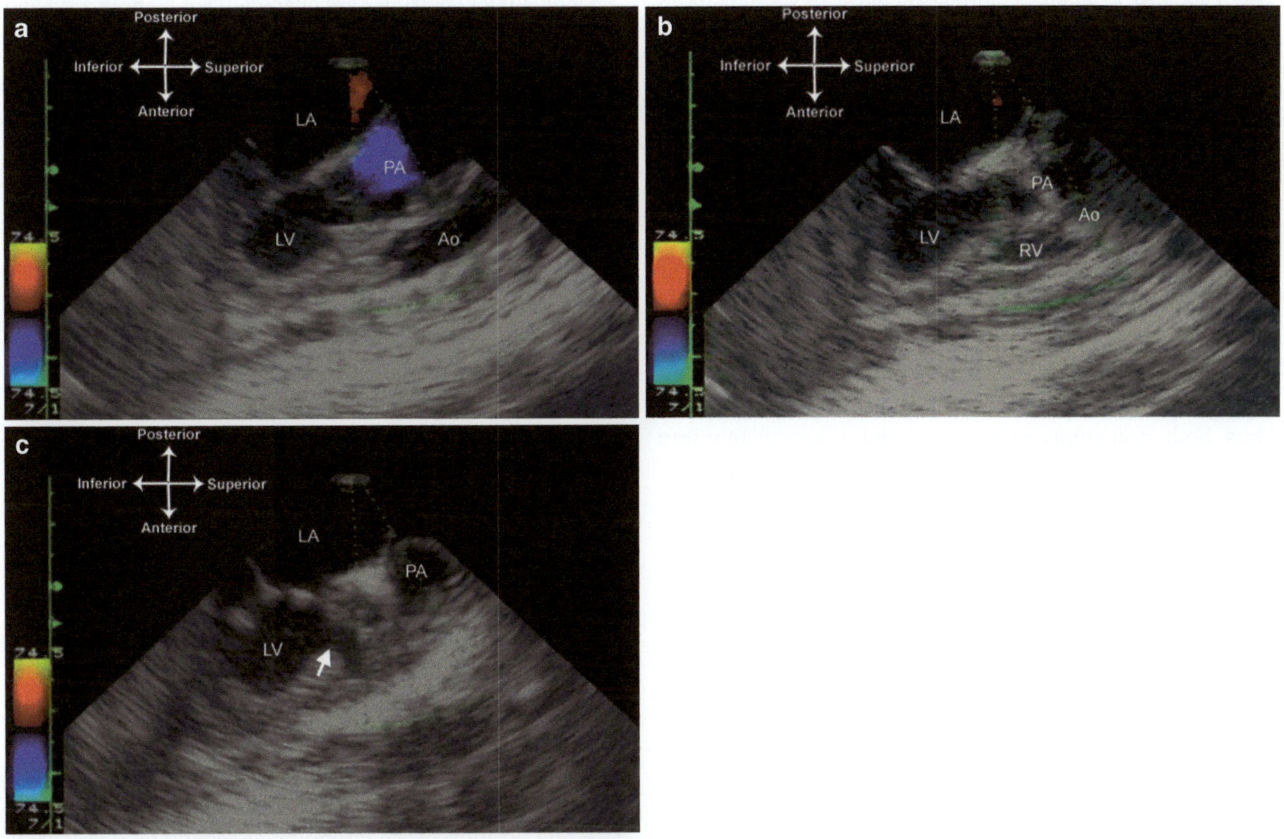

Fig. 10.4 Tricuspid atresia with D-transposed great arteries. Images taken from the mid esophageal aortic valve long axis view, multiplane angle 90°, showing the relationship of the great arteries with the pulmonary artery arising from the left ventricle, and the aorta arising from a small anterior right ventricular outflow chamber (**a**). The ventricular septal defect (bulboventricular foramen) is noted by the *arrow* (**b**). *LA* left atrium, *LV* left ventricle, *PA* pulmonary artery, *Ao* Aorta

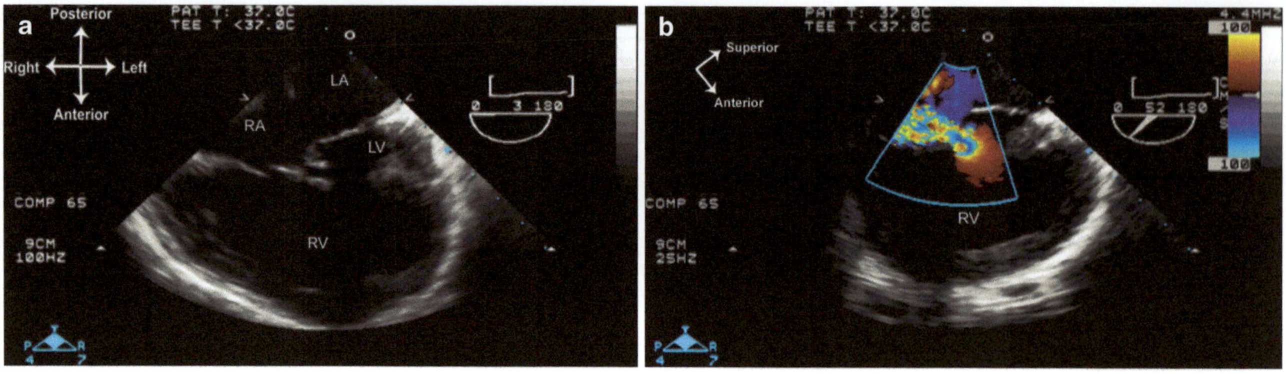

Fig. 10.5 Unbalanced atrioventricular (*AV*) septal defect. (**a**) Mid esophageal four chamber view demonstrates an extremely right dominant AV septal defect with a tiny left ventricle. The large common AV valve empties almost completely into the large right ventricle. (**b**) Significant central AV valve regurgitation as documented with a multiplane angle of 52°. *LA* left atrium, *LV* left ventricle, *RA* right atrium, *RV* right ventricle

Such patients might not require any intervention for the first few months of their life, although ultimately they will require the same surgeries used for all single ventricle patients—namely, the Glenn and Fontan procedures (discussed below).

Univentricular Atrioventricular (AV) Connection

This category of single ventricle includes those defects in which both atria empty completely (or almost completely) into one large ventricle. A second ventricle might or might not be present; if present, it is generally quite hypoplastic. This group of defects includes unbalanced AV septal defect, double inlet ventricle (DILV), as well as the rare double inlet right ventricle (DIRV) and true single (or solitary) ventricular chamber of indeterminate morphology.

Patients with unbalanced AV septal defects have similar characteristics to a large AV septal defect (Chap. 8—AV septal defects and AV valve anomalies), but the common AV valve—instead of being balanced equally over both ventricles—is oriented significantly toward one ventricle. Thus, both atria empty primarily or almost completely into that chamber, and there is usually some degree of hypoplasia of the other ventricle (Fig. 10.5). In some patients, the degree of AV valve unbalance is so pronounced, and/or the degree of ventricular hypoplasia so apparent, that it is clear that the defect cannot be septated — i.e. the patient must be treated as a functional single ventricle. In others, this assessment is more difficult, and various criteria are utilized to determine whether a biventricular repair is feasible [29, 30]. Unbalanced AV septal defect is a common accompanying feature of heterotaxy syndrome (discussed below). The TEE evaluation of such patients is very much the same as for any patient with an AV septal defect, with particular attention paid to the degree of common AV valve distribution or commitment to the underlying ventricular chambers, AV valve function, ventricular hypoplasia, and possible aortic or pulmonary outflow tract obstruction. A combination of mid esophageal views (ME 4 Ch, ME 2 Ch, ME LAX) are best for evaluating the common AV valve and ventricular chambers, and also the degree of AV valve regurgitation (if present). When available, the deep transgastric views (DTG LAX, DTG Sagittal) can be used to evaluate the AV valve *en face* and its balance over both ventricles, similar to the views obtained with a subcostal sagittal view [29, 31]. The TEE evaluation of AV septal defects is discussed extensively in Chap. 8.

Double inlet ventricles are characterized by both atria and AV valves emptying into a large ventricle of either left or right ventricle morphology. The vast majority of these are DILV: both AV valves empty into a large ventricle of LV morphology, and there is generally a smaller RV outflow chamber located anteriorly. In many cases of DILV, it is very difficult to determine which AV valve is tricuspid, and which is mitral. There are three general classes of DILV: (1) normally related great arteries; (2) D-transposed great arteries; (3) L-transposed great arteries. The patient with DILV and normally related great arteries, also known as a Holmes' heart [32], has a normal aortic valve and aorta arising from the large LV, with the pulmonary artery arising from the RV outflow chamber with a variable degree of subpulmonary stenosis (Fig. 10.6, Video 10.5). The patient with DILV and D-transposed great arteries has the aorta arising from a rightward, RV outflow chamber; with L-transposed great arteries the aorta arises from a leftward RV outflow chamber. Of the three types of DILV, the L-transposed is the most common type (60–65 % of all DILV), followed by the D-transposed form (20–25 %), and lastly the normally related great arteries variation (15 %). In both forms of DILV with transposed great arteries, there is either significant subaortic narrowing (often with ascending aorta and aortic arch hypoplasia) or subpulmonary narrowing, depending on the size of the VSD/BVF and position of the infundibular septum [1, 33]. This is analogous to tricuspid atresia and transposed great arteries, as described above.

DIRV is a rare defect in which both AV valves empty into a chamber of RV morphology [34]. In these instances, there

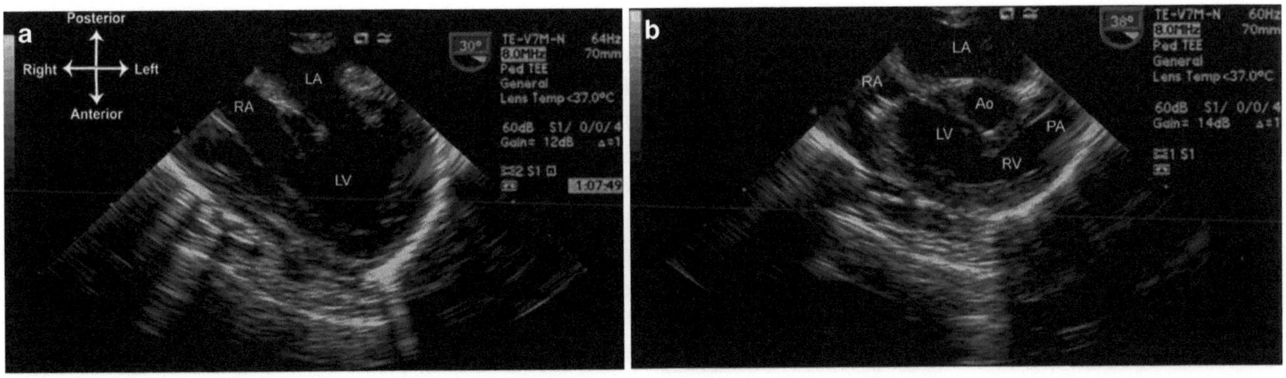

Fig. 10.6 Double inlet left ventricle, normally related great arteries (Holmes' heart) as viewed from the mid esophageal four chamber view. (**a**) A multiplane angle of 30° is used to visualize both atrioventricular valves. (**b**) Rotation of multiplane angle to approximately 40° and probe tip anteflexion demonstrate the origin of the pulmonary artery from the hypoplastic right ventricular outflow chamber (*RV*). *Ao* aorta, *LA* left atrium, *LV* left ventricle, *PA* pulmonary artery, *RA* right atrium

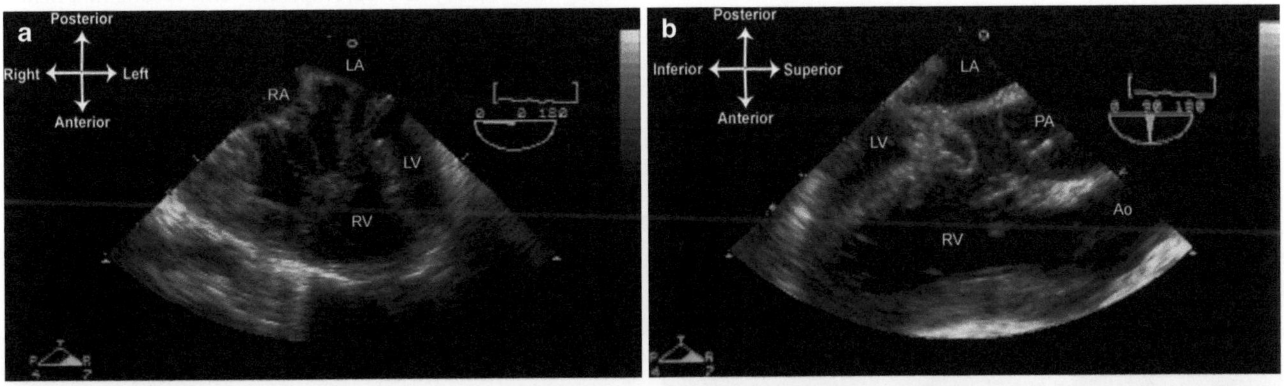

Fig. 10.7 Double inlet, double outlet right ventricle. (**a**) This image is obtained from the mid esophageal four chamber view. Both right and left atrioventricular valves drain into the large right ventricle (*RV*), inserting into a large, bizarre RV papillary muscle. There is a hypoplastic left sided left ventricle (*LV*). (**b**) Equivalent of the mid esophageal aortic valve long axis (90°) view. Both great arteries are seen to arise from the RV, with the aorta anterior to pulmonary artery. *Ao* aorta, *LA* left atrium, *PA* pulmonary artery, *RA* right atrium

are prominent muscle bundles in the large RV chamber; occasionally a large muscle bar is present that can be confused for a remnant of ventricular septum [35]. Usually, both great arteries also emerge from the same large RV, thus this lesion is often termed a double inlet, double outlet RV [35]. However unlike DILV, no anterior outflow chamber is visible. Instead, a rudimentary LV chamber may or may not be present; when present, it is located posteriorly, with no outflow to either great artery (Fig. 10.7, Video 10.6). Varying degrees of obstruction to one of the great arteries (generally the pulmonary trunk) can also be seen [36].

In the true single ventricle, there is no visible second chamber, and the large solitary ventricle has a very primitive morphology that eludes definitive identification as either an RV or LV [4, 33, 37]. There can be either one or two AV valves emptying into the large chamber, or there can even be one large common AV valve (i.e. a large common AV canal). Often, the heart has a very primitive appearance, with bizarre and loose muscular trabeculations seen in the large ventricular cavity. The great arteries have a variable relationship, generally with either stenosis of the aortic or pulmonary artery outflow tracts. There is a higher prevalence of atrial isomerism with indeterminate ventricular morphology [38].

Evaluation of the univentricular heart by TEE is similar to the evaluation of tricuspid atresia. The views of the inflows are best obtained beginning with the lower esophageal situs short axis (LE Situs SAX), first using a multiplane angle of 0–20°, then withdrawing the probe to visualize the junction between IVC and right atrium. Further withdrawal of the probe to the ME 4 Ch view demonstrates the AV valve(s) by imaging. Both color flow and spectral Doppler are necessary to evaluate AV valve function. When two AV valves are present, if either AV valve is stenotic or atretic, patency of the atrial septum must be assessed both by imaging and color flow Doppler. The relationship of the great arteries must also be determined; if one of these arises from a smaller outflow chamber, the VSD/BVF size and patency also need to be evaluated, preferably from several multiplane angles between 0 and 90°. Any subpulmonary or subaortic stenosis can be well visualized from a ME RV In-Out, ME AV LAX, and ME LAX views, multiplane angles between 70° and 120°, optimized to yield the best longitudinal view of

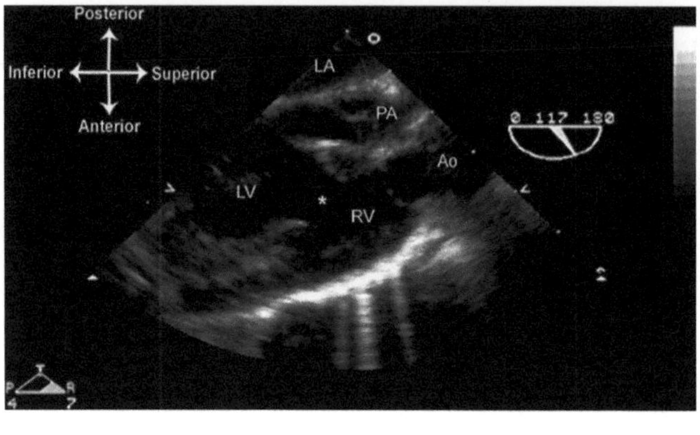

Fig. 10.8 Double inlet left ventricle, D-transposed great arteries, following pulmonary artery band placement. The mid esophageal aortic valve long axis view, multiplane angle of 117°, optimally demonstrates the long axis of both outflow tracts, and also shows the ventricular septal defect/bulboventricular foramen (*). This view also captures the left atrium and both ventricles in the same cross-sectional plane as the two outflow tracts. *Ao* aorta, *LA* left atrium, *LV* left ventricle, *PA* pulmonary artery, *RV* right ventricle

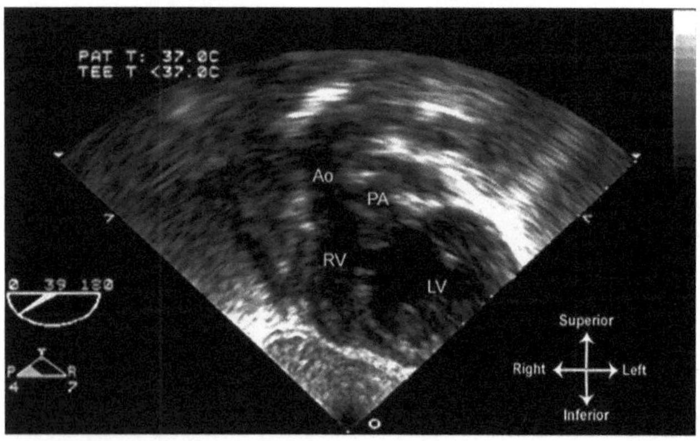

Fig. 10.9 Image from same patient as depicted in Fig. 10.8 obtained from a deep transgastric long axis view, multiplane angle of 39°. Both outflow tracts are displayed. This view offers an excellent angle for spectral Doppler evaluation of the outflow tracts. *Ao* aorta, *LV* left ventricle, *PA* pulmonary artery, *RV* right ventricle

the outflow tract (Fig. 10.8, Video 10.7). When available, the deep transgastric windows (DTG LAX, DTG Sagittal) provide good visualization of a number of structures, including the VSD/BVF, as well as excellent angles of Doppler interrogation for gradients across either the aortic or pulmonary outflow tracts (Fig. 10.9).

As with tricuspid atresia, left juxtaposition of the atrial appendages is also associated with DILV and D-transposed great arteries, and care should be taken not to confuse this entity with a large atrial septal defect.

Heterotaxy

Despite an external appearance of right-left symmetry, much of the human body's internal organ layout is in fact asymmetric, and this asymmetry leads to a definition of normal (and abnormal) sidedness. In *situs solitus* (which typifies most humans), the liver and IVC are on the right, the stomach and aorta on the left. The heart, being an asymmetric organ, also lateralizes to lie in the left chest. In *situs inversus*, the organs lateralize to the opposite side, producing a "mirror image" layout of the heart, lungs, and abdominal viscera. The term *heterotaxy* denotes an abnormality of laterality, or sidedness, in which there is (paradoxically) bilateral visceroatrial symmetry. Hence this condition is known as *situs ambiguous* or *atrial isomerism* and involves multiple organ systems in the body, including the heart. From a genetic standpoint, it is now known that heterotaxy belongs to a class of abnormalities known as "ciliopathies", characterized by abnormalities or dysfunction of primary cilia. During cardiac embryogenesis, primary cilia on the embryonic node are required for generation of the left-right axis. Ciliary dysfunction abnormalities are responsible for disorders of left-right axis determination during early embryonic development. This results in a disorder of laterality, manifested by abnormalities of any internal organ that is asymmetrically position—including the heart. Significant phenotypic variation can result [39, 40].

Patients with heterotaxy generally have significant cardiac abnormalities, often affecting multiple segments of the heart [41–43]. However despite the myriad potential variations in cardiac anatomy, heterotaxy patients tend to fall into one of two categories: (1) right isomerism (bilateral right-sidedness), or **asplenia**; (2) left isomerism (bilateral left-sidedness), or **polysplenia**. The visceral and cardiac variants most commonly seen with each category are listed in Table 10.2. It is important to note, however, that this table lists only the most commonly associated features seen with each category, and a number of exceptions have been reported, as well as considerable overlap between the two categories.

For most heterotaxy patients, especially those with right isomerism (asplenia), the preponderance of cardiac abnormalities—particularly hypoplasia of one ventricle—dictates that a single ventricle pathway be chosen [44, 45]. However in a small percentage of patients (mainly those with left isomerism, or polysplenia), a two ventricle approach can be contemplated [46, 47]. Therefore when a TEE evaluation of either right or left isomerism is performed, a very careful and comprehensive evaluation is recommended in consideration of the implications regarding patient management. Because of potential for anatomic abnormalities at multiple levels, a complete, segmental examination (Chap. 4) should be performed, particularly in those patients with unknown or uncertain anatomy. Using the many available TEE views discussed in Chap. 4 as well as this chapter, careful attention should be paid to systemic and pulmonary venous drainage, number and function of the AV valves, ventricular size and function, great artery position, and possible outflow tract stenosis. In the intraoperative setting, the examination also needs to be tailored to the important surgical questions that must be answered for the proposed surgery. For example, if Fontan surgery is contemplated, evaluation of systemic and pulmonary venous drainage is paramount (Fig. 10.10, Video 10.8)

Table 10.2 Right vs. left isomerism: common anatomic features

	Right isomerism (asplenia)	Left isomerism (polysplenia)
Liver	Midline, symmetric	Asymmetric or symmetric
Lungs	Bilateral tri-lobe	Bilateral bi-lobe
	Eparterial bronchi	Hyparterial bronchi
Spleen	Usually absent, but rarely can be multiple	Usually multiple, but can be only one or absent
Cardiac position	Dextrocardia (36–41 %)	Dextrocardia (33–42 %)
Systemic venous drainage	Bilateral SVCs are common	Interrupted hepatic segment of IVC; azygous or hemiazygous continuation to right or left SVC
	Coronary sinus usually unroofed	One or both SVCs can be present; if two SVCs, one generally drains into a coronary sinus
	IVC usually present; IVC and hepatic veins return together to common atrium	Separate hepatic drainage to atrium
	There can be separate drainage of hepatic veins	
Pulmonary venous drainage	Anomalous pulmonary venous drainage to systemic vein (62–88 %)	Usually to back of common atrium; abnormal position of atrial septum results in right veins to right side, left veins to left side
	Can return directly to heart, often via a common collector	
Atria and atrial septum	Bilatral right atrial appendages	Bilateral left atrial appendages
	Usually common atrium; small remaining atrial septal remnants	Usually common atrium; if atrial septum present, usually primum atrial septal defects
AV valve	Large common AV valve, often RV dominant	Two AV valves (common AV valve can also be seen)
Ventricles	Usually large RV, hypoplastic LV	Can be two balanced ventricles or one dominant ventricle
Ventricular outflow tracts	Often subvalvar/valvar pulmonary stenosis or atresia (88–96 %)	Valvar/subvalvar pulmonary stenosis (about 40 %) and aortic obstruction/atresia (17–22 %)
	Rarely, aortic stenosis/atresia/coarctation	
Ventriculo-arterial relationships	DORV (82 %)/TGA (9 %); often subvalvar/valvar pulmonary stenosis or atresia (88–96 %)	Normally related great arteries (50–84 %); DORV or ventriculo-arterial discordance (16–37 %);
	Rarely, aortic stenosis/atresia/coarctation	

AV atrioventricular, *DORV* double outlet right ventricle, *IVC* inferior vena cava, *LV* left ventricle, *RV* right ventricle, *SVC* superior vena cava

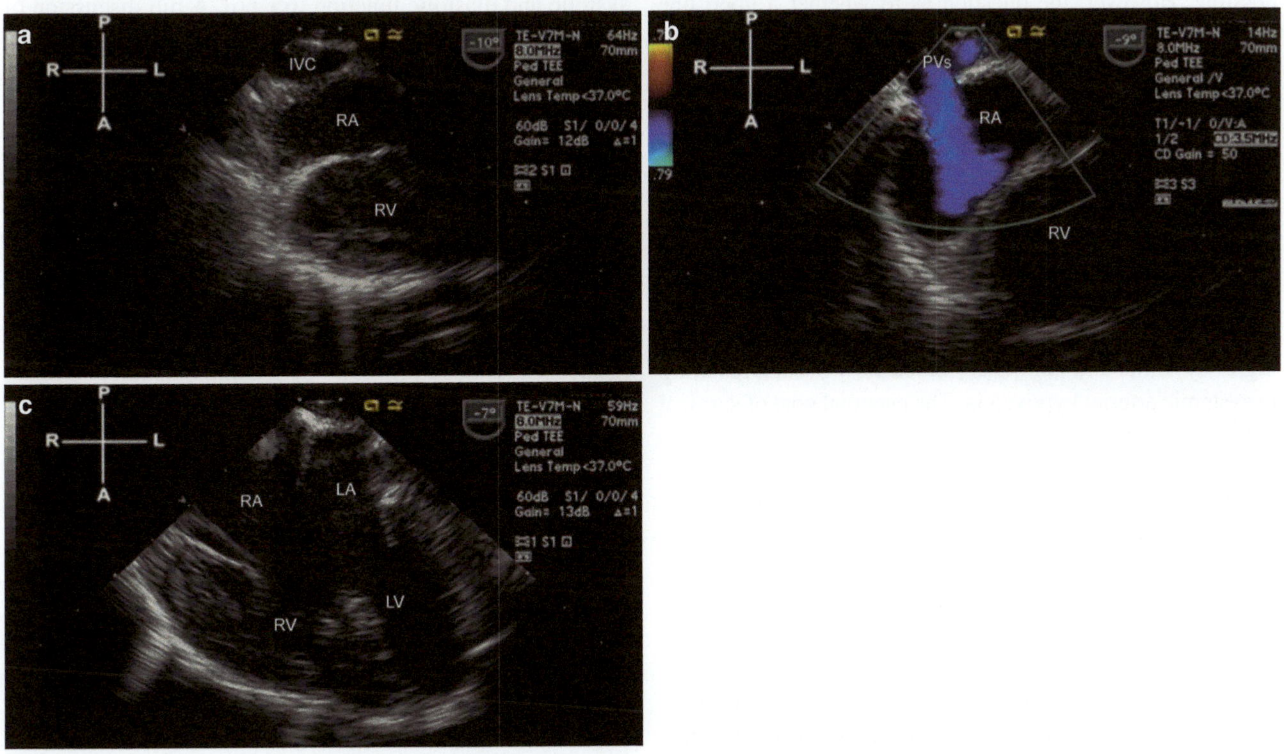

Fig. 10.10 Pre-Fontan study in a patient with right isomerism (asplenia) and double outlet right ventricle/pulmonary atresia. (**a**) Is obtained using multiplane angle 0° after withdrawal of the TEE probe from a lower to mid esophageal position. The inferior vena cava (*IVC*) receives the right hepatic veins and returns to the right atrium. In (**b**) the pulmonary veins are shown as they also return to the right sided atrium. (**c**) Demonstrates the presence of an unbalanced atrioventricular septal defect, right dominant. *LA* left atrium, *LV* left ventricle, *PVs* pulmonary veins, *RA* right atrium, *RV* right ventricle

Other Types of Single Ventricle

There are a number of other forms of complex congenital heart disease that—for one reason or another—fall under the "single ventricle" umbrella, even if they have two AV valves and two ventricles. In some patients, both ventricles are well-formed but other intracardiac features make a two ventricle repair unfeasible or undesirable, and therefore these patients are placed on a single ventricle pathway. Such complicating features include straddling/overriding AV valves, or double outlet RV with a VSD that is remote from either semilunar valve and makes two ventricle repair a high-risk proposition [48–50]. There are also some rare, complex cardiac defects that historically do not lend themselves well to a two ventricle repair. These include some forms of double outlet LV [51], superior-inferior ventricles with criss-cross AV relations [52, 53], etc. In many of these cases, there exist significant intracardiac abnormalities in addition to right or left ventricular hypoplasia.

When TEE is performed in patients with one of these complex cardiac lesions, a complete evaluation should be performed, with specific attention paid to AV valve size and orientation, ventricular chamber size and location of ventricular septal defect(s), and great artery relationships. In some cases, information from the TEE will be utilized to render an assessment as to whether a two ventricle repair is feasible. Currently, the bias for most clinicians caring for CHD patients is to perform a two ventricle repair whenever possible. However, the question as to whether a good one ventricle repair is better than a marginal two ventricle repair remains unanswered and is, in many instances, controversial [54–56].

Surgery for the Single Ventricle

With a single ventricle and single ventricle physiology, there is only one functioning pump that must serve both systemic and pulmonary circulations. Because of this, obligatory mixing of systemic and pulmonary blood flow occurs, resulting in systemic arterial hypoxemia. The eventual goal of surgical management of the single ventricle is to restore normal systemic arterial oxygenation by separating the circulations; this is performed by rerouting systemic venous (deoxygenated) blood directly into the pulmonary arteries, thereby bypassing the heart. Deoxygenated blood is expected to flow directly to the pulmonary arteries without the aid of a cardiac pumping chamber [57]. This is known as the Fontan procedure, which is named and based upon the original surgery described in 1971 by Fontan and Baudet for treatment of tricuspid atresia [58]. Over the past 40+ years the Fontan procedure has undergone a number of modifications and improvements, and has gained widespread acceptance as the preferred surgical management strategy for all forms of single ventricle [59]. It has been clearly established that, even without the aid of a right-sided pumping chamber, Fontan physiology is compatible with long-term survival and good functional status [60]. There are still a number of ongoing questions regarding long-term morbidity (arrhythmias, protein-losing enteropathy, liver dysfunction, ventricular dysfunction, plastic bronchitis, etc.) and survivability into late adulthood; these topics are beyond the scope of the current chapter but are fully discussed in many other references [59, 61–64].

While the ultimate goal for all single ventricle patients is the Fontan procedure and achievement of Fontan physiology, the complete Fontan operation cannot be performed in neonates or young infants because of a still immature pulmonary vascular bed, and still developing neonatal myocardium. The ideal timing for the Fontan procedure is generally felt to be after 2–3 years of age [65, 66]. Therefore, assuming single ventricle patients are correctly diagnosed in early infancy, almost all will require one or more staging surgeries prior to the Fontan procedure. The purpose of these staging surgeries is to ensure that patients are optimally prepared for their eventual Fontan procedure. For successful Fontan physiology, certain key anatomic and physiologic factors should ideally be present, including adequate size pulmonary arteries, low pulmonary arteriolar resistance, no more than mild AV valve regurgitation, and normal ventricular systolic and diastolic function [65, 66]. A full discussion of these important factors can be found in many references [59, 63, 67–70].

Different institutions utilize TEE to varying degrees for the various surgical procedures performed as part of single ventricle surgical pathway. Nonetheless, TEE can provide useful and important information. Preoperative evaluation of single ventricle patients by TEE is generally excellent due to its superior imaging capabilities. However, most preoperative single ventricle patients will have already undergone extensive imaging by several different modalities, hence TEE is used primarily as a complementary imaging technique, e.g. when assessment of AV valve function is desired in a larger patient with poor transthoracic imaging. For postoperative assessment, TEE can play a more prominent role. It is well known that postoperative single ventricle patients, particularly Fontan patients, are notoriously difficult to image by transthoracic echocardiography. Therefore TEE can provide a much greater contribution in the assessment of such patients, most notably in the immediate postoperative period. The following section discusses the important preoperative and postoperative features that can and should be assessed by TEE, whenever it is performed in single ventricle patients.

Preoperative Assessment

The preceding sections of this chapter detailed individual defects considered part of the single ventricle spectrum, including specific anatomic characteristics that should be evaluated. While considerable anatomic heterogeneity exists among the different classes of defects, what becomes evident is that certain common anatomic and functional characteristics must be explored whenever a TEE is performed for preoperative assessment. These characteristics are relevant not only for the patient's current clinical condition, but also for any future palliative surgeries that might be contemplated. The list of potential surgeries for single ventricle palliation is limited (as will be discussed below), thus certain key anatomic features carry great weight—and therefore assume particular relevance—in the preoperative evaluation of these patients. Some of the features were mentioned previously for the individual cardiac lesions, but the following list summarizes the essential elements that should be addressed during preoperative assessment of all such patients:

- **Systemic venous return**. The goal of single ventricle palliation is the return of all systemic venous blood directly to the pulmonary arteries. Thus, detailed knowledge of systemic venous return is essential. Although in most cases systemic venous drainage will have been adequately delineated prior to surgery, in many instances TEE can provide helpful confirmatory information. The presence/absence of the hepatic portion of IVC and the drainage of the hepatic veins should be verified. In some patients, particularly those with visceral heterotaxy, some hepatic veins can drain separately from the IVC and directly into the atrium (Fig. 10.11, Video 10.9). In others, particularly those patients with polysplenia (left isomerism), the hepatic portion of the IVC can be absent (interrupted IVC with azygos continuation) and there can be separate entrances of right and left hepatic veins into the atria. Advancing the TEE probe to the lower esophageal position (LE Situs SAX, multiplane angle 0–20°), with careful withdrawal and clockwise/counterclockwise turning of the TEE probe, can demonstrate the sites of IVC and hepatic vein drainage. Identification of the SVC drainage is also very important: both the number of SVCs (one vs. two), and their sites of drainage, should be determined. This can be performed by withdrawing the TEE probe to the mid/upper esophagus, including the mid esophageal ascending aortic short axis (ME Asc Ao SAX) and UE PA LAX views (both using a multiplane angle 0°), and rotating clockwise and counterclockwise. It is important to search directly for a separate right and left SVC and not rely upon the presence/absence of a dilated coronary sinus, because the coronary sinus could be unroofed or absent, allowing left SVC return directly to the atrium. Sagittal views of both SVCs can then be obtained in the mid to upper esophageal position, multiplane angle at approximately 80–90°, using a combination of views including ME Bicaval, mid esophageal ascending aortic long axis (ME Asc Ao LAX) with rightward rotation to visualize a right SVC, and ME 2 Ch, ME Asc Ao LAX, and UE Ao Arch (all with leftward rotation) to visualize a left SVC. With these sagittal views, azygos or hemiazygos drainage to the SVC can sometimes be seen coursing posteriorly and over the corresponding branch pulmonary artery.
- **Pulmonary venous return**. In general, pulmonary venous drainage will have been established with imaging studies performed prior to the TEE. Nonetheless, in some single ventricle patients the drainage of the pulmonary veins might not be completely clear. The role of the preoperative TEE is to confirm the drainage of all pulmonary veins, and establish that this drainage is unobstructed. Because of the close proximity of the esophagus to the atria, TEE generally provides excellent visualization of pulmonary venous return, both for imaging and color

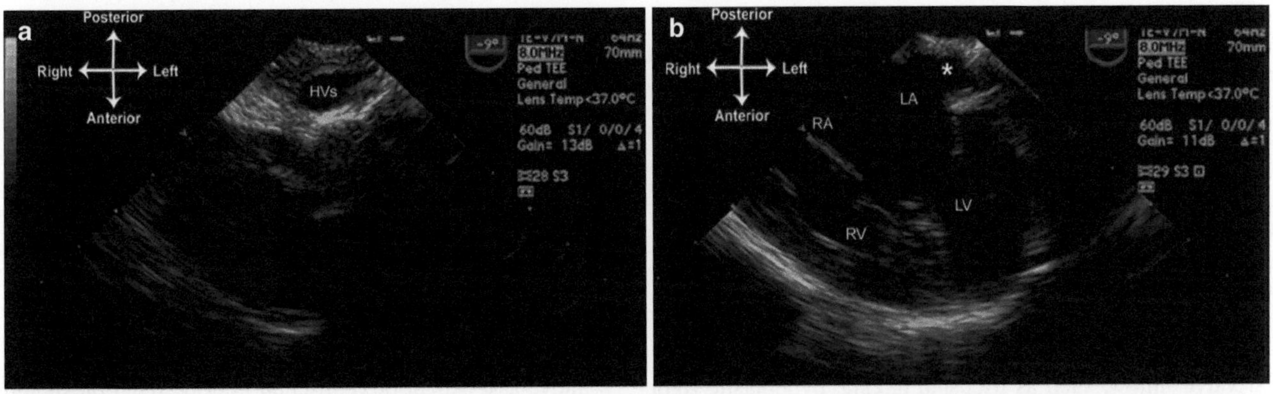

Fig. 10.11 Image from patient in Fig. 10.10. The left sided hepatic veins return separately to the left sided atrium (**a**). The entrance of these veins into the left atrium is marked by an asterisk (**b**). *HVs* left hepatic veins, *LA* left atrium, *LV* left ventricle, *RA* right atrium, *RV* right ventricle

flow/spectral Doppler evaluation (Chaps. 4 and 6). Any obstruction to pulmonary venous flow must be noted, because it will have negative consequences for further single ventricle palliation [71, 72]. The relationship of the pulmonary venous return to the systemic veins should also be noted, as the placement of a Fontan conduit could potentially interfere with pulmonary venous return, and surgical adjustments might be required [73].

- **Patency of the atrial septum**. An unrestrictive atrial septal defect is essential in those patients in whom systemic or pulmonary venous return empties into an atrial chamber associated with a stenotic or absent AV valve, or a hypoplastic/nonfunctional ventricular chamber (e.g. tricuspid atresia or HLHS). In such cases, the only pathway for egress of blood from the chamber is through the atrial communication. Using TEE, this can be evaluated both by imaging as well as color flow/spectral Doppler interrogation. Midesophageal views with a multiplane angle of 0–90° (ME 4 Ch, ME Bicaval) can be used, combined with other probe maneuvers such as advancement/withdrawal and left/right rotation. There are two types of restrictive atrial communication: with left to right shunting, and with right to left shunting. A restrictive *left to right* atrial communication is found in those defects in which there is left sided obstruction, such as HLHS and DILV with left AV valve stenosis/atresia. In these cases, atrial restriction is characterized by a number of findings, including: (a) small size (diameter <3 mm); (b) color flow Doppler aliasing of the atrial shunt and a mean gradient >5 mmHg [74]; (c) dilated pulmonary veins, along with prominent flow reversal in these structures; (e) dilated left atrium, with an atrial septum bowing toward the right (although a large left atrium does not always indicate a restrictive atrial communication); (f) in HLHS patients, a small left atrium with thick atrial septum [75]. The incidence of atrial septal restriction in HLHS patients is estimated between 6 and 20 % [75–78]. When the atrial septal communication is felt to be restrictive, it often requires enlargement, either by interventional cardiology procedures such as balloon dilation/stenting of the septum, or an atrial septectomy at the time of surgery. In HLHS patients with a restrictive atrial septal defect, emergent atrial septostomy is sometimes necessary, though mortality is much higher in this subset of patients [76, 78, 79]. This has led to development of *in utero* atrial septoplasty in HLHS patients prenatally diagnosed as having a restrictive atrial septal defect [80].

  A restrictive *right to left* atrial communication is found in those defects in which there is obstruction to right AV valve inflow, such as tricuspid atresia, hypoplastic right heart syndrome, or DILV with right AV valve stenosis/atresia. In these cases the restriction can be more challenging to determine; unlike HLHS and other left sided obstruction, the atrial septum is often redundant and it can be difficult to define accurately the margins of the atrial defect. Moreover, in some patients restriction might not be apparent immediately after birth, but can increase with time [81]. This type of atrial septal restriction occurs in 5–15 % of tricuspid atresia patients [82, 83]. Overall, less data is available in this group of patients. One study has shown that an atrial septal aneurysm (defined as bulging >6 mm beyond the plane of the atrial septum) and atrial septal defect diameter <5 mm (measured on the 2D echocardiographic image) places tricuspid atresia patients at higher risk for atrial septal restriction [83].
- **Atrioventricular valve (AV) function**. The AV valve(s) should be examined structurally in terms of the leaflets, support apparatus, and annular size. The function of the valves should be assessed as well. This is accomplished by two-dimensional imaging as well as color flow mapping and spectral Doppler. In single ventricle patients, the presence and degree of AV valve regurgitation can have significant bearing on clinical outcomes [84]. In patients with two AV valves (e.g. double inlet LV), the function of both valves should be examined. If one valve is excessively regurgitant, and the other valve competent and of adequate size, the regurgitant valve can be repaired or even oversewn. If one AV valve is significantly stenotic or atretic, a large atrial defect is mandatory to allow atrial blood to pass unobstructed to the other AV valve (as noted above). For the TEE evaluation of the AV valves, the mid esophageal views (ME 4 Ch, ME 2 Ch, ME Mitral, ME LAX) are useful to evaluate valve morphology and function. Additional information regarding chordal and papillary muscle architecture can be provided by the transgastric views: the "short axis" transgastric views (TG Basal SAX, TG Mid SAX) and "long axis" transgastric views (TG 2 Ch, TG LAX, and transgastric RV inflow or TG RV In) views. Given the unusual orientation of the AV valve(s) in many forms of single ventricles, variation in multiplane angle between 0° and 120° in many of these views might be necessary to facilitate optimal visualization. In some instances the deep transgastric views (DTG LAX, DTG Sagittal) can be useful for *en face* evaluation of the AV valves.
- **Ventricular systolic and diastolic function**. Ventricular function plays an essential role in the short and long-term viability of the patient with a single ventricle. However given the unusual and often distorted geometry of many forms of single ventricle, it can be difficult if not impossible to provide accurate quantification of ventricular systolic function, particularly within the time constraints of the intraoperative setting. Nonetheless some type of qualitative assessment of ventricular systolic function should be performed, even if it falls under a somewhat subjective assessment range of "*normal*" to "*mild-moderate-severely depressed*". Any regional wall motion abnormality, including segmental ventricular hypokinesis or dyskinesis,

should be recorded and noted. If time permits, assessment of diastolic and global cardiac function can be performed by analysis of AV valve inflow and tissue Doppler analysis, and other measurements such as the myocardial performance (Tei) index [85–88]. Again, given the abnormal geometry in many single ventricle patients, the utility of standard two-dimensional echocardiographic measurements remains to be determined. The TEE analysis of ventricular function is discussed in detailed in Chap. 5.

- **Ventricular septal defect (VSD) or bulboventricular foramen (BVF)**. Very rarely does a single ventricle patient actually possess only one ventricular chamber. More commonly, there is a large functional ventricular chamber and a smaller, nonfunctional chamber. The connection between these two chambers occurs via a VSD of variable size. In many instances the small ventricular chamber derives solely from the embryologic bulbus cordis, and accepts no AV valve tissue, hence the communication is termed the "bulboventricular foramen" or BVF as previously noted. In those cases in which the aorta arises from the smaller ventricular chamber (e.g. tricuspid atresia or DILV with transposed great arteries), a small VSD/BVF can result in significant subaortic obstruction which, if not addressed, can lead to significant ventricular hypertrophy as well as systolic/diastolic dysfunction (all negative risk factors for subsequent Fontan physiology). Progression of VSD/BVF obstruction can also occur over time after palliative interventions and even after the Fontan procedure [89]. Therefore a careful assessment of the VSD/BVF and subaortic anatomic region must be performed to determine whether this issue needs to be addressed, either by enlargement of the VSD/BVF, a palliative arterial switch operation, or a Damus-Kaye-Stansel procedure (see below). The TEE assessment of the VSD/BVF consists of anatomic evaluation from the mid esophageal window (Fig. 10.8), and linear measurements of diameter should be obtained in at least two orthogonal planes (for example, ME 4 Ch at 0° and ME 2 Ch at 90°). Using measurements of a major and minor axis, Matitiau et al. found that the cross-sectional area of the VSD/BVF can be estimated using the formula of an ellipse (major diameter × minor diameter × $\pi/4$); a cross-sectional area <2 cm^2/m^2 was found to be predictive of subsequent VSD/BVF obstruction [90]. However, this formula might be simplistic because in many cases, the cross-sectional profile of the defect is asymmetric and irregular. Depending upon the location and orientation of the defect, the Doppler gradient across the VSD/BVF can also be obtained by the mid esophageal views (ME 4 Ch, ME LAX, ME AV LAX, etc.), generally with multiplane angles approximating 80–90°, or from the deep transgastric window (DTG LAX, DTG Sagittal) with probe anteflexion. The Doppler-derived gradient can be quantified using the simplified Bernoulli equation: **maximum instantaneous pressure gradient** $= 4V^2$, with V equal to the maximum velocity (meters/second) obtained by continuous wave Doppler (see also Chaps. 1 and 5). However spectral Doppler evaluation across a VSD/BVF can be misleading, because in the presence of a large unobstructed pulmonary valve, there might not be increased flow velocity across the VSD/BVF, even with a potentially restrictive ventricular communication. The reason for this is that an elevated pressure will not develop in the ventricular chamber proximal to the VSD/BVF, as blood flow "decompresses" through the large pulmonary valve. Thus 2D anatomic evaluation of the VSD/BVF is much more valuable for assessment. The native aortic valve annulus and ascending aorta (if visible) can also be visualized and measured using ME AV LAX, ME Asc Ao LAX and UE Ao Arch SAX views (multiplane angle 80–110°). Concurrent aortic and aortic arch anomalies (hypoplasia, interruption) are associated with significantly smaller VSD/BVF areas, however other imaging modalities (transthoracic echocardiography, MRI) are often needed to assess these [91].
- **Outflow tract and semilunar valve patency and function**. The size and patency of the outflow tracts and semilunar valves should be assessed during the TEE examination. Standard mid-esophageal views—ME 4 Ch, ME LAX, ME AV LAX, ME AV SAX, ME RV In-Out—are usually adequate to provide evaluation of these structures. Deep transgastric views (DTG LAX, DTG Sagittal) are useful for Doppler interrogation of flow across the valves. If one semilunar valve is hypoplastic or stenotic, the flow across the valve should be evaluated by color flow Doppler and the Doppler-derived gradient quantified by spectral Doppler, using the simplified Bernoulli equation described above. It should be noted that the gradient estimated by continuous wave Doppler represents a maximum instantaneous gradient, and therefore tends to overestimate the true peak to peak gradient as obtained by direct manometric measurement. Nonetheless it serves as a reasonable approximation. With the heterogeneity of single ventricle anatomy, it is impossible to stipulate a "best" view for spectral Doppler; the best window is the one that provides the most favorable Doppler angle of interrogation. Color flow Doppler should also be used for evaluation of the presence/degree of regurgitation of either semilunar valve, particularly in those cases in which a Damus-Kaye-Stansel or Norwood repair is contemplated, or in those patients who have already undergone these procedures.
- **Main and branch pulmonary artery architecture**. Pulmonary artery size and anatomy are two of the most important factors related to the eventual outcome of the single ventricle patient [65, 69, 92, 93]. Unfortunately the visualization of the pulmonary arteries by TEE is quite variable, and therefore TEE should not be the expected or preferred method for evaluation of pulmonary artery size or stenoses. When TEE does provide visualization of the

branch pulmonary arteries, features such as ductus arteriosus flow, and the sizes of the proximal right and left branch pulmonary arteries can be measured and compared. However, one cannot expect to rely consistently upon TEE assessment of pulmonary artery size and anatomy when planning surgical management.

Surgical Interventions for Single Ventricle and Their Assessment by TEE

Modified Blalock-Taussig and Central Shunts

The modified Blalock-Taussig shunt and its related variant, the central shunt, are mainstays of palliation for both one and two ventricle repairs. The purpose of these procedures is to augment pulmonary blood flow in patients with significant pulmonary stenosis or pulmonary atresia, thereby enhancing systemic arterial saturation. The original or classic Blalock-Taussig shunt involved ligation and division of the right subclavian artery, with the proximal portion turned down and anastomosed to the right pulmonary artery [94]. The modified Blalock-Taussig shunt was subsequently designed to preserve the blood flow to the distal right subclavian artery [95]. This modification involves a tube made of prosthetic material (generally 3.5–5 mm) anastomosed between the right subclavian or innominate artery at one end, and one of the branch pulmonary arteries at the other. The central shunt utilizes the same approach, but the connection of the shunt to the pulmonary artery is much more centrally placed; generally it is located on the main pulmonary artery at the bifurcation point of the two branch pulmonary arteries.

As noted previously, TEE visualization of the branch pulmonary arteries is highly variable. Moreover, visualization of the aortic head and neck vessels by TEE can be difficult. Therefore, TEE may have limited utility in the evaluation of the Blalock-Taussig or central shunt. The upper esophageal window must be used to visualize the shunt, using the upper esophageal aortic arch long axis (UE Ao Arch LAX) and UE PA LAX views; continuous color flow Doppler into a main or branch pulmonary artery confirms shunt patency (Fig. 10.12, Video 10.10). Continuous wave Doppler can be used to evaluate the gradient across the shunt, using the simplified

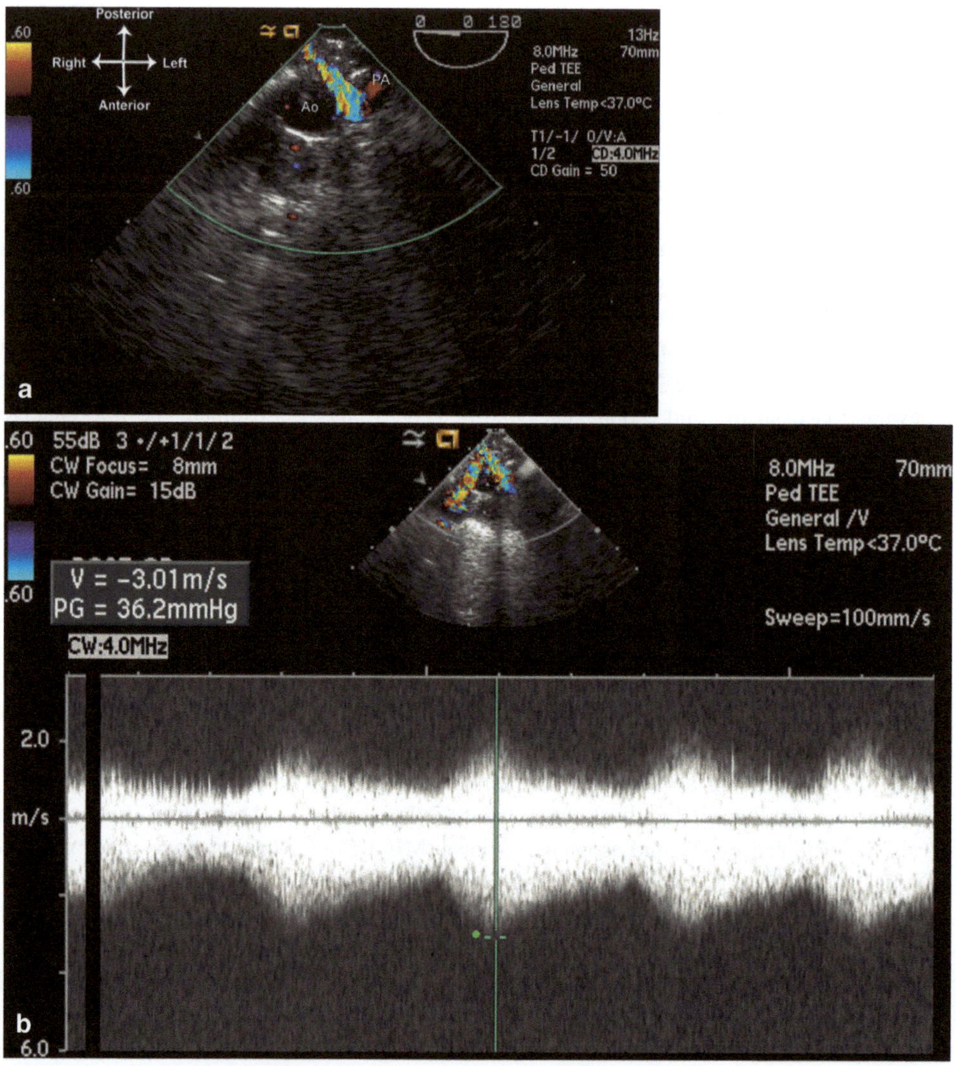

Fig. 10.12 Right modified Blalock-Taussig shunt, visualized from an upper esophageal pulmonary artery long axis view, multiplane angle 0°. (**a**) Flow entering the small right pulmonary artery by color Doppler. (**b**) Continuous flow as displayed by spectral Doppler. *Ao* ascending aorta, *PA* pulmonary artery

Bernoulli equation described above. The systolic pulmonary artery pressure can be estimated by the following equation:

$$\mathbf{PASP} = \mathbf{SBP} - 4V^2$$

PASP = Pulmonary artery systolic pressure (mmHg)
SBP = Systemic systolic pressure (mmHg)
V = Peak velocity (meters/second) across the shunt

As noted previously, the gradient estimated by continuous wave Doppler represents a maximal instantaneous gradient, and therefore tends to overestimate the true peak to peak gradient as obtained by direct manometric measurement. Moreover, because of sometimes unfavorable angles of interrogation, the calculated gradient might underestimate the true gradient across the shunt. Nonetheless with an optimally positioned spectral Doppler angle of interrogation, it can provide a reasonable approximation of the systolic pulmonary arterial pressure. A high gradient is generally desirable because it indicates a low pulmonary artery pressure (i.e. no pulmonary hypertension), while a low gradient could be indicative of elevated pulmonary artery pressure. With a change of the multiplane angle to 80–90° (UE Ao Arch LAX with rightward probe rotation), the length of the shunt can sometimes be visualized by a combination of imaging and color flow Doppler.

Pulmonary Artery Band

Banding of the pulmonary artery can be utilized in the surgical management of patients with biventricular circulations as well as those with a single ventricle. This procedure is performed to limit pulmonary blood flow in single ventricle patients with unobstructed antegrade flow into the main and branch pulmonary arteries. Such patients generally have pulmonary overcirculation leading to congestive heart failure, as well as high pressures in the pulmonary arteries. These two factors can lead to significant muscularization of the pulmonary arterioles and elevation of the pulmonary vascular resistance and pulmonary arterial pressures; these are known risk factors for subsequent single ventricle palliation [57, 70, 89]. Thus, the pulmonary artery band is placed both to limit pulmonary blood flow and to "protect" the pulmonary arteries from potentially detrimental exposure to high pressure and shear stress. The technical aspects of pulmonary artery band placement are relatively straightforward: a small length of material is placed around the main pulmonary artery, between the valve and pulmonary artery bifurcation, and restricts flow across the artery. Pressure gradients across the pulmonary artery band can be estimated by echocardiography or measured directly. One of the benefits of this surgical technique is that it can be performed quickly, without the use of cardiopulmonary bypass.

Band adjustments can be guided by TEE. This is best performed in the mid esophageal window (ME LAX, ME AV LAX, ME AV SAX, ME Asc Ao SAX, ME Asc Ao LAX), and upper esophageal window (UE Ao Arch SAX, UE Ao Arch LAX), with probe anteflexion and variable multiplane angles of interrogation from 0° to 90° depending upon the anatomy (Fig. 10.13a, b, Video 10.11). Alignment of the spectral Doppler cursor guided by two-dimensional and color flow mapping allows for estimation of the band gradient by continuous wave Doppler, using the simplified Bernoulli equation given above (peak velocity across the band is used for *V*). The deep transgastric window (DTG LAX, DTG Sagittal) can also be used for this evaluation (Fig. 10.13c–e, Video 10.11) Depending upon the spatial position of pulmonary artery in relation to the aorta (anterior vs. posterior), the most effective TEE view to obtain a band gradient will vary, and therefore the TEE probe will need to be manipulated accordingly to optimize Doppler interrogation of the band. Effective pulmonary artery banding produces a distal pulmonary artery systolic pressure about 30–50 % of systemic systolic arterial pressure [96]. Obviously the gradient across the band will depend upon systemic arterial pressure, but in general the gradient in a neonate will be between 40 and 70 mmHg (Doppler velocity about 3.2–4.2 m/s) [97]. For balanced single ventricle physiology (pulmonary: systemic flow ratio about 1:1), an optimal systemic arterial oxygen saturation is between 75 and 85 % [97, 98]. Also, with effective banding, there is often a shift in ventricular septal position that can be noted (if sufficient ventricular septum is present). Other features to evaluate include ventricular and AV valve function, which can be influenced by loading conditions. Longer-term issues to be assessed following pulmonary artery band placement include pulmonary valve competency (which can be adversely affected by a pulmonary artery band in close proximity), and possible migration of the pulmonary artery band distally, potentially impinging on one or both branch pulmonary arteries.

Damus-Kaye-Stansel Procedure

The Damus-Kaye-Stansel (DKS) procedure is considered for a single ventricle patient when there is potential or actual obstruction to blood flow through the native ascending aorta [99–101]. This could occur in patients such as those with transposition of great arteries and origin of the aorta from a small outflow chamber in the presence of a restrictive BVF (e.g. patients with tricuspid atresia or DILV), or in those with origin of the aorta from the larger ventricle, but with significant aortic or subaortic stenosis, or aortic atresia [102]. The DKS procedure involves transection of the native main pulmonary artery, and end to side anastomosis of the proximal main pulmonary artery to the ascending aorta, enabling unobstructed systemic output. The distal main pulmonary artery is oversewn, and pulmonary blood flow provided by either an aortopulmonary shunt or cavopulmonary connection (see below).

A standard preoperative TEE study is performed to evaluate intracardiac anatomy and the position and function of the semilunar valves, using the mid esophageal windows (ME

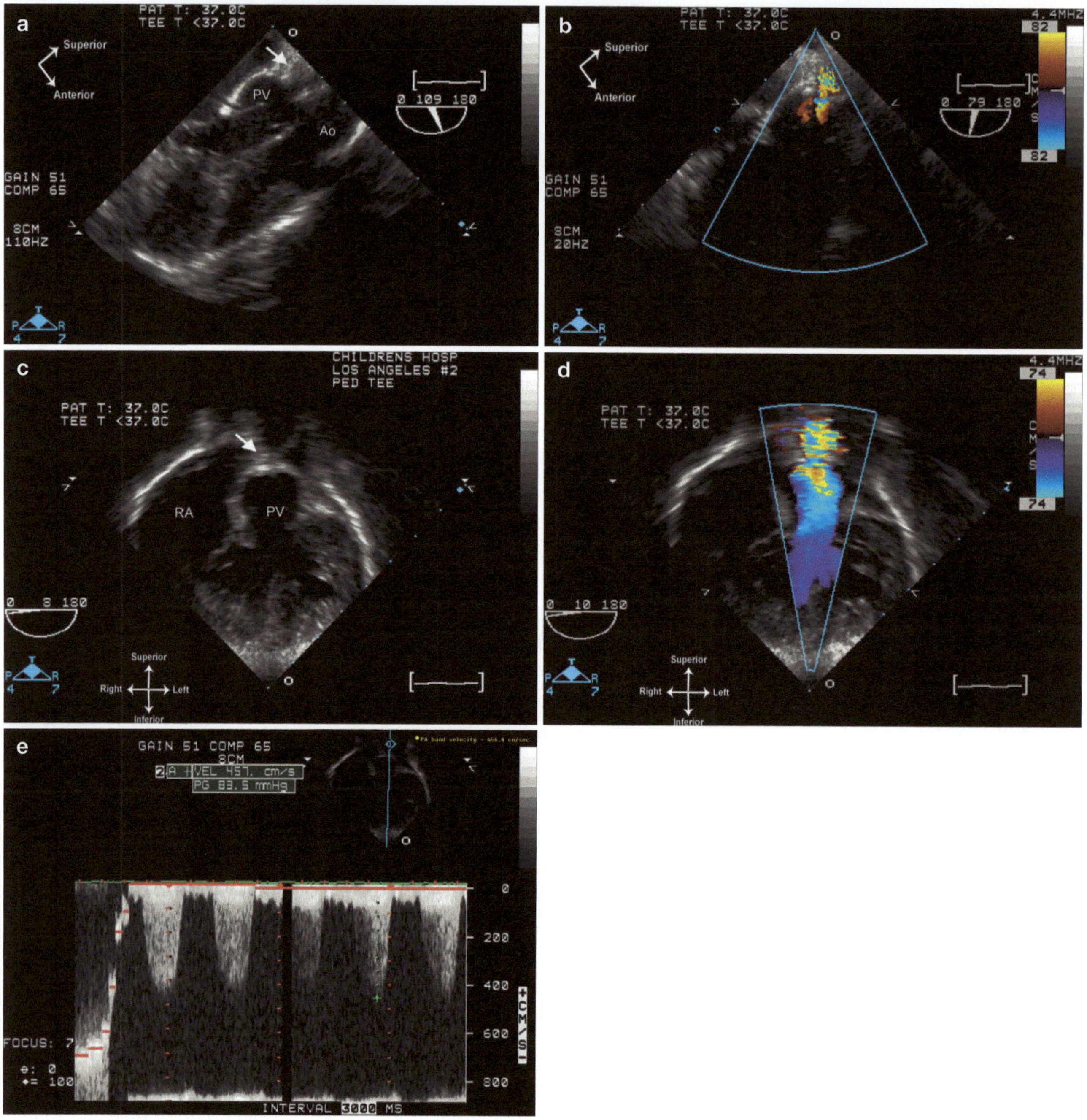

Fig. 10.13 Evaluation of pulmonary artery band. Two-dimensional image and color flow Doppler as seen from the mid esophageal long axis view (**a**, **b**) and deep transgastric long axis view (**c**, **d**). In both views, the location of the band above the pulmonary valve is indicated by the *arrow*. Note the excellent angle provided by the deep transgastric view for Doppler interrogation of the pulmonary band (**e**). *Ao* aorta, *PV* pulmonary valve, *RA* right atrium

LAX, ME AV SAX, ME AV LAX, ME LAX, ME RV In-Out) and varying multiplane angle to best display semilunar valve motion and function. Postoperatively, TEE can be used to assess patency of the great artery anastomosis as well as semilunar valve competence, which can sometimes be compromised during the procedure. Mid to upper esophageal views (ME Asc Ao LAX, ME Asc Ao SAX, UE PA LAX, UE Ao Arch SAX) obtained by multiplane imaging are useful for this evaluation (Fig. 10.14, Video 10.12) Significant semilunar valve regurgitation can prove detrimental to patient survival [103] (Fig. 10.15, Video 10.13). Ventricular and AV valve function should also be assessed.

As an alternative to the DKS procedure, a palliative arterial switch can be performed. This procedure, which is applicable when there are transposed great arteries with the aorta arising from the small outflow chamber (usually in the setting of tricuspid atresia or DILV), involves performing an arterial switch operation including a LeCompte maneuver to

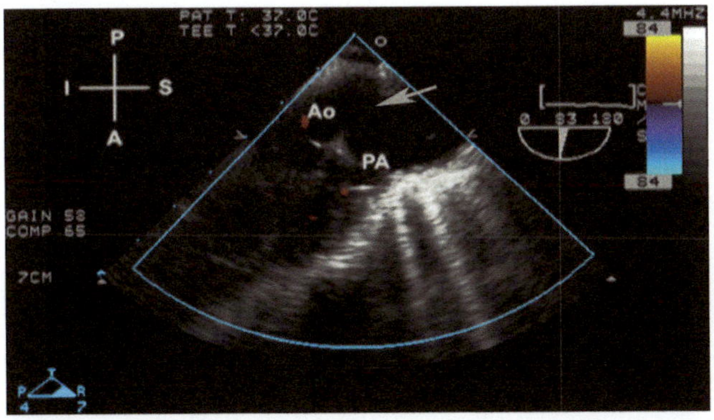

Fig. 10.14 Damus-Kaye-Stansel anastomosis as viewed from a mid esophageal ascending aortic long axis view, multiplane angle 80–90°. The widely patent anastomosis (shown by the *arrow*) lies just above the semilunar valves. *Ao* native aorta, *PA* native pulmonary artery

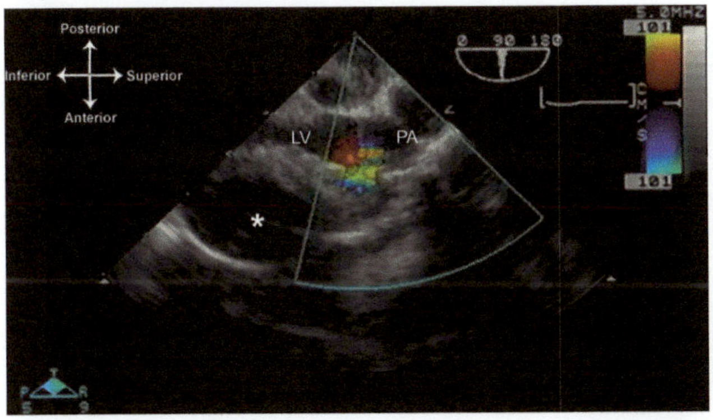

Fig. 10.15 Problematic Damus-Kaye-Stansel (DKS) in a patient with situs inversus, congenitally corrected transposition of the great arteries and hypoplastic right ventricle, as viewed from the equivalent of the mid esophageal aortic valve long axis view, multiplane angle about 90°. The creation of the DKS anastomosis resulted in distortion of the native pulmonary valve, producing significant regurgitation as shown by the color Doppler signal. The ventricular function was severely depressed. A large subpepicardial hematoma (*) occurred as the result of external cardiac massage. *LV* left ventricle, *PA* native pulmonary artery

"relocate" the aorta back to the larger ventricle [104, 105]. Control of pulmonary blood flow can be either from an aorto-pulmonary shunt (e.g. Blalock-Taussig or central shunt), or pulmonary artery band, as dictated by oxygen saturations. In some instances neither is required, as the degree of subpulmonary stenosis after the palliative arterial switch (formerly native subaortic stenosis) is adequate to provide enough pulmonary blood flow for acceptable systemic oxygenation, while at the same time maintaining low pulmonary arterial pressure.

Norwood Procedure

The Norwood procedure utilizes and extends the principle of the DKS procedure to those patients with significant hypoplasia of the ascending aorta and aortic arch. This procedure was initially developed for hypoplastic left heart syndrome patients [106], and has undergone a number of different modifications. The basic principle, however, remains as follows: the main pulmonary artery is disconnected

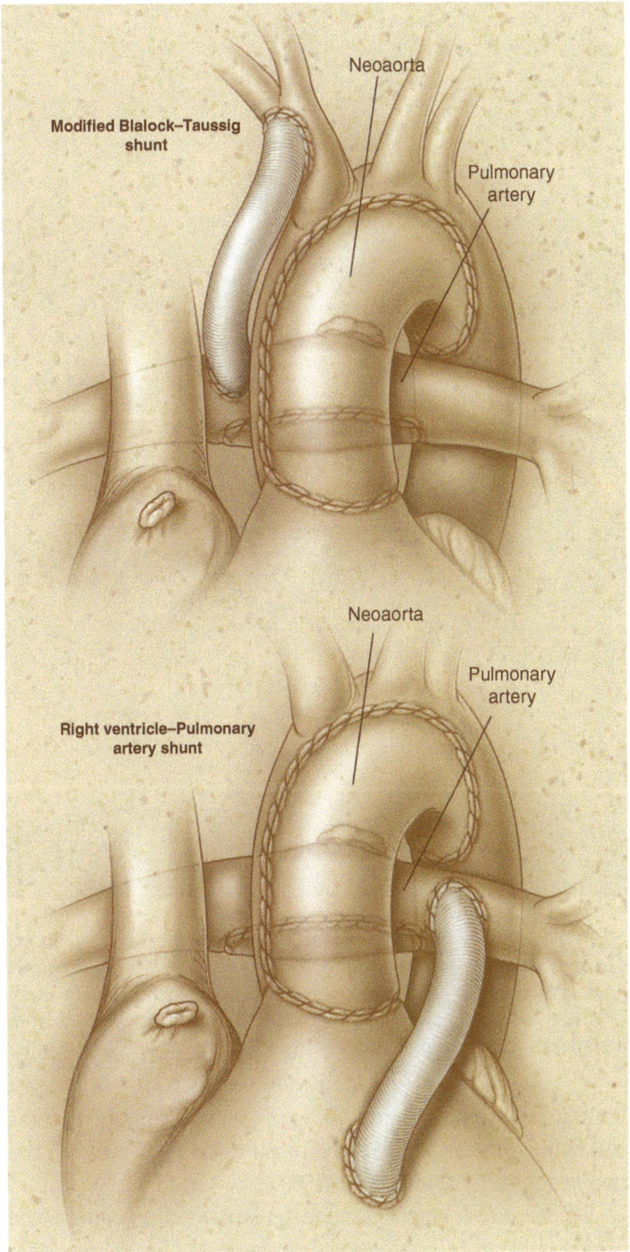

Fig. 10.16 Graphic of the Norwood procedure displaying modified Blalock-Taussig shunt in the *upper panel* and right ventricular to pulmonary artery (Sano) conduit in the *lower panel* (From: Ohye et al. [109]; Reprinted by permission, Massachusetts Medical Society)

from its branches and utilized to augment the hypoplastic ascending aorta and aortic arch, in essence creating a "neo-aorta". An atrial septectomy is performed, the disconnected branch pulmonary arteries are repaired, and pulmonary blood flow provided by either by a modified Blalock-Taussig shunt or a conduit placed between RV infundibulum and the main pulmonary artery (Sano modification) (Fig. 10.16) [107, 108]. Currently, institutions vary in their preference for the type of shunt (Blalock-Taussig vs. Sano modification). A recent randomized multicenter study comparing both shunt types showed better transplantation-free survival

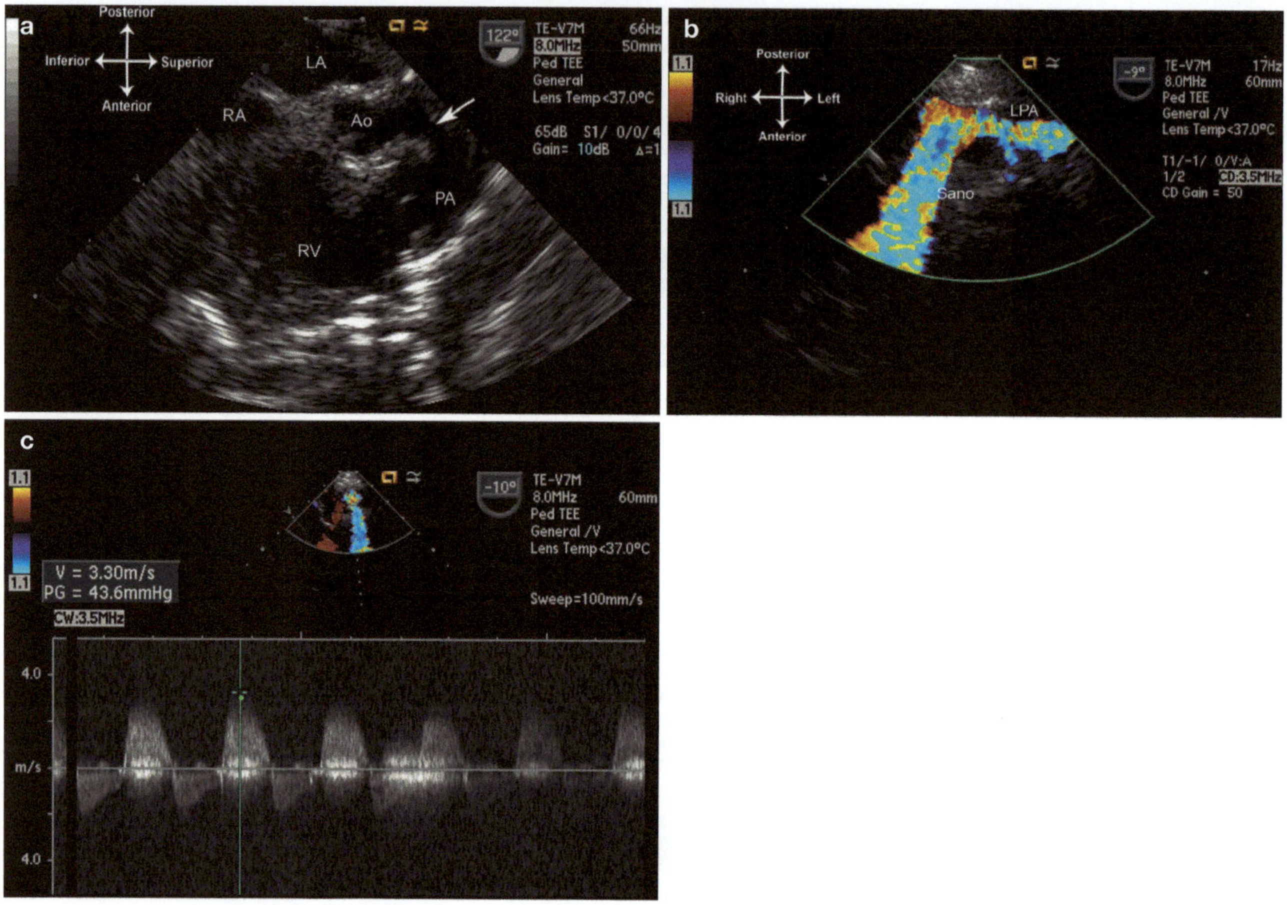

Fig. 10.17 Image of a patient with hypoplastic left heart syndrome variant following Norwood-Sano procedure. (**a**) The anastomosis (*arrow*) between a smaller native aorta (*Ao*) and native pulmonary artery (*PA*) from mid esophageal long axis view. (**b**, **c**) Images obtained from the upper esophageal pulmonary artery long axis view, demonstrating color Doppler aliasing in the distal Sano and to and fro flow by the spectral Doppler tracing of the Sano shunt. *Ao* native aorta, *LA* left atrium, *PA* native pulmonary artery (now neo-aorta), *RA* right atrium, *RV* right ventricle, *LPA* left pulmonary artery

for the Sano modification group within the first 12 months following surgery, but no significant difference between the two groups after that period [109].

When TEE is performed for the Norwood procedure, the preoperative examination serves to provide a baseline assessment of the anatomy, as well as an evaluation of tricuspid valve competency and ventricular systolic function. The postoperative TEE focuses on the following: determination of atrial communication adequacy from ME 4 Ch and ME Bicaval views, reevaluation of tricuspid and "neo-aortic" valves using ME 4 Ch and ME LAX views using both imaging and color flow Doppler, and assessment of ventricular systolic function in the ME 4 Ch, ME 2 Ch, and transgastric views. The neo-aortic root, as well as the anastomosis of the native ascending aorta to the neo-aorta, are best visualized with a ME LAX or ME AV LAX view (Fig. 10.17a, Video 10.14). The reconstructed transverse aortic arch and descending aorta can be visualized by withdrawal of the probe from the mid to the upper esophageal position (ME Asc Ao LAX and SAX, UE Ao Arch LAX, and UE Ao Arch SAX) and concomitant leftward rotation. This can be done with multiplane angles of 0° or 100°. It is rare to be able to visualize the entire arch in a single plane. Instead, the complete arch can be visualized in sections, with gradual leftward rotation of the TEE probe. However the evaluation of potential residual aortic arch gradients may or may not be feasible from these views, due to suboptimal angle of Doppler interrogation. The Blalock Taussig/central shunt can be visualized in the manner described above. If an RV to pulmonary artery conduit (Sano modification) was placed, this is best seen from the UE PA LAX or UE Ao Arch SAX positions, either 0° or 90°, with prominent anteflexion of the TEE probe (Fig. 10.17b, Video 10.15). Continuous wave Doppler can be used to interrogate the conduit (Fig. 10.17c). However its orientation can produce unfavorable Doppler angles of interrogation and sometimes an incomplete spectral signal (Fig. 10.17c).

A more recent alternative to the Norwood procedure, known as the "Hybrid procedure", has received increasing attention [110–112]. The name of this procedure derives from an approach that combines a catheter-based intervention with surgery. This procedure involves catheter-based stent placement across the ductus arteriosus in order to maintain ductal patency and systemic output, and surgical bilateral pulmonary artery banding to limit pulmonary blood flow. A balloon atrial septostomy (and/or stenting of the atrial communication) is performed either at the same time or deferred for a few days. When a hybrid Norwood procedure is performed, definitive aortic arch reconstruction is delayed until a later time in infancy (usually 4–6 months later) at which time removal of the ductal stent, pulmonary artery debanding and possible pulmonary arterioplasties are performed. This operation constitutes the equivalent to the standard second stage (Stage II) of single ventricle palliation, and a bidirectional Glenn anastomosis (discussed below) is also done at that time. In most institutions, TEE is not performed during a Hybrid procedure. However, if a TEE is considered necessary, the evaluation should focus on the specific questions and relevant aspects of the anatomy, applying similar principles as for the standard Norwood procedure.

In neonates with HLHS and intact or a severely restrictive atrial communication, radiofrequency perforation of the atrial septum, followed by balloon dilation and possible stenting of the interatrial communication, can be guided by TEE imaging in combination with fluoroscopy.

Bidirectional Cavopulmonary (Glenn) Anastomosis

The bidirectional cavopulmonary anastomosis, also known as the bidirectional Glenn procedure, represents an intermediate stage (sometimes called "Stage II") for single ventricle palliation prior to the Fontan completion. It is generally performed about 6 months of age, though the exact timing can vary; some centers report successful results with an early bidirectional Glenn (2–4 months) [113]. The original or classic Glenn procedure involved an end to end anastomosis between upper SVC and right pulmonary artery (RPA) after transection of the lower SVC and division of the more proximal RPA, thus the SVC provided flow only to the RPA. In contrast, the bidirectional Glenn anastomosis connects the SVC to the RPA but no transection of the RPA is performed, allowing SVC blood to flow directly into both pulmonary arteries. When bilateral SVCs are present, each is anastomosed to its respective branch pulmonary artery, and the procedure is then known as a *bilateral* bidirectional Glenn anastomosis [59]. An alternative method of directing SVC blood to the right pulmonary artery is known as the hemi-Fontan procedure, in which the SVC blood is redirected using a portion of right atrium into the right pulmonary artery, and a barrier is created at the SVC/right atrial junction using an imperforate disc. This procedure was created to facilitate the completion of the lateral tunnel Fontan procedure.

The bidirectional Glenn can also be used as part of the "one and a half" repair, described in the section for hypoplastic right heart syndrome. The one and a half repair is used when there are two ventricles, but the pulmonary ventricle—generally the morphologic RV—is judged incapable of carrying a full cardiac output. Usually, this is due to RV hypoplasia or a tricuspid valve abnormality. The one and a half procedure retains IVC blood return to the RV, from which it is ejected into the pulmonary artery; however SVC blood is channeled directly to the pulmonary arteries via a bidirectional Glenn anastomosis. Hence, the volume load on the RV is reduced by 25–50 % [13]. In some patients, a small atrial communication is left in place and can be closed (via transcatheter approach) at a later time [114, 115]. The one and a half repair is pertinent not just for hypoplastic right syndrome, but for a number of other forms of CHD in which partial bypassing of the RV might be useful, such as Ebstein's anomaly of the tricuspid valve, straddling tricuspid valve, and hypoplastic tricuspid valve associated with other forms of CHD [115–117]. In addition, it has been described in association with the anatomic repair of congenitally corrected transposition of the great arteries, in which an inferior hemi-Mustard repair is performed in conjunction with a bidirectional Glenn procedure and arterial switch or Rastelli operation (discussed in Chap. 12) [118]. Whatever the indication, when contemplating a one and a half repair, the same physiologic considerations apply as for any prospective bidirectional Glenn or Fontan patient—namely, there must be low pulmonary artery pressure and pulmonary vascular resistance, low systemic ventricular end diastolic pressure, good systemic ventricular function, and low probability of post-Glenn pulmonary hypertension due to factors such extra pulmonary blood flow from multiple VSDs [117].

Another important variation of the bidirectional Glenn operation worth mentioning is the Kawashima procedure. This procedure is generally performed in the setting of left isomerism (polysplenia), when there is interruption of the hepatic portion of IVC and azygos or hemiazygos continuation to the right or left SVC. In the Kawashima procedure, a bidirectional Glenn (or bilateral bidirectional Glenn) is performed, but the azygos or hemiazygos is not ligated allowing systemic venous blood from the lower body to return to the pulmonary arteries [119]. This nearly creates a complete Fontan repair, with only hepatic venous and coronary sinus blood continuing to drain into the heart. It is estimated that, after a Kawashima procedure, 80–85 % of total systemic venous blood returns directly to the lungs [120]. In general, the Kawashima procedure is performed within 6–12 months of life. While it would seem that patients might be too young for the near-Fontan physiology that results at such a young age, in fact most institutions report excellent outcomes following the Kawashima procedure [120]. However this group of patients is notoriously prone to the development of pulmonary arteriovenous malformations, felt to be due to the lack of hepatic venous blood (containing an as yet unidentified "hepatic factor") returning directly into the pulmonary arteries [121–123]. Largely because of this complication, completion of the Fontan circuit is now generally performed at several years of age, with the hepatic veins redirected into the

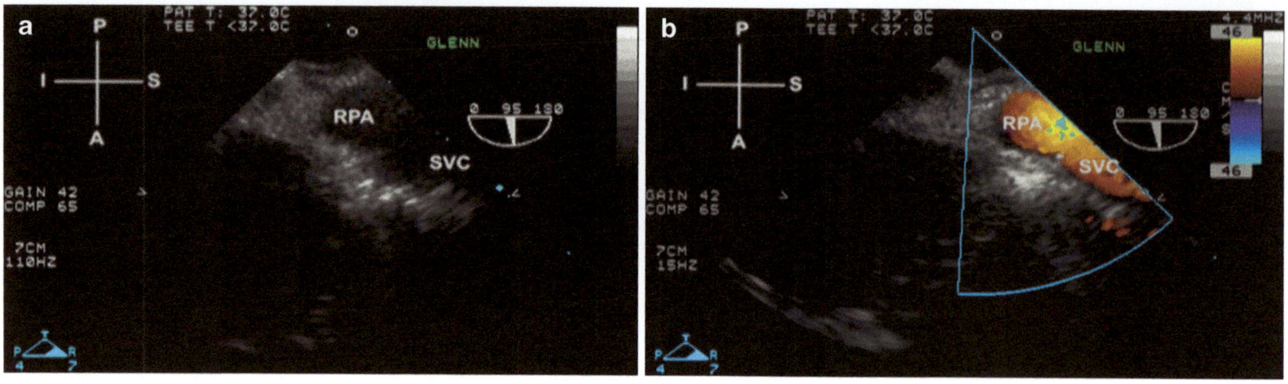

Fig. 10.18 Right bidirectional cavopulmonary (Glenn) anastomosis as viewed from the mid to upper esophageal position, multiplane angle 95°. A mid esophageal ascending aortic long axis view is first obtained, then the probe is turned to the right and slightly withdrawn. The anastomosis is well seen by two-dimensional imaging (**a**), and color flow Doppler (**b**). Potential narrowing at the anastomotic region and/or Doppler flow acceleration can be seen in this view. *RPA* right pulmonary artery, *SVC* superior vena cava

pulmonary artery in a manner similar to standard Fontan completion [120, 124]. This generally results in normal systemic oxygen saturations, likely due to (a) elimination of the hepatic venous right to left shunt into the atrium; (b) return of "hepatic factor" directly into the pulmonary arteries, leading to resolution of the arteriovenous malformations [125].

There is limited utility for TEE in patients with bidirectional Glenn surgery. Given the variability in pulmonary artery visualization by TEE, the Glenn anastomosis cannot always be optimally seen. Withdrawal to a mid to upper esophageal position (ME Asc Ao LAX, UE Ao arch SAX), along with rightward rotation of the TEE probe (in the case of a right sided Glenn) and slight anteflexion while using a multiplane angle of 90° will best show this connection. Color flow and spectral Doppler demonstrate the low velocity, undulating nature of the venous return into the pulmonary arteries (Fig. 10.18, Video 10.16). Any narrowing of the Glenn anastomosis will result in a narrowed appearance and turbulence at the site.

Fontan Procedure

The Fontan procedure was initially described for patients with tricuspid valve atresia [58]. Since then, it has undergone a significant number of changes and modifications, but the underlying, basic concept of Fontan physiology remains the same—diversion of systemic venous blood directly to the pulmonary arteries without the aid of an RV pumping chamber, thereby separating the systemic and pulmonary circulations. The Fontan procedure has become the cornerstone and ultimate goal in the management and surgical planning of any patient with single ventricle physiology, irrespective of ventricular anatomy. In this section, the most common variations of the Fontan are discussed, along with the applications of TEE for its evaluation.

The initial description and early modifications of the Fontan procedure were characterized by one important constant: the anatomic right atrium remained an integral part of the Fontan circuit. The atrial septum was closed, and all right atrial blood was directed in some manner to the pulmonary artery (the right atrium was connected either directly to the pulmonary artery or to the RV outflow tract) [126–128]. This was known as an *atriopulmonary connection* (Fig. 10.19a), or in the case of connection to the RV outflow tract, and *atrioventricular connection* [63]. Over time, problems arose in these patients due to the development of right atrial dilation, atrial arrhythmias, and sinus node dysfunction as well as systemic ventricular dysfunction. Even though it is no longer performed, it should be recognized that there continue to be a large a number of surviving adult CHD patients who have undergone this type of Fontan procedure. Some of these patients have required, or will require, surgical revision to a more contemporary Fontan modification, to allow for a more favorable hemodynamic result [129–132].

To improve upon the energetics of flow in the Fontan circuit, the concept of the *total cavopulmonary connection* was subsequently conceived [133, 134]. In this operation, an intra-atrial tunnel (lateral tunnel Fontan) is constructed directing flow from the inferior vena cava through the inferior portion of the SVC that is connected direct to the RPA, thereby channeling IVC blood into the pulmonary arteries. With the lateral tunnel Fontan, part of the patient's right atrial lateral wall serves as a portion of the tunnel (Fig. 10.19b). An alternate option more recently favored by many institutions consists of placement of an external conduit allowing for flow between the IVC and pulmonary arteries, but avoiding suture lines in the right atrium (a potential source of arrhythmias); this is known as the *extracardiac* Fontan [135, 136] (Fig. 10.19c).

An important added variation to the modified Fontan procedure involves placement of a small fenestration, usually between the Fontan pathway and the anatomic right atrium [137]. The original concept was to improve the immediate postoperative course in high risk Fontan patients by providing a controlled right to left shunt that helps to preserve systemic cardiac output in the presence of factors that may have resulted in elevated pulmonary vascular resistance. This

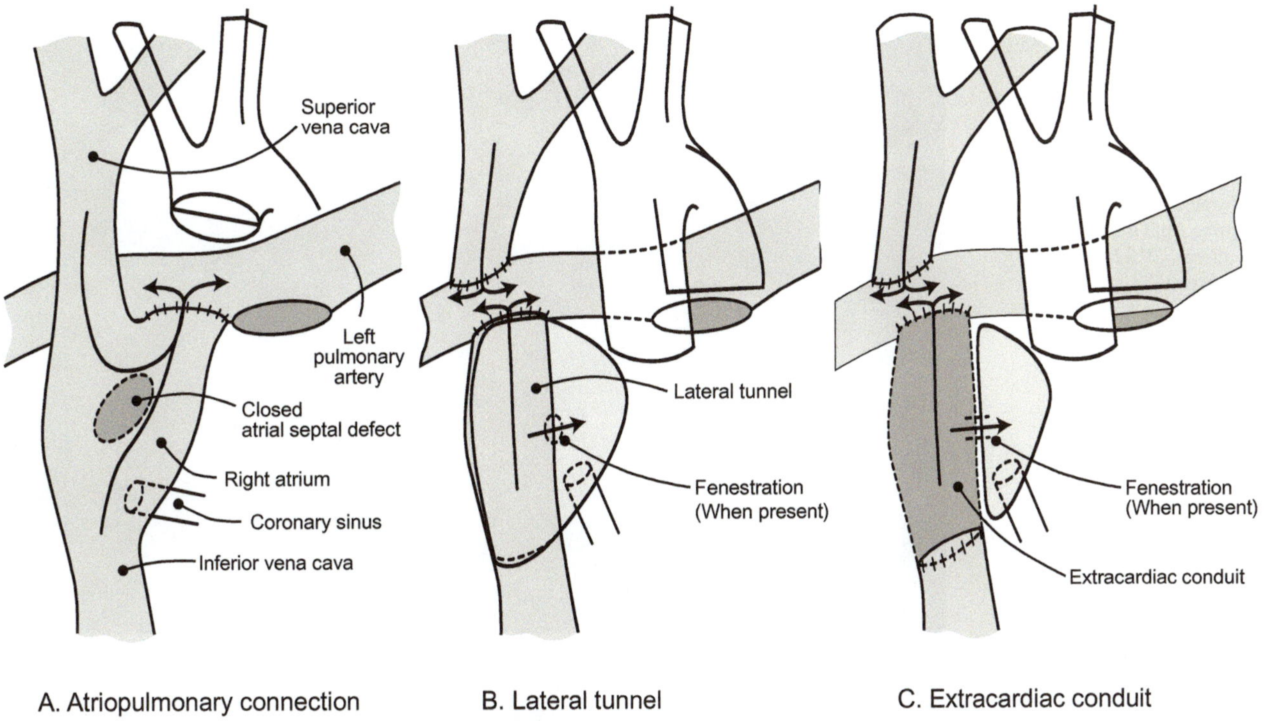

Fig. 10.19 The different types of Fontan circulation (Diagram modified from de Leval [67]. Permission obtained from Nature Publishing Group. Adapted by permission from Macmillan Publishers Ltd: copyright 2005)

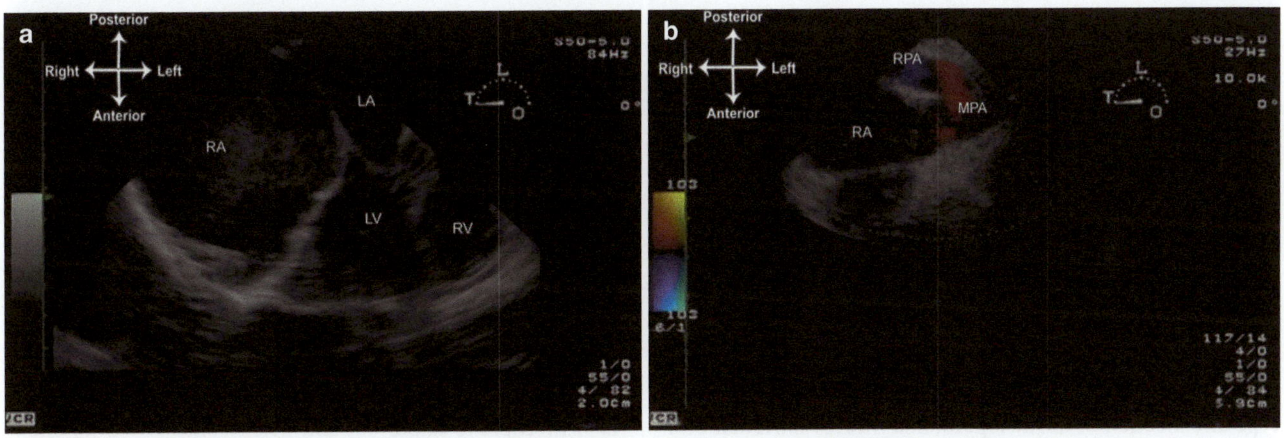

Fig. 10.20 Atriopulmonary Fontan connection, as seen from the mid esophageal four chamber view in a patient with double inlet left ventricle and L-malposed great arteries. The right atrioventricular valve was surgically obliterated as part of the original Fontan procedure. (**a**) The severely dilated right atrium with swirling of flow and spontaneous echo contrast seen. (**b**) The atriopulmonary connection by color Doppler. *LA* left atrium, *LV* left ventricle, *MPA* main pulmonary artery, *RA* right atrium, *RPA* right pulmonary artery, *RV* right ventricle

application was subsequently expanded to all Fontan patients at a number of CHD centers. Over time, the fenestration may close spontaneously, or patients can undergo catheter closure of the fenestration if it is no longer considered necessary [138]. Significant debate remains regarding the routine need for Fontan fenestration, patient selection, and eventual management of a patent fenestration (whether to leave or occlude) [62, 139–141].

The TEE evaluation of the Fontan patient varies based upon the procedure performed. In the case of the atriopulmonary/atrioventricular Fontan connection, the systemic venous return to the right atrium can be visualized sagittally using the ME Bicaval view, or in cross section with probe withdrawal from LE Situs SAX to ME 4 Ch views along with slight anteflexion (multiplane angle 0°). In general, such patients will have a distended atrium, and sluggish blood flow often creates the appearance of "smoke" (spontaneous echo contrast due to red cell aggregation) in the atrium [142, 143] (Fig. 10.20a, Video 10.17). In the ME 4 Ch view (multiplane angle 0–30°), the atrial septum is well-seen; it usually

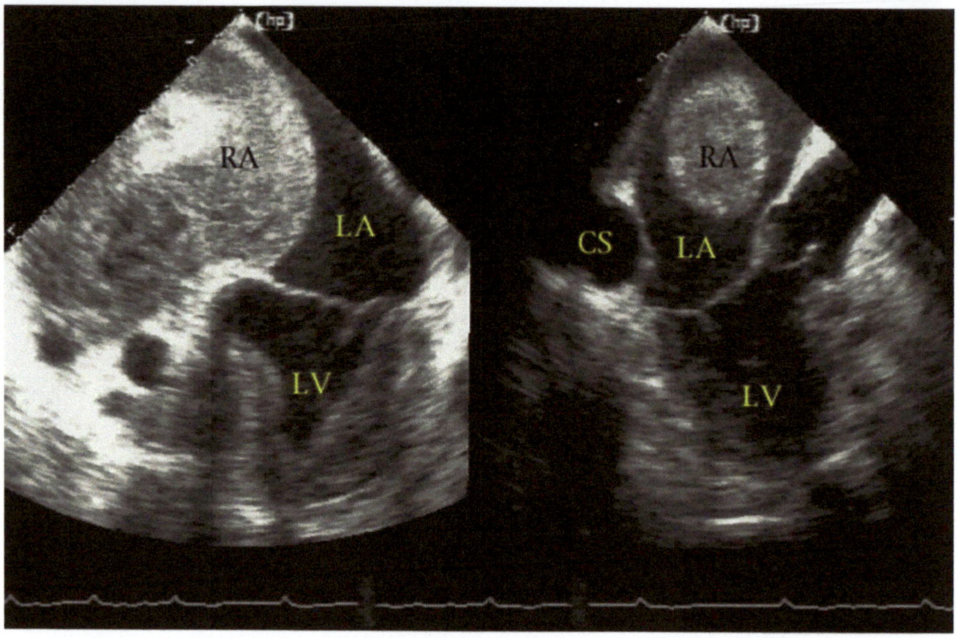

Fig. 10.21 Atriopulmonary Fontan in a patient with tricuspid atresia, showing a severely dilated right atrium completely filled with thrombus, in orthogonal views. Note the dilated coronary sinus (*CS*) due to elevated right atrial pressure resulting from the thrombus. *LA* left atrium, *LV* left ventricle, *RA* right atrium

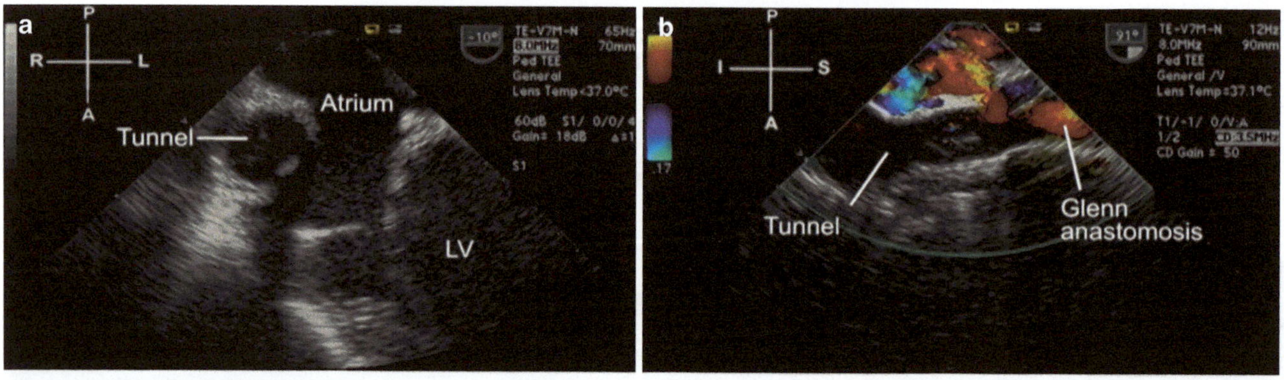

Fig. 10.22 Lateral tunnel Fontan in a patient with double inlet left ventricle, as seen from the mid esophageal views. (**a**) The tunnel in cross-section in the mid esophageal four chamber view. (**b**) The length of the tunnel and the Glenn anastomosis shown more superiorly by color flow Doppler. This view is the equivalent of the mid esophageal bicaval view, with the probe withdrawn slightly to visualize the tunnel and Glenn anastomosis. *LV* left ventricle

bows toward the left, and can be inspected for any residual right to left leaks by color flow Doppler. Depending on the type and location of the atriopulmonary/atrioventricular connection, the mid esophageal views (ME 4 Ch, ME RV In-Out, ME AV SAX, ME Asc Ao SAX) can be used to evaluate patency of the connection (Fig. 10.20b). The branch pulmonary arteries can be visualized in the manner described previously. Flow into the branch pulmonary arteries will be low velocity and phasic in nature. Atrioventricular valve and semilunar valve function, and ventricular systolic function, should be examined carefully. Intra-atrial thrombi can sometimes result from the sluggish blood flow in the right atrium, and these can be seen as irregular echogenic structures. In some cases, there can be near complete thrombosis of the right atrium (Fig. 10.21, Video 10.18)

For the total cavopulmonary connection (modified Fontan procedure), IVC and hepatic drainage should be inspected, and with either the lateral tunnel or extracardiac conduit, the anastomosis of the Fontan pathway to the IVC should be visualized. This is best initiated from the LE Situs SAX view, multiplane angle 0°, and often some probe anteflexion and rightward rotation is necessary (Fig. 10.22a, Video 10.19). The probe is withdrawn to the ME 4 Ch view, and a cross-sectional "sweep" of the Fontan pathway is inspected for any possible narrowing or masses/thrombosis. With further withdrawal to a higher mid esophageal position (ME Asc Ao SAX), the entrance into the pulmonary artery can be seen. If the pulmonary arteries can be visualized, the flow into both branches should be evaluated. Also in the mid-esophageal position the multiplane angle can be rotated to 80–90° to a ME Bicaval view and the probe rotated rightward to reveal a sagittal view of the Fontan pathway, and to evaluate for possible narrowing (Fig. 10.22b, Video 10.19). When a fenestration has been placed, the location can be highly variable. Generally, a fenestration is best seen in the ME 4 Ch view with the transducer angle about 0°

(Fig. 10.23, Video 10.20). Color flow Doppler demonstrates the site of fenestration flow and right to left shunting, and a gradient can be estimated using spectral and/or continuous wave Doppler. Again, as with any Fontan modification, it is important to evaluate overall ventricular function, as well as AV and semilunar valve function. In the patient with an external conduit, the entrance of the pulmonary veins should also be examined for possible compression by the conduit (Fig. 10.24, Video 10.21). However it is also important to remember that temporary pulmonary vein stenosis can be created by compression from the TEE probe, and therefore TEE findings of pulmonary vein stenosis should be corroborated with postoperative imaging studies as well as surgical findings [144, 145].

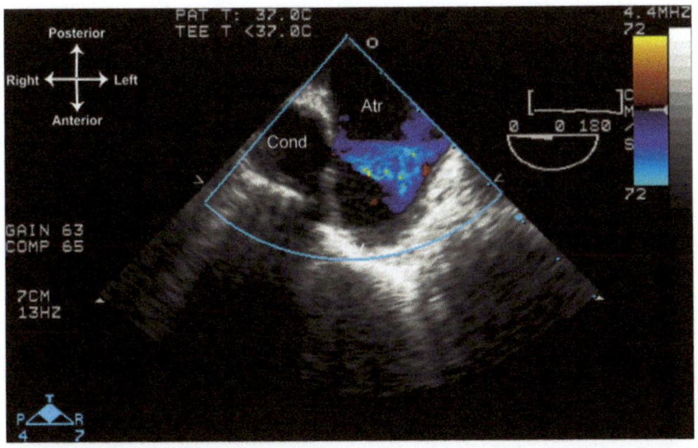

Fig. 10.23 Extracardiac Fontan with fenestration, as viewed from a mid esophageal four chamber view. The Fontan conduit (Cond) is located just outside and to the right of the physiologic "left" atrium, and seen in cross-section. Right to left shunting through the fenestration is clearly seen by color flow Doppler entering the atrium. *Atr* atrium

The use of TEE to evaluate Fontan patients has application in multiple settings [146]. In the operating room, preoperative TEE is used to confirm intracardiac anatomy and function (as noted above), and postoperatively to evaluate patency of the Fontan pathway, characterize flow across a fenestration if present, assess AV and semilunar valve function, and evaluate cardiac function. It should be noted that the extracardiac Fontan can be difficult to visualize immediately following surgery if a polytetrafluoroethylene (PTFE, or Gore-Tex) conduit is used, due to the shadowing and reverberation produced by the microscopic air contained in the walls of the conduit. Over time, the conduit becomes more readily visible. In the outpatient setting, TEE becomes

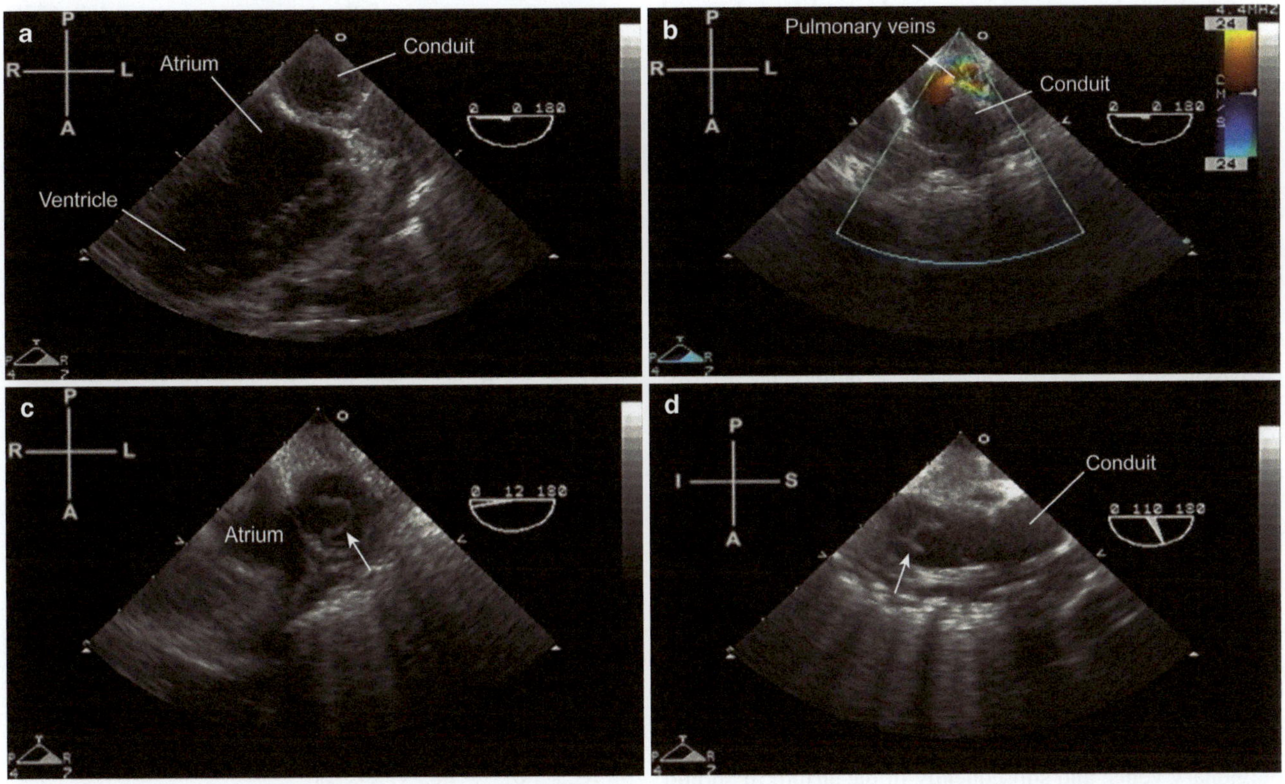

Fig. 10.24 Extracardiac Fontan conduit placed between a right sided IVC and the left pulmonary artery in a patient with heterotaxy and dextrocardia. (**a**) The equivalent of a mid esophageal four chamber view, with the probe rotated slightly rightward (clockwise). Dextrocardia is seen as well as the large conduit passing behind and slightly to the left of the atrium. As the conduit passes from right to left behind the heart, it compresses the pulmonary veins (**b**), causing pulmonary venous obstruction as shown by mosaic color flow next to the conduit. This resulted in a low cardiac output state that likely contributed to the development of a thrombus within the conduit, identified by the *arrow* (**c**). (**d**) The multiplane angle has been rotated to 110° in order to optimize visualization of the length of the conduit. The thrombus is seen toward the more inferior portion (*arrow*)

increasingly more useful in older, larger patients, in whom transthoracic echocardiographic imaging can be quite challenging. When atrial fibrillation is present, TEE is very useful for the assessment of possible thrombosis in the atrial appendage(s), analogous to its utility in the adult patient with atrial fibrillation [147]. Thus TEE can play an important role in ambulatory assessment of adults who have undergone a Fontan procedure. In the intensive care setting, TEE can be useful in those situations in which transthoracic imaging is compromised [148]. In addition, in patients undergoing transcatheter closure of a Fontan fenestration or creation of a fenestration in the patient with a failing Fontan circulation, TEE can be used for monitoring and procedural guidance.

Additional Evaluation

Excessive cyanosis following the bidirectional Glenn, hemi-Fontan, or non fenestrated Fontan procedures raises the possibility of a right to left shunt somewhere in the circulation. In such cases, the underlying cardiac anatomy and repair should be reviewed, and the TEE evaluation performed accordingly, for potential intracardiac shunts. For the atriopulmonary, atrioventricular, and lateral tunnel Fontan procedures, the possibility of a residual intracardiac shunt (across the intra-atrial baffle, atrial septum, or other structure) should be considered. Injection of agitated saline contrast into the systemic venous circuit can be helpful in revealing occult right to left shunts. The examiner should keep an open mind to all possibilities, because surprising findings are occasionally encountered [149]. In addition, excessive cyanosis following the Fontan procedure also raises the question of collateral vessels arising from the systemic venous system and returning directly to the heart (bypassing the lungs), or alternatively, pulmonary arteriovenous malformations. These possibilities can be evaluated during a TEE study by the use of an agitated saline contrast injection. Because agitated saline is filtered in the lungs, none or a minimal amount should return to the atrium [150]. For a possible venous collateral returning to the heart, agitated saline is injected into a systemic vein (preferably through a central line) at a site proximal to the potential site of the collateral. If contrast is seen returning directly to the atrium immediately after injection, the presence of a collateral should be strongly suspected. For pulmonary arteriovenous malformation, contrast will first be visualized in the pulmonary veins, and subsequently in the atrium. It should be noted that these techniques are useful but not fully diagnostic, and there can be false positive results [151]. Cardiac catheterization and angiography are often necessary to provide more definitive anatomic evaluation, particularly in the case of venous collaterals returning to the heart.

Summary

The terms "single ventricle" and "functional single ventricle" refer to a broad, heterogeneous group of congenital cardiac lesions differing markedly in terms of their anatomy and physiology. However despite their great diversity, all of these cardiac defects are distinguished by a simple, common, and unifying characteristic: a biventricular intracardiac repair cannot be performed. For these patients, the management is relatively straightforward: the ultimate goal is to separate the systemic and pulmonary circulations such that deoxygenated systemic venous blood returns passively to the pulmonary arteries without the assistance of a separate pump. Optimizing such patients for this unique physiology—known as Fontan physiology—forms the basis of all current management strategies for the single ventricle patient. This is a very important group of patients, and their diagnosis, evaluation, and management represents one of the most active and topical areas in contemporary pediatric cardiovascular medicine. Moreover, due to the great advances and successes with medical and surgical therapies, particularly with the Fontan procedure, a significant proportion of single ventricle patients are now reaching adulthood. Thus, this group constitutes an ever-growing and increasingly important proportion of the patients seen by adult CHD specialists. In this chapter we discussed the major types of cardiac defects producing single ventricle physiology, as well as their surgical management. For such patients, TEE is very useful both in terms of preoperative diagnosis and intraoperative assessment; moreover it can be helpful as well in a number of other clinical scenarios.

References

1. VanPraagh R, Ongley PA, Swan HJ. Anatomic types of single or common ventricle in man. Morphologic and geometric aspects of 60 necropsied cases. Am J Cardiol. 1964;13:367–86.
2. Van Praagh R, Plett JA, Van Praagh S. Single ventricle. Pathology, embryology, terminology and classification. Herz. 1979;4:113–50.
3. Jacobs ML, Mayer JE. Congenital heart surgery nomenclature and database project: single ventricle. Ann Thorac Surg. 2000;69:S197–204.
4. Jacobs ML, Anderson RH. Nomenclature of the functionally univentricular heart. Cardiol Young. 2006;16 Suppl 1:3–8.
5. Noonan JA, Nadas AS. The hypoplastic left heart syndrome; an analysis of 101 cases. Pediatr Clin North Am. 1958;5:1029–56.
6. Tchervenkov CI, Jacobs JP, Weinberg PM, et al. The nomenclature, definition and classification of hypoplastic left heart syndrome. Cardiol Young. 2006;16:339–68.
7. Beckman CB, Moller JH, Edwards JE. Alternate pathways to pulmonary venous flow in left-sided obstructive anomalies. Circulation. 1975;52:509–16.
8. Satou GM, Perry SB, Gauvreau K, Geva T. Echocardiographic predictors of coronary artery pathology in pulmonary atresia with intact ventricular septum. Am J Cardiol. 2000;85:1319–24.

9. Giglia TM, Mandell VS, Connor AR, Mayer JE, Lock JE. Diagnosis and management of right ventricle-dependent coronary circulation in pulmonary atresia with intact ventricular septum. Circulation. 1992;86:1516–28.
10. Najm HK, Williams WG, Coles JG, Rebeyka IM, Freedom RM. Pulmonary atresia with intact ventricular septum: results of the Fontan procedure. Ann Thorac Surg. 1997;63:669–75.
11. Kouchoukos NT, Blackstone EH, Doty DB, Hanley FL, Karp RB. Pulmonary atresia and intact ventricular septum. In: Kirklin/Barratt-Boyes cardiac surgery. 3rd ed. Philadelphia: Churchill Livingstone; 2003. p. 1095–112.
12. Ashburn DA, Blackstone EH, Wells WJ, et al. Determinants of mortality and type of repair in neonates with pulmonary atresia and intact ventricular septum. J Thorac Cardiovasc Surg. 2004;127:1000–7; discussion 1007–8.
13. Al-Radi OO, Kim S, Van Arsdell GS. Surgery for the small right ventricle. In: Redington AN, Anderson RH, editors. Congenital diseases in the right heart. London: Springer London; 2009. p. 173–9.
14. Chubb H, Pesonen E, Sivasubramanian S, et al. Long-term outcome following catheter valvotomy for pulmonary atresia with intact ventricular septum. J Am Coll Cardiol. 2012;59:1468–76.
15. Yoshimura N, Yamaguchi M. Surgical strategy for pulmonary atresia with intact ventricular septum: initial management and definitive surgery. Gen Thorac Cardiovasc Surg. 2009;57:338–46.
16. Bull C, Kostelka M, Sorensen K, de Leval M. Outcome measures for the neonatal management of pulmonary atresia with intact ventricular septum. J Thorac Cardiovasc Surg. 1994;107:359–66.
17. Li S, Chen W, Zhang Y, et al. Hybrid therapy for pulmonary atresia with intact ventricular septum. Ann Thorac Surg. 2011;91:1467–71.
18. Ovaert C, Qureshi SA, Rosenthal E, Baker EJ, Tynan M. Growth of the right ventricle after successful transcatheter pulmonary valvotomy in neonates and infants with pulmonary atresia and intact ventricular septum. J Thorac Cardiovasc Surg. 1998;115:1055–62.
19. Kreutzer C, Mayorquim RC, Kreutzer GO, et al. Experience with one and a half ventricle repair. J Thorac Cardiovasc Surg. 1999;117:662–8.
20. Hanley FL, Sade RM, Blackstone EH, Kirklin JW, Freedom RM, Nanda NC. Outcomes in neonatal pulmonary atresia with intact ventricular septum. A multiinstitutional study. J Thorac Cardiovasc Surg. 1993;105:406–23, 424–7; discussion 423–4.
21. Castañeda AR, Jonas RA, Mayer JE, Hanley FL. Single-ventricle tricuspid atresia. In: Cardiac surgery of the neonate and infant. Philadelphia: W.B. Saunders; 1994. p. 249–72.
22. Moniotte SL, Barrea C. Functionally univentricular heart. In: Lai W, Mertens L, Cohen MS, Geva T, editors. Echocardiography in pediatric and congenital heart disease: from fetus to adult. Illustrated Ed. Chichester/Hoboken: Wiley; 2009. p. 459–75.
23. Tandon R, Edwards JE. Tricuspid atresia. A re-evaluation and classification. J Thorac Cardiovasc Surg. 1974;67:530–42.
24. Epstein ML. Tricuspid atresia, stenosis, and regurgitation. In: Allen HD, Dricoll DJ, Shaddy RE, Feltes TF, editors. Moss and Adams' heart disease in infants, children, and adolescents: including the fetus and young adult. 7th ed. Philadelphia: Lippincott Williams & Wilkins; 2008. p. 817–34.
25. Weinberg PM. Anatomy of tricuspid atresia and its relevance to current forms of surgical therapy. Ann Thorac Surg. 1980;29:306–11.
26. Rice MJ, Seward JB, Hagler DJ, Edwards WD, Julsrud PR, Tajik AJ. Left juxtaposed atrial appendages: diagnostic two-dimensional echocardiographic features. J Am Coll Cardiol. 1983;1:1330–6.
27. Van Praagh S, O'Sullivan J, Brili S, Van Praagh R. Juxtaposition of the morphologically right atrial appendage in solitus and inversus atria: a study of 35 postmortem cases. Am Heart J. 1996;132:382–90.
28. Stümper O, Rijlaarsdam M, Vargas-Barron J, Romero A, Hess J, Sutherland GR. The assessment of juxtaposed atrial appendages by transoesophageal echocardiography. Int J Cardiol. 1990;29:365–71.
29. Cohen MS, Jacobs ML, Weinberg PM, Rychik J. Morphometric analysis of unbalanced common atrioventricular canal using two-dimensional echocardiography. J Am Coll Cardiol. 1996;28:1017–23.
30. Jegatheeswaran A, Pizarro C, Caldarone CA, et al. Echocardiographic definition and surgical decision-making in unbalanced atrioventricular septal defect: a Congenital Heart Surgeons' Society multiinstitutional study. Circulation. 2010;122:S209–15.
31. Snider AR, Ritter SB, Serwer GA. Echocardiography in pediatric heart disease. 2nd ed. St Louis: Mosby; 1997.
32. Dobell AR, Van Praagh R. The Holmes heart: historic associations and pathologic anatomy. Am Heart J. 1996;132:437–45.
33. Hagler DJ, Edwards WD. Univentricular atrioventricular connections. In: Allen HD, Dricoll DJ, Shaddy RE, Feltes TF, editors. Moss and Adams' heart disease in infants, children, and adolescents: including the fetus and young adult. 7th ed. Philadelphia: Lippincott Williams & Wilkins; 2008. p. 1128–49.
34. Shinebourne EA, Lau KC, Calcaterra G, Anderson RH. Univentricular heart of right ventricular type: clinical, angiographic and electocardiographic features. Am J Cardiol. 1980;46:439–45.
35. Saleeb SF, Juraszek A, Geva T. Anatomic, imaging, and clinical characteristics of double-inlet, double-outlet right ventricle. Am J Cardiol. 2010;105:542–9.
36. Weinberg PM. Morphology of the single ventricle. Prog Pediatr Cardiol. 2002;16:1–9.
37. Anderson RH, Ho SY. What is a ventricle? Ann Thorac Surg. 1998;66:616–20.
38. Kouchoukos NT, Blackstone EH, Doty DB, Hanley FL, Karp RB. Double inlet ventricle and atretic atrioventricular valve. In: Kirklin/Barratt-Boyes cardiac surgery. 3rd ed. Philadelphia: Churchill Livingstone; 2003. p. 1585–608.
39. Ware SM, Aygun MG, Hildebrandt F. Spectrum of clinical diseases caused by disorders of primary cilia. Proc Am Thorac Soc. 2011;8:444–50.
40. Shiraishi I, Ichikawa H. Human heterotaxy syndrome. Circ J. 2012;76:2066–75.
41. Van Mierop LHS, Gessner IH, Schiebler GL. Asplenia and polysplenia syndromes. Birth Defects Orig Artic Ser. 1972;8:36–44.
42. Bartram U, Wirbelauer J, Speer CP. Heterotaxy syndrome—asplenia and polysplenia as indicators of visceral malposition and complex congenital heart disease. Biol Neonate. 2005;88:278–90.
43. Van Praagh S. Cardiac malpositions and the heterotaxy syndromes. In: Keane JF, Lock JE, Fyler DC, editors. Nadas' pediatric cardiology. 2nd ed. Philadelphia: Saunders Elsevier; 2006. p. 675–95.
44. Lim JSL, McCrindle BW, Smallhorn JF, et al. Clinical features, management, and outcome of children with fetal and postnatal diagnoses of isomerism syndromes. Circulation. 2005;112:2454–61.
45. Anagnostopoulos PV, Pearl JM, Octave C, et al. Improved current era outcomes in patients with heterotaxy syndromes. Eur J Cardiothorac Surg. 2009;35:871–7; discussion 877–8.
46. Lim HG, Bacha EA, Marx GR, et al. Biventricular repair in patients with heterotaxy syndrome. J Thorac Cardiovasc Surg. 2009;137:371–379.e3.
47. Serraf A, Bensari N, Houyel L, et al. Surgical management of congenital heart defects associated with heterotaxy syndrome. Eur J Cardiothorac Surg. 2010;38:721–7.
48. Freedom RM, Van Arsdell GS. Biventricular hearts not amenable to biventricular repair. Ann Thorac Surg. 1998;66:641–3.
49. Jacobs ML, Pelletier G, Wearden PD, Morell VO. The role of Fontan's procedure and aortic translocation in the surgical management of patients with discordant atrioventricular connections, interventricular communication, and pulmonary stenosis or atresia. Cardiol Young. 2006;16 Suppl 3:97–102.
50. Ruzmetov M, Rodefeld MD, Turrentine MW, Brown JW. Rational approach to surgical management of complex forms of double

outlet right ventricle with modified Fontan operation. Congenit Heart Dis. 2008;3:397–403.
51. Van Praagh R, Weinberg PM, Srebro JP. Double-outlet left ventricle. In: Adams FH, Emmanouilides GC, Riemenschneider TA, editors. Moss' heart disease in infants, children and adolescents. 4th ed. Baltimore: Williams and Wilkins; 1989. p. 461–85.
52. Anderson RH, Shinebourne EA, Gerlis LM. Criss-cross atrioventricular relationships producing paradoxical atrioventricular concordance or discordance. Their significance to nomenclature of congenital heart disease. Circulation. 1974;50:176–80.
53. Van Praagh S, LaCorte M, Fellows KE, et al. Supero-inferior ventricles: anatomic and angiographic findings in ten postmortem cases. In: Takao A, editor. Etiology and morphogenesis of congenital heart disease. Mt. Kisco: Futura; 1980. p. 317–78.
54. Delius RE, Rademecker MA, de Leval MR, Elliott MJ, Stark J. Is a high-risk biventricular repair always preferable to conversion to a single ventricle repair? J Thorac Cardiovasc Surg. 1996;112:1561–8; discussion 1568–9.
55. Hickey EJ, Caldarone CA, Blackstone EH, et al. Critical left ventricular outflow tract obstruction: the disproportionate impact of biventricular repair in borderline cases. J Thorac Cardiovasc Surg. 2007;134:1429–36; discussion 1436–7.
56. Jonas RA. Fontan or septation: when I abandon septation in complex lesions with two ventricles. Semin Thorac Cardiovasc Surg Pediatr Card Surg Annu. 2009;12:94–8.
57. de Leval MR. The Fontan circulation: what have we learned? What to expect? Pediatr Cardiol. 1998;19:316–20.
58. Fontan F, Baudet E. Surgical repair of tricuspid atresia. Thorax. 1971;26:240–8.
59. de Leval MR, Deanfield JE. Four decades of Fontan palliation. Nat Rev Cardiol. 2010;7:520–7.
60. d'Udekem Y, Cheung MM, Setyapranata S, et al. How good is a good Fontan? Quality of life and exercise capacity of Fontans without arrhythmias. Ann Thorac Surg. 2009;88:1961–9.
61. Chin AJ, Whitehead KK, Watrous RL. Insights after 40 years of the Fontan operation. World J Pediatr Congenital Heart Surg. 2010;1:328.
62. Atz AM, Travison TG, McCrindle BW, et al. Late status of Fontan patients with persistent surgical fenestration. J Am Coll Cardiol. 2011;57:2437–43.
63. Davies RR, Chen JM, Mosca RS. The Fontan procedure: evolution in technique; attendant imperfections and transplantation for "failure". Semin Thorac Cardiovasc Surg Pediatr Card Surg Annu. 2011;14:55–66.
64. Deal BJ, Jacobs ML. Management of the failing Fontan circulation. Heart. 2012;98:1098–104.
65. Gentles TL, Mayer JE, Gauvreau K, et al. Fontan operation in five hundred consecutive patients: factors influencing early and late outcome. J Thorac Cardiovasc Surg. 1997;114:376–91.
66. Driscoll DJ. Long-term results of the Fontan operation. Pediatr Cardiol. 2007;28:438–42.
67. de Leval MR. The Fontan circulation: a challenge to William Harvey? Nat Clin Pract Cardiovasc Med. 2005;2:202–8.
68. Sundareswaran KS, Pekkan K, Dasi LP, et al. The total cavopulmonary connection resistance: a significant impact on single ventricle hemodynamics at rest and exercise. Am J Physiol Heart Circ Physiol. 2008;295:H2427–35.
69. Dasi LP, Krishnankuttyrema R, Kitajima HD, et al. Fontan hemodynamics: importance of pulmonary artery diameter. J Thorac Cardiovasc Surg. 2009;137:560–4.
70. Gewillig M, Brown SC, Eyskens B, et al. The Fontan circulation: who controls cardiac output? Interact Cardiovasc Thorac Surg. 2010;10:428–33.
71. Gaynor JW, Collins MH, Rychik J, Gaughan JP, Spray TL. Long-term outcome of infants with single ventricle and total anomalous pulmonary venous connection. J Thorac Cardiovasc Surg. 1999;117:506–13; discussion 513–4.
72. Foerster SR, Gauvreau K, McElhinney DB, Geva T. Importance of totally anomalous pulmonary venous connection and postoperative pulmonary vein stenosis in outcomes of heterotaxy syndrome. Pediatr Cardiol. 2008;29:536–44.
73. Sakurai T, Kado H, Nakano T, et al. The impact of extracardiac conduit-total cavopulmonary connection on apicocaval juxtaposition. Eur J Cardiothorac Surg. 2010;38:439–44.
74. Photiadis J, Urban AE, Sinzobahamvya N, et al. Restrictive left atrial outflow adversely affects outcome after the modified Norwood procedure. Eur J Cardiothorac Surg. 2005; 27:962–7.
75. Rychik J, Rome JJ, Collins MH, DeCampli WM, Spray TL. The hypoplastic left heart syndrome with intact atrial septum: atrial morphology, pulmonary vascular histopathology and outcome. J Am Coll Cardiol. 1999;34:554–60.
76. Vlahos AP, Lock JE, McElhinney DB, van der Velde ME. Hypoplastic left heart syndrome with intact or highly restrictive atrial septum: outcome after neonatal transcatheter atrial septostomy. Circulation. 2004;109:2326–30.
77. Divanović A, Hor K, Cnota J, Hirsch R, Kinsel-Ziter M, Michelfelder E. Prediction and perinatal management of severely restrictive atrial septum in fetuses with critical left heart obstruction: clinical experience using pulmonary venous Doppler analysis. J Thorac Cardiovasc Surg. 2011;141:988–94.
78. Lowenthal A, Kipps AK, Brook MM, Meadows J, Azakie A, Moon-Grady AJ. Prenatal diagnosis of atrial restriction in hypoplastic left heart syndrome is associated with decreased 2-year survival. Prenat Diagn. 2012;32:485–90.
79. Vida VL, Bacha EA, Larrazabal A, et al. Hypoplastic left heart syndrome with intact or highly restrictive atrial septum: surgical experience from a single center. Ann Thorac Surg. 2007;84:581–5; discussion 586.
80. Marshall AC, Levine J, Morash D, et al. Results of in utero atrial septoplasty in fetuses with hypoplastic left heart syndrome. Prenat Diagn. 2008;28:1023–8.
81. Seliem MA, Shahab RA, Palileo M. Spontaneous obstruction of interatrial communication in infants with atrioventricular valve atresia or stenosis in the neonatal period: serial Echocardiographic-Doppler study. Echocardiography. 1998;15:459–66.
82. Thoele DG, Ursell PC, Ho SY, et al. Atrial morphologic features in tricuspid atresia. J Thorac Cardiovasc Surg. 1991;102:606–10.
83. Tzifa A, Gauvreau K, Geggel RL. Factors associated with development of atrial septal restriction in patients with tricuspid atresia involving the right-sided atrioventricular valve. Am Heart J. 2007;154:1235–41.
84. Menon SC, Dearani JA, Cetta F. Long-term outcome after atrioventricular valve surgery following modified Fontan operation. Cardiol Young. 2011;21:83–8.
85. Hershenson JA, Zaidi AN, Texter KM, et al. Differences in tissue Doppler imaging between single ventricles after the Fontan operation and normal controls. Am J Cardiol. 2010;106:99–103.
86. Mahle WT, Coon PD, Wernovsky G, Rychik J. Quantitative echocardiographic assessment of the performance of the functionally single right ventricle after the Fontan operation. Cardiol Young. 2001;11:399–406.
87. Vitarelli A, Conde Y, Cimino E, et al. Quantitative assessment of systolic and diastolic ventricular function with tissue Doppler imaging after Fontan type of operation. Int J Cardiol. 2005;102:61–9.
88. Williams RV, Ritter S, Tani LY, Pagoto LT, Minich LL. Quantitative assessment of ventricular function in children with single ventricles using the Doppler myocardial performance index. Am J Cardiol. 2000;86:1106–10.
89. Finta KM, Beekman RH, Lupinetti FM, Bove EL. Systemic ventricular outflow obstruction progresses after the Fontan operation. Ann Thorac Surg. 1994;58:1108–12; discussion 1112–3.

90. Matitiau A, Geva T, Colan SD, et al. Bulboventricular foramen size in infants with double-inlet left ventricle or tricuspid atresia with transposed great arteries: influence on initial palliative operation and rate of growth. J Am Coll Cardiol. 1992; 19:142–8.
91. Shiraishi H, Silverman NH. Echocardiographic spectrum of double inlet ventricle: evaluation of the interventricular communication. J Am Coll Cardiol. 1990;15:1401–8.
92. Fontan F, Fernandez G, Costa F, et al. The size of the pulmonary arteries and the results of the Fontan operation. J Thorac Cardiovasc Surg. 1989;98:711–9; discussion 719–24.
93. Knott-Craig CJ, Julsrud PR, Schaff HV, Puga FJ, Danielson GK. Pulmonary artery size and clinical outcome after the modified Fontan operation. Ann Thorac Surg. 1993;55:646–51.
94. Blalock A, Taussig HB. The surgical treatment of malformations of the heart in which there is pulmonary stenosis or pulmonary atresia. JAMA. 1945;251:2123–38.
95. Klinner W, Pasini M, Schaudig A. Anastomosis between systemic and pulmonary arteries with the aid of plastic prostheses in cyanotic heart diseases. Thoraxchirurgie. 1962;10:68–75.
96. Laks H, Odim JN, Sadeghi AM, Allada V. The incisional pulmonary artery band. Ann Thorac Surg. 1999;67:1813–4.
97. Kouchoukos NT, Blackstone EH, Doty DB, Hanley FL, Karp RB. Tricuspid atresia and management of single-ventricle physiology. In: Kirklin/Barratt-Boyes cardiac surgery. 3rd ed. Philadelphia: Churchill Livingstone; 2003. p. 1113–75.
98. Tibby S, Durward A. Interpretation of the echocardiographic pressure gradient across a pulmonary artery band in the setting of a univentricular heart. Intensive Care Med. 2008;34:203–7.
99. Damus PS. Correspondence. Ann Thoracic Surg. 1975;20:724–5.
100. Kaye MP. Anatomic correction of transposition of great arteries. Mayo Clin Proc. 1975;50:638–40.
101. Stansel HC. A new operation for d-loop transposition of the great vessels. Ann Thorac Surg. 1975;19:565–7.
102. Brawn WJ, Sethia B, Jagtap R, et al. Univentricular heart with systemic outflow obstruction: palliation by primary Damus procedure. Ann Thorac Surg. 1995;59:1441–7.
103. Huddleston CB, Canter CE, Spray TL. Damus-Kaye-Stansel with cavopulmonary connection for single ventricle and subaortic obstruction. Ann Thorac Surg. 1993;55:339–45; discussion 346.
104. Ceresnak SR, Quaegebeur JM, Pass RH, Hordof AJ, Liberman L. The palliative arterial switch procedure for single ventricles: are these patients suitable Fontan candidates? Ann Thorac Surg. 2008;86:583–7.
105. Fraser CD. Management of systemic outlet obstruction in patients undergoing single ventricle palliation. Semin Thorac Cardiovasc Surg Pediatr Card Surg Annu. 2009;12:70–5.
106. Norwood WI, Lang P, Casteneda AR, Campbell DN. Experience with operations for hypoplastic left heart syndrome. J Thorac Cardiovasc Surg. 1981;82:511–9.
107. Sano S, Ishino K, Kawada M, et al. Right ventricle-pulmonary artery shunt in first-stage palliation of hypoplastic left heart syndrome. J Thorac Cardiovasc Surg. 2003;126:504–9; discussion 509–10.
108. Sano S, Ishino K, Kado H, et al. Outcome of right ventricle-to-pulmonary artery shunt in first-stage palliation of hypoplastic left heart syndrome: a multi-institutional study. Ann Thorac Surg. 2004;78:1951–7; discussion 1957–8.
109. Ohye RG, Sleeper LA, Mahony L, et al. Comparison of shunt types in the Norwood procedure for single-ventricle lesions. N Engl J Med. 2010;362:1980–92.
110. Akintuerk H, Michel-Behnke I, Valeske K, et al. Stenting of the arterial duct and banding of the pulmonary arteries: basis for combined Norwood stage I and II repair in hypoplastic left heart. Circulation. 2002;105:1099–103.
111. Galantowicz M, Cheatham JP. Lessons learned from the development of a new hybrid strategy for the management of hypoplastic left heart syndrome. Pediatr Cardiol. 2005;26:190–9.
112. Bacha EA, Daves S, Hardin J, et al. Single-ventricle palliation for high-risk neonates: the emergence of an alternative hybrid stage I strategy. J Thorac Cardiovasc Surg. 2006;131:163–71.
113. Petrucci O, Khoury PR, Manning PB, Eghtesady P. Outcomes of the bidirectional Glenn procedure in patients less than 3 months of age. J Thorac Cardiovasc Surg. 2010;139:562–8.
114. Chowdhury UK, Airan B, Sharma R, et al. One and a half ventricle repair with pulsatile bidirectional Glenn: results and guidelines for patient selection. Ann Thorac Surg. 2001;71:1995–2002.
115. Stellin G, Vida VL, Milanesi O, et al. Surgical treatment of complex cardiac anomalies: the 'one and one half ventricle repair'. Eur J Cardiothorac Surg. 2002;22:431–6; discussion 436–7.
116. Anderson RH, Ho SY. Pathologic substrates for 1 1/2 ventricular repair. Ann Thorac Surg. 1998;66:673–7.
117. Chowdhury UK, Airan B, Talwar S, et al. One and one-half ventricle repair: results and concerns. Ann Thorac Surg. 2005;80:2293–300.
118. Malhotra SP, Reddy VM, Qiu M, et al. The hemi-Mustard/bidirectional Glenn atrial switch procedure in the double-switch operation for congenitally corrected transposition of the great arteries: rationale and midterm results. J Thorac Cardiovasc Surg. 2011;141:162–70.
119. Kawashima Y, Kitamura S, Matsuda H, Shimazaki Y, Nakano S, Hirose H. Total cavopulmonary shunt operation in complex cardiac anomalies. A new operation. J Thorac Cardiovasc Surg. 1984;87:74–81.
120. Nath DS, Carden AJ, Nussbaum DP, et al. Can the Kawashima procedure be performed in younger patients? Ann Thorac Surg. 2009;88:581–6; discussion 586–7.
121. Srivastava D, Preminger T, Lock JE, et al. Hepatic venous blood and the development of pulmonary arteriovenous malformations in congenital heart disease. Circulation. 1995;92:1217–22.
122. Kawashima Y. Cavopulmonary shunt and pulmonary arteriovenous malformations. Ann Thorac Surg. 1997;63:930–2.
123. Brown JW, Ruzmetov M, Vijay P, Rodefeld MD, Turrentine MW. Pulmonary arteriovenous malformations in children after the Kawashima operation. Ann Thorac Surg. 2005;80:1592–6.
124. Setyapranata S, Brizard CP, Konstantinov IE, Iyengar A, Cheung M, d'Udekem Y. Should we always plan a Fontan completion after a Kawashima procedure? Eur J Cardiothorac Surg. 2011;40:1011–5.
125. McElhinney DB, Kreutzer J, Lang P, Mayer JE, del Nido PJ, Lock JE. Incorporation of the hepatic veins into the cavopulmonary circulation in patients with heterotaxy and pulmonary arteriovenous malformations after a Kawashima procedure. Ann Thorac Surg. 2005;80:1597–603.
126. Kreutzer G, Galíndez E, Bono H, De Palma C, Laura JP. An operation for the correction of tricuspid atresia. J Thorac Cardiovasc Surg. 1973;66:613–21.
127. Björk VO, Olin CL, Bjarke BB, Thorén CA. Right atrial-right ventricular anastomosis for correction of tricuspid atresia. J Thorac Cardiovasc Surg. 1979;77:452–8.
128. Bull C, de Leval MR, Stark J, Taylor JF, Macartney FJ. Use of a subpulmonary ventricular chamber in the Fontan circulation. J Thorac Cardiovasc Surg. 1983;85:21–31.
129. Ninan M, Myers JL. Conversion of the atriopulmonary Fontan connection to a total cavopulmonary connection. Semin Thorac Cardiovasc Surg Pediatr Card Surg Annu. 1998;1:23–30.
130. Giardini A, Pace Napoleone C, Specchia S, et al. Conversion of atriopulmonary Fontan to extracardiac total cavopulmonary connection improves cardiopulmonary function. Int J Cardiol. 2006; 113:341–4.
131. Mavroudis C, Backer CL, Deal BJ. Late reoperations for Fontan patients: state of the art invited review. Eur J Cardiothorac Surg. 2008;34:1034–40.

132. Sridhar A, Giamberti A, Foresti S, et al. Fontan conversion with concomitant arrhythmia surgery for the failing atriopulmonary connections: mid-term results from a single centre. Cardiol Young. 2011;21:665–9.
133. de Leval MR, Kilner P, Gewillig M, Bull C. Total cavopulmonary connection: a logical alternative to atriopulmonary connection for complex Fontan operations. Experimental studies and early clinical experience. J Thorac Cardiovasc Surg. 1988;96:682–95.
134. Jonas RA, Castaneda AR. Modified Fontan procedure: atrial baffle and systemic venous to pulmonary artery anastomotic techniques. J Card Surg. 1988;3:91–6.
135. Marcelletti CF, Iorio FS, Abella RF. Late results of extracardiac Fontan repair. Semin Thorac Cardiovasc Surg Pediatr Card Surg Annu. 1999;2:131–42.
136. Azakie A, McCrindle BW, Van Arsdell G, et al. Extracardiac conduit versus lateral tunnel cavopulmonary connections at a single institution: impact on outcomes. J Thorac Cardiovasc Surg. 2001;122:1219–28.
137. Bridges ND, Lock JE, Castaneda AR. Baffle fenestration with subsequent transcatheter closure. Modification of the Fontan operation for patients at increased risk. Circulation. 1990;82: 1681–9.
138. Goff DA, Blume ED, Gauvreau K, Mayer JE, Lock JE, Jenkins KJ. Clinical outcome of fenestrated Fontan patients after closure: the first 10 years. Circulation. 2000;102:2094–9.
139. Thompson LD, Petrossian E, McElhinney DB, et al. Is it necessary to routinely fenestrate an extracardiac Fontan? J Am Coll Cardiol. 1999;34:539–44.
140. Salazar JD, Zafar F, Siddiqui K, et al. Fenestration during Fontan palliation: now the exception instead of the rule. J Thorac Cardiovasc Surg. 2010;140:129–36.
141. Bradley SM. Use of a fenestration should be routine during the Fontan procedure: PRO. Semin Thorac Cardiovasc Surg Pediatr Card Surg Annu. 2010;13:55–9.
142. Black IW. Spontaneous echo contrast: where there's smoke there's fire. Echocardiography. 2000;17:373–82.
143. Kwaan HC, Sakurai S, Wang J. Rheological abnormalities and thromboembolic complications in heart disease: spontaneous echo contrast and red cell aggregation. Semin Thromb Hemost. 2003;29:529–34.
144. Kostolny M, Schreiber C, Henze R, Vogt M, Lange R. Temporary pulmonary vein stenosis during intraoperative transesophageal echocardiography in total cavopulmonary connection. Pediatr Cardiol. 2006;27:134–6.
145. Altarabsheh SE, Burkhart HM, Deo S, Cetta F. The transesophageal echocardiography probe: an unusual source of pulmonary venous obstruction. World J Pediatr Congenital Heart Surg. 2011;2:662–3.
146. Fyfe DA, Kline CH, Sade RM, Greene CA, Gillette PC. The utility of transesophageal echocardiography during and after Fontan operations in small children. Am Heart J. 1991;122:1403–15.
147. Manning WJ, Weintraub RM, Waksmonski CA, et al. Accuracy of transesophageal echocardiography for identifying left atrial thrombi. A prospective, intraoperative study. Ann Intern Med. 1995;123:817–22.
148. Wolfe LT, Rossi A, Ritter SB. Transesophageal echocardiography in infants and children: use and importance in the cardiac intensive care unit. J Am Soc Echocardiogr. 1993;6:286–9.
149. Marcus B, Wong PC. Transesophageal echocardiographic diagnosis of right atrioventricular valve patch dehiscence causing intracardiac right-to-left shunting after Fontan operation. Am Heart J. 1993;126:1482–4.
150. Marianeschi SM, McElhinney DB, Reddy VM. Pulmonary arteriovenous malformations in and out of the setting of congenital heart disease. Ann Thorac Surg. 1998;66:688–91.
151. Gazzaniga P, Buscarini E, Leandro G, et al. Contrast echocardiography for pulmonary arteriovenous malformations screening: does any bubble matter? Eur J Echocardiogr. 2009;10:513–8.

Outflow Tract Anomalies

11

Leo Lopez, Roque Ventura, and Nadine F. Choueiter

Abstract

Anomalies of the aortic and pulmonary outflow tracts are usually associated with obstruction, regurgitation, and/or aneurysmal dilation of the proximal great arteries, and they represent some of the conditions most frequently encountered by congenital heart disease specialists. In most instances, a full preoperative diagnosis is performed by standard transthoracic echocardiography and other imaging modalities such as cardiac catheterization and magnetic resonance imaging. However, transesophageal echocardiography (TEE) serves an important role in the perioperative management of these patients. Preoperative TEE can provide information regarding the morphology of the outflow tracts and the degree of obstruction and regurgitation; postoperative TEE can evaluate the success of a surgical procedure and exclude residual obstruction, regurgitation, or other potential complications. In addition, TEE is sometimes necessary outside of the operating room setting for older patients with poor transthoracic echocardiographic windows, particularly if the patient has undergone prior surgery. This chapter discusses the use of TEE for the evaluation of both right and left sided outflow tract anomalies.

Keywords

Aortic stenosis, valvar • Aortic stenosis, subvalvar • Aortic stenosis, supravalvar • Aortic regurgitation • Sinus of Valsalva aneurysm • Pulmonary stenosis, valvar • Double-chambered right ventricle • Pulmonary regurgitation

Introduction

Anomalies of the outflow tracts are usually associated with obstruction, regurgitation, and/or aneurysmal dilation of the proximal great arteries. Based on an analysis of almost 40 published articles on the incidence of congenital heart disease spanning many decades, pulmonary stenosis (PS), the most common anomaly of the right ventricular outflow tract (RVOT), ranks as the 4th most common congenital heart disease with a mean incidence of 0.73 per 1,000 live births, and aortic stenosis (AS), the most common anomaly of the left ventricular outflow tract (LVOT), ranks as the 7th most common with a mean incidence of 0.40 per 1,000 live births [1]. Among almost 60,000 patients evaluated at the Cardiovascular Program of Children's Hospital Boston from 1988 to 2002, a pulmonary valve (PV) abnormality was the 4th most common diagnosis with a frequency of 5.7 %, and an aortic valve (AoV) abnormality was the 5th most common with a frequency of 5.5 % [2]. A bicuspid AoV is in fact the most common congenital heart disease with an incidence of 0.4–2 % in the general population [3–5].

L. Lopez, MD (✉) • N.F. Choueiter, MD
Department of Pediatrics,
Albert Einstein College of Medicine,
Children's Hospital at Montefiore,
3415 Bainbridge Ave – Rosenthal 1,
Bronx, NY 10467, USA
e-mail: llmd@llmd.net

R. Ventura, RCS
Department of Pediatrics,
Miami Children's Hospital, 3100 Southwest 62nd Avenue,
Miami, FL 33155, USA

The online version of this chapter (doi:10.1007/978-1-84800-064-3_11) contains supplementary material, which is available to authorized users.

P.C. Wong, W.C. Miller-Hance (eds.), *Transesophageal Echocardiography for Congenital Heart Disease*,
DOI 10.1007/978-1-84800-064-3_11, © Springer-Verlag London 2014

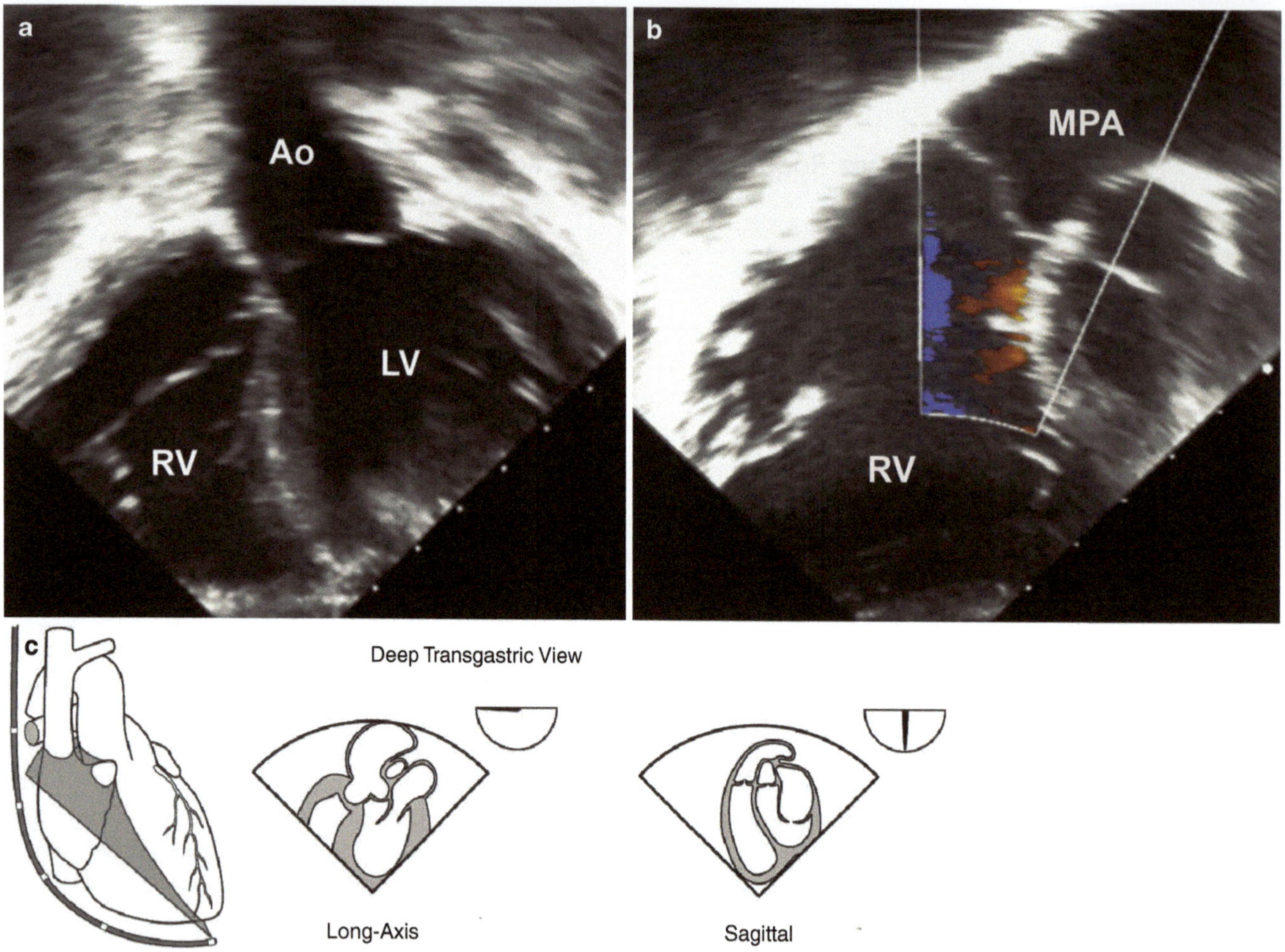

Fig. 11.1 (**a**) Deep transgastric long axis view at 0° showing the LV outflow tract; (**b**) Deep transgastric sagittal view at 90° showing the RV outflow tract; (**c**) Illustration depicting how the LV and RV outflow tracts are evaluated in deep transgastric views (*Ao* aorta, *LV* left ventricle, *MPA* main pulmonary artery, *RV* right ventricle)

Because isolated obstruction at the valvar level in both outflow tracts is generally treated in the catheterization laboratory rather than in the operating room, intraoperative transesophageal echocardiography (TEE) is not frequently performed for valvar stenosis. However, if the obstruction occurs at the subvalvar or supravalvar level or if the primary lesion is regurgitation and/or aneurysmal dilation of the proximal great artery, surgical intervention is often necessary, thereby requiring intraoperative TEE before and after the surgery.

Utility of Transesophageal Echocardiography

Patients with significant outflow tract anomalies other than valvar AS or PS do not usually require surgery during the first year of life, and they often do not undergo any intervention until they are toddlers, adolescents, or adults. Outflow tract obstruction and semilunar valve regurgitation are usually associated with a morphologic abnormality at or near the semilunar valves. During the preoperative evaluation in the operating room, TEE can usually provide information regarding the morphology of the outflow tracts from the mid and upper esophageal views, and the degree of obstruction and regurgitation, if present, from the deep transgastric (Fig. 11.1, Video 11.1a and 11.1b) and mid esophageal views (see Chap. 4) [6]. Postoperative TEE can evaluate the success of a surgical procedure and exclude residual obstruction, regurgitation, or other potential complications. However it is important to note that intraoperative TEE data will always reflect the patient's hemodynamics, which can be affected by general anesthesia, inotropic support, volume status, and ventricular function. For example, the degree of residual obstruction or regurgitation across a semilunar valve can be underestimated in the setting of general anesthesia, hypovolemia, tachycardia, or poor ventricular function. In contrast, the degree of dynamic obstruction, as seen in tetralogy of Fallot or hypertrophic cardiomyopathy secondary to muscular hypertrophy in the subarterial region, can be overestimated in the presence of hypovolemia or hyperdynamic ventricular function, especially with inotropic support.

Occasionally, TEE is necessary outside of the operating room for older patients with poor transthoracic echocardiographic windows, particularly if the patient has undergone prior surgery.

Normal Anatomy

The term conotruncus (from the Greek words conus for cone and truncus for trunk or body) represents the outflow tracts of both ventricles. It is composed of the subarterial regions, the semilunar valves, the great arterial roots, and the proximal trunks. The conus (also known as the infundibulum from the Latin word for funnel) defines the subarterial muscular chamber, which prevents fibrous continuity between the semilunar valve and the corresponding atrioventricular valve. In the normal heart, the subpulmonary conus prevents fibrous continuity between the tricuspid valve and the PV. The supraventricular crest is the prominent muscular shelf along the posterior aspect of the subpulmonary conus, and it is composed of the conal septum (or infundibular septum) separating the RVOT from the LVOT, the right ventriculo-infundibular fold separating the tricuspid valve leaflets from the PV leaflets, and the subpulmonary muscular sleeve supporting the PV leaflets. The subpulmonary conus is separated from the trabecular segment of the RV chamber at the infundibular os, an area defined by the moderator band, the septal band (also known as the septomarginal trabeculation), and the parietal band of the RV. The subaortic conus regresses *in utero*, resulting in varying degrees of fibrous continuity between the mitral valve and AoV. This fibrous area, known as the mitral-aortic intervalvular fibrosa, is measured as the shortest distance from the anterior mitral leaflet to the base of the non-coronary or left coronary AoV leaflet and can be elongated in cases of subvalvar AS and tetralogy of Fallot.

The normal semilunar valve is a three-dimensional structure wherein three leaflets (or cusps) are attached to the arterial root and supporting ventricular muscle in a semilunar or crown-like fashion. The leaflets are separated by three commissures that extend during diastole from the center of the valve at the level of the ventriculo-arterial junction to the periphery at the level of the sino-tubular junction (Fig. 11.2, Video 11.2). It is important to recognize that the semilunar valve "annulus" is in fact a diagnostician construct without a true anatomic correlate since the semilunar valve leaflet attachments extend from the anatomic ventriculo-arterial junction up to the sino-tubular junction; the so-called "annulus" as defined in echocardiography represents only the most proximal attachment of the semilunar valve and not its attachment in entirety [7] (Fig. 11.3, Video 11.3).

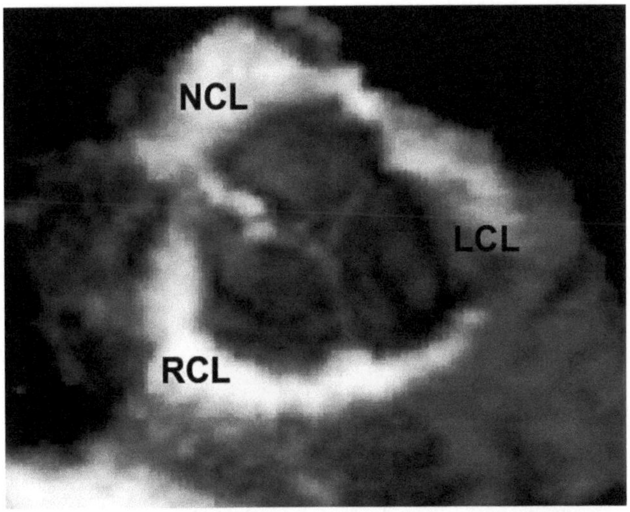

Fig. 11.2 Three-dimension mid esophageal aortic valve short axis view depicting the three-dimensional nature of a normal tri-leaflet aortic valve (*LCL* left coronary leaflet, *NCL* non-coronary leaflet, *RCL* right coronary leaflet)

Left Ventricular Outflow Tract Anomalies

Valvar Aortic Stenosis

Congenital valvar AS results from a bicuspid or unicuspid AoV, a dysplastic tricuspid AoV, or a hypoplastic aortic "annulus". Acquired valvar AS usually results from calcification secondary to degenerative or post-inflammatory causes [8], though a bicuspid AoV is also a risk factor for calcification [5]. A bicuspid AoV is the most common cause of valvar AS, although the presence of a bicuspid AoV does not necessarily mean a patient has (or will develop) valvar AS. As noted previously, a bicuspid AoV is the most common congenital heart defect, with an incidence of 0.4–2 % in the general population [3–5]. There are several distinct anatomic variations. It is rare to encounter a bicuspid AoV with only two well-developed leaflets (Fig. 11.4, Video 11.4); instead, it usually involves fusion of two of the three leaflets or underdevelopment of one of the commissures (known as a raphé) [9]. It is because of the absence of one of the three commissures that the lesion is often referred to as a bicommissural AoV. Among these, fusion occurs most commonly at the intercoronary commissure between the right and left coronary leaflets with a frequency of 70 % (Fig. 11.5, Video 11.5), followed by the commissure between the right and non-coronary leaflets with a frequency of 28 % (Fig. 11.6, Video 11.6); fusion at the commissure between the left and non-coronary leaflets is very rare [10]. In adults, the rate of AS progression appears to be higher in those valves with fusion of the intercoronary commissure [11], though studies in children have revealed more rapid progression of AS and regurgitation as well as shorter time from diagnosis to

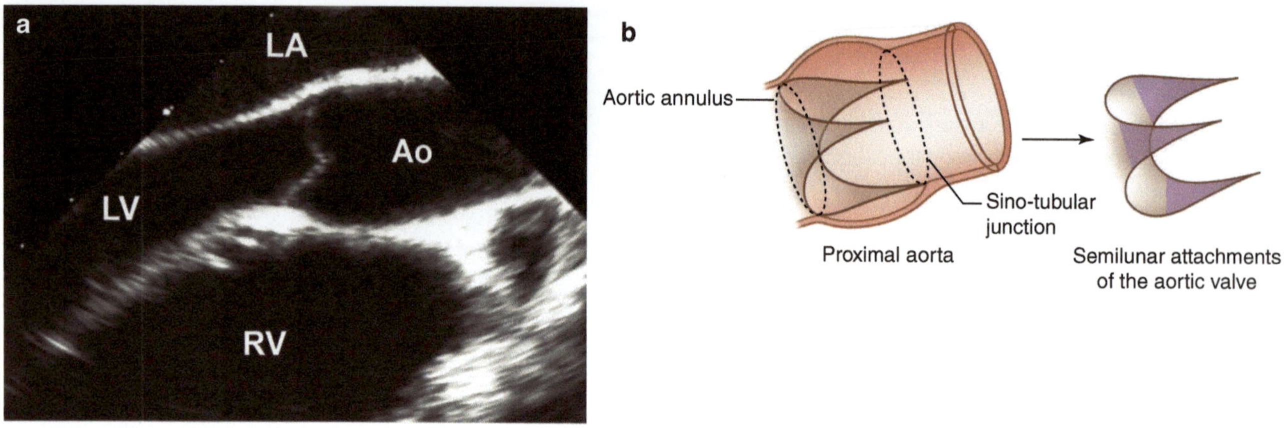

Fig. 11.3 (**a**) Mid esophageal aortic valve long axis view at 120° showing the LV outflow tract; (**b**) Illustration of the aortic valve and its semilunar attachments within the aortic root from the ventriculo-arterial junction to the sino-tubular junction (*Ao* aorta, *LA* left atrium, *LV* left ventricle, *RV* right ventricle)

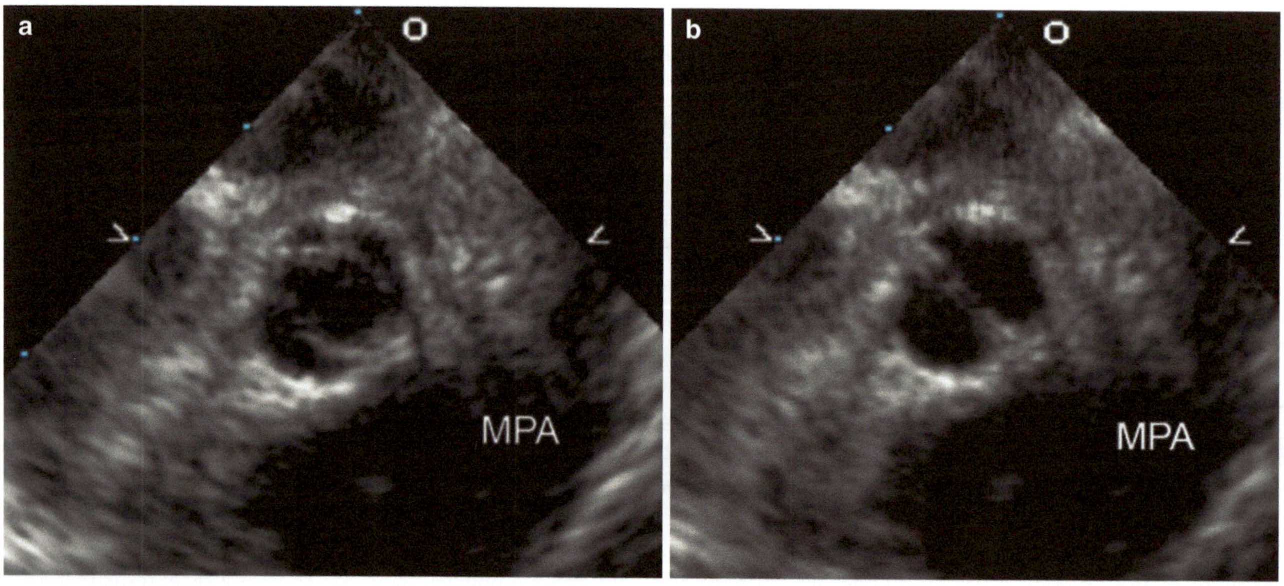

Fig. 11.4 Mid esophageal aortic valve short axis view at 30° shows a true bicuspid aortic valve with only two leaflets (the right and left coronary leaflets) and absent non-coronary leaflet, in the open (**a**) and closed (**b**) positions. This gives a "fishmouth" appearance to the valve orifice (*MPA* main pulmonary artery)

intervention in valves with fusion of the commissure between the right and non-coronary leaflets [12]. Associations with a bicuspid AoV include aortic coarctation [3] or interrupted aortic arch, subvalvar AS, a ventricular septal defect (VSD), a coronary anomaly, Turner syndrome [13], and aortic dilation or aneurysm formation [14–16]. Valvar AS can be an evolving pathology and the degree of progression may be associated with age at presentation and/or severity at the time of presentation [17]. Although it occurs rarely, sudden death in this patient population appears to be related to significant stenosis and regurgitation [18]. In addition, the chronic pressure load experienced by the LV leads to hypertrophy with the potential for permanent muscular damage and fibrosis. Therefore, management of these patients must focus on prevention of these sequelae.

Over the past several decades, transcatheter balloon valvotomy in the catheterization laboratory has become a more popular management approach for patients with valvar AS, superseding surgical valvotomy as the primary mode of treatment. TEE is not often needed during this procedure, though occasionally it is helpful in determining the appropriate intervention and/or assessing its efficacy. Echocardiography for valvar AS should always include assessment of leaflet and commissural morphology, degree of obstruction, degree of LV

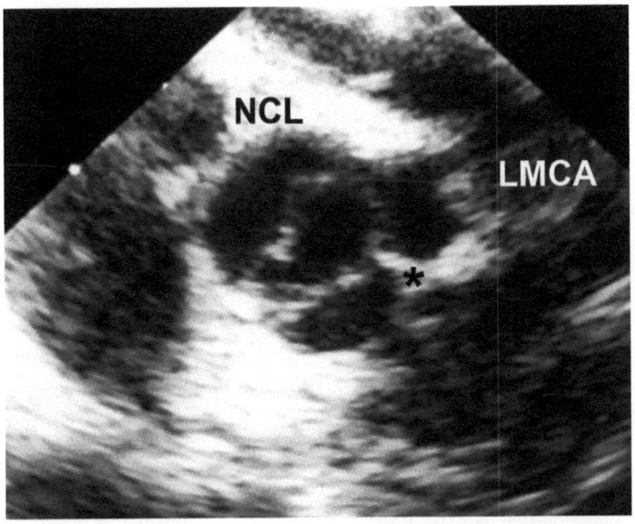

Fig. 11.5 Mid esophageal aortic valve short axis view at 30° showing a bicuspid aortic valve with fusion or underdevelopment of the intercoronary commissure (*black asterisk*) (*NCL* non-coronary leaflet, *LMCA* left main coronary artery)

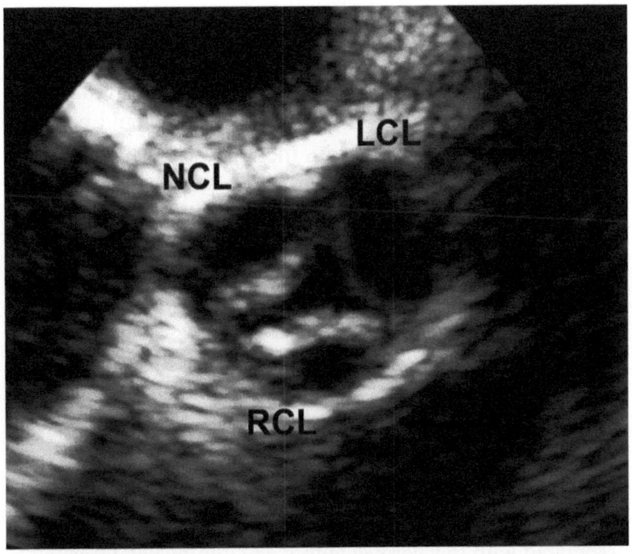

Fig. 11.7 Mid esophageal aortic valve short axis view at 30° showing a dysplastic aortic valve with thickened right and non-coronary leaflets (*LCL* left coronary leaflet, *NCL* non-coronary leaflet, *RCL* right coronary leaflet)

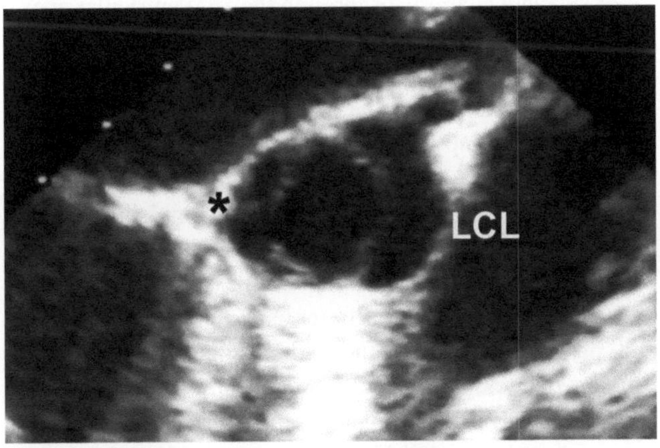

Fig. 11.6 Mid esophageal aortic valve short axis view at 30° showing a bicuspid aortic valve with fusion or underdevelopment of the commissure between the right and non-coronary leaflets (*black asterisk*) (*LCL* left coronary leaflet)

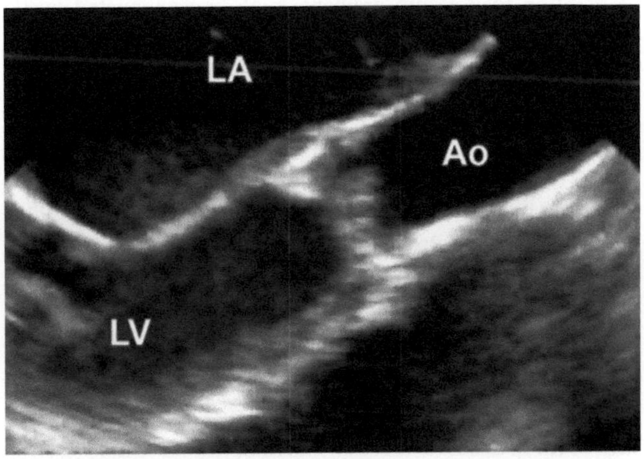

Fig. 11.8 Mid esophageal aortic valve long axis view at 120° showing a dysplastic aortic valve associated with valvar aortic stenosis (*Ao* aorta, *LA* left atrium, *LV* left ventricle)

hypertrophy, ascending aortic size, and left atrial dilation. Aortic measurements (aortic valve, aortic root, and ascending aorta) are often helpful. Leaflet and commissural morphology are best evaluated in the mid esophageal views, usually at 30–45° for the mid esophageal aortic valve short axis (ME AV SAX) images (Figs. 11.4, 11.5, 11.6, and 11.7, Videos 11.4, 11.5, 11.6, and 11.7) and at ~120° for the mid esophageal aortic valve long axis (ME AV LAX) images (Fig. 11.8, Video 11.8). It is, however, important to recognize that pure short and long axis images can be difficult to obtain—even with multiplane TEE—because of the fixed spatial relationship between the esophagus and the aortic outflow tract. When a pure short axis image is available (that is, when the AoV annular plane is completely perpendicular to the axis of the beam), the relative sizes of the leaflets should be evaluated, and failure of commissural opening in the setting of a bicuspid or unicuspid valve can be displayed. Long axis imaging of the AoV can reveal thickened and doming leaflets. More recently, three-dimensional echocardiography has emerged as an important tool for the assessment of aortic valve anatomy and pathology (Chaps. 19 and 20).

The degree of obstruction is generally assessed by estimation of the pressure gradient across the stenotic valve, using continuous wave Doppler interrogation along the aortic outflow tract. This is best performed in the deep transgastric long axis (DTG LAX) view with multiplane angle between 0° and 30° (Fig. 11.1a, Video 11.1a), or sometimes from the deep transgastric sagittal (DTG Sagittal) view with multiplane angle between 80° and 110° (Fig. 11.1b, Video 11.1b).

Because of the distance from the probe to the outflow tract, imaging from this view often requires using the lowest possible frequency for improved penetration as well as minimizing the image and color sector size. Every effort should be made to align the Doppler beam with the LVOT. As an alternative, the transgastric long axis view (TG LAX) can be used for interrogation of the LVOT because it generally provides favorable angles for continuous wave Doppler interrogation (Chap. 4) with a shorter distance from the probe to the aortic valve. Both peak and mean pressure gradients should be measured [19–21]. It is important to recognize that echocardiographically derived Doppler gradients often do not correspond to the peak-to-peak gradient measured in the catheterization laboratory, a common discrepancy which results from several factors, including a phenomenon called pressure recovery [22]. In addition, severe LV dysfunction in the setting of valvar AS is associated with low cardiac output and diminished transvalvar flow, and Doppler interrogation may reveal a low gradient despite severe obstruction at the valvar level. Similarly, the degree of LVOT obstruction can be artificially decreased in the setting of general anesthesia, deep sedation, or hypovolemia. In addition to pressure gradient, some use calculated aortic valve area to evaluate the degree of obstruction as derived by the continuity equation, which states that the stroke volume in the subaortic region is the same as the stroke volume at the valvar level (see Chap. 1). Since stroke volume is equal to the velocity-time integral multiplied by cross-sectional area at a particular location, the effective aortic valve area can be calculated if the LVOT cross-sectional area and the velocity-time integrals at the LVOT and at the aortic valve are known [23]. However, the LVOT is frequently not circular in shape, precluding accurate assessment of LVOT cross-sectional areas using LVOT diameters, and some have suggested that three-dimensional TEE may be preferable to two-dimensional imaging for more accurate assessments of aortic valve area [24].

It is important to note that AS represents a disease continuum, and severity cannot be defined by a single value [21]. With these considerations in mind, the following echocardiographic criteria for classification of AoV stenosis severity were recently given by a 2008 American College of Cardiology/American Heart Association (ACC/AHA) task force on valvular heart disease [21].

- Mild: peak velocity <3 m/s, mean gradient <25 mmHg, valve area >1.5 cm^2
- Moderate: peak velocity 3.0–4.0 m/s, mean gradient 25–40 mmHg, valve area 1.0–1.5 cm^2
- Severe: peak velocity >4 m/s, mean gradient >40 mmHg, valve area <1.0 cm^2

Similar guidelines have not been written specifically for the pediatric population. At present, the above criteria are generally applied to this group of patients as well [25–27].

LV hypertrophy is best evaluated in the transgastric basal short axis (TG Basal SAX) and transgastric mid short axis (TG Mid SAX) views at 0°, though a quantitative assessment of the degree of hypertrophy may not be reliable with TEE, again because pure short axis images of the LV in transgastric views at 0° may not always be available. The size of the aortic root and ascending aorta are best measured in mid esophageal aortic valve long axis (ME AV LAX) and mid esophageal ascending aortic long axis (ME Asc Ao LAX) views at 90–120°; important measurements that should be obtained in early to mid systole include the diameters of the aortic valve annulus, aortic root diameter, sino-tubular junction, and ascending aorta [28]. These measurements are analogous to those obtained by transthoracic echocardiography, and they can be compared to published normal values [29, 30]. Left atrial dilation can be easily visualized in mid esophageal fourchamber (ME 4 Ch) and twochamber (ME 2 Ch) views at 0° and 90° respectively.

Recently, a new procedure for the nonsurgical treatment of severe valvar AS has garnered widespread interest. Known as transcatheter AoV replacement/implantation, or TAVR/TAVI, this procedure is performed in the cardiac catheterization laboratory and involves the implantation of a bovine or porcine pericardial valve mounted upon a metal support frame [31]. Delivered transarterially (access by percutaneous femoral or subclavian artery, or through the left ventricular apex), the balloon-mounted valve is advanced to the AoV position, and the balloon expanded within the diseased AoV, displacing the diseased native valve leaflets. During the procedure, TEE is utilized and serves a number of important functions: (a) pre-procedure evaluation of anatomy and function; (b) monitoring of valve implantation; (c) post-implantation evaluation of valve function and valve regurgitation (Fig. 11.9, Video 11.9). The post-implantation TEE is particularly useful in that it enables accurate differentiation between transvalvar and paravalvar aortic regurgitation, something not easily visualized by angiography or fluoroscopy [32]. At present, two major valves are available—the Edwards SAPIEN XT heart valve (Edwards Lifesciences Inc., Irvine, California) and the CoreValve ReValving system (Medtronic Inc., Minneapolis, Minnesota)—but a number of other valves are undergoing early clinical evaluation [33]. Currently, the procedure is performed only in adults; candidates are generally patients with severe valvar AS felt to be too high risk for surgical intervention [34, 35] (see also Chap. 16).

Subvalvar Aortic Stenosis

Subvalvar AS is rarely diagnosed *in utero* or in the newborn period, prompting many people to classify this lesion as an acquired heart disease rather than a congenital one [36, 37]. It is a progressive disease, particularly in children, and some have suggested that its development may involve the following mechanisms: abnormal LVOT morphology leads to increased septal shear stress, which because of some genetic predisposition leads in turn to cellular proliferation [38, 39]. Some of the abnormalities in LVOT morphology that are

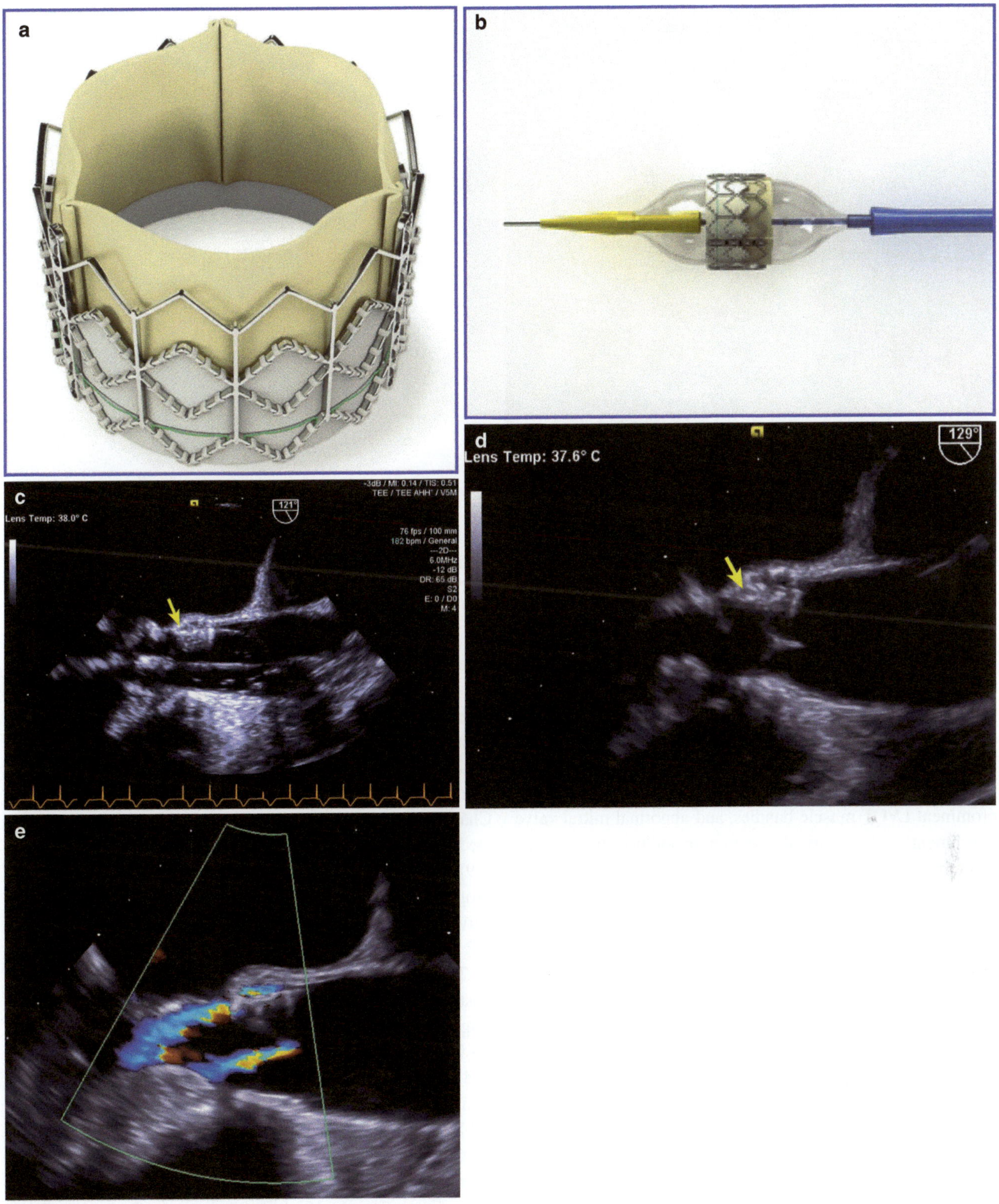

Fig. 11.9 Transcatheter aortic valve replacement/implantation (TAVR/TAVI). (**a**) Shows the Edwards SAPIEN valve (Edwards Lifesciences Inc., Irvine, California), a bovine pericardial valve mounted on a stainless steel frame. (**b**) Shows the same valve mounted on a balloon catheter that is used for valve delivery. (**c–e**) Are transesophageal echocardiographic images obtained from the mid esophageal aortic valve long axis view at 120–130°. (**c**) Shows the balloon being inflated (device indicated with *arrow*), and (**d**) Shows the valve (*arrow*) after implantation. In (**e**), following valve implantation color flow Doppler shows two small jets of regurgitation: one a central transvalvar jet, the other a peripheral paravalvar jet (Echocardiographic images provided courtesy of Siemens Medical Systems USA, Inc. © 2012–13 Siemens Medical Solutions USA, Inc. All rights reserved)

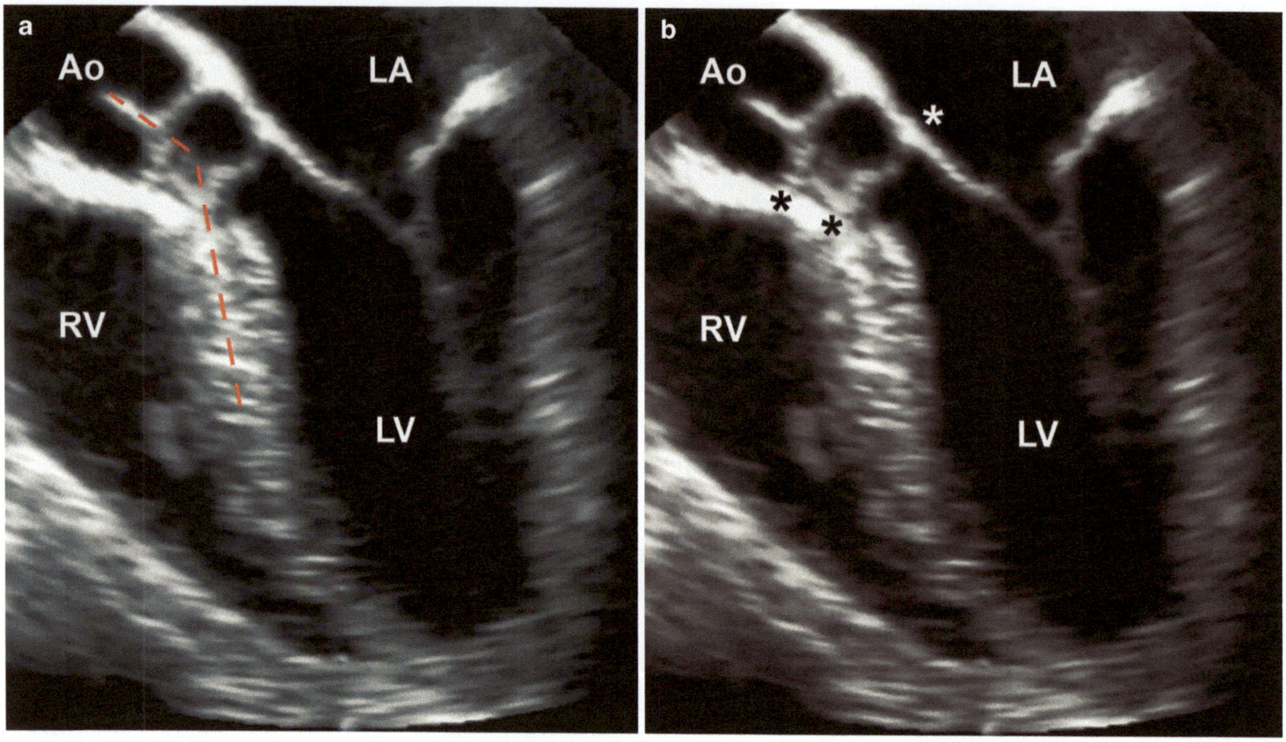

Fig. 11.10 Mid esophageal four chamber view with probe anteflexion to visualize the left ventricular outflow tract, showing a subaortic fibromuscular ridge associated with subvalvar aortic stenosis. The two figures depict (**a**) a steep aorto-septal angle (*dashed red lines*), and (**b**) the distance between the ridge and the aortic annulus (*black asterisk*) and extension of the fibromuscular ridge to the anterior mitral leaflet (*white asterisk*) (*Ao* aorta, *LA* left atrium, *LV* left ventricle, *RV* right ventricle)

associated with subvalvar AS include a steep aorto-septal angle (Fig. 11.10a, Video 11.10), an elongated mitral-aortic intervalvular fibrosa, exaggerated aortic override [40, 41], prominent LVOT muscle bundles, and abnormal mitral valve attachments to the ventricular septum. In addition, the distance from the level of the obstruction to the AoV appears to be one of the major predictors of significantly progressive obstruction [42] (Fig. 11.10b, Video 11.10). Subvalvar AS can occur without or with a VSD. Examples of subvalvar AS in the absence of a VSD include: (a) a discrete fibrous or fibromuscular subaortic ridge protruding from the ventricular septum and sometimes extending to the anterior mitral leaflet (Fig. 11.10b, Video 11.10); (b) an extensive muscular shelf creating a tunnel-like LVOT; (c) hypertrophic cardiomyopathy with dynamic obstruction secondary to diffuse septal hypertrophy and systolic anterior motion of the mitral valve and/or its tensor apparatus (Fig. 11.11, Video 11.11). Subvalvar AS without a VSD can also develop postoperatively after mitral valve replacement with a mechanical prosthesis [43–45]. The most common type of subvalvar AS in the setting of a VSD occurs with posterior deviation of the conal septum, a lesion that is often associated with aortic coarctation or interrupted aortic arch [46, 47]. (see Chaps. 9 and 13) Other examples of subvalvar AS include endocardial folds or fibromuscular ridges at the crest of the muscular septum (Fig. 11.12, Video 11.12), often without significant obstruction [48], and abnormal mitral valve attachments to the ventricular septum, often in the setting of an atrioventricular canal (atrioventricular septal) defect (see Chap. 8) Aside from a VSD, subvalvar AS can also be associated with a bicuspid AoV, a double-chambered RV (DCRV) [49], and aortic regurgitation (AR). In fact, the risk for rapidly progressive AR is frequently the reason that children with subvalvar AS require early surgical intervention [50], although AR in adults with subvalvar AS is rarely progressive [51, 52].

TEE is especially useful in delineating the mechanism of obstruction in patients with subvalvar AS. A fibromuscular ridge with or without extension to the anterior mitral leaflet, posterior deviation of the conal septum, a tunnel-like LVOT, and abnormal mitral valve attachments to the ventricular septum can usually be characterized in the ME 4 Ch and ME AV LAX (at ~120°) views or in the DTG LAX view at 0–30° and DTG Sagittal view at 80–110°. In addition, the distance from a fibromuscular ridge to the AoV leaflets can be measured in these views (Fig. 11.10b). The degree of AR can usually be assessed in multiple mid esophageal and deep transgastric views (as discussed later in this chapter). The AoV leaflet and commissural morphology should always be evaluated in the ME AV SAX view at ~30° (Figs. 11.4, 11.5, 11.6, and 11.7), especially in the setting of significant AR. The utility and limitations of the DTG LAX view at 0–30° in quantifying the

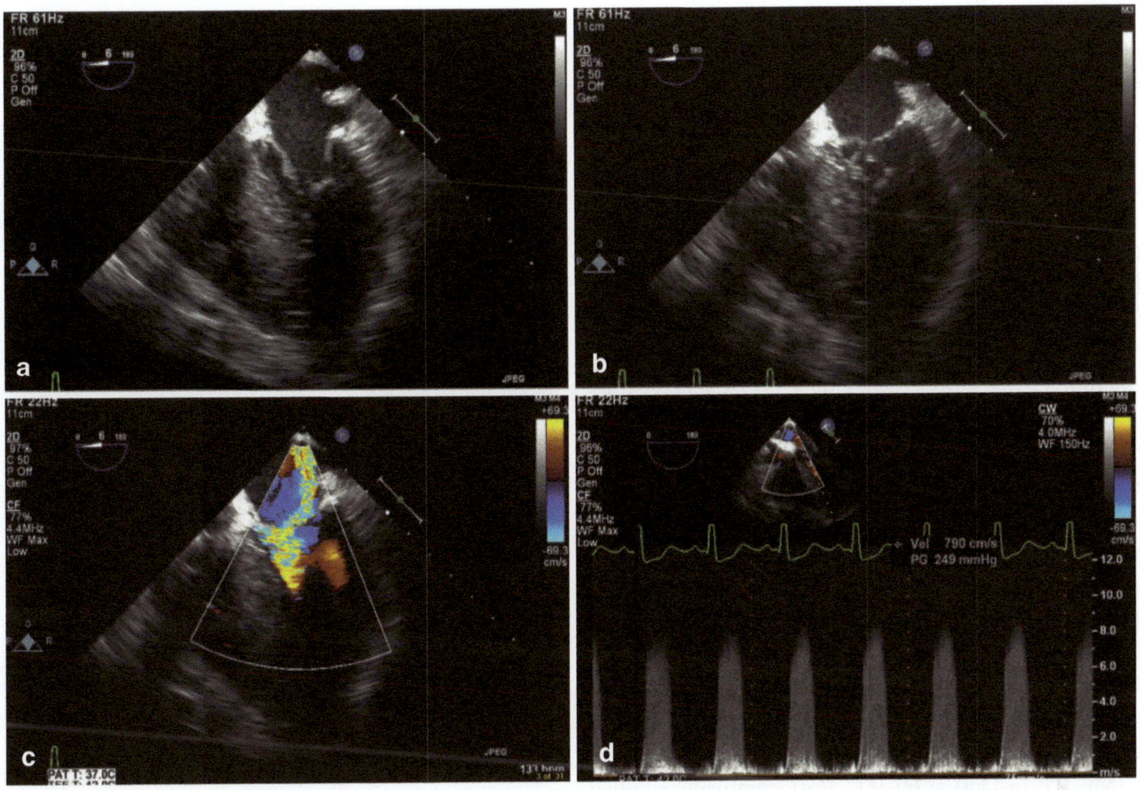

Fig. 11.11 Mid esophageal four chamber view showing subaortic stenosis causing systolic anterior motion (SAM) of the mitral valve, in a patient with significant ventricular septal hypertrophy. This is characterized by systolic displacement of the anterior mitral leaflet into the left ventricular outflow tract. In diastole (**a**) the mitral valve opens normally. However during systole there is a "drag" effect produced by the underfilled, hyperdynamic left ventricle that pulls the anterior leaflet into the left ventricular outflow tract (**b**). This prevents the mitral valve from effective coaptation and produces significant mitral regurgitation (**c**). The SAM also results in dynamic left ventricular outflow tract obstruction, producing a gradient that can be very high; in this patient there is a late-peaking, dagger-shaped spectral Doppler tracing, with a peak velocity measured at nearly 8 m/s, or 256 mmHg (**d**)

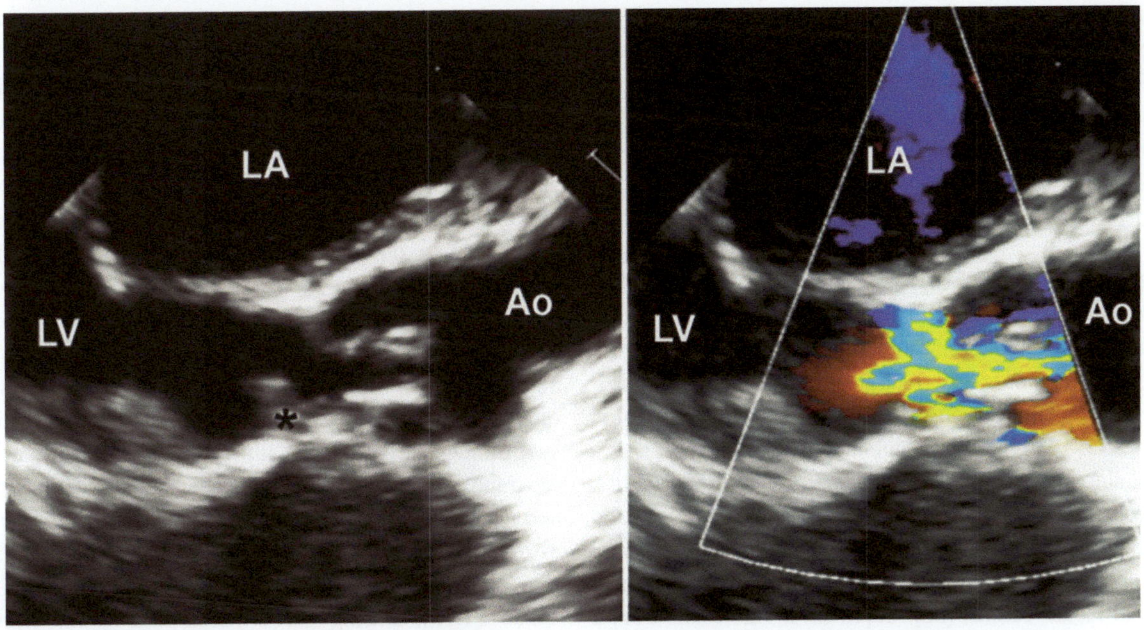

Fig. 11.12 Mid esophageal aortic valve long axis view at 120° showing a subaortic fibromuscular ridge (*black asterisk*) and a dysplastic aortic valve resulting in combined subvalvar and valvar aortic stenosis in addition to a small membranous ventricular septal defect (not well-seen on the image, but readily visible on Video 11–12). The fibromuscular ridge is located at the crest of the muscular septum. *Ao* aorta, *LA* left atrium, *LV* left ventricle

degree of obstruction have been discussed previously. Occasionally a ME Asc Ao LAX view at ~120°, or higher view such as the upper esophageal aortic arch long axis (UE Ao Arch LAX) at 0° or upper esophageal aortic arch short axis (UE Ao Arch SAX) at ~120° can provide an adequate Doppler angle to measure the gradient arising from the subaortic region. In some instances of subvalvar AS, a favorable angle for spectral Doppler interrogation can even be obtained from a modified ME 4 Ch view (Fig. 11.11, Video 11.11), though care must be taken not to contaminate the continuous wave Doppler tracing with a mitral regurgitation jet present along the same scan line. After mitral valve replacement with a mechanical prosthesis, the mid esophageal window can be ineffective because the mechanical prosthesis is located between the TEE probe and the LVOT, and acoustic interference by the prosthesis can partially or completely inhibit visualization of the outflow tract. In these instances, the TG LAX and deep transgastric views (DTG LAX, DTG Sagittal) can be helpful since the probe is positioned beyond the prosthesis, allowing for unobstructed imaging and Doppler interrogation. Associations such as a VSD or a DCRV should be excluded in the preoperative TEE, and these are usually visualized in the mid esophageal views: the ME 4 Ch view at 0° and the mid esophageal right ventricular inflow-outflow (ME RV In-Out) at 60–90°. Postoperatively, residual LVOT obstruction should be excluded qualitatively in the ME AV LAX and mid esophageal long axis (ME LAX) views (multiplane angle for both at ~120°), and quantitatively (by spectral Doppler evaluation) in the DTG LAX, DTG Sagittal, and TG LAX views. The AoV leaflets should be re-evaluated in the ME AV SAX view at 30–45°, and the presence of post-interventional AR should be assessed in multiple mid esophageal and deep transgastric views. Finally, inadvertent VSD creation and/or mitral valve injury are known complications following surgical intervention of subvalvar aortic stenosis [53, 54]. These areas should be evaluated carefully by postoperative TEE using a variety of mid esophageal and deep transgastric views, as described above and in Chap. 4.

Supravalvar Aortic Stenosis

Supravalvar AS is the least common type of LVOT obstruction, representing only 7 % of all patients undergoing surgical repair for LVOT obstruction at Children's Hospital Boston from 1956 to 1976 [55]. Although it occasionally presents as a familial autosomal dominant lesion or as a sporadic idiopathic disorder, it is usually associated with Williams syndrome, a constellation of clinical features which include developmental delay, calcium metabolism problems, failure to thrive, and abnormal facial features [56]. Supravalvar AS results from a mutation or deletion of the elastin gene on chromosome 7 [57, 58]. The obstruction occurs at the sino-tubular junction, and three anatomic subtypes have been described: the hourglass type (most common) involving dilation of the aortic root proximal to the narrowing and the ascending aorta distal to the narrowing (Fig. 11.13, Video 11.13), the membranous or diaphragmatic type, and the rare tubular type with diffuse hypoplasia of the ascending aorta [59, 60]. Patients with Williams syndrome can also have branch pulmonary artery stenosis, aortic coarctation, and renal artery stenosis in addition to supravalvar AS. Other associations include subvalvar AS, an abnormal AoV, and coronary abnormalities such as coronary artery dilation, coronary thickening, ostial stenosis, and ostial entrapment by a tethered AoV (Fig. 11.13). Obstruction can occur at more than one level, and the degree of obstruction usually progresses over time. Surgical intervention is generally undertaken when significant obstruction is present in order to prevent irreversible left ventricular myocardial damage. In many cases, TEE is superior to transthoracic echocardiography in the evaluation of the entire extent of the ascending aorta. The aortic root and proximal ascending aorta are best assessed by TEE in a ME AV LAX view at ~120° wherein the long axis of the proximal aorta can be displayed (Fig. 11.13, Video 11.13). During probe withdrawal in this view, the ascending aorta can be further evaluated with the ME Asc Ao LAX view. The degree of obstruction can be quantified with

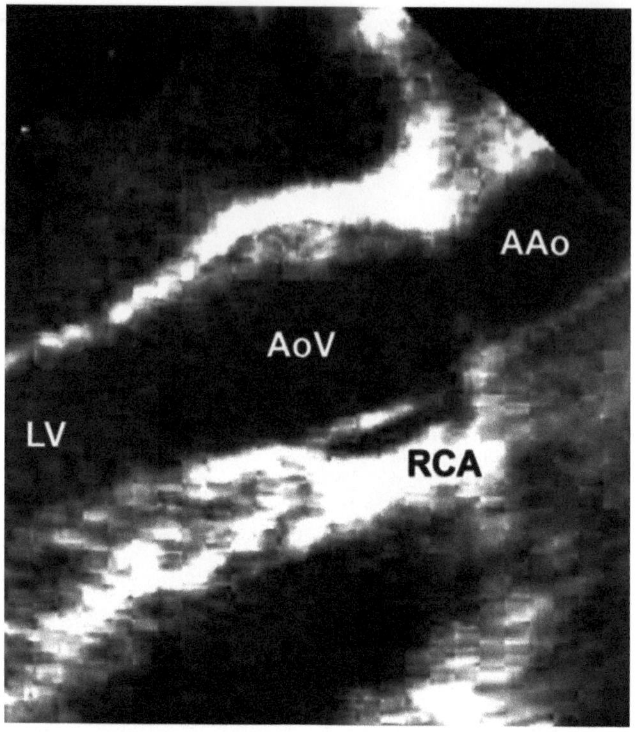

Fig. 11.13 Mid esophageal aortic valve long axis view at 120° showing discrete narrowing at the sino-tubular junction resulting in supravalvar aortic stenosis and entrapment of the right coronary ostium (*AAo* ascending aorta, *AoV* aortic valve, *LV* left ventricle, *RCA* right coronary artery)

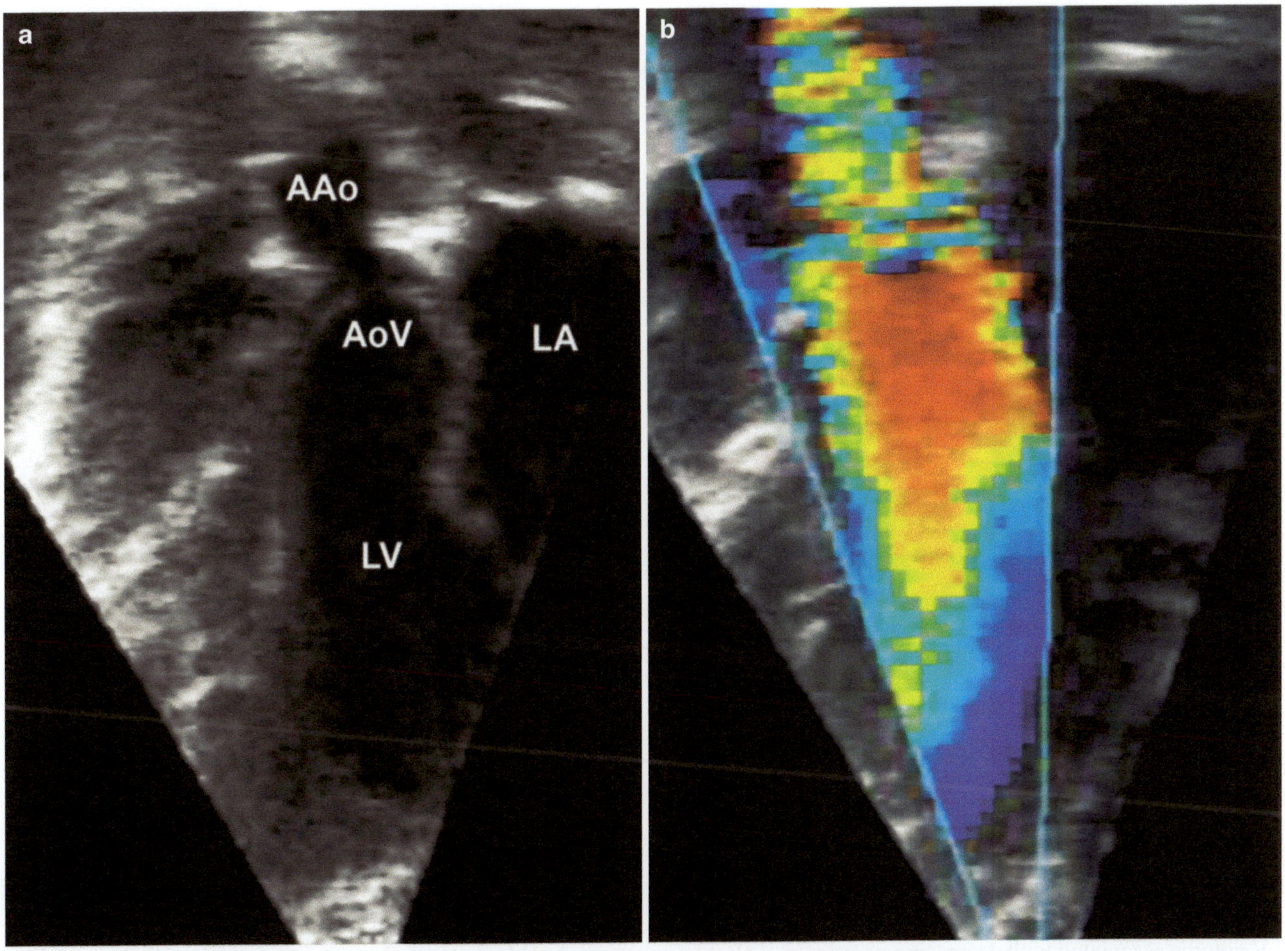

Fig. 11.14 Deep transgastric long axis view at 30° showing discrete narrowing of the sino-tubular junction resulting in supravalvar aortic stenosis (**a**) two-dimensional imaging and (**b**) color flow mapping (*AAo* ascending aorta, *AoV* aortic valve, *LA* left atrium, *LV* left ventricle)

DTG LAX (Fig. 11.14, Video 11.14), DTG Sagittal, and TG LAX views. In some cases, withdrawing the probe to an UE Ao Arch LAX or UE Ao Arch SAX view will provide an adequate Doppler angle of interrogation to quantify the degree of obstruction. TEE imaging, color mapping, and Doppler interrogation should also exclude other associations such as subvalvar AS (ME 4 Ch, ME AV LAX views), an abnormal AoV (ME AV SAX, ME AV LAX views), and coronary artery dilation and coronary ostial obstruction (ME AV SAX, ME AV LAX views). Evaluation of possible coronary ostial obstruction is best performed with color mapping looking for turbulence in the area of stenosis [61–63]. The TG Mid and Basal SAX views can also be used to evaluate for segmental wall motion abnormalities, supporting the possibility of coronary artery obstruction. The branch pulmonary arteries should also be evaluated for possible stenosis using the mid esophageal ascending aorta short axis (ME Asc Ao SAX), upper esophageal pulmonary artery LAX (UE PA LAX), and UE Ao Arch SAX views. The branch pulmonary arteries can be difficult to evaluate by TEE, though color mapping can be quite helpful in ascertaining the presence and location of the stenosis (Chaps. 4 and 13).

Aortic Regurgitation

Isolated congenital AR, defined loosely as diastolic flow from the aortic root into the LV, is a rare lesion [64]. Congenital etiologies causing AR in childhood include a bicuspid or quadricuspid AoV (Fig. 11.15, Video 11.15), a dysplastic tricuspid AoV, an aortico-left ventricular tunnel, absence of one or more AoV leaflets, a coronary-cameral fistula into the LV, and a ruptured sinus of Valsalva aneurysm into the LV. Occasionally AR occurs in the setting of subvalvar AS (as discussed previously), AoV prolapse into a membranous or doubly-committed subarterial VSD, or a ruptured sinus of Valsalva aneurysm into the right atrium (Fig. 11.16, Video 11.16a and 11.16b) or RV. It can also be seen with aortic root dilation in association with neonatal Marfan syndrome, tetralogy of Fallot, or truncus arteriosus.

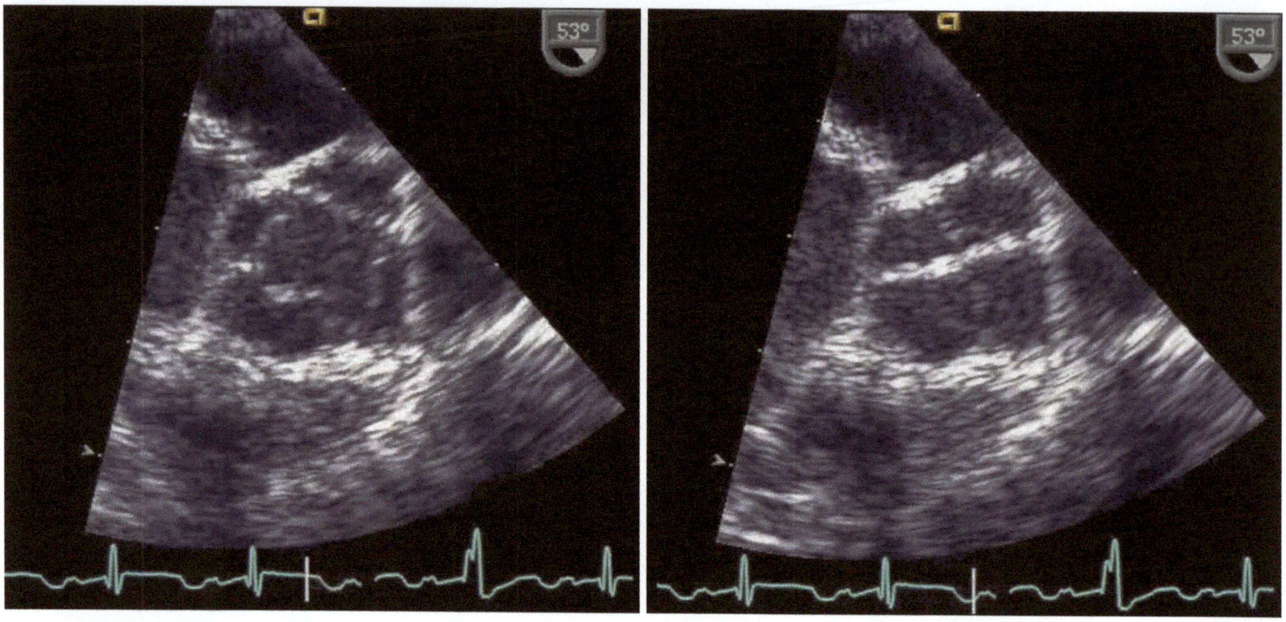

Fig. 11.15 Quadricuspid aortic valve as seen from the mid esophageal aortic valve short axis view, in systole (*left figure*) and diastole (*right figure*)

Acquired AR generally occurs with endocarditis, rheumatic fever, or after surgical or transcatheter balloon valvotomy for valvar AS. AR is a progressive disease. The increased volume load on the LV initially results in compensatory hypertrophy, though the degree of hypertrophy becomes inadequate as regurgitation worsens (decompensated AR). Increasing LV volume associated with decreasing ventricular wall thickness results in increased afterload; eventually this increased afterload leads to myocardial damage and diminished contractility. In an effort to prevent irreversible myocardial damage, some echocardiographic guidelines have been established regarding the timing for intervention. In 2006, the ACC/AHA Task Force on Practice Guidelines recommended an end-diastolic diameter of 75 mm and an end-systolic diameter of 55 mm (as measured in transthoracic parasternal short axis views of the LV) as thresholds for intervention in asymptomatic adults with significant AR [65]. Comparable guidelines for the pediatric population have not yet been established.

The utility of transthoracic echocardiography in assessing the degree of AR and the appropriate timing for intervention has been discussed extensively [66]. Once a patient is in the operating room, TEE provides a highly accurate assessment of all types of AR lesions, whether it is annular dilation, leaflet prolapse (in the setting of a VSD), or leaflet deficiency as in a bicommissural aortic valve or in rheumatic heart disease [67]. This is especially important if surgical repair of the valve is a consideration as valves with bicommissural morphology and those after rheumatic fever tend to be better candidates for surgical repair [68]. Therefore, TEE should evaluate the AoV and aortic root morphology in multiple mid esophageal views. The ME AV SAX view at 30–45° will display abnormalities in AoV commissural morphology, discrepancies among the individual leaflet sizes, absence of one or more of the leaflets, dilation of a coronary artery in the setting of a significant coronary-cameral fistula into the LV, disruption of one or more AoV leaflets (flail segment) secondary to endocarditis or after valvotomy, or rupture of a sinus of Valsalva into one of the intracardiac chambers (Fig. 11.16a, Video 11.16a). The ME AV LAX view at ~120° and ME RV In-Out view between 60° and 90° will display abnormally thickened AoV leaflets after rheumatic fever, an aortico-left ventricular tunnel, or a ruptured sinus of Valsalva aneurysm (Fig. 11.16b, Video 11.16b). The location of the regurgitant jet should be assessed from multiple TEE windows, including the mid esophageal (ME AV SAX, ME AV LAX, ME LAX), deep transgastric (DTG LAX, DTG Sagittal), and transgastric (TG LAX) views. Regarding assessment of AR severity, a 2003 report from the American Society of Echocardiography task force on valvular regurgitation suggested that a vena contracta width for the regurgitant jet >0.6 cm and a ratio between the color flow jet width and the LVOT diameter >65 % represent severe AR [69]. Both of these measurements are best obtained from the ME AV LAX view. In keeping with these recommendations, the 2008 ACC/AHA task force [21] listed the following echocardiographic criteria for classification of AR:

- Mild: Vena contracta width <0.3 cm, jet width/LVOT diameter <25 %
- Moderate: Vena contracta width 0.3–0.6 cm, jet width/LVOT diameter 25–65 %

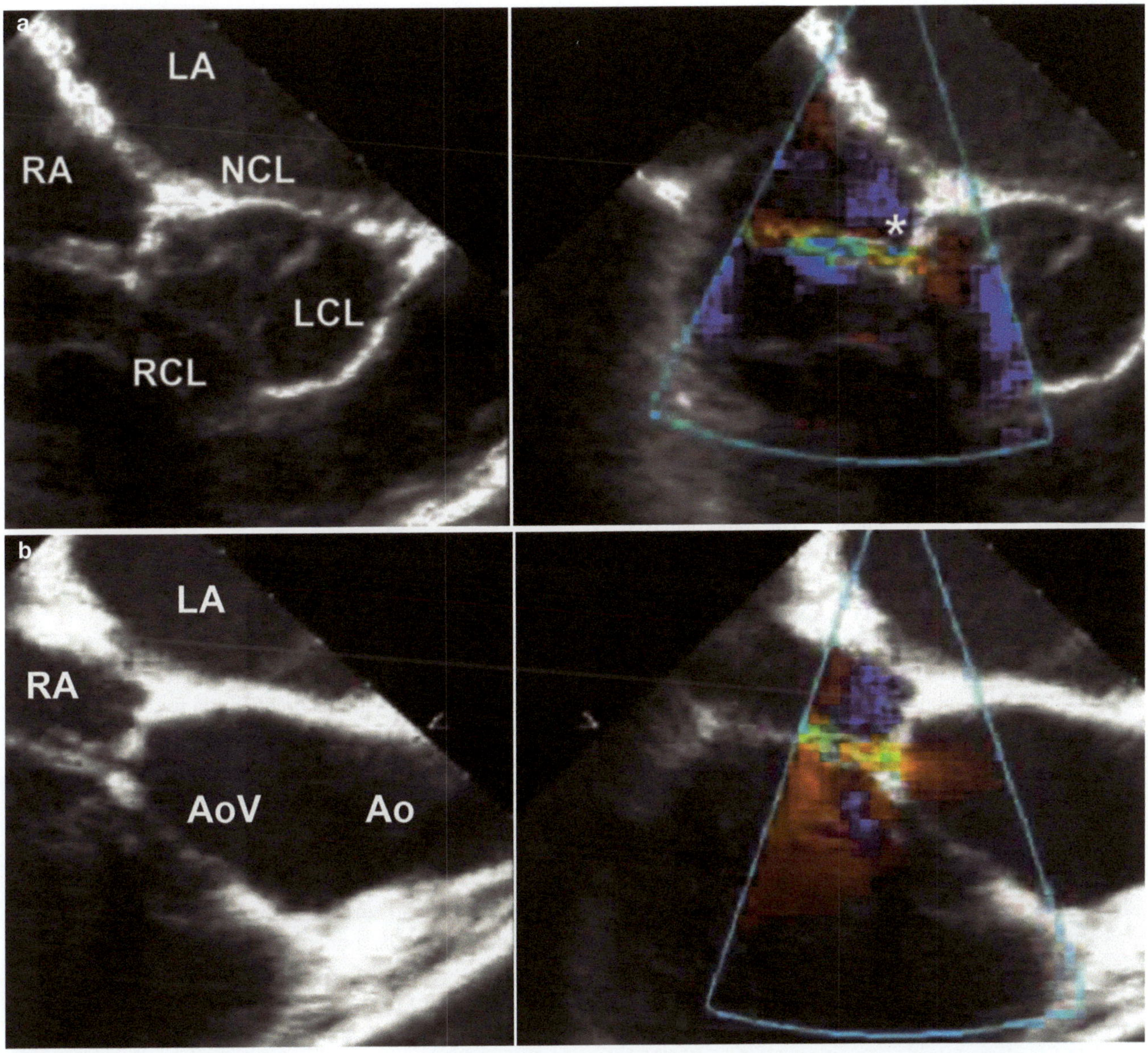

Fig. 11.16 (**a**) Mid esophageal aortic valve short axis view at 45° showing a short axis view of the aortic valve and a ruptured non-coronary sinus of Valsalva aneurysm (*asterisk*) into the right atrium; (**b**) Modified mid esophageal right ventricular inflow-outflow view at 90° showing the same ruptured of sinus of Valsalva aneurysm into the right atrium (*Ao* aorta, *AoV* aortic valve, *LA* left atrium, *LCL* left coronary leaflet, *NCL* non-coronary leaflet, *RA* right atrium, *RCL* right coronary leaflet)

- Severe: Vena contracta width >0.6 cm, jet width/LVOT diameter >65 %.

Other supportive data that can indicate at least moderate AR include prominent retrograde diastolic flow in the descending aorta, as noted by both color flow and pulsed wave Doppler [19, 20, 70]. This can best be evaluated using a combination of upper esophageal (UE Ao Arch LAX, SAX) and descending aorta long axis (Desc Ao LAX) and descending aortic short axis (Desc Ao SAX) views. There are few data on the utility of TEE to evaluate other indices of AR severity such as pressure half-time (which reflects the rate of equalization of aortic and LV diastolic pressures in the setting of AR), especially since this index can be affected by LV compliance, LV diastolic pressures, aortic compliance, and any therapy which changes ventricular afterload [70, 71]. In general, a pressure half-time > 500 ms is usually compatible with mild AR, while a value < 200 ms is consistent with severe AR [69]. Methods that have been discussed in other sources, but are rather difficult and time-consuming to perform in the intraoperative setting, include the calculation of effective regurgitant orifice area (EROA) by the flow convergence method (PISA) [69, 72]. If used, the following grading system (EROA in cm^2) has been suggested: mild AR <0.10, moderate AR 0.10–0.30 severe AR >0.30 [21]. It should be noted that the degree of AR can be difficult to assess by TEE, particularly in the operating room in which changing hemodynamics and general anesthesia could artificially alter its severity. However, in a cohort of pediatric patients who had undergone aortic valve repair, Honjo *et al.* found that, using the jet width/LVOT criteria, there was reasonable agreement between the degree of AR found by intraoperative TEE and subsequently by pre-discharge transthoracic echocardiogram [73].

In addition to the evaluation of AR, LV size and function should be assessed qualitatively in the transgastric short axis views (TG Mid SAX, TG Basal SAX) at 0°. Associated abnormalities such as subvalvar AS, a VSD, and aortic dilation can be assessed in multiple views as discussed above.

Surgical intervention generally involves aortic valvuloplasty (occasionally involving the use of autologous pericardium), a Ross procedure (involving replacement of the aortic root with the patient's pulmonary root and placement of a homograft from the RV to the pulmonary artery), or AoV replacement with a mechanical valve, bioprosthesis, or homograft valve. The postoperative TEE should exclude residual LVOT obstruction using the transgastric LAX and deep transgastric views: DTG LAX at 0–30°, and DTG Sagittal view at ~90°. Residual AR can be evaluated in multiple mid esophageal, transgastric, and deep transgastric views. After aortic valvuloplasty, a maximum instantaneous gradient >45 mmHg or degree of AR ≥ moderate are considered indications to return to cardiopulmonary bypass for a repeat AoV repair or replacement [74]. After a Ross procedure, any neo-AR is a highly sensitive predictor of ≥ moderate neo-AR at the time of hospital discharge [75] If a prosthetic aortic valve is present, symmetric motion of the valve leaflets can usually be seen in the mid esophageal views, particularly the ME AV SAX and ME AV LAX views (Fig. 11.17, Video 11.17), though this can become difficult secondary to acoustic interference from the prosthetic valve annular ring. The transgastric and deep transgastric views are helpful here: since they visualize the valve from the left ventricular aspect, they avoid shadowing and reverberation artifacts, allowing evaluation of the "upstream" portion of the prosthetic valve and leaflet motion. Doppler evaluation of the prosthetic valve should be performed from the transgastric or deep transgastric views, as described above and discussed in Chap. 16.

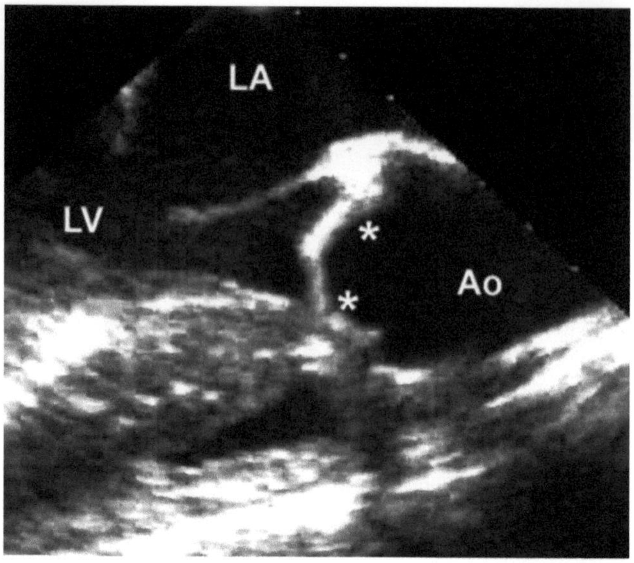

Fig. 11.17 Mid esophageal aortic valve long axis view at 120° showing a prosthetic aortic valve with symmetric positioning of the prosthetic hemidisc leaflets (*asterisks*) (*Ao* aorta, *LA* left atrium, *LV* left ventricle)

Aneurysm of the Proximal Aorta

Formation of an aortic root aneurysm and aneurysmal dilation of the proximal aorta result from an intrinsic aortopathy, usually involving smooth muscle cell loss and extracellular matrix disruption (cystic medial necrosis). These structural abnormalities in the muscular and elastic components lead to thinned and weakened aortic walls. As seen in supravalvar AS, abnormalities in elastin homeostasis may play a major role in the development of aortic root aneurysms and a dilated proximal aorta. For example, Marfan syndrome, with its predilection for aortic root dilation, is caused by mutations in the fibrillin gene on chromosome 15 [76], and fibrillin is an important glycoprotein necessary for elastin production and maintenance [77]. Associations with dilation of the proximal aorta include Marfan syndrome, Loeys-Dietz syndrome, Ehlers-Danlos syndrome, Turner syndrome, a bicuspid AoV, systemic hypertension, and aortic coarctation. Congenital cardiac defects known to be associated include tetralogy of Fallot, D-transposition of the great arteries, and truncus arteriosus [78]. Because of the intrinsic weakness in the aortic wall, a sinus of Valsalva aneurysm is at risk for rupture into the right and left heart chambers (most frequently into the RV) [79] (Fig. 11.16, Video 11.16a and 11.16b), and a dilated aortic root or ascending aorta is at risk for dissection and rupture [80] (Fig. 11.18, Video 11.18). Both of these problems are frequently associated with AR [79, 81]. In addition, aortic root aneurysms are also frequently associated with a VSD [79]. TEE is frequently superior to transthoracic echocardiography in the evaluation of the entire extent of the proximal aorta, particularly in older children and in adults, and occasionally a TEE study is performed before the decision to intervene surgically is made. Mid esophageal views at multiple angles can display a sinus of Valsalva aneurysm as well as its spatial relationship to surrounding cardiac structures. Color mapping can easily display the continuous restrictive jet of a ruptured aneurysm into the right atrium, RV, and left atrium; when the aneurysm ruptures into the LV, color mapping can display the diastolic jet. The location and degree of AR can also be evaluated with color mapping in multiple mid esophageal views.

Aneurysmal dilation of the aortic root and ascending aorta is best evaluated with ME AV LAX and ME Asc Ao LAX views between 90° and 130° (Fig. 11.19, Video 11.19). One should always look for the characteristic parallel lines of dissection along the aortic wall in these patients from multiple mid esophageal views (Fig. 11.18, Video 11.18), and color mapping will occasionally show the connection between the dissection and the aortic lumen. The more superior portion of the ascending aorta, as well as aortic arch and proximal descending aorta, can also be evaluated for dilation and possible dissection using the upper esophageal TEE views (UE Ao Arch LAX at 90–120°, UE Ao Arch SAX at 0°). See Chap. 16 for further discussion on the TEE evaluation of aortic dissection.

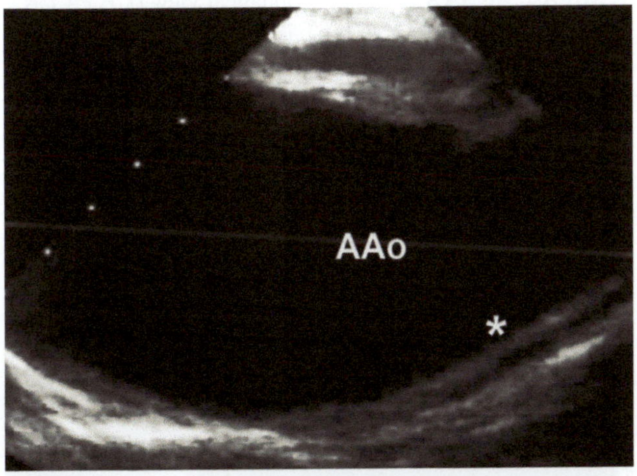

Fig. 11.18 Mid esophageal ascending aortic long axis view at 120° showing a markedly dilated aortic root and ascending aorta with associated aortic dissection along the anterior wall of the ascending aorta (the double linear density representing the aortic dissection along the anterior ascending aortic wall is indicated by the *asterisk*) in a patient with Marfan syndrome (*AAo* ascending aorta)

Right Ventricular Outflow Tract Anomalies

Valvar Pulmonary Stenosis

Valvar PS is one of the most commonly occurring types of congenital heart disease [1, 2]. It can present either as thin but doming leaflets with tricuspid or bicuspid morphology or as dysplastic leaflets with thickened edges. The former represents the more common presentation and is often associated with post-stenotic dilation of the main pulmonary trunk (Fig. 11.20, Video 11.20). Because one or more of the commissures can be partially or completely fused or underdeveloped (with formation of a raphé), the thickened raphé can appear tethered to the arterial wall at the sino-tubular junction, giving the lesion the appearance of supravalvar narrowing (Fig. 11.20, Video 11.20). As discussed previously, the semilunar valve attachments extend up to the sino-tubular junction [82] (Fig. 11.3b), and this particular variant of valvar PS can sometimes be difficult to distinguish from discrete narrowing of the pulmonary sino-tubular junction (supravalvar stenosis) without valvar obstruction. Because of the underdeveloped distal segments of the commissures, the leaflets are often attached in a more circular fashion at the pulmonary root rather than the normal semilunar arrangement discussed previously [83]. The dysplastic form of valvar PS is not as common and is often associated with pulmonary annular hypoplasia and a small pulmonary trunk. The leaflets are usually attached to the pulmonary root in a semilunar fashion. Occasionally there is separate but discrete narrowing of the pulmonary sino-tubular junction resulting in combined valvar and supravalvar PS. Valvar PS places excess pressure load on the RV, often resulting in significant RV hypertrophy, which in turn can contribute to the total obstruction along the RVOT. An atrial septal defect or patent foramen ovale is also commonly found in these patients [84].

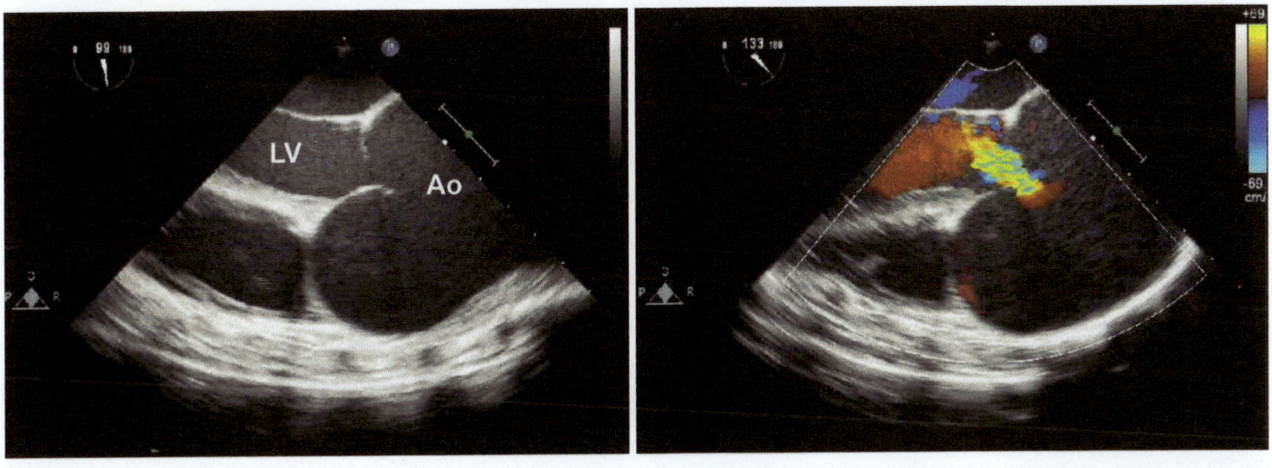

Fig. 11.19 Markedly dilated aortic root as seen from the mid esophageal aortic valve long axis view without color mapping (*left panel*) and with color mapping, showing central aortic regurgitation (*right panel*). *Ao* aorta, *LV* left ventricle

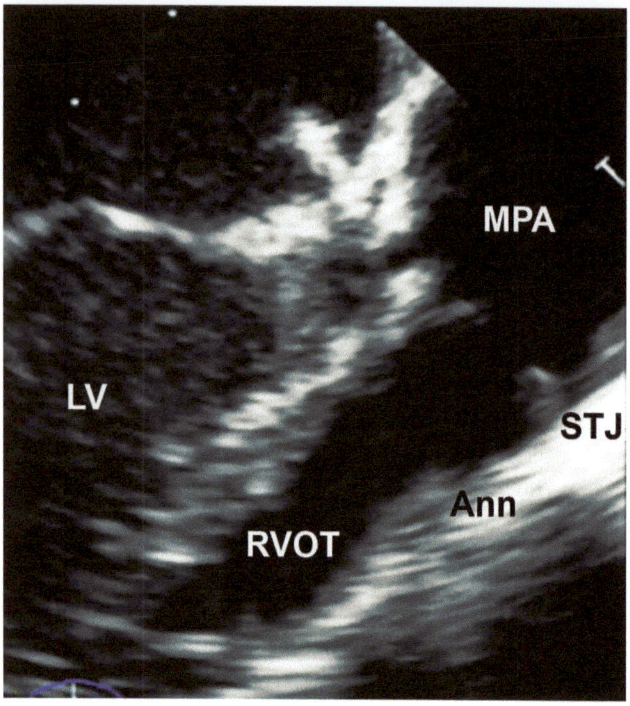

Fig. 11.20 Mid esophageal aortic valve long axis view with multiplane angle at 90° and slight leftward probe rotation. This image shows valvar pulmonary stenosis with thin but doming pulmonary valve leaflets abutting against the sino-tubular junction and post-stenotic dilation of the main pulmonary artery (*Ann* pulmonary annulus, *LV* left ventricle, *MPA* main pulmonary artery, *RVOT* right ventricular outflow tract, *STJ* pulmonary sino-tubular junction)

Because the majority of these patients undergo intervention when necessary in the catheterization laboratory, TEE is rarely needed to evaluate the pulmonary valve morphology and degree of obstruction. However, TEE is frequently used during transcatheter device closure of atrial septal defects, and the excess pulmonary blood flow associated with these lesions often results in turbulence across the pulmonary valve without true valvar PS (relative PS). TEE performed in the catheterization laboratory can help determine whether intervention is necessary at the pulmonary valve. The RVOT, and particularly the pulmonary valve, can easily be evaluated with the ME AV SAX at 0°, the ME RV In-Out view at 60°–90°, and a modified ME AV LAX at 90° with leftward probe rotation to visualize the pulmonary outflow tract (Fig. 11.20, Video 11.20). Occasionally, a higher esophageal view, such as ME Asc Ao SAX or upper esophageal view (UE PA LAX at 0°, UE Ao Arch SAX at 90°), is necessary in patients with an elongated subpulmonary conus. Quantitative assessment of the degree of valvar PS can be performed in the DTG Sagittal view at 90° (Fig. 11.1b, Video 11.1b) in the same way that LVOT obstruction is evaluated by Doppler interrogation, usually requiring slight rotation of the probe to visualize the RVOT. Occasionally, the degree of valvar PS can be assessed in ME Asc Ao SAX and UE PA LAX view at 0° by interrogating the high velocity flow into the main pulmonary trunk (Figs. 11.21 and 11.22; Video 11.21). This view also allows for measurements of the main and proximal branch

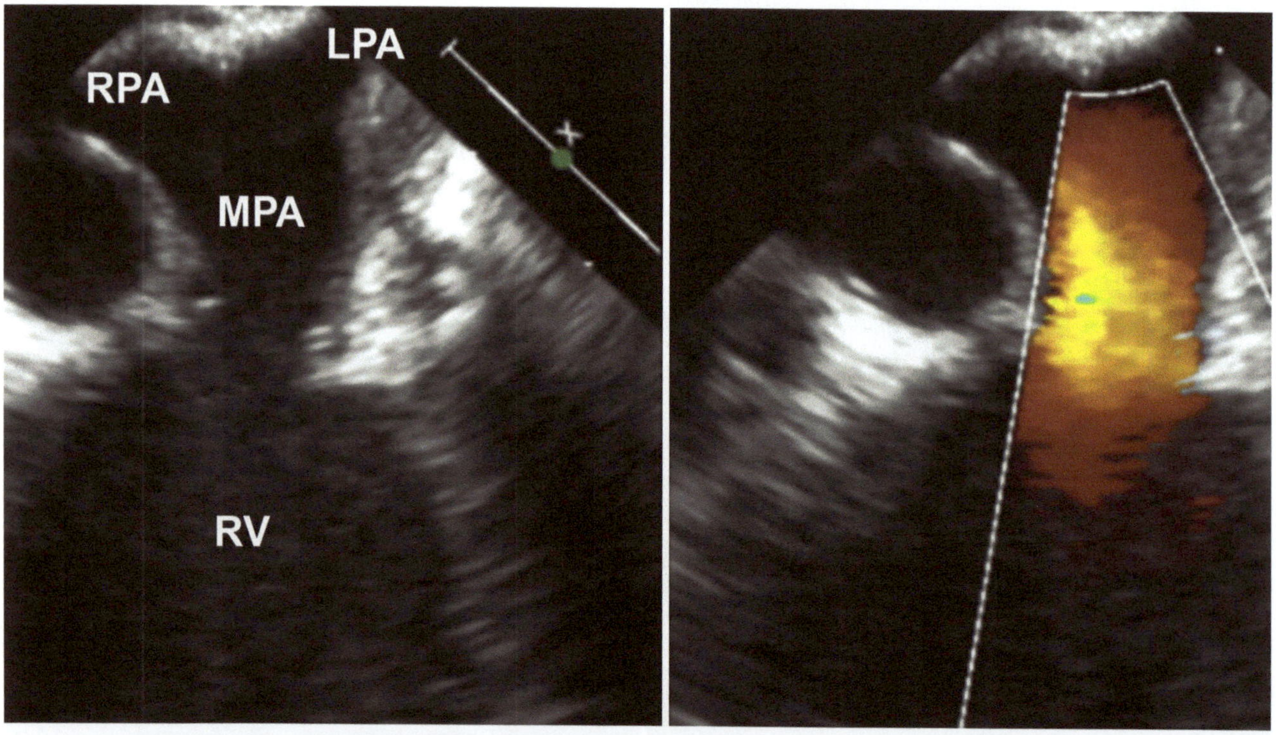

Fig. 11.21 Upper esophageal pulmonary artery long axis view at 0° showing the main pulmonary artery in the setting of mild valvar pulmonary stenosis with thin doming pulmonary valve leaflets, and minimal flow acceleration across the valve. In this image the bifurcation of the branch pulmonary arteries can also be seen (*LPA* left pulmonary artery, *MPA* main pulmonary artery, *RPA* right pulmonary artery, *RV* right ventricle)

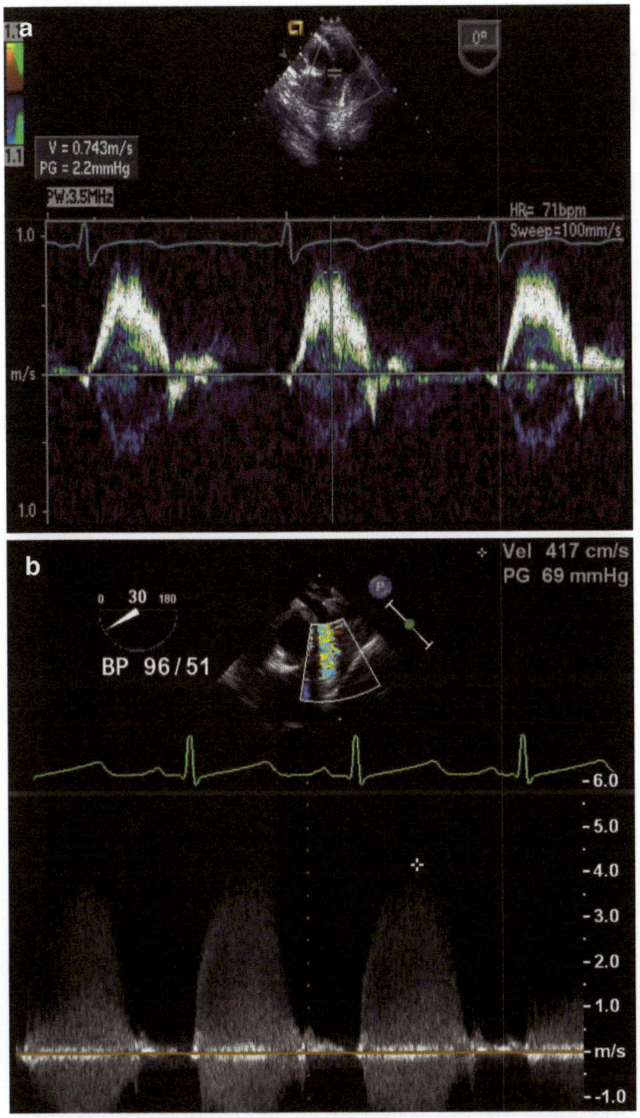

Fig. 11.22 Spectral Doppler recordings of flow across the pulmonary valve, as obtained from the mid esophageal ascending aortic short axis view at 0°. In (**a**), there is normal, low velocity laminar flow seen in the main pulmonary artery through a normal pulmonary valve. In (**b**), high velocity flow is obtained by continuous wave Doppler across a pulmonary valve that is stenotic

pulmonary artery diameters. In many instances, the UE PA LAX and UE Ao Arch SAX views provide an excellent angle for Doppler interrogation of the high velocity jet arising from the pulmonary valve (Video 11.20).

There are a number of congenital heart defects in which pulmonary stenosis (subvalvar, valvar, and sometimes supravalvar) is a frequent finding. At times, pulmonary outflow obstruction is an important and integral part of the anatomic spectrum of the cardiac defect. Examples of such anomalies include tetralogy of Fallot, double outlet right ventricle, tricuspid atresia, and transposition of the great arteries, and these cardiac defects are discussed in other chapters in this textbook. Nonetheless, the TEE evaluation of the pulmonary outflow tract in those conditions mirrors that described in this chapter and should be performed using a similar approach.

Subvalvar Pulmonary Stenosis (Double-Chambered Right Ventricle)

A double-chambered RV (DCRV) is a type of RVOT obstruction involving anomalously prominent RV muscle bundles that divide the RV into two chambers: a proximal high-pressure inflow chamber and a distal low-pressure outflow chamber (Fig. 11.23, Video 11.22). Some prefer to use the term divided RV for this lesion [85], although a divided RV does not always involve anomalous RV muscle bundles [86]. The division in a DCRV usually occurs at the infundibular os, with the distal outflow chamber corresponding to a well-developed subpulmonary infundibulum. Like subvalvar AS, the obstruction associated with a DCRV is not always present early in life, prompting some people to classify the lesion as an acquired disease [87]. However, others suggest that a congenital anatomic substrate for a DCRV is present before obstruction develops and can actually be predicted echocardiographically by measuring the distance from the moderator band to the PV [88]. In this setting, DCRV is thought to result from superior displacement and hypertrophy of the moderator band, contributing to progressive obstruction at the infundibular os. Others suggest, however, that the anomalously prominent muscle bundles in a DCRV are in fact distinct from the moderator band since the septal attachment of a normal moderator band is located more apically than the usual attachments of these anomalous muscle bundles [89]. The most common association is a VSD, usually a small or moderate membranous VSD, occurring in at least 67 % of these patients [90]. Viewed in another manner, a DCRV can be present in up to 10 % of patients who require VSD surgery [91], necessitating careful assessment of the RVOT in all patients with a VSD. Another common association is a fixed subaortic ridge or echo dense area at the crest of the ventricular septum, occurring in up to 88 % of patients with a DCRV and a VSD, although some degree of subvalvar AS is present in only a quarter of these patients [49]. This lesion must be distinguished from tetralogy of Fallot, wherein anterior and superior deviation of the conal septum results in a large VSD and an underdeveloped subpulmonary infundibulum.

The RVOT obstruction in DCRV is usually progressive, presenting during childhood or adolescence, although cases of adult presentation have been reported [90, 92]. Almost all cases require surgical intervention. TEE is useful in the preoperative evaluation, and the infundibular os and RVOT are easily visualized in the ME RV In-Out view with multiplane angle between 60° and 90°. However, the anterior location of

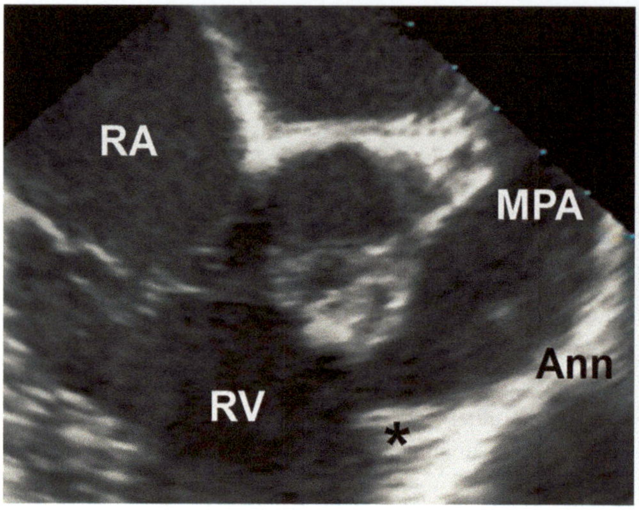

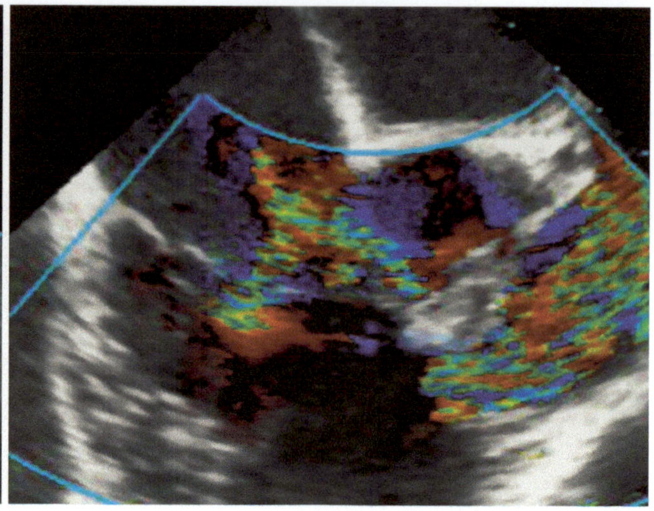

Fig. 11.23 Mid esophageal right ventricular inflow-outflow view at 60° showing a double-chambered right ventricle with prominent muscle bundles at the infundibular os (*asterisk*) separating the proximal right ventricular chamber from the well-developed right ventricular infundibular chamber and resulting in subvalvar pulmonary stenosis (the pulmonary annulus is within normal limits in size). (Moderate tricuspid regurgitation is also present *Ann* pulmonary annulus, *MPA* main pulmonary artery, *RA* right atrium, *RV* right ventricle)

the prominent muscle bundles and their proximity to the probe often makes qualitative assessment of the extent of the muscle bundles difficult. Thus this area should be examined carefully as it is easy to overlook RVOT obstruction at this level. In addition, the orientation of blood flow across the muscle bundles is often directly perpendicular to the echocardiographic beam in the mid esophageal views, precluding adequate color mapping and quantitative spectral Doppler interrogation of the area (Fig. 11.23, Video 11.22). Quantitative assessment of the degree of RVOT obstruction is best performed in the DTG Sagittal view at 90° as discussed in the previous section (Fig. 11.24, Video 11.23). Postoperative evaluation after resection of the muscle bundles should exclude residual obstruction in the DTG Sagittal view at 90°; the TEE study should evaluate for the development of pulmonary regurgitation in multiple mid esophageal views. Occasionally, resection of the muscle bundles results in the development of tiny coronary-cameral fistulae along the RV anterior free wall, and these are easily visualized with color mapping in multiple mid esophageal views.

Pulmonary Regurgitation

Pulmonary regurgitation (PR) is a common finding during routine echocardiographic evaluation with a prevalence of up to 88 % in normal healthy children and up to 68 % in healthy adults [93]. The prevalence may decrease later in adulthood, though this trend may be more related to technical limitations in adults with poor echocardiographic windows rather than a true decrease in the frequency of the lesion. Among the 3,370 subjects with pulmonary outflow tract anomalies evaluated by echocardiography at Children's Hospital Boston from 1988 to 2002, over 40 % (1403) had PR and almost 24 % of these (335) had ≤ mild PR without associated cardiac structural abnormalities [94]. Isolated PR as a congenital anomaly is extremely rare and has been associated with aneurysmal dilation of the pulmonary arteries secondary to cystic medial necrosis (as seen in the aortopathy of Marfan syndrome and bicuspid AoV) [95]. Many of these patients do not require intervention, unless the severity of the PR results in significant RV dilation and dysfunction. Occasionally, isolated PR with idiopathic dilation of the pulmonary arteries is associated with absence of one or more PV leaflets [95, 96]. Although this is seen more frequently in the setting of tetralogy of Fallot with absent or dysplastic PV leaflets, it can occur as an isolated abnormality, and marked dilation of the pulmonary arteries can also occur, resulting in significant airway compression that requires surgical intervention.

Quantification of PR is not as well established by echocardiography (either transthoracic or transesophageal). Doppler methods, both color flow and spectral, are generally used, though variable hemodynamic conditions (RV diastolic properties and filling pressures, driving pressure between pulmonary artery and RV, etc.) will influence the Doppler evaluation. Pulsed wave Doppler assessment of the forward and reverse flow in the main pulmonary artery (using the velocity time integral) could theoretically be used to estimate the percent and volume of regurgitant flow; however this method has not been standardized and also is not valid in patients with pulmonary valve stenosis. Criteria for vena contracta width (which would seem to be more accurate than jet width) and regurgitant orifice area width to assess PR

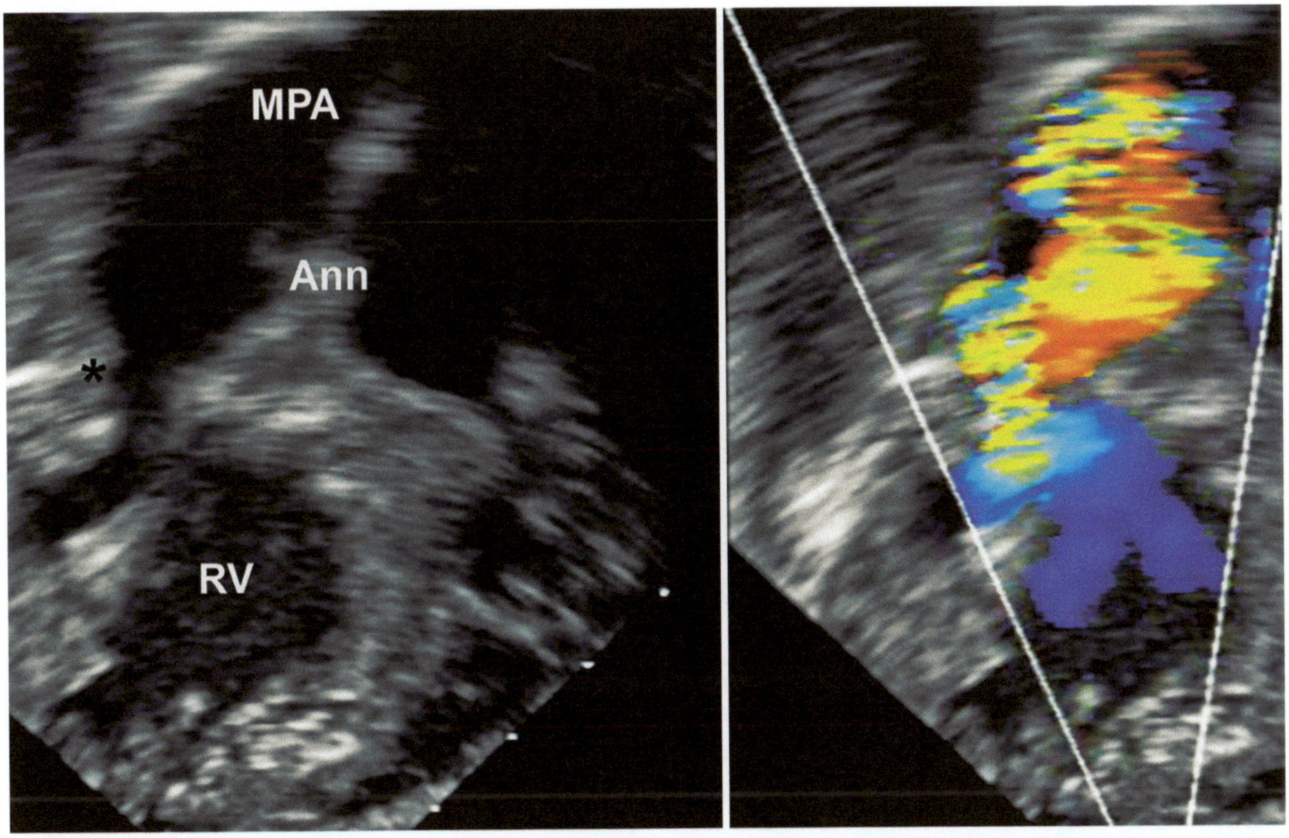

Fig. 11.24 Deep transgastric sagittal view at 90° showing a double-chambered right ventricle with prominent muscle bundles at the infundibular os (*asterisk*) separating the proximal right ventricular chamber from the well-developed right ventricular infundibular chamber and resulting in subvalvar pulmonary stenosis (the pulmonary annulus is within normal limits in size); this is an ideal view to measure the gradient along the right ventricular outflow tract (*Ann* pulmonary annulus, *MPA* main pulmonary artery, *RV* right ventricle)

Table 11.1 Echocardiographic and Doppler parameters used in grading pulmonary regurgitation severity

Parameter	Mild	Moderate	Severe
Pulmonary valve	Normal	Normal or abnormal	Abnormal
RV size	Normal[a]	Normal or dilated	Dilated
Jet size by color flow Doppler[b]	Thin (usually <10 mm in length) with a narrow origin	Intermediate	Usually large, with a wide origin; may be brief in duration
Jet density and deceleration rate—CW[c]	Soft; slow deceleration	Dense; variable deceleration	Dense; steep deceleration, early termination of diastolic flow
Pulmonic systolic flow compared to systemic flow—PW[d]	Slightly increased	Intermediate	Greatly increased

Reprinted from Zoghbi et al [69]; with permission from Elsevier
CW continuous wave Doppler, *PR* pulmonic regurgitation, *PW* pulsed wave Doppler, *RA* right atrium, *RF* regurgitant fraction, *RV* right ventricle
[a]Unless there are other reasons for RV enlargement
[b]At a Nyquist limit of 50–60 cm/s
[c]Steep deceleration is not specific for severe PR
[d]Cut-off values for regurgitant volume and fraction are not well validated

severity have not been well established [70]. Indirect evidence of PR severity can be obtained by evaluating RV size and function, though with by echocardiography this can be more challenging due to the more complex shape of the RV. Also, the RV diastolic properties (specifically the stiffness) can affect the degree of RV dilation. Some of the features commonly used to grade PR severity are listed in Table 11.1 [73]. Overall, it is clear that the grading of PR severity is more difficult because standards for its quantification are less well defined than for AR [70, 97]. Thus when assessing severity of PR, an integrated approach is probably best, utilizing color flow Doppler, continuous and pulsed wave spectral Doppler, as well as evaluations of the pulmonary valve and RV sizes and RV function [73].

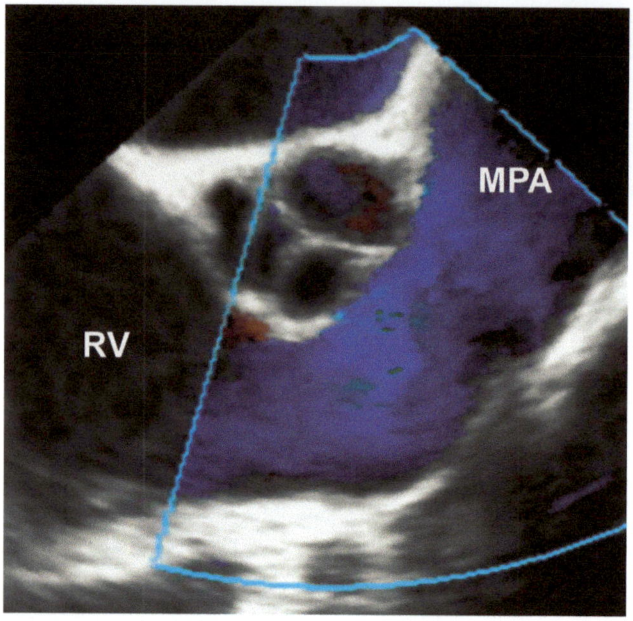

Fig. 11.25 Mid esophageal right ventricular inflow-outflow view at 60° showing free pulmonary regurgitation in the setting of tetralogy of Fallot repair with a transannular right ventricular outflow tract patch (*MPA* main pulmonary artery, *RV* right ventricle)

The most common scenarios for significant PR occur after some type of intervention: after surgical repair of tetralogy of Fallot (Fig. 11.25, Video 11.24), after surgical or transcatheter balloon valvotomy for valvar PS, and after surgical placement of a homograft from the RV to the pulmonary artery for lesions such as tetralogy of Fallot (with or without pulmonary atresia), truncus arteriosus, transposition of the great arteries with a VSD, and pulmonary atresia with intact ventricular septum. As in patients with significant AR, significant PR is associated initially with an increase in RV end-diastolic volume, followed by an increase in RV end-systolic volume, followed by a decrease in RV function and contractility. Symptoms of right-sided heart failure appear, signaling the development of irreversible RV myocardial damage. In many postoperative instances, there are markedly akinetic segments of the RV due to outflow tract patch augmentation and aggressive muscular resection, contributing to the progressive RV systolic and diastolic dysfunction. In addition, newly acquired, significant postoperative PR is not well tolerated by older patients, unlike neonates and children who respond better to this postoperative problem. Strategies for timing of intervention in these patients necessarily involves echocardiographic evaluation, and some of the echocardiographic indices for PR include pressure half-time of the regurgitant jet, presence of flow reversal in the branch pulmonary arteries, and RV size and function [98]. Other echocardiographic indicators are listed above. Restrictive RV physiology can also be identified when diastolic forward flow is seen in the main pulmonary artery during atrial systole by Doppler interrogation [99]. More recently, magnetic resonance imaging and its ability to quantitatively assess RV size and function have superseded echocardiography in determining the timing of intervention [100–102].

Intraoperative assessment of PR by TEE involves color mapping in mid esophageal views along multiple planes such as the ME AV SAX and ME RV In-Out views (Fig. 11.25, Video 11.24). Occasionally a somewhat higher esophageal view, such as the ME Asc Ao SAX and upper esophageal views (UE PA LAX, UE Ao Arch SAX), can provide better color mapping display of the to-and-fro flow across the PV; these views can also display diastolic reversal in the proximal branch pulmonary arteries by color mapping and pulsed wave Doppler interrogation. The DTG Sagittal view of the RVOT at 90° can also display the PR, especially since the direction of flow is parallel to the echocardiographic beam. However, the distance from the probe to the RVOT often limits color mapping in this view for larger patients. Following implantation of a PV, the postoperative TEE examination should exclude residual PR in multiple mid esophageal views and in the DTG Sagittal view at 90°. The new PV, whether it is a mechanical prosthetic valve, a bioprosthetic valve, or part of a valved homograft, should also be evaluated in mid esophageal views using multiple planes such as the ME RV In-Out and MV AV LAX with slight leftward rotation of the probe. The deep transgastric views (DTG Sagittal and LAX) can also be useful in evaluating the flow across the pulmonary valve, both with color flow and spectral Doppler.

Summary

This chapter discusses the common congenital defects affecting the right and left ventricular outflow tracts in both children and adults. While the semilunar valves are most commonly involved, pathology can be seen at any level—subvalvar, valvar, supravalvar, or a combination of one or more levels. Stenosis and/or regurgitation at either or both outflow tracts can occur. Thus a careful echocardiographic evaluation must be undertaken to define precisely the nature, location, and severity of the abnormality/abnormalities. For evaluation of the outflow tracts, TEE excels by providing excellent anatomic imaging and color mapping. It plays a vital role in the perioperative evaluation of outflow tract abnormalities with precise characterization of the pathology preoperatively and assessment of the adequacy of surgical repair postoperatively. It is also important in the evaluation of interventional procedures such as TAVR/TAVI. In addition, TEE can also be valuable in the ambulatory setting, such as the evaluation of subaortic stenosis in older patients. Thus for the assessment and treatment of outflow tract abnormalities, TEE serves as an important and extremely valuable tool.

References

1. Hoffman JI, Kaplan S. The incidence of congenital heart disease. J Am Coll Cardiol. 2002;39:1890–900.
2. Triedman JK. Methodological issues for database development: trends. In: Keane JF, Fyler DC, Lock J, editors. Nadas' pediatric cardiology. 2nd ed. Philadelphia: Saunders; 2006. p. 323–36.
3. Campbell M. Calcific aortic stenosis and congenital bicuspid aortic valves. Br Heart J. 1968;30:606–16.
4. Roberts WC. The congenitally bicuspid aortic valve. A study of 85 autopsy cases. Am J Cardiol. 1970;26:72–83.
5. Ward C. Clinical significance of the bicuspid aortic valve. Heart. 2000;83:81–5.
6. Shanewise JS, Cheung AT, Aronson S, et al. ASE/SCA guidelines for performing a comprehensive intraoperative multiplane transesophageal echocardiography examination: recommendations of the American Society of Echocardiography Council for Intraoperative Echocardiography and the Society of Cardiovascular Anesthesiologists Task Force for Certification in Perioperative Transesophageal Echocardiography. J Am Soc Echocardiogr. 1999;12:884–900.
7. Anderson RH, Freedom RM. Normal and abnormal structure of the ventriculo-arterial junctions. Cardiol Young. 2005;15 Suppl 1:3–16.
8. Dare AJ, Veinot JP, Edwards WD, Tazelaar HD, Schaff HV. New observations on the etiology of aortic valve disease: a surgical pathologic study of 236 cases from 1990. Hum Pathol. 1993;24:1330–8.
9. Angelini A, Ho SY, Anderson RH, et al. The morphology of the normal aortic valve as compared with the aortic valve having two leaflets. J Thorac Cardiovasc Surg. 1989;98:362–7.
10. Fernandes SM, Sanders SP, Khairy P, et al. Morphology of bicuspid aortic valve in children and adolescents. J Am Coll Cardiol. 2004;44:1648–51.
11. Beppu S, Suzuki S, Matsuda H, Ohmori F, Nagata S, Miyatake K. Rapidity of progression of aortic stenosis in patients with congenital bicuspid aortic valves. Am J Cardiol. 1993;71:322–7.
12. Fernandes SM, Khairy P, Sanders SP, Colan SD. Bicuspid aortic valve morphology and interventions in the young. J Am Coll Cardiol. 2007;49:2211–4.
13. Miller MJ, Geffner ME, Lippe BM, et al. Echocardiography reveals a high incidence of bicuspid aortic valve in Turner syndrome. J Pediatr. 1983;102:47–50.
14. Fedak PW, Verma S, David TE, Leask RL, Weisel RD, Butany J. Clinical and pathophysiological implications of a bicuspid aortic valve. Circulation. 2002;106:900–4.
15. Nistri S, Sorbo MD, Basso C, Thiene G. Bicuspid aortic valve: abnormal aortic elastic properties. J Heart Valve Dis. 2002;11:369–73; discussion 373–4.
16. Nkomo VT, Enriquez-Sarano M, Ammash NM, et al. Bicuspid aortic valve associated with aortic dilatation: a community-based study. Arterioscler Thromb Vasc Biol. 2003;23:351–6.
17. Wagner HR, Ellison RC, Keane JF, Humphries OJ, Nadas AS. Clinical course in aortic stenosis. Circulation. 1977;56:I47–56.
18. Keane JF, Driscoll DJ, Gersony WM, et al. Second natural history study of congenital heart defects. Results of treatment of patients with aortic valvar stenosis. Circulation. 1993;87:I16–27.
19. Mehta Y, Singh R. Quantification of AS and AR. Ann Card Anaesth. 2009;12:166.
20. Savino JS. Transesophageal echocardiographic evaluation of native valvular disease and repair. Crit Care Clin. 1996;12:321–81.
21. Bonow RO, Carabello BA, Chatterjee K, et al. 2008 Focused update incorporated into the ACC/AHA 2006 guidelines for the management of patients with valvular heart disease: a report of the American College of Cardiology/American Heart Association Task Force on Practice Guidelines (Writing Committee to Revise the 1998 Guidelines for the Management of Patients With Valvular Heart Disease): endorsed by the Society of Cardiovascular Anesthesiologists, Society for Cardiovascular Angiography and Interventions, and Society of Thoracic Surgeons. Circulation. 2008;118:e523–661.
22. Heinrich RS, Fontaine AA, Grimes RY, et al. Experimental analysis of fluid mechanical energy losses in aortic valve stenosis: importance of pressure recovery. Ann Biomed Eng. 1996; 24:685–94.
23. Baumgartner H, Hung J, Bermejo J, et al. Echocardiographic assessment of valve stenosis: EAE/ASE recommendations for clinical practice. Eur J Echocardiogr. 2009;10:1–25.
24. Nakai H, Takeuchi M, Yoshitani H, Kaku K, Haruki N, Otsuji Y. Pitfalls of anatomical aortic valve area measurements using two-dimensional transoesophageal echocardiography and the potential of three-dimensional transoesophageal echocardiography. Eur J Echocardiogr. 2010;11:369–76.
25. Schneider DJ, Moore JW. Aortic stenosis. In: Allen HD, Driscoll DJ, Shaddy RE, Feltes TF, editors. Moss and Adams' heart disease in infants, children, and adolescents: including the fetus and young adult. 7th ed. Philadelphia: Lippincott Williams & Wilkins; 2008. p. 968–87.
26. Simpson JM. Anomalies of left ventricular outflow tract and aortic valve. In: Lai W, Mertens L, Cohen MS, Geva T, editors. Echocardiography in pediatric and congenital heart disease: from fetus to adult. Illustrated Ed. Chichester/Hoboken: Wiley; 2009. p. 297–314.
27. Lopez L. Abnormalities of left ventricular outflow. In: Eidem BW, Ceteta F, O'Leary PW, editors. Echocardiography in pediatric and adult congenital heart disease. Philadelphia: Lippincott Williams & Wilkins; 2010. p. 215–36.
28. Lopez L, Colan SD, Frommelt PC, et al. Recommendations for quantification methods during the performance of a pediatric echocardiogram: a report from the Pediatric Measurements Writing Group of the American Society of Echocardiography Pediatric and Congenital Heart Disease Council. J Am Soc Echocardiogr. 2010;23:465–95.
29. Daubeney PE, Blackstone EH, Weintraub RG, Slavik Z, Scanlon J, Webber SA. Relationship of the dimension of cardiac structures to body size: an echocardiographic study in normal infants and children. Cardiol Young. 1999;9:402–10.
30. Pettersen MD, Du W, Skeens ME, Humes RA. Regression equations for calculation of z scores of cardiac structures in a large cohort of healthy infants, children, and adolescents: an echocardiographic study. J Am Soc Echocardiogr. 2008;21:922–34.
31. Leon MB, Smith CR, Mack M, et al. Transcatheter aortic-valve implantation for aortic stenosis in patients who cannot undergo surgery. N Engl J Med. 2010;363:1597–607.
32. Billings FT, Kodali SK, Shanewise JS. Transcatheter aortic valve implantation: anesthetic considerations. Anesth Analg. 2009;108:1453–62.
33. Webb JG, Wood DA. Current status of transcatheter aortic valve replacement. J Am Coll Cardiol. 2012;60:483–92.
34. Makkar RR, Fontana GP, Jilaihawi H, et al. Transcatheter aortic-valve replacement for inoperable severe aortic stenosis. N Engl J Med. 2012;366:1696–704.
35. Gilard M, Eltchaninoff H, Iung B, et al. Registry of transcatheter aortic-valve implantation in high-risk patients. N Engl J Med. 2012;366:1705–15.
36. Leichter DA, Sullivan I, Gersony WM. "Acquired" discrete subvalvular aortic stenosis: natural history and hemodynamics. J Am Coll Cardiol. 1989;14:1539–44.
37. Vogt J, Dische R, Rupprath G, de Vivie ER, Kotthoff S, Kececioglu D. Fixed subaortic stenosis: an acquired secondary obstruction? A twenty-seven year experience with 168 patients. Thorac Cardiovasc Surg. 1989;37:199–206.
38. Cape EG, Vanauker MD, Sigfusson G, Tacy TA, del Nido PJ. Potential role of mechanical stress in the etiology of pediatric heart disease: septal shear stress in subaortic stenosis. J Am Coll Cardiol. 1997;30:247–54.

39. Cilliers AM, Gewillig M. Rheology of discrete subaortic stenosis. Heart. 2002;88:335–6.
40. Kleinert S, Geva T. Echocardiographic morphometry and geometry of the left ventricular outflow tract in fixed subaortic stenosis. J Am Coll Cardiol. 1993;22:1501–8.
41. Sigfusson G, Tacy TA, Vanauker MD, Cape EG. Abnormalities of the left ventricular outflow tract associated with discrete subaortic stenosis in children: an echocardiographic study. J Am Coll Cardiol. 1997;30:255–9.
42. Bezold LI, Smith EO, Kelly K, Colan SD, Gauvreau K, Geva T. Development and validation of an echocardiographic model for predicting progression of discrete subaortic stenosis in children. Am J Cardiol. 1998;81:314–20.
43. Melero JM, Rodriguez I, Such M, Porras C, Olalla E. Left ventricular outflow tract obstruction with mitral mechanical prosthesis. Ann Thorac Surg. 1999;68:255–7.
44. Rietman GW, van der Maaten JMAA, Douglas YL, Boonstra PW. Echocardiographic diagnosis of left ventricular outflow tract obstruction after mitral valve replacement with subvalvular preservation. Eur J Cardiothorac Surg. 2002;22:825–7.
45. Wu Q, Zhang L, Zhu R. Obstruction of left ventricular outflow tract after mechanical mitral valve replacement. Ann Thorac Surg. 2008;85:1789–91.
46. Geva T, Hornberger LK, Sanders SP, Jonas RA, Ott DA, Colan SD. Echocardiographic predictors of left ventricular outflow tract obstruction after repair of interrupted aortic arch. J Am Coll Cardiol. 1993;22:1953–60.
47. Salem MM, Starnes VA, Wells WJ, et al. Predictors of left ventricular outflow obstruction following single-stage repair of interrupted aortic arch and ventricular septal defect. Am J Cardiol. 2000;86:1044–7.
48. Silverman NH, Gerlis LM, Ho SY, Anderson RH. Fibrous obstruction within the left ventricular outflow tract associated with ventricular septal defect: a pathologic study. J Am Coll Cardiol. 1995;25:475–81.
49. Vogel M, Smallhorn JF, Freedom RM, Coles J, Williams WG, Trusler GA. An echocardiographic study of the association of ventricular septal defect and right ventricular muscle bundles with a fixed subaortic abnormality. Am J Cardiol. 1988;61:857–60.
50. Coleman DM, Smallhorn JF, McCrindle BW, Williams WG, Freedom RM. Postoperative follow-up of fibromuscular subaortic stenosis. J Am Coll Cardiol. 1994;24:1558–64.
51. Oliver JM, Gonzalez A, Gallego P, Sanchez-Recalde A, Benito F, Mesa JM. Discrete subaortic stenosis in adults: increased prevalence and slow rate of progression of the obstruction and aortic regurgitation. J Am Coll Cardiol. 2001;38:835–42.
52. Stassano P, Di Tommaso L, Contaldo A, et al. Discrete subaortic stenosis: long-term prognosis on the progression of the obstruction and of the aortic insufficiency. Thorac Cardiovasc Surg. 2005; 53:23–7.
53. Kuralay E, Ozal E, Bingöl H, Cingöz F, Tatar H. Discrete subaortic stenosis: assessing adequacy of myectomy by transesophageal echocardiography. J Card Surg. 1999;14:348–53.
54. Darcin OT, Yagdi T, Atay Y, et al. Discrete subaortic stenosis: surgical outcomes and follow-up results. Tex Heart Inst J. 2003; 30:286–92.
55. Bernhard WF, Keane JF, Fellows KE, Litwin SB, Gross RE. Progress and problems in the surgical management of congenital aortic stenosis. J Thorac Cardiovasc Surg. 1973;66:404–19.
56. Williams JC, Barratt-Boyes BG, Lowe JB. Supravalvular aortic stenosis. Circulation. 1961;24:1311–8.
57. Brooke BS, Bayes-Genis A, Li DY. New insights into elastin and vascular disease. Trends Cardiovasc Med. 2003;13:176–81.
58. Ewart AK, Jin W, Atkinson D, Morris CA, Keating MT. Supravalvular aortic stenosis associated with a deletion disrupting the elastin gene. J Clin Invest. 1994;93:1071–7.
59. O'Connor WN, Davis JB, Geissler R, Cottrill CM, Noonan JA, Todd EP. Supravalvular aortic stenosis. Clinical and pathologic observations in six patients. Arch Pathol Lab Med. 1985;109: 179–85.
60. Stamm C, Li J, Ho SY, Redington AN, Anderson RH. The aortic root in supravalvular aortic stenosis: the potential surgical relevance of morphologic findings. J Thorac Cardiovasc Surg. 1997; 114:16–24.
61. Jureidini SB, Marino CJ, Singh GK, Fiore A, Balfour IC. Main coronary artery and coronary ostial stenosis in children: detection by transthoracic color flow and pulsed Doppler echocardiography. J Am Soc Echocardiogr. 2000;13:255–63.
62. Firstenberg MS, Greenberg NL, Lin SS, Garcia MJ, Alexander LA, Thomas JD. Transesophageal echocardiography assessment of severe ostial left main coronary stenosis. J Am Soc Echocardiogr. 2000;13:696–8.
63. Sobkowicz B, Hirnle T, Dobrzycki S, Frank M, Sawicki R. Intraoperative echocardiographic assessment of the severe isolated ostial stenosis of left main coronary artery before and after surgical patch angioplasty. Eur J Echocardiogr. 2005;6:280–5.
64. Donofrio MT, Engle MA, O'Loughlin JE, et al. Congenital aortic regurgitation: natural history and management. J Am Coll Cardiol. 1992;20:366–72.
65. Bonow RO, Carabello BA, Chatterjee K, et al. ACC/AHA 2006 guidelines for the management of patients with valvular heart disease: a report of the American College of Cardiology/American Heart Association Task Force on Practice Guidelines (writing Committee to Revise the 1998 guidelines for the management of patients with valvular heart disease) developed in collaboration with the Society of Cardiovascular Anesthesiologists endorsed by the Society for Cardiovascular Angiography and Interventions and the Society of Thoracic Surgeons. J Am Coll Cardiol. 2006;48:e1–148.
66. Enriquez-Sarano M, Tajik AJ. Clinical practice. Aortic regurgitation. N Engl J Med. 2004;351:1539–46.
67. le Polain de Waroux J-B, Pouleur A-C, Goffinet C, et al. Functional anatomy of aortic regurgitation: accuracy, prediction of surgical repairability, and outcome implications of transesophageal echocardiography. Circulation. 2007;116:I264–9.
68. Tweddell JS, Pelech AN, Frommelt PC, et al. Complex aortic valve repair as a durable and effective alternative to valve replacement in children with aortic valve disease. J Thorac Cardiovasc Surg. 2005;129:551–8.
69. Zoghbi WA, Enriquez-Sarano M, Foster E, et al. Recommendations for evaluation of the severity of native valvular regurgitation with two-dimensional and Doppler echocardiography. J Am Soc Echocardiogr. 2003;16:777–802.
70. Lancellotti P, Tribouilloy C, Hagendorff A, et al. European Association of Echocardiography recommendations for the assessment of valvular regurgitation. Part 1: aortic and pulmonary regurgitation (native valve disease). Eur J Echocardiogr. 2010;11:223–44.
71. Friedrich AD, Shekar PS. Interrogation of the aortic valve. Crit Care Med. 2007;35:S365–71.
72. Tribouilloy CM, Enriquez-Sarano M, Fett SL, Bailey KR, Seward JB, Tajik AJ. Application of the proximal flow convergence method to calculate the effective regurgitant orifice area in aortic regurgitation. J Am Coll Cardiol. 1998;32:1032–9.
73. Honjo O, Kotani Y, Osaki S, et al. Discrepancy between intraoperative transesophageal echocardiography and postoperative transthoracic echocardiography in assessing congenital valve surgery. Ann Thorac Surg. 2006;82:2240–6.
74. Tweddell JS, Pelech AN, Jaquiss RDB, et al. Aortic valve repair. Semin Thorac Cardiovasc Surg Pediatr Card Surg Annu. 2005:112–21.
75. Marino BS, Pasquali SK, Wernovsky G, et al. Accuracy of intraoperative transesophageal echocardiography in the prediction of future neo-aortic valve function after the Ross procedure in children and young adults. Congenit Heart Dis. 2008;3:39–46.

76. Dietz HC, Pyeritz RE, Hall BD, et al. The Marfan syndrome locus: confirmation of assignment to chromosome 15 and identification of tightly linked markers at 15q15-q21.3. Genomics. 1991;9:355–61.
77. Boileau C, Jondeau G, Mizuguchi T, Matsumoto N. Molecular genetics of Marfan syndrome. Curr Opin Cardiol. 2005;20: 194–200.
78. Yetman AT, Graham T. The dilated aorta in patients with congenital cardiac defects. J Am Coll Cardiol. 2009;53:461–7.
79. Abe T, Komatsu S. Surgical repair and long-term results in ruptured sinus of Valsalva aneurysm. Ann Thorac Surg. 1988; 46:520–5.
80. Davies RR, Goldstein LJ, Coady MA, et al. Yearly rupture or dissection rates for thoracic aortic aneurysms: simple prediction based on size. Ann Thorac Surg. 2002;73:17–27; discussion 27–8.
81. Thenabadu PN, Steiner RE, Cleland WP, Goodwin JF. Observations on the treatment of dissection of the aorta. Postgrad Med J. 1976;52:671–7.
82. Martinez RM, Anderson RH. Echocardiographic features of the morphologically right ventriculo-arterial junction. Cardiol Young. 2005;15 Suppl 1:17–26.
83. Stamm C, Anderson RH, Ho SY. Clinical anatomy of the normal pulmonary root compared with that in isolated pulmonary valvular stenosis. J Am Coll Cardiol. 1998;31:1420–5.
84. Roberts WC, Shemin RJ, Kent KM. Frequency and direction of interatrial shunting in valvular pulmonic stenosis with intact ventricular septum and without left ventricular inflow or outflow obstruction. An analysis of 127 patients treated by valvulotomy. Am Heart J. 1980;99:142–8.
85. Freedom RM, Yoo SJ. The divided right ventricle. In: Freedom RM, Yoo SJ, Mikailian H, Williams WG, editors. The natural and modified history of congenital heart disease. New York: Blackwell Publishing; 2004. p. 232–5.
86. Restivo A, Cameron AH, Anderson RH, Allwork SP. Divided right ventricle: a review of its anatomical varieties. Pediatr Cardiol. 1984;5:197–204.
87. Pongiglione G, Freedom RM, Cook D, Rowe RD. Mechanism of acquired right ventricular outflow tract obstruction in patients with ventricular septal defect: an angiocardiographic study. Am J Cardiol. 1982;50:776–80.
88. Wong PC, Sanders SP, Jonas RA, et al. Pulmonary valve-moderator band distance and association with development of double-chambered right ventricle. Am J Cardiol. 1991;68:1681–6.
89. Lucas RV, Varco RL, Lillehei CW, Adams P, Anderson RC, Edwards JE. Anomalous muscle bundle of the right ventricle. Hemodynamic consequences and surgical considerations. Circulation. 1962;25:443–55.
90. Hachiro Y, Takagi N, Koyanagi T, Morikawa M, Abe T. Repair of double-chambered right ventricle: surgical results and long-term follow-up. Ann Thorac Surg. 2001;72:1520–2.
91. Simpson WFJ, Sade RM, Crawford FA, Taylor AB, Fyfe DA. Double-chambered right ventricle. Ann Thorac Surg. 1987; 44:7–10.
92. McElhinney DB, Chatterjee KM, Reddy VM. Double-chambered right ventricle presenting in adulthood. Ann Thorac Surg. 2000;70:124–7.
93. Yoshida K, Yoshikawa J, Shakudo M, et al. Color Doppler evaluation of valvular regurgitation in normal subjects. Circulation. 1988;78:840–7.
94. Keane JF, Fyler DC. Pulmonary stenosis. In: Keane JF, Fyler DC, Lock J, editors. Nadas' pediatric cardiology. 2nd ed. Philadelphia: Saunders; 2006. p. 549–58.
95. Veldtman GR, Dearani JA, Warnes CA. Low pressure giant pulmonary artery aneurysms in the adult: natural history and management strategies. Heart. 2003;89:1067–70.
96. Sayger P, Lewis M, Arcilla R, Ilbawi M. Isolated congenital absence of a single pulmonary valve cusp. Pediatr Cardiol. 2000;21:487–9.
97. Mercer-Rosa L, Yang W, Kutty S, Rychik J, Fogel M, Goldmuntz E. Quantifying pulmonary regurgitation and right ventricular function in surgically repaired tetralogy of Fallot: a comparative analysis of echocardiography and magnetic resonance imaging. Circ Cardiovasc Imaging. 2012;5(5):637–43.
98. Bouzas B, Chang AC, Gatzoulis MA. Pulmonary insufficiency: preparing the patient with ventricular dysfunction for surgery. Cardiol Young. 2005;15 Suppl 1:51–7.
99. Gatzoulis MA, Clark AL, Cullen S, Newman CG, Redington AN. Right ventricular diastolic function 15 to 35 years after repair of tetralogy of Fallot. Restrictive physiology predicts superior exercise performance. Circulation. 1995;91:1775–81.
100. Bouzas B, Kilner PJ, Gatzoulis MA. Pulmonary regurgitation: not a benign lesion. Eur Heart J. 2005;26:433–9.
101. Oosterhof T, van Straten A, Vliegen HW, et al. Preoperative thresholds for pulmonary valve replacement in patients with corrected tetralogy of Fallot using cardiovascular magnetic resonance. Circulation. 2007;116:545–51.
102. Geva T. Repaired tetralogy of Fallot: the roles of cardiovascular magnetic resonance in evaluating pathophysiology and for pulmonary valve replacement decision support. J Cardiovasc Magn Reson. 2011;13:1–24.

Evaluation of Conotruncal Abnormalities

12

Laura M. Mercer-Rosa and Meryl S. Cohen

Abstract

Conotruncal malformations encompass a group of congenital heart defects with abnormal ventriculo-arterial connections. The conotruncal abnormalities are often seen in association with other cardiac defects, and the intracardiac anatomy can be quite complex. Cardiac surgery is almost always required to repair the anatomic abnormalities and restore normal physiology. As such, transesophageal echocardiography (TEE) is often required in the intraoperative setting in order to evaluate and confirm preoperatively the cardiac abnormalities, and to assess the cardiac repair postoperatively. Moreover, patients with a conotruncal malformation (operated and sometimes unoperated) will survive into adulthood, and in the ambulatory setting, TEE can provide important anatomic and physiologic information superior to that available by transthoracic echocardiography. This chapter discusses the TEE evaluation of the most common and important conotruncal defects, including tetralogy of Fallot, double outlet right ventricle, truncus arteriosus, transposition of the great arteries (also known as complete, or D-transposition of the great arteries), and congenitally corrected transposition of the great arteries.

Keywords

Transesophageal echocardiography • Heart defects • Congenital • Tetralogy of Fallot • Double outlet right ventricle • Transposition of the great arteries, complete • Truncus arteriosus • Transposition of the great arteries, corrected

Introduction

Conotruncal malformations encompass a group of defects with abnormal ventriculo-arterial connections. Cardiac surgery is almost always required for conotruncal abnormalities and therefore transesophageal echocardiography (TEE) is essential in the evaluation of most patients with these defects.

This chapter will review the application of TEE in the evaluation of conotruncal anomalies including: tetralogy of Fallot, double outlet right ventricle, truncus arteriosus, transposition of the great arteries (also known as complete or D-transposition of the great arteries), and congenitally corrected transposition of the great arteries. These cardiac defects comprise the vast majority of conotruncal abnormalities encountered by congenital heart disease specialists; extremely rare conditions including anatomically corrected malposition of the great arteries and double outlet left ventricle will not be addressed.

L.M. Mercer-Rosa, MD, MSCE • M.S. Cohen, MD (✉)
Division of Cardiology, Department of Pediatrics,
The Children's Hospital of Philadelphia,
Perelman School of Medicine at the University of Pennsylvania,
34th St. & Civic Center Blvd., Philadelphia, PA 19104, USA
e-mail: cohenm@email.chop.edu

The online version of this chapter (doi:10.1007/978-1-84800-064-3_12) contains supplementary material, which is available to authorized users.

P.C. Wong, W.C. Miller-Hance (eds.), *Transesophageal Echocardiography for Congenital Heart Disease*,
DOI 10.1007/978-1-84800-064-3_12, © Springer-Verlag London 2014

General Comments

TEE is an important diagnostic tool in patients diagnosed with conotruncal abnormalities in a variety of settings. Conotruncal malformations are usually diagnosed prenatally, or in the neonatal period, therefore diagnostic echocardiography is generally performed using transthoracic echocardiography (TTE). TEE becomes a powerful tool in the intraoperative setting. Preoperative TEE often provides additional anatomic information that allows the echocardiographer to determine the best views for imaging after surgical intervention; this is particularly important when complex baffling procedures are being considered. Postoperative TEE is an invaluable tool used to assess the adequacy of surgical repair for many of these lesions. This includes evaluation of: residual intracardiac shunts, residual outflow obstruction, evaluation of atrioventricular (AV) and semilunar valve function, and assessment of ventricular performance. TEE is also essential in the evaluation of patients (particularly adults) with poor transthoracic acoustic windows. Moreover, TEE is largely used in the evaluation of infective endocarditis, suspicion for intracardiac thrombus, and suspected aortic dissection [1], as discussed in Chap. 16. TEE is also helpful to assist in catheter-directed interventions (Chap. 17).

Specific Lesions

In this section, we discuss the anatomy, echocardiographic evaluation, and surgical considerations for: tetralogy of Fallot, double outlet right ventricle, truncus arteriosus, transposition of the great arteries, and congenitally corrected transposition of the great arteries.

Tetralogy of Fallot

Anatomy

The four morphologic abnormalities that constitute the term "tetralogy" of Fallot (TOF) include a ventricular septal defect (VSD), override of the aorta over the ventricular septum, subpulmonary stenosis, and right ventricle (RV) hypertrophy. Yet the fundamental anatomic defect in TOF is anterior malalignment of the infundibular (conal) septum. This malalignment results in a large, typically unrestrictive VSD with concurrent override of the aorta over the ventricular septum. Furthermore, the infundibulum (conal muscle under the pulmonary valve) is hypoplastic with variable degrees of subpulmonary and pulmonary stenosis. RV hypertrophy is a consequence of the large VSD (the RV being at systemic pressure) [2].

TOF displays wide anatomic variation: from mild pulmonary stenosis to the most severe form, pulmonary atresia. In TOF with pulmonary atresia (TOF/PA), the anatomy of the pulmonary arteries has a wide spectrum: from normal-sized, confluent pulmonary arteries to diminutive or even non-existent pulmonary arteries with pulmonary blood flow supplied by way of aorto–pulmonary collateral vessels.

Known genetic abnormalities occur in 20 % of patients with TOF. 22q11.2 deletion syndrome (including the DiGeorge and velo-cardio-facial syndromes) is seen in 15 % of patients with TOF and is particularly common in those with associated arch sidedness abnormalities. TOF is the third most common lesion in children with Down syndrome (trisomy 21) and is sometimes seen in association with endocardial cushion defect in those patients. Other conditions associated with TOF include VACTERL association and CHARGE syndrome. Patients with TOF and chromosomal anomalies have worse outcome than those without genetic defects [3].

With the most common form of TOF (malalignment VSD and subvalvar/valvar pulmonic stenosis), surgery is usually performed within the first 6 months of life. Some patients with only a mild to moderate amount of pulmonary outflow tract obstruction will have relatively balanced shunting across the VSD, with only a mild degree of cyanosis, and acceptable oxygen saturations that can sometimes be higher than 90 % (so-called "pink TOF"). In this group, complete, one-stage surgical repair can be electively performed at any time, usually 5–6 months, sometimes even later. In other patients, surgical intervention is necessary at a younger age; indications for this include significant cyanosis and/or "*tetralogy spells*" (acute, severe hypercyanosis). For such patients, many institutions utilize a staged surgical approach. Surgical palliation is first performed to augment pulmonary blood flow, usually with a modified Blalock-Taussig shunt. When pulmonary stenosis is primarily at pulmonary valve level, a few institutions will utilize balloon dilation of the pulmonary valve (performed in the catheterization laboratory) as an alternative form of palliation to increase pulmonary blood flow [4–6]. In either case, complete repair is undertaken several months later. However some centers prefer to perform a complete, one-stage repair of TOF at a very young age, even as a neonate [7–9].

The surgical management of patients with TOF/PA is variable. Most will require some type of surgical intervention, and the timing of surgery can vary from the neonatal period to infancy or even older. The surgical intervention is dependent on the anatomical subtype. Some patients are staged to complete repair: a modified Blalock-Taussig shunt or other type of aorto-pulmonary connection is performed in the neonatal period, followed by a complete repair (often with an RV to pulmonary artery conduit) within the first year of life. In some cases, initial palliation to establish reliable pulmonary blood flow can be performed without surgery. This is achieved by interventional catheterization methods such as stenting of the ductus arteriosus [10–12] and, when membranous pulmonary valve atresia is present, radiofrequency perforation of a pulmonary valve [13]. In more severe cases such as TOF/PA with multiple aorto-pulmonary collateral arteries (MAPCAS), complex staged surgical palliation is required including *unifocalization* of the pulmonary arteries and collateral vessels to a central location with a reliable source of pulmonary blood flow (Blalock-Taussig shunt or RV to pulmonary artery conduit). It should also be noted that some patients with TOF/PA and MAPCAS do not undergo any intervention throughout their lifetime. They continue to have lower than normal arterial oxygen saturations, but these remain compatible with survival because the aorto-pulmonary collaterals provide enough pulmonary blood flow to maintain adequate systemic arterial oxygenation.

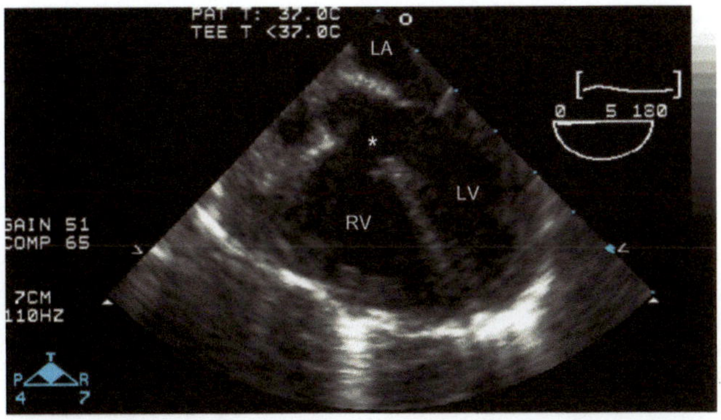

Fig. 12.1 Tetralogy of Fallot. Mid esophageal four chamber view showing right ventricular hypertrophy, the large malalignment ventricular septal defect (*asterisk*), and overriding aorta. *LA* left atrium, *LV* left ventricle, *RV* right ventricle

TEE Evaluation

There are pertinent findings in TOF to keep in mind when performing a TEE:

- Additional VSDs, which are typically seen in the muscular septum. Some patients may have absence or hypoplasia of the conal septum in addition to malalignment.
- Restrictive VSD due to accessory tricuspid valve tissue
- Coronary anomalies, particularly a coronary artery crossing the RV outflow tract, which occur in approximately 5 % of TOF patients. This includes variations such as origin of the left anterior descending coronary artery from the right coronary artery, and right coronary artery from the left anterior descending [14, 15].
- Persistent left superior vena cava (SVC), seen in 9–12 % of patients [16, 17]. In these cases the left SVC usually drains into a dilated coronary sinus, but in rare instances it can return directly to the left atrium.
- Discontinuous pulmonary arteries, whereby one pulmonary artery originates from a ductus arteriosus or collateral vessel.
- Common AV canal defect (complete AV septal defect), seen almost exclusively in Down syndrome.
- Absent pulmonary valve syndrome, A subtype of TOF, the main features of this condition include an unguarded pulmonary valve annulus with massively dilated main and proximal branch pulmonary arteries. Free pulmonary insufficiency is the norm, as well as compression of the right and left mainstem bronchi and/or as distal bronchioles.
- Atrial septal defect or patent foramen ovale (the so-called pentalogy of Fallot).

Though the diagnosis of TOF is generally made using TTE, TEE can be used for confirmation of diagnosis or in those patients with poor transthoracic acoustic windows. This includes the rare adult with unrepaired TOF. The starting point is generally the mid esophageal four chamber (ME 4 Ch) view which displays the four cardiac chambers and two AV valves along with the large malalignment VSD. This view also confirms RV hypertrophy. In addition, the atrial septum can be inspected for any defects. As the probe is advanced, the coronary sinus is viewed; it can be enlarged when it is connected to a left SVC. As the probe is withdrawn, the VSD is again seen with the aorta overriding the ventricular septum (Fig. 12.1, Video 12.1). Further withdrawal demonstrates the hypoplastic pulmonary outflow tract. The atrial septum is interrogated for a communication from inferior to superior in the 0–30° ME 4 Ch view. The mid esophageal bicaval (ME Bicaval) 90° view establishes the systemic venous connections (in a sagittal plane) and confirms the presence of an atrial communication, if present. As the probe sweeps to the left (counterclockwise), the VSD is seen with the anterior malalignment of the conal septum, in a view known as the mid esophageal right ventricular inflow-outflow (ME RV In-Out) view, multiplane angle 60°–90°. (Fig. 12.2, Video 12.2). From here, forward rotation of the multiplane angle setting to 90°–110° produces the mid esophageal long axis (ME LAX) and mid esophageal aortic valve long axis (ME AV LAX) views. Both of these views can also be used to evaluate the relationship of the overriding aorta to the VSD. If the TEE probe can be advanced into the stomach and anteflexed, the deep transgastric long axis (DTG LAX) and deep transgastric sagittal (DTG Sagittal) views provide excellent visualization of the overriding aorta, malalignment VSD, anteriorly malaligned infundibular septum, and narrowed RV outflow tract (Fig. 12.3, Video 12.3). These views are similar to those obtained with the standard transthoracic subcostal coronal and sagittal sweeps.

Color Doppler evaluation prior to surgical intervention includes assessment of flow across the atrial septum (typical flow pattern is from the left atrium to the right atrium). The ventricular septum can be interrogated in all views to assess for additional ventricular communications in the muscular septum. Spectral Doppler assessment of the gradient across the RV outflow tract is best performed in the mid esophageal

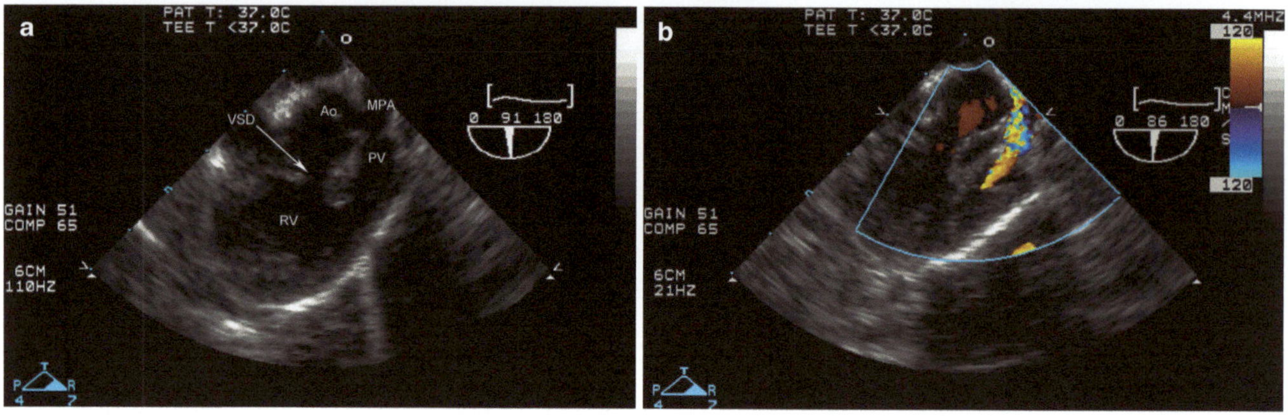

Fig. 12.2 Tetralogy of Fallot. (**a**) Modified mid esophageal right ventricular inflow-outflow view (multiplane angle about 90°) showing the malalignment ventricular septal defect (*VSD*), as well as narrowing of the right ventricular outflow due to a malaligned conal septum. (**b**) Color flow Doppler shows aliasing beginning at subpulmonary level, and continuing across the hypoplastic pulmonary valve. *Ao* aorta, *MPA* main pulmonary artery, *PV* pulmonary valve, *RV* right ventricle

ascending aortic short axis (ME Asc Ao SAX), ME RV In-Out or DTG LAX and Sagittal views—whichever yields a more favorable angle for Doppler evaluation (Figs. 12.2 and 12.3, Videos 12.2 and 12.3). To evaluate flow in the branch pulmonary arteries, and to search for a possible patent ductus arteriosus, color Doppler can be performed using the upper esophageal pulmonary artery long axis (UE PA LAX) and upper esophageal aortic arch short and long axis (UE Ao Arch SAX, UE Ao Arch LAX) views. It should be remembered that a significant proportion of TOF patients with a right-sided aortic arch (which occurs in about 25 % of TOF) will have a *left* sided ductus arteriosus originating from the left subclavian or innominate artery, and entering the main/left pulmonary artery [18].

Surgical Considerations

The operative repair of tetralogy of Fallot involves closure of the ventricular septal defect (Fig. 12.4, Video 12.4) and relief of the RV outflow tract obstruction. The outflow tract surgery is dependent upon the severity of infundibular and pulmonary valvar hypoplasia. A transannular outflow tract patch is

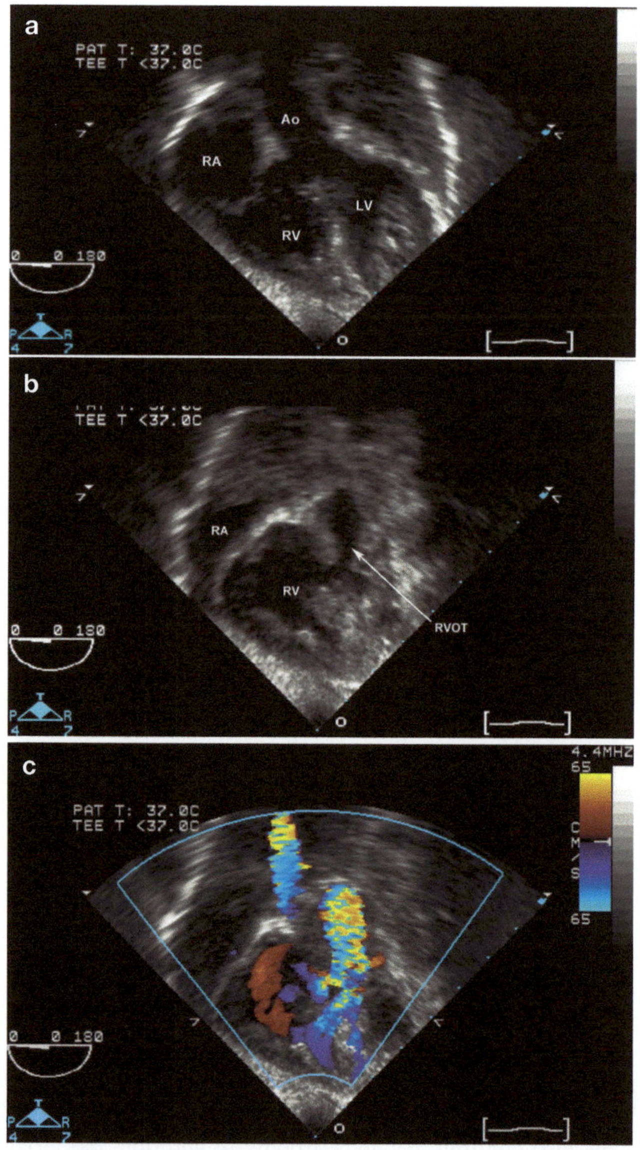

Fig. 12.3 Tetralogy of Fallot: deep transgastric long axis (**a–c**) and sagittal views (**d**, **e**) that simulate transthoracic subcostal coronal and sagittal views. (**a–c**) Shows the overriding aorta and malalignment ventricular septal defect (**a**). With slight probe withdrawal, the anteriorly malaligned infundibular septum is seen (**b**), producing subpulmonary stenosis, with color flow aliasing at this level (**c**). (**d**, **e**) Also show the anteriorly malaligned infundibular septum with color flow Doppler aliasing, as well as the ventricular septal defect with *right* to *left* shunting. The spectral Doppler tracing shows the typical "dagger" shape seen with subpulmonary stenosis. *Ao* aorta, *LV* left ventricle, *MPA* pulmonary artery, *RA* right atrium, *RV* right ventricle, *RVOT* right ventricular outflow tract

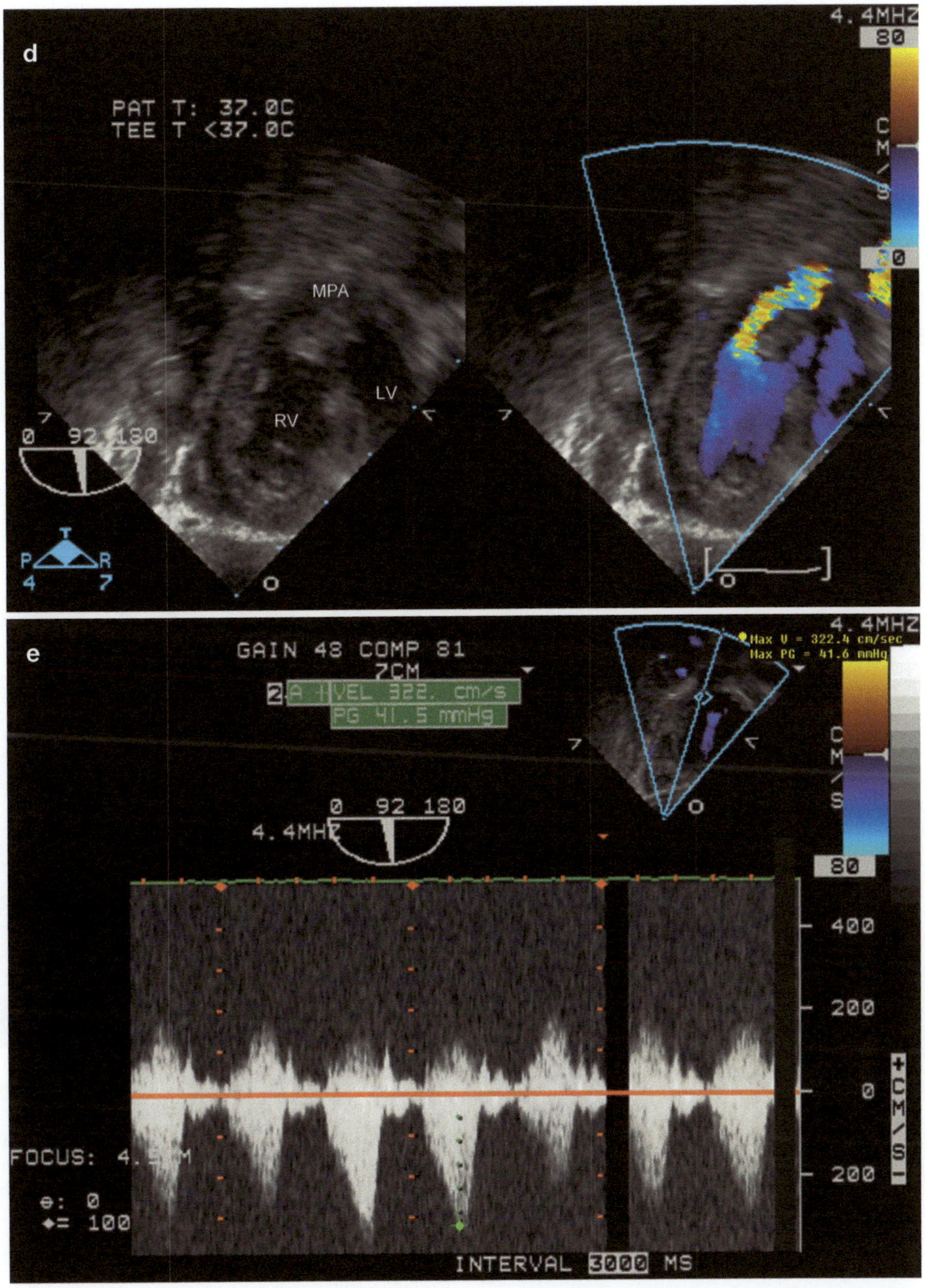

Fig. 12.3 (continued)

used when the outflow tract obstruction is severe, with significant pulmonary valve annular hypoplasia. In milder forms of TOF, patch enlargement of the hypoplastic infundibulum (a non transannular patch), if required, is performed while the pulmonary valve is preserved to avoid long-term severe pulmonary regurgitation. In some centers, a transatrial approach is employed, in which the VSD is closed and RV muscle is resected from the right atrium, thereby minimizing or avoiding a right ventriculotomy [19]. Conduits from the RV to the pulmonary artery are required in many cases of pulmonary atresia or when a coronary (typically a left anterior descending from the right coronary) crosses the RV outflow tract. The coronary arteries can be evaluated preoperatively using the mid esophageal aortic valve short axis (ME AV SAX) view, as discussed in Chap. 4. With probe anteflexion and careful evaluation, it is possible to visualize a coronary crossing the RV outflow tract (Fig. 12.5, Video 12.5).

Postoperative TEE is indicated to evaluate for (1) residual RV outflow tract obstruction, (2) residual VSDs (Figs. 12.6 and 12.7, Video 12.6), (3) assessment of ventricular performance, (4) severity of pulmonary regurgita-

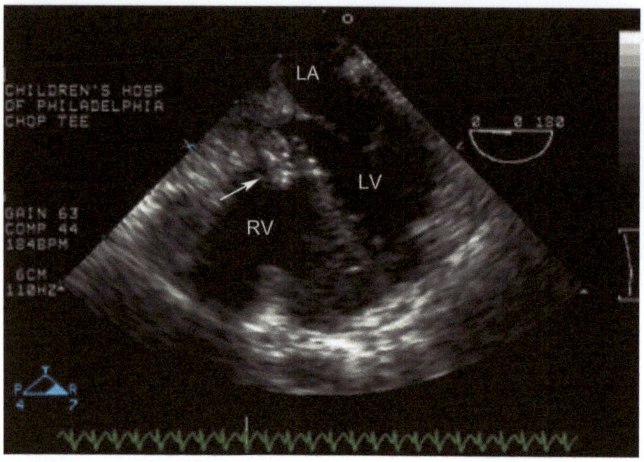

Fig. 12.4 Mid esophageal four chamber view demonstrating right ventricular hypertrophy in a patient with tetralogy of Fallot. Also note the presence of a ventricular septal defect patch (*arrow*), in good position

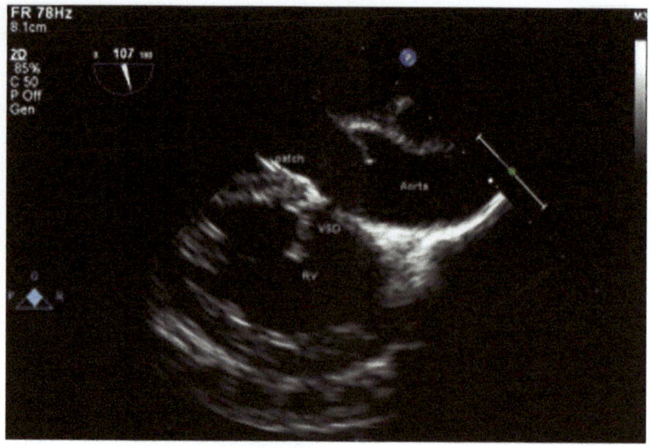

Fig. 12.6 Modified mid esophageal long axis view, with multiplane angle 107° in a patient with tetralogy of Fallot demonstrating a residual ventricular septal defect (*VSD*). The defect is located in the superior aspect of the VSD patch just under the aortic valve. *RV* right ventricle

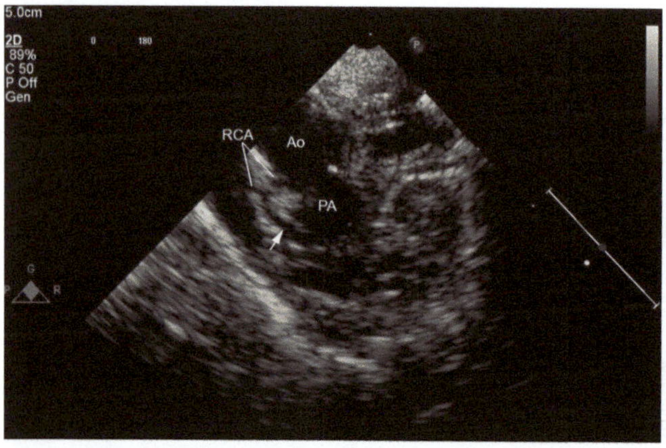

Fig. 12.5 Preoperative study in a patient with tetralogy of Fallot. A prominent anterior descending coronary artery (*arrow*) arises from the right coronary artery (*RCA*) and courses anterior to the right ventricular outflow tract, thereby precluding a transannular patch. *Ao* aorta, *PA* main pulmonary artery

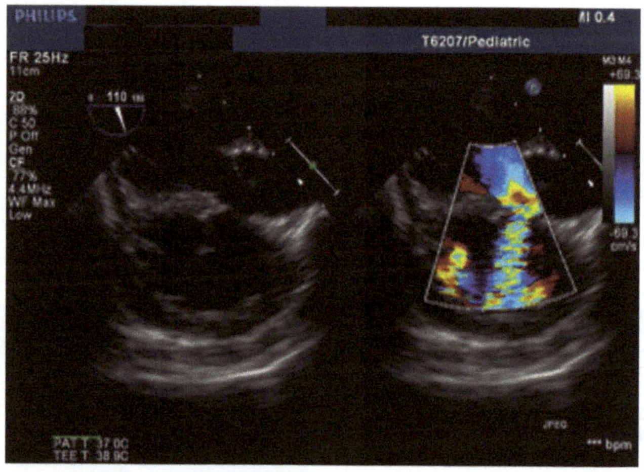

Fig. 12.7 Modified mid esophageal long axis view, with multiplane angle 110°. This color compare image illustrates the presence of a residual ventricular septal defect after repair of tetralogy of Fallot; the defect is located immediately inferior to the aorta. The etiology of the defect is attributed to patch dehiscence. Here, the ventricular shunt direction is left to right

tion, and (5) flow direction across the atrial septum (if an intentional small communication is present). Branch pulmonary artery stenosis can be difficult to diagnose using TEE [20], but in some instances useful information about the branch pulmonary arteries can be obtained using the mid and upper esophageal views, using the techniques and views discussed in Chap. 4 (Fig. 12.8, Video 12.7). As in all forms of conotruncal malformations, all TEE views should be used to assess for residual VSD. The most common type of residual defect is a peri-patch leak between sutures (Figs. 12.6 and 12.7). Defects less than 3 mm tend to have minimal hemodynamic impact, though some defects of that size can be a concern, particularly in very small infants [21]. Determination of RV pressure either by Doppler interrogation of the tricuspid regurgitation jet (if present) or by the residual VSD jet, particularly when the RV outflow tract is unobstructed, is of utmost importance in assessment of hemodynamic significance of the residual VSD. By definition, a restrictive VSD is associated with RV pressure that is subsystemic. If RV pressure cannot be estimated by TEE, an assessment of pulmonary to systemic blood flow ratio (Qp/Qs), in which the surgeon directly obtains blood samples from the SVC and pulmonary and systemic arteries for oximetry, is helpful to determine the significance of the residual VSD.

One of the most challenging types of residual VSDs to assess is the intramural defect. This type of defect occurs in the setting of conotruncal malformations, when the VSD

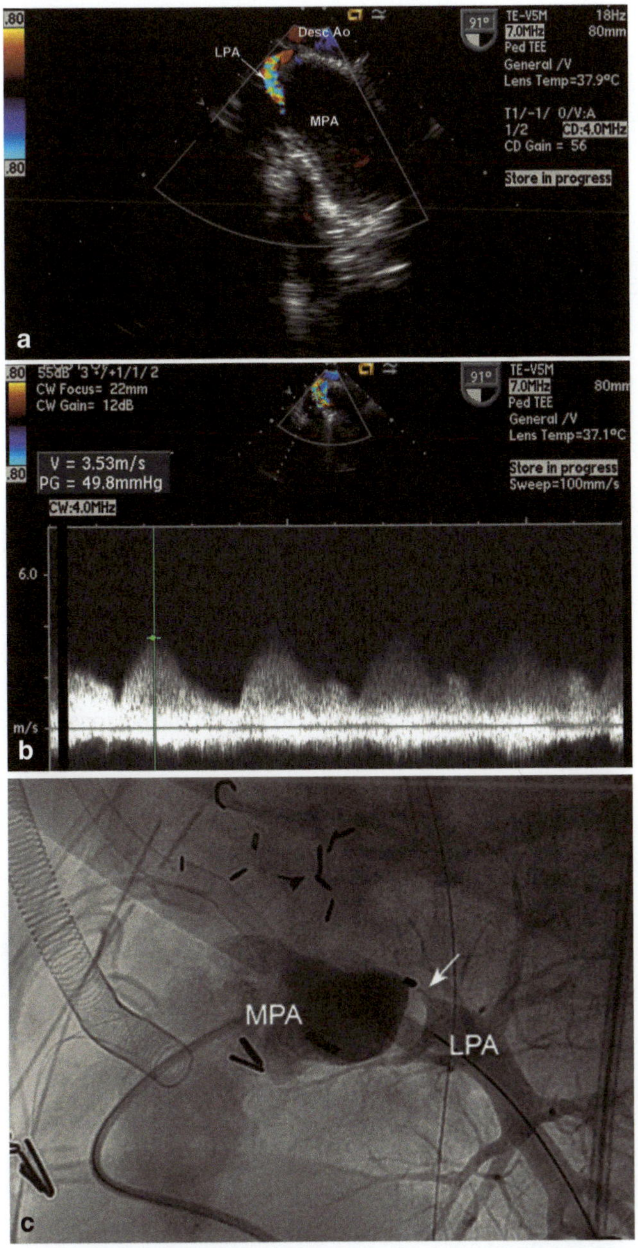

Fig. 12.8 (**a**) Upper esophageal aortic arch short axis with counterclockwise rotation, demonstrating significant left pulmonary artery stenosis in this patient with tetralogy of Fallot who underwent complete correction, including unifocalization of discontinuous pulmonary arteries. (**b**) Spectral continuous wave Doppler tracing showing the significant gradient across the stenotic area. (**c**) Postoperative pulmonary artery angiogram confirming the marked stenosis (*arrow*) of the proximal left pulmonary artery. *Desc Ao* descending aorta, *LPA* left pulmonary artery, *MPA* main pulmonary artery

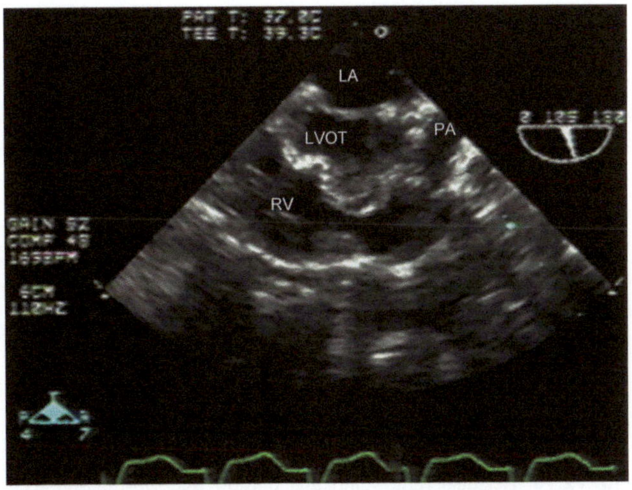

Fig. 12.9 Residual right ventricular outflow tract narrowing is seen in a patient after tetralogy of Fallot repair in a modified mid esophageal right ventricular inflow-outflow view, with slight probe withdrawal to display the outflow tract more clearly *LA* left atrium, *LVOT* left ventricular outflow tract, *PA* pulmonary artery, *RV* right ventricle

patch attaches to the trabeculated right ventricular free wall related to the ventriculoinfundibular fold (parietal band), creating a communication through the intertrabeculated spaces to the right ventricular cavity [21–23]. This area of the heart is difficult for the surgeon to visualize during the repair. Importantly, these defects can increase in size over time. The ME 4 Ch view highlights this type of residual defect well but it can also be seen with a modified ME RV In-Out view, in which the multiplane angle has been rotated to about 90°. Intramural residual VSDs should be looked for in all patients undergoing repair of conotruncal anomalies that include VSD closure.

Assessment of the RV outflow tract for residual obstruction is best performed in a modified ME RV In-Out view with rotation of the multiplane angle to 90–110° (Figs. 12.9 and 12.10, Video 12.8). Doppler interrogation of the RV outflow tract can be performed with this view, and withdrawal of the probe enables evaluation of the more distal portion of the outflow tract. In some cases where the outflow obstruction is more inferior, the DTG LAX and DTG Sagittal views can be used for optimal Doppler evaluation. A peak Doppler velocity that exceeds 3 m/s (36 mmHg) is considered potentially significant [24]. However, it should be noted that a hypercontractile state exists immediately following TOF repair, due in part to inotropic support and hypovolemia, which can accentuate a dynamic RV outflow tract gradient. Indeed, a study by Kaushal et al. evaluating 166 TOF patients immediately following transatrial repair (median age 7 years) found that 35 % had "significant" residual obstruction (gradient >40 mmHg, right:left ventricular pressure ratio >85 %). Most of these patients (88 %) had a dynamic, rather than fixed, obstruction as defined by TEE; patients with fixed obstruction underwent immediate surgical revision, while those with dynamic obstruction did not. Operative mortality and morbidity were not related to

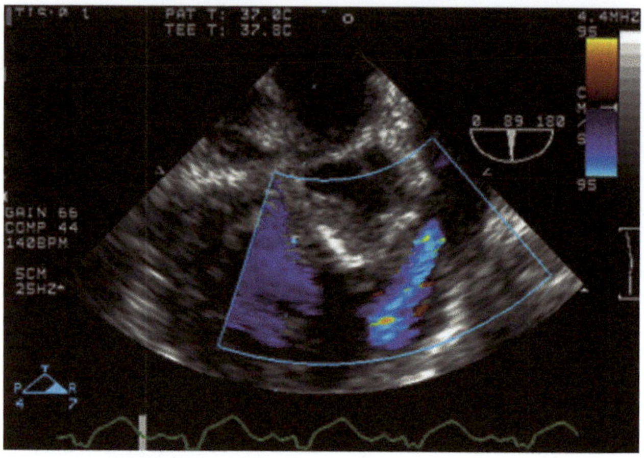

Fig. 12.10 Residual right ventricular outflow tract obstruction seen following tetralogy of Fallot surgery, with color Doppler interrogation in a modifed mid esophageal right ventricular inflow-outflow view. Following surgery, increased velocity in the right ventricular outflow tract is present (manifested by color flow Doppler aliasing), mostly related to dynamic subpulmonary obstruction

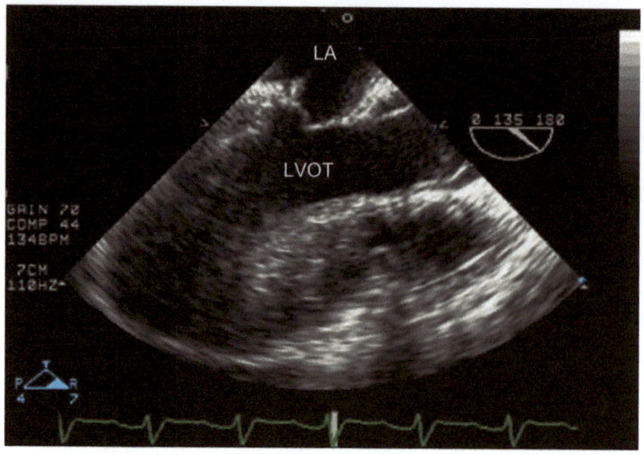

Fig. 12.11 Mid esophageal aortic valve long axis view demonstrating an unobstructed left ventricular outflow tract (*LVOT*) after repair of tetralogy of Fallot. The aortic valve is in the open position. *LA* left atrium

higher residual gradients, and on follow-up (mean 18.5 months) outflow gradients had declined sharply (mean 16 mmHg) irrespective of the severity of intraoperative gradients [25]. Thus a "significant" gradient in the immediate postoperative study should be viewed carefully; the nature of the obstruction (fixed vs. dynamic), and other intraoperative factors, should be considered when deciding to reoperate.

In the immediate postoperative hemodynamic assessment of the TOF patient, several other factors should be evaluated. Detection of intracardiac air and monitoring of cardiac de-airing can be performed using the ME 4 Ch and ME LAX views. Evaluation of right and left ventricular function can be performed with a number of mid esophageal and transgastric TEE views, including ME 4 Ch, mid esophageal two chamber (ME 2 Ch), ME RV In-Out, and the transgastric basal and mid short axis (TG Basal SAX, TG Mid SAX) views. The LV outflow tract is well visualized in both the ME AV LAX, multiplane angle 120–135° (Fig. 12.11, Video 12.9), and ME 4 Ch view (Fig. 12.12, Video 12.10) but this is rarely obstructed after TOF repair. Assessment of severity of pulmonary regurgitation can also be performed using the same views used to evaluate the RV outflow tract, including the ME RV In-Out view and the DTG Sagittal and LAX views. Some degree of pulmonary regurgitation can be expected after TOF repair, particularly following transannular patch. Several methods can be used to evaluate the degree of pulmonary regurgitation, including width of the color Doppler jet compared to outflow tract diameter (mild ≤1/3, moderate 1/3 to 2/3, severe ≥2/3) and presence of diastolic flow reversal in the branch pulmonary arteries [26]. However, changing hemodynamic and ventilatory conditions following TOF surgery can alter the amount of pulmonary regurgitation noted in the immediate postoperative period, compared to later in the postoperative course.

In some TOF patients, a small atrial communication (usually a patent foramen ovale) is left patent as a "pop off" to facilitate cardiac output in the immediate postoperative period. The Doppler flow pattern across the foramen ovale is typically from right atrium to left atrium after surgery as a result of poor RV compliance (from the right ventriculotomy and RV hypertrophy) (Fig. 12.13). The atrial septum can be evaluated by sweeping from the inferior vena cava (IVC) to the superior vena cava. This sweep is performed by starting with the lower esophageal situs short axis (LE Situs SAX) view to image the IVC and hepatic veins, then slowly withdrawing the probe to the ME 4 Ch view (with slight rightward probe rotation) to visualize the atria, atrial septum and superior vena cava, while maintaining the multiplane angle between 0 and 30°.

In the case of a patient with TOF and AV canal defect, both atrial and ventricular septal patches should be evaluated for residual shunts. As with all AV canal repairs (Chap. 8), both AV valves (particularly the mitral valve) must be evaluated for possible regurgitation (Fig. 12.14, Video 12.11). However in addition, the RV outflow tract must be evaluated in the same manner as other TOF patients

In older patients, TEE can be used to assess TOF repair including adults with poor acoustic windows. The long-term impact of severe pulmonary regurgitation can be gauged by evaluation of RV size and performance. When there appears to be significant negative impact of the regurgitation (manifested by marked RV dilation and/or deteriorating RV systolic function), prosthetic pulmonary valve implantation is indicated. This is usually performed

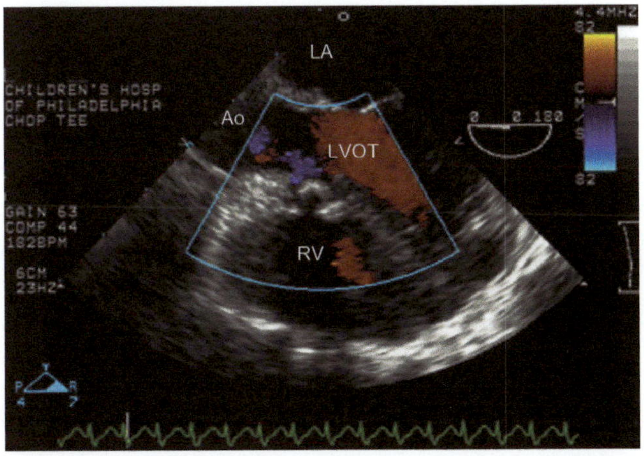

Fig. 12.12 Mid esophageal four chamber view with probe withdrawn to image the left ventricular outflow tract (*LVOT*) demonstrates that there is no residual VSD by color Doppler interrogation after tetralogy of Fallot repair. In addition, flow is laminar into the left ventricular outflow tract. *Ao* aorta, *LA* left atrium, *RV* right ventricle

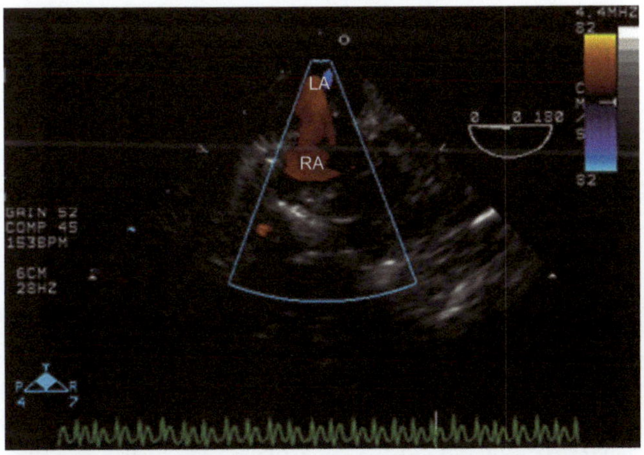

Fig. 12.13 Mid esophageal four chamber view, with probe withdrawn superiorly to the level of the atrial septum and rotated clockwise toward the patient's right side. Color Doppler interrogation demonstrates a residual right to left shunt (*red*) through an atrial communication that was intentionally left patent during surgery. This type of shunting typically occurs in the early postoperative period after tetralogy of Fallot repair. *LA* left atrium, *RA* right atrium

surgically but in some instances, a transcatheter approach (notably using the Melody valve) can be employed (Chap. 16). In addition, tricuspid valve replacement might be indicated in cases of severe tricuspid regurgitation (Fig. 12.15, Video 12.12). RV systolic pressure estimate can be performed if tricuspid regurgitation is present. Aortic root dilation is a common finding in adults with TOF and can be associated with the development of aortic regurgitation over time. Patients with TOF can also develop important arrhythmias such as ventricular tachycardia. In some cases, TEE can help distinguish the type of arrhythmia.

Double Outlet Right Ventricle

Anatomy

Double outlet right ventricle (DORV) is not a specific congenital malformation, but rather, an abnormal ventriculo-

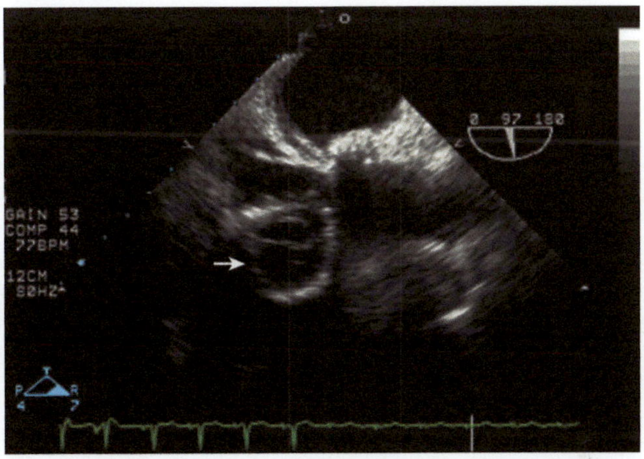

Fig. 12.15 Severe tricuspid regurgitation prompted tricuspid valve replacement in this adult long after tetralogy of Fallot repair; as seen here in a modified mid esophageal right ventricular inflow-outflow view (multiplane angle 97°), the prosthetic valve appears in cross section as indicated by the *arrow*

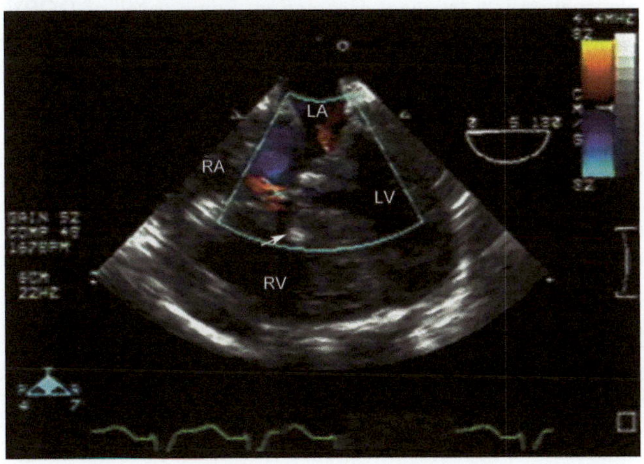

Fig. 12.14 Mid esophageal four chamber view in a patient who has undergone tetralogy of Fallot and atrioventricular canal repair. A large ventricular septal defect patch is seen (*arrow*). Minimal residual atrioventricular valve regurgitation is seen across the right and left atrioventricular valves. *LA* left atrium, *LV* left ventricle, *RA* right atrium, *RV* right ventricle

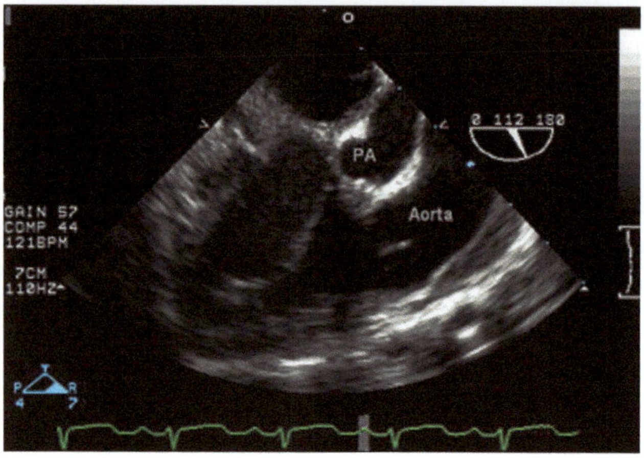

Fig. 12.16 Modified mid esophageal right ventricular inflow-outflow view (multiplane angle 110°) in a patient with double outlet right ventricle with posterior malalignment of the conal septum and subaortic ventricular septal defect, demonstrating that the aorta is anterior to the smaller pulmonary artery (*PA*). Both great vessels arise from the anterior right ventricle. The conal septum is seen between the aorta and PA

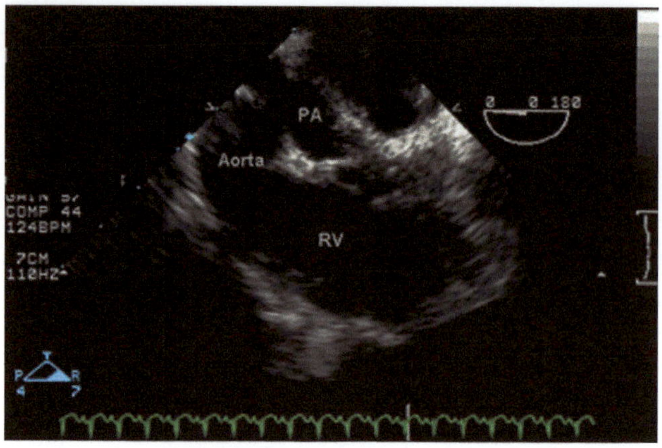

Fig. 12.17 Mid esophageal four chamber view with the probe withdrawn towards the base of the heart in the same patient displayed in Fig. 12.16 with double outlet right ventricle, posterior malalignment of the conal septum with subaortic ventricular septal defect; in this image, the aorta and pulmonary artery (*PA*) come into view, both arising from the right ventricle (*RV*). The PA is smaller than the aorta because of the conal septal malalignment

arterial alignment whereby both great arteries arise from the morphologic RV (Figs. 12.16 and 12.17, Video 12.13). By most criteria, both great vessels must sit more than 50 % over the RV [27]. Typically, there is *bilateral conus*, with myocardium separating both great vessels from the AV valves. However, other conal anatomy can occur in DORV [28]. A VSD is present in almost all cases and usually acts as the "outlet" from the left ventricle (LV). There are rare reports of DORV with an intact ventricular septum [29, 30]. In DORV, the ventricular loop may be "D" (normal) or "L" (inverted) and this will affect the relationship of the great arteries to the ventricle and to each other.

The anatomic and physiologic spectrum of DORV is wide. Associated anomalies are common and include ventricular hypoplasia, superior/inferior ventricles, mitral valve anomalies (including mitral atresia, straddling or parachute mitral valve), common AV canal (in heterotaxy syndrome) and outflow obstruction [28, 31, 32].

The pathophysiology can be similar to TOF, transposition of the great arteries, or a large VSD. This physiology is determined by the location of the great vessels in relationship to the VSD and the degree of outflow obstruction. Of critical importance is the type and location of the VSD: it often determines the type of surgical repair as well as, in some instances, the viability for two-ventricle versus a single ventricle surgical strategy. By far, the most common type of VSD in DORV is the malalignment type, however any type of VSD (such as AV canal, mid muscular, or apical muscular) can occur [33]. The VSD is also classified as one of four types, based upon its relationship to the great vessels: subaortic, subpulmonary, noncommitted, and doubly committed. In those patients with DORV with malalignment type VSD, the most common location of the VSD is subaortic. This is seen on echocardiography as muscle between the mitral and aortic valves. If there is no pulmonary stenosis, the physiology is similar to a large unrestrictive VSD because the blood flow streams from the LV into the aorta. If there is pulmonary stenosis, the physiology is similar to TOF. However, the distinction between DORV and TOF is of utmost importance because those patients with TOF-like DORV have complete subaortic conus that can result in subaortic obstruction after surgery [34]. Subaortic stenosis is extremely rare in TOF.

DORV with subpulmonary VSD is classically termed a "Taussig-Bing" anomaly. In this defect, the great vessels are spatially oriented side-by-side, bilateral conus is present, and the aorta is to the right of the pulmonary artery. The blood from the LV streams into the pulmonary artery so that the physiology is similar to transposition of the great arteries (see below). The subaortic conus is usually small, thus arch obstruction is a frequent association. Some cases of DORV with subpulmonary VSD are not classic Taussig-Bing anomalies but rather fall within the spectrum of that anatomic description. The distinction is critically important when determining surgical strategy.

More uncommon locations of the VSD in DORV include non-committed or doubly-committed subtypes. In DORV with non-committed VSD, the VSD is usually a muscular or a canal (inlet) type VSD. Since it is far from both outflow tracts, baffling procedures may pose a significant challenge. Often, AV valve tissue is obstructing the potential pathway from the LV to the aorta. Moreover, straddling tricuspid valve can occur in association with a canal type VSD. When a muscular VSD is present, there is a tendency for the defect to get smaller over time because it is surrounded by muscle; therefore in general, muscular VSDs are not considered reliable pathways to a great artery. In the rare doubly-committed type, both great vessels sit directly over the VSD.

Other variations of DORV exist, most commonly including those with mitral atresia or hypoplasia associated with left ventricular hypoplasia. When there is significant ventricular hypoplasia, the single ventricle surgical strategy is usually indicated. DORV is often seen in patients with superior/inferior ventricles with criss-cross AV valves. In this rare anomaly, the RV is situated superior to the LV and it is typically hypoplastic. The VSD is usually a canal (inlet) type.

Genetic syndromes can be seen with DORV but there is not one particular association. Transforming growth factor (TGF)-beta 2 knockout mice have been observed to develop DORV in the majority of cases [35]. Heterotaxy syndrome often has DORV as one of its cardiac components.

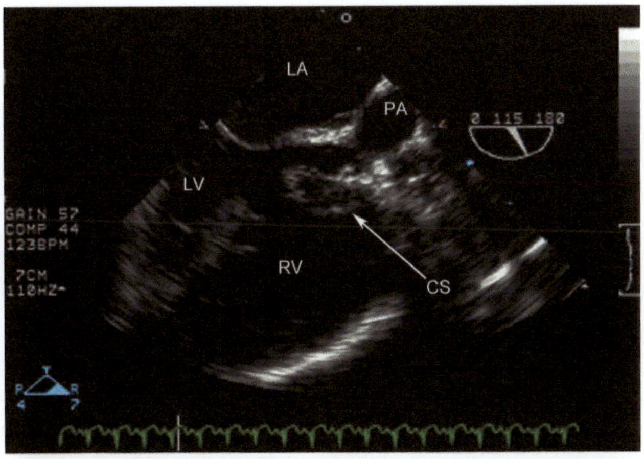

Fig. 12.18 Mid esophageal aortic valve long axis view in the same patient as Figs. 12.16 and 12.17 with double outlet right ventricle, posterior malalignment of the conal septum (*CS*), and subpulmonary ventricular septal defect, highlighting the posterior deviation of the conal septum that results in severe subpulmonary stenosis. The conal septum is also hypertrophied. *LA* left atrium, *LV* left ventricle, *PA* pulmonary artery, *RV* right ventricle

TEE Evaluation

There are pertinent findings seen with DORV to keep in mind when performing a TEE:

- Location and size of the VSD.
- Relationship of great vessels to the VSD.
- Presence of additional VSDs.
- Restrictive VSD due to accessory AV valve tissue.
- Anatomy and size of AV valves.
- Presence and severity of outflow tract obstruction (and to which great vessel).
- Coronary anomalies, particularly if the arterial switch operation is being considered.

One of the most important aspects of the pre-operative evaluation of the patient with DORV is assessment of location and size of the VSD and its relationship to the great vessels (Fig. 12.18, Video 12.14). This, along with the other echocardiographic goals mentioned above, can often help in the determination of the optimal surgical strategy. TEE is an excellent tool to assess for AV valve abnormalities that might preclude a biventricular repair. For example, a straddling AV valve over a VSD usually obstructs the pathway from the LV to a great artery. TEE can also assess whether a VSD is restrictive and the mechanism of the restriction (i.e. AV valve tissue, conal muscle) [36]. Moreover, important anatomic features to help determine a surgical strategy include prominence of the conal septum, presence of tricuspid valve attachments to conal septum, and the distance between the pulmonary and tricuspid valves [37].

The standard ME 4 Ch view may not show evidence of pathology other than RV hypertrophy. However, probe withdrawal and anteflexion will demonstrate that both great vessels arise mostly or completely from the anatomic RV (Fig. 12.16 and 12.17). The anatomy of the AV valves can be seen in this view, as well as in a sweep of the multiplane angle from 0 to 90° that incorporates both the ME RV In-Out and ME 2 Ch views. Alignment of the great vessels is dependent on their position; therefore no single TEE view will be adequate for all patients with DORV. The advantage of the multiplane probe is that the best view of the outflow tracts can be determined as the study is performed. The DTG LAX and DTG Sagittal views are also useful to visualize the great arteries and their relationship to the VSD (Fig. 12.19, Video 12.15). Additional VSDs can be viewed in the ME 4 Ch and ME RV In-Out views, with variation of multiplane angle between 0 and 90° and axial probe rotation to perform a complete sweep of the ventricular septum. The transgastric short axis views (TG Basal SAX, TG Mid SAX) are also useful to evaluate for additional VSDs. Other associated anomalies can be demonstrated using TEE, including AV canal defect (as is common in heterotaxy syndrome), as well as juxtaposition of the atrial appendages, which can be seen from a modified ME 4 Ch view as well as ME AV SAX view (Fig. 12.20, Video 12.16). Systemic venous connections can be evaluated with the LE Situs SAX and lower esophageal IVC long axis (LE IVC LAX) views, as well as the ME Bicaval view (Chap. 4). Pulmonary venous connections can be evaluated using the modified ME 4 Ch and ME Bicaval/ME 2Ch views, as described in Chaps. 4 and 6.

Color Doppler can be used to assess for preoperative AV and semilunar valve regurgitation as well as restriction of flow across the VSD. Color interrogation can also be useful to assess inflow into each ventricle, particularly when straddling or overriding AV valves are suspected. Pulsed and continuous wave Doppler assessment of outflow tract obstruction is dependent on the angle of interrogation. The DTG LAX and DTG Sagittal views can be very helpful for this purpose. LV systolic pressure estimate (as measured by

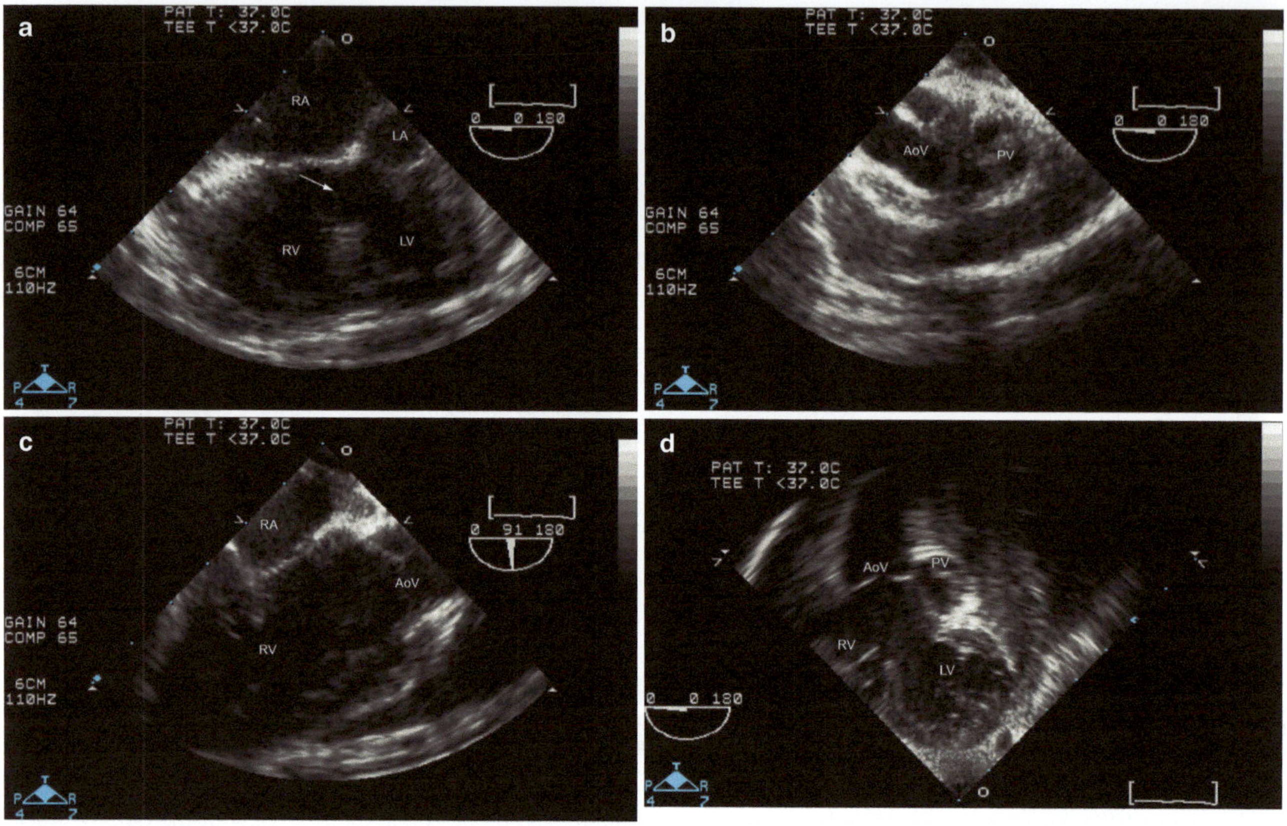

Fig. 12.19 Double outlet right ventricle with pulmonary outflow tract obstruction. Mid esophageal four chamber view (**a**) shows a large ventricular septal defect (*arrow*). With probe withdrawal and anteflexion, the semilunar valves are visualized (**b**). However the pathway from left ventricle (*LV*) to aortic valve (*AoV*) is not clearly shown. Rotation of multiplane angle to about 90° (**c**) shows right atrium (*RA*) and right ventricle (*RV*) as well as AoV, but it is still unclear whether the pathway from LV to AoV is unobstructed. The deep transgastric long axis view (**d**) shows that this pathway is unobstructed. This patient successfully underwent a patch closure of the ventricular septal defect and relief of pulmonary outflow tract stenosis.

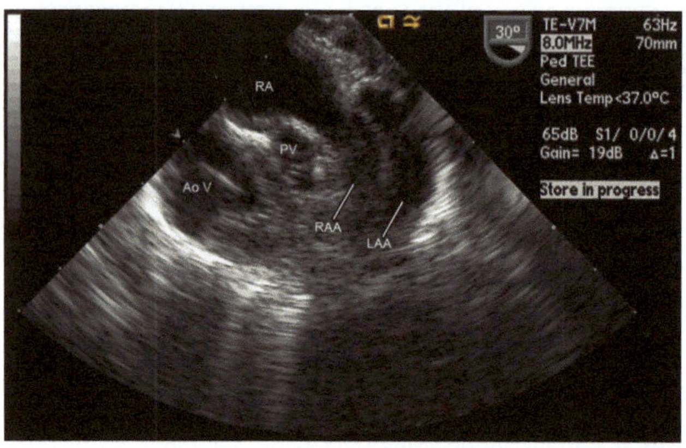

Fig. 12.20 Left juxtaposition of the atrial appendages in a patient with double outlet right ventricle and pulmonary stenosis. This image was obtained from a mid esophageal aortic valve short axis view. Note how the right atrial appendage (*RAA*) crosses posterior to the great arteries to lie just anterior to the left atrial appendage (*LAA*). *AoV* aortic valve, *RA* right atrium, *PV* pulmonary valve

mitral regurgitation jet) is important if a restrictive VSD is suspected. The LV may be at suprasystemic pressure in these instances. This method of assessment, performed in the ME 4 Ch and ME 2 Ch views, is particularly important when the VSD jet is not at an appropriate angle for interrogation.

Surgical Considerations

When both ventricles and both AV valves are well developed, the goal of surgical repair is to utilize the VSD to baffle the LV to one of the great arteries. If baffled to the aorta, a "physiologic repair" is achieved. If baffled to the pulmonary artery, an arterial switch operation is required. In cases where the VSD is remote from the great arteries, septation might not be possible. In addition, presence of a straddling tricuspid valve over a canal type VSD or straddling mitral valve over a malalignment VSD may also preclude septation into two ventricles. In these cases, staged surgical palliation culminating in the Fontan operation is usually performed [38].

For those undergoing a biventricular repair, selection of the appropriate operation depends upon an assessment of great artery relationship in relation to the ventricles and VSD, whether outflow tract obstruction is present and if so, which outflow tract is obstructed and to what degree. Based upon these assessments, a determination can be made as to

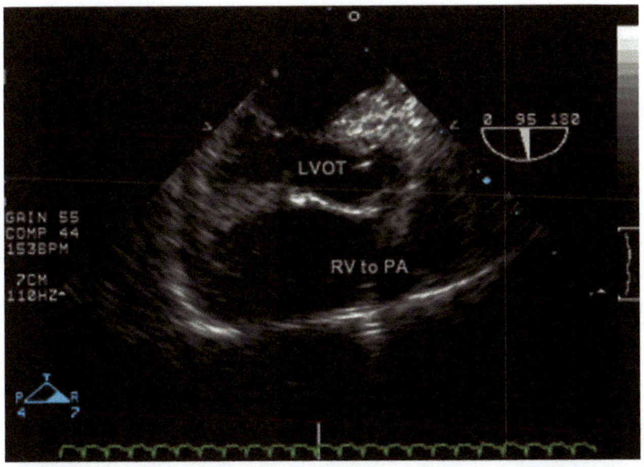

Fig. 12.21 Mid esophageal aortic valve long axis view in the patient from Figs. 12.16, 12.17, and 12.18 with double outlet right ventricle, posterior malalignment of the conal septum with subpulmonary ventricular septal defect after the Nikaidoh procedure (aortic translocation). The translocation of the aorta has placed the aortic valve closer to the left ventricle, improving left ventricle to aortic valve alignment and reducing the possibility of subaortic obstruction once the ventricular septal defect has been closed by a patch. This image demonstrates the "physiologic" repair achieved by baffling the ventricular septal defect to the aorta in its new position and the right ventricle to pulmonary artery conduit. *LVOT* left ventricular outflow tract, *PA* pulmonary artery, *RV* right ventricle

the most suitable operation to effect a complete biventricular repair. The most common operations include:

- Patch closure of VSD (baffle to the aorta).
- Rastelli type procedure: Baffle closure of VSD to aorta, with repair of obstructed RV outflow tract (outflow patch or RV to pulmonary artery conduit).
- Arterial switch operation with closure of VSD to neo-aorta.
- Nikaidoh operation with translocation of the aorta into the pulmonary position over the LV, VSD closure and placement of an RV to pulmonary artery conduit [39, 40]. This operation is designed to bring the aorta and aortic valve closer to the LV, thus reducing the risk of postoperative LV outflow tract obstruction (Fig. 12.21, Video 12.17).

Postoperative assessment is dependent upon the surgical intervention. In those patients with a subaortic VSD, the two most important issues for intraoperative TEE are assessment for a residual VSD and determination of possible LV outflow tract obstruction from the baffle to the aorta. Subaortic conus as well as VSD patch position may result in significant subaortic obstruction. The best view to assess the LV outflow tract is variable, depending on the relationship of the aorta to the LV. Though the ME AV LAX view with a multiplane angle of 120° is best for a normal LV outflow tract, this may not be the case in DORV, thus trying different TEE views, probe rotations, and multiplane angles, will often be required to obtain the best image. Doppler interrogation of the outflow tracts can also be challenging. A variety of different TEE views will often be necessary to obtain the optimal Doppler angle of interrogation; these usually include a combination of mid esophageal, transgastric, and (when available) deep transgastric views. Severity of obstruction may also have to be determined by other methods such as smallest diameter. In some cases, direct pressure measurements in the LV and the aorta might be required.

Assessment for residual ventricular communications is very important in patients undergoing repair of DORV. Intramural type defects can occur in this lesion as well (See section "Tetralogy of Fallot"). In patients with Taussig-Bing anatomy that undergo the arterial switch operation, intraoperative TEE assesses adequacy of the neo-aortic and neo-pulmonic anastomoses (see section "Transposition of the Great Arteries") as well as the adequacy of the repair of associated defects.

Truncus Arteriosus

Anatomy

Truncus arteriosus communis, also known more simply as truncus arteriosus (TA) or common arterial trunk, is characterized by the following anatomic features: a solitary great vessel arises from the heart, giving rise to the aorta, at least one pulmonary artery, and at least one coronary artery. Almost always, there is a large VSD in which the septal band (septomarginal trabeculation) forms the "floor" of the VSD, and the truncal root overrides the crest of the ventricular septum so that the solitary truncal valve forms the "roof" of the VSD [41]. The morphology of the VSD in TA is virtually identical in to that of TOF [42], however in TA the infundibular septum is absent. TA must be distinguished from TOF/PA. In TOF/PA a remnant of the main pulmonary artery and valve can often be seen. In the most extreme form of TOF/PA, the pulmonary circulation may be supplied directly from the aorta. Thus, the distinction between TOF/PA and TA is sometimes difficult. In TA, the solitary semilunar valve, the truncal valve, is often morphologically abnormal. Though a tricuspid truncal valve is the most common anatomic subtype (69 %), other variations can occur including (in order of frequency), quadricuspid (22 %), bicuspid (9 %), and rarely valves with five leaflets (0.3 %) [43]. Because of these frequent abnormalities in valvar anatomy, truncal valve stenosis and/or regurgitation are common, and if clinically significant, they may need to be addressed surgically. Approximately 25 % of patients with TA have a right aortic arch. Other associated cardiac anomalies include aberrant origin of a subclavian artery from the descending aorta, persistent left superior vena cava to coronary sinus connection, coronary anomalies, and an atrial communication in the

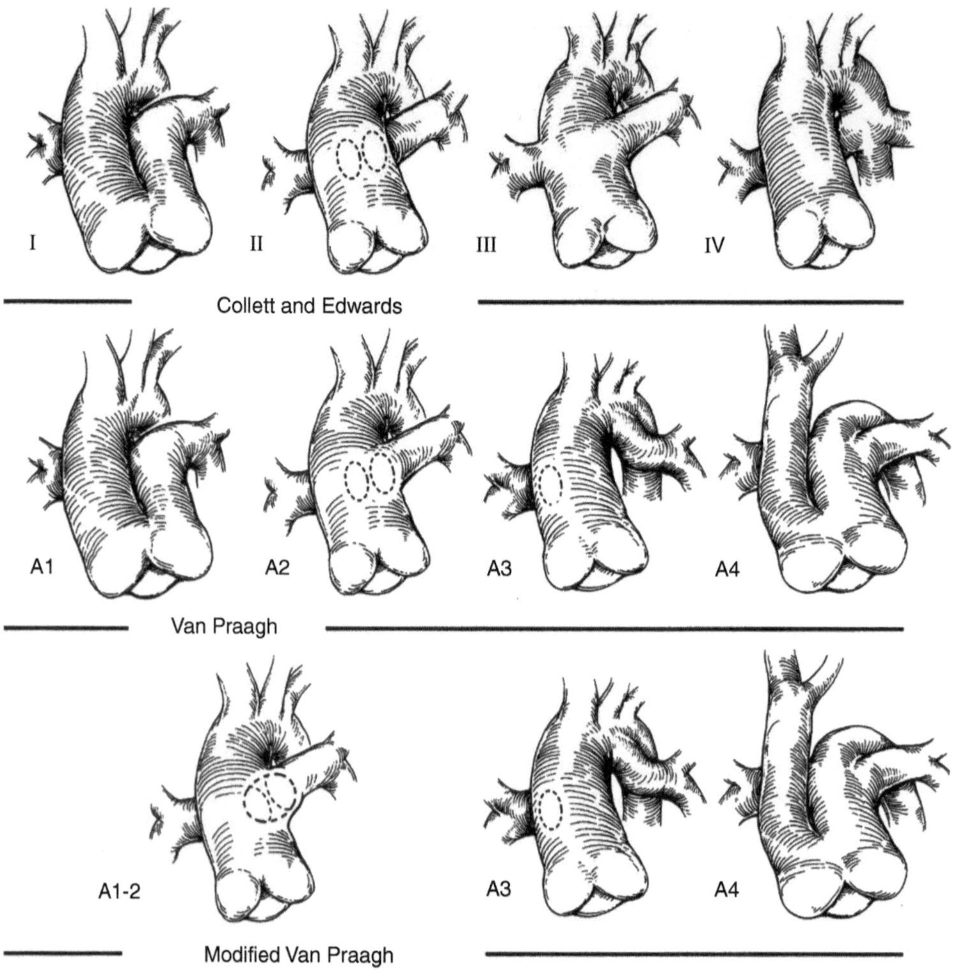

Fig. 12.22 The two common classification systems for truncus arteriosus: Collett and Edwards (*first row*) and Van Praagh (*second row*). A modified Van Praagh classification system is shown on the *third row*. See text for details (Reprinted from: Jacobs [46] with permission from Elsevier)

form of a patent foramen ovale or secundum atrial septal defect. There have been rare reports of TA with single ventricle. In the absence of aortic arch obstruction a ductus is rarely seen in this lesion.

Two classification schemes have been proposed for this malformation: one described by Collett and Edwards [44], the other by Van Praagh [42, 45]. Both are based principally upon the manner in which the pulmonary arteries arise. The classifications share similarities although there are also some important differences (Fig. 12.22).

The Collett and Edwards classification is listed as follows:

Type 1: There is partial absence of the aorto-pulmonary artery septum, and a short main pulmonary artery segment (of variable length) that arises from the common trunk and gives rise to the branch pulmonary arteries. This is the most common type, comprising 48–68 % of all TA [43].

Type 2: There is total absence of the aorto-pulmonary septum and the pulmonary arteries arise directly from the posterior aspect of the common trunk. This type comprises 29–48 % of all TA [43].

Type 3: The branch pulmonary arteries arise separately from the common trunk and are remote from each other. This type comprises 6–10 % of all TA [43].

Type 4: The pulmonary circulation derives from the collateral arteries arising from the descending aorta. This type is now considered a form of TOF/PA with aortopulmonary collaterals, and is not generally used as a classification for TA.

The Van Praagh classification is listed below:

Type A1: There is partial absence of the aorto-pulmonary artery septum: there is a main pulmonary artery segment (of variable length) that arises from the common trunk and gives rise to the branch pulmonary arteries.

Type A2: There is total absence of the aorto-pulmonary septum and the pulmonary arteries arise directly from the posterior aspect of the common trunk.

Type A3: One of the pulmonary arteries arises directly from the common trunk and one arises directly from a collateral supply (usually the ductus arteriosus). This is also known as truncus with absent pulmonary artery.

Type A4: Truncus arteriosus in association with interruption of the aortic arch. The common trunk gives rise to the ascending aorta and a main pulmonary artery, from which the ductus arteriosus and the branch pulmonary arteries arise. The transverse arch is absent, thus there is an interrupted aortic arch. The ductus arteriosus provides blood to the descending aorta, thus this type of TA is a ductal-dependent lesion. The interruption is usually type B (between the left carotid and the left subclavian arteries). This type occurs in 13 % of cases.

Of note, the original Van Praagh classification provided a subclassification of each type: **A** (with a VSD) and **B** (no VSD). Thus a Type 1 TA could be divided into Type A1 and Type B1, depending upon the presence/absence of a VSD [42]. However given the fact that a VSD is almost always present, the Type B subclassifications are rarely seen. The reader will also note that the first two types of TA for both classification schemes are essentially identical; these are by far the common types of TA encountered. Another important point is that many TA patients are classified as "Type 1" when, in reality, the two pulmonary artery orifices are located so close together that no main pulmonary artery segment is present. This type is often referred to as "truncus arteriosus Type 1–2" or "Type 1½" (Fig. 12.22) [46].

Genetic syndromes are quite common in association with TA. In fact, 40 % of patients have 22q11 deletion syndrome; this association is particularly high in those with a right aortic arch [47]. Other chromosomal defects such as isochromosome 8q have been implicated as well [48].

TEE Evaluation

The pertinent aspects of cardiac anatomy and function that should be evaluated in a patient with TA includes the following:

- Assessment of the VSD and evaluation for potential additional VSDs.
- Evaluation of truncal valve anatomy and function.
- Determination of the origin of both pulmonary arteries from the common trunk as well as their anatomy.
- Evaluation of AV valve function.
- Evaluation of ventricular systolic function.
- Comparison of ascending aorta to main pulmonary artery size. In Type 1 TA (Type A1 of Van Praagh), the ascending aorta is generally much larger than the main pulmonary artery segment. However in TA patients with an interrupted aortic arch (Type A4 of Van Praagh), the ascending aortic diameter will usually be smaller than that of the main pulmonary artery [42, 45, 49].
- Assessment of other possible cardiac abnormalities, including atrial septal defects, systemic/pulmonary venous anomalies, and possible coronary artery anomalies.

TEE can be very helpful in the pre-operative evaluation of the patient with TA. A careful TEE study can be used to evaluate all of the elements listed above. The ME 4 Ch view provides for evaluation of AV valve function and global assessment of ventricular performance. Withdrawal of the probe with anteflexion will demonstrate the truncal valve. Forward rotation of the multiplane angle to 30–45° will often reveal the truncal valve anatomy *en face* (Fig. 12.23, Video 12.18). Similar to all conotruncal defects, complementary TEE views (modified ME 4 Ch, ME Bicaval, LE Situs SAX and LE IVC LAX) establish the systemic venous connections and confirm the presence of an atrial communication, if present. The VSD can be visualized in orthogonal planes in the ME 4 Ch view (using probe anteflexion) or the ME AV LAX view (Fig. 12.24, Video 12.19). In Type 1 or 2 TA, the mid ME Asc Ao SAX and mid esophageal ascending aortic long axis (ME Asc Ao LAX) views, will often demonstrate the pulmonary arteries originating from the posterior aspect of the trunk (Fig. 12.24, Video 12.19). It can be difficult to see the entire length of the branch pulmonary arteries by TEE, but significant portions can be visualized using the aforementioned TEE views as well as the upper esophageal views (UE PA LAX, UE Ao Arch SAX).

It is important to consider that TEE probe placement can be difficult in small infants with TA especially when there is associated 22q11 deletion syndrome (Chap. 3).

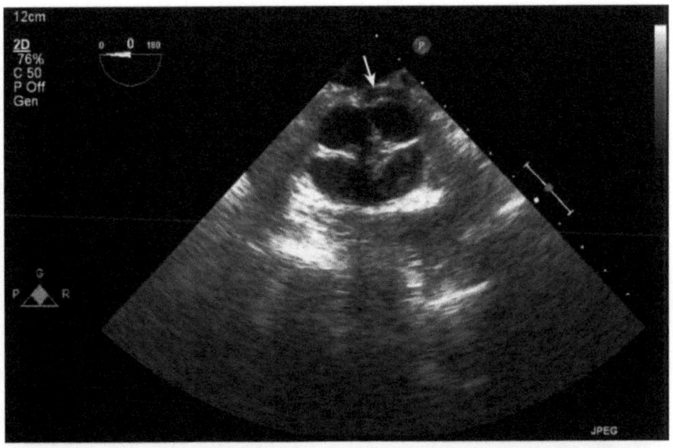

Fig. 12.23 Truncal valve seen *en face* from a modified mid esophageal aortic valve short axis view. This shows a quadricuspid truncal valve with thickened edges and a central area of noncoaptation. Note the left main coronary artery arising from the rightward, posterior cusp (*arrow*)

Surgical Considerations

Surgery for TA is usually performed in the neonatal period because most patients become symptomatic with congestive symptoms and pulmonary vascular obstructive disease can develop early. The type of surgical approach is dictated by the truncal anatomy. For the common forms of TA (Types 1 and 2) surgical repair consists of closure of the VSD to the truncal valve, establishing continuity between the LV and truncal valve, removal of the pulmonary arteries from the common trunk, and in most cases, placement of a conduit between the RV and the pulmonary arteries. In TA Type A4

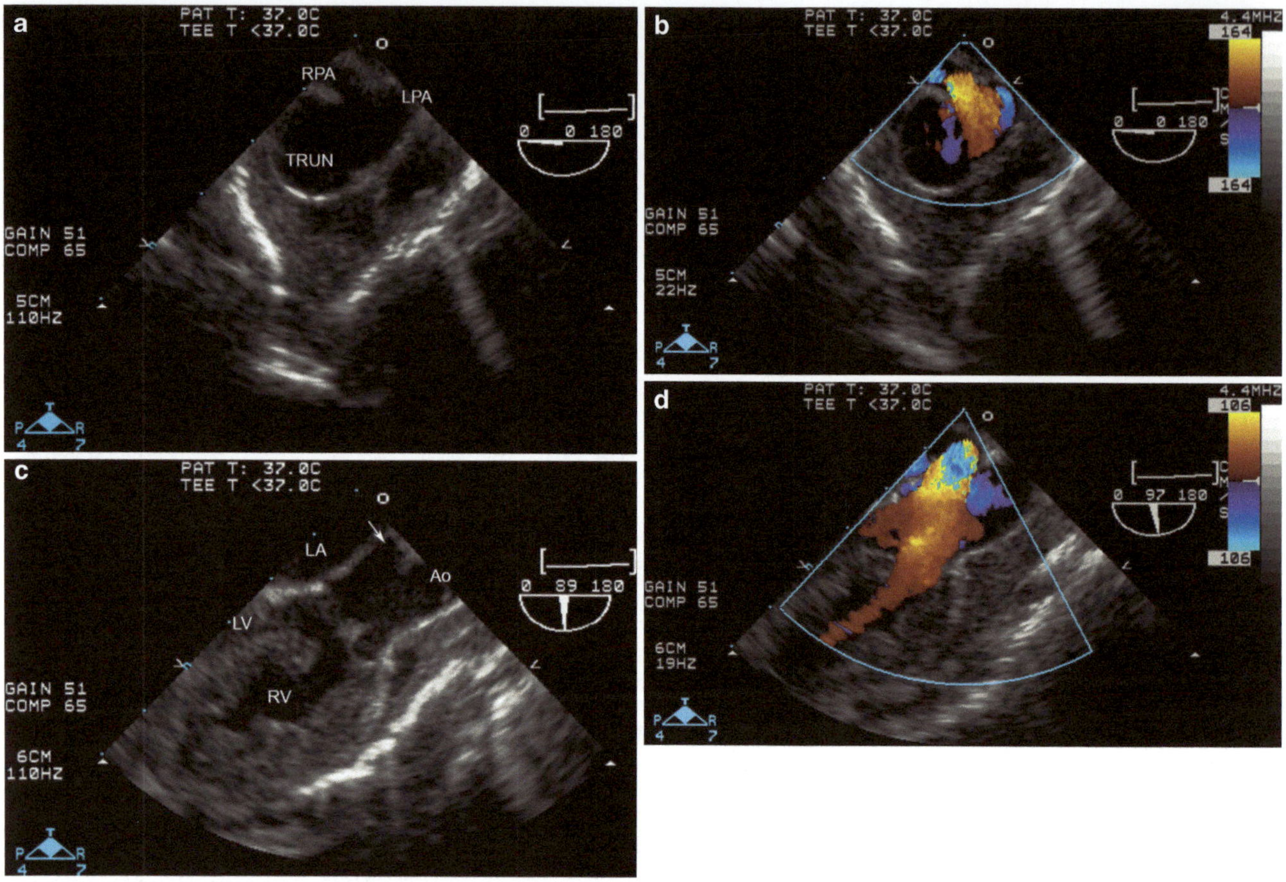

Fig. 12.24 Truncus arteriosus Type "1½" as seen from the mid esophageal ascending aortic short axis (**a**, **b**) and mid esophageal aortic valve long axis (**c**, **d**) views. From the short axis view, the right pulmonary artery (*RPA*) and left pulmonary artery (*LPA*) origins are seen immediately adjacent to each other, arising from the posterior aspect of the trunk (*TRUN*). From the long axis view this posterior origin of the pulmonary arteries is also seen (*arrow*), and the truncal valve shown to override the ventricular septal defect. *Ao* ascending aorta, *LA* left atrium, *LV* left ventricle, *RV* right ventricle

(of Van Praagh), the interrupted arch is addressed in addition to VSD closure and RV to pulmonary artery conduit, as noted above. For all TA repairs, if the truncal valve manifests significant stenosis and/or regurgitation, surgical intervention might be necessary.

Postoperative TEE helps determine adequacy of the repair. The goals of this imaging are to assure that there is unobstructed flow from the LV to the truncal root, no significant residual VSD and unobstructed flow from the RV to the branch pulmonary arteries. Evaluation of the interatrial septum should be undertaken for residual shunting. It should be noted that in some cases, an intentional small interatrial communication remains, allowing for potential right to left shunting and the maintenance of cardiac output during the immediate postoperative period. In addition, the postbypass examination is of benefit in the evaluation of truncal valve function (estimation of residual severity of obstruction and/or regurgitation) in cases where concomitant valve interventions were performed.

The ME 4 Ch view sweeping from inferior to superior demonstrates that the VSD patch is in the correct position and color flow Doppler can be used to determine whether there is residual shunting (Fig. 12.25, Video 12.20). The intramural type VSD previously described can also occur with TA repair [23]. Assessment for a residual VSD should always occur in more than one view. The ME RV In-Out view is quite useful to demonstrate a peri-patch residual leak. In addition, the RV to pulmonary artery pathway is best seen in this view with a counterclockwise turn of the probe toward the left side of the patient. Doppler interrogation of this pathway can also be performed to assess for outflow tract obstruction. The LV to truncal valve pathway can be seen well in the ME AV LAX view along with assessment of truncal stenosis and regurgitation (Fig. 12.26, Video 12.21) [50]. When available, the deep transgastric views (DTG LAX, DTG Sagittal) can provide visualization of the LV outflow tract and proximal RV to pulmonary artery conduit, as well as excellent angles of insonation for spectral

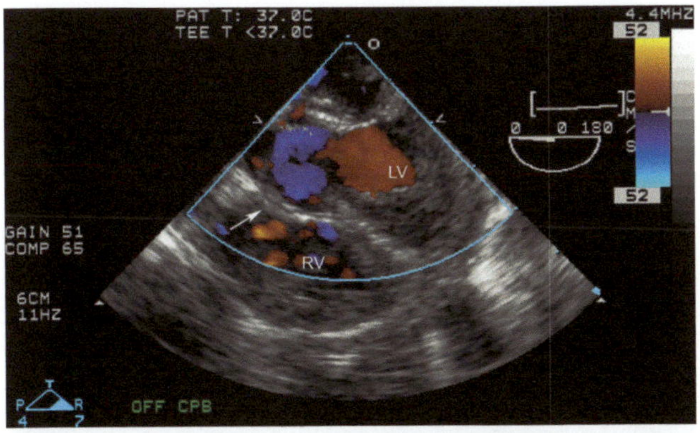

Fig. 12.25 Postop truncus arteriosus repair, seen from mid esophageal four chamber view with probe anteflexion. The ventricular septal defect patch is shown by the *arrow*; no residual defect is present by color flow imaging. *LV* left ventricle, *RV* right ventricle,

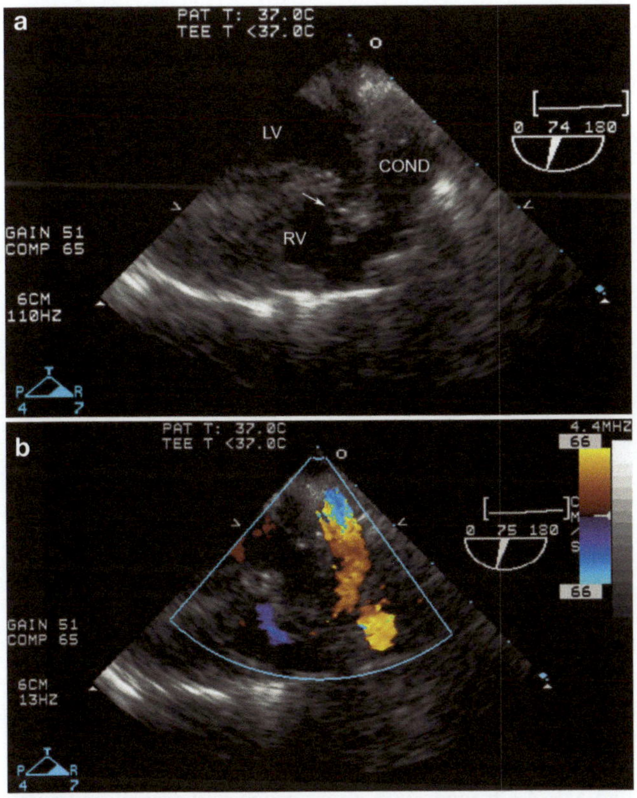

Fig. 12.26 Postop truncus arteriosus repair, seen from a modified mid esophageal aortic valve long axis view, multiplane angle about 75°, with imaging (**a**) and color flow Doppler (**b**). The ventricular septal defect patch (*arrow*) is seen as well as the origin of the conduit (*COND*) from the right ventricle (*RV*) to the pulmonary artery. *LV* left ventricle

Doppler assessment. The ME 4 Ch and ME Bicaval views can be used to assess the atrial septum, and the ME 4 Ch, ME RV In-Out, and ME 2 Ch views can facilitate the evaluation AV valve function.

Transposition of the Great Arteries

Anatomy

Transposition of the great arteries, also known as D-transposition of the great arteries, or complete or physiologically uncorrected transposition of the great arteries, is defined as an abnormal ventriculoarterial alignment whereby the aorta arises from the RV and the pulmonary artery from the LV. This results in ventriculoarterial *discordance*. However, there remains atrioventricular *concordance* (right atrium connected with RV, left atrium with LV). This anatomy produces a clinical picture of parallel circulations, in which deoxygenated systemic venous blood returns predominantly back to the aorta, and oxygenated pulmonary venous blood predominantly back to the pulmonary arteries. Thus these patients are usually cyanotic, sometimes profoundly so. Transposition of the great arteries is generally seen in combination with visceroatrial situs solitus and a D-ventricular loop (the 'normal' ventricular loop for situs solitus), hence the widely used abbreviation D-TGA, which will also be used for the remainder of this chapter. In its most common form, subaortic conus is present with absence of subpulmonary conus; thus there is mitral valve to pulmonary valve fibrous continuity. However, the conal anatomy may vary: in a series of 117 patients with D-TGA and VSD, subaortic conus was present in almost 90 % of patients, while bilateral conus, subpulmonary conus only and bilaterally deficient conus (extremely rare) were present in the remaining 10 % of patients [51]. In most patients with D-TGA, the aorta is spatially oriented anterior and rightward to the pulmonary artery [52]. In some cases the great vessels are side by side. In more unusual cases, the aorta is leftward or posterior to the pulmonary artery. Also, this entity occurs rarely in the setting of visceroatrial situs inversus [53]. For the purposes of this chapter, we will address the most common anatomic manifestation of D-TGA. Those familiar with the nomenclature of Van Praagh will recognize this as transposition of the great arteries with cardiac segments {S,D,D}: situs solitus of the atria, D-ventricular loop and D-position of the great arteries (with an anterior and rightward aorta) [54].

D-TGA occurs in three principal anatomic manifestations: (a) with an intact ventricular septum; (b) with a VSD; (c) with a VSD and LV outflow tract obstruction. D-TGA with an intact ventricular septum and no other cardiac abnormalities (other than a patent foramen ovale or patent ductus arteriosus) is the most frequent anatomic manifestation of D-TGA, occurring in approximately 50 % of all patients. Of the remaining 50 %, the most commonly associated cardiac defect is a VSD, occurring in 40–45 % of all patients. Any type of VSD is possible in D-TGA; the most common type is the perimembranous/conoventricular defect (33 %), but other types are possible including muscular (27 %), malalignment (30 %), AV canal (5 %), and conal septal hypoplasia (5 %) [55]. When there is malalignment of the conal septum in D-TGA, two anatomic subtypes are seen: (1) anterior malalignment results in subaortic narrowing in association with distal arch obstruction, (2) posterior malalignment results in LV outflow tract obstruction consisting of subpulmonic obstruction and often, valvar pulmonary stenosis. The combination of VSD and LV outflow tract obstruction is seen in about 10–12 % of D-TGA patients; isolated LV outflow tract obstruction (without a VSD) occurs in only about 5 % of all patients [55, 56].

Coronary anatomy in D-TGA is variable. The so called "usual" coronary anatomy occurs in approximately two thirds of cases: the right coronary artery (RCA) arises from the right-sided sinus of Valsalva and the left main coronary artery (LCA) (anterior descending coronary and circumflex artery) arises from the left-sided sinus of Valsalva. In approximately 20 % of cases, the circumflex artery comes off the RCA and courses posterior to the pulmonary artery. Rarer anatomical subtypes include single RCA, single LCA, or inverted coronaries. In some patients, a portion of the coronary artery may take an intramural course in the wall of the aorta. This anatomy may complicate surgical repair [57].

Other cardiac anomalies that can be seen with D-TGA include aortic arch abnormalities such as coarctation (seen in about 5 % of all patients), as well as tricuspid and mitral valve abnormalities which have been reported in 20–30 % of autopsy series, though most of these AV abnormalities are functionally insignificant [55]. However AV abnormalities must be evaluated carefully, particularly when a VSD is present: overriding or straddling AV valve tissue can present problems from a cardiac surgery standpoint. Left juxtaposition of the atrial appendages (discussed above) occurs in about 2–5 % of D-TGA patients; when present, it often heralds more significant pathology such as dextrocardia, RV hypoplasia, and tricuspid valve stenosis or atresia [56].

Genetic causes of D-TGA are poorly defined and likely multifactorial. Environmental factors such as maternal diabetes or fetal exposure to retinoic acids have been implicated. In contrast to other conotruncal defects, isolated D-TGA is not usually linked to genetic syndromes such as 22q11.2 deletion syndrome [58].

TEE Evaluation

There are pertinent associated cardiac lesions seen with D-TGA that need to be kept in mind when performing a TEE:

- Size, location, and shunting pattern across the atrial communication
- Size and location of VSD(s), if present, and shunting pattern across the defect(s). It is important to remember that, in D-TGA/VSD and no pulmonary outflow obstruction, VSD shunting pattern is generally from the RV to LV, which is the reverse of that expected with a VSD and normally related (nontransposed) great arteries.
- Anatomy and size of AV valves.
- Presence and severity of outflow tract obstruction.
- Semilunar valve anatomy.
- Coronary anomalies, particularly if the arterial switch operation is being considered.

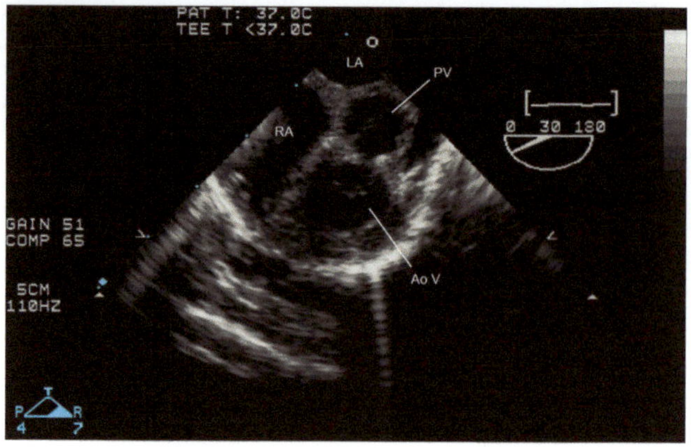

Fig. 12.27 D-transposition of the great arteries. Using a mid esophageal aortic valve short axis view, both semilunar valves are seen *en face*, with the aortic valve (*AoV*) anterior and rightward to the pulmonary valve (*PV*). *LA* left atrium, *RA* right atrium

In D-TGA with an intact ventricular septum, a pre-operative TEE is rarely needed for diagnostic assessment. However, it can still be very useful for confirmation of the pre-operative findings, for the assessment of AV and semilunar valve function, for evaluation of ventricular performance prior to surgical intervention, and as a reference for comparison with the post-operative examination. The ME 4 Ch sweep provides a good global view of these aspects of D-TGA evaluation. In some cases, the coronary anatomy can be well-delineated by TEE. The ME AV SAX view with multiplane angle 30–45° can be used to determine semilunar valve anatomy (Fig. 12.27, Video 12.22). Because both great vessels are parallel, rather than the normal criss-cross orientation, both semilunar valves can generally be seen in the same plane. The coronary artery origins can sometimes be seen from this view (Fig. 12.28, Video 12.23). Using a modified ME 4 Ch view with slight probe withdrawal and anteflexion, the outflow tracts, semilunar valves and great arteries can be shown (Fig. 12.29, Video 12.24); these structures can also be displayed in an orthogonal manner using the ME RV In-Out, ME 2 Ch, ME LAX, and ME AV LAX views (Fig. 12.30, Video 12.25). A very abnormal pulmonary valve and/or narrowed pulmonary outflow tract may preclude the ability to perform an arterial switch procedure (Fig. 12.31, Video 12.26). In such cases, a Rastelli procedure (discussed below) might be necessary; the pre-operative TEE can be used to help determine the pathway from the LV to the aorta and to find the best view to evaluate this after surgery.

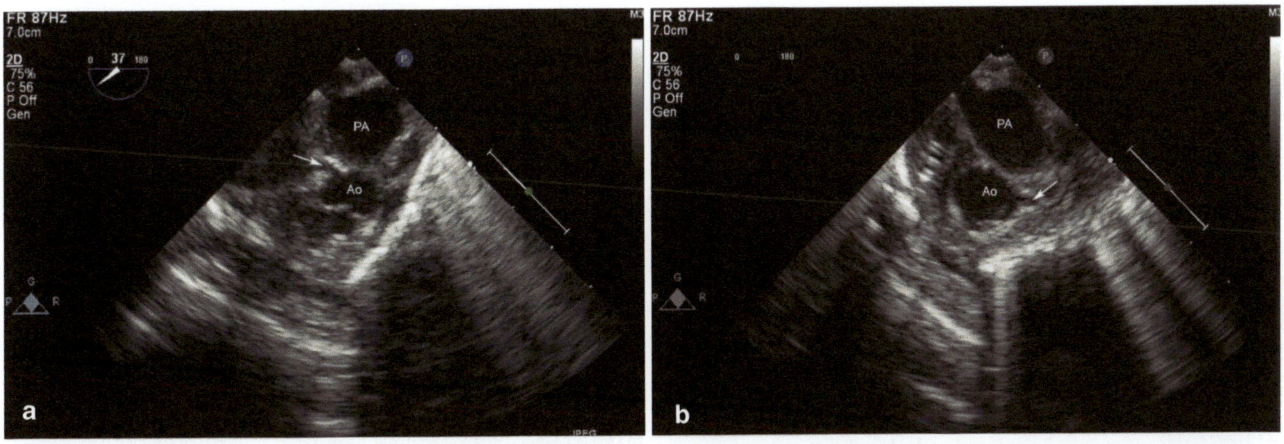

Fig. 12.28 Origins of the right (**a**) and left (**b**) coronary arteries (*arrows*) from the opposite aortic valve sinuses facing the pulmonary artery in transposition of the great arteries, as seen from the mid esophageal aortic valve short axis view. This coronary pattern is the most common type seen in this cardiac defect. *Ao* aorta, *PA* pulmonary artery

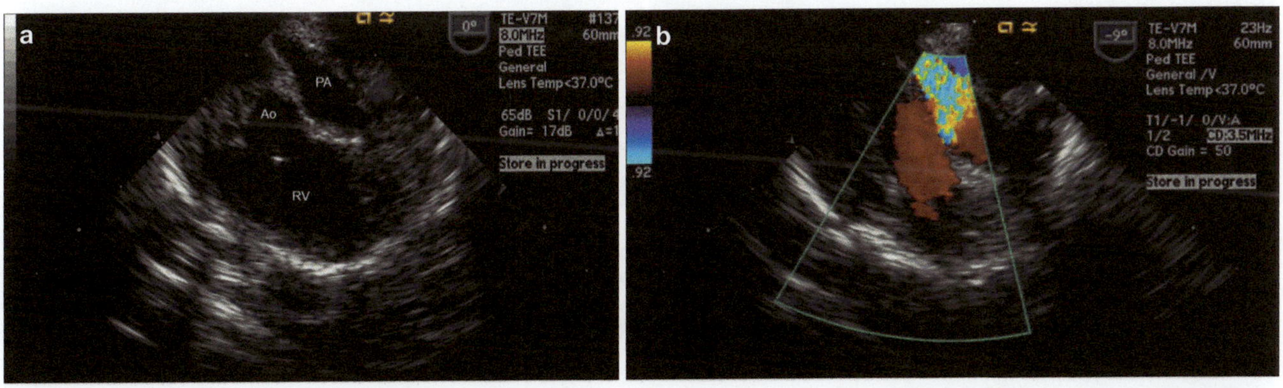

Fig. 12.29 Transposition of the great arteries, as viewed from a mid esophageal view. With anteflexion and slight probe withdrawal from the mid esophageal four chamber view, both great arteries are seen in parallel, with the aorta (*Ao*) arising from the right ventricle (*RV*), and the pulmonary artery (*PA*) from the left ventricle (**a**). Color flow Doppler shows continuous flow in the PA from ductal shunting (**b**)

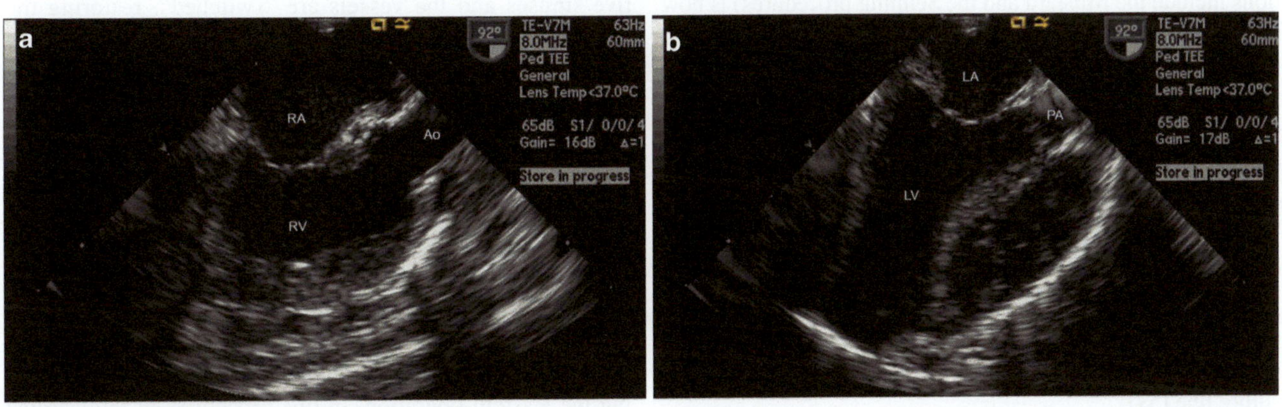

Fig. 12.30 Transposition of the great arteries, as viewed from a mid esophageal right ventricular inflow-outflow/long axis view, multiplane angle about 90°. The aorta arises from the right ventricle (**a**), and the pulmonary artery from the left ventricle. (**b**) Both great arteries have the same alignment, and therefore take a parallel course. *Ao* aorta, *LA* left atrium, *LV* left ventricle, *PA* pulmonary artery, *RA* right atrium, *RV* right ventricle

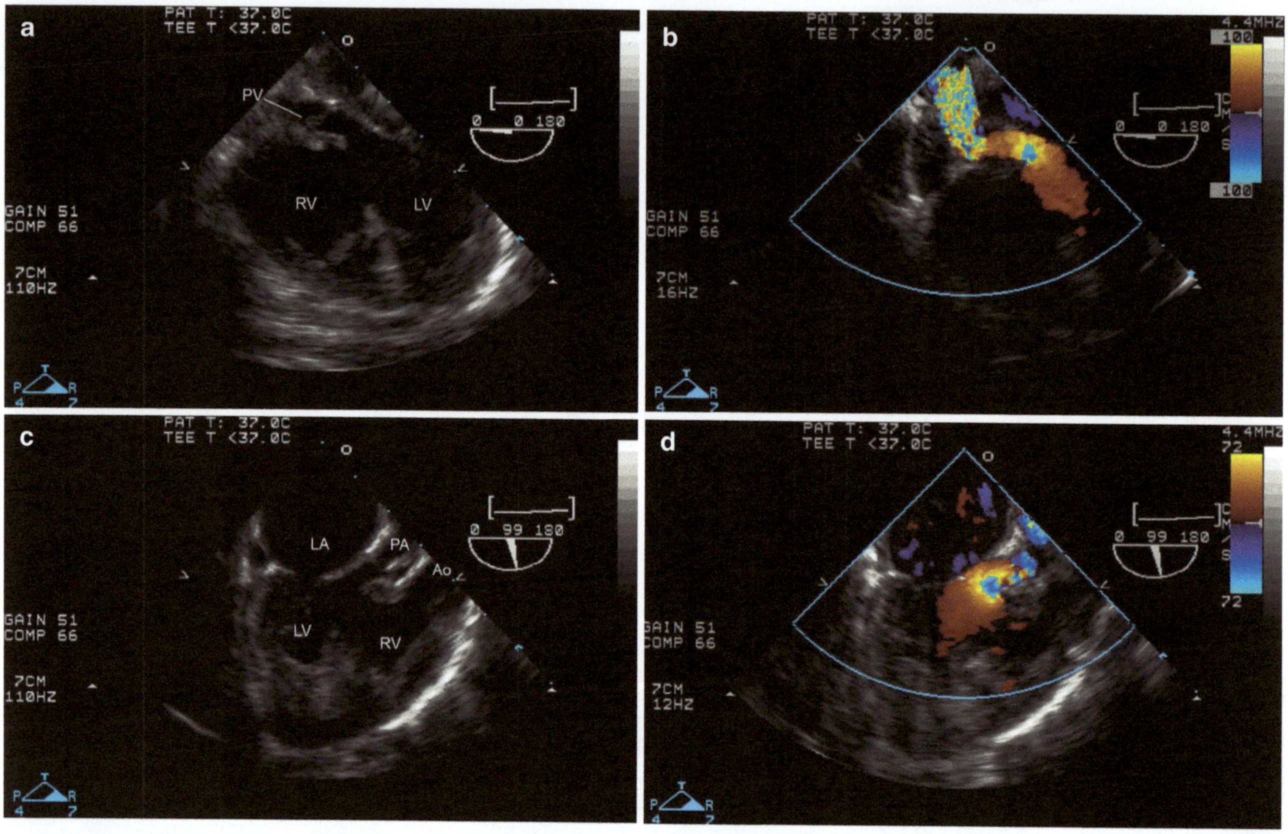

Fig. 12.31 D-transposition of the great arteries, with a large ventricular septal defect and pulmonary outflow obstruction, as seen from a modified mid esophageal four chamber view (**a**, **b**) and mid esophageal long axis view (**c**, **d**). Posteriorly malaligned infundibular septum produces prominent subpulmonary narrowing, and turbulence is seen by color flow Doppler across the pulmonary outflow tract. *Ao* aorta, *LA* left atrium, *LV* left ventricle, *PA* pulmonary artery, *PV* pulmonary valve, *RV* right ventricle

Surgical Considerations

Surgical intervention for D-TGA has progressed from the atrial switch operation to the arterial switch operation over the course of the last 25 years. The atrial switch procedure (variations include the Mustard and the Senning procedures) is now performed in very rare circumstances (late presentation, significantly abnormal pulmonary valve, isolated ventricular inversion, and in those with congenitally corrected TGA, see below). In this procedure, superior and inferior vena caval venous return are baffled directly to the mitral valve, while the pulmonary venous blood is channeled into the tricuspid valve. This procedure has been abandoned as the favored surgical option for D-TGA because of many long-term complications including: RV failure (the RV must act as the systemic ventricle), tricuspid regurgitation, as well as sinus node dysfunction and significant atrial arrhythmias from the extensive atrial suture line [59].

The arterial switch operation is now the preferred corrective surgical repair in those patients with isolated D-TGA or in those with a VSD but without significant narrowing of the pulmonary outflow tract. It is also the suitable surgical intervention for patients with the Taussig-Bing-type of DORV where there is a subpulmonary VSD (see section "Double Outlet Right Ventricle"). In this procedure, both great arteries are transected above their respective sinuses and the vessels are "switched", restoring the normal ventricular-arterial connection. The pulmonary artery is brought in front of the aorta by means of the "Lecompte maneuver" (both the right and left pulmonary artery lie anterior to the aorta) and the coronary arteries are translocated to the neo-aorta [60]. Associated defects are addressed at the time of surgery, included intracardiac communications, if present [61].

In cases of D-TGA with posterior malalignment VSD and LV outflow tract stenosis (subpulmonary/pulmonary valve stenosis), an arterial switch operation is not feasible. For these cases, other surgical options may be considered including the Rastelli operation. In this procedure an intracardiac tunnel is created to allow ejection of left ventricular blood through the VSD into the rightward aorta, while at the same time eliminating ventricular level shunting, and a conduit is placed from the RV to the pulmonary artery [61].

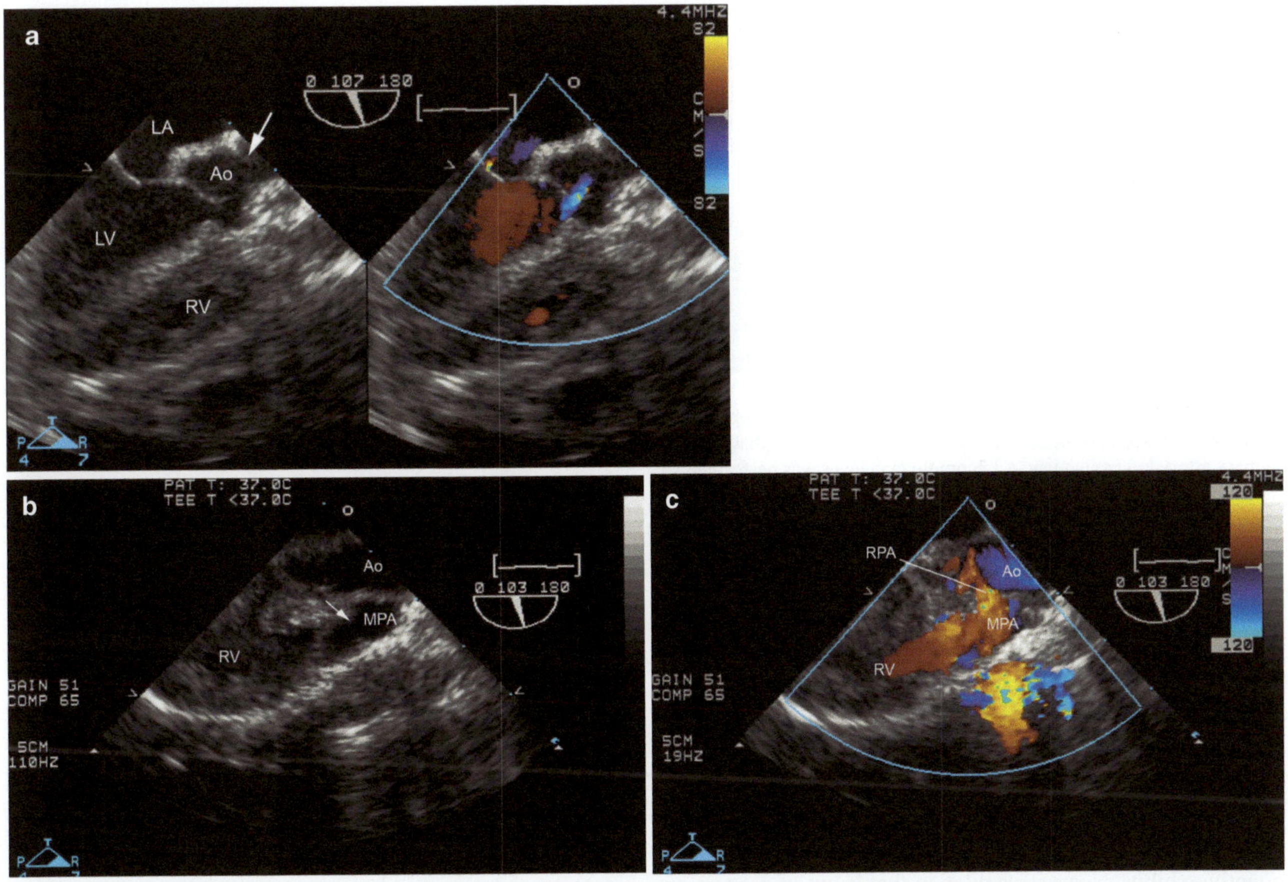

Fig. 12.32 Postoperative study following arterial switch operation. (**a**) From the mid esophageal long axis view, the figure shows the neo-aortic valve with a small amount of regurgitation. The aortic anastomosis is shown by the *arrow*. (**b**) From the mid esophageal ascending aorta long axis view, the figure shows the pulmonary artery anastomosis (*arrow*); the branch pulmonary arteries arise just above (superior to) the anastomosis. In (**c**) the right pulmonary artery is seen. *Ao* aorta, *LA* left atrium, *LV* left ventricle, *MPA* main pulmonary artery, *RPA* right pulmonary artery, *RV* right ventricle

TEE Evaluation Following Cardiac Surgery

Arterial Switch Operation

Postoperative TEE for the arterial switch operation has several goals including: (1) assuring patent right and left ventricular outflow tracts after transection and "switch" of the great arteries, (2) determination of regional and global systolic ventricular function after transfer of the coronary arteries, (3) assessment for residual intracardiac shunts (if present pre-operatively), (4) assessment of semilunar (particularly neo-aortic valve) competency. The ME 4 Ch view provides a good cross section for global assessment of ventricular performance. The TG Basal SAX and transgastric two chamber (TG 2 Ch) views provide excellent images to determine if there are regional wall motion abnormalities consistent with coronary obstruction during the transfer to the neo-aorta. The ME RV In-Out and ME AV LAX views demonstrate the right and left ventricular outflow tracts (Fig. 12.32, Video 12.27). The supravalvar regions are seen as the probe is withdrawn to the upper esophagus; this is important because the suture lines can cause obstruction or semilunar valve regurgitation might be present. Often the branch pulmonary arteries are difficult to image because they are the most anterior structures, however, withdrawal to the UE PA LAX view can visualize the branch pulmonary arteries anterior to, and straddling the ascending aorta (Fig. 12.33, Video 12.28).

Color Doppler can be used to assess for AV valve regurgitation, which can occur in the presence of ventricular dysfunction. Coronary ischemia can also result in papillary muscle dysfunction leading to mitral regurgitation. If tricuspid regurgitation is present, an RV systolic pressure estimate can be performed in the ME 4 Ch view to determine the pulmonary artery pressure (assuming that the branch pulmonary arteries are unobstructed). Pulsed and continuous wave Doppler are used to assess the severity of outflow tract obstruction, if this is present. The deep transgastric views (DTG LAX, DTG Sagittal), when available, are particularly helpful in this regard. Neo-aortic and neo-pulmonary valve function should be determined, because valve distortion can occur with the procedure. With the color flow at low-scale,

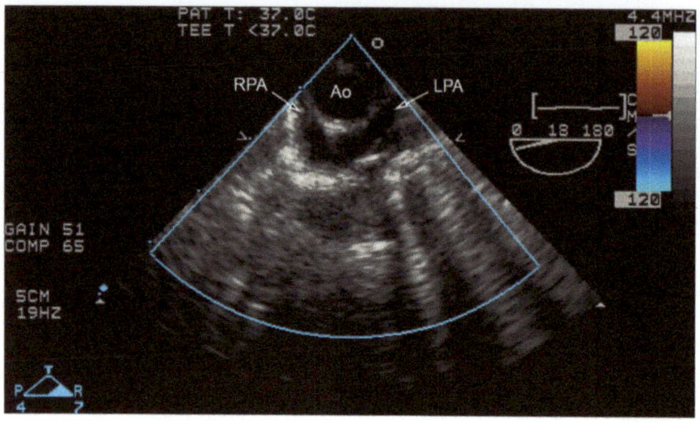

Fig. 12.33 Postoperative study following arterial switch operation, showing the branch pulmonary arteries from the upper esophageal pulmonary artery long axis view. A Lecompte maneuver was performed so the main and branch pulmonary arteries are situated anterior to the aorta (*Ao*). *LPA* left pulmonary artery, *RPA* right pulmonary artery

coronary blood flow in diastole can also be seen in some cases.

In the longer term, TEE provides information on potential sequelae of the arterial switch operation: supravalvar pulmonary stenosis, supravalvar aortic stenosis, dilation of the neoaortic root, and neoaortic regurgitation. At midterm follow-up, trivial to mild neoaortic regurgitation develops in the majority of patients. A smaller percentage of patients develop more significant regurgitation. Importantly, the neoaortic root frequently exhibits progressive dilation that is out of proportion to somatic growth [62]. The extent of this dilation into adulthood and the risk for dissection or rupture remain to be seen.

Rastelli Procedure

The postoperative TEE for the Rastelli procedure differs in its objectives from the arterial switch operation. Goals for this study include (1) surveillance for residual VSD, (2) assurance of an unobstructed pathway from the LV to the aorta, (3) assessment of the function of the RV to pulmonary artery conduit. Multiple sweeps are used to assess for a residual VSD. It is important to sweep from the most posterior aspect of the heart to the great vessels to assure that a residual VSD is not missed. This should be performed in the ME 4 Ch, ME RV In-Out, and ME AV SAX views. Intramural VSDs (discussed under TOF) can occur with this procedure as well. In the ME RV In-Out view, the conduit can be assessed in the most anterior region. Withdrawal of the probe to the ME Asc Ao LAX and UE Ao Arch SAX will demonstrate the most distal portion of the conduit as it is connected to the branch pulmonary arteries. Rotating the multiplane angle to 0–10°, using the ME AV SAX and UE PA LAX views, the right pulmonary artery is usually seen well. The left pulmonary artery can be difficult to visualize with TEE, but it can be seen in some patients using the UE PA LAX view and leftward probe rotation. The ME AV LAX view is an important view after a Rastelli procedure to assure that there is an unobstructed pathway from the LV to the aorta. If the angle of interrogation is appropriate, pulsed and continuous wave Doppler can also be performed in this view. The angle to image the pathway may need to be altered depending on the relationship of the aorta to the LV. As with the other outflow tract abnormalities mentioned above, DTG LAX and DTG Sagittal views can provide important additional information of the LV to aorta pathway, as well as excellent angles for spectral Doppler interrogation. Alternatively, the transgastric long axis (TG LAX) view, multiplane angle 90°-120°, is also excellent to evaluate this pathway and also allows for spectral Doppler evaluation. This view can be used in older patients and/or when the DTG views are not available (see Chap. 4 for a detailed description of the TG LAX view).

Long-term assessment of the Rastelli operation primarily involves evaluation of conduit patency and regurgitation. Almost all patients who undergo the Rastelli operation during infancy or childhood require reoperation for conduit failure later in life [63]. Subaortic obstruction can develop late after repair as well.

Atrial Switch Operation

Prior to the 1980s, surgical management for D-TGA was achieved using a procedure that rerouted the systemic venous return to the LV, and pulmonary venous return to the RV. These procedures were known as the atrial switch operation or atrial baffle procedure, and venous flow redirection was accomplished by the use of two principal surgical variations: the Mustard and Senning procedures [56, 61]. TEE is a very important tool to assess the long-term outcome after the atrial switch. Many regions of concern are difficult to visualize using TTE, particularly the venous baffles. Surveillance by TEE in these patients provides superior visualization, particularly in older patients with marginal TTE imaging [64]. In addition, TEE is frequently used in patients with atrial flutter or fibrillation prior to cardioversion to assure that there is no thrombus present. Other long-term complications after the atrial switch that can be diagnosed using TEE include: residual intracardiac shunts, baffle leaks, pulmonary or systemic venous pathway obstruction, tricuspid and/or mitral valve regurgitation, thrombi/vegetations on pacing leads, right and/or left ventricular outflow tract obstruction, and semilunar valve insufficiency [59]. Contrast injection into the venous circulation during the TEE can help discern baffle leaks. TEE guidance can be used for device closure of such leaks (Figs. 12.34 and 12.35, Videos 12.29 and 12.30). The TG Basal SAX will give an excellent view of overall ventricular performance. It is important to keep in mind that the ventricular septum will be shifted toward the LV because of the systemic RV pressure. The pulmonary venous baffle can best be viewed in ME 4 Ch view (Fig. 12.36, Video 12.31) and with the probe rotated counterclockwise to the left the entrance of

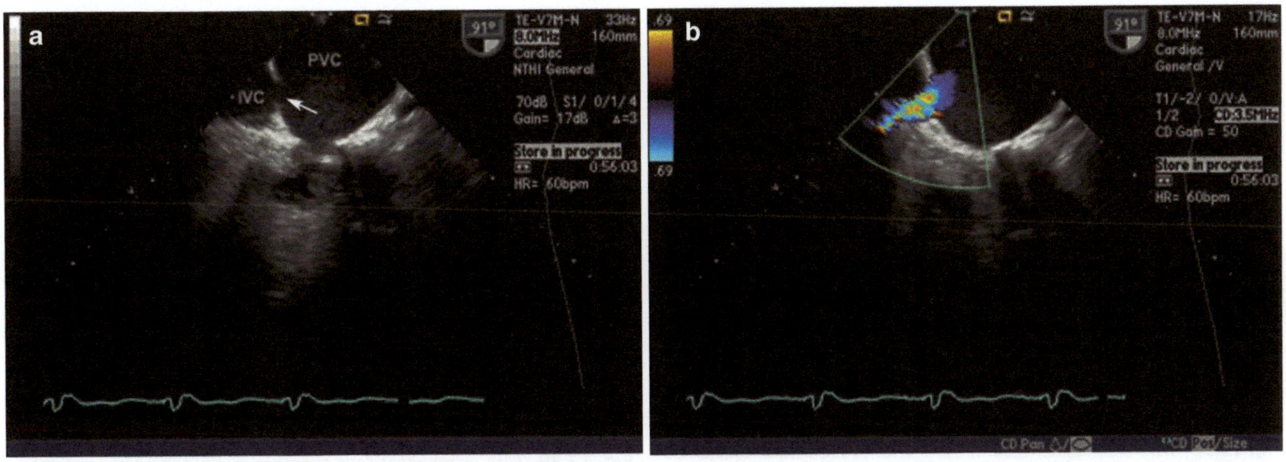

Fig. 12.34 Modified mid esophageal bicaval view with the probe advanced toward the liver in an adult who has undergone an atrial switch operation for D-transposition of the great arteries. (**a**) A communication (*baffle leak*) between the inferior vena cava (*IVC*) and pulmonary venous channel (*PVC*) is seen by two-dimensional imaging (*arrow*). (**b**) The color flow demonstrates flow from the pulmonary venous channel to the IVC (*left* to *right shunt*)

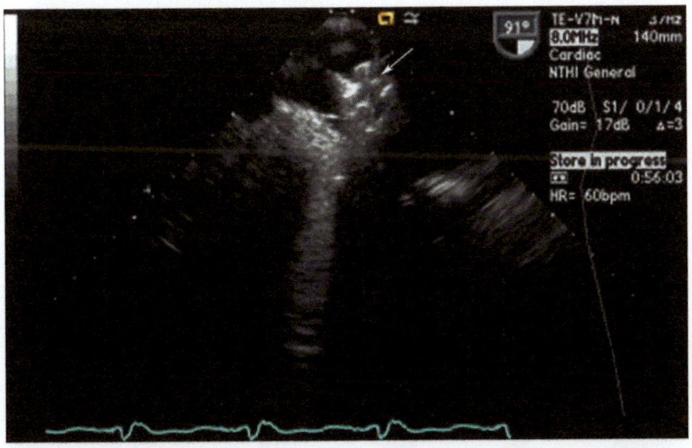

Fig. 12.35 Modified mid esophageal bicaval view with the probe advanced toward the liver in the same patient as Fig. 12.34 with the atrial switch and baffle leak. This image is obtained during transcatheter device deployment. The image demonstrates an Amplatzer device (*arrow*) just prior to its release

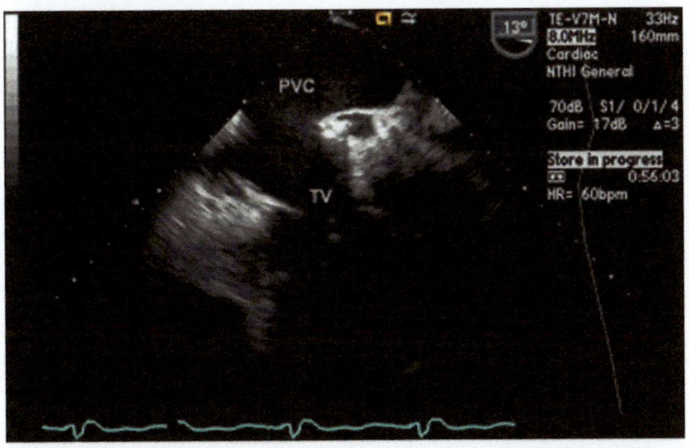

Fig. 12.36 Mid esophageal four chamber view of a patient after atrial switch operation demonstrating the pulmonary venous channel (*PVC*) as it makes its way to the tricuspid valve (*TV*). In this patient, the pathway is unobstructed

the left pulmonary veins can be seen. In the same plane, tilting the probe clockwise, toward the right, the entrance of the right pulmonary veins can be seen. The LE Situs SAX allows identification of the IVC within the liver. Withdrawal of the TEE probe shows the IVC entering into the inferior limb of the intra-atrial baffle and subsequent counterclockwise rotation connects the baffle to the mitral valve (ME 4 Ch view). Turning the multiplane angle to 90°, the superior limb of the systemic venous pathway is best seen in ME Bicaval view (Fig. 12.37, Video 12.32). With rotation of the probe toward the left, the baffle can be seen as it leads to the mitral valve. Obstruction is more common in the superior limb of the baffle because of the remnant of septum secundum along the pathway (Figs. 12.38 and 12.39, Video 12.33). Some patients have pacemaker wires in the superior limb that further contribute to narrowing along this venous pathway (Figs. 12.37, 12.38, and 12.39, Videos 12.32 and 12.33).

Congenitally Corrected Transposition of the Great Arteries

Anatomy

Congenitally corrected transposition of the great arteries (CCTGA), also known as physiologically corrected or L-transposition of the great arteries, is a cardiac defect in which there is both atrioventricular (AV) *and* ventriculoarterial discordance. The AV discordance results from ventricular inversion, in which the looping is the opposite of normal: in situs solitus, the RV ventricle assumes an L-loop (left hand) configuration, and in situs inversus, a D-loop (right hand). Thus, the right atrium empties into the morphologic LV, and the left atrium into the morphologic RV. In addition, the great arteries are transposed so that there is ventriculoarterial

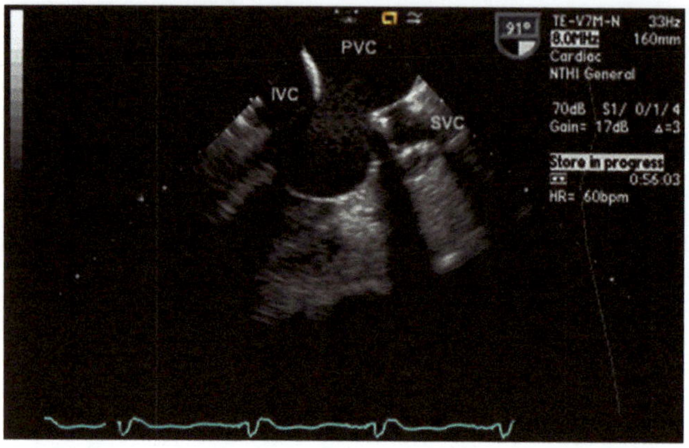

Fig. 12.37 Mid esophageal bicaval view with probe turned clockwise toward the patient's right side. This image is from a patient who has superior systemic venous limb obstruction after atrial switch operation. In this view, both inferior (*IVC*) and superior (*SVC*) limbs of the systemic venous channel are seen with the pulmonary venous channel (*PVC*) coursing in between. Pacing wires (echobright structures) are seen in the superior limb

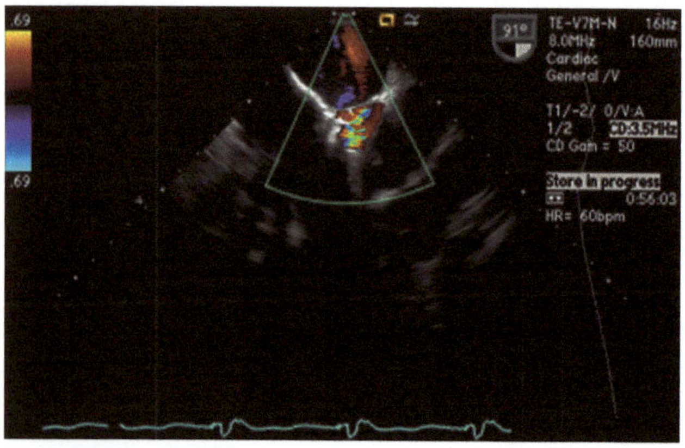

Fig. 12.38 Modified mid esophageal right ventricular inflow-outflow view using color Doppler in the same patient as Fig. 12.37 after atrial switch operation with superior limb obstruction. Aliasing of the color flow is seen in the superior limb of the channel

discordance: similar to D-TGA, the aorta arises from the morphologic RV, and pulmonary artery from the morphologic LV, and there is generally subaortic conus present with absence of subpulmonary conus, and mitral valve to pulmonary valve fibrous continuity. With situs solitus, great artery spatial positioning is such that the aorta is situated leftward and anterior to the pulmonary artery, and both great arteries are oriented parallel to each other (Fig. 12.40). Because of the "double discordance", CCTGA patients are physiologically corrected (systemic venous blood flows to the pulmonary artery, pulmonary venous blood to the aorta) and generally have normal systemic arterial oxygen saturation, unlike D-TGA. Most cases of CCTGA are seen with situs solitus, although CCTGA can definitely be seen with situs inversus. For the purposes of this chapter, we will address only the more common form of CCTGA with visceroatrial situs solitus. Again, those familiar with the nomenclature of

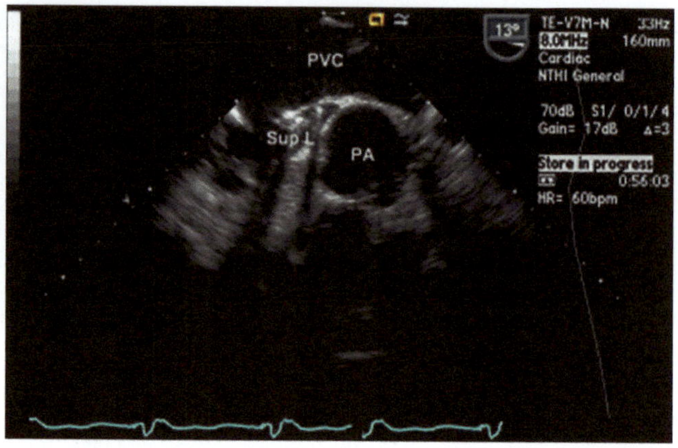

Fig. 12.39 Mid esophageal four chamber view in the same patient as Figs. 12.37 and 12.38 who has superior limb obstruction after atrial switch operation. This image demonstrates significant narrowing of the superior limb of the systemic venous channel as it crosses posterior to the pulmonary artery (*PA*). Transvenous pacing wires are seen (echobright structures) within the superior limb of the systemic venous channel (*Sup L*), which likely contribute to the obstruction. *PVC* pulmonary venous channel

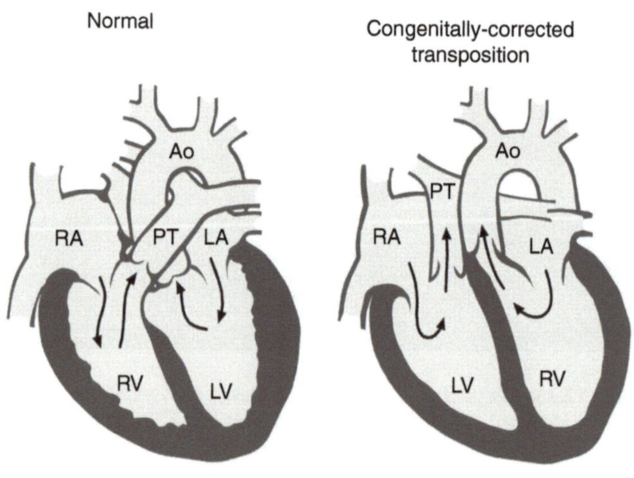

Fig. 12.40 Side by side schematic drawings of a normal heart and a heart with congenitally corrected transposition of the great arteries (*CCTGA*). The left diagram (*normal heart*) demonstrates normal atrioventricular (*AV*) and ventriculoarterial (*VA*) relationships; the right diagram (*CCTGA*) demonstrates both AV and VA discordance. In CCTGA, the normal great arterial relationships are lost; the aorta is situated anterior and leftward to the pulmonary trunk (*PT*), and the great arteries are oriented parallel to each other. *Ao* indicates aorta, *LA* morphological left atrium, *LV* morphological LV, *RA* morphological right atrium, *RV* morphological RV (From Warnes [65]; used with permission)

Van Praagh will recognize this as transposition of the great arteries with cardiac segments {S,L,L}: situs solitus of the atria, L-ventricular loop, and L-position of the great arteries (aorta anterior and leftward to the pulmonary artery) [54].

While CCTGA can occur without other cardiac defects, this is usually not the case. Most cases of CCTGA have associated defects, which include the following:

- A VSD is present in approximately 80 % of patients [66]. It is usually a perimembranous defect but can occur in any portion of the ventricular septum. The VSD can be variable in size and physiologic significance; when moderate to large, there can be hemodynamically significant left to right shunting and pulmonary overcirculation. With perimembranous VSDs, it is not unusual to have AV valve tissue and/or chordae (from either AV valve) attached to the crest of the ventricular septum, and sometimes confluent with tissue covering the VSD. This may have surgical implications.

- Left ventricular (pulmonary) outflow tract obstruction is seen in 40–50 % of patients [66]. It can be valvar, subvalvar, or both. Subvalvar pulmonary obstruction is usually the result of fibrous tissue originating from the membranous septum and attaching to the mitral valve, creating a fibrous collar. Subpulmonary stenosis can also be caused by an excrescence (or "windsock") of tissue protruding from the membranous septum into the pulmonary outflow tract [67, 68].
- Abnormalities of the systemic AV (tricuspid) valve have been described in 90 % of patients evaluated by autopsy [66]; these usually manifest as an Ebstein-type malformation of the valve, characterized by inferiorly displaced leaflets with impaired mobility. The valve anatomy differs from that of a true right sided Ebstein anomaly: there is little to no atrialized portion of the RV, adherence of the septal/posterior leaflets is limited, and the anterior leaflet is not sail-like [65, 69, 70]. Other tricuspid valve abnormalities, such as deficient leaflet tissue and thickened valve leaflets, as well as abnormal papillary musculature, can be seen in CCTGA [71]. The abnormal tricuspid valve presents with a variable degree of valvar regurgitation. In some patients, despite a very abnormal appearance to the valve, the degree of regurgitation can be surprisingly mild.
- Other abnormalities seen in association with CCTGA include subaortic stenosis and atrial septal defects. Aortic insufficiency can develop and progress over time [72]. The coronary arteries are the reverse of normal: the anterior descending and circumflex arise from the right facing sinus of Valsalva, the "right" coronary artery from the left facing sinus of Valvalva. Patients with CCTGA are also at increased risk for spontaneous development of complete heart block, and this risk increases with time at the rate of approximately 2 % per year [65].

The clinical presentation of CCTGA is variable, depending upon whether associated cardiac lesions are present, and the severity of these lesions. If other cardiac defects are present, such as a moderate VSD or significant AV valve regurgitation, patients can present in childhood with signs/symptoms of congestive heart failure. If significant pulmonary outflow tract obstruction is present, patients can present with cyanosis. When CCTGA occurs without any associated cardiac lesions, patients can be asymptomatic for decades [73]. However in many of these patients, systemic AV valve regurgitation can develop with time and patients can eventually become symptomatic. Of concern is that, by the fourth and fifth decades of life, a significant proportion of patients with or without associated cardiac lesions will have developed congestive heart failure and systemic ventricular (RV) dysfunction. This complication is particularly seen in those patients with important tricuspid (systemic AV valve) regurgitation [72, 74]. Thus CCTGA is one of the cardiac defects commonly encountered by specialists who treat adults with congenital heart disease (Chap. 18).

The genetic basis of CCTGA is still unknown [75]. There appears to be an increased incidence among families [76, 77], with a recurrence risk given between 2.6 and 5.2 % [78].

TEE Evaluation

Evaluation of the CCTGA patient should begin with a careful segmental analysis. In order to establish the diagnosis of atrioventricular and ventriculoarterial discordance, it is first necessary to identify the morphology of the three principal segments (atria, ventricles, great arteries), and then determine the manner in which these individual segments connect to each other (Chap. 4). This analysis can be further complicated by the high incidence of cardiac malposition in CCTGA patients (mesocardia in 15 %, dextrocardia in 30 %), despite the fact that most of these patients will have visceroatrial *situs solitus*. Thus the methods outlined in Chap. 4 for segmental evaluation hold an even greater importance in the assessment of these patients.

There are particular anatomic features of CCTGA that should be evaluated by TEE. These include the following:

- Anatomy of the AV valves, particularly the systemic (tricuspid) AV valve.
- Ventricular septum, and if a VSD is present, its size and location. In many CCTGA patients the ventricular septum is oriented in a straight sagittal (antero-posterior) plane, which differs from the angled orientation of the septum in normal patients.
- Evaluation of the pulmonary outflow tract, particularly in regard to subpulmonary and pulmonary valve obstruction.
- Relationship of the AV valves to the VSD (if present) and any pulmonary outflow tract obstruction (fibrous tissue, excrescences, etc.)
- Aortic valve anatomy.
- Atrial septal defect.
- Systemic and pulmonary venous return.
- Morphology and size of the ventricles.

Atrial situs can be evaluated using the techniques outlined in Chap. 4. The LE Situs SAX and LE IVC LAX views are useful for localizing the entrance of the IVC and coronary sinus, two markers that identify the morphologic right atrium. This evaluation also becomes important in identifying the location of the inferior systemic venous pathway when a double switch operation (discussed below) is planned. The ME 4 Ch view and its modifications (clockwise/counterclockwise rotation), is the most useful TEE view for evalua-

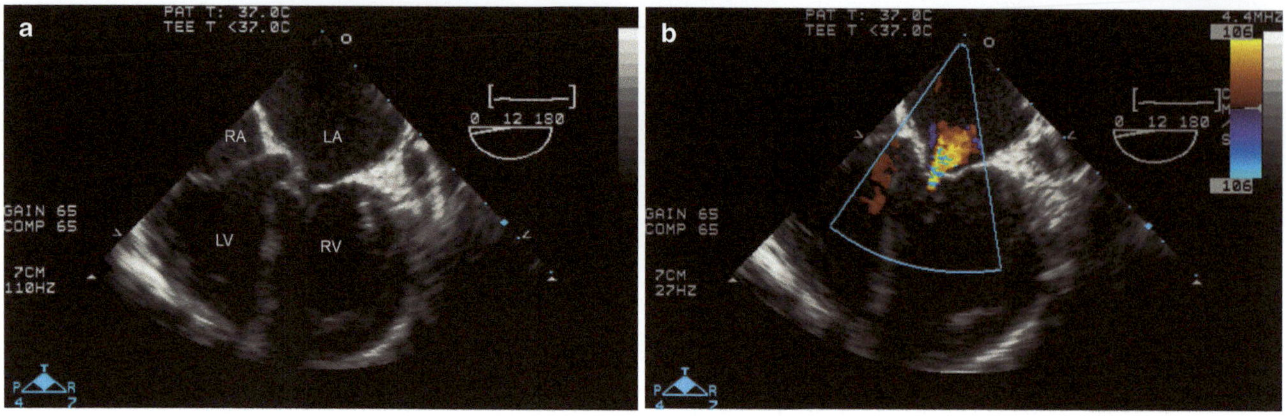

Fig. 12.41 Congenitally corrected transposition of the great arteries. Using a mid esophageal four chamber view (**a**), marked inferior displacement of the septal leaflet of the left sided tricuspid valve is seen, compared with the right sided mitral valve. Incomplete coaptation of this valve results in a mild to moderate degree of tricuspid insufficiency, as noted in (**b**). *LA* left atrium, *LV* left ventricle, *RA* right atrium, *RV* right ventricle

tion of CCTGA, as a number of important structures can be visualized: (1) the atrial appendages and systemic/pulmonary venous return; (2) the atrial septum; (3) the AV valves and the offset between tricuspid and mitral valves (reverse of normal); (4) the inlet, membranous, and trabecular portions of the ventricular septum; (5) the pulmonary outflow tract and, with probe withdrawal and slight anteflexion, the pulmonary valve. Thus the ME 4 Ch view allows evaluation of the defects most commonly seen in CCTGA [79]. The degree of inferior tricuspid valve displacement is very well shown with the ME 4 Ch, and color flow Doppler will provide an excellent profile of the degree of AV valve insufficiency (if any) (Fig. 12.41, Video 12.34). Further views of the left sided tricuspid valve can be provided with rotation of the multiplane angle between 0° and 90°, along with slight counterclockwise rotation, to obtain the equivalent of the ME 2 Ch and ME LAX views (Fig. 12.42, Video 12.35). The ventricular septum will also be well seen using the ME 4 Ch view. Again, given the straight sagittal orientation of the ventricular septum in many CCTGA patients, the ME 4 Ch, with varying amounts of retroflexion and anteflexion, provides the best sweep of this structure. This view also provides excellent depiction of perimembranous VSDs, along with detail regarding AV valve chordal attachments to the crest of ventricular septum and/or straddling across the septum (Fig. 12.43, Video 12.36). Additional views of the ventricular septum and ventricular morphology can be provided by the TG Basal and TG Mid SAX views; the ventricular inversion will be apparent with the two LV papillary muscles on the patient's right, and the trabeculated RV on the patient's left (Fig. 12.44, Video 12.37). In the transgastric position, additional views of the tricuspid valve can be obtained by rotating the multiplane angle to 90° and slight counterclockwise rotation to obtain the TG 2 Ch view.

The pulmonary outflow tract can be evaluated with several views. It can be visualized with the ME 4 Ch view and

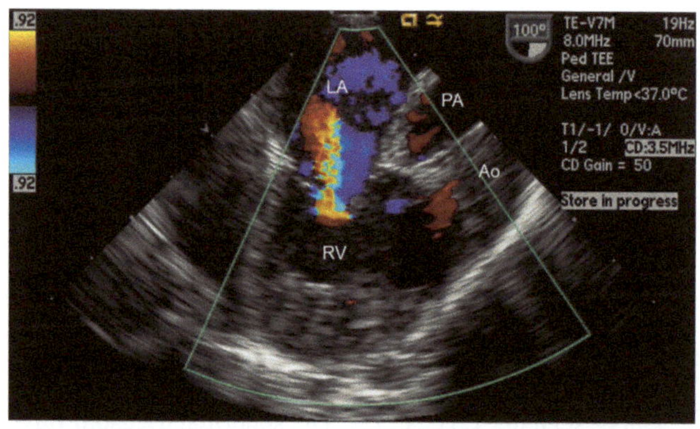

Fig. 12.42 Congenitally corrected transposition of the great arteries. Using the mid esophageal long axis view, the left sided tricuspid valve is seen, with significant regurgitation. *Ao* aorta, *LA* left atrium, *PA* pulmonary artery, *RV* right ventricle

slight probe withdrawal, as well as a small amount of probe anteflexion. However, the best views of the outflow tract will be obtained by a small amount of clockwise rotation as well as rotation of the multiplane angle to 90°–110°. This sagitally oriented view more fully displays the long axis of the pulmonary outflow tract, and provides anatomic detail regarding subpulmonary stenosis (if present) [67, 80, 81], including the distance between area of stenosis and the pulmonary valve (Fig. 12.45, Video 12.38). This view also provides excellent color flow Doppler visualization for evaluation of outflow tract stenosis, and fair to good angles for spectral Doppler quantification. Supplementary cross-sections from the transgastric (TG LAX) and deep transgastric views (DTG LAX, DTG Sagittal) offer additional angles for Doppler interrogation of the pulmonary outflow tract (Fig. 12.46, Video 12.39).

Like D-TGA, the great arteries of CCTGA arise in parallel fashion from the ventricles. From the ME 4 Ch view, a sweep using both probe withdrawal and anteflexion will

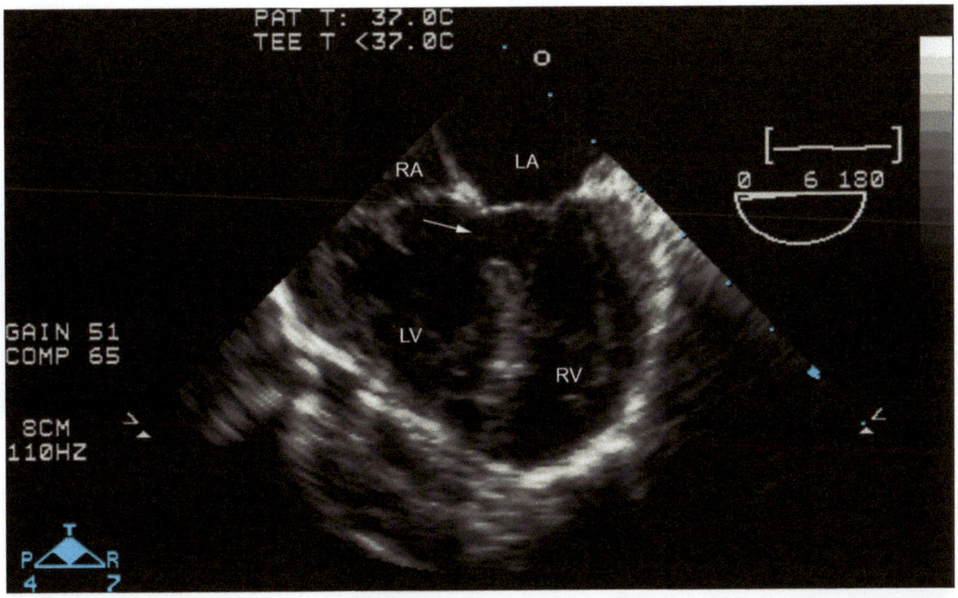

Fig. 12.43 Mid esophageal four chamber view shows a large perimembranous ventricular septal defect (*arrow*) in a patient with congenitally corrected transposition of the great arteries. Note the left sided tricuspid valve chordal attachment to ventricular septum, as well as the presence of a moderator band in the left sided right ventricle (*RV*). *LA* left atrium, *LV* left ventricle, *RA* right atrium

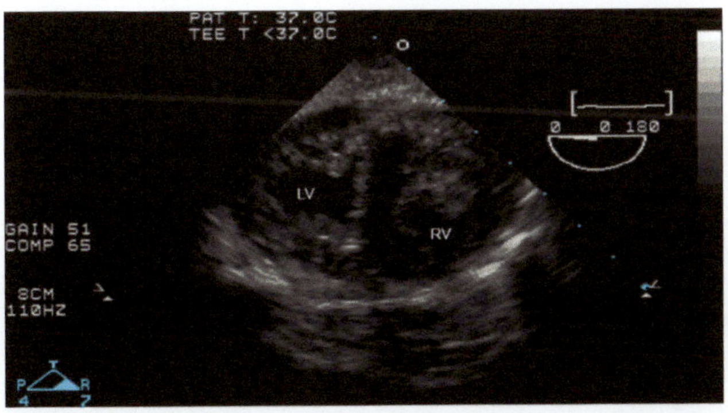

Fig. 12.44 Congenitally corrected transposition of the great arteries. Transgastric mid short axis view shows the inverted ventricles in cross section. Note the smooth walled septal surface in the left ventricle (*LV*), and the prominent moderator band in the right ventricle (*RV*)

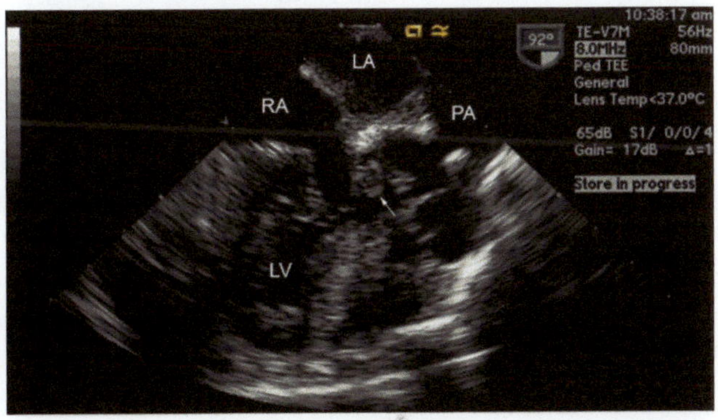

Fig. 12.45 Congenitally corrected transposition of the great arteries, as seen from the mid esophageal window in an approximately 90° sagittal plane. There is a "windsock" aneurysm of tissue (*arrow*) originating from the anterior leaflet of mitral valve and protruding into the pulmonary outflow tract, just below the pulmonary valve. In addition fibrous tissue from the mitral valve extends across the outflow tract and attaches to the ventricular septum. Neither of these was obstructive. A pulmonary artery band is seen in the main pulmonary artery, with flow acceleration noted across it. *LA* left atrium, *LV* left ventricle, *PA* pulmonary artery, *RA* right atrium

display both semilunar valves arising from their respective ventricles, and (because of the parallel great artery arrangement) an *en face* view of both semilunar valves in the same plane (Fig. 12.47, Video 12.40). Most commonly, the aortic valve will be seen anterior and leftward to the pulmonary valve. At this point, if the multiplane angle is rotated between 80° and 100° (a view approximating the ME AV LAX view), both semilunar valves and great arteries will be seen in parallel, with slight clockwise/counterclockwise rotation bringing each great artery into view [80]. These views are useful to measure semilunar valve annular diameters and also to observe the motion of the valves, including evaluation by color flow Doppler (Fig. 12.48, Video 12.41). When the aortic valve is visualized, the inflow and outflow portions of the RV can be seen, along with subaortic conus and tricuspid/aortic fibrous discontinuity. The deep transgastric views (DTG LAX, DTG Sagittal) also provide additional visualization of the intracardiac anatomy, including the semilunar valves. Given the higher incidence of cardiac malposition and sagittal orientation of the ventricular septum, the DTG LAX views generally provide more useful information regarding the intracardiac anatomy and ventricular outflow tracts (Figs. 12.46 and 12.49, Videos 12.39 and 12.42). For CCTGA, it should be noted that the more sagitally oriented views (ME LAX, ME AV LAX, DTG Sagittal, sometimes ME RV In-Out) can be confusing, because the ventriculoarterial discordant connections, along with the parallel alignment of the great arteries from the ventricles, very much resembles that of D-TGA (as described earlier). Without proper left-right orientation, it can be difficult to discern visceroatrial situs,

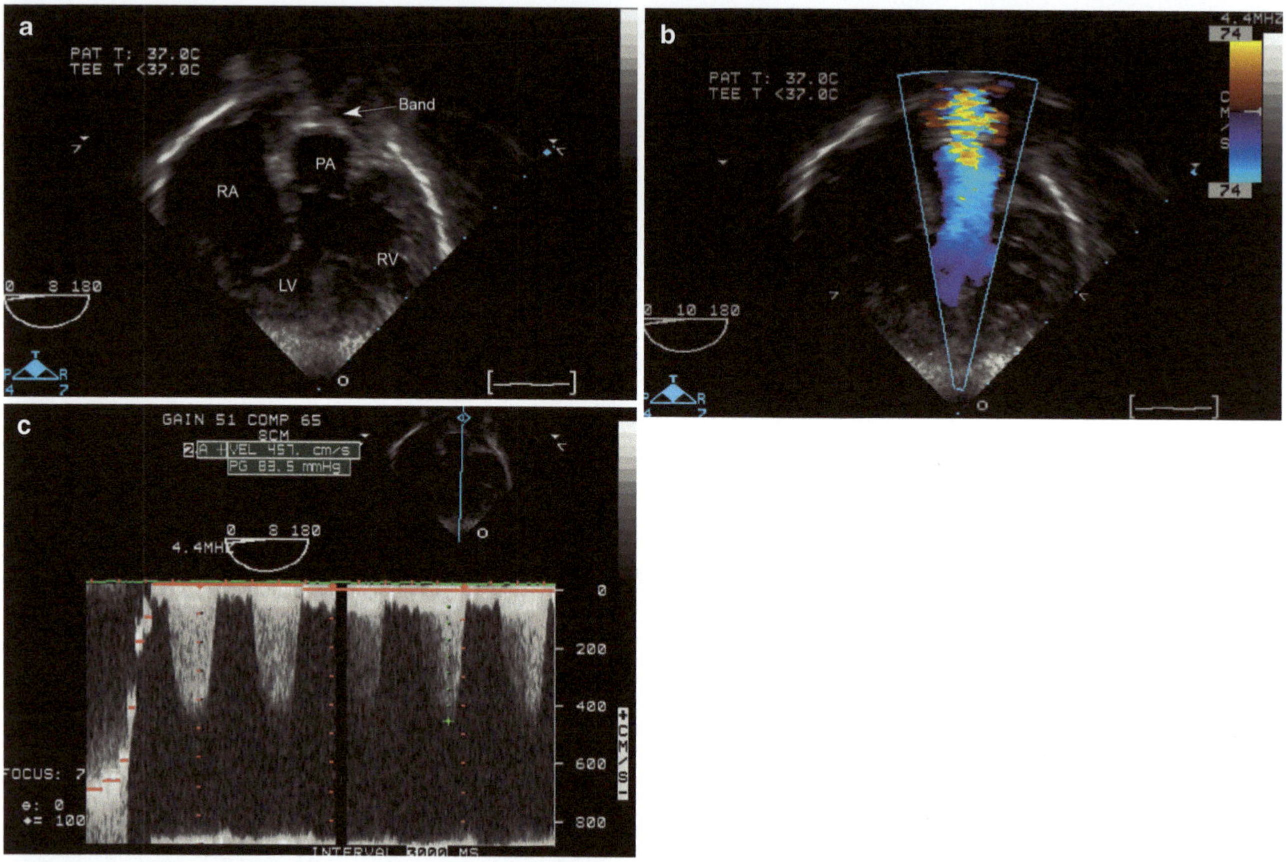

Fig. 12.46 Deep transgastric long axis view in a patient with congenitally corrected transposition of the great arteries and ventricular septal defect, in whom a pulmonary artery band (*Band*) was placed. (**a**) Shows the band well above the pulmonary valve. (**b**) Shows significant aliasing across the band, and (**c**) Displays the corresponding spectral Doppler tracing, with a peak gradient of 84 mmHg. Note the excellent angle for Doppler interrogation. *LV* left ventricle, *PA* pulmonary artery, *RA* right atrium, *RV* right ventricle

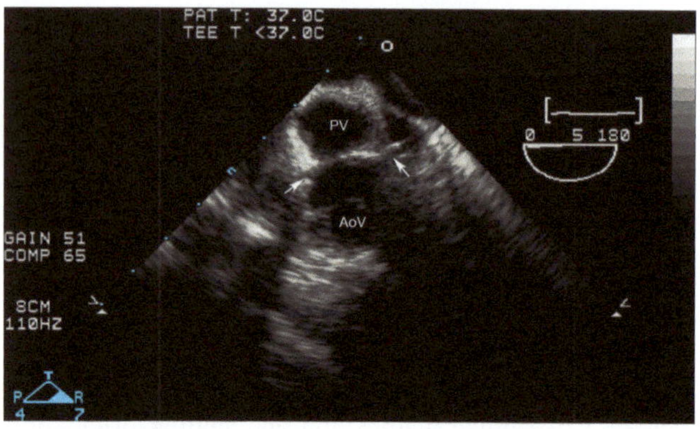

Fig. 12.47 Mid esophageal aortic valve short axis view in a patient with congenitally corrected transposition of the great arteries. Note the position of the aortic valve (*AoV*) anterior and slightly to the left of the pulmonary valve (*PV*). Coronary arteries (*arrows*) are seen to arise from the right and left facing sinuses of Valsalva

AV concordance/discordance, or relationship of the great arteries to each other. Thus in CCTGA (as well as D-TGA), the more sagittal views should always be used in conjunction with those that display left-right orientation, such as ME 4 Ch, ME AV SAX, DTG LAX, etc. Alternatively, the examiner can perform a careful right/left or left/right sweep, but meticulous attention and notation must be made as to the direction of the sweep, and the structures visualized at each point (Video 12.43).

Returning to 0° in the mid esophagus, further probe withdrawal to the upper esophageal windows (UE Ao Arch LAX, UE PA LAX) will display the branch pulmonary arteries and ascending aorta, as well as the aortic arch, and descending aorta. A ductus arteriosus, if patent, can also be seen from these views. These same structures can also be evaluated from a more sagittal perspective by turning the multiplane angle to approximately 90° (producing the UE Ao Arch SAX view), and rotating the TEE probe clockwise/counterclockwise to visualize the different vascular structures.

Surgical Considerations

The first important determination in a patient with CCTGA is whether a biventricular repair is feasible. If biventricular surgery can be performed, several options are available. The remainder of this section discusses biventricular repair of CCTGA; the surgical approach to the single ventricle is discussed in Chap. 10.

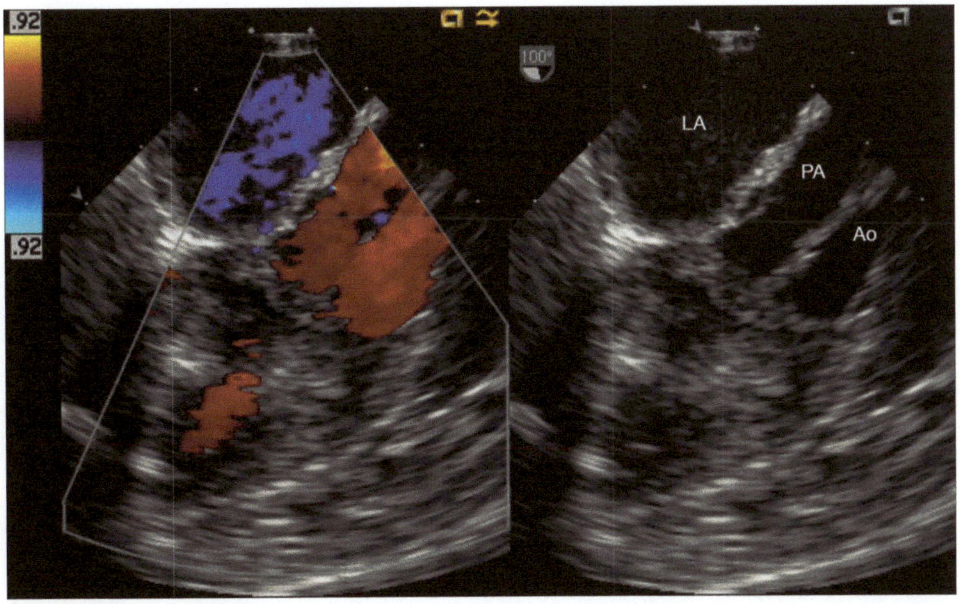

Fig. 12.48 Mid esophageal long axis view in congenitally corrected transposition of the great arteries, showing the parallel course of both aorta (*Ao*) and pulmonary artery (*PA*) as they arise from the heart. In this view, the ventriculoarterial discordance, and parallel arrangement of the great arteries, is very similar to that seen in D-transposition of the great arteries. Thus complementary views and sweeps are necessary to determine visceroatrial situs and atrioventricular connections. *LA* left atrium

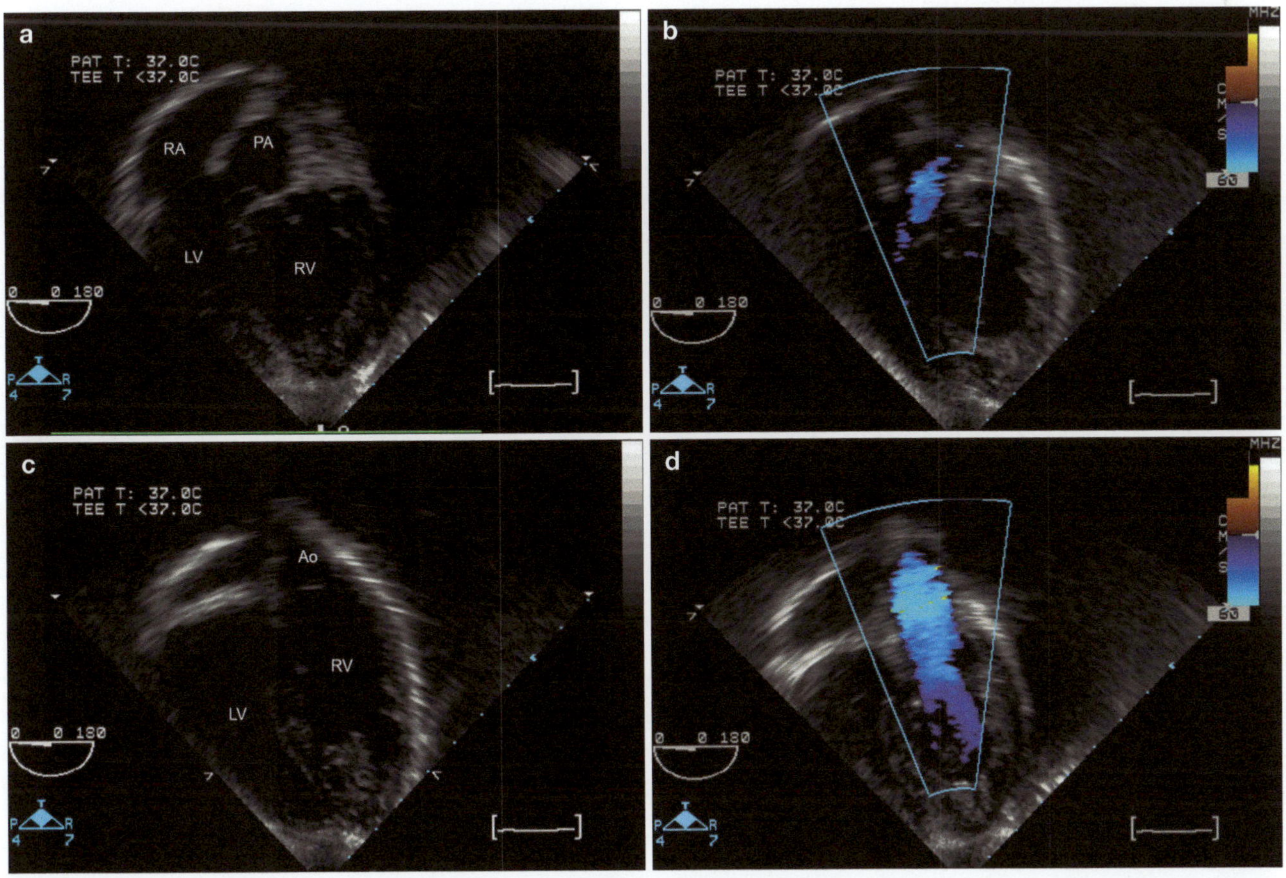

Fig. 12.49 Deep transgastric long axis view in a patient with congenitally corrected transposition of the great arteries. (**a**, **b**) show the right atrium (*RA*), left ventricle (*LV*), and pulmonary artery (*PA*), with ventricular septum bowing toward the LV. Unobstructed flow is seen across the pulmonary outflow tract. In (**c**) the probe has been withdrawn slightly to point the tip more anteriorly, visualizing the anterior aorta (*Ao*) arising from the right ventricle (*RV*). Unobstructed flow is seen into the aorta (**d**)

Biventricular surgery for CCTGA can be divided into two major classes, depending upon which morphologic ventricle assumes the role of the systemic ventricle.

Physiologic Repair

In this type of repair, also referred to as 'classic repair for CCTGA', the RV remains the systemic ventricle. Surgery is directed toward addressing important associated cardiac defects, including closure of atrial and ventricular septal defects, and tricuspid valve repair or replacement if significant tricuspid regurgitation is present. Pulmonary outflow obstruction (if present) is addressed either by direct relief of the subpulmonary obstruction, or via alternate pulmonary ventricle (LV) to pulmonary artery connection using either a conduit or direct pulmonary artery to ventricle anastomosis (*réparation à l'étage ventriculaire*, or REV procedure) [82]. In these types of surgeries, postoperative TEE is used to assess the adequacy of the repairs, using the ME 4 Ch view and its modifications to focus upon tricuspid valve anatomy/function, pulmonary outflow tract, and the atrial/ventricular septa. If an LV to pulmonary artery conduit has been placed, it can be visualized using mid and upper esophageal views with rotation of the multiplane angle between 80° and 110°, the imaging plane depending upon the exact placement of the conduit (which generally lies to the right of the aorta). The REV procedure can also be visualized in a similar manner.

Anatomic Repair

This type of repair has gained popularity over recent years, as preferences for surgical repair of CCTGA have been influenced by recent studies demonstrating a high incidence of deterioration of systemic AV valve and morphologic RV function in adulthood [72, 74, 83], and also suboptimal outcomes with physiologic repair [84, 85]. The anatomic repair for CCTGA is designed to redirect blood flow in such a manner that the LV becomes the systemic ventricle [86]. There are two principal forms of anatomic repair. In the first, both an atrial switch (Senning, Mustard) and arterial switch operation are performed at the same time. This surgery, also known as a "double switch", re-routes pulmonary venous blood through the LV to the aorta, and systemic venous blood through the RV to the pulmonary arteries (Fig. 12.50). All other cardiac lesions (e.g. atrial and ventricular septal defects) are addressed at the same time. In those patients with an intact ventricular septum or a pressure-restrictive VSD, LV "retraining" is necessary due to the fact that the LV, adapted to low pulmonary artery pressures, lacks sufficient muscle mass to maintain cardiac output against higher systemic arterial afterload. Thus a preparatory pulmonary arterial band is placed and after a sufficient period of time (months to years in most cases), the double switch is performed [87]. The second type of anatomic repair is utilized when there is pulmonary outflow obstruction (precluding an arterial switch), as well as an adequate size VSD. In these cases an atrial switch procedure is performed, along with

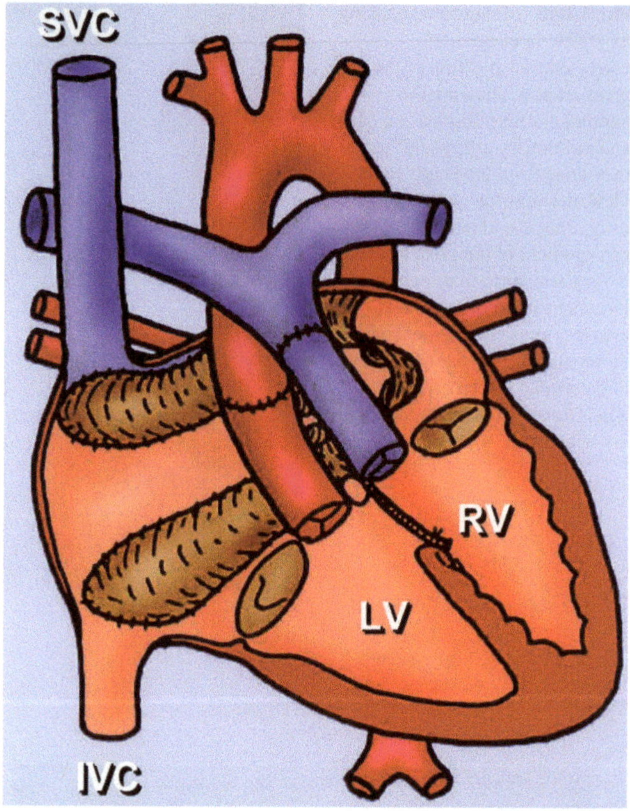

Fig. 12.50 Double-switch operation for congenitally corrected transposition of the great arteries, using the Mustard atrial baffle technique and arterial switch procedure. Venous blood from the superior and inferior vena cava (*SVC, IVC*) is directed to the right ventricle (*RV*) and then to the pulmonary trunk, and pulmonary venous blood is directed to the left ventricle (*LV*) and then to the aorta. The ventricular septal defect has been closed with a patch (From Warnes [65]; used with permission)

VSD closure to the aorta and an RV to pulmonary connection (usually a conduit). No coronary artery transfer is performed. This second type of operation is often referred to as an "atrial switch-Rastelli" and does not require a preparatory pulmonary artery band. In some institutions, for both the "double switch" as well as "atrial switch-Rastelli", a bidirectional cavopulmonary anastomosis (Glenn procedure) is performed along with an intra-atrial baffle redirecting IVC blood return to the morphologic RV (hemi-Mustard). This procedure, performed to partially unload the RV [82, 88, 89], this is procedure is akin to the "one and a half" ventricle strategy used for patients with pulmonary atresia/intact ventricular septum (hypoplastic right heart) or severe forms of Ebstein anomaly [90–92].

It should be noted that, in those cases with significant pulmonary outflow obstruction and intact ventricular septum or a small or remote VSD, neither anatomic repair is feasible. In these cases a physiologic repair must be performed, with or without the need for a "one and a half" ventricle modification.

The postoperative TEE evaluation of the anatomic correction of CCTGA is essentially the same as that described for the repairs described earlier in this chapter. Specifically, TEE

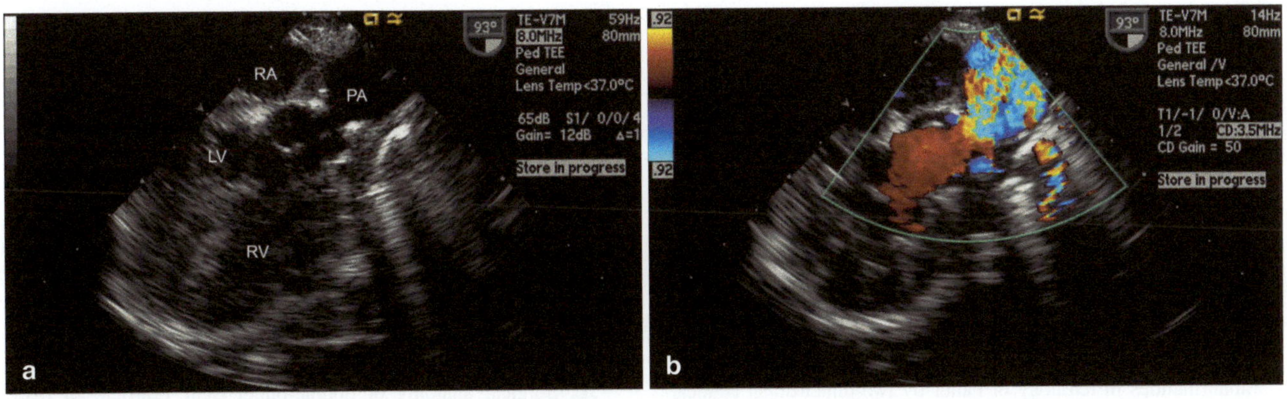

Fig. 12.51 Same patient as Fig. 12.44. The pulmonary artery band is clearly seen well above the pulmonary valve (**a**), and color flow Doppler demonstrates significant aliasing across the band (**b**). *LV* left ventricle, *PA* pulmonary artery, *RA* right atrium, *RV* right ventricle

evaluation of the atrial switch, arterial switch, and Rastelli repairs should be performed in a similar manner, with TEE views and multiplane angle adjustments made to accommodate the alterations in anatomy seen with CCTGA. It is important for the TEE examiner to have a complete understanding of the surgery that has been performed. For those patients who have undergone a preparatory pulmonary artery band, postoperative TEE can be used to evaluate LV size and function, pulmonary valve function, band placement, and the gradient across the pulmonary artery band. A combination of deep transgastric, mid and upper esophageal views can be used to assess the gradient across the band (Figs. 12.46 and 12.51, Videos 12.39 and 12.44). In some of these cases, tricuspid regurgitation significantly lessens after band placement, as the ventricular septum shifts toward the RV and decreases tricuspid annular diameter [89, 93]. This change in tricuspid regurgitation can be compared between pre and postoperative TEE studies. The altered septal geometry may also impact the systolic function of the systemic RV.

It remains to be seen whether the anatomic repair for CCTGA will eventually result in improved long-term outcomes as compared to the natural history of unoperated patients, and to those patients who have undergone physiologic repairs. The short to intermediate term results are promising, but long-term data are still lacking [93]. Specifically, there is the potential for arrhythmias and sinus node dysfunction from the atrial switch, and late LV dysfunction, neo-aortic root dilation, and neo-aortic valve insufficiency from the arterial switch [94]. Close long-term follow-up will be required to determine the actual incidence and severity of these potential complications.

Summary

The majority of conotruncal defects require surgical intervention. TEE evaluation of these malformations can be performed prior to surgery, during intra-operative repair and in the assessment of the long-term outcome of surgery for these defects. The flexibility of the multi-plane probe allows for unusual angles of interrogation when standard views are not adequate. Outcomes for conotruncal malformations have been improved by our ability to assess repairs in the operating room and to perform surveillance long after repair particularly when TTE windows are inadequate. Three-dimensional TEE is a new application that has the potential to help determine the most appropriate surgical pathway for patients with complex anatomy.

References

1. Snider AR, Ritter SB, Serwer GA. Abnormalities within the cardiac chambers, proximal vessels, and thorax. In: Echocardiography in pediatric heart disease. 2nd ed. St Louis: Mosby; 1997. p. 497–511.
2. Anderson RH, Weinberg PM. The clinical anatomy of tetralogy of Fallot. Cardiol Young. 2005;15 Suppl 1:38–47.
3. Michielon G, Marino B, Formigari R, et al. Genetic syndromes and outcome after surgical correction of tetralogy of Fallot. Ann Thorac Surg. 2006;81:968–75.
4. Kohli V, Azad S, Sachdev MS, et al. Balloon dilation of the pulmonary valve in premature infants with tetralogy of Fallot. Pediatr Cardiol. 2008;29:946–9.
5. Massoud I, Imam A, Mabrouk A, et al. Palliative balloon valvoplasty of the pulmonary valve in tetralogy of Fallot. Cardiol Young. 1999;9:24–36.
6. Sluysmans T, Neven B, Rubay J, et al. Early balloon dilatation of the pulmonary valve in infants with tetralogy of Fallot. Risks and benefits. Circulation. 1995;91:1506–11.
7. Hirsch JC, Mosca RS, Bove EL. Complete repair of tetralogy of Fallot in the neonate: results in the modern era. Ann Surg. 2000;232:508–14.
8. Kolcz J, Pizarro C. Neonatal repair of tetralogy of Fallot results in improved pulmonary artery development without increased need for reintervention. Eur J Cardiothorac Surg. 2005;28:394–9.
9. Reddy VM, Liddicoat JR, McElhinney DB, Brook MM, Stanger P, Hanley FL. Routine primary repair of tetralogy of Fallot in neonates and infants less than three months of age. Ann Thorac Surg. 1995;60:S592–6.

10. Schneider M, Zartner P, Sidiropoulos A, Konertz W, Hausdorf G. Stent implantation of the arterial duct in newborns with duct-dependent circulation. Eur Heart J. 1998;19:1401–9.
11. Alwi M, Choo KK, Latiff HA, Kandavello G, Samion H, Mulyadi MD. Initial results and medium-term follow-up of stent implantation of patent ductus arteriosus in duct-dependent pulmonary circulation. J Am Coll Cardiol. 2004;44:438–45.
12. Alwi M. Stenting the ductus arteriosus: case selection, technique and possible complications. Ann Pediatr Cardiol. 2008;1:38–45.
13. Walsh MA, Lee KJ, Chaturvedi R, Van Arsdell GS, Benson LN. Radiofrequency perforation of the right ventricular outflow tract as a palliative strategy for pulmonary atresia with ventricular septal defect. Catheter Cardiovasc Interv. 2007;69:1015–20.
14. Jureidini SB, Appleton RS, Nouri S. Detection of coronary artery abnormalities in tetralogy of Fallot by two-dimensional echocardiography. J Am Coll Cardiol. 1989;14:960–7.
15. Need LR, Powell AJ, del Nido P, Geva T. Coronary echocardiography in tetralogy of fallot: diagnostic accuracy, resource utilization and surgical implications over 13 years. J Am Coll Cardiol. 2000; 36:1371–7.
16. Suzuki A, Ho SY, Anderson RH, Deanfield JE. Further morphologic studies on tetralogy of Fallot, with particular emphasis on the prevalence and structure of the membranous flap. J Thorac Cardiovasc Surg. 1990;99:528–35.
17. Postema PG, Rammeloo LAJ, van Litsenburg R, Rothuis EGM, Hruda J. Left superior vena cava in pediatric cardiology associated with extra-cardiac anomalies. Int J Cardiol. 2008;123:302–6.
18. Knight L, Edwards JE. Right aortic arch. Types and associated cardiac anomalies. Circulation. 1974;50:1047–51.
19. Padalino MA, Vida VL, Stellin G. Transatrial-transpulmonary repair of tetralogy of Fallot. Semin Thorac Cardiovasc Surg Pediatr Card Surg Annu. 2009;12(1):48–53.
20. Joyce JJ, Hwang EY, Wiles HB, Kline CH, Bradley SM, Crawford FA. Reliability of intraoperative transesophageal echocardiography during tetralogy of Fallot repair. Echocardiography. 2000;17:319–27.
21. Yang SG, Novello R, Nicolson S, et al. Evaluation of ventricular septal defect repair using intraoperative transesophageal echocardiography: frequency and significance of residual defects in infants and children. Echocardiography. 2000;17:681–4.
22. Belli E, Houyel L, Serraf A, Lacour-Gayet F, Petit J, Planché C. Transaortic closure of residual intramural ventricular septal defect. Ann Thorac Surg. 2000;69:1496–8.
23. Preminger TJ, Sanders SP, van der Velde ME, Castañeda AR, Lock JE. "Intramural" residual interventricular defects after repair of conotruncal malformations. Circulation. 1994;89:236–42.
24. Motta P, Miller-Hance WC. Transesophageal echocardiography in tetralogy of Fallot. Semin Cardiothorac Vasc Anesth. 2012;16(2):70–87.
25. Kaushal SK, Radhakrishanan S, Dagar KS, et al. Significant intraoperative right ventricular outflow gradients after repair for tetralogy of Fallot: to revise or not to revise? Ann Thorac Surg. 1999;68:1705–12; discussion 1712–3.
26. Zoghbi WA, Enriquez-Sarano M, Foster E, et al. Recommendations for evaluation of the severity of native valvular regurgitation with two-dimensional and Doppler echocardiography. J Am Soc Echocardiogr. 2003;16:777–802.
27. Bradley TJ, Karamlou T, Kulik A, et al. Determinants of repair type, reintervention, and mortality in 393 children with double-outlet right ventricle. J Thorac Cardiovasc Surg. 2007;134: 967–973.e6.
28. Keane JF, Fyler DC. Double-outlet right ventricle. In: Keane JF, Lock JE, Fyler DC, Nadas AS, editors. Nadas' pediatric cardiology. 2nd ed. Philadelphia: Saunders; 2006. p. 735–41.
29. Ikemoto Y, Nogi S, Teraguchi M, Imamura H, Kobayashi Y. Double-outlet right ventricle with intact ventricular septum. Acta Paediatr Jpn. 1997;39:233–6.
30. Vairo U, Tagliente MR, Fasano ML, Adurno G, Serino W. Double-outlet right ventricle with intact ventricular septum. Ital Heart J. 2001;2:397–400.
31. Geva T, Van Praagh S, Sanders SP, Mayer JE, Van Praagh R. Straddling mitral valve with hypoplastic right ventricle, crisscross atrioventricular relations, double outlet right ventricle and dextrocardia: morphologic, diagnostic and surgical considerations. J Am Coll Cardiol. 1991;17:1603–12.
32. Hagler DJ. Double-outlet right ventricle and double outlet left ventricle. In: Allen HD, Dricoll DJ, Shaddy RE, Feltes TF, editors. Moss and Adams' heart disease in infants, children, and adolescents: including the fetus and young adult. 7th ed. Philadelphia: Lippincott Williams & Wilkins; 2008. p. 1100–27.
33. Anderson RH, Becker AE, Wilcox BR, Macartney FJ, Wilkinson JL. Surgical anatomy of double-outlet right ventricle—a reappraisal. Am J Cardiol. 1983;52:555–9.
34. Belli E, Serraf A, Lacour-Gayet F, et al. Surgical treatment of subaortic stenosis after biventricular repair of double-outlet right ventricle. J Thorac Cardiovasc Surg. 1996;112:1570–8.
35. Bartram U, Molin DG, Wisse LJ, et al. Double-outlet right ventricle and overriding tricuspid valve reflect disturbances of looping, myocardialization, endocardial cushion differentiation, and apoptosis in TGF-beta(2)-knockout mice. Circulation. 2001;103:2745–52.
36. Kleinert S, Sano T, Weintraub RG, Mee RB, Karl TR, Wilkinson JL. Anatomic features and surgical strategies in double-outlet right ventricle. Circulation. 1997;96:1233–9.
37. Castaneda AR, Jonas RA, Mayer JE, Hanley FL. Double-outlet right ventricle. In: Cardiac surgery of the neonate and infant. Philadelphia: W.B. Saunders; 1994. p. 445–59.
38. Artrip JH, Sauer H, Campbell DN, et al. Biventricular repair in double outlet right ventricle: surgical results based on the STS-EACTS International Nomenclature classification. Eur J Cardiothorac Surg. 2006;29:545–50.
39. Morell VO, Jacobs JP, Quintessenza JA. Aortic translocation in the management of transposition of the great arteries with ventricular septal defect and pulmonary stenosis: results and follow-up. Ann Thorac Surg. 2005;79:2089–92; discussion 2092–3.
40. Yeh T, Ramaciotti C, Leonard SR, Roy L, Nikaidoh H. The aortic translocation (Nikaidoh) procedure: midterm results superior to the Rastelli procedure. J Thorac Cardiovasc Surg. 2007;133:461–9.
41. Penny DJ, Anderson RH. Common arterial trunk. In: Anderson RH, Baker EJ, Redington A, Rigby ML, Penny D, Wernovsky G, editors. Paediatric cardiology. 3rd ed. Philadelphia: Churchill Livingstone/Elsevier; 2009. p. 859–74.
42. Van Praagh R, Van Praagh S. The anatomy of common aorticopulmonary trunk (truncus arteriosus communis) and its embryologic implications. A study of 57 necropsy cases. Am J Cardiol. 1965;16: 406–25.
43. Cabalka AK, Edwards WD, Dearani JA. Truncus arteriosus. In: Allen HD, Driscoll DJ, Shaddy RE, Feltes TF, editors. Moss and Adams' heart disease in infants, children, and adolescents: including the fetus and young adult. 7th ed. Philadelphia: Lippincott Williams & Wilkins; 2008. p. 911–22.
44. Collett RW, Edwards JE. Persistent truncus arteriosus; a classification according to anatomic types. Surg Clin North Am. 1949;29: 1245–70.
45. Van Praagh R. Truncus arteriosus: what is it really and how should it be classified? Eur J Cardiothorac Surg. 1987;1:65.
46. Jacobs ML. Congenital heart surgery nomenclature and database project: truncus arteriosus. Ann Thorac Surg. 2000;69:S50–5.
47. McElhinney DB, Driscoll DA, Emanuel BS, Goldmuntz E. Chromosome 22q11 deletion in patients with truncus arteriosus. Pediatr Cardiol. 2003;24:569–73.
48. Silengo M, Rulli I, Delmonaco AG, Ferrero GB, Pucci A, Sanna R. Truncus arteriosus and isochromosome 8q. Am J Med Genet A. 2005;133A:223–4.

49. Calder L, Van Praagh R, Van Praagh S, et al. Truncus arteriosus communis. Clinical, angiocardiographic, and pathologic findings in 100 patients. Am Heart J. 1976;92:23–38.
50. Kalavrouziotis G, Purohit M, Ciotti G, Corno AF, Pozzi M. Truncus arteriosus communis: early and midterm results of early primary repair. Ann Thorac Surg. 2006;82:2200–6.
51. Pasquini L, Sanders SP, Parness IA, et al. Conal anatomy in 119 patients with d-loop transposition of the great arteries and ventricular septal defect: an echocardiographic and pathologic study. J Am Coll Cardiol. 1993;21:1712–21.
52. Norwood WI, Dobell AR, Freed MD, Kirklin JW, Blackstone EH. Intermediate results of the arterial switch repair. A 20-institution study. J Thorac Cardiovasc Surg. 1988;96:854–63.
53. Van Praagh R, Weinberg PM, Smith SD, Foran RB, Van Praagh S. Malpositions of the heart. In: Adams FH, Emmanouilides GC, Riemenschneider TA, editors. Moss' heart disease in infants, children and adolescents. 4th ed. Baltimore: Williams and Wilkins; 1989. p. 530–80.
54. Van Praagh R. Segmental approach to diagnosis. In: Keane JF, Lock JE, Fyler DC, editors. Nadas' pediatric cardiology. 2nd ed. Philadelphia: Saunders Elsevier; 2006. p. 39–46.
55. Kouchoukos NT, Blackstone EH, Hanley FL, Doty DB, Karp RB. Complete transposition of the great arteries. In: Kirklin/Barratt-Boyes cardiac surgery. 3rd ed. Philadelphia: Churchill Livingstone; 2003. p. 1438–507.
56. Wernovsky G. Transposition of the great arteries. In: Allen HD, Dricoll DJ, Shaddy RE, Feltes TF, editors. Moss and Adams' heart disease in infants, children, and adolescents: including the fetus and young adult. 7th ed. Philadelphia: Lippincott Williams & Wilkins; 2008. p. 1038–87.
57. Pasquini L, Sanders SP, Parness IA, et al. Coronary echocardiography in 406 patients with d-loop transposition of the great arteries. J Am Coll Cardiol. 1994;24:763–8.
58. Frohn-Mulder IM, Wesby Swaay E, Bouwhuis C, et al. Chromosome 22q11 deletions in patients with selected outflow tract malformations. Genet Couns. 1999;10:35–41.
59. Kirjavainen M, Happonen JM, Louhimo I. Late results of Senning operation. J Thorac Cardiovasc Surg. 1999;117:488–95.
60. Lecompte Y, Neveux JY, Leca F, et al. Reconstruction of the pulmonary outflow tract without prosthetic conduit. J Thorac Cardiovasc Surg. 1982;84:727–33.
61. Castaneda AR, Jonas RA, Mayer JE, Hanley FL. D-Transposition of the great arteries. In: Cardiac surgery of the neonate and infant. Philadelphia: W.B. Saunders; 1994. p. 409–38.
62. Marino BS, Wernovsky G, McElhinney DB, et al. Neo-aortic valvar function after the arterial switch. Cardiol Young. 2006;16:481–9.
63. Vouhé PR, Tamisier D, Leca F, Ouaknine R, Vernant F, Neveux JY. Transposition of the great arteries, ventricular septal defect, and pulmonary outflow tract obstruction. Rastelli or Lecompte procedure? J Thorac Cardiovasc Surg. 1992;103:428–36.
64. Kaulitz R, Stümper OF, Geuskens R, et al. Comparative values of the precordial and transesophageal approaches in the echocardiographic evaluation of atrial baffle function after an atrial correction procedure. J Am Coll Cardiol. 1990;16:686–94.
65. Warnes CA. Transposition of the great arteries. Circulation. 2006;114:2699–709.
66. Allwork SP, Bentall HH, Becker AE, et al. Congenitally corrected transposition of the great arteries: morphologic study of 32 cases. Am J Cardiol. 1976;38:910–23.
67. Rodrigues AG, Mercier LA, Tardif JC, de Guise P. Aneurysm of the membranous ventricular septum and accessory valvular tissue causing obstruction of the pulmonary outflow tract in corrected transposition. J Am Soc Echocardiogr. 1995;8:957–60.
68. Anderson RH, Becker AE, Gerlis LM. The pulmonary outflow tract in classically corrected transposition. J Thorac Cardiovasc Surg. 1975;69:747–57.
69. Anderson KR, Danielson GK, McGoon DC, Lie JT. Ebstein's anomaly of the left-sided tricuspid valve: pathological anatomy of the valvular malformation. Circulation. 1978;58:I87–91.
70. Castaneda AR, Jonas RA, Mayer JE, Hanley FL. Corrected transposition of the great arteries. In: Cardiac surgery of the neonate and infant. Philadelphia: W.B. Saunders; 1994. p. 445–59.
71. Jaffe RB. Systemic atrioventricular valve regurgitation in corrected transpositon of the great vessels. Angiographic differentiation of operable and nonoperable valve deformities. Am J Cardiol. 1976; 37:395–402.
72. Graham TP, Bernard YD, Mellen BG, et al. Long-term outcome in congenitally corrected transposition of the great arteries: a multi-institutional study. J Am Coll Cardiol. 2000;36:255–61.
73. Presbitero P, Somerville J, Rabajoli F, Stone S, Conte MR. Corrected transposition of the great arteries without associated defects in adult patients: clinical profile and follow up. Br Heart J. 1995;74:57–9.
74. Connelly MS, Liu PP, Williams WG, Webb GD, Robertson P, McLaughlin PR. Congenitally corrected transposition of the great arteries in the adult: functional status and complications. J Am Coll Cardiol. 1996;27:1238–43.
75. Brawn WJ, Jones TI, Anderson RH, Barron DJ. Congenitally corrected transposition. In: Anderson RH, Baker EJ, Redington A, Rigby ML, Penny D, Wernovsky G, editors. Paediatric cardiology. 3rd ed. Philadelphia: Churchill Livingstone/Elsevier; 2009. p. 819–35.
76. Piacentini G, Digilio MC, Capolino R, et al. Familial recurrence of heart defects in subjects with congenitally corrected transposition of the great arteries. Am J Med Genet A. 2005;137:176–80.
77. Digilio MC, Casey B, Toscano A, et al. Complete transposition of the great arteries: patterns of congenital heart disease in familial precurrence. Circulation. 2001;104:2809–14.
78. Wallis GA, Debich-Spicer D, Anderson RH. Congenitally corrected transposition. Orphanet J Rare Dis. 2011;6:1–12.
79. Sreeram N, Stümper OF, Kaulitz R, Hess J, Roelandt JR, Sutherland GR. Comparative value of transthoracic and transesophageal echocardiography in the assessment of congenital abnormalities of the atrioventricular junction. J Am Coll Cardiol. 1990;16:1205–14.
80. Caso P, Ascione L, Lange A, Palka P, Mininni N, Sutherland GR. Diagnostic value of transesophageal echocardiography in the assessment of congenitally corrected transposition of the great arteries in adult patients. Am Heart J. 1998;135:43–50.
81. Vargas-Barron J, Rijlaarsdam M, Romero-Cardenas A, Keirns C, Diaz-Moncada S. Transesophageal echocardiography in adults with congenital cardiopathies. Am Heart J. 1993;126:426–32.
82. Lim H-G, Lee JR, Kim YJ, et al. Outcomes of biventricular repair for congenitally corrected transposition of the great arteries. Ann Thorac Surg. 2010;89:159–67.
83. Rutledge JM, Nihill MR, Fraser CD, Smith OE, McMahon CJ, Bezold LI. Outcome of 121 patients with congenitally corrected transposition of the great arteries. Pediatr Cardiol. 2002;23:137–45.
84. Hraska V, Duncan BW, Mayer JE, Freed M, del Nido PJ, Jonas RA. Long-term outcome of surgically treated patients with corrected transposition of the great arteries. J Thorac Cardiovasc Surg. 2005;129:182–91.
85. Bogers AJJC, Head SJ, de Jong PL, Witsenburg M, Kappetein AP. Long term follow up after surgery in congenitally corrected transposition of the great arteries with a right ventricle in the systemic circulation. J Cardiothorac Surg. 2010;5:74.
86. Ilbawi MN, DeLeon SY, Backer CL, et al. An alternative approach to the surgical management of physiologically corrected transposition with ventricular septal defect and pulmonary stenosis or atresia. J Thorac Cardiovasc Surg. 1990;100:410–5.
87. Murtuza B, Barron DJ, Stumper O, et al. Anatomic repair for congenitally corrected transposition of the great arteries: a single-institution 19-year experience. J Thorac Cardiovasc Surg. 2011;142:1348–57.

88. Zias EA, Mavroudis C, Cook KE, Makarewicz AJ, Backer CL, Hernandez JM. The effect of pulmonary circulation hemodynamics on right ventricular unloading via the bidirectional Glenn shunt: implications for congenitally corrected transposition repair. Semin Thorac Cardiovasc Surg Pediatr Card Surg Annu. 2003;6:27–32.
89. Malhotra SP, Reddy VM, Qiu M, et al. The hemi-Mustard/bidirectional Glenn atrial switch procedure in the double-switch operation for congenitally corrected transposition of the great arteries: rationale and midterm results. J Thorac Cardiovasc Surg. 2011; 141:162–70.
90. Chowdhury UK, Airan B, Sharma R, et al. One and a half ventricle repair with pulsatile bidirectional Glenn: results and guidelines for patient selection. Ann Thorac Surg. 2001;71:1995–2002.
91. Lee YO, Kim YJ, Lee JR, Kim W-H. Long-term results of one-and-a-half ventricle repair in complex cardiac anomalies. Eur J Cardiothorac Surg. 2011;39:711–5.
92. Kreutzer C, Mayorquim RC, Kreutzer GO, et al. Experience with one and a half ventricle repair. J Thorac Cardiovasc Surg. 1999;117:662–8.
93. Hraška V, Mattes A, Haun C, et al. Functional outcome of anatomic correction of corrected transposition of the great arteries. Eur J Cardiothorac Surg. 2011;40:1227–34.
94. Quinn DW, McGuirk SP, Metha C, et al. The morphologic left ventricle that requires training by means of pulmonary artery banding before the double-switch procedure for congenitally corrected transposition of the great arteries is at risk of late dysfunction. J Thorac Cardiovasc Surg. 2008;135:1137–44.

Great Artery and Other Vascular Abnormalities

13

Wanda C. Miller-Hance

Abstract

Echocardiography is the diagnostic modality of choice in the initial evaluation and serial assessment of most types of pediatric heart disease. The anomalies of a congenital nature that most often affect the great arteries and related vascular structures are frequently first suspected and identified by high-resolution imaging provided by transthoracic echocardiography. Technological advances made during the last several decades allow for complementary noninvasive imaging modalities to be applied when further characterization of these congenital cardiovascular malformations or variants is required. Transesophageal echocardiography (TEE) plays a limited diagnostic role in these anomalies but nonetheless provides major contributions in the care of affected patients. In the intraoperative setting, TEE is able to confirm the presence of selected abnormal vascular structure(s) or connection(s). More importantly, TEE facilitates the detailed evaluation of associated defects, provides for intraoperative monitoring, and allows for assessment of the surgical intervention(s). This chapter discusses the most frequently encountered great artery and vascular anomalies of a congenital nature, focusing on the applications of TEE in the evaluation of these lesions.

Keywords

Great artery anomalies • Vascular anomalies • Patent ductus arteriosus • Aortopulmonary window • Pulmonary artery anomalies • Anomalous origin of a branch pulmonary artery from the aorta • Pulmonary artery sling • Anomalous origin of the left pulmonary artery from the right pulmonary artery • Aortic arch anomalies • Coarctation of the aorta • Interrupted aortic arch

Introduction

In congenital heart disease (CHD), abnormalities of the great arteries and related vascular connections are commonly encountered. Transthoracic echocardiography (TTE) serves as the initial and primary diagnostic tool for their identification and assessment, particularly in the pediatric population. Additional complementary and noninvasive imaging modalities, such as cardiac magnetic resonance imaging (MRI) and computerized tomography (CT), can also be used to characterize these pathologies further, while at the same time providing information regarding related intracardiac and extracardiac structures.

In most, if not all, cases, TTE alone or in combination with these other imaging studies is able to define fully the abnormalities that affect the great arteries and delineate abnormal vascular connections. Thus, transesophageal echocardiography (TEE) generally does not play a major diagnostic role in these malformations. However despite certain challenges, the assessment of the great arteries and vascular

W.C. Miller-Hance, MD, FACC, FASE
Divisions of Pediatric Anesthesiology and Pediatric Cardiology, Departments of Pediatrics and Anesthesiology, Texas Children's Hospital, Baylor College of Medicine, 6621 Fannin, Suite W17417, Houston, TX 77030, USA
e-mail: wmh@bcm.edu

The online version of this chapter (doi:10.1007/978-1-84800-064-3_13) contains supplementary material, which is available to authorized users.

P.C. Wong, W.C. Miller-Hance (eds.), *Transesophageal Echocardiography for Congenital Heart Disease*, DOI 10.1007/978-1-84800-064-3_13, © Springer-Verlag London 2014

anomalies is feasible by TEE. In the operating room setting, in addition to providing confirmation of the abnormalities affecting these structures, TEE allows for evaluation of associated pathology, exclusion of suspected defects, and intraoperative monitoring. TEE can also provide a method for the assessment of an intervention or surgical procedure affecting the great arteries or related vascular structures; at the same time it serves a very important role in determining the adequacy of repair of any coexisting lesion(s). In this setting, TEE functions to identify and correct (or at least limit) residual pathology of hemodynamic significance that might negatively impact patient outcome.

This chapter addresses selected malformations that primarily affect the great arteries and highlights the most commonly found abnormal connections between these vascular structures. The discussion focuses on the role of TEE in the assessment of these anomalies with an emphasis on perioperative applications. As an introduction to the subject, the reader is referred to Chap. 4 for a detailed discussion of TEE imaging of the great arteries. The overview presented there should serve as a foundation for this chapter and will facilitate understanding of the lesions/variants discussed. Anomalies of venous structures are presented in Chap. 6 and will not be addressed here.

Abnormal Vascular Connections

Patent Ductus Arteriosus

Anatomic Features

The ductus arteriosus is a vascular channel that connects the pulmonary trunk to the proximal descending aorta. Anatomically, the ductus arteriosus typically originates from the posterosuperior aspect of the junction between the main and left pulmonary artery, and inserts into the anterolateral or ventral aspect of the descending thoracic aorta, just distal to the origin of the left subclavian artery (Fig. 13.1). Among individuals, the ductus arteriosus may vary in its position, course, size, and length.

In most patients with a left aortic arch, the ductus arteriosus is a left-sided structure. A right or left-sided ductus may be present in patients with a right aortic arch. In some cases, the ductus arteriosus originates from the innominate or subclavian arteries or may even be duplicated (bilateral ductus). Two important issues merit mention: (1) anatomic factors such as aortic arch sidedness, aortic arch branching pattern, and ductal origin/position may result in anomalies causing a vascular ring [1] and (2) an abnormal location, course or shape of the ductus arteriosus, as well as bilateral ductus, are more likely to occur in the setting of complex CHD.

In the normal fetal circulation, the right ventricle generates approximately two-thirds of the fetal cardiac output.

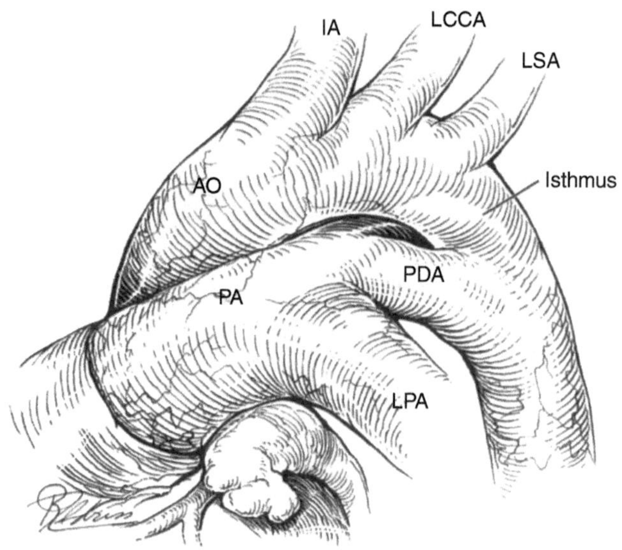

Fig. 13.1 Patent ductus arteriosus. Graphic depiction of patent ductus arteriosus (*PDA*) as visualized from a left anterior oblique view. The typical ductus extends as illustrated from the junction of the main pulmonary artery (*PA*) with the left pulmonary artery (*LPA*) to the descending thoracic aorta just distal to the left subclavian artery (*LSA*). *AO* aorta, *IA* innominate artery, *LCCA* left common carotid artery (Reproduced with permission from Hillman et al. [130])

The majority of this blood is ejected into the descending aorta through the ductus arteriosus, as only a small fraction of the right ventricular output (5–10 %) passes through the lungs. Thus, this communication is an essential component of normal fetal life, allowing for right ventricular ejection into the descending aorta within the context of a high-resistance pulmonary circulation.

In the normal full-term infant, functional closure of the ductus arteriosus occurs several hours after birth. Anatomic closure of this channel takes place in the first few weeks of life. Failure of the ductus arteriosus to close, a process not completely understood, results in persistent ductal patency (*patent ductus arteriosus* or PDA). As an isolated lesion, it accounts for between 4 and 12 % of all cases of CHD.

Associated Defects

A PDA can be found in isolation or in association with other cardiovascular anomalies (e.g., atrial septal defect, ventricular septal defect, atrioventricular septal defect, coarctation of the aorta). A high incidence is found in premature neonates, infants with respiratory distress syndrome, patients affected by rubella syndrome, and children living at high altitudes. Ductal-dependency for either pulmonary or systemic blood flow may be part of the physiology of moderate to severe forms of CHD. The discussion that follows focuses primarily on the PDA as an isolated lesion. The presence and role of the PDA in association with other cardiac defects is also briefly addressed.

Pathophysiology

In the isolated PDA, shunt magnitude is determined by the physical size of the communication (length and internal diameter) and the relationship between the systemic and pulmonary vascular resistances. A small PDA may have little to no physiologic impact. However, the hemodynamic effects of moderate-to-large communications are those of a classic left-to-right shunt manifested by increased pulmonary blood flow, resulting in left atrial and left ventricular volume overload. In a moderate size PDA, an element of ductal constriction is present, so shunting is restrictive to some extent and the pulmonary artery pressure is mildly elevated or may even be normal. Large communications are associated with a greater degree of pulmonary artery pressure elevation. In this setting, shunting can be bidirectional and dictated primarily by the resistances of the vascular beds at either sides of the PDA. The increased left atrial pressure associated with large shunts may lead to stretching of the foramen ovale and result in an additional shunt at this level, further compounding the volume load presented to the pulmonary arteries.

Management Considerations

The management options in the infant beyond prematurity or in the older child who requires ductal closure are occlusion of the communication in the cardiac catheterization laboratory or surgical closure. Various approaches have been used for surgical closure of the isolated PDA, including closed procedures via thoracoscopy (either robotically or video assisted) and open interventions, in most cases, via a thoracotomy. The adult or older patient with a PDA presents a challenge as friable tissue, aneurysmal dilation, or ductal calcification increases the likelihood of procedural complications.

Applications of Transesophageal Echocardiography

TEE has been used for diagnostic applications in the detection and characterization of flow across a PDA [2–8]. However, the use of TEE for this sole purpose is relatively rare. As previously noted, a ductus or ligamentum arteriosum may be part of a vascular ring. In these cases transesophageal instrumentation is generally avoided as probe placement or manipulation can lead to airway compromise due to compression of the trachea by surrounding vascular structures.

In the current era, transcatheter interventions aimed at ductal occlusion are guided primarily by fluoroscopy and angiography. Although TEE has been used in this setting [8, 9], and more recently, three-dimensional (3D) TEE has also been applied [10, 11], its role in these procedures is limited. The use of TEE has also been documented during interventions involving thoracoscopic surgery for the PDA, as well as open procedures in both children and adults [12–16]. The primary role is that of evaluation of shunt flow and magnitude, as well as the success of surgery in obliterating the communication. Currently, TEE is not considered an indication solely for monitoring or assessing the results of surgical closure of an isolated PDA. As such, the discussion that follows is relevant mostly to the use of TEE in the evaluation of patients undergoing surgical ligation or division of a PDA in the setting in which additional cardiac defects are also being addressed.

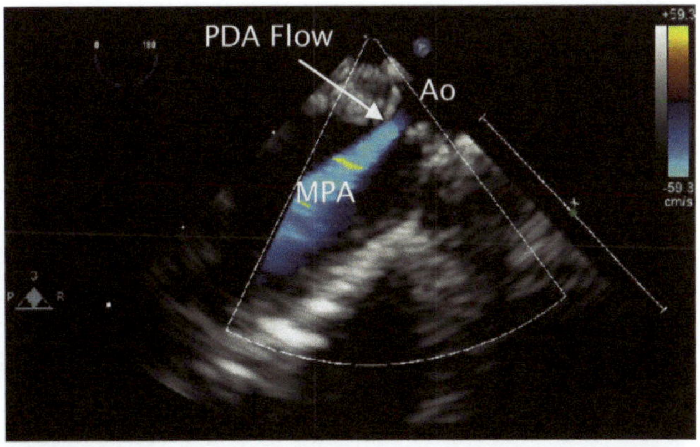

Fig. 13.2 Patent ductus arteriosus. Upper esophageal pulmonary artery long axis view demonstrating flow by color Doppler (*blue signal* away from imaging probe) corresponding to left-to-right shunting across a patent ductus arteriosus (*PDA flow*). *Ao* aorta, *MPA* main pulmonary artery

Goals of TEE Prior to Catheter or Surgical Intervention

Visualization of a PDA and Detection of Ductal Shunting

Direct imaging of the ductus arteriosus to assess patency can be challenging by two-dimensional (2D) transesophageal imaging alone. The examination of a PDA relies to a significant extent on the use of Doppler ultrasound techniques that interrogate flow across the pulmonary artery and descending aorta. The upper esophageal views, particularly the upper esophageal pulmonary artery long axis (UE PA LAX) and the upper esophageal aortic arch short axis (UE Ao Arch SAX), are essential for this evaluation (Fig. 13.2, Video 13.1). These views allow direct visualization of the ductal communication between the aorta and pulmonary artery. In addition, the mid esophageal ascending aortic short axis (ME Asc Ao SAX) with probe anteflexion and counterclockwise rotation, and the mid esophageal right ventricular inflow-outflow (ME RV In-Out) views (Fig. 13.3, Video 13.2), can also provide evidence of left-to-right ductal shunting into the pulmonary artery. As described below, views of the descending aorta that allow for the characterization of flow are also helpful. The combination of these different TEE views for the typical left-sided PDA enables visualization of the communication, including detection of ductal shunting,

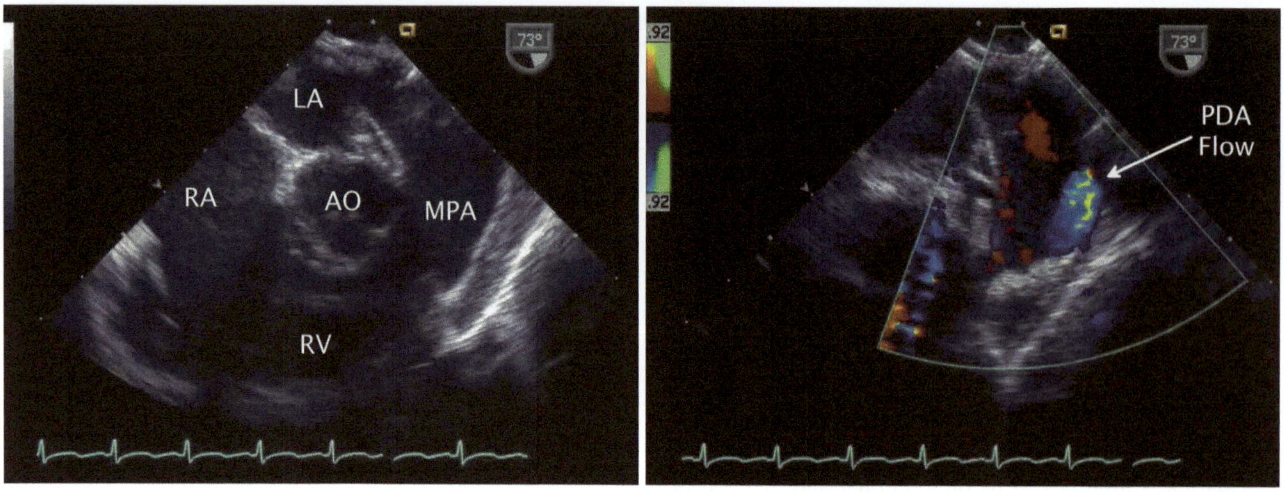

Fig. 13.3 Patent ductus arteriosus. *Left panel*, two-dimensional image of mid esophageal right ventricular inflow-outflow view. *Right panel*, corresponding color Doppler image depicts flow (blue signal) from patent ductus arteriosus (*PDA*) into main pulmonary artery (*MPA*). *AO* aorta, *LA* left atrium, *RA* right atrium, *RV* right ventricle

determination of shunt direction, and gross estimation of shunt magnitude.

Characterization of Flow Across a PDA

In the setting of a restrictive ductus arteriosus and relatively normal pulmonary artery pressures, the higher systemic arterial pressure results in continuous left-to-right shunting into the pulmonary artery throughout the cardiac cycle. This communication can be demonstrated by spectral Doppler assessment and color flow mapping in the upper esophageal, ME Asc Ao SAX, and ME RV In-Out views as previously described. Sampling near the pulmonary end in this case displays continuous high velocity flow, peaking in late systole directed away from the transducer. Color flow Doppler mapping increases the sensitivity of the interrogation and demonstrates turbulent or aliased flow (seen as a mosaic color pattern) from the PDA into the distal main pulmonary artery (Fig. 13.4, Video 13.3). The ductal flow can extend to the level of the pulmonary valve, or beyond into the right ventricular outflow tract, in the presence of pulmonary regurgitation.

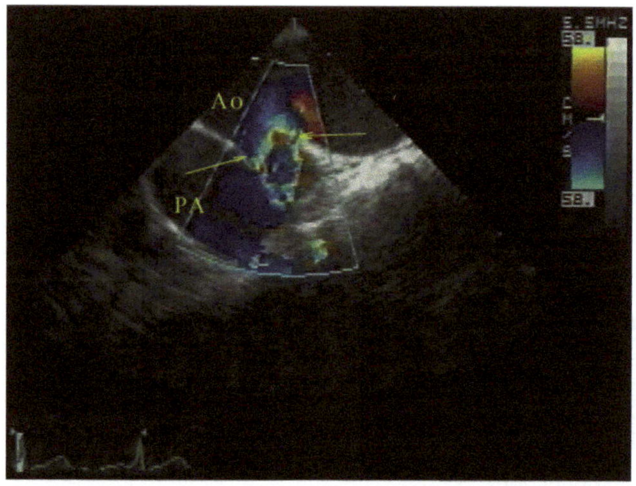

Fig. 13.4 Patent ductus arteriosus. Upper esophageal aortic arch short axis view with color mapping demonstrating aliased flow from the aorta (*Ao*) into the pulmonary artery (*PA*) across a patent ductus arteriosus (*arrows*) (Reproduced with permission from Russell et al. [131])

In the setting of pulmonary hypertension, shunting across the ductus is continuous and of low velocity, peaking in late systole [17, 18]. As the pulmonary artery pressure and pulmonary vascular resistance increase, there will be blunting of the left-to-right shunt in diastole, so that systolic left-to-right shunting predominates. Further increases in pulmonary artery pressure/vascular resistance result in low velocity bidirectional ductal shunting (right-to-left during systole and left-to-right in late systole extending into late diastole) [19]. This flow pattern can also be seen in ductal-dependent left-sided obstructive lesions such as hypoplastic left heart syndrome or interrupted aortic arch (see below) and can also be a normal finding in the neonate [20]. Increasing levels of pulmonary artery pressures and the development of increased pulmonary vascular resistance are characterized by blunting of the left-to-right shunt in diastole. In some cases, exclusive right-to-left ductal shunting is present (reverse ductal shunting), peaking in early systole; this pattern is generally seen with significant elevation in pulmonary artery pressure/vascular resistance (such as obstructed total anomalous pulmonary venous return), and in many cases can be difficult to detect by TEE. Injection of agitated saline into a peripheral or central venous catheter while imaging the descending aorta may demonstrate microcavitations distal to the level of the left subclavian artery, consistent with ductal level right-to left shunting. [6]

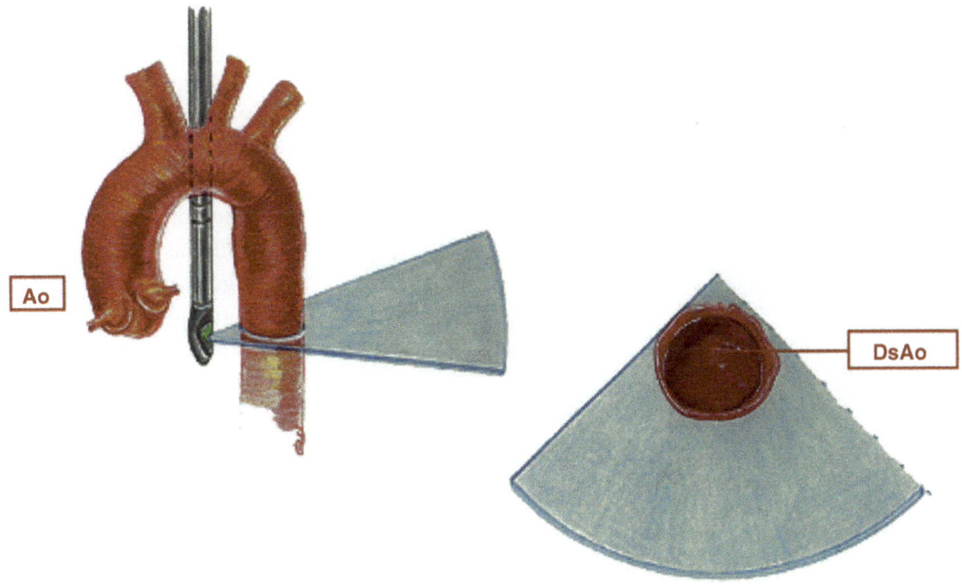

Fig. 13.5 Descending aorta. Graphic illustration of imaging probe position and cross-section displayed in the mid esophageal descending aortic short axis view. *Ao* ascending aorta, *DsAo* descending aorta (Reproduced with permission from Cahalan [132])

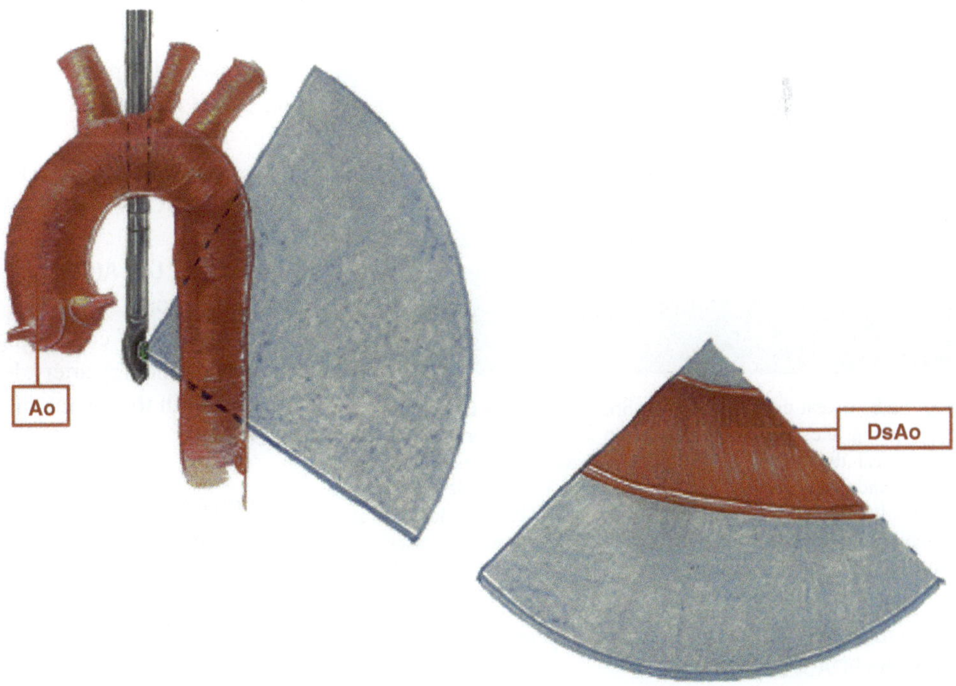

Fig. 13.6 Descending aorta. Graphic illustration of imaging probe position and cross-section displayed in the mid esophageal descending aortic long axis view. *Ao* ascending aorta, *DsAo* descending aorta (Reproduced with permission from Cahalan [132])

Doppler Interrogation of Descending Aorta

The presence of a PDA in association with a large amount of shunt flow may also be suggested by an increase in the caliber of the descending aortic pulsations. Spectral Doppler analysis in the descending aorta demonstrates both antegrade systolic flow and diastolic flow reversal. They are best appreciated in the descending aortic short (Desc Ao SAX, Fig. 13.5) and long axis (Desc Ao LAX, Fig. 13.6) views, in the areas distal to the ductus arteriosus. The retrograde flow represents diastolic runoff into the pulmonary circulation within the context of low pulmonary artery diastolic pressures (Figs. 13.7 and 13.8). The presence and magnitude of holodiastolic flow reversal in the distal descending aorta also provide clues regarding the extent of ductal shunting, as increasing degrees of retrograde flow are present with larger shunts. A parameter that has been examined by transthoracic imaging to estimate shunt size is the ratio of the areas corresponding to retrograde and forward flows [21]. Although not yet validated for TEE, this may also provide a crude index of shunt magnitude.

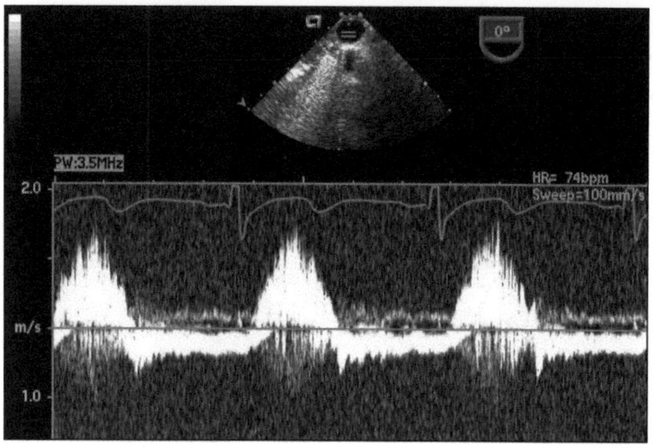

Fig. 13.7 Patent ductus arteriosus. Spectral Doppler interrogation in the mid esophageal descending aortic short axis view demonstrating systolic forward flow as well flow reversal that continues throughout diastole in a patient with a patent ductus arteriosus

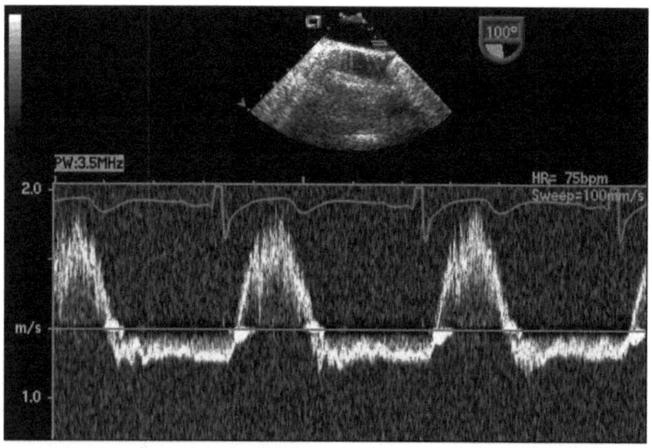

Fig. 13.8 Patent ductus arteriosus. Spectral Doppler tracing obtained by rotating the imaging plane to an orthogonal orientation (mid esophageal descending aorta long axis view) with respect to same patient and probe position as shown in Fig. 13.7. This view provides a more suitable angle for Doppler interrogation and likewise demonstrates holodiastolic flow reversal in the distal descending aorta in association with a patent ductus arteriosus

Estimation of Pulmonary Artery Systolic Pressure from the PDA Jet

The use of Doppler ultrasound facilitates the assessment of systolic pressure gradients between the systemic and pulmonary circulations and estimation of the pulmonary artery systolic pressure (PASP) [22, 23]. This can be accomplished by examining the velocity from the left-to-right jet across the ductus as follows [24]:

$$\text{PASP} = \text{SBP} - 4\text{V}^2$$

V, represents the peak flow velocity (in meters per second) across the ductus in late systole; SBP, systolic blood pressure

Several limitations have been described in the assessment of PASP using this approach [23]. Although they have been reported for transthoracic imaging, these issues are also relevant to TEE. These limitations include potential errors related to position of the spectral sample volume, possible contamination of the continuous wave Doppler signal by flow from adjacent structures, and a PDA shape that does not allow for optimal Doppler cursor alignment for determination of maximal flow velocity, resulting in underestimation of the true pressure drop across the communication. This last issue may be more significant during TEE imaging, as movement of the probe is confined within the esophagus/stomach, in contrast to one's ability to move a transthoracic probe freely across multiple windows to optimize the Doppler evaluation.

Estimation of PASP from the Tricuspid Regurgitant Jet Velocity

Right ventricular systolic pressure (RVSP) also can be estimated from the peak velocity of a tricuspid regurgitant jet, if present (Fig. 13.9, Video 13.4), using the following equation:

$$\text{PASP or RVSP} = 4\text{V}^2 + \text{RAp}(\text{if available})$$

V, represents the peak flow velocity of the tricuspid regurgitant jet (in meters/second); RAp, mean right atrial pressure [25].

In the absence of right ventricular outflow tract obstruction, RVSP equals PASP.

Evaluation of Left Atrial and Left Ventricular Size for Dilation

In the absence of co-existing structural defects, the size of the main pulmonary artery, left atrium, and left ventricle may correlate with the degree of the ductal shunting (Fig. 13.10, Video 13.5).

Additional Applications

The assessment of associated cardiovascular defects (e.g., atrioventricular septal defect, subaortic stenosis) represents the main indication for the use of intraoperative TEE in patients with a PDA. The approach suggested in Chap. 4 for the structural evaluation of the heart by TEE should be followed. Depending upon the nature of the associated defects, suitable TEE planes should be obtained to assess the details of the anatomy. Aspects to be examined as part of a comprehensive examination include (but are not limited to) interrogation of atrioventricular and semilunar valves, outflow tracts, and assessment of ventricular systolic function. However even when evaluation of other defects is the primary objective, the mid and upper esophageal TEE views (as noted above) should still be obtained to evaluate the PDA. Of note, it is good practice to utilize these views on a regular basis whenever a comprehensive study is performed; occasionally one can discover a PDA that had previously been unsuspected.

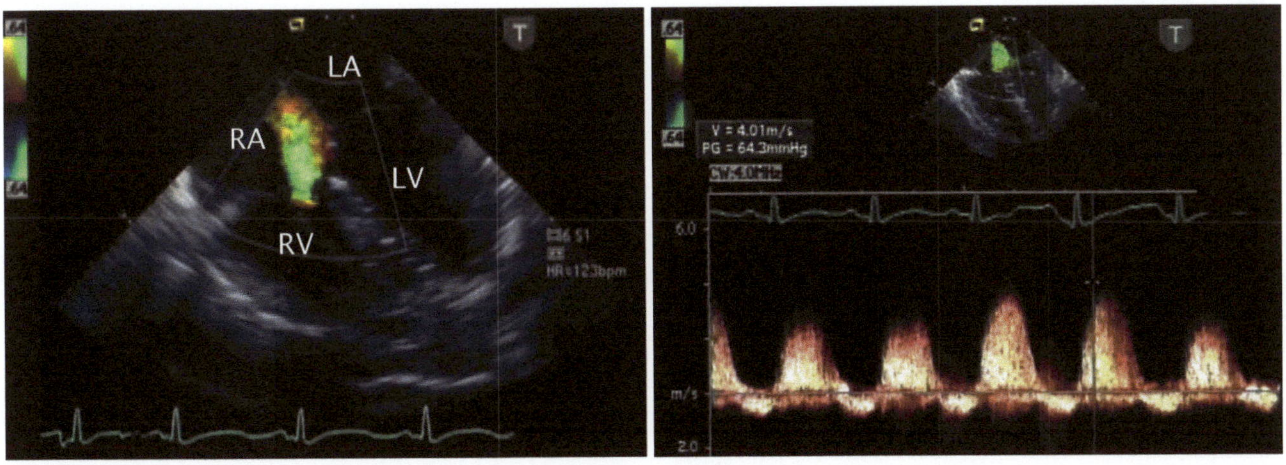

Fig. 13.9 Tricuspid regurgitation. Mid esophageal four chamber view illustrating the jet of tricuspid regurgitation displayed by color flow imaging (*left panel*) and the corresponding spectral Doppler tracing (*right panel*). Note that the peak velocity of the regurgitant jet reaches nearly 4 m/s. The peak velocity predicts an elevated right ventricular and pulmonary artery pressure in this infant. *LA* left atrium, *LV* left ventricle, *RA* right atrium, *RV* right ventricle

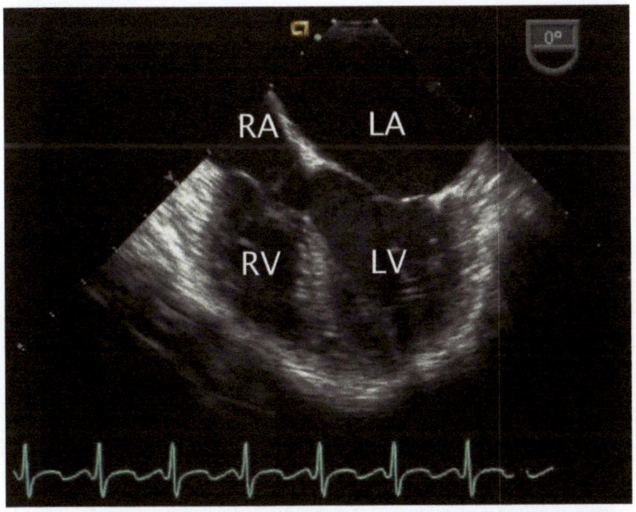

Fig. 13.10 Left heart dilation resulting from a patent ductus arteriosus. Image depicts a mid esophageal four chamber view in a patient with a volume-loaded left heart corresponding to left-to-right ductal level shunting as manifested by dilation of left-sided structures, particularly the left atrium in this case. A tricuspid valve aneurysm is seen. *LA* left atrium, *LV* left ventricle, *RA* right atrium, *RV* right ventricle

Goals of TEE After Catheter or Surgical Intervention

Detection of Residual Ductal Shunting

The magnitude of residual ductal shunting during transcatheter closure or surgery is likely to be relatively small, if at all present. Under these circumstances, a signal representing high velocity, disturbed flow with shunting in the left-to-right direction may be detected in the distal aspect of the main pulmonary artery, near the origin of the left pulmonary artery (in the presence of a left aortic arch).

Additional Applications

Depending on the nature of associated cardiovascular lesions and the catheter-based or surgical intervention(s) performed, TEE should be applied to the post procedure evaluation, as pertinent for the pathology as discussed throughout this textbook.

Aortopulmonary Window

Anatomic Features

Aortopulmonary (AP) window, also referred to as *aortopulmonary septal defect, aortopulmonary fenestration*, and *aorticopulmonary window/septal defect*, is a malformation characterized by a defect in the wall between the ascending aorta and the pulmonary artery, creating a communication between these structures [26]. It is thought to be the result of abnormal development of the AP septum. Anatomically and physiologically, an AP window can resemble a truncus arteriosus; however unlike, truncus arteriosus, two distinct semilunar valves are present. It represents a rare defect, accounting for 0.1 % of all congenital cardiovascular anomalies.

The size and location of the communication can vary related to the extent of faulty partitioning of the AP septum. Mori and colleagues classified the AP window into three types (Fig. 13.11) [27]:

- Type I: found in the proximal aspect of the AP septum, located just above the sinuses of Valsalva; it represents the most common type of the defect (referred to as *proximal defect*)
- Type II: found in the most distal part of the AP septum or most superior aspect of the ascending aorta, adjacent to the right pulmonary artery (referred to as *distal defect*)

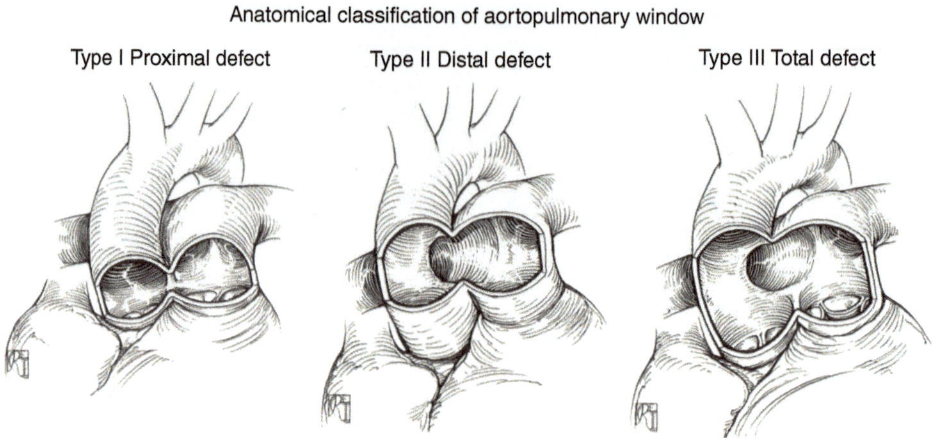

Fig. 13.11 Aortopulmonary window. Classification of aortopulmonary window as per Mori et al. (refer to text) (Reproduced with permission from Gaynor [133])

- Type III: a combination of Types 1 and II, involving the majority of the ascending aorta (referred to as *total defect*)

In a large review of cases, Kutsche and Van Mierop suggested that different developmental mechanisms likely account for the distinct forms of the defect [28]. Their analysis described three morphologic types as follows:

- A defect of small to moderate size with a more or less circular border located at the midpoint between the semilunar valves and pulmonary artery bifurcation
- A similarly located defect in which the border represents a helix
- A usually large defect without posterior (distal) border

Other classification schemes have been reported for anomalies of AP septation [29] and specifically consider the various types of AP windows [30].

Associated Defects

An AP window may occur in isolation, but more than half of the cases are associated with other cardiovascular malformations. Coexistent anomalies include PDA, septal defects at the atrial and/or ventricular levels, tetralogy of Fallot, double outlet right ventricle, type A interrupted aortic arch [31], right aortic arch, anomalous origin of the left coronary artery from the pulmonary artery [32], and coarctation of the aorta.

Pathophysiology

The magnitude of the shunt across an AP window relates to factors such as the size of the defect, pulmonary artery pressures, and relative resistances of the pulmonary and systemic circulations. Left-to-right shunting across the communication results in increased pulmonary blood flow, pulmonary hypertension, left-sided volume overload, and congestive symptoms. This condition is similar to the hemodynamic consequences of any other large abnormal vascular connection such as a PDA. An uncorrected communication can lead to the development of pulmonary vascular disease relatively early in life.

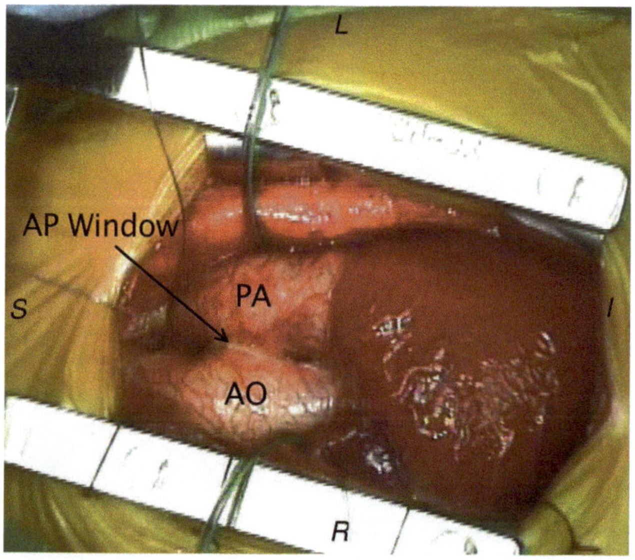

Fig. 13.12 Aortopulmonary window. Intraoperative photograph depicting the anatomical findings of an aortopulmonary (*AP*) window from a surgical perspective. *AO* aorta, *PA* pulmonary artery. *Image orientation*: *I* inferior, *L* left, *R* right, *S* superior

Management Considerations

Although successful transcatheter closure of an AP window has been reported [33–36], the standard treatment for this congenital lesion is considered to be surgical. The approach to this defect has evolved considerably over the years. In the past, simple ligation or division by suture closure was advocated [29, 37]; however, most centers now perform patch closure of the communication, using a median sternotomy and cardiopulmonary bypass (Fig. 13.12) [38, 39].

Applications of Transesophageal Echocardiography

As in many structural defects, the diagnosis of an AP window in the majority of cases is established by TTE alone [40–45]. Recently, the utility of 3D echocardiography has also been reported in the assessment of this anomaly [46].

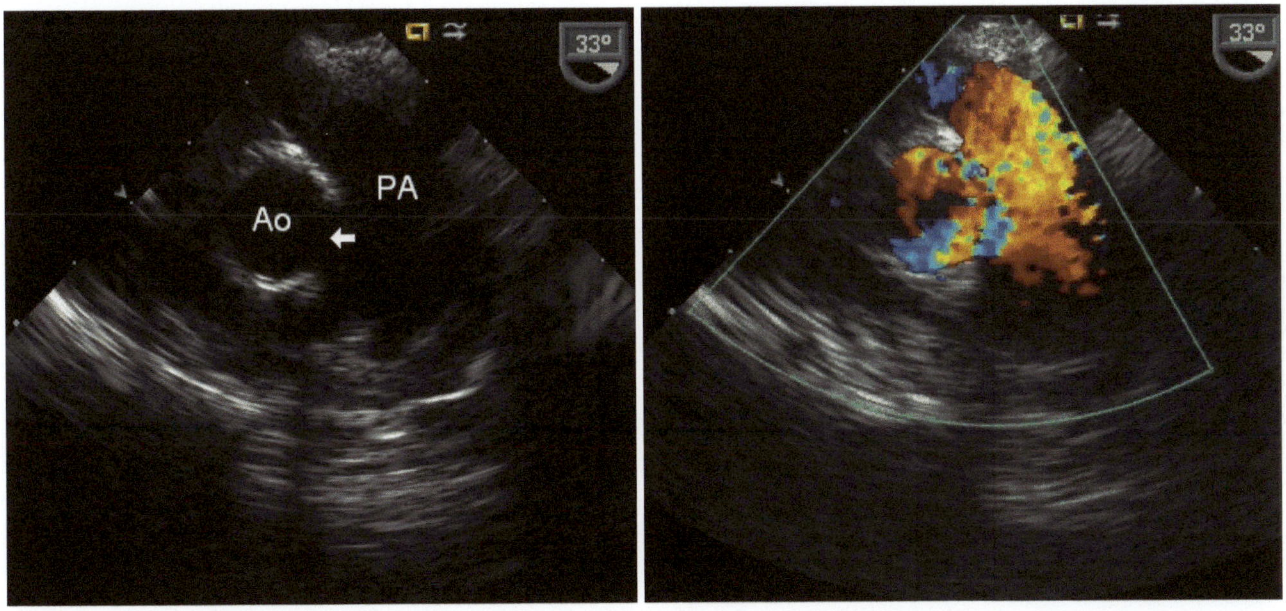

Fig. 13.13 Aortopulmonary window. Mid esophageal ascending aorta short axis view in infant with an aortopulmonary window. Note the echocardiographic drop out in the region between the arterial roots (*arrow*) corresponding to faulty aortopulmonary septation (*left panel*) and shunting across this region by color Doppler (*right panel*). *Ao* aorta, *PA* pulmonary artery

Rarely, additional imaging studies are required to further characterize the defect. TEE has been shown to be of benefit in the perioperative management of patients with AP communications such as an AP window [47].

Goals of TEE Prior to Surgical Intervention

Identification of an AP Window

The AP window is displayed by 2D imaging as a direct communication between the arterial trunks. It appears as a deficiency or absence (echocardiographic "dropout") of the wall normally interposed between the great arteries. The communication is usually large and frequently located along the anterior and leftward aspect of the aorta in the region where the great arteries are normally in apposition. The location and size of the defect, as well as its proximity to the semilunar valves are best evaluated in multiple views. Suggested TEE cross-sections to characterize an AP window are the UE PA LAX, UE Ao Arch SAX, and ME Asc Ao SAX views (Fig. 13.13 **left panel**, Video 13.6). The region of interest is the area of overlap between the great arteries or where they are seen in close proximity. The comprehensive evaluation of this defect may require the use of additional or non-standard TEE imaging planes, as may also be the case with other defects discussed throughout this textbook. For example, from the mid esophageal aortic valve long axis (ME AV LAX), mid esophageal long axis (ME LAX), mid esophageal ascending aortic long axis (ME Asc Ao LAX), and their respective modified views, the probe can be withdrawn slowly and sweeps performed by rotating the transducer in clockwise and counterclockwise fashions to display

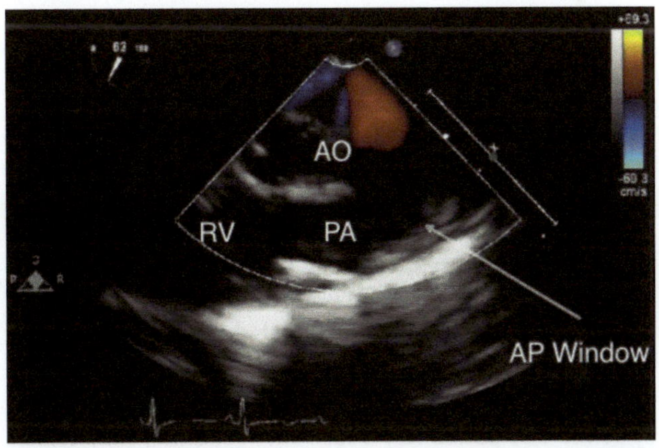

Fig. 13.14 Aortopulmonary window. View of the ascending aorta obtained at the upper esophageal level depicting an aortopulmonary (*AP*) window (*arrow*). *AO* aorta, *PA* pulmonary artery, *RV* right ventricle

the great arteries and the communication (Fig. 13.14, Video 13.7). The deep transgastric long axis (DTG LAX) and sagittal (DTG Sagittal) views, as well as modified respective views that display the great arteries as they cross each other, provide complementary information. It is important to note that an AP window would represent an extremely rare new finding on TEE; therefore, when a presumptive AP window has been identified for the first time on a TEE study, it is important to exclude potential diagnostic pitfalls that can mimic this defect, such as false echocardiographic dropouts in this region. Confirmatory information should be obtained, as discussed below.

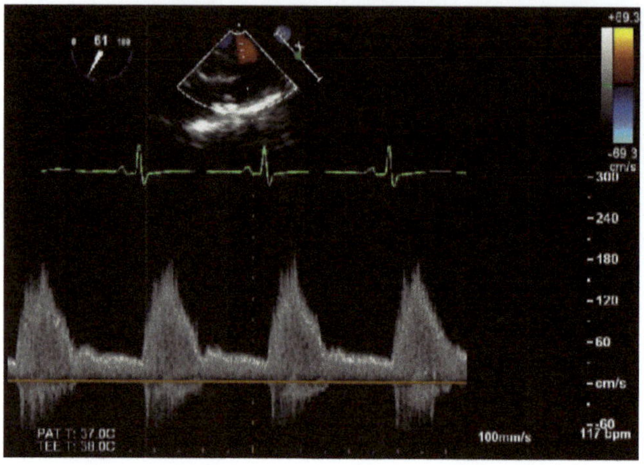

Fig. 13.15 Aortopulmonary window. Spectral Doppler tracing obtained in the same patient and same view as shown in Fig. 13.14. Note the systolic flow and continuous forward flow during diastole into the pulmonary artery

Characterization of Shunting Across AP Window

Color Doppler plays a very important role in the echocardiographic evaluation of an AP window. It verifies and characterizes the flow across the communication, providing qualitative information regarding shunt direction and magnitude. The same TEE views described in the identification of the defect can be used for this evaluation (Fig. 13.13 **right panel**, Videos 13.6 and 13.7). The spectral Doppler examination demonstrates antegrade continuous forward flow into the pulmonary artery near the area of the defect (Fig. 13.15). The presence of pulmonary hypertension at or near systemic levels is the norm for most large defects. In this case, low velocity, laminar, bidirectional (predominantly left-to-right) shunting across the communication reflects the negligible systolic pressure gradient between the systemic and pulmonary beds. This condition may render the identification of shunting somewhat difficult. Adjustment of the Nyquist limit for the color Doppler scale enhances the detection of low velocity flows and can be used to facilitate the detection of shunting across the communication. It is important to distinguish the low velocity color flow signal across an AP window from the "bleeding" of color flow sometimes seen across the walls of the aorta and pulmonary artery in a normal heart. Interrogation of the ascending aorta near the communication or of the descending thoracic aorta may display diastolic flow reversal in the presence of low pulmonary vascular resistance. It is similar to the nature of descending aortic flow in a moderate to large-sized PDA, and serves as indirect evidence of the presence of an AP communication, although it is not specific of the type. Smaller, restrictive defects can display a turbulent color flow Doppler pattern that corresponds to high velocity, continuous left-to-right shunting across the area.

Estimation of Pulmonary Artery Systolic Pressure

As indicated, flow across large communications displays low velocity consistent with elevated pulmonary artery pressures. Smaller defects result in pressure restriction, displaying flow aliasing (mosaic pattern) by color Doppler and high velocity flow by spectral Doppler. The peak velocity of the continuous wave Doppler signal can be used to estimate PASP (as described for a PDA). The peak velocity of the tricuspid regurgitant jet, if present, can also be applied to estimate RVSP, as noted previously. Additional findings that may provide insight into the extent of pulmonary artery pressure elevation include: motion and configuration of the interventricular septum, right ventricular wall thickness, and degree of right ventricular dilation.

Additional Applications

Depending on the presence of associated defects, additional aspects of the anatomy should be examined using corresponding TEE views as necessary. The hemodynamic effects of the volume load result in dilation of the pulmonary arteries and left-sided cardiac structures. The nature of the runoff associated with an AP window may result in low systemic diastolic pressures, low coronary perfusion pressures, and the potential for coronary ischemia and/or myocardial dysfunction. Thus, it is essential to assess both global and segmental left ventricular systolic function in the preoperative evaluation. This assessment is best performed in the transgastric mid short axis (TG Mid SAX), transgastric basal short axis (TG Basal SAX), transgastric two chamber (TG 2 Ch), mid esophageal four chamber (ME 4 Ch), mid esophageal two chamber (ME 2 Ch), and ME LAX views (also refer to Chap. 5).

Intraoperative Monitoring

In rare cases, depending upon the location of the AP window and other factors such as the size and length of the communication, consideration may be given to using a surgical approach that obliterates the communication without the need for cardiopulmonary bypass. In this setting, TEE is valuable for intraoperative monitoring and assessing the results of surgery. In addition, TEE is extremely useful for evaluating global and segmental ventricular function as well as left ventricular preload, and also for excluding the presence of intracardiac/intravascular air.

Goals of TEE After Surgical Intervention

Assessment of the Repair

Obliteration of the abnormal AP connection in most cases requires patch closure (Fig. 13.16, Video 13.8). The post-repair TEE assessment should explore potential residual shunting and patency of the arterial roots to exclude

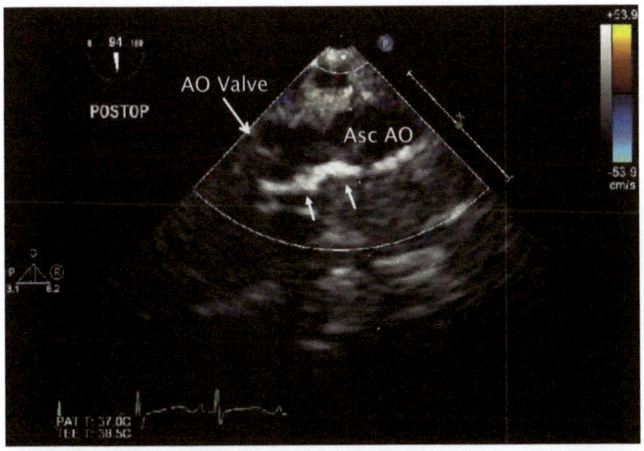

Fig. 13.16 Aortopulmonary window. Postoperative transesophageal echocardiogram in the mid esophageal ascending aortic long axis view depicts the bright region along the wall of the ascending aorta (*Asc AO*) by two-dimensional imaging corresponding to the pericardial patch (*arrows*) utilized to close the aortopulmonary defect in the patient depicted in Figs. 13.14 and 13.15. *AO* aortic

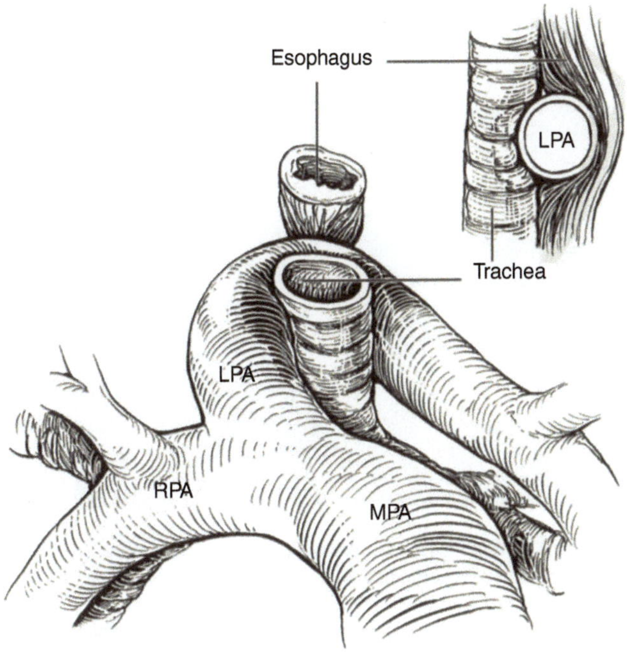

Fig. 13.17 Pulmonary artery sling. Graphic depiction of a pulmonary artery sling. *LPA* left pulmonary artery, *MPA* main pulmonary artery, *RPA* right pulmonary artery. *Inset*, lateral view of anterior compression of esophagus (Reproduced with permission from Backer et al. [134])

obstruction of either the aorta or pulmonary artery. This represents the primary reason for morbidity in this lesion [48]. Semilunar valve competence also should be examined, as regurgitation can result from the repair, particularly if the AP window is proximally located near the semilunar valves.

Additional Applications

The adequacy of the surgical intervention with regard to coexistent lesions should also be examined thoroughly, as well as other relevant aspects of any postbypass evaluation (e.g., ventricular systolic function, atrioventricular and semilunar valve regurgitation).

Anomalies of the Branch Pulmonary Arteries

Anomalous Origin of the Left Pulmonary Artery from the Right Pulmonary Artery

Anatomic Features

In this vascular anomaly, also referred to as a *pulmonary artery sling* [49], the left pulmonary artery originates abnormally from the proximal right pulmonary artery [50]. The course of the left pulmonary artery is such that it arises from the posterior aspect of the right pulmonary artery, crosses above the right mainstem bronchus, and travels posteriorly between the trachea and esophagus towards the left hilum (Fig. 13.17). Hypoplasia of the left pulmonary artery often is seen, whereas some degree of dilation of the right pulmonary artery is the norm. The boundaries of the trachea in this setting consist of the main pulmonary artery anteriorly, the left pulmonary artery to the right and posteriorly, and the ductus or ligamentum arteriosum to the left. In contrast to other vascular anomalies such as a double aortic arch or right aortic arch with a left ductus/ligamentum, a pulmonary artery sling, does not represent a true complete anatomic ring. However, this lesion is frequently considered within the context of vascular anomalies causing a ring. The pathology is attributed to a developmental malformation, although several instances have been reported in patients with a relatively recently described genetic syndrome (Mowat-Wilson) [51, 52].

Associated Defects

A significant number of patients with this malformation (more than 50 %) have complete tracheal rings and/or other tracheobronchial abnormalities (Fig. 13.18) [53, 54]. This condition is associated with tracheal narrowing, and, if significant, the stenosis can result in airway obstruction [53, 55–57]. Tracheomalacia is present in nearly all patients. Additional cardiovascular pathology also is a frequent finding. The most commonly associated defects include intracardiac communications at either the atrial or ventricular levels, PDA, and tetralogy of Fallot [57–59]. Other extracardiac abnormalities, such as hypoplasia and agenesis of the right lung, have also been reported [53].

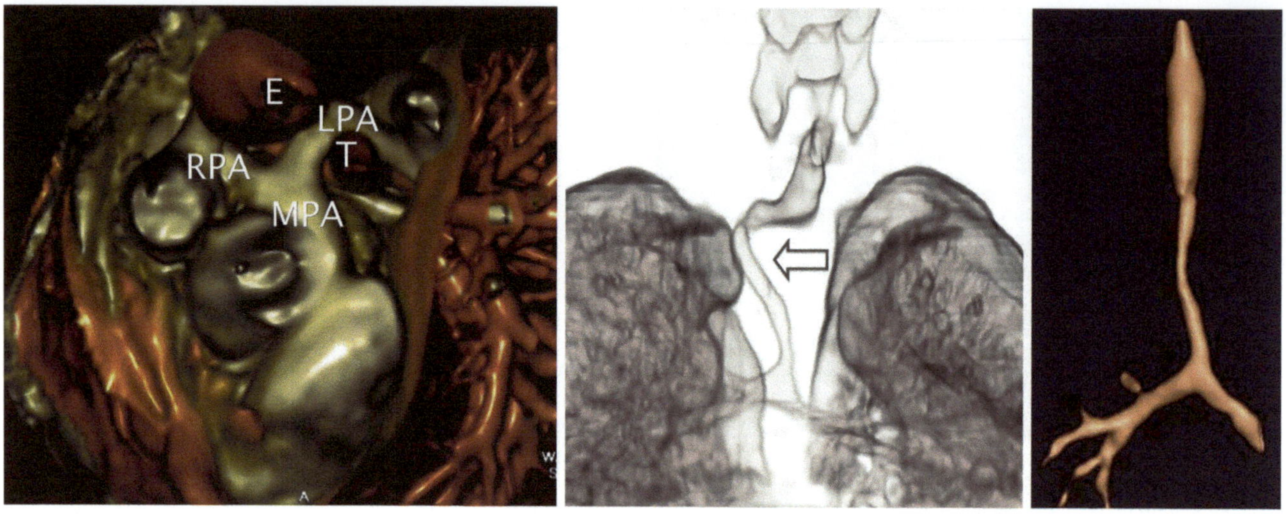

Fig. 13.18 Pulmonary artery sling. Three-dimensional rendered images obtained by computed tomography in a patient with anomalous origin of the left pulmonary artery from the right pulmonary artery. *Left panel*, anomalous left pulmonary artery (*LPA*) as it arises from the posterior aspect of the right pulmonary artery (*RPA*) and courses behind the trachea (*T*) and anterior to the esophagus (*E*) to reach the left hilum. Examples of associated tracheobronchial anomalies that can be seen in this vascular anomaly include a "corkscrew-type" (*arrow*) deformity (*middle panel*) and complete tracheal rings with absence of the membranous trachea causing airway narrowing (*right panel*). Both of these entities frequently result in airway compromise. *MPA* main pulmonary artery (Images by courtesy of Rajesh Krishnamurthy, MD)

Pathophysiology

Although a pulmonary artery sling may present as an incidental finding, the unusual course of the anomalous vessel behind the trachea or right bronchus frequently leads to distortion of the tracheobronchial tree, airway compression, and respiratory symptoms in early infancy. The airway compromise occurs regardless of the presence of associated congenital tracheal stenosis. In some cases, the anomalous left pulmonary artery displays stenosis and/or hypoplasia. The clinical manifestation of this defect can be influenced significantly by the presence of coexistent anomalies.

Management Considerations

The high incidence of tracheal anomalies in this lesion requires comprehensive airway assessment to formulate suitable management plans [53, 60]. The surgical approach in most cases consists of left pulmonary artery division and reimplantation into the main pulmonary artery, allowing for the vessel to be positioned anterior to the trachea. This procedure is now accomplished at most centers via a median sternotomy approach using cardiopulmonary bypass [53, 61]. Concomitant repair of tracheal stenosis and associated intracardiac anomalies is performed as indicated [62–65]. If short-segment tracheal stenosis is present, resection of the involved region is performed; while the trachea is divided, the left pulmonary artery can be translocated anterior to the trachea, obviating the need for surgical division and left pulmonary artery reimplantation.

Applications of Transesophageal Echocardiography

In addition to TTE, other imaging modalities such as chest CT scanning and MRI play important roles in identifying and defining the details of the anatomy in the patient with a pulmonary artery sling prior to surgical intervention [54, 60, 66–74]. At the same time, these additional imaging studies allow for the airway to be examined. The characteristic finding is that of the abnormal origin and course of the vessel. Depending on the particular diagnostic study, an anterior indentation of the esophagus is seen, in contrast to other types of vascular rings, which produce a posterior indentation of the esophagus.

Because of concerns related to frequently associated airway pathology and potential for respiratory decompensation due to esophageal instrumentation, serious consideration of the risk-benefit ratio should be given prior to the use of TEE in affected patients, particularly considering that the anatomic abnormalities usually have been thoroughly outlined. Epicardial imaging should be considered a potentially safer alternative in this case. Another reason for hesitation relates to possible alterations in pulmonary blood flow caused by vascular compression of the anomalous vessel, which can be impinged between the trachea and the esophageal probe. All these factors have discouraged the routine use of TEE in this anomaly and likely account for the limited experience. The discussion that follows highlights known or potential applications of TEE when used in this setting.

Goals of TEE Prior to Surgical Intervention

Characterization of the Anomaly

TEE can confirm or refine the preoperative diagnosis in patients undergoing surgical repair of a pulmonary sling, particularly if concomitant defects are present. The ME Asc Ao SAX and UE PA LAX views using sweeps of the imaging plane obtained by clockwise-counterclockwise rotation

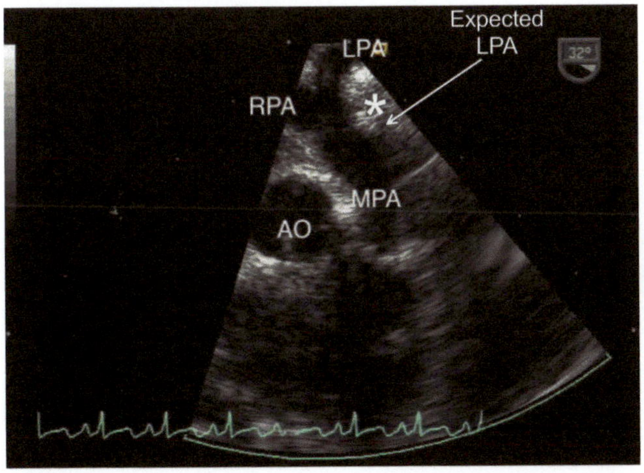

Fig. 13.19 Pulmonary artery sling. Upper esophageal pulmonary artery long axis view of a pulmonary artery sling. The image demonstrates the abnormal takeoff of the left pulmonary artery (*LPA*) from the right pulmonary artery (*RPA*). Note the lack of a normal main pulmonary artery bifurcation that typically would occur more proximally relative to the pulmonary valve (approximate expected site of normal LPA origin noted). The anomalous course of the LPA with respect to the trachea (*white asterisk*) is shown. *AO* aorta, *MPA* main pulmonary artery

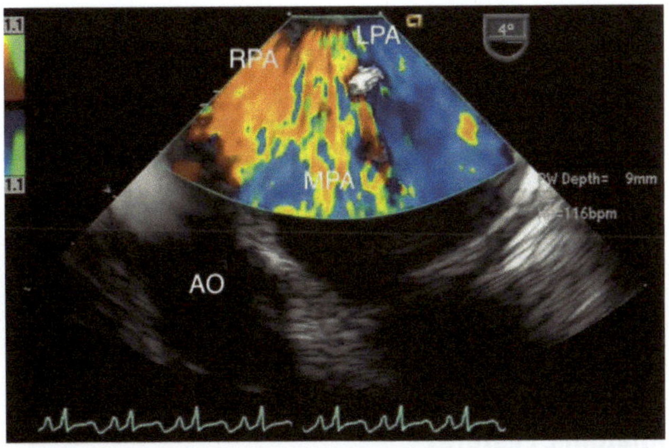

Fig. 13.20 Pulmonary artery sling. Color Doppler image of the same cross-section depicted in Fig. 13.19 obtained in a zoom mode. Note flow into the left pulmonary artery (*LPA*) as it arises from the right pulmonary artery (*RPA*). *AO* aorta, *MPA* main pulmonary artery

to visualize the main and branch pulmonary arteries should display the vascular anomaly. In this interrogation, only the right pulmonary artery origin from the main pulmonary artery is visualized if one scans proximally, in contrast to the normal pulmonary artery bifurcation. If the right pulmonary artery is examined slightly more distally, the origin of the left pulmonary artery might be seen posteriorly (Fig. 13.19, Video 13.9). Although the pulmonary artery bifurcation may appear to have moved rightwards, this finding should not be interpreted as normal. The 2D examination should allow for measurements to be made of the pulmonary arteries to assess for the degree of vessel dilation, stenosis, or possible associated hypoplasia. Doppler interrogation using spectral and color flow modalities facilitates characterization of the anomaly (Fig. 13.20, Video 13.10). In addition to the cross-sections described above, deep transgastric imaging (DTG LAX and DTG Sagittal views) may on occasion assist in the evaluation of a vascular sling, particularly if scanning sweeps are performed.

The findings in a pulmonary artery sling should not to be confused with those of an early takeoff of the right upper lobe pulmonary artery or other vascular anomalies in which the left pulmonary artery originates from the systemic circulation (to be discussed in the section that follows). The demonstration of the origin and course of the left pulmonary artery is essential in this distinction. On TTE, a PDA or left atrial appendage can be mistaken for a normal pulmonary artery, leading to a diagnostic error [67], and it may also confound the TEE evaluation. Partial forms of pulmonary artery sling have been described in which the left pulmonary artery arises from the bifurcation normally, but one of the left lobar branches originates from the right pulmonary artery and courses in anomalous fashion similar to that of the classic form of pulmonary artery sling [75, 76]. This lesion has been identified by transthoracic imaging and, although not yet documented, TEE may also be able to assist in the characterization of this malformation. The finding of a 'normal bifurcation' in this defect may also confound the examination of a partial sling if the echocardiographer is not familiar with this anomaly and the more distal right pulmonary artery is not examined to identify the anomalous origin of the lobar branch.

TEE has been shown to be of benefit in the identification of the abnormal origin and unusual path of the left pulmonary artery in this lesion, but some limitations have been identified [77]. Although color Doppler echocardiography enhances the assessment, the origin of an anomalous vessel or entire course behind the trachea may not be readily delineated, even using the combination of standard and modified scanning planes. Spectral Doppler can be used to provide information regarding severity of pulmonary artery obstruction if present. The caveat to this approach is that optimal beam alignment may not be feasible, and the severity of the obstruction can be underestimated if flow to the distal pulmonary vascular bed is limited.

Additional Applications

TEE in this setting is of value in the evaluation of associated defects (such as tetralogy of Fallot) and for intraoperative monitoring [78].

Goals of TEE After Surgical Intervention

Postsurgical Assessment

If TEE is used, the postoperative study should assess the repair by examining the anastomotic connection of the left pulmonary artery to the main pulmonary artery and the nature of blood flow across the corresponding site. This assessment is important considering that tension can be created at this site or a left pulmonary arterioplasty may be required to address associated branch hypoplasia. The results of additional surgical interventions for coexistent defects should also be examined.

Anomalous Origin of a Branch Pulmonary Artery from the Aorta

Anatomic Features

Anomalous origin of a branch pulmonary artery branch from the aorta is a rare congenital malformation. In this anomaly, a main pulmonary segment arises normally from the right ventricle, but only one branch emerges from the pulmonary artery confluence, and the controlateral branch originates from the ascending aorta, resulting in discontinuity between the pulmonary arteries.

Several theories have been proposed to explain the developmental alterations leading to this anomaly, but no consensus has been reached [79–81]. Although this malformation has also been referred to as *hemitruncus*, anatomically it should be distinguished from truncus arteriosus because, in contrast to a single semilunar valve, two semilunar valves are present in this setting. This anomaly represents less than 0.1 % of all CHD.

Although the anomaly described above of an aortic origin of a branch pulmonary artery represents the most common form of this lesion [82], the anomalous vessel can originate elsewhere [83]. In some cases, the pulmonary artery originates from unusual locations, particularly in the context of complex cardiovascular malformations [84]. It has been proposed that proximal anomalous origin of a pulmonary artery from the ascending aorta and anomalous origin from the innominate artery, also referred to as *absent* or *occult pulmonary artery* [85, 86], are two distinct and separate entities from the standpoint of embryology, clinical presentation, and treatment [87–89].

In a review of the pathologic anatomic features and associated cardiovascular anomalies of patients with anomalous origin of one pulmonary artery, the following observations were made: (1) in most cases, the anomalous origin was that of the right pulmonary artery and (2) the anomalous right pulmonary artery typically arose from the posterior aspect of the ascending aorta in immediate proximity to the aortic valve, or, less commonly, the vessel originated from the lateral aspect of the ascending aorta just proximal to the innominate artery [79]. The anomalous vessel may arise from the left, anterior, or posterior wall of the ascending aorta, innominate/subclavian artery, ductus arteriosus, aortopulmonary collateral vessel, or descending aorta [90].

The discussion that follows focuses primarily on anomalous origin of the pulmonary artery from the ascending aorta, the malformation that most likely benefits from TEE, and briefly addresses related lesions or variants as described above.

Associated Defects

When the right pulmonary artery arises from the ascending aorta, in most instances there is a left aortic arch. In contrast, in the case of an anomalous left pulmonary artery, frequently the arch is right-sided [79]. Associated defects include simple lesions such as a PDA and more complex defects include conotruncal anomalies [91]. Tetralogy of Fallot and aortic arch anomalies have been frequently found in anomalous origin of the left pulmonary artery [79, 90, 92]. Normal cardiac anatomy has been reported in some cases.

Pathophysiology

The clinical features of anomalous origin of a branch pulmonary artery from the ascending aorta usually are those characteristic of pulmonary overcirculation and congestive heart failure [93]. In most infants, evidence of pulmonary hypertension is seen [94]. It is of interest that pulmonary artery pressures are at systemic or suprasystemic levels not only in the bed perfused by the anomalous vessel but also in the controlateral lung supplied by the pulmonary artery that arises from the right ventricle. The rapid development of pulmonary vascular disease, although recognized as a major cause of morbidity in the past [95], rarely occurs in the current era because symptoms prompt medical attention in most affected infants.

If the anomalous pulmonary artery arises near the innominate/subclavian artery, a high incidence of stenosis at the origin of vessel has been observed [82]. If the anomalous vessel has a ductal origin, eventual isolation occurs at the time of ductal closure. The clinical presentation in the latter case varies and may represent an incidental finding in some patients; for example, it may be diagnosed after evaluation of an abnormal chest radiograph in children or it may be identified later in life.

Management Considerations

The management of this malformation depends on the nature of the pathology. If the anomalous vessel arises proximally in the ascending aorta and there is no restriction to blood flow, as is usually the case, early surgical intervention is indicated [91, 94, 96–98]. Primary repair involves reimplantation of the anomalous pulmonary artery into the pulmonary trunk (Fig. 13.21) [90, 99].

If there is evidence of restriction to blood flow and/or associated hypoplasia, or isolation of the vessel, various strategies have been used in order to attempt to 'resuscitate' the anomalous vessel. The main goal is to restore normal antegrade flow to the pulmonary artery [100, 101]. The

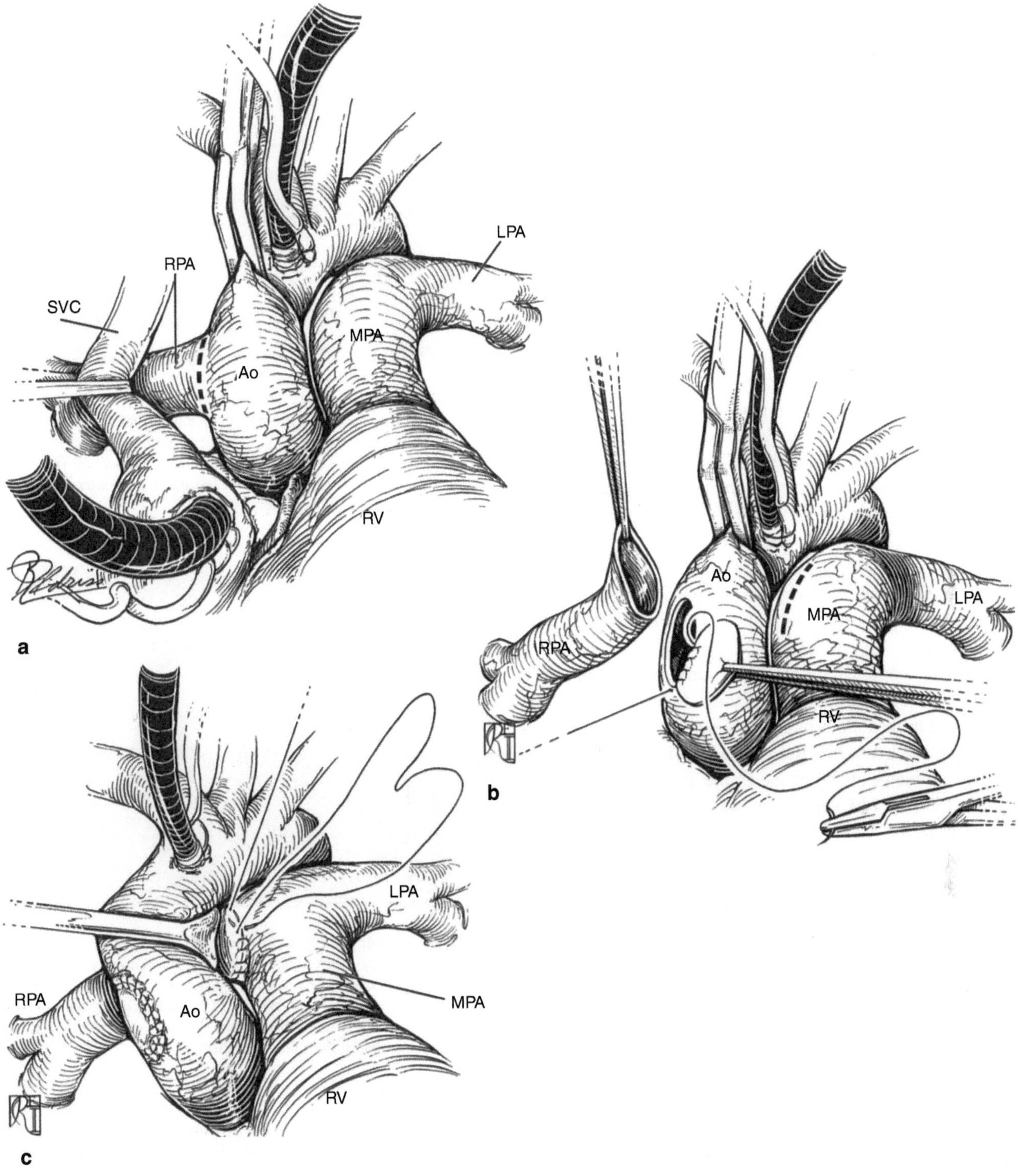

Fig. 13.21 Aortic origin of pulmonary artery. Graphic depiction of surgical repair for aortic origin of right pulmonary artery (RPA). Panel **a** displays the anomaly after cannulation for cardiopulmonary bypass. Panel **b** shows detachment of the RPA from the aorta (Ao) and patch closure of the ensuing wall defect. Panel **c** illustrates the direct anastomosis of the RPA into the main pulmonary artery (MPA) to establish continuity with the left pulmonary artery (LPA). *RV* right ventricle, *SVC* superior vena cava (Reproduced with permission from Gaynor [133])

approach might involve resection of a stenotic segment and/or placement of an interposing aortopulmonary graft to promote growth, followed by eventual takedown of the anomalous vessel and reestablishment of continuity between the pulmonary arteries. In some cases of focal stenosis at the vessel origin, a single-staged approach can be used by resecting the stenotic segment and incorporating the anomalous vessel into the main pulmonary artery.

Applications of Transesophageal Echocardiography

In the classic form of this lesion, the diagnosis usually is established by transthoracic imaging [41, 95, 102]. If the anomalous pulmonary artery cannot be identified by echocardiography, as may be the case in older children with isolation of the aberrant vessel or in adult patients, additional imaging studies are undertaken to confirm the diagnosis and to attempt to delineate the vessel. In some cases, this approach may include cardiac catheterization and angiography [100].

Goals of TEE Prior to Surgical Intervention

Characterization of the Anomaly

In this malformation, 2D TEE demonstrates two distinct outflow tracts and semilunar valves. This condition can be assessed in a combination of planes allowed by the UE PA LAX, mid esophageal aortic valve short axis (ME AV SAX), ME AV LAX, ME LAX, and ME RV In-Out views. In the normal heart, the pulmonary artery bifurcation typically is seen in the ME Asc Ao SAX, UE PA LAX, and transgastric views (Figs. 13.22 and 13.23; Videos 13.11 and 13.12). In the setting of anomalous origin of a pulmonary artery from the ascending aorta, the bifurcation is absent and only a single branch arises from the pulmonary trunk (Fig. 13.24, Video 13.13).

When the anomalous branch originates near the aortic valve or from a relatively proximal site in the aortic root, its origin and immediate proximal course can be demonstrated in the ME AV LAX, ME Asc Ao LAX, ME Asc Ao SAX, or equivalent views if a biplane probe is used (Fig. 13.25, Videos 13.14 and 13.15). In some cases, as the probe is withdrawn from the ME LAX to the ME Asc Ao LAX, a relatively distal origin of an anomalous vessel can be seen (Fig. 13.26, Video 13.16). If the anomalous pulmonary branch originates from the innominate or subclavian arteries or elsewhere, TEE is not adequate to define or characterize the pathology in detail.

The exam is facilitated by color Doppler flow mapping, displaying discontinuity between the pulmonary artery branches and flow from the aorta into the anomalous branch (Fig. 13.26, Video 13.16). Sampling of the aorta distal to the communication demonstrates retrograde flow in diastole, consistent with the runoff physiology.

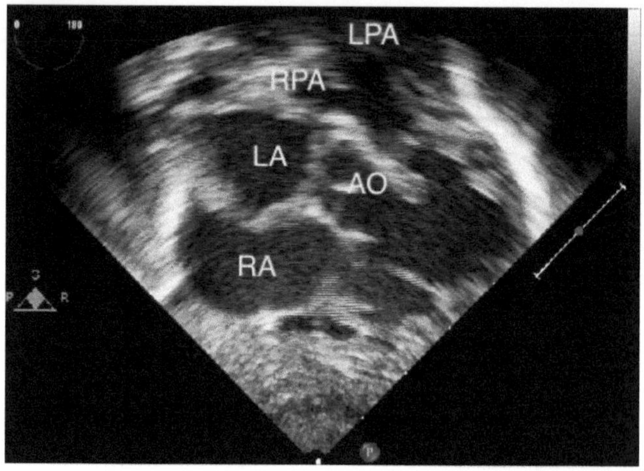

Fig. 13.23 Main pulmonary artery bifurcation. Modified deep transgastric image obtained in an infant with double outlet right ventricle and a subaortic ventricular septal defect to demonstrate the normal main pulmonary artery bifurcation as seen in cross-section from this window. *AO* aorta, *LA* left atrium, *LPA* left pulmonary artery, *RA* right atrium, *RPA* right pulmonary artery

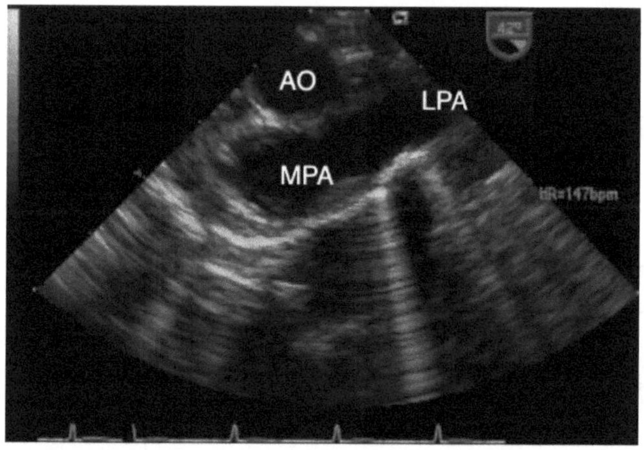

Fig. 13.24 Absent main pulmonary artery bifurcation in aortic origin of right pulmonary artery. Upper esophageal pulmonary artery long axis view displaying the left pulmonary artery (*LPA*) as it arises from the main pulmonary artery (*MPA*). Note the absence of the normal pulmonary artery bifurcation in this patient with anomalous origin of the right pulmonary artery from the aorta (*AO*)

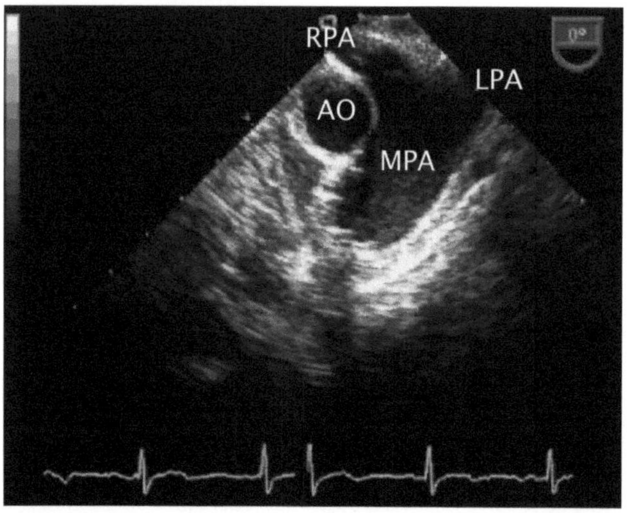

Fig. 13.22 Main pulmonary artery bifurcation. Normal branching of the main pulmonary artery (*MPA*) into the right (*RPA*) and left (*LPA*) pulmonary arteries as imaged from the upper esophageal pulmonary artery long axis view. *AO* aorta

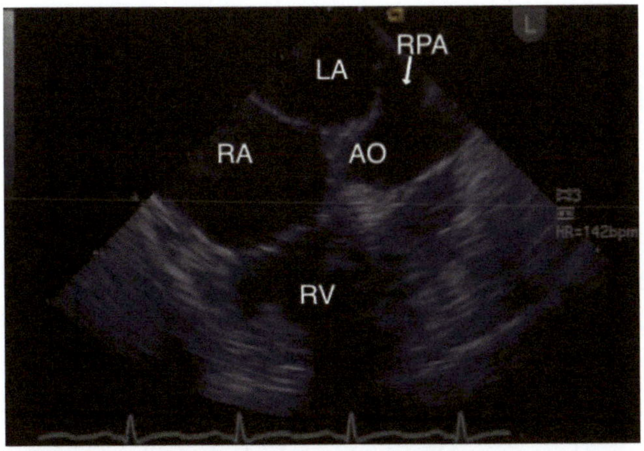

Fig. 13.25 Aortic origin of right pulmonary artery. Image obtained in a long axis plane using a biplane transesophageal probe displaying anomalous origin (*arrow*) of the right pulmonary artery (*RPA*) from the aorta (*AO*). *LA* left atrium, *RA* right atrium, *RV* right ventricle

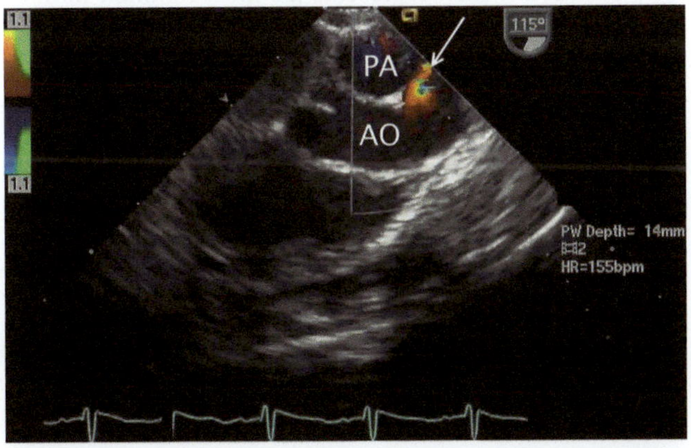

Fig. 13.26 Aortic origin of right pulmonary artery. Mid esophageal ascending aortic long axis view with color Doppler displaying anomalous origin of right pulmonary artery from the ascending aorta (*AO*). Note the more distal origin of the anomalous vessel (*arrow*) as compared to that seen in the patient shown in Fig. 13.25. *PA* main pulmonary artery

The echocardiographic features of anomalous origin of a pulmonary artery from the ascending aorta should be distinguished from those of other lesions. In the case of an AP window, a normal main pulmonary artery bifurcation is present and continuity between the pulmonary arteries is seen. This observation is in contrast to the lack of a pulmonary artery confluence seen when a branch pulmonary artery arises elsewhere. When a pulmonary artery arising anomalously from the aorta is the lone defect, there will still be two arterial roots and two semilunar valves present. This contrasts to truncus arteriosus, in which a single semilunar valve, corresponding to a single arterial root, gives rise to the systemic, pulmonary, and coronary circulations. It is important to remember that discontinuous pulmonary arteries can also exist in the setting of truncus arteriosus, specifically Type A3 of the Van Praagh classification (Chap. 12) in which the right pulmonary artery arises from the truncus arteriosus, but the left pulmonary artery arises from a ductus arteriosus. This underlines the importance of determining whether one or two semilunar valves are present.

Additional Applications

As mentioned, pulmonary hypertension (in both lungs) is a common finding in patients with proximal aortic origin of a branch pulmonary artery. As this is the most frequent variant of this class of defects, the TEE examination should utilize 2D and spectral Doppler to attempt to estimate the pulmonary artery pressures (Fig. 13.9, Video 13.4). This determination can be accomplished by assessing the flow velocities corresponding to the tricuspid or pulmonary regurgitant jets, the gradient across the junction of the aorta and anomalous vessel, the configuration of the interventricular septum, and the thickness of the right ventricular wall. Additional benefits of TEE include intraoperative monitoring and evaluation of associated defects.

Goals of TEE After Surgical Intervention

Postsurgical Assessment

After the anomalous branch pulmonary artery has been reimplanted, the TEE evaluation should focus on 2D imaging and Doppler analysis of the main pulmonary artery, region of newly created confluence, and both branches, particularly the reconstructed anomalous vessel. The same TEE views used for the presurgical examination can be applied. It is important to document patency of the vessel and characterize the nature of the flow both at the site of anastomosis and further distally. If there was significant preoperative pulmonary hypertension, an attempt should be made to reassess the pulmonary artery pressures following surgery, using the methods outlined above. The adequacy of interventions performed for concomitant pathology should also be assessed. All of the standard postoperative monitoring evaluations previously mentioned—such as cardiac function, intracardiac air, ventricular filling—should be carefully performed.

The postoperative assessment can be particularly challenging in the case of a hypoplasic anomalous pulmonary artery. This may be due to factors such as the relatively small size of the vessel, even after arterioplasty, and/or distortion of mediastinal structures due to underdevelopment of the lung parenchyma, that may not allow for optimal 2D imaging. Color Doppler can enhance this examination, although the frequently associated collateral circulation to the corresponding distal pulmonary vasculature can confuse the characterization of flow related to the reconstructed vessel.

Anomalies of the Aortic Arch

When used in patients with aortic arch anomalies, the primary goal of TEE is the evaluation of coexistent defect(s), rather than to focus on the aortic arch pathology itself, because of the limitations of the imaging modality. The difficulty stems from the anterior position of the air-filled trachea relative to the esophagus making the comprehensive examination of the distal ascending aorta and proximal aortic arch challenging, if not impossible. Despite these shortcomings, the discussion that follows highlights the role of TEE in patients with coarctation of the aorta and interrupted aortic arch. Other aortic arch abnormalities/variants are not discussed in this chapter because the applications of TEE for their specific assessment are limited, have not been described, or the use of this imaging approach is considered contraindicated. These anomalies include vascular rings (e.g. double aortic arch), cervical aortic arch, and anomalous origin of a subclavian artery. For these lesions, modalities such as TTE, MRI, chest CT, and angiography are considered diagnostic. In the case of aortic arch laterality variants such as a right aortic arch, although TEE can define/confirm aortic arch sidedness this does not represent a major application of the technology. The branching pattern cannot be well defined due to the fact that the arch vessels are difficult to image adequately and consistently.

Coarctation of the Aorta

Anatomic Features

In coarctation of the aorta (CoA), there is narrowing of the aortic lumen, most frequently in the region of insertion of the ductus arteriosus/ligamentum arteriosum. This defect accounts for 5–8 % of all congenital cardiovascular pathologies and has a higher prevalence in males. The constriction in CoA may take the form of a discrete infolding-like posterior shelf or a diffuse hourglass narrowing of the distal arch. An elongated, narrowed aortic outflow tract is often associated with hypoplasia of the transverse arch and aortic isthmus, in which case other structural cardiac malformations can be present. Thus, CoA is considered to represent a disease spectrum. This malformation occurs in sporadic fashion; however, genetic factors are implicated because CoA is present in more than a third of females with Turner syndrome.

Traditionally, CoA was classified into two types, the preductal (infantile) or postductal (adult) forms (Fig. 13.27). The infantile type of CoA referred to the lesion in the neonate characterized by a long, tubular hypoplastic segment of the aortic arch and large ductus supplying the distal descending aorta. The adult form, presenting after infancy, was described as a shelf-like infolding of the posterior aortic wall into the lumen either at or distal to the ligamentum. This discrete obstructive shelf represents the most common form of this lesion, affecting the region where the isthmus, ductus arteriosus, and descending aorta join together; it is currently referred to as *juxtaductal* CoA.

Associated Defects

CoA may be seen in isolation (with or without PDA), in which case it is referred to as *simple* CoA, or coexisting with other defects, also known as *complex* CoA. Associated malformations include ventricular septal defect(s), bicuspid aortic valve, aortic stenosis, atrioventricular septal defect, double

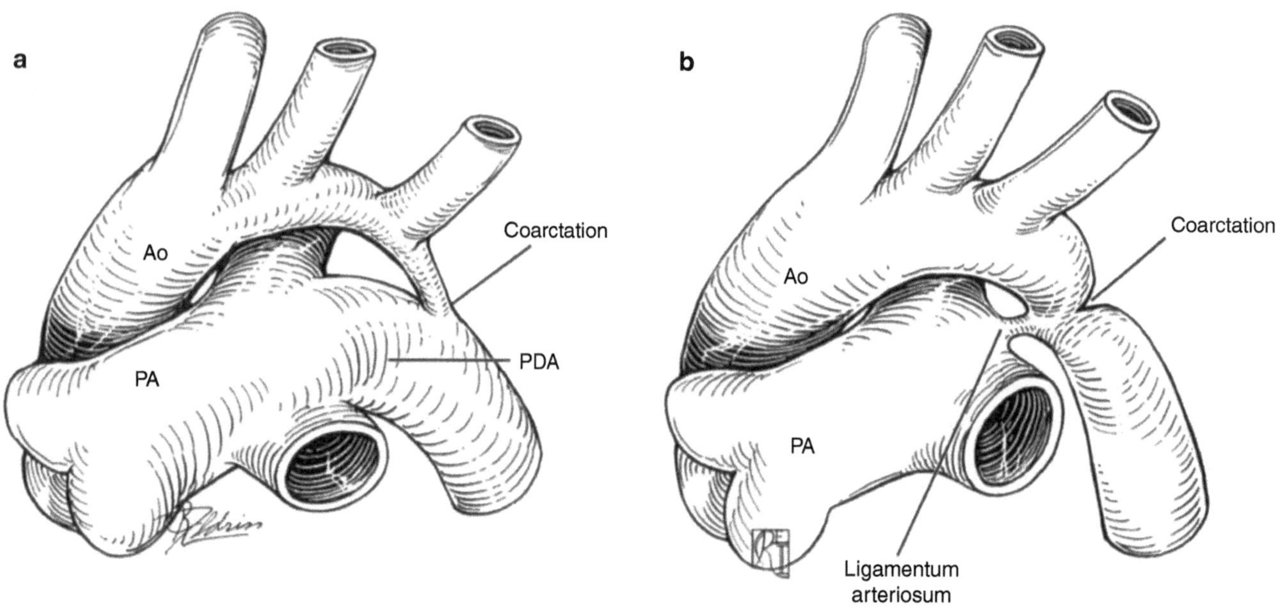

Fig. 13.27 Coarctation of the aorta. Graphic illustration of coarctation of the aorta. (**a**) Infantile, or "preductal", coarctation of the aorta. The patent ductus arteriosus (*PDA*) provides the majority of blood flow to the descending aorta. There is tubular narrowing of the transverse arch and a small aortic isthmus. (**b**) Adult, or "postductal", coarctation of the aorta. The area of narrowing is actually juxtaductal and consists of a prominent posterior ridge projecting into the lumen. The ductus arteriosus has closed and is now a ligamentum arteriosum. *Ao* aorta, *PA* pulmonary artery (Reproduced with permission from Backer et al. [135])

outlet right ventricle, transposition of the great arteries, mitral valve abnormalities, and various other types of left-sided obstructive lesions. Some investigators have proposed that the etiology and pathophysiology of bicuspid aortic valve and CoA are closely related and represent a spectrum of a more generalized arteriopathy rather than discrete pathologies [103]. Dilated aortic root and intracranial aneurysms are known to be associated with coarctation [104]. CoA may also be part of the constellation of defects identified in Shone's complex, characterized in addition by subaortic obstruction, parachute mitral valve, and supravalvar mitral ring [105].

Pathophysiology

The hemodynamic repercussions of this lesion relate to obstruction of systemic blood flow. The main physiologic consequence being that of increased left ventricular afterload and stroke work. The clinical features of patients with CoA vary relative to the timing of presentation (early versus late). An early presentation is considered that in the neonate/infant, whereas a presentation later in life refers to that in childhood, adolescence or adulthood. In the neonatal period, a clinical picture of hemodynamic instability/shock and ductal dependence for systemic blood flow is consistent with a severe or critical CoA. In this setting an element of ventricular dysfunction is frequently present, in many cases, severe. Infants with CoA typically demonstrate evidence of right ventricular dilation and congestive symptoms. Ductal constriction or lack of patency, within the context of severe aortic narrowing, is associated with arterial hypertension proximal to the site of obstruction and an upper to lower extremity blood pressure gradient. In the older child or adult, the diagnosis may follow evaluation for a murmur, upper extremity hypertension, headache, exercise intolerance or leg fatigue. The progressive development of collateral circulation around the region of CoA is typically found with longstanding pathology. In some cases, particularly with significant collateral development, even in the presence of severe aortic arch obstruction, the patient may remain asymptomatic.

Management Considerations

Because the management options in CoA depend on the anatomical features and the presence of coexistent cardiovascular malformations, no single approach is suitable in all patients [106]. Catheter-based interventions consist of balloon angioplasty with or without stent placement. Surgical strategies have evolved over the years and include subclavian flap repair, patch aortoplasty, resection and end-to-end anastomosis, extended end-to-end repair, and aortic arch advancement. The use of prosthetic material such as interposition grafts or extra-anatomical bypass grafts is less favored today, particularly in young children, because of the need for replacement with somatic growth. The optimal strategy for the treatment of native CoA (balloon angioplasty versus surgery) remains a matter of debate.

The surgical approach to alleviate the obstruction in most cases involves a lateral thoracotomy or median sternotomy, depending on the anatomic details and the planned procedure. In regards to the timing of surgery, early interventions are undertaken in neonates with critical disease and more likely in those with associated aortic arch hypoplasia and symptomatic infants; elective procedures are considered in patients with CoA encountered later in life.

Applications of Transesophageal Echocardiography

It is rare that TEE is required for evaluation of an isolated CoA. Imaging modalities such as TTE, MRI, CT, and cardiac catheterization/angiography are better suited to define the site, extent of the aortic narrowing, and severity of obstruction than is TEE. Several case reports have documented the use of TEE in the assessment of CoA; most of these data have been in reference to the adult patient [107–109]. The limited experience indicates that 2D TEE assisted by color and spectral Doppler can aid in the identification and characterization of CoA. Although TEE has been able to recognize some complications related to the native pathology [110] or treatment [111], it has significant limitations [112]. The approaches to this pathology in the cardiac catheterization laboratory are guided by fluoroscopy and angiography; thus, the use of TEE is unlikely in this setting.

Depending upon the surgical approach (thoracotomy versus sternotomy) and the need to address associated defects, TEE may be considered in the patient undergoing CoA repair. If a thoracotomy is planned, TEE rarely is necessary and, if so, its indication is primarily to evaluate ventricular function during the aortic cross-clamp application; however, even then the need for TEE would be unusual. On occasion, if concerns remain regarding the intracardiac anatomy, a TEE examination might be undertaken in the operating room prior to a planned thoracotomy procedure; once the study is completed, the imaging probe often is removed.

If the intervention is performed via a median sternotomy approach, TEE can be used whether the planned intervention is solely to address the CoA or also to repair associated defects. In the former setting, the primary goal of TEE is intraoperative monitoring and, in some cases, reevaluation of the anatomy and hemodynamics of left-sided structures once the distal aortic arch obstruction has been relieved and the ductus has been ligated. If surgery is also undertaken to repair coexistent anomalies, TEE can be applied to the prebypass and postbypass assessments, particularly for ensuring the adequacy of the intervention(s) and for intraoperative monitoring.

The long-term surveillance of complications related to native pathology, residual disease, or problems as a result of catheter or surgical interventions requires imaging modalities other than TEE [113].

Goals of TEE Prior to Surgical Intervention

Evaluation of CoA

As previously noted, despite the limitations of TEE, this modality has been applied in the evaluation of CoA in adult patients. Anatomic and hemodynamic information may be obtained by a combination of multiple planes that display the aorta in long and short axis views [108, 114]. This examination is accomplished by rotating the imaging probe posteriorly behind the heart and advancing the transducer from the upper esophagus to mid esophageal levels. Pertinent cross-sections include the UE Ao Arch SAX, upper esophageal aortic arch long axis (UE Ao Arch LAX), and ME Desc Ao SAX and LAX views (Fig. 13.28, Video 13.17). Sweeps of the TEE imaging probe are also helpful to delineate the anatomy (Fig. 13.29, Video 13.18). Color flow mapping of the descending aorta can display aliasing in the affected region of the thoracic aorta, or identify turbulent, high velocity jets around the area of obstruction. Changes in these flow patterns can be confirmed after the repair is completed. Continuous flow from collateral vessels may also be identified in this region.

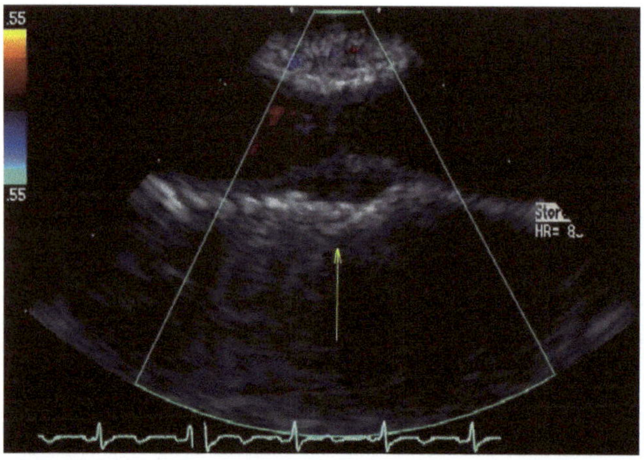

Fig. 13.28 Coarctation of the aorta. Mid esophageal descending aorta long axis view depicting narrowing at the level of the thoracic descending aorta (*arrow*) (Reproduced with permission from Russell et al. [131])

Although optimal alignment of the Doppler beam with the direction of blood flow may not be feasible, precluding an accurate estimation of a peak instantaneous pressure gradient across this region by the simplified Bernoulli equation ($\Delta P = 4V^2$, V = velocity in meters per second), flow acceleration may be detected in this region. A pressure gradient can be obtained across the area of narrowing, with an antegrade spectral flow pattern that extends into diastole, with increasing severity of the obstruction [107]. Blunting of the arterial systolic upstroke and a delay in the mean acceleration rate can also be detected by sampling the descending aorta using the Desc Ao LAX at the level of the abdomen. In some infants a similar evaluation might on occasion be possible using the deep transgastric approach by sampling descending aortic flow at or below the level of the diaphragm.

Characterization and Hemodynamic Assessment of Associated Defects

TEE also can be beneficial in the morphologic and hemodynamic assessment of associated lesions such as a bicuspid aortic valve, ventricular septal defect, left ventricular outflow, or inflow-related pathology [115]. The particular views of interest are dictated by the specific anatomic abnormalities. The reader is referred to other chapters in this textbook that specifically focus on each of the associated pathologies.

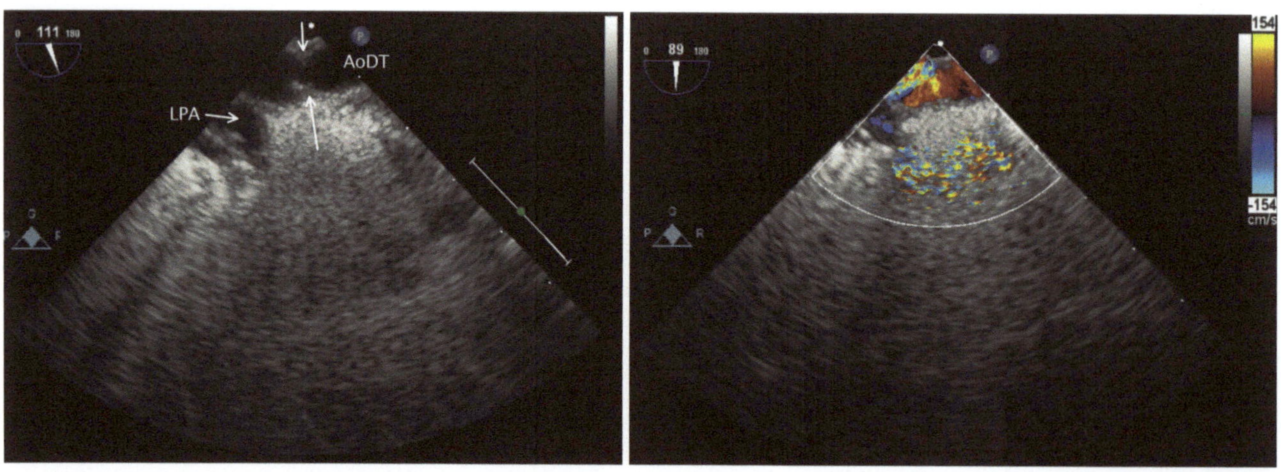

Fig. 13.29 Coarctation of the aorta. *Left panel*, upper esophageal aortic arch short axis view with leftwards transducer rotation demonstrating the descending aorta (*AoDT*) displayed longitudinally as well as the left pulmonary artery (*LPA*). A discrete area of narrowing is noted (*arrows*) corresponding to the area of aortic obstruction. *Right panel*, color Doppler imaging displays turbulent flow across the region of obstruction. These images were obtained in an infant with a ductal-dependent coarctation

Additional Applications

TEE in this setting allows for intraoperative monitoring, evaluation of the left ventricular size and function, estimation of pulmonary artery pressure, and identification of additional anatomic and hemodynamic abnormalities.

Goals of TEE After Surgical Intervention

Postsurgical Assessment

As with the other congenital malformations discussed throughout this textbook, TEE plays an important role in the assessment of the surgical repair, serving to evaluate any hemodynamically significant residual pathology. This should be the focus of the examination. As previously noted, TEE is usually unnecessary for evaluation of aortic arch obstruction alone. However, in postoperative patients with CoA in whom a TEE is performed for evaluation of associated defects, the aortic arch and descending aorta can be investigated both by 2D imaging and color flow Doppler, using TEE views similar to those used in the preoperative evaluation. While these views are not always optimal, they can sometimes provide useful information about the status of the aortic arch/coarctation repair.

Interrupted Aortic Arch

Anatomic Features

Interrupted aortic arch (IAA) is characterized by discontinuity between the proximal and distal segments of the aortic arch. This defect is relatively rare, accounting for less than 1.5 % of all congenital heart defects. The malformation was once thought to result from altered fetal hemodynamics and consequent abnormal development of the aortic arch [116]. The fact that IAA is seen in children with DiGeorge syndrome and related conditions associated with deletions of the chromosome 22q11 [117] has brought into question the theory of fetal hemodynamics and suggested a genetic etiology.

The site of interruption is variable, and as classified by Celoria and Patton [118], may occur at any of three levels as follows (Fig. 13.30):

- In *type A*, the interruption occurs distal to the left subclavian artery at the aortic isthmus. In this case, all the aortic arch vessels are proximal to the interruption, and blood flow in the descending aorta depends on ductal patency. A severe form of aortic coarctation resembles this lesion.
- In *type B*, the interruption occurs at the distal aortic arch between the left common carotid artery and left subclavian artery. It is the most common type of IAA and the one associated with DiGeorge syndrome (at least 15 % of patients).
- In *type C*, the interruption takes place in the proximal aortic arch between the innominate artery (brachiocephalic trunk) and left common carotid artery. This type is quite rare.

Associated Defects

Regardless of the type of interruption, IAA defects are *always* ductal-dependent lesions, thus ductal patency is

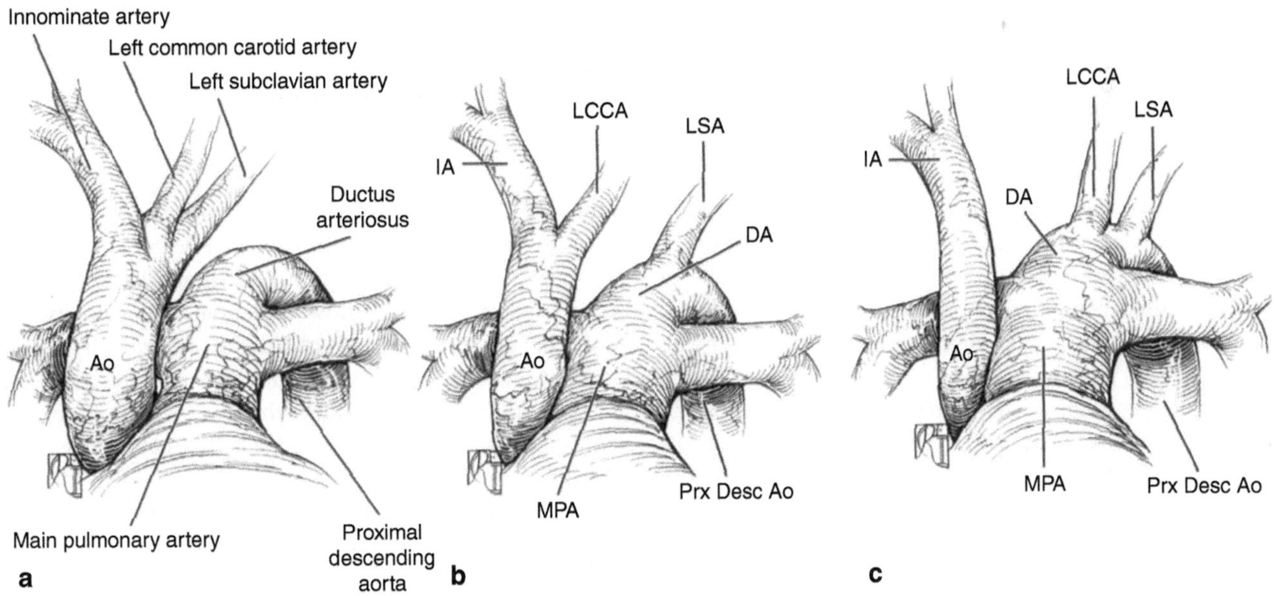

Fig. 13.30 Interrupted aortic arch. Graphic depiction of the various anatomic types of interrupted aortic arch, as described by Celoria and Patton. (**a**) *Type A*, interruption distal to the left subclavian artery. (**b**) *Type B*, interruption between the left carotid and left subclavian arteries. (**c**) *Type C*, interruption between the innominate and left carotid arteries. *Ao* aorta, *DA* ductus arteriosus, *IA* innominate artery, *LCCA* left common carotid artery, *LSA* left subclavian artery, *MPA* main pulmonary artery, *Prx Desc Ao* proximal descending aorta (Reproduced with permission from Jonas [136])

required for perfusion of the descending aorta and any accompanying head and neck vessels arising from the descending aorta. IAA is almost always associated with other intracardiac anomalies such as a ventricular septal defect and subaortic stenosis [119]. A significant number of patients (over 80 %) will have a concomitant ventricular septal defect; this defect is typically large and unrestrictive. The characterization of the ventricular septal defect in this lesion is that of a 'malalignment-type' of defect; the conal (infundibular) or outlet muscular septum is posteriorly deviated relative to the remaining ventricular septum, leading to crowding of the left ventricular outflow tract and resultant variable degrees of subaortic obstruction. It may be present within the context of a bicuspid aortic valve, as well as hypoplasia of the aortic annulus and root. Other important associated lesions include truncus arteriosus, AP, double outlet right ventricle, transposition of the great arteries, and single ventricle malformations. In many of these associated defects, IAA is frequently seen within the context of narrowing or stenosis of the aortic outflow tract; thus the finding of aortic tract narrowing should always prompt a search for arch obstruction/interruption.

An aberrant subclavian artery (arising from the descending thoracic aorta, distal to the PDA) represents a frequent finding in IAA, occurring in approximately 25–30 % of cases [120]. Aortic arch sidedness anomalies can also be seen. In the setting of a left aortic arch, an aberrant subclavian artery, if present, originates distal to the site of interruption as the last vessel (anomalous right subclavian artery). In a right aortic arch, the anomalous subclavian, if present, is the left subclavian artery.

Pathophysiology

The clinical presentation of IAA typically is in the first few days of life. The scenario varies but usually is that of a neonate with respiratory distress, heart failure, cyanosis, or poor cardiac output and impending or overt cardiovascular collapse. Cardiovascular decompensation is the result of ductal closure leading to hypoperfusion of major organs and vascular beds distal to the obstruction. Without treatment, such patients generally expire soon after presentation. Intravenous prostaglandin E_1 therapy is usually necessary to maintain systemic blood flow. In very rare cases, the ductus arteriosus fails to close and patients can survive (clinically undetected) into childhood or beyond.

Management Considerations

The definitive surgical management of this lesion consists of arch reconstruction, at which time associated defects also are addressed [121]. In the current surgical area, the preferred approach is that of a single-stage procedure in the neonate in which aortic continuity is established by end-to-end anastomosis of the proximal and distal arch segments [122, 123]. Patch closure of the ventricular septal defect is accomplished via a transatrial or transpulmonary approach. Depending on the severity of the obstruction, interventions may be required to enlarge the left ventricular outflow tract. This is usually performed by resection of the muscular outlet septum. However in some instances more extensive surgery, such as a Konno-type procedure, Yasui procedure or aortic root replacement, might be necessary to alleviate the subaortic obstruction and/or aortic root hypoplasia [122]. In some patients, the anatomy is not suitable for a biventricular approach and a single ventricle strategy must be undertaken.

Late issues that can lead to morbidity and in some cases require reintervention include outflow tract problems, aortic arch obstruction, and residual intracardiac shunts.

Applications of Transesophageal Echocardiography

In almost all neonates with IAA, TTE provides accurate diagnosis and definition of the anatomic abnormalities, and is sufficient for surgical planning. Occasionally, additional imaging in the form of MRI or chest CT is performed to further delineate the anatomy, particularly details of extracardiac structures such as the aortic arch (sidedness, aberrant subclavian artery, and site of interruption) or associated anomalies [124]. As such, TEE is rarely used strictly for diagnostic evaluation of the great artery abnormalities. However, as is the case with many of the other congenital heart defects discussed in this chapter and throughout this textbook, TEE still plays a significant role in the perioperative setting. Although TEE has limited utility for the assessment of the aortic arch and its reconstruction, it is extremely helpful in the evaluation of the pathologies frequently associated with IAA. These are discussed below.

Goals of TEE Prior to Surgical Intervention

Characterization of the Ventricular Septal Defect

The interventricular communication should be defined in terms of size, location, flow direction, and velocity. In addition, the presence of additional ventricular septal defects should be considered. The approach described in detail in Chap. 9 for the comprehensive evaluation of the ventricular septum is recommended. Particular cross-sections of interest are those allowed by the ME 4 Ch, ME AV SAX, and ME LAX views. The orientation of the outlet septum with respect to the trabecular interventricular septum should be explored to evaluate for potential posterior septal malalignment and concomitant subaortic obstruction. TEE views that allow for this assessment include the ME 4 Ch with probe anteflexion to bring the aorta into view, ME LAX, ME AV LAX, transgastric long axis (TG LAX), and DTG LAX, and DTG Sagittal views (Figs. 13.31, 13.32, and 13.33; Videos 13.19, 13.20, and 13.21). Multiple

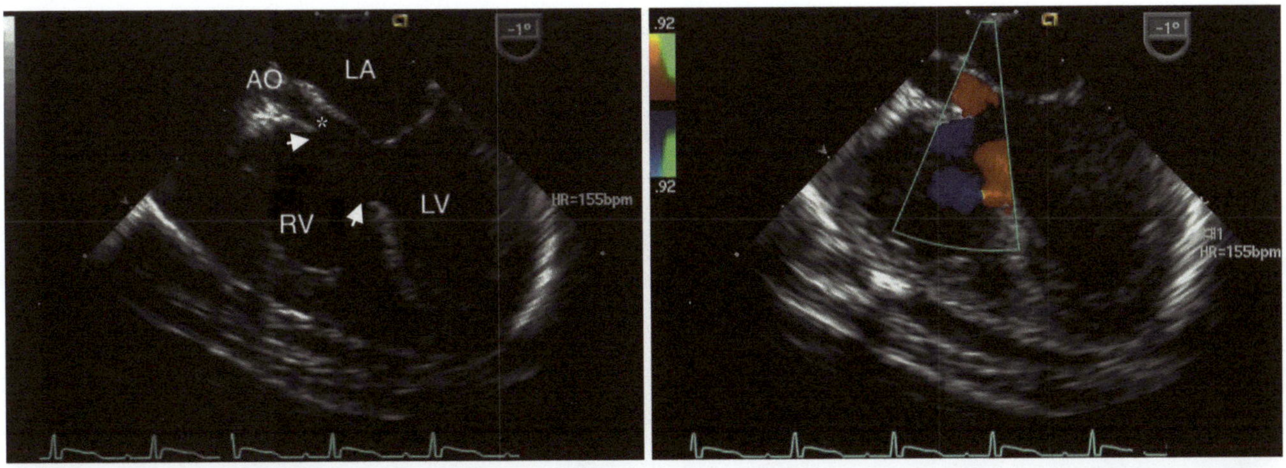

Fig. 13.31 Interrupted aortic arch. Two-dimensional mid esophageal four chamber image (*left panel*) and corresponding color flow mapping (*right panel*) in an infant with interrupted aortic arch demonstrating a large posteriorly malaligned ventricular septal defect as marked by the *arrowheads*. The hypoplastic subaortic region and aortic annulus are also shown (*asterisk*). *AO* aorta, *LA* left atrium, *LV* left ventricle, *RV* right ventricle

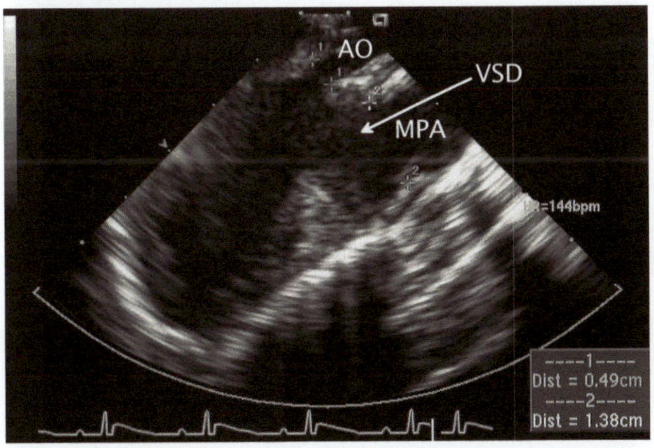

Fig. 13.32 Interrupted aortic arch. Mid esophageal aortic valve long axis view obtained from the same infant as shown in Fig. 13.31, demonstrating the ventricular septal defect (*VSD*) and marked discrepancy in the sizes of the arterial roots. *AO* aorta, *MPA* main pulmonary artery

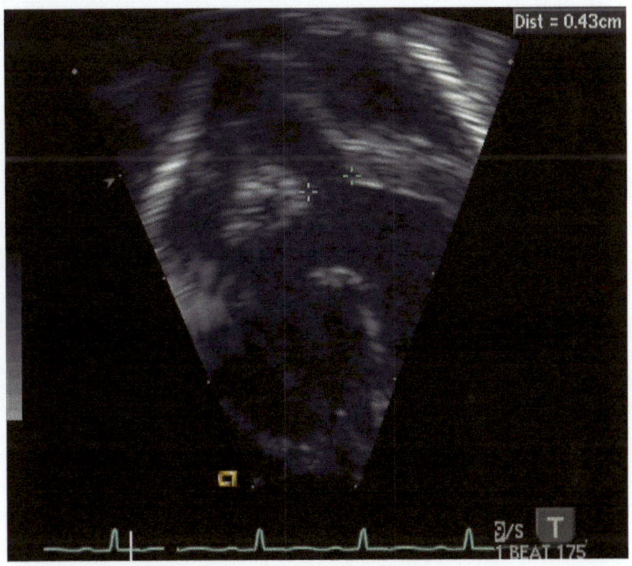

Fig. 13.33 Interrupted aortic arch. Deep transgastric long axis image from infant with interrupted aortic arch demonstrating the ventricular septal defect and subaortic narrowing. The figure indicates measurement of the aortic annulus

sweeps of the ventricular septum are suggested to evaluate the anatomy fully.

Characterization of the Subaortic Region

The left ventricular outflow tract should be fully characterized in terms of size, nature of flow (laminar versus turbulent), and patency. This is best accomplished by a combination of mid esophageal (ME AV LAX, ME LAX) and deep transgastric imaging (Figs. 13.32 and 13.33; Videos 13.20 and 13.21). Doppler interrogation (both pulsed and continuous wave Doppler) should be applied to define the level and severity of an obstruction, if present. The deep transgastric windows provide an optimal angle for spectral Doppler interrogation (Fig. 13.34). This evaluation should include determination of peak and mean velocities for estimation of peak and mean gradients. A caveat to be considered is that flow velocities may underestimate the severity of the obstruction due to: (1) reduced prograde flow across these structures related to the interruption, (2) the presence of left-to-right shunting across the ventricular septal defect, and (3) associated impaired ventricular systolic function. Detailed measurements of the subaortic region, aortic valve annulus, and root should be obtained in multiple views, as this information can impact the surgical intervention and dictate the need for more complex procedures as previously noted (Figs. 13.32 and 13.33). In addition, the information can help to predict left ventricular outflow obstruction after repair of the defect. Parameters that may determine either the likelihood of

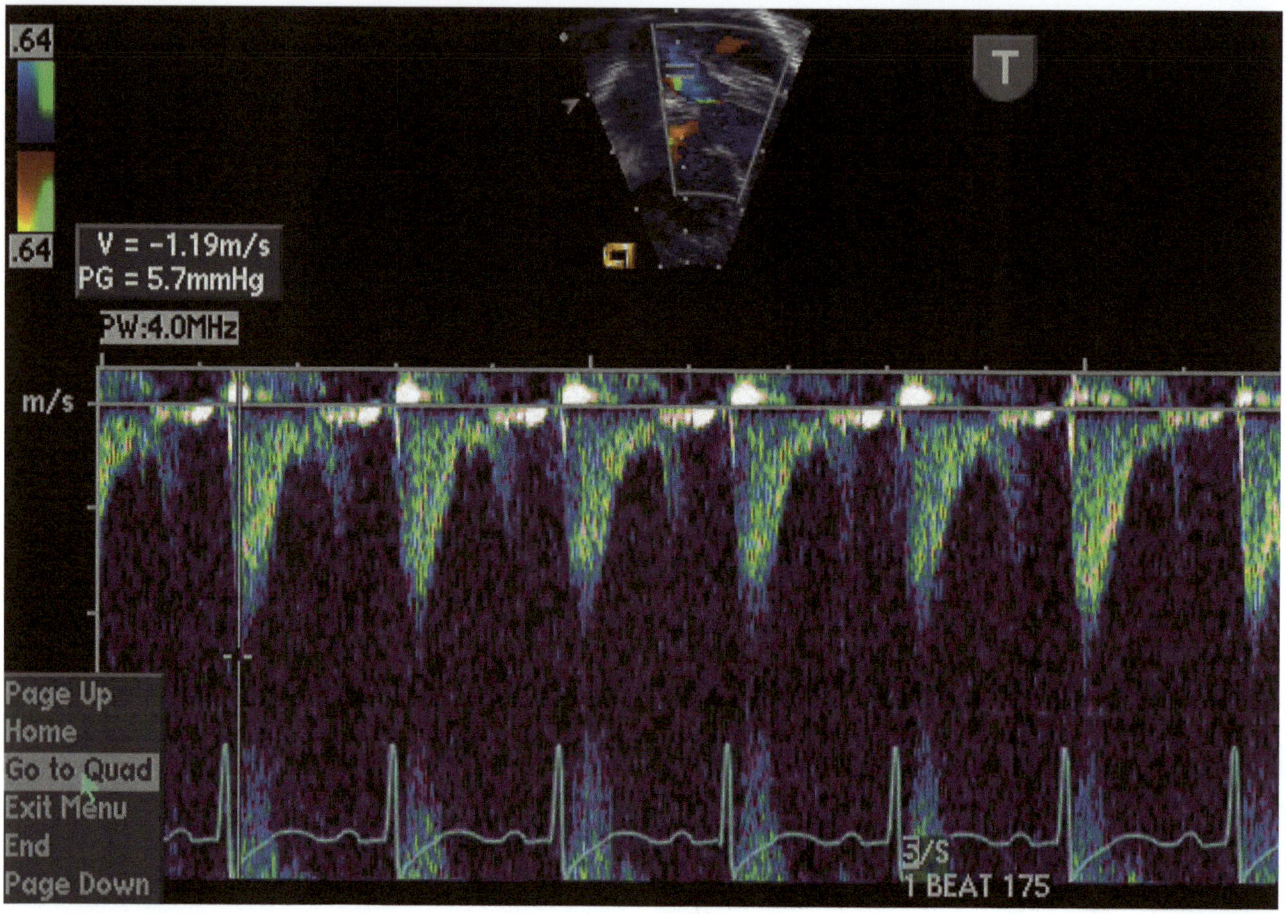

Fig. 13.34 Interrupted aortic arch. Spectral Doppler tracing obtained in the deep transgastric window across the left ventricular outflow tact corresponding to the patient depicted in Fig. 13.33

postoperative subaortic obstruction in IAA (left ventricular outflow tract area <0.7 cm/m^2) or need for a single ventricle strategy (subaortic diameter <3 mm) have been derived from preoperative TTE imaging [125–128]. TEE allows for these measurements to be confirmed and provides further information that could influence the surgical options or predict long-term outcome.

Characterization of the Aortic Valve

The aortic valve should be evaluated to determine morphology, number of cusps, mobility, and competence. The ME AV SAX and LAX, as well as the ME RV In-Out view, are particularly suited for this evaluation. The ME Asc Ao SAX (Video 13.22) and LAX views facilitates the assessment of the ascending aorta. Although pulsed and continuous Doppler analysis allow for determination of flow velocities across the aortic valve, the potentially associated subvalvar narrowing and the presence of an adjacent ventricular septal defect may render this evaluation challenging. As previously noted, these factors could interfere with the assessment of the separate contributions of annular size or concomitant valve pathology to the outflow obstruction. Thus, to a great extent, this determination is qualitative in nature and based primarily on morphologic findings as demonstrated by 2D imaging.

Additional Applications

The prebypass evaluation should include examination of the atrial septum for the presence of a communication, assessment of atrioventricular valve morphology and flows, and baseline determination of ventricular systolic function.

Goals of TEE After Surgical Intervention

Detection of Residual Intracardiac Shunts

The postoperative TEE examination should include 2D and Doppler interrogation for residual VSD patch leaks or other residual shunts at either the atrial or ventricular level (Fig. 13.35, Videos 13.23 and 13.24). The size and direction of blood flow across the communication, as well as hemodynamic significance of any residual intracardiac defect, should be ascertained. The same TEE views described in the preoperative examination should be utilized.

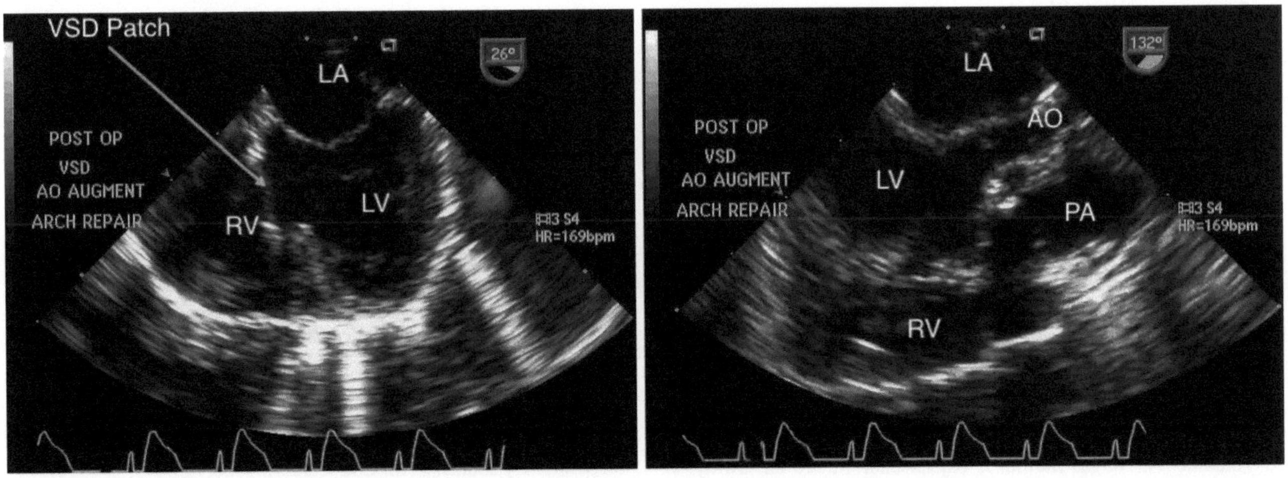

Fig. 13.35 Interrupted aortic arch. Intraoperative images in orthogonal planes (*left* and *right panels*) obtained following aortic arch advancement, subaortic resection, and ventricular septal defect closure in the infant with interrupted aortic arch shown in Figs. 13.31 and 13.32. Note the large pericardial patch across the ventricular septal defect (*VSD patch*) and the relatively small subaortic area, aortic annulus, and aortic root. *AO* aorta, *LA* left ventricle, *LV* left ventricle, *PA* main pulmonary artery, *RV* right ventricle

Assessment of Residual Subaortic Obstruction

In all patients, and particularly in those with concerns regarding left ventricular outflow tract obstruction, a comprehensive multiplane TEE examination should be undertaken after the surgical repair. The same approach applies to the patient undergoing reintervention for residual or recurrent subaortic obstruction in the prebypass and postbypass settings. It is imperative to assess the severity of the left ventricular outflow tract obstruction by both qualitative and quantitative methods (Videos 13.23 and 13.24). The same TEE views used for preoperative 2D evaluation of the subaortic region, and for optimal Doppler assessment, should also be used postoperatively to facilitate this interrogation.

Aortic Arch Evaluation

As with CoA surgery, in some cases portions of the aortic arch and descending aorta can be visualized both by 2D imaging color flow Doppler, using a combination of upper and mid esophageal TEE views (outlined in the CoA section above). Again, while these views are not optimal, they can sometimes provide useful information about the status of the aortic arch repair.

Additional Applications

In the postbypass examination, atrioventricular valve competence and systolic ventricular function should be examined and compared to the preoperative findings (Video 13.25). Patch closure of the VSD may require a radial incision along the tricuspid valve annulus to enhance surgical exposure of the defect. Although on follow-up this intervention has not been associated with tricuspid valve dysfunction [129], the postoperative TEE should evaluate flow across the tricuspid valve to ensure the absence of obstruction and/or regurgitation, or any other changes from the baseline examination. The follow-up assessment and long-term surveillance of aortic arch reconstruction requires modalities other than TEE to exclude recurrent obstruction.

Summary

Congenital anomalies that affect the great arteries and related vascular structures are identified and well defined by noninvasive imaging modalities. High-resolution transthoracic imaging represents the initial, and often the sole, diagnostic approach required to outline medical and surgical management plans in affected patients. In view of limitations related to the TEE imaging approach, which in some cases will not allow adequate or comprehensive definition of vascular structures, the diagnostic role of this modality can be somewhat limited. However, this does not negate the value of TEE in such patients. In the intraoperative setting, TEE may still be able to confirm the presence of abnormal vascular structure(s) or connection(s). Frequently, the malformations that affect the great arteries are associated with coexistent pathology, and not uncommonly these malformations are of a complex nature. TEE facilitates the detailed evaluation of these defects in terms of anatomic and hemodynamic assessment while playing a major role in surgical planning. This imaging modality also provides for intraoperative monitoring, assessment of the adequacy of the surgical intervention(s), and guidance of the revision if required. As such, TEE can provide significant contributions in patients with great artery and other vascular anomalies.

References

1. Knight L, Edwards JE. Right aortic arch. Types and associated cardiac anomalies. Circulation. 1974;50:1047–51.
2. Mugge A, Daniel WG, Lichtlen PR. Imaging of patent ductus arteriosus by transesophageal color-coded Doppler echocardiography. J Clin Ultrasound. 1991;19:128–9.
3. Szulc M, Ritter SB. Patent ductus arteriosus in an infant with atrioventricular septal defect and pulmonary hypertension: diagnosis by transesophageal color flow echocardiography. J Am Soc Echocardiogr. 1991;4:194–8.
4. Takenaka K, Sakamoto T, Shiota T, et al. Diagnosis of patent ductus arteriosus in adults by biplane transesophageal color Doppler flow mapping. Am J Cardiol. 1991;68:691–3.
5. Shyu KG, Lai LP, Lin SC, et al. Diagnostic accuracy of transesophageal echocardiography for detecting patent ductus arteriosus in adolescents and adults. Chest. 1995;108:1201–5.
6. Andrade A, Vargas-Barron J, Rijlaarsdam M, et al. Utility of transesophageal echocardiography in the examination of adult patients with patent ductus arteriosus. Am Heart J. 1995;130:543–6.
7. Krauss D, Weinert L, Lang RM. The role of multiplane transesophageal echocardiography in diagnosing PDA in an adult. Echocardiography. 1996;13:95–8.
8. Chang ST, Hung KC, Hsieh IC, et al. Evaluation of shunt flow by multiplane transesophageal echocardiography in adult patients with isolated patent ductus arteriosus. J Am Soc Echocardiogr. 2002;15:1367–73.
9. Tumbarello R, Sanna A, Cardu G, et al. Usefulness of transesophageal echocardiography in the pediatric catheterization laboratory. Am J Cardiol. 1993;71:1321–5.
10. Chuang YC, Yin WH, Hsiung MC, et al. Successful transcatheter closure of a residual patent ductus arteriosus with complex anatomy after surgical ligation using an amplatzer ductal occluder guided by live three-dimensional transesophageal echocardiography. Echocardiography. 2011;28:E101–3.
11. Marek T, Zelizko M, Kautzner J. Images in cardiovascular medicine. Real-time 3-dimensional transesophageal echocardiography imaging: adult patent ductus arteriosus before and after transcatheter closure. Circulation. 2009;120:e92–3.
12. Wang KY, Hsieh KS, Yang MW, et al. The use of transesophageal echocardiography to evaluate the effectiveness of patent ductus arteriosus ligation. Echocardiography. 1993;10:53–7.
13. Lavoie J, Burrows FA, Gentles TL, et al. Transoesophageal echocardiography detects residual ductal flow during video-assisted thoracoscopic patent ductus arteriosus interruption. Can J Anaesth. 1994;41:310–3.
14. Lavoie J, Javorski JJ, Donahue K, et al. Detection of residual flow by transesophageal echocardiography during video-assisted thoracoscopic patent ductus arteriosus interruption. Anesth Analg. 1995;80:1071–5.
15. Shiota T, Omoto R, Cobanoglu A, et al. Usefulness of transesophageal imaging of flow convergence region in the operating room for evaluating isolated patent ductus arteriosus. Am J Cardiol. 1997;80:1108–12.
16. Ho AC, Tan PP, Yang MW, et al. The use of multiplane transesophageal echocardiography to evaluate residual patent ductus arteriosus during video-assisted thoracoscopy in adults. Surg Endosc. 1999;13:975–9.
17. Hatle L, Anglesen B. Pulsed and continuous wave Doppler in diagnosis and assessment of various heart lesions. In: Hatle L, Anglesen B, editors. Doppler ultrasound in cardiology. Physical principles and clinical applications. Philadelphia: Lea & Febiger; 1985. p. 97–292.
18. Hiraishi S, Horiguchi Y, Misawa H, et al. Noninvasive Doppler echocardiographic evaluation of shunt flow dynamics of the ductus arteriosus. Circulation. 1987;75:1146–53.
19. Cloez JL, Isaaz K, Pernot C. Pulsed Doppler flow characteristics of ductus arteriosus in infants with associated congenital anomalies of the heart or great arteries. Am J Cardiol. 1986;57:845–51.
20. Shiraishi H, Yanagisawa M. Bidirectional flow through the ductus arteriosus in normal newborns: evaluation by Doppler color flow imaging. Pediatr Cardiol. 1991;12:201–5.
21. Serwer GA, Armstrong BE, Anderson PA. Nonivasive detection of retrograde descending aortic flow in infants using continuous wave doppler ultrasonography. Implications for diagnosis of aortic run-off lesions. J Pediatr. 1980;97:394–400.
22. Musewe NN, Smallhorn JF, Benson LN, et al. Validation of Doppler-derived pulmonary arterial pressure in patients with ductus arteriosus under different hemodynamic states. Circulation. 1987;76:1081–91.
23. Snider AR. The ductus arteriosus: a window for assessment of pulmonary artery pressures? J Am Coll Cardiol. 1990;15:457–8.
24. Marx GR, Allen HD, Goldberg SJ. Doppler echocardiographic estimation of systolic pulmonary artery pressure in patients with aortic-pulmonary shunts. J Am Coll Cardiol. 1986;7:880–5.
25. Milan A, Magnino C, Veglio F. Echocardiographic indexes for the non-invasive evaluation of pulmonary hemodynamics. J Am Soc Echocardiogr. 2010;23:225–39; quiz 332–4.
26. Neufeld HN, Lester RG, Adams PJ, et al. Aorticopulmonary septal defect. Am J Cardiol. 1962;9:12–25.
27. Mori K, Ando M, Takao A, et al. Distal type of aortopulmonary window. Report of 4 cases. Br Heart J. 1978;40:681–9.
28. Kutsche LM, Van Mierop LH. Anatomy and pathogenesis of aorticopulmonary septal defect. Am J Cardiol. 1987;59:443–7.
29. Richardson JV, Doty DB, Rossi NP, et al. The spectrum of anomalies of aortopulmonary septation. J Thorac Cardiovasc Surg. 1979; 78:21–7.
30. Ho SY, Gerlis LM, Anderson C, et al. The morphology of aortopulmonary windows with regard to their classification and morphogenesis. Cardiol Young. 1994;4:146–55.
31. Murin P, Sinzobahamvya N, Blaschczok HC, et al. Aortopulmonary window associated with interrupted aortic arch: report of surgical repair of eight cases and review of literature. Thorac Cardiovasc Surg. 2012;60:215–20.
32. Pace Napoleone C, Oppido G, Angeli E, et al. Aortopulmonary window and anomalous coronary artery: an exceptional association. Ann Thorac Surg. 2011;91:1272–4.
33. Stamato T, Benson LN, Smallhorn JF, et al. Transcatheter closure of an aortopulmonary window with a modified double umbrella occluder system. Cathet Cardiovasc Diagn. 1995;35:165–7.
34. Tulloh RM, Rigby ML. Transcatheter umbrella closure of aortopulmonary window. Heart. 1997;77:479–80.
35. Jureidini SB, Spadaro JJ, Rao PS. Successful transcatheter closure with the buttoned device of aortopulmonary window in an adult. Am J Cardiol. 1998;81:371–2.
36. Srivastava A, Radha AS. Transcatheter closure of a large aortopulmonary window with severe pulmonary arterial hypertension beyond infancy. J Invasive Cardiol. 2012;24:E24–6.
37. Doty DB, Richardson JV, Falkovsky GE, et al. Aortopulmonary septal defect: hemodynamics, angiography, and operation. Ann Thorac Surg. 1981;32:244–50.
38. Hew CC, Bacha EA, Zurakowski D, et al. Optimal surgical approach for repair of aortopulmonary window. Cardiol Young. 2001;11:385–90.
39. Jonas RA. Patent ductus arteriosus, aortopulmonary window, sinus of valsalva fistula, aortoventricular tunnel. In: Jonas RA, editor. Comprehensive surgical management of congenital heart disease. New York: Arnold; 2004. p. 195–9.
40. Rice MJ, Seward JB, Hagler DJ, et al. Visualization of aortopulmonary window by two-dimensional echocardiography. Mayo Clin Proc. 1982;57:482–7.
41. Smallhorn JF, Anderson RH, Macartney FJ. Two dimensional echocardiographic assessment of communications between ascending

aorta and pulmonary trunk or individual pulmonary arteries. Br Heart J. 1982;47:563–72.
42. Lau KC, Calcaterra G, Miller GA, et al. Aorto-pulmonary window. J Cardiovasc Surg (Torino). 1982;23:21–7.
43. Alboliras ET, Chin AJ, Barber G, et al. Detection of aortopulmonary window by pulsed and color Doppler echocardiography. Am Heart J. 1988;115:900–2.
44. Balaji S, Burch M, Sullivan ID. Accuracy of cross-sectional echocardiography in diagnosis of aortopulmonary window. Am J Cardiol. 1991;67:650–3.
45. Mahle WT, Kreeger J, Silverman NH. Echocardiography of the aortopulmonary window, aorto-ventricular tunnels, and aneurysm of the sinuses of Valsalva. Cardiol Young. 2010;20 Suppl 3:100–6.
46. Singh A, Mehmood F, Romp RL, et al. Live/Real time three-dimensional transthoracic echocardiographic assessment of aorto-pulmonary window. Echocardiography. 2008;25:96–9.
47. Samdarshi TE, Morrow WR, Nanda NC, et al. Transesophageal echocardiography in aortopulmonary communications. Echocardiography. 1991;8:383–95.
48. Barnes ME, Mitchell ME, Tweddell JS. Aortopulmonary window. Semin Thorac Cardiovasc Surg Pediatr Card Surg Annu. 2011;14:67–74.
49. Contro S, Miller RA, White H, et al. Bronchial obstruction due to pulmonary artery anomalies. I. Vascular sling. Circulation. 1958; 17:418–23.
50. Castaneda AR. Pulmonary artery sling. Ann Thorac Surg. 1979; 28:210–1.
51. Adam MP, Schelley S, Gallagher R, et al. Clinical features and management issues in Mowat-Wilson syndrome. Am J Med Genet A. 2006;140:2730–41.
52. Strenge S, Heinritz W, Zweier C, et al. Pulmonary artery sling and congenital tracheal stenosis in another patient with Mowat-Wilson syndrome. Am J Med Genet A. 2007;143A:1528–30.
53. Backer CL, Russell HM, Kaushal S, et al. Pulmonary artery sling: current results with cardiopulmonary bypass. J Thorac Cardiovasc Surg. 2012;143:144–51.
54. Newman B, Meza MP, Towbin RB, et al. Left pulmonary artery sling: diagnosis and delineation of associated tracheobronchial anomalies with MR. Pediatr Radiol. 1996;26:661–8.
55. Sade RM, Rosenthal A, Fellows K, et al. Pulmonary artery sling. J Thorac Cardiovasc Surg. 1975;69:333–46.
56. Berdon WE, Baker DH, Wung JT, et al. Complete cartilage-ring tracheal stenosis associated with anomalous left pulmonary artery: the ring-sling complex. Radiology. 1984;152:57–64.
57. Gikonyo BM, Jue KL, Edwards JE. Pulmonary vascular sling: report of seven cases and review of the literature. Pediatr Cardiol. 1989;10:81–9.
58. Binet JP, Longlois J. Aortic arch anomalies in children and infants. J Thorac Cardiovasc Surg. 1977;73:248–52.
59. Backer CL. Vascular rings, slings, and tracheal rings. Mayo Clin Proc. 1993;68:1131–3.
60. Zhong YM, Jaffe RB, Zhu M, et al. CT assessment of tracheobronchial anomaly in left pulmonary artery sling. Pediatr Radiol. 2010;40:1755–62.
61. Backer CL, Mavroudis C, Dunham ME, et al. Pulmonary artery sling: results with median sternotomy, cardiopulmonary bypass, and reimplantation. Ann Thorac Surg. 1999;67:1738–44; discussion 1744–5.
62. Jonas RA, Spevak PJ, McGill T, et al. Pulmonary artery sling: primary repair by tracheal resection in infancy. J Thorac Cardiovasc Surg. 1989;97:548–50.
63. Fiore AC, Brown JW, Weber TR, et al. Surgical treatment of pulmonary artery sling and tracheal stenosis. Ann Thorac Surg. 2005; 79:38–46; discussion 38–46.
64. Oshima Y, Yamaguchi M, Yoshimura N, et al. Management of pulmonary artery sling associated with tracheal stenosis. Ann Thorac Surg. 2008;86:1334–8.
65. Huang SC, Wu ET, Wang CC, et al. Surgical management of pulmonary artery sling: trachea diameter and outcomes with or without tracheoplasty. Pediatr Pulmonol. 2012;47:903–8.
66. McCray P, Grandgeorge S, Smith W, et al. Cine CT diagnosis of pulmonary artery sling. Pediatr Radiol. 1986;16:508–10.
67. Yeager SB, Chin AJ, Sanders SP. Two-dimensional echocardiographic diagnosis of pulmonary artery sling in infancy. J Am Coll Cardiol. 1986;7:625–9.
68. Gnanapragasam JP, Houston AB, Jamieson MP. Pulmonary artery sling: definitive diagnosis by colour Doppler flow mapping avoiding cardiac catheterisation. Br Heart J. 1990;63:251–2.
69. Murdison KA, Andrews BA, Chin AJ. Ultrasonographic display of complex vascular rings. J Am Coll Cardiol. 1990;15:1645–53.
70. Lillehei CW, Colan S. Echocardiography in the preoperative evaluation of vascular rings. J Pediatr Surg. 1992;27:1118–20; discussion 1120–1.
71. van Son JA, Julsrud PR, Hagler DJ, et al. Imaging strategies for vascular rings. Ann Thorac Surg. 1994;57:604–10.
72. Backer CL. Diagnostic issues and indications for surgery in patients with pulmonary artery sling. Circulation. 1998;98:188–9.
73. Lee KH, Yoon CS, Choe KO, et al. Use of imaging for assessing anatomical relationships of tracheobronchial anomalies associated with left pulmonary artery sling. Pediatr Radiol. 2001;31:269–78.
74. Newman B, Cho Y. Left pulmonary artery sling—anatomy and imaging. Semin Ultrasound CT MR. 2010;31:158–70.
75. Erickson LC, Cocalis MW, George L. Partial anomalous left pulmonary artery: new evidence on the development of the pulmonary artery sling. Pediatr Cardiol. 1996;17:319–21.
76. Tateishi A, Kawada M. Partial form of a pulmonary artery sling. Ann Thorac Surg. 2009;87:965.
77. Nakajima H, Satomi G, Nakazawa M, et al. Color Doppler and transesophageal echocardiography of vascular sling. Heart Vessels. 1992;7:99–103.
78. Lin CR, Tsai SK, Wang MJ, et al. Airway management and transesophageal echocardiographic monitoring for pulmonary artery sling. J Formos Med Assoc. 1999;98:863–5.
79. Kutsche LM, Van Mierop LH. Anomalous origin of a pulmonary artery from the ascending aorta: associated anomalies and pathogenesis. Am J Cardiol. 1988;61:850–6.
80. Edasery B, Sharma M, Vaddigiri V, et al. Hemitruncus presenting in an adult. A case report. Angiology. 1996;47:1023–6.
81. Aru GM, English WP, Gaymes CH, et al. Origin of the left pulmonary artery from the aorta: embryologic considerations. Ann Thorac Surg. 2001;71:1008–10.
82. Nakamura Y, Yasui H, Kado H, et al. Anomalous origin of the right pulmonary artery from the ascending aorta. Ann Thorac Surg. 1991;52:1285–91.
83. Sotomora RF, Edwards JE. Anatomic identification of so-called absent pulmonary artery. Circulation. 1978;57:624–33.
84. Wu QY, Yang XB. Anomalous origin of the pulmonary artery from the right coronary artery. Ann Thorac Surg. 2001;72:1396–8.
85. Presbitero P, Bull C, Haworth SG, et al. Absent or occult pulmonary artery. Br Heart J. 1984;52:178–85.
86. McCaffrey F. Around pediheart: absent pulmonary artery. Pediatr Cardiol. 2001;22:332.
87. Pfefferkorn JR, Loser H, Pech G, et al. Absent pulmonary artery. A hint to its embryogenesis. Pediatr Cardiol. 1982;3:283–6.
88. Apostolopoulou SC, Kelekis NL, Brountzos EN, et al. "Absent" pulmonary artery in one adult and five pediatric patients: imaging, embryology, and therapeutic implications. AJR Am J Roentgenol. 2002;179:1253–60.
89. Apostolopoulou SC, Kelekis NL. Anomalous origin of pulmonary artery from the innominate artery. Pediatr Cardiol. 2004;25:565.
90. Prifti E, Bonacchi M, Murzi B, et al. Anomalous origin of the left pulmonary artery from the aorta. Our experience and literature review. Heart Vessels. 2003;18:79–84.

91. Peng EW, Shanmugam G, Macarthur KJ, et al. Ascending aortic origin of a branch pulmonary artery—surgical management and long-term outcome. Eur J Cardiothorac Surg. 2004;26:762–6.
92. Morgan JR. Left pulmonary artery from ascending aorta in tetralogy of Fallot. Circulation. 1972;45:653–7.
93. Fontana GP, Spach MS, Effmann EL, et al. Origin of the right pulmonary artery from the ascending aorta. Ann Surg. 1987;206:102–13.
94. Santos MA, Azevedo VM. Anomalous origin of a pulmonary artery from the ascending aorta: surgical repair resolving pulmonary arterial hypertension. Arq Bras Cardiol. 2004;83(503–7):498–502.
95. Fong LV, Anderson RH, Siewers RD, et al. Anomalous origin of one pulmonary artery from the ascending aorta: a review of echocardiographic, catheter, and morphological features. Br Heart J. 1989;62:389–95.
96. Penkoske PA, Castaneda AR, Fyler DC, et al. Origin of pulmonary artery branch from ascending aorta. Primary surgical repair in infancy. J Thorac Cardiovasc Surg. 1983;85:537–45.
97. Mee RB. Surgical repair of hemitruncus: principles and techniques. J Card Surg. 1987;2:247–56.
98. Nathan M, Rimmer D, Piercey G, et al. Early repair of hemitruncus: excellent early and late outcomes. J Thorac Cardiovasc Surg. 2007;133:1329–35.
99. Prifti E, Bonacchi M, Murzi B, et al. Anomalous origin of the right pulmonary artery from the ascending aorta. J Card Surg. 2004;19:103–12.
100. Ishizawa E, Horiuchi T, Tadokoro M, et al. Diagnosis and surgical treatment of "angiographically absent pulmonary artery syndrome". Tohoku J Exp Med. 1978;125:1–9.
101. Moreno-Cabral RJ, McNamara JJ, Reddy VJ, et al. Unilateral absent pulmonary artery: surgical repair with a new technique. J Thorac Cardiovasc Surg. 1991;102:463–5.
102. Duncan WJ, Freedom RM, Olley PM, et al. Two-dimensional echocardiographic identification of hemitruncus: anomalous origin of one pulmonary artery from ascending aorta with the other pulmonary artery arising normally from right ventricle. Am Heart J. 1981;102:892–6.
103. Warnes CA. Bicuspid aortic valve and coarctation: two villains part of a diffuse problem. Heart. 2003;89:965–6.
104. Connolly HM, Jr H, Brown RDJ, et al. Intracranial aneurysms in patients with coarctation of the aorta: a prospective magnetic resonance angiographic study of 100 patients. Mayo Clin Proc. 2003;78:1491–9.
105. Shone JD, Sellers RD, Anderson RC, et al. The developmental complex of "parachute mitral valve," supravalvular ring of left atrium, subaortic stenosis, and coarctation of aorta. Am J Cardiol. 1963;11:714–25.
106. Kenny D, Hijazi ZM. Coarctation of the aorta: from fetal life to adulthood. Cardiol J. 2011;18:487–95.
107. Duffy CI, Plehn JF. Transesophageal echocardiographic assessment of aortic coarctation using color, flow-directed Doppler sampling. Chest. 1994;105:286–8.
108. Engvall J, Sjoqvist L, Nylander E, et al. Biplane transoesophageal echocardiography, transthoracic Doppler, and magnetic resonance imaging in the assessment of coarctation of the aorta. Eur Heart J. 1995;16:1399–409.
109. Trehan VK, Bhardwaj S, Rastogi P, et al. Multiplane transoesophageal echocardiography in an adult with coarctation of aorta. Indian Heart J. 1996;48:707–9.
110. Skinner JR, Bexton R, Wren C. Aortic coarctation endarteritis and aneurysm: diagnosis by transoesophageal echocardiography. Int J Cardiol. 1992;34:216–8.
111. Thwaites BK, Stamatos JM, Crowl FD, et al. Transesophageal echocardiographic diagnosis of intraaortic thrombus during coarctation repair. Anesthesiology. 1992;76:638–9.
112. Chatrath R, Hagler DJ. Improved imaging of aortic coarctation using an intracardiac probe for transesophageal echocardiography. Tex Heart Inst J. 2004;31:194–5.
113. Kinsara A, Chan KL. Noninvasive imaging modalities in coarctation of the aorta. Chest. 2004;126:1016–8.
114. Stern H, Erbel R, Schreiner G, et al. Coarctation of the aorta: quantitative analysis by transesophageal echocardiography. Echocardiography. 1987;4:387–95.
115. Gopal AS, Arora NS, Vardanian S, et al. Utility of transesophageal echocardiography for the characterization of cardiovascular anomalies associated with Turner's syndrome. J Am Soc Echocardiogr. 2001;14:60–2.
116. Rudolph AM, Heymann MA, Spitznas U. Hemodynamic considerations in the development of narrowing of the aorta. Am J Cardiol. 1972;30:514–25.
117. Loffredo CA, Ferencz C, Wilson PD, et al. Interrupted aortic arch: an epidemiologic study. Teratology. 2000;61:368–75.
118. Celoria GC, Patton RB. Congenital absence of the aortic arch. Am Heart J. 1959;58:407–13.
119. Powell CB, Stone FM, Atkins DL, et al. Operative mortality and frequency of coexistent anomalies in interruption of the aortic arch. Am J Cardiol. 1997;79:1147–8.
120. Ramaswamy P, Lytrivi ID, Thanjan MT, et al. Frequency of aberrant subclavian artery, arch laterality, and associated intracardiac anomalies detected by echocardiography. Am J Cardiol. 2008;101:677–82.
121. Schreiber C, Eicken A, Vogt M, et al. Repair of interrupted aortic arch: results after more than 20 years. Ann Thorac Surg. 2000;70:1896–9; discussion 1899–900.
122. Tchervenkov CI, Jacobs JP, Sharma K, et al. Interrupted aortic arch: surgical decision making. Semin Thorac Cardiovasc Surg Pediatr Card Surg Annu. 2005:92–102.
123. Flint JD, Gentles TL, MacCormick J, et al. Outcomes using predominantly single-stage approach to interrupted aortic arch and associated defects. Ann Thorac Surg. 2010;89:564–9.
124. Dillman JR, Yarram SG, D'Amico AR, et al. Interrupted aortic arch: spectrum of MRI findings. AJR Am J Roentgenol. 2008;190:1467–74.
125. Geva T, Hornberger LK, Sanders SP, et al. Echocardiographic predictors of left ventricular outflow tract obstruction after repair of interrupted aortic arch. J Am Coll Cardiol. 1993;22:1953–60.
126. Jacobs ML, Rychik J, Murphy JD, et al. Results of Norwood's operation for lesions other than hypoplastic left heart syndrome. J Thorac Cardiovasc Surg. 1995;110:1555–61; discussion 1561–2.
127. Rychik J, Murdison KA, Chin AJ, et al. Surgical management of severe aortic outflow obstruction in lesions other than the hypoplastic left heart syndrome: use of a pulmonary artery to aorta anastomosis. J Am Coll Cardiol. 1991;18:809–16.
128. Apfel HD, Levenbraun J, Quaegebeur JM, et al. Usefulness of preoperative echocardiography in predicting left ventricular outflow obstruction after primary repair of interrupted aortic arch with ventricular septal defect. Am J Cardiol. 1998;82:470–3.
129. Russell HM, Forsberg K, Backer CL, et al. Outcomes of radial incision of the tricuspid valve for ventricular septal defect closure. Ann Thorac Surg. 2011;92:685–90; discussion 690.
130. Hillman HD, Mavroudis C, Backer CL. Patent ductus ateriousus. In: Mavroudis C, Backer CL, editors. Pediatric cardiac surgery. 3rd ed. Philadelphia: Mosby; 2003. p. 223–33.
131. Russell IA, Rouine-Rapp K, Stratmann G, Miller-Hance WC. Congenital heart disease in the adult: a review with internet-accessible transesophageal echocardiographic images. Anesth Analg. 2006;102(3):694–723.

132. Cahalan MK. Intraoperative transesophageal echocardiography: an interactive text and atlas. New York: Churchill Livingstone Interactive Publication; 1996.
133. Gaynor WJ. Aortopulmonary window and aortic origin of a pulmonary artery. In: Mavroudis C, Backer CL, editors. Pediatric cardiac surgery. 3rd ed. Philadelphia: Mosby; 2003. p. 353–60.
134. Backer CL, Mavroudis C. Vascular rings and pulmonary artery sling. In: Mavroudis C, Backer CL, editors. Pediatric cardiac surgery. 3rd ed. Philadelphia: Mosby; 2003. p. 234–50.
135. Backer CL, Mavroudis C. Coarctation of the aorta. In: Mavroudis C, Backer CL, editors. Pediatric cardiac surgery. 3rd ed. Philadelphia: Mosby; 2003. p. 251–72.
136. Jonas RA. Interrupted aortic arch. In: Mavroudis C, Backer CL, editors. Pediatric cardiac surgery. 3rd ed. Philadelphia: Mosby; 2003. p. 273–82.

Congenital Coronary Artery Anomalies

14

Peter C. Frommelt

Abstract

Assessment of coronary artery anatomy has become an important component of the echocardiographic examination in many forms of congenital heart disease, however the presence of isolated congenital or acquired coronary artery anomalies in an otherwise structurally normal heart has only recently been appreciated. Because of its superior resolution, transesophageal echocardiography (TEE) is recognized as an important diagnostic tool to image coronary artery anomalies. This chapter will focus on the anatomic features and TEE evaluation of isolated congenital coronary anomalies. In addition, this chapter also provides a brief discussion in the use of TEE in patients with Kawasaki disease who have important coronary artery involvement.

Keywords

Coronary artery abnormalities • Anomalous origin of a coronary artery • Intramural coronary artery • Coronary artery fistula • Kawasaki disease • Coronary artery aneurysms

Introduction

Assessment of coronary artery anatomy has become an important component of the echocardiographic examination in many forms of congenital heart disease (CHD), however the presence of isolated congenital or acquired coronary artery anomalies in an otherwise structurally normal heart has only recently been appreciated. Isolated congenital coronary artery anomalies are quite common in the general population [1–3] and the need for careful interrogation by echocardiography has been recognized. Transthoracic echocardiography (TTE) is the ideal technique because it is risk-free, noninvasive, and widely available. Continued improvements in ultrasound technology now allow delineation of coronary artery anatomy in both children and adults using this imaging modality. Confirmation of coronary abnormalities has traditionally been obtained using coronary angiography, however, the higher cost and increased risk associated with this procedure has made it a less attractive technique, particularly in children. Magnetic resonance imaging [4–7] and computer assisted tomography [8] are techniques able to image coronary artery anatomy, however, TTE is considered the initial and most important screening procedure. Reports of prospective identification of isolated coronary anomalies using TTE have become common in the literature and have helped dispel the notion that coronary artery anatomy cannot be well delineated using this technique. Echocardiographic findings in patients with isolated coronary anomalies [9–22] have been well characterized, and the feasibility of detailed coronary imaging in patients greater than 50 kg has been described.

P.C. Frommelt, MD
Division of Pediatric Cardiology, Department of Pediatrics, Medical College of Wisconsin, Children's Hospital of Wisconsin, 9000 W. Wisconsin Avenue, Milwaukee, WI 53122, USA
e-mail: pfrommelt@chw.org

The online version of this chapter (doi:10.1007/978-1-84800-064-3_14) contains supplementary material, which is available to authorized users.

P.C. Wong, W.C. Miller-Hance (eds.), *Transesophageal Echocardiography for Congenital Heart Disease*, DOI 10.1007/978-1-84800-064-3_14, © Springer-Verlag London 2014

Table 14.1 Important congenital coronary anomalies

1. Anomalous origin of a coronary artery from the opposite sinus of Valsalva
(a) Anomalous origin of the left coronary from the right sinus
(b) Anomalous origin of the right coronary from the left sinus
2. Anomalous origin of the left coronary artery from the pulmonary artery
3. Coronary artery fistulae

Transesophageal echocardiography (TEE) has also been recognized as a diagnostic tool to image coronary artery anomalies [23–30]. Since symptoms such as congestive heart failure, exercise-induced chest pain, and syncope can be related to congenital coronary anomalies in children and adults, focused interrogation of coronary anatomy using TEE has become a valuable adjunct tool in the evaluation of any patient presenting with these complaints who has poorly characterized coronary origins or the suspicion of a coronary anomaly has been raised. Although the majority of isolated congenital coronary anomalies are noted as incidental findings, there can be a significant risk of myocardial ischemia, myocardial dysfunction, congestive heart failure, and sudden death in some of the anatomic subtypes of coronary artery anomalies related to the origin and/or course of the anomalous vessel [31–37]. This risk appears to be highest during childhood and adolescence; therefore an understanding of these anomalies and the TEE techniques to optimally image them is important for the pediatric and adult echocardiographer.

This chapter will focus on the anatomic features and TEE evaluation of isolated congenital coronary anomalies associated with myocardial dysfunction and adverse outcomes (Table 14.1): anomalous origin of a coronary artery from the opposite sinus of Valsalva with an interarterial course between the great arteries, anomalous origin of a coronary artery from the pulmonary artery, and coronary artery fistulae. In addition, a brief discussion of Kawasaki disease and implications regarding coronary artery involvement in this condition will conclude the chapter.

Role and Utility of TEE in the Evaluation of Congenital Coronary Artery Anomalies

Aberrant Origin of Coronary Artery (Right or Left) from the Aortic Root

Anatomy

Anomalous aortic origin of a coronary artery (AAOCA) from the opposite sinus of Valsalva has been associated with myocardial ischemia, ventricular arrhythmias, and sudden death, particularly when the vessel courses between the great arteries (Fig. 14.1) [28, 31–49]. Although AAOCA from the non-coronary, or posterior sinus of Valsalva has been described, it is quite rare and usually not associated with myocardial ischemia or sudden death [32]. Similarly, AAOCA can occur from the opposite sinus of Valsalva (either the right coronary arising from the left sinus or the left coronary arising the right sinus of Valsalva) but is usually not associated with myocardial ischemia unless the anomalous coronary courses in between the great arteries [36, 39]. When the anomalous coronary is interarterial, it can course within the myocardial sulcus between the great arteries (intramyocardial) or within the anterior wall of the aorta between the great arteries (intramural) [28, 50]. AAOCA of the left coronary artery from the right sinus of Valsalva with the anomalous vessel coursing between the great arteries is quite rare (with an estimated incidence of 0.03–0.05 %), however, this is frequently associated with sudden cardiac death [31–39]. AAOCA of the right coronary artery from the left sinus of Valsalva is more common (incidence estimated 0.1 %) and is also associated with sudden cardiac death [41–49].

The mechanisms that lead to myocardial ischemia in the patient with AAOCA from the opposite sinus that courses between the pulmonary and aortic roots are unclear, but several theories have been proposed. The ostium of the anomalously arising coronary artery is frequently slit-like, possibly compromising flow reserve [32]. In addition, the anomalous coronary artery usually arises at an acute angle from the aorta, rather than perpendicularly, and this may alter flow patterns into that coronary artery bed [39]. Finally, it has been hypothesized that the interarterial course places the anomalous coronary at risk of compression between the great arteries. This seems unlikely given the low pressure in the pulmonary artery in normal individuals, even during exercise. The ischemia is more likely due to deformation of the anomalous coronary artery within the aortic wall during periods of arterial hypertension with exercise, particularly in patients with an intramural course [51].

Transesophageal Echocardiographic Evaluation

Transesophageal echocardiographic imaging of coronary artery origins is critical and should be a part of the routine complete examination in every patient. This is usually best accomplished from the mid esophageal window, using the mid esophageal aortic valve short axis view (ME AV SAX) as a starting point where both origins can be visualized by scanning superior to the aortic valve with careful interrogation of the aortic sinuses. The left main coronary artery usually arises at approximately 2 o'clock if one considers the aortic root as a clock face (using the image display noted in the American Society of Echocardiography/Society of Cardiovascular Anesthesiologists guidelines), and the right

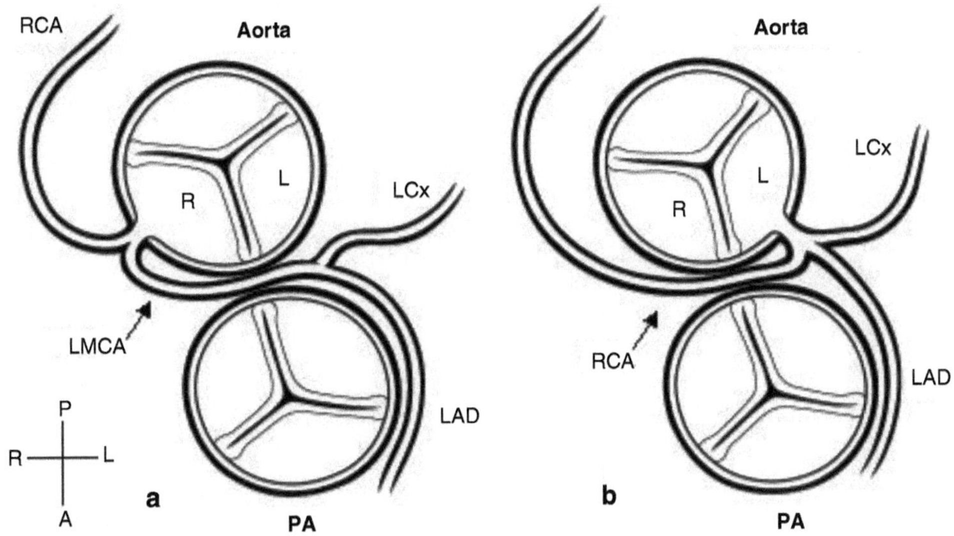

Fig. 14.1 Schematic diagram of the two forms of anomalous origin of a coronary from the opposite sinus potentially associated with myocardial ischemia. Panel **a** anomalous origin of the left coronary artery from the right sinus of Valsalva; Panel **b** anomalous origin of the right coronary artery from the left sinus of Valsalva. In each case, the anomalous coronary artery can be seen coursing between the aorta and pulmonary artery (*PA*). With anomalous origin of the left coronary, the left main coronary artery (*LMCA*) arises from the right aortic sinus (*R*) and courses between the great arteries before dividing into its two usual branches, the left anterior descending (*LAD*) and left circumflex (*LCx*) coronary arteries. With anomalous origin of the right coronary, the right coronary artery (*RCA*) arises from the left aortic sinus (*L*) and passes between the great arteries before coursing in its usual distribution. (Orientation marker: *A* anterior, *L* left, *P* posterior, *R* right) (Reprinted with permission from Frommelt and Frommelt [86])

coronary artery arises at approximately 7 o'clock. Rotation of the multiplane element from the standard short axis position (0°) to 25–70°, along with slight leftward rotation of the TEE transducer, frequently improves imaging of the length of the left main coronary artery and its early branches, the left anterior descending and circumflex coronary arteries. Similarly, slight rightward rotation of the transducer, using the standard short axis view (0°), can facilitate imaging of the origin of the right coronary artery. Color Doppler flow interrogation of the left and right main coronaries is also important, as documentation of both direction and timing of flow is also helpful in diagnosing anomalies (as described below). Spectral Doppler may also facilitate this assessment.

Normal coronary artery flow is predominantly diastolic, since that is the time that aortic pressure (and thus coronary pressure) exceeds ventricular pressure. In order to identify these coronary flow signals, which are usually low velocity, the Nyquist limit of the color Doppler map should be decreased to 20–40 cm/s. Many echocardiographic systems allow presets for coronary imaging to facilitate altering the set-up to better identify the low velocity coronary flow signals.

TEE can be an important tool for prospectively identifying and/or confirming anomalous origin of the left coronary from the right sinus of Valsalva [9–11, 23, 24, 52] and anomalous origin of the right coronary from the left sinus of Valsalva [12–14, 26, 53]. Identification of either anomaly requires focused two-dimensional (2D) and color Doppler imaging of the coronary arteries. This is especially important when the course of the anomalous coronary is interarterial and intramural, because the anomalous vessel can appear to arise normally from the appropriate sinus by 2D imaging as it exits the aortic wall [22]. The anomalous intramural coronary segment can be visualized as an echo-lucent linear space in the anterior aortic wall (Figs. 14.2 and 14.3; Videos 14.1a, 14.1b, 14.2, 14.3, 14.4a, and 14.4b), but a high index of suspicion is usually necessary to recognize this during routine screening of coronary origins. The origin of the anomalous coronary artery must be carefully delineated, particularly in relationship to the aortic sinuses, since anomalous coronary artery origins with an interarterial and intramural course can arise near the commissure between the appropriate sinus and the opposite adjacent sinus. This is especially true for anomalous origin of the right coronary from the left sinus of Valsalva (Fig. 14.3; Video 14.2).

Color Doppler imaging is frequently helpful in making this diagnosis, as it can identify flow in the intramural segment. Color Doppler interrogation of the aortic root will demonstrate an abnormal linear diastolic color Doppler signal in the anterior aortic wall, representing the diastolic flow in the intramural segment. Color Doppler can also be helpful in identifying which coronary artery is anomalous.

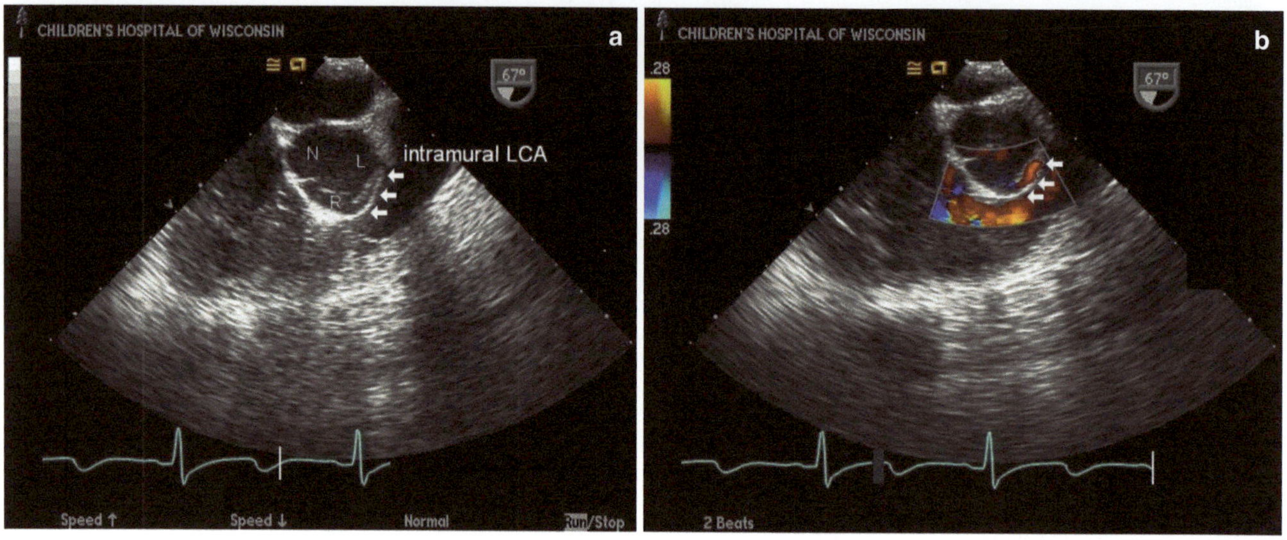

Fig. 14.2 Transesophageal echocardiogram from a mid esophageal right ventricular inflow-outflow view through the aortic root in a patient with anomalous origin of the left coronary artery from the right sinus of Valsalva with an intramural course. The two-dimensional image (**a**) shows the anomalous left main coronary artery (*intramural LCA*) arising from the right sinus of Valsalva (*R*) and running intramurally within the anterior aortic wall (*arrows*) between the aorta and right ventricular outflow tract before exiting the wall in the left sinus of Valsalva (*L*). The non-coronary cusp (*N*) is seen posteriorly. The right coronary artery origin is not visualized in this image. Color Doppler imaging (**b**) shows the linear diastolic flow of the anomalous coronary within the anterior aortic wall (*arrows*); the red color signal confirms anomalous coronary flow towards the transducer, consistent with the coronary originating from the right sinus and coursing towards the more posteriorly positioned left sinus

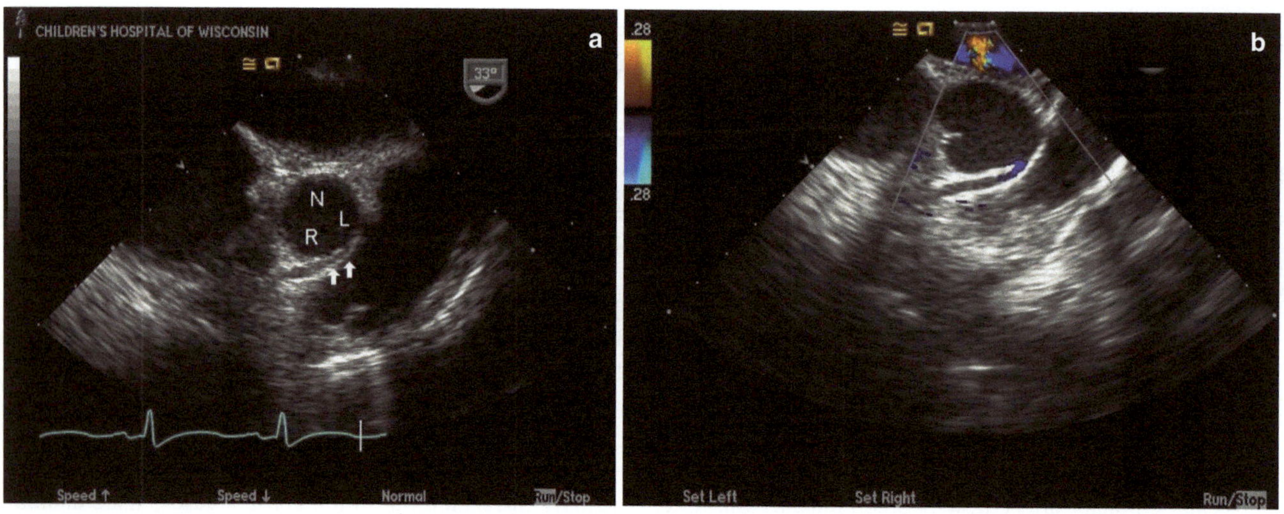

Fig. 14.3 Transesophageal echocardiogram from a mid esophageal aortic valve short axis view in a patient with anomalous origin of the right coronary artery (*RCA*) from the left sinus of Valsalva and an intramural course of the anomalous vessel. The anomalous RCA can be seen arising from the left sinus of Valsalva (*L*) and coursing intramurally within the anterior aortic wall (*arrows*) between the aorta and the right ventricular outflow tract (**a**) towards the right sinus of Valsalva (*R*). The non-coronary cusp (*N*) is seen posteriorly. Color Doppler imaging (**b**) shows the linear diastolic flow of the anomalous RCA within the anterior aortic wall; the blue color signal confirms anomalous coronary flow away from the transducer anteriorly, consistent with the coronary originating from the left sinus and coursing towards the more anteriorly positioned right sinus. The left coronary origin is not visualized

With anomalous origin of the left coronary from the right sinus of Valsalva, a red color Doppler signal will be seen in the anomalous coronary as flow moves away from the right sinus towards the more posterior positioned left sinus of Valsalva (Fig. 14.2; Video 14.4a and 14.4b). This is in contrast to anomalous origin of the right coronary from the left sinus, where a blue color Doppler signal will be seen in the anomalous coronary as flow moves away from the TEE transducer towards the right sinus from its origin in the left sinus (Fig. 14.3; Video 14.1a and 14.1b).

Other TEE views can also provide imaging evidence that a coronary artery has an anomalous origin from the aortic

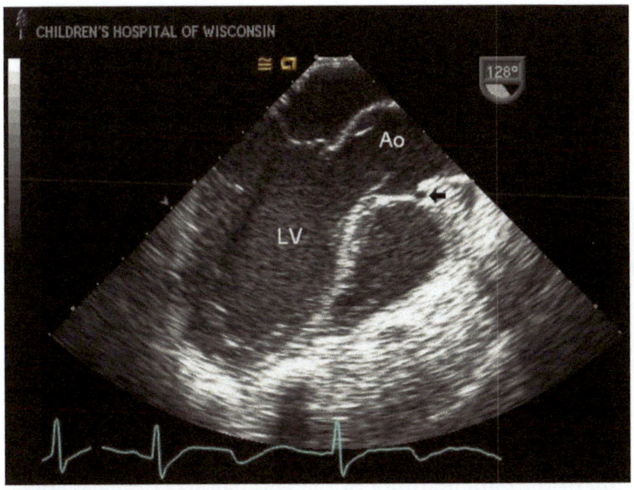

Fig. 14.4 Mid esophageal long axis image through the left ventricle (*LV*) and aortic root in a patient with anomalous origin of left coronary artery from the opposite sinus of Valsalva with an interarterial course. The anomalous coronary is seen coursing anterior to the aorta (*Ao*) between the great arteries as a discrete circle (*arrow*); this may be the first clue that there is a coronary anomaly, as visualization of a coronary anterior to the Ao from this view is never seen with normal coronary anatomy

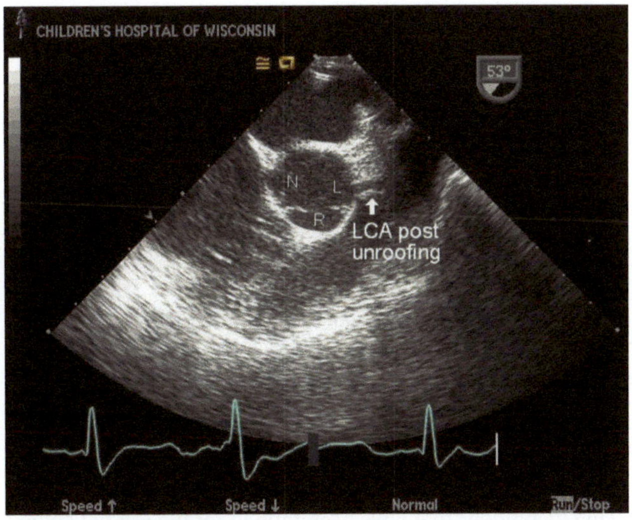

Fig. 14.5 Mid esophageal right ventricular inflow-outflow view displaying the aortic root in a patient with anomalous origin of the left coronary artery (*LCA*) from the right sinus of Valsalva and an intramural course of the anomalous vessel after surgical unroofing of the intramural segment. The anomalous LCA can be seen arising appropriately from the left sinus of Valsalva (*L*) after removal of the intramural segment with creation of large neo-orifice that is oriented perpendicular to the aortic root, similar to the appearance of a normal LCA origin. The right (*R*) and non-coronary (*N*) sinuses are indicated

root. From the mid esophageal long axis view (ME LAX) through the left ventricle and aortic outflow, the anomalous coronary artery can be seen running between the great arteries as a discrete circle anterior to the aortic root as an initial clue (Fig. 14.4). Turning the probe counterclockwise from this position towards the patient's left can allow visualization of the proximal left coronary artery branches as they leave the anterior aortic wall (Video 14.5). In addition, in patients who allow for high quality deep transgastric imaging, scanning from the aortic root more anteriorly to the pulmonary root in the deep transgastric long axis view (DTG LAX) can identify a length of the anomalous coronary artery coursing between the great arteries (Video 14.6).

Surgical repair of AAOCA has generally been reserved for patients with known symptoms of myocardial ischemia, although in some cases consideration may be given for surgical intervention in the absence of symptoms or coronary insufficiency. Multiple surgical techniques have been utilized, including coronary artery bypass grafting [54–58], patch enlargement of the anomalous coronary origin [28], reimplantation of the anomalous coronary to the appropriate sinus [59, 60], and unroofing of the intramural segment of the anomalous vessel [50, 61–64]. The unroofing procedure is performed by removing the common wall between the aorta and anomalous coronary artery to create a neo-orifice of the anomalous vessel in the appropriate sinus that arises perpendicularly, rather than obliquely, from the aortic root. The results of this technique can be easily visualized by TEE after surgery, with both imaging and color Doppler assessment of the neo-orifice (Fig. 14.5; Video 14.7).

Anomalous Origin of Left Coronary Artery from Main Pulmonary Artery

Anatomy

Anomalous origin of the left coronary artery from the pulmonary artery (ALCAPA) is a rare congenital abnormality, occurring in approximately 1 in 300,000 children [65]. An anomalous coronary artery that arises from the pulmonary root is most commonly the left main, although anomalous origin from the right coronary artery has also been described [20, 66]. The anomalous left coronary artery typically courses adjacent to its normal aortic origin near the left aortic sinus before branching in the usual left coronary distribution. Since coronary artery flow is dependent on the diastolic pressure gradient between the vessel supplying the coronary artery and the myocardial bed it perfuses, patients with this anomaly are at risk for left ventricular ischemia. Diastolic pulmonary artery pressure is usually lower than left ventricular diastolic pressure after birth, and so patients develop a myocardial "steal" phenomenon because right coronary blood preferentially flows to the pulmonary artery instead of perfusing the left ventricular myocardium. Perfusion in the left coronary bed in all patients with ALCAPA is retrograde, supplied via collateral circulation from the normally arising right coronary artery off the higher-pressure aorta. Thus, patients with ALCAPA can develop progressive left ventricular dysfunction with signs and symptoms of myocardial ischemia/infarction. The timing of presentation during childhood is quite variable and is related to adequacy of collateralization from the right coronary artery [20]. Surgery to establish a connection of the left coronary artery with the aortic root is indicated in all patients when this lesion is identified, even in the patient with good left ventricular function, in order to normalize perfusion to the left coronary bed. Historically, the favored surgical management of ALCAPA was ligation of the left coronary artery to prevent myocardial steal. Subsequently techniques creating an aortopulmonary window and a tunnel (Takeuchi operation) that directed flow from the aortic root through the pulmonary artery to the anomalous coronary were used. Today, however, almost all patients can have direct reimplantation of the anomalous coronary artery into the aortic root, using techniques that have been refined for the arterial switch procedure for transposition of the great arteries and other coronary translocation procedures.

It should be remembered that, while most cases of anomalous origin of a coronary artery from the pulmonary artery occur with a structurally normal heart, in rare instances this entity can be seen in association with other forms of CHD such as tetralogy of Fallot.

Transesophageal Echocardiographic Evaluation

Prospective identification of ALCAPA using echocardiography has been well described, and this technique should be diagnostic in most patients [20]. Although TTE is usually adequate without the need for additional imaging, TEE can be a useful adjunct modality [67, 68]. Again, careful interrogation of the coronary artery origins and flow patterns are necessary to make the diagnosis. 2D assessment may provide direct visualization of the anomalous coronary artery insertion into the pulmonary artery from mid esophageal long and short axis imaging, with the coronary artery usually inserting into the posterior and leftward aspect of the main pulmonary artery (Fig. 14.6; Video 14.8a and 14.8b). The anomalous left coronary artery frequently courses close to its normal site of origin near the left sinus of Valsalva, however, and therefore recognition of associated echocardiographic findings is critical to the diagnosis in many patients. Because the anomalous coronary artery is perfused in retrograde fashion from the normally arising opposite coronary, spectral and color Doppler is essential. This allows for identification of retrograde filling of the anomalous coronary artery [12] and detection of abnormal diastolic flow signals in the pulmonary artery as the anomalous coronary empties into the pulmonary artery [10, 11] (Figs. 14.6, 14.7, and 14.8; Videos 14.8a, 14.8b, 14.9, 14.10, and 14.11). Color Doppler interrogation is useful in documenting the direction of flow in the coronary arteries, with the expectation that normal coronary flow is always away from, and not towards the aortic root. The normally arising coronary artery can have significant dilatation because of the obligate collateral circulation needed to perfuse the anomalous coronary system retrograde (Fig. 14.8; Video 14.9). The degree of dilatation can be dramatic in older patients who have survived with this anomalous coronary circulation for several years. As in all cases of suspected coronary artery anomalies, additional echocardiographic parameters to be obtained include the assessment of global and

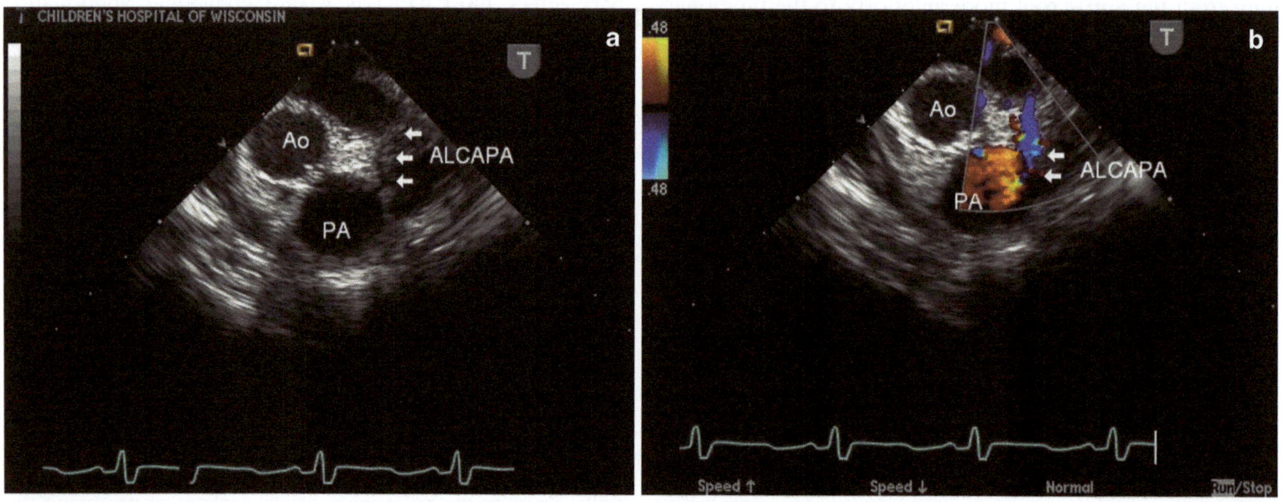

Fig. 14.6 Mid esophageal aortic valve short axis TEE images of the anomalous insertion of the left main coronary artery (*LCA*) into the posterior aspect of the proximal main pulmonary artery (*PA*) in a patient with anomalous left coronary artery from the pulmonary artery (*ALCAPA*). In (**a**) the LCA is seen entering the PA through a short coronary segment and then bifurcating into the left anterior descending and circumflex branches (*arrows*), clearly a long distance from the normal entrance into the aortic root (*Ao*). Color Doppler interrogation in (**b**) shows a *blue color* signal in the LCA (*arrows*), consistent with coronary flow towards the PA, indicating retrograde filling of the anomalous vessel that empties into the PA

segmental ventricular systolic function. In addition, atrioventricular valve competency should be assessed as children with ALCAPA can have various degrees of mitral regurgitation resulting from papillary muscle ischemia or infarction. The analysis of regional ventricular function is facilitated by the transgastric mid short axis (TG Mid SAX) and mid esophageal four chamber (ME 4 Ch) views. These TEE windows allow for examination of myocardial segments supplied by the right, circumflex, and left anterior descending coronary arteries from cross sections at the basal, mid, and apical ventricular levels (refer to Chap. 5). This analysis is important not only in the pre-cardiopulmonary bypass setting, but also immediately following the surgical intervention.

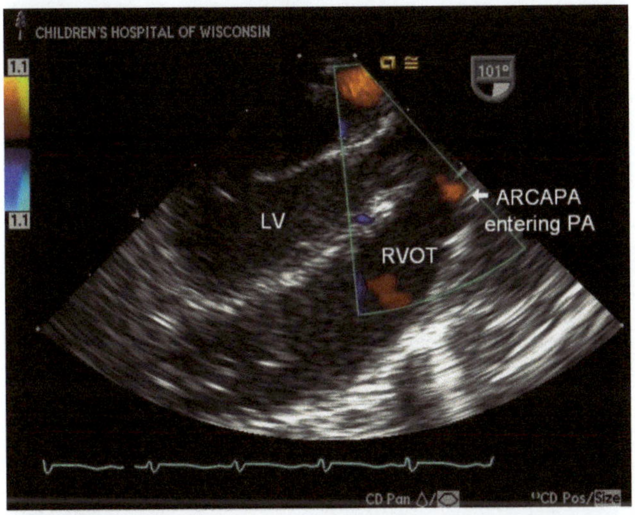

Fig. 14.7 Mid esophageal long axis image through the left ventricle (*LV*) in a patient with anomalous origin of the right coronary from the pulmonary artery (*ARCAPA*). There is a diastolic color Doppler flow signal entering the pulmonary artery (*PA*) anteriorly above the right ventricular outflow tract (*RVOT*). This flow signal may be the first clue that there is an anomalous coronary arising from the PA, as direct visualization of a coronary entering the PA can sometimes be difficult to obtain

Coronary Artery Fistula

Anatomy

Congenital coronary artery fistula (CAF) is a rare isolated anomaly of the coronary artery system defined as a direct communication between a coronary artery and another vascular structure or cardiac cavity. The involved coronary artery usually arises normally from the aorta and connects to one of the intracardiac chambers, systemic veins, or pulmonary artery via a tortuous anomalous branch. It more frequently involves the right coronary artery and the fistula usually drains into one of the right heart chambers [69]. Symptoms and signs are dependent on the size of the fistulous connection; rarely, large fistulas can have a significant left-to-right shunt with resultant congestive heart failure and cardiomegaly in infancy [70]. Surgical closure is safe and effective [71, 72]. Recent advances in interventional techniques now allow closure of CAF in the cardiac catheterization laboratory using devices such as detachable coils and balloons, and this has become the initial treatment of choice in children and adults [73–75].

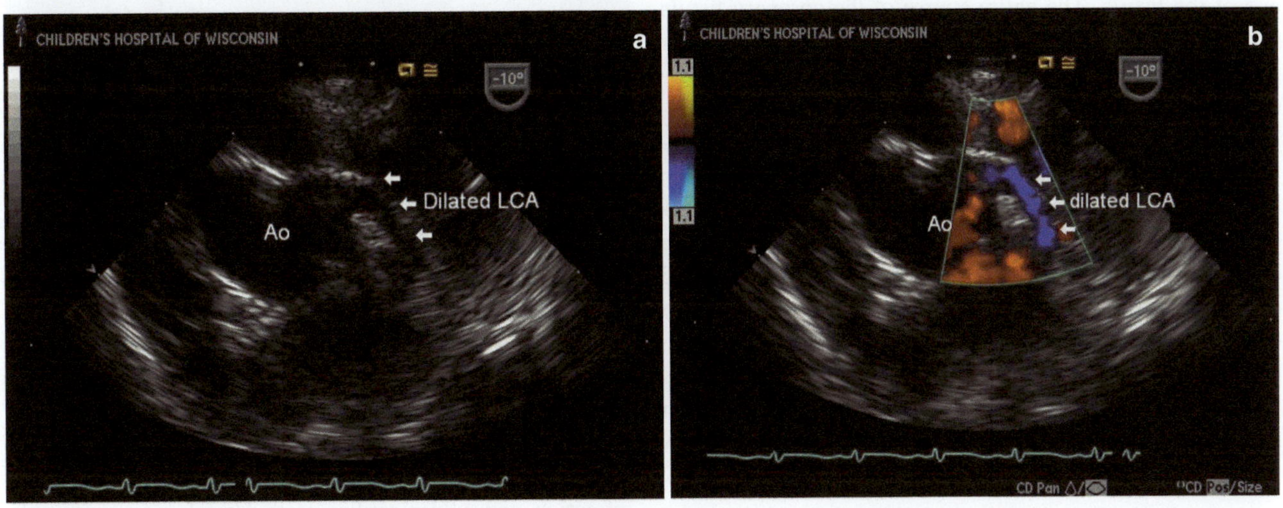

Fig. 14.8 Transesophageal images at the level of the mid esophagus displaying the aortic root (*Ao*) and a dilated left coronary artery (*LCA*) in a child with anomalous right coronary artery (*RCA*) from the pulmonary artery; the LCA measured 3.5 mm at its origin, which is significantly abnormal for age. (**a**) The LCA arises normally from the Ao; the anomalous RCA is not seen. Color Doppler documents flow in the dilated LCA, even without lowering the Nyquist limit (**b**), due to the increased flow into the left coronary bed as it functions as the single vessel supplying the entire myocardium with steal of coronary flow from the anomalous RCA emptying into the low pressure pulmonary bed

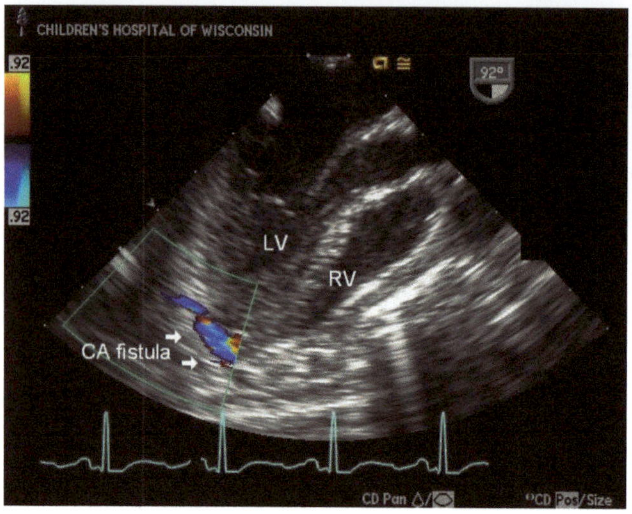

Fig. 14.9 Mid esophageal long axis image through the left ventricle (*LV*) in a patient with a left coronary artery to right ventricular fistula with color Doppler imaging of the fistula as it courses along the cardiac apex. A turbulent jet of flow can be seen at the apex where the coronary artery fistula (*CA fistula*) empties into the right ventricle (*RV*) (*arrows*)

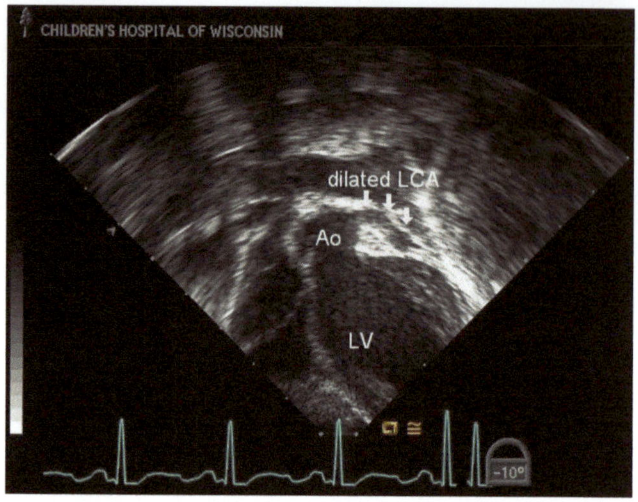

Fig. 14.10 Transesophageal imaging from a deep transgastric long axis position through the left ventricle (*LV*) and aortic outflow (*Ao*) from a patient with a left coronary artery (*LCA*) fistula. Because of the increased flow into the LCA to supply the fistula, the proximal LCA is easily seen and appears dilated (*arrows*)

Transesophageal Echocardiographic Evaluation

TTE is usually diagnostic and can identify the involved coronary artery and its site of drainage, but many reports exist detailing the value of TEE in diagnosing coronary fistulae [76–82]. The hallmark is identifying the site of drainage of the fistula into the heart or vascular bed (Fig. 14.9; Video 14.12); a continuous turbulent jet of flow is usually present where the fistula empties (since all chambers except the aorta and left ventricle are at lower pressures than the coronary bed). Color Doppler is critical in identifying the site of drainage of the fistula. The entire course of the coronary fistula can sometimes be tracked using imaging and color Doppler interrogation and the site of drainage is best identified by color Doppler because a high velocity continuous color signal is evident where the coronary artery empties into the usually lower pressure chamber. Because of low resistance into the affected coronary artery secondary to steal of flow through the fistula as it empties into the lower pressure chamber where it terminates, the coronary artery supplying the fistula will be dilated (Fig. 14.10). The coronary artery can be quite dilated, ectatic, and tortuous, depending upon the amount of fistula flow (Figs. 14.11 and 14.12; Videos 14.13a and 14.14a), and results in easily identifiable flow in the vessel by color Doppler (Videos 14.13b and 14.14b).

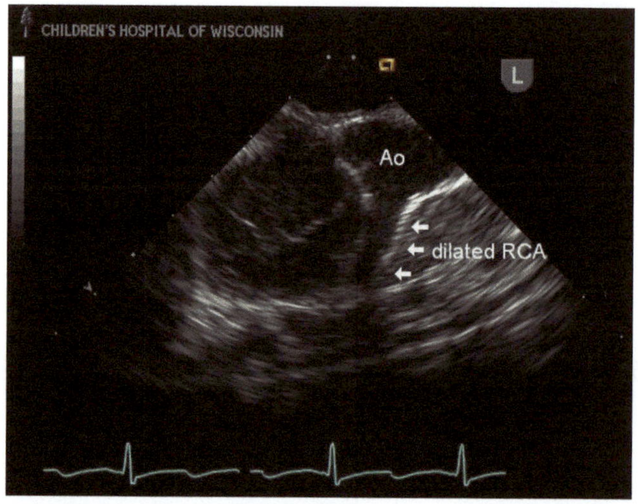

Fig. 14.11 Mid esophageal long axis view of the aorta (*Ao*) displaying the right coronary artery (*RCA*) in a patient with a right coronary artery fistula. Because of the increased flow into the RCA to supply the fistula, the proximal RCA is easily seen and appears markedly dilated (*arrows*) measuring 5 mm in diameter proximally

Kawasaki Disease

Anatomy

Kawasaki disease is a systemic vasculitis of unclear etiology that may be associated with coronary artery changes. This is considered the most common form of acquired pediatric heart disease. Coronary involvement includes ectasia and aneurysm formation that may result in myocardial ischemia, myocardial infarction, and sudden cardiac death. Vessels most commonly affected (in decreasing order of incidence) are the proximal left anterior descending and proximal right coronary arteries, followed by the left main coronary artery, then left circumflex, and finally the distal right coronary artery [83]. Thrombi formation can be associated with giant aneurysms (> 8 mm).

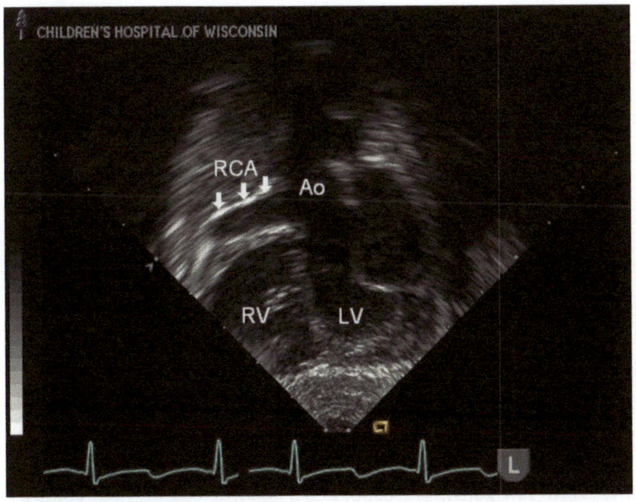

Fig. 14.12 Transesophageal imaging from a deep transgastric sagittal position (longitudinal plane) through the left ventricle (*LV*) and aortic outflow (*Ao*), from the same patient as depicted in Fig. 14.11 with a right coronary artery (*RCA*) fistula. In this view the markedly dilated RCA is also seen (*arrows*). The distal termination site of the fistula into the right atrium is not visualized in this image. The right ventricle is seen anteriorly (*RV*) and appears dilated, secondary to the fistula shunt

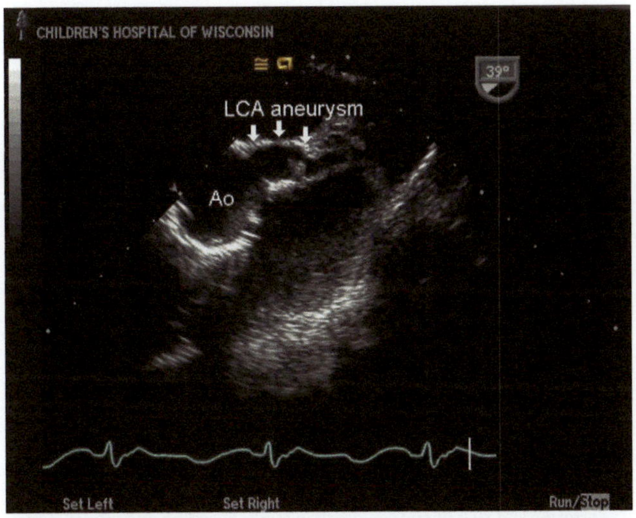

Fig. 14.13 Mid esophageal aortic valve short axis view displays the aortic root in a patient with Kawasaki disease and a left coronary artery (*LCA*) aneurysm. The aneurysm can be seen in the LCA immediately adjacent to the vessel origin (*arrows*). A small echodensity in the aneurysmal coronary segment raises the concern of intraluminal thrombus. The more distal left main coronary artery also appears dilated

Transesophageal Echocardiographic Evaluation

TTE is the technique of choice in identifying and serially following coronary artery changes associated with Kawasaki disease. In some cases valvar pathology, myocardial, and/or pericardial involvement may be present, also amenable to transthoracic imaging. TEE may optimize coronary imaging in patients with limited transthoracic windows, and the

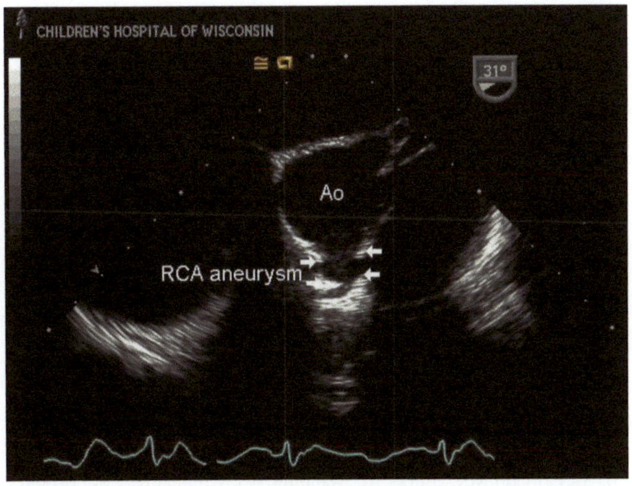

Fig. 14.14 Mid esophageal aortic valve short axis imaging displays the aortic root (*Ao*) in a patient with Kawasaki disease and a right coronary artery (*RCA*) aneurysm. The aneurysm can be seen in the proximal vessel immediately adjacent to the RCA origin (*arrows*). The more distal RCA is of normal caliber

techniques described above should allow evaluation of the proximal right and left coronary beds (Figs. 14.13 and 14.14). Although a comprehensive examination of the distal coronary vasculature for pathologic changes may be challenging, in some cases this assessment may be enhanced by obtaining complementary TEE views (ME 4 Ch, mid esophageal two chamber, mid esophageal right ventricular inflow-outflow). Criteria for diagnosis of coronary artery ectasia has been described and varies with patient size [84]; aneurysms have also been classified by size with the largest ones clearly associated with late development of coronary insufficiency and myocardial ischemia [85].

Summary

Coronary artery anomalies can coexist with many forms of congenital heart disease, may be found in isolation, or can represent an acquired pathology in the otherwise structurally normal heart. TEE can play an important role as an adjunct in the diagnostic evaluation of these anomalies. This imaging tool also contributes significantly to the care of affected patients during surgical or catheter-based interventions by confirming the coronary artery anatomy, associated functional abnormalities, providing for intraoperative/procedural monitoring, and facilitating optimization of hemodynamic management as necessary. As such, it is important for the pediatric and adult practitioner involved in echocardiography to have an in-depth understanding of the characteristic features of the most common anomalies that affect the coronary arteries and their detailed TEE evaluation.

References

1. Yamanaka O, Hobbs RE. Coronary artery anomalies in 126,595 patients undergoing coronary arteriography. Cathet Cardiovasc Diagn. 1990;21:28–40.
2. Topaz O, DeMarchena EJ, Perin E, et al. Anomalous coronary arteries: angiographic findings in 80 patients. Int J Cardiol. 1992;34:129–38.
3. Angelini P, Velasco JA, Flamm S. Coronary anomalies: incidence, pathophysiology, and clinical relevance. Circulation. 2002;105:2449–54.
4. McConnell MV, Ganz P, Selwyn AP, et al. Identification of anomalous coronary arteries and their anatomic course by magnetic resonance coronary angiography. Circulation. 1995;92:3158–62.
5. Taylor AM, Thorne SA, Rubens MB, et al. Coronary artery imaging in grown up congenital heart disease: complementary role of magnetic resonance and x-ray coronary angiography. Circulation. 2000;101:1670–8.
6. McConnell MV, Stuber M, Manning WJ. Clinical role of coronary magnetic resonance angiography in the diagnosis of anomalous coronary arteries. J Cardiovasc Magn Reson. 2000;2:217–24.
7. White CS, Laskey WK, Stafford JL, et al. Coronary MRA: use in assessing anomalies of coronary artery origin. J Comput Assist Tomogr. 1999;23:203–7.
8. Sevrukov A, Aker N, Sullivan C, et al. Identifying the course of an anomalous left coronary artery using contrast-enhanced electron beam tomography and three-dimensional reconstruction. Catheter Cardiovasc Interv. 2002;57:532–6.
9. Koike K, Musewe NN, Smallhorn JF, et al. Distinguishing between anomalous origin of the left coronary artery from the pulmonary trunk and dilated cardiomyopathy: role of echocardiographic measurement of the right coronary artery diameter. Br Heart J. 1989;61:192–7.
10. King DH, Danford DA, Huhta JC, et al. Noninvasive detection of anomalous origin of the left main coronary artery from the pulmonary trunk by pulsed Doppler echocardiography. Am J Cardiol. 1985;55:608–9.
11. Sanders SP, Parness IA, Colan SD. Recognition of abnormal connections of coronary arteries with the use of Doppler color flow mapping. J Am Coll Cardiol. 1989;13:922–6.
12. Holley DG, Sell JE, Hougen TJ, et al. Pulsed Doppler echocardiographic and color flow imaging detection of retrograde filling of anomalous left coronary artery from the pulmonary artery. J Am Soc Echocardiogr. 1992;5:85–8.
13. Salzer-Muhar U, Proll E, Kronik G. Intercoronary collateral flow detected by Doppler colour flow mapping is an additional diagnostic sign in children with anomalous origin of the left coronary artery from the pulmonary artery. Br Heart J. 1993;70:558–9.
14. Frommelt MA, Miller E, Williamson J, et al. Detection of septal coronary collaterals by color flow Doppler mapping is a marker for anomalous origin of a coronary artery from the pulmonary artery. J Am Soc Echocardiogr. 2002;15:259–63.
15. Frommelt PC, Friedberg DZ, Frommelt MA, et al. Anomalous origin of the right coronary artery from the left sinus of Valsalva: transthoracic echocardiographic diagnosis. J Am Soc Echocardiogr. 1999;12:221–4.
16. Stefanelli CB, Stevenson JG, Jones TK, et al. A case for routine screening of coronary artery origins during echocardiography: fortuitous discovery of a life-threatening coronary anomaly. J Am Soc Echocardiogr. 1999;12:769–72.
17. Nowak B, Voigtlander T, Kolsch B, et al. Echocardiographic visualization of anomalous left main coronary arteries originating from the right sinus of Valsalva. Int J Cardiol. 1994;46:67–73.
18. Daliento L, Fasoli G, Mazzucco A. Anomalous origin of the left coronary artery from the anterior aortic sinus: role of echocardiography. Int J Cardiol. 1993;38:89–91.
19. Zeppilli P, dello Russo A, Santini C, et al. In vivo detection of coronary artery anomalies in asymptomatic athletes by echocardiographic screening. Chest. 1998;114:89–93.
20. Maron BJ, Leon MB, Swain JA, et al. Prospective identification by two-dimensional echocardiography of anomalous origin of the left main coronary artery from the right sinus of Valsalva. Am J Cardiol. 1991;68:140–2.
21. Erol C, Candan I, Sonel A, et al. Anomalous origin of the right coronary artery from the left sinus of Valsalva: echocardiographic diagnosis—a case report. Angiology. 1987;38:268–70.
22. Frommelt PC, Berger S, Pelech AN, et al. Prospective identification of anomalous origin of left coronary artery from the right sinus of Valsalva using transthoracic echocardiography: importance of color Doppler flow mapping. Pediatr Cardiol. 2001;22:327–32.
23. Gaither NS, Rogan KM, Stajduhar K, et al. Anomalous origin and course of coronary arteries in adults: identification and improved imaging utilizing transesophageal echocardiography. Am Heart J. 1991;122:69–75.
24. Hsieh YK, Fu M, Wu CJ, et al. Anomalous origin of left coronary artery from right coronary artery (single coronary artery): diagnosis by transesophageal echocardiography. J Ultrasound Med. 1996;15:169–71.
25. Alam M, Brymer J, Smith S. Transesophageal echocardiographic diagnosis of anomalous left coronary artery from the right aortic sinus. Chest. 1993;103:1617–8.
26. Koh KK. Confirmation of anomalous origin of the right coronary artery from the left sinus of Valsalva by means of transesophageal echocardiography. Am Heart J. 1991;122:851–4.
27. Henson KD, Geiser EA, Billett J, et al. Use of transesophageal echocardiography to visualize an anomalous right coronary artery arising from the left main coronary artery (single coronary artery). Clin Cardiol. 1992;15:462–5.
28. Smolin MR, Gorman PD, Gaither NS, et al. Origin of the right coronary artery from the left main coronary artery identified by transesophageal echocardiography. Am Heart J. 1992;123:1062–5.
29. Kasprzak JD, Kratochwil D, Peruga JZ, et al. Coronary anomalies diagnosed with transesophageal echocardiography: complementary clinical value in adults. Int J Card Imaging. 1998;14:89–95.
30. Fernandes F, Alam M, Smith S, et al. The role of transesophageal echocardiography in identifying anomalous coronary arteries. Circulation. 1993;88:2532–40.
31. Liberthson RR, Dinsmore RE, Fallon JT. Aberrant coronary artery origin from the aorta. Report of 18 patients, review of literature and delineation of natural history and management. Circulation. 1979;59:748–54.
32. Roberts WC. Major anomalies of coronary arterial origin seen in adulthood. Am Heart J. 1986;111:941–63.
33. Frescura C, Basso C, Thiene G, et al. Anomalous origin of coronary arteries and risk of sudden death: a study based on an autopsy population of congenital heart disease. Hum Pathol. 1998;29:689–95.
34. Taylor AJ, Rogan KM, Virmani R. Sudden cardiac death associated with isolated congenital coronary artery anomalies. J Am Coll Cardiol. 1992;20:640–7.
35. Lipsett J, Byard RW, Carpenter BF, et al. Anomalous coronary arteries arising from the aorta associated with sudden death in infancy and early childhood. An autopsy series. Arch Pathol Lab Med. 1991;115:770–3.
36. Kragel AH, Roberts WC. Anomalous origin of either the right or left main coronary artery from the aorta with subsequent coursing between aorta and pulmonary trunk: analysis of 32 necropsy cases. Am J Cardiol. 1988;62:771–7.
37. Wesselhoeft H, Fawcett JS, Johnson AL. Anomalous origin of the left coronary artery from the pulmonary trunk. Its clinical spectrum, pathology, and pathophysiology, based on a review of 140 cases with seven further cases. Circulation. 1968;38:403–25.

38. Herrmann MA, Dousa MK, Edwards WD. Sudden infant death with anomalous origin of the left coronary artery. Am J Forensic Med Pathol. 1992;13:191–5.
39. Roberts WC, Shirani J. The four subtypes of anomalous origin of the left main coronary artery from the right aortic sinus (or from the right coronary artery). Am J Cardiol. 1992;70:119–21.
40. Barth CW, Roberts WC. Left main coronary artery originating from the right sinus of Valsalva and coursing between the aorta and pulmonary trunk. J Am Coll Cardiol. 1986;7:366–73.
41. Aoyagi S, Suzuki S, Kosuga K, et al. Anomalous origin of the right coronary artery associated with congenital bicuspid aortic valve. Kurume Med J. 1991;38:199–202.
42. Roberts WC, Siegel RJ, Zipes DP. Origin of the right coronary artery from the left sinus of Valsalva and its functional consequences: analysis of 10 necropsy patients. Am J Cardiol. 1982;49:863–8.
43. Isner JM, Shen EM, Martin ET, et al. Sudden unexpected death as a result of anomalous origin of the right coronary artery from the left sinus of Valsalva. Am J Med. 1984;76:155–8.
44. Berdoff R, Haimowitz A, Kupersmith J. Anomalous origin of the right coronary artery from the left sinus of Valsalva. Am J Cardiol. 1986;58:656–7.
45. McManus BM, Gries LA, Ness MJ, et al. Anomalous origin of the right coronary artery from the left sinus of Valsalva. Pediatr Pathol. 1990;10:987–91.
46. Barth CW, Bray M, Roberts WC. Sudden death in infancy associated with origin of both left main and right coronary arteries from a common ostium above the left sinus of Valsalva. Am J Cardiol. 1986;57:365–6.
47. Liberthson RR, Gang DL, Custer J. Sudden death in an infant with aberrant origin of the right coronary artery from the left sinus of Valsalva of the aorta: case report and review of the literature. Pediatr Cardiol. 1983;4:45–8.
48. Mantovani E, Carraro R, Thiene G. Another case of juvenile sudden death caused by anomalous origin of the right coronary from the left anterior sinus of Valsalva. G Ital Cardiol. 1987;17:791–9.
49. Hanzlick R, Stivers RR. Sudden death in a marathon runner with origin of right coronary artery from the left sinus of Valsalva. Am J Cardiol. 1983;51:1467.
50. Frommelt PC, Frommelt MA, Tweddell JS, et al. Prospective echocardiographic diagnosis and surgical repair of anomalous origin of a coronary artery from the opposite sinus with an interarterial course. J Am Coll Cardiol. 2003;42:148–54.
51. Angelini P. Coronary artery anomalies: an entity in search of an identity. Circulation. 2007;115:1296–305.
52. Kaku B, Shimizu M, Kita Y, et al. Detection of anomalous origin of the left coronary artery by transesophageal echocardiography and magnetic resonance imaging. Jpn Heart J. 1994;35:383–8.
53. Sasson Z, Grande P, Lorette I, et al. Proximal narrowing of anomalous right coronary artery from the left coronary sinus: delineation by omniplane transesophageal echocardiogram. Can J Cardiol. 1996;12:529–31.
54. Mavroudis C, Backer CL, Muster AJ, et al. Expanding indications for pediatric coronary artery bypass. J Thorac Cardiovasc Surg. 1996;111:181–9.
55. Thomas D, Salloum J, Montalescot G, et al. Anomalous coronary arteries coursing between the aorta and pulmonary trunk: clinical indications for coronary artery bypass. Eur Heart J. 1991;12:832–4.
56. Kucera RF, Bowden WD, Thomas HMJ, et al. Anomalous origin of the right coronary artery from the left sinus of Valsalva: a case report. Cathet Cardiovasc Diagn. 1986;12:334–6.
57. Brandt B, Martins JB, Marcus ML. Anomalous origin of the right coronary artery from the left sinus of Valsalva. N Engl J Med. 1983;309:596–8.
58. Ghosh PK, Agarwal SK, Kumar R, et al. Anomalous origin of right coronary artery from left aortic sinus. J Cardiovasc Surg (Torino). 1994;35:65–70.
59. Bucsenez D, Messmer BJ, Gillor A, et al. Management of anomalous origin of the left coronary artery from the right sinus of Valsalva. J Thorac Cardiovasc Surg. 1994;107:1370–3.
60. Di Lello F, Mnuk JF, Flemma RJ, et al. Successful coronary reimplantation for anomalous origin of the right coronary artery from the left sinus of Valsalva. J Thorac Cardiovasc Surg. 1991;102:455–6.
61. Mustafa I, Gula G, Radley-Smith R, et al. Anomalous origin of the left coronary artery from the anterior aortic sinus: a potential cause of sudden death. Anatomic characterization and surgical treatment. J Thorac Cardiovasc Surg. 1981;82:297–300.
62. Donaldson RM, Raphael MJ, Yacoub MH, et al. Hemodynamically significant anomalies of the coronary arteries. Surgical aspects. Thorac Cardiovasc Surg. 1982;30:7–13.
63. Van Son JA, Haas GS. Anomalous origin of left main coronary artery from right sinus of Valsalva: modified surgical treatment to avoid neo-coronary ostial stenosis. Eur J Cardiothorac Surg. 1996;10:467–9.
64. Nelson-Piercy C, Rickards AF, Yacoub MH. Aberrant origin of the right coronary artery as a potential cause of sudden death: successful anatomical correction. Br Heart J. 1990;64:208–10.
65. Keith J. Diseases of coronary arteries and aorta. In: Keith J, Rowe R, Vlad P, editors. Heart disease in infancy and childhood. New York: Macmillan; 1978. p. 278–9.
66. Tingelstad JB, Lower RR, Eldredge WJ. Anomalous origin of the right coronary artery from the main pulmonary artery. Am J Cardiol. 1972;30:670–3.
67. Hsu SY, Lin FC, Chang HJ, et al. Multiplane transesophageal echocardiography in diagnosis of anomalous origin of the left coronary artery from the pulmonary artery: a case report. J Am Soc Echocardiogr. 1998;11:668–72.
68. Kececioglu D, Kotthoff S, Konertz W, et al. Pulmonary artery origin of the left coronary artery: diagnosis by transesophageal echocardiography in infancy. Eur Heart J. 1993;14:1006–7.
69. Lowe JE, Oldham HNJ, Sabiston DCJ. Surgical management of congenital coronary artery fistulas. Ann Surg. 1981;194:373–80.
70. Hsieh KS, Huang TC, Lee CL. Coronary artery fistulas in neonates, infants, and children: clinical findings and outcome. Pediatr Cardiol. 2002;23:415–9.
71. Kamiya H, Yasuda T, Nagamine H, et al. Surgical treatment of congenital coronary artery fistulas: 27 years' experience and a review of the literature. J Card Surg. 2002;17:173–7.
72. Cheung DL, Au WK, Cheung HH, et al. Coronary artery fistulas: long-term results of surgical correction. Ann Thorac Surg. 2001;71:190–5.
73. Dorros G, Thota V, Ramireddy K, et al. Catheter-based techniques for closure of coronary fistulae. Catheter Cardiovasc Interv. 1999;46:143–50.
74. Reidy JF, Anjos RT, Qureshi SA, et al. Transcatheter embolization in the treatment of coronary artery fistulas. J Am Coll Cardiol. 1991;18:187–92.
75. Hartnell GG. Embolization in the treatment of acquired and congenital abnormalities of the heart and thorax. Radiographics. 1993;13:1349–62; quiz 1363–4.
76. Arazoza EA, Bowser M, Obeid AI. Coronary artery fistula: diagnosis by biplane transesophageal echocardiography. J Am Soc Echocardiogr. 1992;5:277–80.
77. Prewitt KC, Smolin MR, Coster TS, et al. Coronary artery fistula diagnosed by transesophageal echocardiography. Chest. 1994;105:959–61.
78. Lin FC, Chang HJ, Chern MS, et al. Multiplane transesophageal echocardiography in the diagnosis of congenital coronary artery fistula. Am Heart J. 1995;130:1236–44.
79. Tsai LM, Chen JH, Teng JK, et al. Right coronary artery-to-left ventricle fistula identified by transesophageal echocardiography. Am Heart J. 1992;124:1106–9.

80. Aude YW, Rosado A, Vignola P, et al. Coronary arteriovenous fistula with a giant aneurysm: role of transesophageal echocardiography. J Am Soc Echocardiogr. 1999;12:1104–6.
81. Okwuosa TM, Gundeck EL, Ward RP. Coronary to pulmonary artery fistula—diagnosis by transesophageal echocardiography. Echocardiography. 2006;23:62–4.
82. Vitarelli A, De Curtis G, Conde Y, et al. Assessment of congenital coronary artery fistulas by transesophageal color Doppler echocardiography. Am J Med. 2002;113:127–33.
83. Newburger JW, Takahashi M, Gerber MA, et al. Diagnosis, treatment, and long-term management of Kawasaki disease: a statement for health professionals from the Committee on Rheumatic Fever, Endocarditis and Kawasaki Disease, Council on Cardiovascular Disease in the Young, American Heart Association. Circulation. 2004;110:2747–71.
84. de Zorzi A, Colan SD, Gauvreau K, et al. Coronary artery dimensions may be misclassified as normal in Kawasaki disease. J Pediatr. 1998;133:254–8.
85. Research Committee on Kawasaki Disease. Report of subcommittee on standardization of diagnostic criteria and reporting of coronary artery lesions in Kawasaki disease. Tokyo: Ministry of Health and Welfare; 1984.
86. Frommelt PC, Frommelt MA. Congenital coronary anomalies. Pediatr Clin N Am. 2004;51:1275.

Intraoperative and Postoperative Transesophageal Echocardiography in Congenital Heart Disease

15

Wanda C. Miller-Hance and Isobel A. Russell

Abstract

The early experience with epicardial imaging in patients undergoing surgery for congenital heart disease (CHD) provided strong evidence to the idea that intraoperative echocardiography could guide specific surgical and anesthetic adjustments during this critical period. Since the introduction of transesophageal echocardiography (TEE) to the intraoperative setting in the late 1980s, numerous publications have documented the utility of this imaging modality in the care of patients with CHD. Technologic advances over the years that have included miniaturization of probes and multiplane imaging now allows for comprehensive assessment of structural abnormalities, evaluation of hemodynamics, and very importantly, appraisal of the surgical results in nearly all patients with CHD. The recognition of residual pathology of hemodynamic significance during congenital surgery and the ability of TEE to guide the surgical revision as necessary, represent major contributions to perioperative care. Additional important benefits of this technology in the perioperative period include its role as a monitoring adjunct to facilitate hemodynamic and pharmacologic management and to influence treatment strategies. TEE also provides a framework to assist in the formulation of management plans in the immediate postoperative period and the further characterization of postoperative unexpected/unusual findings or problems.

This chapter provides an overview of the applications of TEE in the intraoperative care of patients with CHD with an emphasis on impact on surgical, medical, and anesthetic management. Data on cost effectiveness, pitfalls, and limitations of intraoperative TEE are reviewed. Lastly, the role of TEE in the postoperative setting in the patient with CHD is addressed.

Keywords

Intraoperative transesophageal echocardiography in congenital heart disease • Postoperative transesophageal echocardiography in congenital heart disease • Applications of intraoperative TEE in congenital heart disease • Intraoperative TEE in children • TEE in the postoperative patient with congenital heart disease • Limitations of TEE in congenital heart disease

W.C. Miller-Hance, MD, FACC, FASE (✉)
Divisions of Pediatric Anesthesiology and Pediatric Cardiology,
Departments of Pediatrics and Anesthesiology,
Texas Children's Hospital, Baylor College of Medicine,
6621 Fannin, Suite W17417, Houston, TX 77030, USA
e-mail: wmh@bcm.edu

I.A. Russell, MD, PhD, FACC
Department of Cardiovascular Anesthesiology,
Kaiser Permanente, 2425 Geary Blvd,
San Francisco, CA 94115, USA

P.C. Wong, W.C. Miller-Hance (eds.), *Transesophageal Echocardiography for Congenital Heart Disease*,
DOI 10.1007/978-1-84800-064-3_15, © Springer-Verlag London 2014

Technological Evolution of Intraoperative Imaging in Congenital Heart Disease

Initial efforts in intraoperative echocardiography in children with congenital heart disease (CHD) explored the benefits of epicardial imaging. Standard transthoracic imaging probes covered in a sterile sheath were directly applied to the surface of the heart in order to assess cardiac anatomy and function prior to the initiation and after separation from cardiopulmonary bypass. This allowed for confirmation of preoperative diagnoses and assessment of the adequacy of the surgical repair [1–3]. Clinical experience over several years supported the benefits of the epicardial imaging approach in the perioperative management of patients with CHD [4–7].

Reports regarding the intraoperative applications of transesophageal echocardiography (TEE) in CHD can be traced to the late 1980s when Cyran and colleagues documented one of the earliest experiences [8]. While using an adult-sized probe, the potential benefits of TEE were examined in older children and young adults undergoing surgical interventions for a variety of structural heart defects. The report noted that TEE was valuable and could be performed safely and reliably in this patient group.

Kyo and associates in conjunction with Aloka Company in Japan developed the first TEE probe with specific applications to infants and young children [9, 10]. This was a single plane, 28-element, 5.0 MHz phased array device mounted on a flexible gastroscope of an external diameter of 6.8 mm. Although the transducer was limited to only transverse (horizontal, 0°) plane scanning, worldwide reports using this probe documented its accuracy and feasibility in the assessment of CHD [11–16].

It was observed that in some cases, TEE had superior diagnostic capabilities as compared to the transthoracic approach, and accuracy equivalent to epicardial imaging in the intraoperative setting [17–20]. Initial reports on the benefits of TEE during surgery for CHD ranged from the assessment of septal defects to complex lesions [21–23].

A major limitation of the technology during the early experience however, was the suboptimal image quality provided by a small probe with a relatively low number of elements and the inability to adequately interrogate the ventricular outflow tracts [24]. Despite these shortcomings, several studies highlighted the fact that when compared to epicardial echocardiography, transesophageal imaging did not interrupt surgery or caused potential distortion of cardiac structures. This imaging modality was also less likely to trigger rhythm abnormalities, produce hemodynamic alterations, or influence the infection risk. Efforts thus continued into improving the TEE technology for pediatric applications.

In the early 1990s a new single plane TEE transducer was introduced (5.0 MHz phased array, 48-element). This allowed for superior image resolution to that provided by previous hardware, in addition to continuous wave Doppler capabilities [25]. Concurrent refinements in Doppler technology allowed for improved assessment of blood flow velocities, jet direction, and overall evaluation of the severity of obstructive/regurgitant pathology.

The subsequent development of biplane probes (48 and 64-elements) for pediatric use enhanced the transesophageal examination by allowing for imaging not only in the transverse plane, as had been the case with single plane devices, but also in the longitudinal or vertical plane (90°) [26, 27]. The additional plane of interrogation improved the diagnostic accuracy of TEE, particularly for pathology affecting the ventricular outflow tracts [28]. The benefits of biplane imaging were not limited to children, but were also reported in adults with congenital cardiovascular malformations [29].

Despite the advantages offered by biplane imaging, several limitations of the technology were recognized at the time. One of these related to the inability to optimally align the spectral Doppler angle of interrogation with the direction of blood flow while imaging from the esophageal windows. This limitation was partly addressed by transgastric imaging, which provided much more favorable angles for Doppler interrogation of ventricular outflow tracts and great arteries using existing single and biplane TEE devices [30, 31].

The introduction of multiplane TEE imaging for children in the mid 1990s represented a major technological advancement. At the time, experience had suggested superiority of multiplane over biplane imaging in adults [32, 33]. This development provided the opportunity for the acquisition of high-resolution images in an unlimited number of planes, a necessity for the comprehensive assessment of complex cardiovascular pathology. The initial pediatric multiplane probe (mini-multiplane device) was a 48-element, phased array, single crystal 5-MHz transducer with two-dimensional, M-mode and full Doppler capabilities [34–36]. The probe was mounted on a transducer shaft of 7 mm, with tip dimensions of 27 mm (length) by 10.6 mm (width) by 7.9 mm (thickness). Steering from an arc ranging from 0° to 180° was performed manually, in contrast to the electronic control then available in the adult multiplane probe. A second knob allowed for flexion of the transducer tip anteriorly and posteriorly (anteflexion and retroflexion respectively). This device, originally designed by Odelft BV (Delft, The Netherlands), was marketed soon thereafter and adapted for use on a number of echocardiographic platforms produced by different manufacturers (refer to Chap. 2).

There has been ongoing interest in further miniaturizing the TEE technology to provide allow for a larger margin of safety. Sporadic reports have acknowledged potential benefits and shortcomings of these imaging probes [37, 38]. Limited experience with an imaging device more suitable for use in neonates and small infants (Odelft micro-multiplane

TEE probe) was reported several years ago. An 8 mm diameter probe tip mounted on a 5 mm gastroscope characterized this 7.5 MHz, 48-element transducer [39–41]. The device allowed the examination of infants as small as 2.5 kg of weight without major complications. Unfortunately, technological challenges stalled the development of this device.

In recent years a miniaturized multiplane device became commercially available (Philips Medical, Andover, MA, USA, micro TEE transducer). This probe has a shaft width of 5.2 mm, transducer tip width of 7.5 mm, and height of 5.5 mm. The 32-element phased array multiplane transducer incorporates two-dimensional, color, full spectral Doppler modalities, and M-Mode. The center frequency of this device is 6 MHz (range 3.2–7.4 MHz). The experience with this probe thus far has demonstrated a highly successful insertion rate in tiny neonates and high-quality diagnostic imaging without respiratory or hemodynamic compromise (refer to Chap. 2) [42].

A prospective study assessed the image quality of the micro-multiplane TEE probe and compared it with that obtained using the standard pediatric or adult probe [43]. A total of 24 studies were performed (23 patients, median weight of 11.7 kg, median age of 3 years). The micro-multiplane TEE probe was found to provide diagnostic image quality in the neonatal age group, however, in children between 10 and 30 kg, standard-sized pediatric probes allowed for better imaging.

A catheter approved for intracardiac echocardiography (ICE) has been used off label for transesophageal intraoperative imaging in tiny infants. This miniaturized device (AcuNav™ Ultrasound Catheter, Siemens Medical), with a diameter of 3.3 mm, carries a 64-element phased-array multifrequency transducer (5.5–10 MHz). Capabilities include longitudinal plane imaging, as well as spectral and color Doppler modalities. The handle controls allow for four-way steering in two planes: anterior-posterior, left-right; with 160° rotation in each direction. A report noted a group of 17 infants (weight between 2.1 and 5.6 kg) undergoing 22 examinations with this device [44]. Most studies were of diagnostic quality and no complications were identified. A case report in an infant with single ventricle also demonstrated the diagnostic utility of this catheter when used for imaging via the esophagus [45].

The principal advantage of this catheter is its slender profile, which allows safe esophageal placement in very small babies, with excellent imaging quality and full Doppler capabilities. The major disadvantage is that there is only a single, longitudinal (90°) imaging plane; a second orthogonal transverse plane (0°) is not available, nor are there multiplane capabilities. This limits the imaging effectiveness of this catheter for certain types of CHD in which the transverse plane is important. Also, no temperature sensing is available on this device raising concerns regarding safety.

Currently, most centers prefer the use of multiplane imaging in patients with CHD as this enables detailed assessment of anatomy, hemodynamics, and function. Biplane imaging may be considered an acceptable, though less desirable option if multiplane interrogation is not feasible.

Impact of TEE on Intraoperative Care

Influences on Surgical Management

An extensive experience over a period of many years has documented the utility of intraoperative imaging in the care of patients with CHD, as well as in children with acquired pathologies. It is well recognized that intraoperative imaging provides detailed anatomic and hemodynamic information prior to the planned surgical procedure, assists in the assessment of the quality of the repair, and allows for real-time monitoring of ventricular loading and performance.

One of the initial reports regarding the utility of echocardiography during surgery for CHD was by Ungerleider and colleagues [46]. Their experience consisted of 1,000 patients at Duke University Medical Center from a period spanning between the years of 1987 and 1994. Surgery in the majority of cases was performed using cardiopulmonary bypass. Intraoperative imaging made use of the epicardial approach during the early years due to lack of miniaturized TEE transducers. Subsequently, the use of TEE was favored, and in many cases, both imaging modalities were employed. The authors reported that during the later years of their experience it was extremely unlikely for the intraoperative prebypass examination to reveal new findings or provide information leading to an alteration in the surgical plan. However, they continued to subjectively perceive value in performing the examination as it provided for baseline images to be obtained for later comparison to the postbypass study and allowed the identification of optimal planes of interrogation that could later be applied to facilitate the postrepair assessment. Regarding the need for surgical revisions, there was a 4.4 % incidence of return to bypass based on the echocardiographic findings. Most patients underwent a successful revision, with success being defined by the fact that the residual defect being revised was either eliminated or considered "acceptable". In recognition of the utility of intraoperative echocardiography, the authors indicated, "it was not possible for the surgeon to predict the need for a revision based on his confidence of the repair".

Numerous reports of the early TEE experience for CHD followed, documenting the benefits of this technology in the intraoperative setting as a diagnostic tool and in regards to surgical decision-making [5, 15, 17, 21–26, 28, 29, 47–57]. Subsequent publications have continued to support the major impact of this modality during surgery not only for congenital pathology but also for pediatric acquired heart disease [58, 59].

The overall incidence of alteration in surgical plan with the aid of preoperative TEE has been reported to be in the range of 3–15 %. A retrospective review of the first 341 intraoperative studies performed at Texas Children's Hospital during the years of 1990–1995, noted that the prebypass TEE resulted in alteration of the planned surgical procedure in as many as 9.4 % of cases [56]. Diagnostic categories in which TEE had the most impact on surgical procedures included ventricular septal defect in association with double-chambered right ventricle or subaortic membrane, isolated subaortic stenosis, atrioventricular valve dysfunction, single ventricle, and pulmonary atresia with ventricular septal defect. More likely, however, was the detection of minor TEE diagnostic findings that did not influence the surgical plan. This was noted in 13.2 % of the cohort. The need for immediate reoperation based on the TEE findings was reported in 8.2 % of patients.

Several years later, Randolph and colleagues at the Mayo Clinic reported the results of their study on a large number of patients, undertaken to further define the impact of intraoperative TEE during congenital heart surgery and determine appropriate indications for the use of this modality [60]. The investigation included patients encompassing a wide age range spectrum, from the neonate to the elderly. A major impact was identified in 13.8 % of cases; findings were considered to have had a major impact when unique prebypass information altered the planned surgical procedure or prompted immediate revision of hemodynamically significant defects. This was more likely to occur in younger patients, during reoperations, and in those undergoing valve repairs or complex outflow tract reconstructions.

Sloth and associates in Denmark described their experience with the use of TEE in 532 consecutive children over a period of 5 years [61]. In this series, findings on TEE led to return to bypass in approximately 3 % of patients. Ma and colleagues from the Paediatric Heart Center in Shanghai examined transesophageal recordings in 350 children with CHD [62]. Preoperative TEE added additional findings or altered prior diagnoses in 9.4 % of patients. The findings modified the planned surgical procedure in 6.6 % of the study group. Residual problems or sequelae were detected by postoperative TEE in 16.3 %, with a total of 3.7 % of patients requiring immediate intervention or return to bypass for revision of the surgical procedure.

Bettex and colleagues in Switzerland, in a two-center observational study, provided further support for the use of TEE during congenital heart surgery in children [63]. Among 865 patients under 17 years of age, alterations in surgical management were reported in 12.7 % of cases and included the need for reinstitution of cardiopulmonary bypass in 7.3 %. Changes in medical management resulting from TEE findings were required in 19.4 % of cases during the intraoperative period.

The contemporary experience among institutions that routinely utilize intraoperative imaging during congenital heart surgery suggests a return to bypass rate as guided by TEE in the range of approximately 3–7 %. Even more compelling is the observation that failure to address significant residual pathology may lead to high morbidity in these patients and in some cases account for perioperative mortality [63, 64].

While the benefits of TEE for assessing the adequacy of the surgical intervention in congenital heart surgery have been well documented, several isolated case reports describe additional benefits of intraoperative TEE in patients with CHD as well as in children with acquired cardiovascular disorders. These include: the detection of complications associated with cannulation during cardiopulmonary bypass, resection of cardiac tumors, evaluation of pulmonary artery flow after the Fontan procedure, identification and guided drainage of pericardial and pleural effusions, and others [65–70].

In addition to the utility of TEE during cases requiring cardiopulmonary bypass, the benefits of this imaging approach have also been reported during other interventions such as in video assisted thoracoscopic procedures for CHD [71–74]. Transesophageal imaging has also been utilized for guiding interventions that involve placement of devices, such as septal occluders or stents via the perventricular or direct approach in the operating room as a hybrid or combined effort by the cardiothoracic surgeon and interventional cardiologist (refer to Chap. 17) [75, 76].

The cumulative experience validates the ability of intraoperative TEE to improve the quality of the surgical interventions in CHD, both in children and adults, as well as other pediatric cardiovascular interventions. This has resulted in imaging during cardiac surgery representing the most common indication for TEE in this patient group. Although formal, rigorous scientific data regarding the impact of intraoperative TEE on clinical outcomes is lacking, this modality is now considered to be of significant benefit, evolving into an important part of perioperative management in patients with CHD, as well as other acquired cardiovascular pathologies in children. As such, TEE has become standard of care practice in many centers that specialize in CHD, in agreement with the indications outlined by various clinical practice guidelines [77–83].

Influences on Medical Management

In addition to the impact of TEE on surgical care, the literature has documented the many contributions of TEE to medical management and other aspects of anesthetic care during congenital heart surgery. Several of these benefits are described in the sections that follow.

Catheter Placement and Guidance

Central venous catheterization is considered an important aspect of perioperative care, providing for vascular access and hemodynamic monitoring. Reports have documented the use of TEE to facilitate percutaneous central venous catheter placement, allowing for visualization of guidewire position prior to the insertion of large bore central venous catheters. This may prevent repeated attempts at cannulation and potential complications, particularly in young patients [84, 85].

The utility of TEE for optimization of catheter tip placement has been reported in adults as well as in children undergoing cardiovascular interventions [86–88]. A prospective, randomized, controlled clinical trial in children examined the role of TEE in guiding proper depth of central venous catheter insertion and confirming superior vena cava cannulation [89]. The study comprised 145 patients (ages 1 day to 29 years) undergoing surgery for CHD. Correct central line catheter placement was defined as a catheter tip visible in the superior vena cava at or above the superior vena cava to right atrial junction and parallel to the wall of the superior vena cava, as determined by either TEE or chest radiograph (CXR). TEE-guided catheter placement resulted in 100 % correct placement when assessed by TEE, versus 86 % in the control group (catheter depth based on external landmarks). If the CXR was used to determine correct position, there were no differences in proper catheter positioning. The investigators concluded that TEE can be use to guide central catheter placement in patients undergoing congenital heart surgery, significantly improving the success rate of proper placement.

The placement of transthoracic intracardiac catheters may be necessary for hemodynamic monitoring in infants and children with congenital or acquired heart disease [90, 91]. Although the utility of TEE in guiding placement of these catheters has not been documented in detail, the confirmation of appropriate catheter position is facilitated and can be verified by TEE. This is also the case with placement and optimal positioning of circulatory support hardware (aortic and venous cannulae, mechanical support devices) and pulmonary artery catheters [92].

Cardiac Dealring and Identification of Intracardiac Air

The bright reflections produced by the presence of air bubbles within the heart and vasculature can be readily identified by echocardiography due to the unique acoustic properties that characterize air, in contrast to other media such as blood. Retained intracardiac air may account for significant morbidity during cardiac surgery, negatively impacting clinical outcomes. Air embolization to the coronary circulation may have immediate and/or late effects that can lead to myocardial dysfunction. This is turn can necessitate prolongation of cardiopulmonary bypass and require interventions such as institution or adjustment of inotropic support or other therapies [93, 94]. Other serious complications include those related to the presence of air in the systemic circulation and potential neurologic injury [95, 96].

Echocardiography has been shown to be exquisitely sensitive in the detection of intracardiac air and TEE provides significant benefit in facilitating cardiac deairing [97–106]. During congenital heart surgery, ensuring the adequacy of cardiac deairing prior to discontinuation of cardiopulmonary bypass is of particular relevance, given that interventions frequently require cardiotomy. Greeley and associates reported the observation of intramyocardial air in patients undergoing repair of congenital heart defects. This was described as the presence of air within the wall of a myocardial segment supplied by a coronary artery branch, suggesting air embolization of this vessel. The relevance of this observation was that this finding could lead to ventricular dysfunction after separation from bypass, regional wall motion abnormalities, and potential hemodynamic instability [107]. The report underscored the fact that the identification of intramyocardial air by intraoperative imaging may allow for the development of a specific management plan because the likely etiology for the functional and hemodynamic alterations can be readily recognized.

Additional contributions of TEE regarding the detection of air apply to procedures performed on a beating heart when aortic cross-clamping is not required or can be avoided. These procedures may involve interventions in the right-heart (e.g., right ventricular to pulmonary artery conduit replacement), left heart (e.g., insertion of inflow cannula during placement of ventricular assist device), or single ventricle (e.g., placement of graft in the right ventricle during the Sano modification of the Norwood procedure). The concern during right-heart surgery is entrainment of air into left-sided cardiac structures across an intracardiac communication (right-to-left shunting) and the risk for paradoxical air embolization. Similarly, air entrained by the left ventricle during coring of the apex for placement of a mechanical support cannula, or in the single ventricle, during right ventricular graft placement, represents a potential risk for paradoxical emboli when/if the aortic (or neoartic) valve opens.

For the reasons discussed above, in patients with a biventricular circulation undergoing 'beating right-heart surgery' the exclusion of intracardiac communications is of relevance and TEE plays an important role in this assessment. Color flow mapping and contrast echocardiography facilitates the detection of intracardiac shunting. The use of contrast imaging, for example with agitated saline or albumin, in combination with a simulated Valsalva maneuver in intubated and mechanically ventilated patients, increases the detection of intracardiac communications as right-to-left intracardiac shunting can be identified (refer to Chap. 4). Because the reliability of contrast TEE in the detection of intracardiac communications in patients with CHD has been questioned, continuous monitoring for the presence of intracardiac air should be considered during these procedures in order to enhance their safety [108]. A similar vigilant approach applies to interventions on the left ventricle or single ventricle patient during beating heart surgery.

Assessment of Ventricular Loading Conditions

Manipulation of ventricular preload represents a key element in the optimization of cardiac performance and a major focus of hemodynamic management in the care of patients with CHD. Various parameters and techniques have been utilized in clinical practice to provide an estimation of ventricular filling, including TEE [109–111].

The determination of ventricular preload by TEE has mostly focused on the left ventricle [112–114]. Several studies have compared/correlated the assessment of left ventricular preload by TEE with measurements of filling pressures. Echocardiographic indices frequently examined have included the estimation of left ventricular end-diastolic area and/or volume. TEE has been shown to provide a more sensitive method for detecting hypovolemia than traditional hemodynamic parameters of ventricular preload, such as central venous pressure and pulmonary artery capillary wedge pressure [115]. However, a number of limitations are recognized in this assessment, including the fact that measured volumes by two-dimensional TEE are known to be significantly smaller than those obtained by angiography [115, 116].

Data regarding TEE-guided manipulations of ventricular preload in young patients with CHD is extremely limited. An investigation by Reich and co-workers recruited a small number of patients undergoing elective repair of various defects, ranging in weight from 3 to 15 kg in order to determine whether TEE could identify alterations in cardiac filling resulting from manipulations of blood volume. Changes in left ventricular end-diastolic and end-systolic areas were assessed in the transgastric left ventricular midpapillary short axis view (TG Mid SAX). At the same time, hemodynamic data were recorded while several interventions were performed after sternal closure. Measurements were obtained at baseline, upon phlebotomy, and after the reinfusion of blood. The study demonstrated that decreases in blood volume as small as 5–8 % were associated with a reduction in left ventricular end-diastolic area, as well as central venous and systemic arterial pressures. Thus both the qualitative and quantitative measurements documented changes in left ventricular filling, thereby validating the application of TEE as a useful monitor of cardiac preload in pediatric patients.

Estimation of ventricular areas and volumes, however, is known to be time-consuming and impractical in the operating room setting, representing a potential distraction for healthcare providers. In addition, the abnormal and highly variable geometry of structurally abnormal hearts imposes significant limitations upon this assessment. These factors account for the fact that the routine intraoperative evaluation of ventricular filling mostly takes place through a qualitative assessment from the echocardiographic display of the ventricular chamber of interest in multiple planes. For the left ventricle, this translates to the evaluation of changes in end-diastolic area in the TG Mid SAX view, in addition to gross assessment of left ventricular cavity size in the mid esophageal four chamber view (ME 4 Ch). For the right ventricle, a combination of views may be used including the ME 4 Ch, mid esophageal right ventricular inflow-outflow, and additional views at the transgastric and deep transgastric levels.

Assessment of Ventricular Function

The evaluation of ventricular performance is one of the most relevant applications of intraoperative echocardiography since clinical outcomes are greatly influenced by myocardial function. Ventricular performance can be described in terms of global or regional function and can also be considered in reference to the systolic and diastolic contributions.

Echocardiography provides for qualitative and quantitative measurements of ventricular systolic function and contractility (for an in depth discussion on the subject the reader is referred to Chap. 5). The applications of TEE in the determination of left ventricular ejection phase indices such as fractional shortening, fractional area change, ejection fraction, and others have been well described [117]. However, validation of these measurements, have not been thoroughly performed, with a potential error in the measurement of fractional area change in the range of 10 % under optimal conditions [118]. The abnormal ventricular geometry associated with many structural heart defects further complicates this assessment. A study of left ventricular performance in children determined that M-mode indices derived from transthoracic echocardiography and TEE were not directly comparable, presumably because of regional non-uniformity of function [119]. This is not a surprising finding considering that these measurements cannot be obtained in exactly the same plane by the two imaging modalities.

Over the last several years there has been increasing interest in the routine evaluation of diastolic function by echocardiography in both, pediatric and adult age groups, since abnormalities of ventricular relaxation and compliance are known to contribute to perioperative morbidity [120–125]. This effort has relied heavily on the use of Doppler modalities, particularly spectral analysis, in order to examine left ventricular filling alterations that may correlate with diastolic function.

It is well recognized that diastolic dysfunction plays a major role in many congenital and acquired pathologies in the pediatric age group [126–129]. Unfortunately, the evaluation of diastolic function in young patients has met several challenges, including the many confounding variables that influence appropriate Doppler assessment and interpretation of findings. Using criteria developed for transthoracic echocardiography to the transesophageal approach further magnifies these difficulties [130]. Thus the use of TEE to assess diastolic function in children with CHD remains, up to the time of this writing, of limited utility and an important area of future investigation.

Another area that has received limited attention and may benefit from further insight is the evaluation of right ventricular and single ventricular function by TEE [131, 132]. As with diastolic function, limited information is currently available in these areas and they remain important subjects for ongoing research.

Detection of Myocardial Ischemia

TEE has been shown to be a sensitive tool for the detection and monitoring of myocardial ischemia in adults. The sensitivity of TEE for intraoperative ischemia detection is known to be superior to electrocardiography-detected ST segment changes or elevations of pulmonary artery wedge pressure during pulmonary artery catheter monitoring [133]. As such, the qualitative assessment of regional myocardial function by TEE has become a widely used modality in the perioperative care of adult patients at risk for compromised coronary blood flow, either during cardiac or noncardiac surgery [134].

Although limited data is available, a few investigations have focused on the potential applications of this monitor for the detection of myocardial ischemia in children undergoing interventions that involve manipulation of the coronary arteries [135]. Rouine-Rapp and associates prospectively studied a group of neonates undergoing an arterial switch operation to determine if segmental wall motion abnormalities, as identified by intraoperative TEE, represented myocardial ischemia [136]. The investigation demonstrated that when multiple segmental wall motion abnormalities were present, the regional wall dysfunction tended to persist at the time of chest closure. Relative to those with normal wall motion after surgical repair, this group of infants had more postoperative ischemic events based on Holter monitoring (ST segment changes) and elevated cardiac troponin I levels, confirming the correlation between TEE detected regional wall motion abnormalities and myocardial ischemia.

These observations validate the benefits of TEE in the early diagnosis of compromised myocardial blood flow and support the perioperative use of this modality in infants and children at increased risk of myocardial ischemia or infarction during congenital heart surgery. This application likely extends to pediatric patients undergoing interventions for acquired pathology and also to the adult population with CHD who may in addition have comorbidities that impact coronary blood flow.

Impact on Anesthetic and Hemodynamic Management

An extensive literature supports the role of TEE in clinical decision-making in adult patients. Several studies have also demonstrated the benefits of this technology regarding hemodynamic monitoring and modifications of medical management in patients with CHD and children with acquired cardiovascular pathologies. These reports include experiences worldwide.

Two investigations that included large number of patients focused on changes in medical care as a result of intraoperative TEE. Sloth and associates in Denmark evaluated the monitoring value of intraoperative TEE in 532 consecutive children, over a 5-year period undergoing heart surgery [61]. New information was identified by TEE in 45 % of the cohort. This information was judged to have been instrumental in directing, altering or changing medical management in 8 % of cases (43 out of 532). The most frequent interventions included changes in inotropic strategy related to ventricular dysfunction and volume replacement. Bettex and coworkers analyzed reports from 865 intraoperative examinations between two specialized congenital heart surgery centers [63]. Medical management was assisted by TEE in 19.4 % of cases, leading to changes that included optimization of ventricular filling and pharmacologic therapy.

The overall data, although limited, provide support for the extended role of intraoperative TEE outside of its impact on the surgery itself. The data demonstrate the utility of perioperative TEE as a monitoring adjunct to facilitate anesthetic care, hemodynamic and pharmacologic management, medical decision making, and influence on treatment strategies. Moreover, this imaging approach also provides a framework to assist in the formulation of care plans during the immediate postoperative period.

Cost Effectiveness of Intraoperative TEE

The early experience using epicardial imaging during congenital heart surgery acknowledged not only the impact of this technology on surgical management but also suggested that the benefits of this approach justified the associated costs [1]. Ungerleider et al. noted that the costs involved in the performance of the intraoperative studies was justified by savings in operating room time and possible prevention of reoperations because of less than optimal results [3]. In a subsequent report, a more formal cost benefit analysis was performed comparing hospital costs between patients requiring a reoperation versus those undergoing immediate revision of the repair based on echocardiographic data [46]. Not surprisingly, hospital costs were substantially lower in the latter group. These findings provided clear and compelling evidence of the financial benefits of intraoperative TEE.

Other studies have also examined the issue of cost-effectiveness of intraoperative TEE. Relatively early in the experience a cost-benefit analysis was reported by Benson and Cahalan that included various cardiac surgical settings, including surgery for CHD [137]. Based upon published data regarding the impact of TEE in identifying residual defects that required immediate revision during interventions for CHD in infants and children, their analysis estimated a definite financial patient benefit per TEE study performed. In fact, in their assessment, among patients undergoing cardiac surgery, those with CHD derived the greatest overall financial benefits. Their analysis indicated that the financial gain of TEE was substantial, frequently outweighing the costs of repeat surgery.

Siwik and colleagues examined the costs and resources required in performing routine TEE services as an adjunct to congenital heart surgery in a case-controlled analysis of 63 children undergoing elective, complex intracardiac repairs [138]. Their study concluded that the routine use of TEE in these children was cost-effective, based on the observation that it did not significantly increase echocardiography costs in the combined operative and postoperative periods. There was a trend toward fewer echocardiographic studies in the TEE group suggesting that the routine use of TEE avoided the need for some additional postoperative studies in the intensive care unit. It was emphasized that the cost benefit was independent of any impact of TEE on clinical outcomes. No patient in this cohort required return to cardiopulmonary bypass and surgical therapy was altered by TEE findings in 3 % of patients (2 out of 63). Complications were rare, self-limited, and when they occurred these were associated with probe placement or manipulation in smaller patients.

Randolph and co-workers, in a large study defining the impact of TEE, estimated that an intraoperative TEE service would pay for itself, even without considering any benefits derived from the preoperative examination [60]. A retrospective review of a 10-year experience by a European center sought to examine the cost-effectiveness of routine intraoperative TEE in pediatric cardiac surgery [139]. The report comprised 580 studies performed in patients younger than 17 years of age undergoing surgery (mean age 35 months). Thirty-three patients required reinitiation of cardiopulmonary bypass based on TEE findings. The study proposed a savings of $690–$2,190 per patient based on conservative calculations. It was emphasized that this calculation likely represented an underestimate of the true cost-effectiveness of routine intraoperative TEE. The estimates were based upon assumptions regarding the cost of reoperation and complications related to a residual defect.

In summary, although the number of formal investigations that have explored this issue is relatively small, all published work to date has demonstrated substantial cost-benefit regarding the use of TEE during congenital heart surgery, particularly in the pediatric population.

Limitations and Pitfalls of Intraoperative TEE

TEE provides high-resolution images and hemodynamic information that may not be obtainable with other diagnostic tools during the perioperative period. Although the benefits of this approach are widely recognized, the limitations of the technology should also be appreciated [140, 141]. Whereas transthoracic imaging provides for transducer interrogation through various locations over the chest wall, the TEE imaging windows are constrained by the confines of the esophagus and stomach, thus restricting transducer mobility. This also results in limited potential for optimal Doppler angle alignment. Other challenges relate to suboptimal far field imaging, particularly of anterior structures and less than expected image quality in some patients. The air-filled tracheobronchial tree can present difficulties in the evaluation of certain cardiovascular structures, such as the left pulmonary artery beyond its proximal region, the distal ascending aorta, and the transverse aortic arch. In addition, comprehensive evaluation of vascular structures within the thorax, such as high superior vena cava, innominate vein, anomalous systemic or pulmonary venous return, may not be feasible.

Other limitations should also be recognized including the fact that, in the majority of cases, the ultrasound examination is performed under suboptimal ambient lighting that can be challenging. Time constraints or clinical conditions may also limit the time available to undertake a comprehensive study.

The literature extensively documents the utility of TEE in the detection of residual abnormalities that may require immediate revision in congenital heart surgery. Regarding return to bypass decisions to address residual pathology or suboptimal results, it is important to consider that a number of factors, including the level of inotropic support, immediate postbypass catecholamine state, loading conditions, and functional state of the myocardium can influence the echocardiographic findings. These factors may lead to under or overestimation of the hemodynamic severity of the condition in question. The optimal setting for hemodynamic assessment in most postoperative patients is one in which conditions reflect an equilibrium, or steady state. Given the changing and dynamic nature of the respiratory, hemodynamic, pharmacologic, and anesthesia-related management interventions that occur continuously in the operating room, it is not surprising that accurate assessment of a patient's hemodynamic status represents a significant challenge, if not an impossibility, in this setting. Thus, the findings from intraoperative TEE should be interpreted within this context.

A report by Kausal and coworkers highlights some of the difficulties regarding return to bypass decisions [142]. This group explored the question as to whether significant intraoperative right ventricular outflow gradients after repair of tetralogy of Fallot represented an indication for revision. The study population included 166 patients (median age 7 years) undergoing a transatrial repair. A "significant" right ventricular outflow obstruction was identified in 35 % of patients following the repair (gradient greater than 40 mmHg, right ventricular to left ventricular pressure ratio over 85 %). Fixed obstruction, requiring immediate surgical revision, was present in only 12 % of these cases. The remaining 88 % of patients with a "significant" gradient were felt to have dynamic right ventricular outflow obstruction and did not undergo reoperation. It is of interest that, irrespective of the severity of the obstruction detected intraoperatively, outflow gradients declined sharply on follow-up (mean 18.5 months after surgery). No reoperations or late deaths were reported. The authors concluded that intraoperative echocardiography was helpful in distinguishing "fixed" from "dynamic" obstruction, thereby obviating needless revisions. The finding of a decline in dynamic right ventricular outflow tract gradient regardless of initial postoperative severity suggested that this should not be considered in isolation to determine the need for surgical revision in this patient population.

Although TEE plays a significant role in assessing the adequacy of the surgical intervention, it needs to be emphasized that return to bypass decisions should consider an assessment of the overall risk versus benefit ratio. In most cases this decision involves clinical judgment based not only upon the echocardiographic findings, but also a number of other factors, including the likelihood of an adequate or improved result balanced against the risk of potential morbidity related to additional surgery/cardiopulmonary bypass/ischemic time.

Although data regarding the correlation between intraoperative and postoperative echocardiographic data is scarce, there is literature suggesting that in some cases a discrepancy may be found. Lee and associates examined the validity of intraoperative TEE in predicting the severity of mitral regurgitation at follow up in patients after complete repair of atrioventricular septal defects [143]. The assessment of mitral regurgitation was performed using a biplane TEE probe after weaning from cardiopulmonary bypass but prior to chest closure. The ratio of the maximum regurgitant jet area by color Doppler flow imaging, to the left atrial area on two-dimensional imaging was used for quantification of mitral regurgitation. A discrepancy in the grade of mitral regurgitation was noted in 47 % of patients, in most of cases, with a higher grade of valvar regurgitation on follow-up. This suggested that the grade on intraoperative mitral regurgitation by TEE may not predict the degree of regurgitation at follow up. Subsequently, Honjo and colleagues evaluated 42 consecutive children undergoing valve repairs [144]. Significant discrepancies were identified between the assessment of residual atrioventricular valve regurgitation and stenosis between the intraoperative TEE and predischarge transthoracic echocardiogram (disagreement rate of 64 %). The authors noted that in most cases the residual regurgitation was underestimated in the operating room. In contrast, there was reasonable agreement for the evaluation of aortic valve regurgitation. It is not altogether surprising that a discrepancy might exist between intraoperative and postoperative echocardiographic findings. Factors such as the level of sedation/depth of anesthesia and changing hemodynamic conditions likely influence study results, particularly the assessment of valvar stenosis/regurgitation. Moreover, the quality of echocardiographic imaging can differ substantially between TEE and postoperative transthoracic studies. Finally, there are occasionally changes that can occur in a surgical repair, even within a few days postoperatively, and these might also affect the echocardiographic appearance.

Potential pitfalls of TEE, including misinterpretation of findings leading to erroneous diagnoses, should be recognized. The use of TEE in the evaluation of CHD and the assessment of the surgical results requires an advanced level of both skills and knowledge. This assumes a combination of training, experience, and expertise in the field. Unlike most adult cardiovascular disease, the vast majority of abnormalities in children are structural in nature and their characterization require extensive familiarity with the wide spectrum of congenital cardiac pathologies. There is a need for an in-depth and wide-ranging skill set: three-dimensional understanding of normal and abnormal cardiovascular anatomy/pathology, structural variants, physiologic impact and hemodynamic consequences, natural history of the defects, and medical and surgical approaches/options. Furthermore, an understanding of TEE technology is essential, including indications, contraindications, optimization of system settings, benefits and limitations of the modality, and the recognition of artifacts. Finally, a thorough knowledge of the TEE techniques and views/probe manipulations used to evaluate CHD is essential, along with a solid understanding of the echocardiographic appearance of the many different forms of unoperated and operated CHD.

In his review of clinical outcomes in children, Stevenson highlighted the importance of physician skills in intraoperative echocardiography during congenital heart surgery [145]. A positive impact on clinical outcomes was noted when TEE examinations were performed by physicians who met the published guidelines. This publication, accompanied by a thought provoking editorial entitled "*Transesophageal*

Echocardiography Guidelines: *Return to Bypass or to Bypass the Guidelines*?" and several subsequent letters to the editor, outlined the critical importance of sufficient training and expertise by intraoperative echocardiographers regardless of specialty.

Evaluation of Congenital Heart Disease by TEE in the Postoperative Setting

The use of TEE has been extensively documented in the cardiac intensive care unit and other postoperative settings at many centers [146–153]. The fact that the applications of TEE in the critically ill have been reported more frequently in adult patients is likely an indication that children generally have more favorable transthoracic windows and adequate information can usually be obtained by standard transthoracic echocardiography. However in the subset of postoperative pediatric patients (with both congenital and acquired cardiovascular pathology) in whom transthoracic imaging is suboptimal in the intensive care setting, the superior resolution of TEE may facilitate morphologic and functional assessment. In such patients, TEE can overcome limitations related to poor windows, suboptimal image quality due to lung interference, and/or the presence of bandages [154]. In some cases, an open sternum does not allow for accessible transthoracic diagnostic imaging and in this setting TEE may be extremely helpful [155].

In the pediatric age group, mechanical support of the circulation is receiving increasing attention as hardware appropriate for patient-size has become available. Existing technologies continue to be applied, and novel devices are being considered to address circulatory failure in those with CHD and other pathologies. The use of TEE in the operating room and/or intensive care unit may facilitate the care of these patients by providing assistance in cannulae/device positioning, assessment of cardiac chamber decompression, evaluation of ventricular loading conditions, and determination of recovery of myocardial function [156]. In addition, TEE can assist in the optimization of pharmacologic and other medical therapies, and it can provide information regarding the suitability of weaning from support.

Although several investigations have reported on the role of TEE in the assessment of cardiac output and systemic vascular resistance in critically ill adult patients, these types of assessments have not yet been validated in children [157, 158].

TEE may assist in the further characterization of unexpected/unusual findings or pathology following congenital cardiac surgery—findings identified or suspected but not adequately defined by transthoracic imaging. Examples of possible postoperative clinical situations in which TEE can provide significant additional information include (but are not limited to) the evaluation of:

- Residual atrial shunting, particularly in patients with unexplained cyanosis
- Possible pulmonary venous obstruction
- Residual ventricular septal defects
- Atrioventricular and semilunar valve abnormalities
- Mechanism of right or left ventricular outflow tract obstruction
- Prosthetic valve function
- Possible infective endocarditis

Although a subset of patients with a complicated or unanticipated immediate postoperative course may necessitate further diagnostic evaluation, in a number of cases the diagnostic capabilities of TEE can obviate the need for alternate (and sometimes more invasive) imaging studies.

The American College of Cardiology Foundation and the American Society of Echocardiography, in combination with key specialty and subspecialty societies, conducted an appropriateness review for transthoracic and transesophageal echocardiographic imaging in adult patients (18 years of age or older) [159]. This effort assumed that TEE would be used as an adjunct or as a subsequent test to transthoracic echocardiography, when suboptimal images precluded an adequate diagnostic study. With respect to potential applications of TEE in adult patients with CHD in the intraoperative and postoperative settings, indications generally acceptable and considered reasonable by members of the working group included:

- Assessment of known or suspected adult CHD including anomalies of great vessels and cardiac chambers and valves, or suspected intracardiac shunt following repair/operation
- Evaluation of hypotension or hemodynamic instability of uncertain or suspected cardiac etiology
- Evaluation of pericardial conditions including but not limited to pericardial mass, effusion, constrictive pericarditis, effusive-constrictive conditions, patients post-cardiac surgery, or suspected pericardial tamponade
- Evaluation of known or suspected pulmonary hypertension including evaluation of right ventricular function and estimated pulmonary artery pressure
- Re-evaluation of patients with prosthetic valve with suspected dysfunction or thrombosis or a change in clinical status
- Evaluation for cardiovascular source of embolic event (patent foramen ovale/atrial septal defect, thrombus, neoplasm)
- Re-evaluation of infective endocarditis in patients with any of the following: virulent organism, severe hemodynamic lesion, aortic involvement, persistent bacteremia, a change in clinical status, or symptomatic deterioration

Data regarding the applications of TEE in children in the immediate postoperative period are quite limited. Thus, indications comparable to those discussed above have not yet been clearly defined. Nonetheless, many situations are analogous to those encountered in adults, and the clinical experience suggests that TEE, when used in a judicious and appropriate manner, can also provide real and important benefits in the postoperative setting in the pediatric age group.

Summary

The overwhelming contributions of TEE have led to this imaging approach being considered the standard of care for intraoperative assessment of most congenital heart repairs by many centers. Extensive experience has documented significant benefits in patients with CHD that include surgical planning, evaluation of the intervention, guidance of the surgical revision as necessary, and a major overall impact in surgical decision-making. Contributions to anesthetic care include real time monitoring of ventricular filling, myocardial performance, ensuring adequate cardiac deairing, in addition to optimization of hemodynamic management strategies. Intraoperative TEE assists in the formulation and optimization of plans for postoperative care and provides important contributions in this setting. Although not formally assessed in a rigorous scientific manner, the experience regarding the perioperative contributions of TEE is compelling enough to assume a major impact of this technology on clinical outcome in CHD.

References

1. Gussenhoven EJ, van Herwerden LA, Roelandt J, Ligtvoet KM, Bos E, Witsenburg M. Intraoperative two-dimensional echocardiography in congenital heart disease. J Am Coll Cardiol. 1987;9:565–72.
2. Ungerleider RM, Kisslo JA, Greeley WJ, Van Trigt P, Sabiston Jr DC. Intraoperative prebypass and postbypass epicardial color flow imaging in the repair of atrioventricular septal defects [see comments]. J Thorac Cardiovasc Surg. 1989;98:90–9; discussion 99–100.
3. Ungerleider RM, Greeley WJ, Sheikh KH, et al. Routine use of intraoperative epicardial echocardiography and Doppler color flow imaging to guide and evaluate repair of congenital heart lesions. A prospective study. J Thorac Cardiovasc Surg. 1990;100:297–309.
4. Ungerleider R. Decision making in pediatric cardiac surgery using intraoperative echo. Int J Card Imaging. 1989;4:33–5.
5. Hsu YH, Santulli Jr T, Wong AL, Drinkwater D, Laks H, Williams RG. Impact of intraoperative echocardiography on surgical management of congenital heart disease. Am J Cardiol. 1991;67:1279–83.
6. Ungerleider RM. The use of intraoperative epicardial echocardiography with color flow imaging during the repair of complete atrioventricular septal defects. Cardiol Young. 1992;2:56–64.
7. Papagiannis J, Kanter RJ, Armstrong BE, Greeley WJ, Ungerleider RM. Intraoperative epicardial echocardiography during repair of tetralogy of Fallot. J Am Soc Echocardiogr. 1993;6:366–73.
8. Cyran SE, Kimball TR, Meyer RA, et al. Efficacy of intraoperative transesophageal echocardiography in children with congenital heart disease. Am J Cardiol. 1989;63:594–8.
9. Kyo S, Koike K, Takanawa E, et al. Impact of transesophageal Doppler echocardiography on pediatric cardiac surgery. Int J Card Imaging. 1989;4:41–2.
10. Omoto T, Kyo S, Matsumura M. Recent technological progress in transesophageal color Doppler flow imaging with special reference to newly developed biplane and pediatric probes. In: Erbel R, Khandheria BK, Brennecke R, editors. Transesophageal echocardiography: a new window to the heart. Berlin: Springer; 1989. p. 21–6.
11. Ritter SB, Thys D. Pediatric transesophageal color flow imaging: smaller probes for smaller hearts. Echocardiography. 1989;6: 431–40.
12. Ritter SB, Hillel Z, Narang J, Lewis D, Thys D. Transesophageal real time Doppler flow imaging in congenital heart disease: experience with a new pediatric transducer probe. Dyn Cardiovasc Imaging. 1989;2:92–6.
13. Ritter SB. Transesophageal echocardiography in children: new peephole to the heart. J Am Coll Cardiol. 1990;16:447–50.
14. Ritter SB. Pediatric transesophageal color flow imaging 1990: the long and short of it. Echocardiography. 1990;7:713–25.
15. Stumper OF, Elzenga NJ, Hess J, Sutherland GR. Transesophageal echocardiography in children with congenital heart disease: an initial experience. J Am Coll Cardiol. 1990;16:433–41.
16. Ritter SB. Transesophageal real-time echocardiography in infants and children with congenital heart disease. J Am Coll Cardiol. 1991;18:569–80.
17. Muhiudeen IA, Roberson DA, Silverman NH, Haas G, Turley K, Cahalan MK. Intraoperative echocardiography in infants and children with congenital cardiac shunt lesions: transesophageal versus epicardial echocardiography. J Am Coll Cardiol. 1990;16:1687–95.
18. Stumper O, Kaulitz R, Sreeram N, et al. Intraoperative transesophageal versus epicardial ultrasound in surgery for congenital heart disease. J Am Soc Echocardiogr. 1990;3:392–401.
19. Sreeram N, Stumper OF, Kaulitz R, Hess J, Roelandt JR, Sutherland GR. Comparative value of transthoracic and transesophageal echocardiography in the assessment of congenital abnormalities of the atrioventricular junction. J Am Coll Cardiol. 1990;16:1205–14.
20. Wienecke M, Fyfe DA, Kline CH, et al. Comparison of intraoperative transesophageal echocardiography to epicardial imaging in children undergoing ventricular septal defect repair. J Am Soc Echocardiogr. 1991;4:607–14.
21. Roberson DA, Muhiudeen IA, Cahalan MK, Silverman NH, Haas G, Turley K. Intraoperative transesophageal echocardiography of ventricular septal defect. Echocardiography. 1991;8:687–97.
22. Roberson DA, Muhiudeen IA, Silverman NH, Turley K, Haas GS, Cahalan MK. Intraoperative transesophageal echocardiography of atrioventricular septal defect. J Am Coll Cardiol. 1991;18: 537–45.
23. Muhiudeen IA, Roberson DA, Silverman NH, Haas GS, Turley K, Cahalan MK. Intraoperative echocardiography for evaluation of congenital heart defects in infants and children. Anesthesiology. 1992;76:165–72.
24. Roberson DA, Muhiudeen IA, Silverman NH. Transesophageal echocardiography in pediatrics: technique and limitations. Echocardiography. 1990;7:699–712.
25. Muhiudeen I, Silverman N. Intraoperative transesophageal echocardiography using high resolution imaging in infants and children with congenital heart disease. Echocardiography. 1993;10:599–608.
26. Gentles TL, Rosenfeld HM, Sanders SP, Laussen PC, Burke RP, van der Velde ME. Pediatric biplane transesophageal echocardiography: preliminary experience. Am Heart J. 1994;128:1225–33.
27. Lam J, Neirotti RA, Lubbers WJ, et al. Usefulness of biplane transesophageal echocardiography in neonates, infants and children with congenital heart disease [published erratum appears in Am J Cardiol 1994 Mar 15;73(8):625]. Am J Cardiol. 1993;72:699–706.
28. Xu J, Shiota T, Ge S, et al. Intraoperative transesophageal echocardiography using high-resolution biplane 7.5 MHz probes with continuous-wave Doppler capability in infants and children with tetralogy of Fallot. Am J Cardiol. 1996;77:539–42.

29. O'Leary PW, Hagler DJ, Seward JB, et al. Biplane intraoperative transesophageal echocardiography in congenital heart disease. Mayo Clin Proc. 1995;70:317–26.
30. Hoffman P, Stumper O, Rydelwska-Sadowska W, Sutherland GR. Transgastric imaging: a valuable addition to the assessment of congenital heart disease by transverse plane transesophageal echocardiography. J Am Soc Echocardiogr. 1993;6:35–44.
31. Muhiudeen IA, Silverman NH, Anderson RH. Transesophageal transgastric echocardiography in infants and children: the subcostal view equivalent. J Am Soc Echocardiogr. 1995;8:231–44.
32. Tardif JC, Schwartz SL, Vannan MA, Cao QL, Pandian NG. Clinical usefulness of multiplane transesophageal echocardiography: comparison to biplanar imaging. Am Heart J. 1994;128:156–66.
33. Yvorchuk KY, Sochowski RA, Chan KL. A prospective comparison of the multiplane probe with the biplane probe in structure visualization and Doppler examination during transesophageal echocardiography. J Am Soc Echocardiogr. 1995;8:111–20.
34. Djoa KK, De Jong N, Cromme-Dijkhuis AH, Lancee CT, Bom N. Two decades of transesophageal phased array probes. Ultrasound Med Biol. 1996;22:1–9.
35. Cromme-Dijkhuis AH, Djoa KK, Bom N, Hess J. Pediatric transesophageal echocardiography by means of a miniature 5-MHz multiplane transducer. Echocardiography. 1996;13:685–9.
36. Sloth E, Hasenkam JM, Sorensen KE, et al. Pediatric multiplane transesophageal echocardiography in congenital heart disease: new possibilities with a miniaturized probe. J Am Soc Echocardiogr. 1996;9:622–8.
37. Lam J, Neirotti RA, Hardjowijono R, Blom-Muilwijk CM, Schuller JL, Visser CA. Transesophageal echocardiography with the use of a four-millimeter probe. J Am Soc Echocardiogr. 1997;10:499–504.
38. Kawahito S, Kitahata H, Tanaka K, Nozaki J, Oshita S. Intraoperative transoesophageal echocardiography in a low birth weight neonate with atrioventricular septal defect. Paediatr Anaesth. 2003;13:735–8.
39. Shiota T, Lewandowski R, Piel JE, et al. Micromultiplane transesophageal echocardiographic probe for intraoperative study of congenital heart disease repair in neonates, infants, children, and adults. Am J Cardiol. 1999;83:292–5.
40. Rice MJ, Sahn DJ. Transesophageal echocardiography for congenital heart disease—who, what, and when [editorial]. Mayo Clin Proc. 1995;70:401–2.
41. Scohy TV, Gommers D, Jan ten Harkel AD, Deryck Y, McGhie J, Bogers AJ. Intraoperative evaluation of micromultiplane transesophageal echocardiographic probe in surgery for congenital heart disease. Eur J Echocardiogr. 2007;8:241–6.
42. Zyblewski SC, Shirali GS, Forbus GA, et al. Initial experience with a miniaturized multiplane transesophageal probe in small infants undergoing cardiac operations. Ann Thorac Surg. 2010;89:1990–4.
43. Pushparajah K, Miller OI, Rawlins D, Barlow A, Nugent K, Simpson JM. Clinical application of a micro multiplane transoesophageal probe in congenital cardiac disease. Cardiol Young. 2012;22:170–7.
44. Bruce CJ, O'Leary P, Hagler DJ, Seward JB, Cabalka AK. Miniaturized transesophageal echocardiography in newborn infants. J Am Soc Echocardiogr. 2002;15:791–7.
45. Cannesson M, Henaine R, Metton O, et al. Images in cardiovascular medicine. Intraoperative transesophageal echocardiography using a miniaturized transducer in a neonate undergoing Norwood procedure for hypoplastic left heart syndrome. Circulation. 2008;117:702–3.
46. Ungerleider RM, Kisslo JA, Greeley WJ, et al. Intraoperative echocardiography during congenital heart operations: experience from 1,000 cases. Ann Thorac Surg. 1995;60:S539–42.
47. Stumper O, Fraser AG, Elzenga N, et al. Assessment of ventricular septal defect closure by intraoperative epicardial ultrasound. J Am Coll Cardiol. 1990;16:1672–9.
48. Stumper O. Transesophageal echocardiography: a new diagnostic method in paediatric cardiology. Arch Dis Child. 1991;66:1175–7.
49. Lam J, Neirotti RA, Nijveld A, Schuller JL, Blom-Muilwijk CM, Visser CA. Transesophageal echocardiography in pediatric patients: preliminary results. J Am Soc Echocardiogr. 1991;4:43–50.
50. Fyfe DA, Kline CH. Transesophageal echocardiography for congenital heart disease. Echocardiography. 1991;8:573–86.
51. Fyfe DA, Kline CH, Sade RM, Greene CA, Gillette PC. The utility of transesophageal echocardiography during and after Fontan operations in small children. Am Heart J. 1991;122:1403–15.
52. Stumper O, Kaulitz R, Elzenga NJ, et al. The value of transesophageal echocardiography in children with congenital heart disease. J Am Soc Echocardiogr. 1991;4:164–76.
53. Tee SD, Shiota T, Weintraub R, et al. Evaluation of ventricular septal defect by transesophageal echocardiography: intraoperative assessment. Am Heart J. 1994;127:585–92.
54. Shuler CO, Fyfe DA, Sade R, Crawford FA. Transesophageal echocardiographic evaluation of cor triatriatum in children. Am Heart J. 1995;129:507–10.
55. Stevenson JG. Role of intraoperative transesophageal echocardiography during repair of congenital cardiac defects. Acta Paediatr Suppl. 1995;410:23–33.
56. Bezold LI, Pignatelli R, Altman CA, et al. Intraoperative transesophageal echocardiography in congenital heart surgery. The Texas Children's Hospital experience. Tex Heart Inst J. 1996;23:108–15.
57. Bengur AR, Li JS, Herlong JR, Jaggers J, Sanders SP, Ungerleider RM. Intraoperative transesophageal echocardiography in congenital heart disease. Semin Thorac Cardiovasc Surg. 1998;10:255–64.
58. Kavanaugh-McHugh A, Tobias JD, Doyle T, Heitmiller ES, Meagher C. Transesophageal echocardiography in pediatric congenital heart disease. Cardiol Rev. 2000;8:288–306.
59. Lim DS, Dent JM, Gutgesell HP, Matherne GP, Kron IL. Transesophageal echocardiographic guidance for surgical repair of aortic insufficiency in congenital heart disease. J Am Soc Echocardiogr. 2007;20:1080–5.
60. Randolph GR, Hagler DJ, Connolly HM, et al. Intraoperative transesophageal echocardiography during surgery for congenital heart defects. J Thorac Cardiovasc Surg. 2002;124:1176–82.
61. Sloth E, Pedersen J, Olsen KH, Wanscher M, Hansen OK, Sorensen KE. Transoesophageal echocardiographic monitoring during paediatric cardiac surgery: obtainable information and feasibility in 532 children. Paediatr Anaesth. 2001;11:657–62.
62. Ma XJ, Huang GY, Liang XC, et al. Transoesophageal echocardiography in monitoring, guiding, and evaluating surgical repair of congenital cardiac malformations in children. Cardiol Young. 2007;17:301–6.
63. Bettex DA, Schmidlin D, Bernath MA, et al. Intraoperative transesophageal echocardiography in pediatric congenital cardiac surgery: a two-center observational study. Anesth Analg. 2003;97:1275–82.
64. Stevenson JG, Sorensen GK, Gartman DM, Hall DG, Rittenhouse EA. Transesophageal echocardiography during repair of congenital cardiac defects: identification of residual problems necessitating reoperation. J Am Soc Echocardiogr. 1993;6:356–65.
65. Chen TH, Chan KC, Cheng YJ, Wang MJ, Tsai SK. Bedside pericardiocentesis under the guidance of transesophageal echocardiography in a 13-month-old boy. J Formos Med Assoc. 2001;100:620–2.
66. Kawahito S, Kitahata H, Tanaka K, et al. Intraoperative management of a pediatric patient undergoing cardiac tumor resection with the aid of transesophageal and epicardial echocardiography. Anesth Analg. 1999;88:1048–50.
67. Komai H, Naito Y, Fujiwara K, Uemura S. The benefits of surgical atrial septostomy guided by transesophageal echocardiography in pediatric patients. J Thorac Cardiovasc Surg. 1999;118:758–9.
68. Kawahito S, Kitahata H, Tanaka K, Nozaki J, Oshita S. Intraoperative evaluation of pulmonary artery flow during the

Fontan procedure by transesophageal Doppler echocardiography. Anesth Analg. 2000;91:1375–80.
69. Boddu K, Vavilala MS, Stevenson JG, Lam AM. The use of transesophageal echocardiography to facilitate removal of a thoracic nail. Anesth Analg. 2002;95:624–6.
70. Nitta K, Kawahito S, Kitahata H, Nozaki J, Katayama T, Oshita S. Two unusual complications associated with cardiopulmonary bypass for pediatric cardiac surgery detected by transesophageal echocardiography after decannulation. Paediatr Anaesth. 2008;18:325–9.
71. Lavoie J, Burrows FA, Gentles TL, Sanders SP, Burke RP, Javorski JJ. Transoesophageal echocardiography detects residual ductal flow during video-assisted thoracoscopic patent ductus arteriosus interruption. Can J Anaesth. 1994;41:310–3.
72. Lavoie J, Javorski JJ, Donahue K, Sanders SP, Burke RP, Burrows FA. Detection of residual flow by transesophageal echocardiography during video-assisted thoracoscopic patent ductus arteriosus interruption. Anesth Analg. 1995;80:1071–5.
73. Ho AC, Tan PP, Yang MW, et al. The use of multiplane transesophageal echocardiography to evaluate residual patent ductus arteriosus during video-assisted thoracoscopy in adults. Surg Endosc. 1999;13:975–9.
74. Ho AC, Chen CK, Yang MW, Chu JJ, Lin PJ. Usefulness of intraoperative transesophageal echocardiography in the assessment of surgical repair of pediatric ventricular septal defects with video-assisted endoscopic techniques in children. Chang Gung Med J. 2004;27:646–53.
75. Bacha EA, Cao QL, Galantowicz ME, et al. Multicenter experience with perventricular device closure of muscular ventricular septal defects. Pediatr Cardiol. 2005;26:169–75.
76. Gan C, An Q, Lin K, et al. Perventricular device closure of ventricular septal defects: six months results in 30 young children. Ann Thorac Surg. 2008;86:142–6.
77. Fyfe DA, Ritter SB, Snider AR, et al. Guidelines for transesophageal echocardiography in children. J Am Soc Echocardiogr. 1992;5:640–4.
78. Practice guidelines for perioperative transesophageal echocardiography. A report by the American Society of Anesthesiologists and the Society of Cardiovascular Anesthesiologists Task Force on Transesophageal Echocardiography. Anesthesiology. 1996;84:986–1006.
79. Cheitlin MD, Alpert JS, Armstrong WF, et al. ACC/AHA Guidelines for the Clinical Application of Echocardiography. A report of the American College of Cardiology/American Heart Association Task Force on Practice Guidelines (Committee on Clinical Application of Echocardiography). Developed in collaboration with the American Society of Echocardiography. Circulation. 1997;95:1686–744.
80. Cheitlin MD, Armstrong WF, Aurigemma GP, et al. ACC/AHA/ASE 2003 guideline update for the clinical application of echocardiography: summary article: a report of the American College of Cardiology/American Heart Association Task Force on Practice Guidelines (ACC/AHA/ASE Committee to Update the 1997 Guidelines for the Clinical Application of Echocardiography). Circulation. 2003;108:1146–62.
81. Stevenson JG. Utilization of intraoperative transesophageal echocardiography during repair of congenital cardiac defects: a survey of North American centers. Clin Cardiol. 2003;26:132–4.
82. Ayres NA, Miller-Hance W, Fyfe DA, et al. Indications and guidelines for performance of transesophageal echocardiography in the patient with pediatric acquired or congenital heart disease: report from the task force of the Pediatric Council of the American Society of Echocardiography. J Am Soc Echocardiogr. 2005;18:91–8.
83. Practice guidelines for perioperative transesophageal echocardiography. An updated report by the American Society of Anesthesiologists and the Society of Cardiovascular Anesthesiologists Task Force on Transesophageal Echocardiography. Anesthesiology. 2010;112:1084–1096.
84. Sawchuk C, Fayad A. Confirmation of internal jugular guide wire position utilizing transesophageal echocardiography. Can J Anaesth. 2001;48:688–90.
85. Mahmood F, Sundar S, Khabbaz K. Misplacement of a guidewire diagnosed by transesophageal echocardiography. J Cardiothorac Vasc Anesth. 2007;21:420–1.
86. Andropoulos DB. Transesophageal echocardiography as a guide to central venous catheter placement in pediatric patients undergoing cardiac surgery. J Cardiothorac Vasc Anesth. 1999;13:320–1.
87. Chaney MA, Minhaj MM, Patel K, Muzic D. Transoesophageal echocardiography and central line insertion. Ann Card Anaesth. 2007;10:127–31.
88. Hsu JH, Wang CK, Hung CW, Wang SS, Cheng KI, Wu JR. Transesophageal echocardiography and laryngeal mask airway for placement of permanent central venous catheter in cancer patients with radiographically unidentifiable SVC-RA junction: effectiveness and safety. Kaohsiung J Med Sci. 2007;23:435–41.
89. Andropoulos DB, Stayer SA, Bent ST, et al. A controlled study of transesophageal echocardiography to guide central venous catheter placement in congenital heart surgery patients. Anesth Analg. 1999;89:65–70.
90. Gold JP, Jonas RA, Lang P, Elixson EM, Mayer JE, Castaneda AR. Transthoracic intracardiac monitoring lines in pediatric surgical patients: a ten-year experience. Ann Thorac Surg. 1986;42:185–91.
91. Flori HR, Johnson LD, Hanley FL, Fineman JR. Transthoracic intracardiac catheters in pediatric patients recovering from congenital heart defect surgery: associated complications and outcomes. Crit Care Med. 2000;28:2997–3001.
92. Rimensberger PC, Beghetti M. Pulmonary artery catheter placement under transoesophageal echocardiography guidance. Paediatr Anaesth. 1999;9:167–70.
93. Eguchi S, Bosher LHJ. Myocardial dysfunction resulting from coronary air embolism. Surgery. 1962;51:103–11.
94. Goldfarb D, Bahnson HT. Early and late effects on the heart of small amounts of air in the coronary circulation. J Thorac Cardiovasc Surg. 1963;46:368–78.
95. Fearn SJ, Pole R, Burgess M, Ray SG, Hooper TL, McCollum CN. Cerebral embolisation during modern cardiopulmonary bypass. Eur J Cardiothorac Surg. 2001;20:1163–7.
96. Borger MA, Peniston CM, Weisel RD, Vasiliou M, Green RE, Feindel CM. Neuropsychologic impairment after coronary bypass surgery: effect of gaseous microemboli during perfusionist interventions. J Thorac Cardiovasc Surg. 2001;121:743–9.
97. Duff HJ, Buda AJ, Kramer R, Strauss HD, David TE, Berman ND. Detection of entrapped intracardiac air with intraoperative echocardiography. Am J Cardiol. 1980;46:255–60.
98. Oka Y, Moriwaki KM, Hong Y, et al. Detection of air emboli in the left heart by M-mode transesophageal echocardiography following cardiopulmonary bypass. Anesthesiology. 1985;63:109–13.
99. Topol EJ, Humphrey LS, Borkon AM, et al. Value of intraoperative left ventricular microbubbles detected by transesophageal two-dimensional echocardiography in predicting neurologic outcome after cardiac operations. Am J Cardiol. 1985;56:773–5.
100. Diehl JT, Ramos D, Dougherty F, Pandian NG, Payne DD, Cleveland RJ. Intraoperative, two-dimensional echocardiography-guided removal of retained intracardiac air. Ann Thorac Surg. 1987;43:674–5.
101. Meloni L, Abbruzzese PA, Cardu G, et al. Detection of microbubbles released by oxygenators during cardiopulmonary bypass by intraoperative transesophageal echocardiography. Am J Cardiol. 1990;66:511–4.
102. Orihashi K, Matsuura Y, Hamanaka Y, et al. Retained intracardiac air in open heart operations examined by transesophageal echocardiography. Ann Thorac Surg. 1993;55:1467–71.
103. Tingleff J, Joyce FS, Pettersson G. Intraoperative echocardiographic study of air embolism during cardiac operations. Ann Thorac Surg. 1995;60:673–7.

104. Orihashi K, Matsuura Y, Sueda T, Shikata H, Mitsui N, Sueshiro M. Pooled air in open heart operations examined by transesophageal echocardiography. Ann Thorac Surg. 1996;61:1377–80.
105. Dalmas JP, Eker A, Girard C, et al. Intracardiac air clearing in valvular surgery guided by transesophageal echocardiography. J Heart Valve Dis. 1996;5:553–7.
106. Hoka S, Okamoto H, Yamaura K, Takahashi S, Tominaga R, Yasui H. Removal of retained air during cardiac surgery with transesophageal echocardiography and capnography. J Clin Anesth. 1997;9:457–61.
107. Greeley WJ, Kern FH, Ungerleider RM, Kisslo JA. Intramyocardial air causes right ventricular dysfunction after repair of a congenital heart defect. Anesthesiology. 1990;73:1042–6.
108. Cassorla L, Miller-Hance WC, Rouine-Rapp K, Reddy VM, Hanley FL, Silverman NH. Reliability of intraoperative contrast transesophageal echocardiography for detecting interatrial communications in patients with other congenital cardiovascular malformations. Am J Cardiol. 2003;91:1027–31, A8–9.
109. Clements FM, Harpole DH, Quill T, Jones RH, McCann RL. Estimation of left ventricular volume and ejection fraction by two-dimensional transoesophageal echocardiography: comparison of short axis imaging and simultaneous radionuclide angiography. Br J Anaesth. 1990;64:331–6.
110. Tousignant CP, Walsh F, Mazer CD. The use of transesophageal echocardiography for preload assessment in critically ill patients. Anesth Analg. 2000;90:351–5.
111. Buhre W, Buhre K, Kazmaier S, Sonntag H, Weyland A. Assessment of cardiac preload by indicator dilution and transoesophageal echocardiography. Eur J Anaesthesiol. 2001;18:662–7.
112. Swenson JD, Harkin C, Pace NL, Astle K, Bailey P. Transesophageal echocardiography: an objective tool in defining maximum ventricular response to intravenous fluid therapy. Anesth Analg. 1996;83:1149–53.
113. Stoddard MF, Longaker RA, Calzada N. Left atrial inflow propagation rate: a new transesophageal echocardiographic index of preload. J Am Soc Echocardiogr. 2002;15:1057–64.
114. Hofer CK, Ganter MT, Rist A, Klaghofer R, Matter-Ensner S, Zollinger A. The accuracy of preload assessment by different transesophageal echocardiographic techniques in patients undergoing cardiac surgery. J Cardiothorac Vasc Anesth. 2008;22:236–42.
115. Swenson JD, Bull D, Stringham J. Subjective assessment of left ventricular preload using transesophageal echocardiography: corresponding pulmonary artery occlusion pressures. J Cardiothorac Vasc Anesth. 2001;15:580–3.
116. Smith MD, MacPhail B, Harrison MR, Lenhoff SJ, DeMaria AN. Value and limitations of transesophageal echocardiography in determination of left ventricular volumes and ejection fraction. J Am Coll Cardiol. 1992;19:1213–22.
117. Poortmans G, Schupfer G, Roosens C, Poelaert J. Transesophageal echocardiographic evaluation of left ventricular function. J Cardiothorac Vasc Anesth. 2000;14:588–98.
118. Bailey JM, Shanewise JS, Kikura M, Sharma S. A comparison of transesophageal and transthoracic echocardiographic assessment of left ventricular function in pediatric patients with congenital heart disease. J Cardiothorac Vasc Anesth. 1995;9:665–9.
119. Martins TC, Rigby ML, Redington AN. Left ventricular performance in children: transthoracic versus transoesophageal measurement of M mode derived indices. Br Heart J. 1992;68:485–7.
120. Schmitz L, Koch H, Bein G, Brockmeier K. Left ventricular diastolic function in infants, children, and adolescents. Reference values and analysis of morphologic and physiologic determinants of echocardiographic Doppler flow signals during growth and maturation. J Am Coll Cardiol. 1998;32:1441–8.
121. Nishimura RA, Tajik AJ. Evaluation of diastolic filling of left ventricle in health and disease: Doppler echocardiography is the clinician's Rosetta Stone. J Am Coll Cardiol. 1997;30:8–18.
122. Mirsky I, Pasipoularides A. Clinical assessment of diastolic function. Prog Cardiovasc Dis. 1990;32:291–318.
123. Oh JK, Appleton CP, Hatle LK, Nishimura RA, Seward JB, Tajik AJ. The noninvasive assessment of left ventricular diastolic function with two-dimensional and Doppler echocardiography. J Am Soc Echocardiogr. 1997;10:246–70.
124. Bernard F, Denault A, Babin D, et al. Diastolic dysfunction is predictive of difficult weaning from cardiopulmonary bypass. Anesth Analg. 2001;92:291–8.
125. Border WL, Michelfelder EC, Glascock BJ, et al. Color M-mode and Doppler tissue evaluation of diastolic function in children: simultaneous correlation with invasive indices. J Am Soc Echocardiogr. 2003;16:988–94.
126. Gidding SS, Snider AR, Rocchini AP, Peters J, Farnsworth R. Left ventricular diastolic filling in children with hypertrophic cardiomyopathy: assessment with pulsed Doppler echocardiography. J Am Coll Cardiol. 1986;8:310–6.
127. Olivier M, O'leary PW, Pankratz VS, et al. Serial Doppler assessment of diastolic function before and after the Fontan operation. J Am Soc Echocardiogr. 2003;16:1136–43.
128. McMahon CJ, Nagueh SF, Pignatelli RH, et al. Characterization of left ventricular diastolic function by tissue Doppler imaging and clinical status in children with hypertrophic cardiomyopathy. Circulation. 2004;109:1756–62.
129. McMahon CJ, Chang AC, Pignatelli RH, et al. Left ventricular noncompaction cardiomyopathy in association with trisomy 13. Pediatr Cardiol. 2005;26:477–9.
130. Castello R, Pearson AC, Lenzen P, Labovitz AJ. Evaluation of pulmonary venous flow by transesophageal echocardiography in subjects with a normal heart: comparison with transthoracic echocardiography [see comments]. J Am Coll Cardiol. 1991;18:65–71.
131. Gardeback M, Settergren G, Brodin LA. Hepatic blood flow and right ventricular function during cardiac surgery assessed by transesophageal echocardiography. J Cardiothorac Vasc Anesth. 1996;10:318–22.
132. Mishra M, Swaminathan M, Malhotra R, Mishra A, Trehan N. Evaluation of right ventricular function during CABG: transesophageal echocardiographic assessment of hepatic venous flow versus conventional right ventricular performance indices. Echocardiography. 1998;15:51–8.
133. Smith JS, Cahalan MK, Benefiel DJ, et al. Intraoperative detection of myocardial ischemia in high-risk patients: electrocardiography versus two-dimensional transesophageal echocardiography. Circulation. 1985;72:1015–21.
134. Moises VA, Mesquita CB, Campos O, et al. Importance of intraoperative transesophageal echocardiography during coronary artery surgery without cardiopulmonary bypass. J Am Soc Echocardiogr. 1998;11:1139–44.
135. Balaguru D, Auslender M, Colvin SB, Rutkowski M, Artman M, Phoon CK. Intraoperative myocardial ischemia recognized by transesophageal echocardiography monitoring in the pediatric population: a report of 3 cases. J Am Soc Echocardiogr. 2000; 13:615–8.
136. Rouine-Rapp K, Rouillard KP, Miller-Hance W, et al. Segmental wall-motion abnormalities after an arterial switch operation indicate ischemia. Anesth Analg. 2006;103:1139–46.
137. Benson MJ, Cahalan MK. Cost-benefit analysis of transesophageal echocardiography in cardiac surgery. Echocardiography. 1995;12:171–83.
138. Siwik ES, Spector ML, Patel CR, Zahka KG. Costs and cost-effectiveness of routine transesophageal echocardiography in congenital heart surgery. Am Heart J. 1999;138:771–6.
139. Bettex DA, Pretre R, Jenni R, Schmid ER. Cost-effectiveness of routine intraoperative transesophageal echocardiography in pediatric cardiac surgery: a 10-year experience. Anesth Analg. 2005;100:1271–5.

140. Seward JB, Khandheria BK, Oh JK, Freeman WK, Tajik AJ. Critical appraisal of transesophageal echocardiography: limitations, pitfalls, and complications. J Am Soc Echocardiogr. 1992;5:288–305.
141. Khandheria BK, Seward JB, Tajik AJ. Critical appraisal of transesophageal echocardiography: limitations and pitfalls. Crit Care Clin. 1996;12:235–51.
142. Kaushal SK, Radhakrishanan S, Dagar KS, et al. Significant intraoperative right ventricular outflow gradients after repair for tetralogy of Fallot: to revise or not to revise? Ann Thorac Surg. 1999;68:1705–12; discussion 1712–3.
143. Lee HR, Montenegro LM, Nicolson SC, Gaynor JW, Spray TL, Rychik J. Usefulness of intraoperative transesophageal echocardiography in predicting the degree of mitral regurgitation secondary to atrioventricular defect in children. Am J Cardiol. 1999;83:750–3.
144. Honjo O, Kotani Y, Osaki S, et al. Discrepancy between intraoperative transesophageal echocardiography and postoperative transthoracic echocardiography in assessing congenital valve surgery. Ann Thorac Surg. 2006;82:2240–6.
145. Stevenson JG. Adherence to physician training guidelines for pediatric transesophageal echocardiography affects the outcome of patients undergoing repair of congenital cardiac defects. J Am Soc Echocardiogr. 1999;12:165–72.
146. Oh JK, Seward JB, Khandheria BK, et al. Transesophageal echocardiography in critically ill patients. Am J Cardiol. 1990;66: 1492–5.
147. Font VE, Obarski TP, Klein AL, et al. Transesophageal echocardiography in the critical care unit. Cleve Clin J Med. 1991;58:315–22.
148. Foster E, Schiller NB. The role of transesophageal echocardiography in critical care: UCSF experience. J Am Soc Echocardiogr. 1992;5:368–74.
149. Poelaert J, Schmidt C, Van Aken H, Colardyn F. Transoesophageal echocardiography in critically ill patients. A comprehensive approach. Eur J Anaesthesiol. 1997;14:350–8.
150. Khoury AF, Afridi I, Quinones MA, Zoghbi WA. Transesophageal echocardiography in critically ill patients: feasibility, safety, and impact on management. Am Heart J. 1994;127:1363–71.
151. Huttemann E, Schelenz C, Kara F, Chatzinikolaou K, Reinhart K. The use and safety of transoesophageal echocardiography in the general ICU—a minireview. Acta Anaesthesiol Scand. 2004;48:827–36.
152. Huttemann E. Transoesophageal echocardiography in critical care. Minerva Anestesiol. 2006;72:891–913.
153. Ananthasubramaniam K, Jaffery Z. Postoperative right atrial compression by extracardiac hematoma: transesophageal echocardiographic diagnosis in the critically ill patient. Echocardiography. 2007;24:661–3.
154. Wolfe LT, Rossi A, Ritter SB. Transesophageal echocardiography in infants and children: use and importance in the cardiac intensive care unit. J Am Soc Echocardiogr. 1993;6:286–9.
155. Marcus B, Wong PC, Wells WJ, Lindesmith GG, Starnes VA. Transesophageal echocardiography in the postoperative child with an open sternum. Ann Thorac Surg. 1994;58:235–6.
156. Scheinin SA, Radovancevic B, Ott DA, Nihill MR, Cabalka A, Frazier OH. Postcardiotomy LVAD support and transesophageal echocardiography in a child. Ann Thorac Surg. 1993;55:529–31.
157. Feinberg MS, Hopkins WE, Davila-Roman VG, Barzilai B. Multiplane transesophageal echocardiographic doppler imaging accurately determines cardiac output measurements in critically ill patients. Chest. 1995;107:769–73.
158. Baillard C, Cohen Y, Fosse JP, Karoubi P, Hoang P, Cupa M. Haemodynamic measurements (continuous cardiac output and systemic vascular resistance) in critically ill patients: transoesophageal Doppler versus continuous thermodilution. Anaesth Intensive Care. 1999;27:33–7.
159. Douglas PS, Khandheria B, Stainback RF, et al. ACCF/ASE/ACEP/ASNC/SCAI/SCCT/SCMR 2007 appropriateness criteria for transthoracic and transesophageal echocardiography: a report of the American College of Cardiology Foundation Quality Strategic Directions Committee Appropriateness Criteria Working Group, American Society of Echocardiography, American College of Emergency Physicians, American Society of Nuclear Cardiology, Society for Cardiovascular Angiography and Interventions, Society of Cardiovascular Computed Tomography, and the Society for Cardiovascular Magnetic Resonance endorsed by the American College of Chest Physicians and the Society of Critical Care Medicine. J Am Coll Cardiol. 2007;50:187–204.

Additional Applications of Transesophageal Echocardiography

16

Pierre C. Wong

Abstract
While the majority of this book addresses the use of transesophageal echocardiography (TEE) for the evaluation of patients with congenital heart disease (CHD), there are a number of other conditions in which TEE can play a significant role in pediatric and young adult patients. Some conditions, such as infective endocarditis, can occur in patients with a history of CHD. Other pathologies, such as cardiac tumors, can be seen in the absence of coexisting CHD. This chapter addresses additional applications of TEE in the pediatric and young adult population.

Keywords
Endocarditis • Bacterial • Heart valve prosthesis • Heart neoplasms • Heart-assist devices • Heart transplantation • Lung transplantation • Aneurysm • Dissecting • Echocardiography • Transesophageal

Introduction

While the majority of this book addresses the use of transesophageal echocardiography (TEE) for the evaluation of congenital heart disease (CHD), there are other conditions in which TEE can prove beneficial in pediatric and young adult patients with and without CHD. This chapter discusses some of the more common clinical scenarios in which this might occur, and how TEE can contribute useful (and sometimes invaluable) additional information. Some situations will require TEE to be performed both in and out of the intraoperative setting.

Infective Endocarditis

Infective endocarditis (IE) is defined as a microbial infection of the endocardial (endothelial) surface of the heart, primarily involving the valves but also affecting other endocardial surfaces, including any prosthetic or foreign material in the heart. Infection can also occur on the endothelial surfaces of the great vessels (including the great arteries), and in this case it is known as infective endarteritis. Infective endocarditis can be caused by a number of different organisms, mainly bacteria and fungae (Table 16.1), and the clinical course ranges in severity from indolent to fulminant [1, 2]. Despite the fact that

P.C. Wong, MD
Division of Cardiology, Children's Hospital Los Angeles, Department of Pediatrics, Keck School of Medicine, University of Southern California, 4650 Sunset Blvd, Mailstop #34, Los Angeles, CA 90027, USA
e-mail: pwong@chla.usc.edu

The online version of this chapter (doi:10.1007/978-1-84800-064-3_16) contains supplementary material, which is available to authorized users.

P.C. Wong, W.C. Miller-Hance (eds.), *Transesophageal Echocardiography for Congenital Heart Disease*, DOI 10.1007/978-1-84800-064-3_16, © Springer-Verlag London 2014

Table 16.1 Organisms commonly associated with infectious endocarditis

Bacteria	
	Viridans group streptococci (alpha-hemolytic)—*S. mitis, S. sanguis, S. mutans,* etc.
	Staphylococcus aureus
	Coagulase-negative staphylococcus
	Streptococcus pneumonia
	Streptococcus bovis and other streptococci
	Enterococcus species
	HACEK (*Hemophilus* species, *Aggregatibacter actinomycetemcomitans, Cardiobacterium hominis, Eikinella* species, *Kingella kingae)*
	Pseudomonas species
	Culture negative (*Chlamydia* species, *Coxiella burnetii, Abiotrophia* species, *Bartonella* species, *Brucella* species, *Legionella* species, etc.)
Fungal	
	Candida albicans
	Candida tropicalis
	Histoplasma capsulatum
	Aspergillus
	Cryptococcus neoformans

IE begins as an infection of the endocardial surface, the infectious process can be highly invasive, causing extensive destruction of heart valve and surrounding tissue, as well as intramyocardial abscesses. Some of the most severe complications resulting from IE include congestive heart failure (due to valvar regurgitation), systemic and pulmonary embolic phenomena, sepsis, arrhythmias, myocardial failure, and death [3].

A number of conditions can predispose to IE, including mitral valve prolapse, rheumatic heart disease, indwelling catheters, intravenous drug abuse, prosthetic valves, and both unrepaired and repaired CHD [1]. The role of congenital cardiac disease as a predisposing factor for IE continues to increase in developed countries; CHD now appears to be the predominant underlying condition for IE in children over the age of 2 years [4]. Certain congenital heart lesions are recognized to have an association with IE, including ventricular septal defects, patent ductus arteriosus, aortic valve abnormalities, and tetralogy of Fallot [5]. Furthermore, increasing numbers of children with IE have had previous palliative or corrective surgery for CHD [4, 6]. However, IE can occur in the absence of any structural heart disease; this is seen in approximately 2–5 % of younger pediatric IE cases (2 months to 15 years of age), and 25–45 % of older IE patients (15–60 years of age) [1, 7].

Because of the variability in clinical presentation, the diagnosis of IE is not always straightforward. To assist in diagnosis, a set of criteria—known as the Duke criteria—were proposed in 1994 as a diagnostic schema for patients with suspected IE [8]. Several refinements were made in 2000, resulting in the modified Duke criteria [9]. These criteria incorporate clinical, laboratory, pathologic and

Table 16.2 Modified Duke criteria: definition of terms used for the diagnosis of infective endocarditis (IE)

Major criteria
Blood culture positive for IE
Typical microorganisms consistent with IE from two separate blood cultures:
Viridans streptococci, *Streptococcus bovis,* HACEK group, *Staphylococcus aureus;* or
Community-acquired enterococci, in the absence of a primary focus; or
Microorganisms consistent with IE from persistently positive blood cultures, defined as follows:
At least two positive cultures of blood samples drawn >12 h apart; or
All of three or a majority of ≥4 separate cultures of blood (with first and last sample drawn at least 1 h apart)
Single positive blood culture for Coxiella burnetii or antiphase I IgG antibody titer >1:800
Evidence of endocardial involvement
Echocardiogram positive for IE (**TEE recommended in patients with prosthetic valves, rated at least "possible IE" by clinical criteria, or complicated IE [paravalvular abscess]; TTE as first test in other patients),** defined as follows:
Oscillating intracardiac mass on valve or supporting structures, in the path of regurgitant jets, or on implanted material in the absence of an alternative explanation; or
Abscess; or
New partial dehiscence of prosthetic valve
New valvular regurgitation (worsening or changing of pre-existing murmur not sufficient)
Minor criteria
Predisposition, predisposing heart condition or injection drug use
Fever, temperature >38 °C
Vascular phenomena, major arterial emboli, septic pulmonary infarcts, mycotic aneurysm, intracranial hemorrhage, conjunctival hemorrhages, and Janeway's lesions
Immunologic phenomena: glomerulonephritis, Osler's nodes, Roth's spots, and rheumatoid factor
Microbiological evidence: positive blood culture but does not meet a major criterion as noted above[a] or serological evidence of active infection with organism consistent with IE
Echocardiographic minor criteria eliminated

From: Li et al [9]; reproduced with permission, Oxford University Press. **(Modifications shown in boldface)**

TEE transesophageal echocardiography, *TTE* transthoracic echocardiography

[a]Excludes single positive cultures for coagulase-negative staphylococci and organisms that do not cause endocarditis

echocardiographic criteria, and stratify patients into three main categories—definite IE, possible IE, and rejected—based upon the presence of major and minor criteria (Tables 16.2 and 16.3). "Definite" IE is defined by the presence of two major criteria, or one major and three minor, or five minor criteria. "Possible" IE is defined by one major and one minor criterion, or three minor criteria. "Rejected" indicates absence of evidence supporting the diagnosis of IE. For diagnosis, microbiologic confirmation (as demonstrated by positive blood cultures) is a principal

Table 16.3 Definition of endocarditis from modified Duke criteria

Definite infective endocarditis
Pathologic criteria
1. Microorganisms demonstrated by culture or histologic examination of a vegetation, a vegetation that has embolized, or an intracardiac abscess specimen; or
2. Pathologic lesions; vegetation or intracardiac abscess confirmed by histologic examination showing active endocarditis
Clinical criteria [a]
1. Two major criteria; or
2. One major criterion and three minor criteria; or
3. Five minor criteria
Possible infective endocarditis
1. One major criterion and one minor criterion; or
2. Three minor criteria
Rejected
1. Firm alternate diagnosis explaining evidence of infective endocarditis; or
2. Resolution of infective endocarditis syndrome with antibiotic therapy for ≤4 days; or
3. No pathologic evidence of infective endocarditis at surgery or autopsy, with antibiotic therapy for ≤4 days; or
4. Does not meet criteria for possible infective endocarditis, as above

From: Li JS et al [9]*; reproduced with permission, Oxford University Press*
(Modifications shown in boldface)
[a]See Table 16.2 for definitions of major and minor criteria

criterion. However, the Duke criteria clearly recognize and acknowledge the importance of echocardiography (with special mention of TEE) in the diagnosis of IE, as evidenced by the inclusion of echocardiographic findings as a major criterion for diagnosis. Indeed, echocardiography is now considered essential in the diagnostic workup and continuing evaluation of IE [10]. The utility of the Duke criteria have been validated by a number of studies in both the adult and pediatric populations [11–14]. They are now widely accepted guidelines for the evaluation of possible IE, both in adults as well as children [4, 15, 16].

The full diagnostic evaluation and management of IE encompasses a wide variety of aspects, including microbiology, antimicrobial therapy/duration, ongoing assessment, extracardiac complications, and indications and timing of surgical management [1, 17]. Therapy of IE is aimed at (a) eradication of the infecting microorganism; (b) treatment of cardiac complications; (c) prevention and/or treatment of extracardiac (particularly embolic) complications [1]. Antimicrobial therapy (selection/duration) is based upon the microbiology and susceptibility of the causative organism, and continues to evolve as new therapeutic agents are introduced. The role of surgery for IE also continues to evolve, and it is clear that this role has expanded; a recent European survey revealed that >50 % of adult patients with IE underwent surgery [18]. Controversy still exists as to the exact indications and timing for surgery; in most instances surgery is performed for left sided endocarditis, severe valvular involvement, and/or evidence of embolic phenomena [19]. Recently, there has also been published evidence that early surgery for severe left sided endocarditis in adults results in significantly better outcomes than conventional medical therapy [20]. Proposed indications and timing of surgery in adults are listed in Tables 16.4 and 16.5 [19]. In children, the indications for surgery are not as straightforward; surgery tends to be performed less frequently because 80–90 % of children with IE are expected to survive solely with conservative medical treatment [21, 22]. Nonetheless several published series of IE in children have reported an important percentage (between 16–67 %) of cases that required surgical intervention—in patients with and without CHD. In most published reports, the indications for cardiac surgery in pediatric IE patients tend to be similar to those of adults—valve dysfunction, congestive heart failure, septic embolization, and large vegetations. In addition, surgery is performed in CHD patients to repair the underlying cardiac defect (if still present), and also to remove or replace infected prosthetic material such as homografts and aortopulmonary shunts [7, 18, 21, 23–25].

Despite advances in medical and surgical management, IE remains a serious medical condition, with important risks of morbidity and mortality. A thorough and complete review of this multifaceted topic, including diagnosis, antimicrobial considerations, and medical/surgical therapy, would require its own separate chapter. For the purposes of this chapter, it is important to understand the integral role that echocardiography—and particularly TEE—plays in the many different aspects of the diagnosis and management of IE. This will be discussed below.

Echocardiographic Manifestations of IE

There are several ways in which IE can appear by echocardiography. The principal echocardiographic manifestations of IE include the following.

Vegetations

Vegetations are the most characteristic finding associated with endocarditis. They represent a mass of pathologic organisms nestled within a weave of platelets, red blood cells, and fibrin. Vegetations often develop in an area where the endothelium has been injured or disrupted by an abnormal high velocity jet or intravenous catheter; this usually occurs on a valvar surface, but can also be seen on a cardiac chamber wall when the endothelial surface has been injured. Vegetations also have the propensity to develop on foreign material such as a prosthetic valve or patch. The surface of the damaged endothelium or prosthetic material serves as a nidus for

Table 16.4 Indications for surgery in IE

Congestive heart failure[a]	
	Congestive heart failure caused by severe aortic or mitral regurgitation or, more rarely, by valve obstruction caused by vegetations
	Severe acute aortic or mitral regurgitation with echocardiographic signs of elevated left ventricular end-diastolic pressure or significant pulmonary hypertension
	Congestive heart failure as a result of prosthetic dehiscence or obstruction
Periannular extension	
	Most patients with abscess formation or fistulous tract formation
Systemic embolism[b]	
	Recurrent emboli despite appropriate antibiotic therapy
	Large vegetations (>10 mm) after one or more clinical or silent embolic events after initiation of antibiotic therapy
	Large vegetations and other predictors of a complicated course
	Very large vegetations (>15 mm) without embolic complications, especially if valve-sparing surgery is likely (remains controversial)
Cerebrovascular complications[c]	
	Silent neurological complication or transient ischemic attack and other surgical indications
	Ischemic stroke and other surgical indications, provided that cerebral hemorrhage has been excluded and neurological complications are not severe (e.g., coma)
Persistent sepsis	
	Fever or positive blood cultures persisting for >5–7 days despite an appropriate antibiotic regimen, assuming that vegetations or other lesions requiring surgery persist and that extracardiac sources of sepsis have been excluded
	Relapsing IE, especially when caused by organisms other than sensitive streptococci or in patients with prosthetic valves
Difficult organisms	
	S aureus IE involving a prosthetic valve and most cases involving a left-sided native valve
	IE caused by other aggressive organisms (Brucella, Staphylococcus lugdunensis)
	IE caused by multiresistant organisms (e.g., methicillin-resistant staphylococcus aureus or vancomycin-resistant enterococci) and rare infections caused by Gram-negative bacteria
	Pseudomonas aeruginosa or Fungal IE
	Q fever IE and other relative indications for intervention
Prosthetic valve endocarditis	
	Virtually all cases of early prosthetic valve endocarditis
	Virtually all cases of prosthetic valve endocarditis caused by staphylococcus aureus
	Late prosthetic valve endocarditis with heart failure caused by prosthetic dehiscence or obstruction, or other indications for surgery

From: Prendergast and Tornos [19]; reprinted with permission from Walters Kluwer

[a]Surgery should be performed immediately, irrespective of antibiotic therapy, in patients with persistent pulmonary edema or cardiogenic shock. If congestive heart failure disappears with medical therapy and there are no other surgical indications, intervention can be postponed to allow a period of days or weeks of antibiotic treatment under careful clinical and echocardiographic observation. In patients with well tolerated severe valvular regurgitation or prosthetic dehiscence and no other reasons for surgery, conservative therapy under careful clinical and echocardiographic observation is recommended with consideration of deferred surgery after resolution of the infection, depending upon tolerance of the valve lesion

[b]In all cases, surgery for the prevention of embolism must be performed very early since embolic risk is highest during the first days of therapy

[c]Surgery is contraindicated for at least 1 month after intracranial hemorrhage unless neurosurgical or endovascular intervention can be performed to reduce bleeding risk

platelet/fibrin deposition, producing a thrombus (vegetation) at the site. This vegetation is at first sterile, but with bacteremia, circulating microorganisms can become adherent to the meshwork, resulting in an infected vegetation. Infection triggers further deposition of platelets and fibrin over the microorganisms; the organisms embedded within the vegetation are then shielded from host defense mechanisms, allowing them to proliferate rapidly and produce further growth of the vegetation [26]. Vegetations can have a number of detrimental effects: (a) they can grow and destroy adjacent tissue; (b) organisms can be released continuously into the bloodstream, leading to persistent bacteremia and hematogenous seeding of remote sites; (c) pieces of the vegetation can break off and embolize to other organs (brain, lung, kidney), sometimes producing serious and even devastating complications; (d) antibody response to the infecting organisms leads to subsequent tissue injury by immune complex deposition [1].

By echocardiography, vegetations are echogenic masses, generally irregular in shape and variable in size. They can localize anywhere on an affected valve or nonvalvar structure, though they tend to arise on a valve or endothelial surface "downstream" to a high velocity jet, e.g. adjacent to a ventricular septal defect or valvar regurgitant jet. They are usually freely mobile, oscillating with the cardiac cycle, and can move back and forth within the plane of a valve.

Table 16.5 Timing of Surgery

Emergency surgery (within 24 h)
Native (aortic or mitral) or prosthetic valve endocarditis and severe congestive heart failure or cardiogenic shock caused by:
Acute valvular regurgitation
Severe prosthetic dysfunction (dehiscence or obstruction)
Fistula into a cardiac chamber or the pericardial space
Urgent surgery (within days)
Native valve endocarditis with persisting congestive heart failure, signs of poor hemodynamic tolerance, or abscess
Prosthetic valve endocarditis with persisting congestive heart failure, signs of poor hemodynamic tolerance, or abscess
Prosthetic valve endocarditis caused by staphylococci or Gram-negative organisms
Large vegetation (>10 mm) with an embolic event
Large vegetation (>10 mm) with other predictors of a complicated course
Very large vegetation (>15 mm), especially if conservative surgery is available
Large abscess and/or periannular involvement with uncontrolled infection
Early elective surgery (during the in-hospital stay)
Severe aortic or mitral regurgitation with congestive heart failure and good response to medical therapy
Prosthetic valve endocarditis with valvular dehiscence or congestive heart failure and good response to medical therapy
Presence of abscess or periannular extension
Persisting infection when extracardiac focus has been excluded
Fungal or other infections resistant to medical cure

From Prendergast et al [19]; reprinted with permission from Walters Kluwer

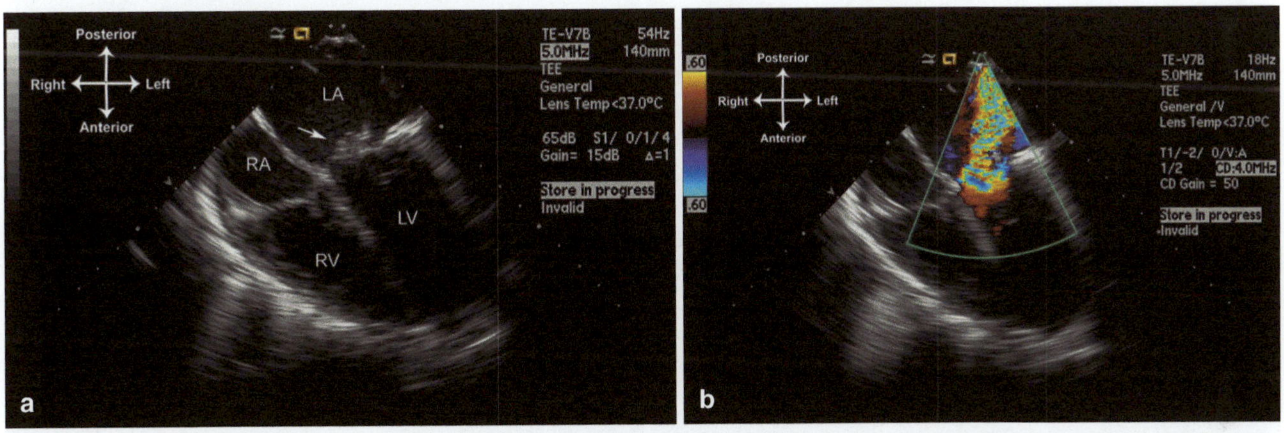

Fig. 16.1 Large vegetation (*arrow*) on the anterior leaflet of mitral valve (**a**), which resulted in chordal destruction and severe mitral regurgitation (**b**). Mid esophageal view four chamber (multiplane angle 0°). *LA* left atrium, *LV* left ventricle, *RA* right atrium, *RV* right ventricle

Intracardiac vegetations are generally very well seen by TEE (Fig. 16.1, Video 16.1).

Valvar Dysfunction

The echocardiographic manifestations of valvar dysfunction include ruptured chordae with prolapsing or flail leaflets, fenestrations in the valve cusps, and torn leaflets. All of these lead to disruption of valvar function and resultant valvar regurgitation, often to a significant degree. The amount of regurgitation, and the area of origin, can be well-seen using color flow Doppler. It is not uncommon to see vegetations in association with valvar disruption, as evidence of the destructive process from IE. Such patients not only appear toxic from their infection, but might also suffer symptoms of congestive heart failure if valvar incompetence is significant. Examples of valve disruption and accompanying vegetation are shown in Figs. 16.1 and 16.2, Videos 16.1 and 16.2.

Intracardiac Abscesses

Intracardiac abscess formation results from suppurative extension of the infective process. Purulent cavities form as the infection spreads into adjacent tissue. Most commonly, this occurs with native aortic valve IE, as infection extends into the weakest portion of the annulus—the membranous septum and atrioventricular node. When this occurs, heart block is a frequent sequela. Perivalvar abscess formation occurs in 10–40 % of all native IE; as noted, it is most common in native aortic valve IE, less common with native tricuspid or mitral IE [10]. Perivalvar abscesses are seen even

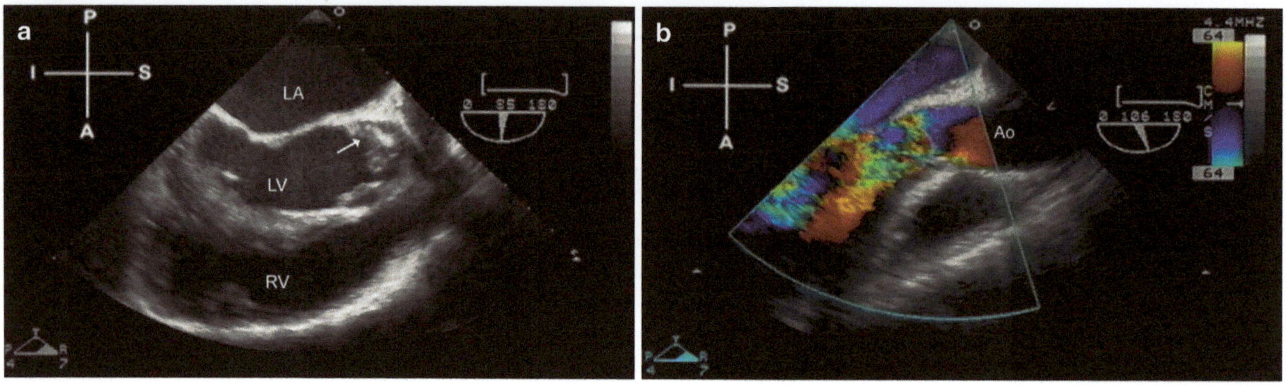

Fig. 16.2 Aortic valve endocarditis, seen from a mid esophageal aortic valve long axis view (multiplane angle 85°–106°). Figure **a** shows a prominent vegetation (*arrow*) on the left coronary cusp, which has caused significant cusp destruction and resulted in severe aortic valve regurgitation (**b**). *Ao* ascending aorta, *LA* left atrium, *LV* left ventricle, *RV* right ventricle

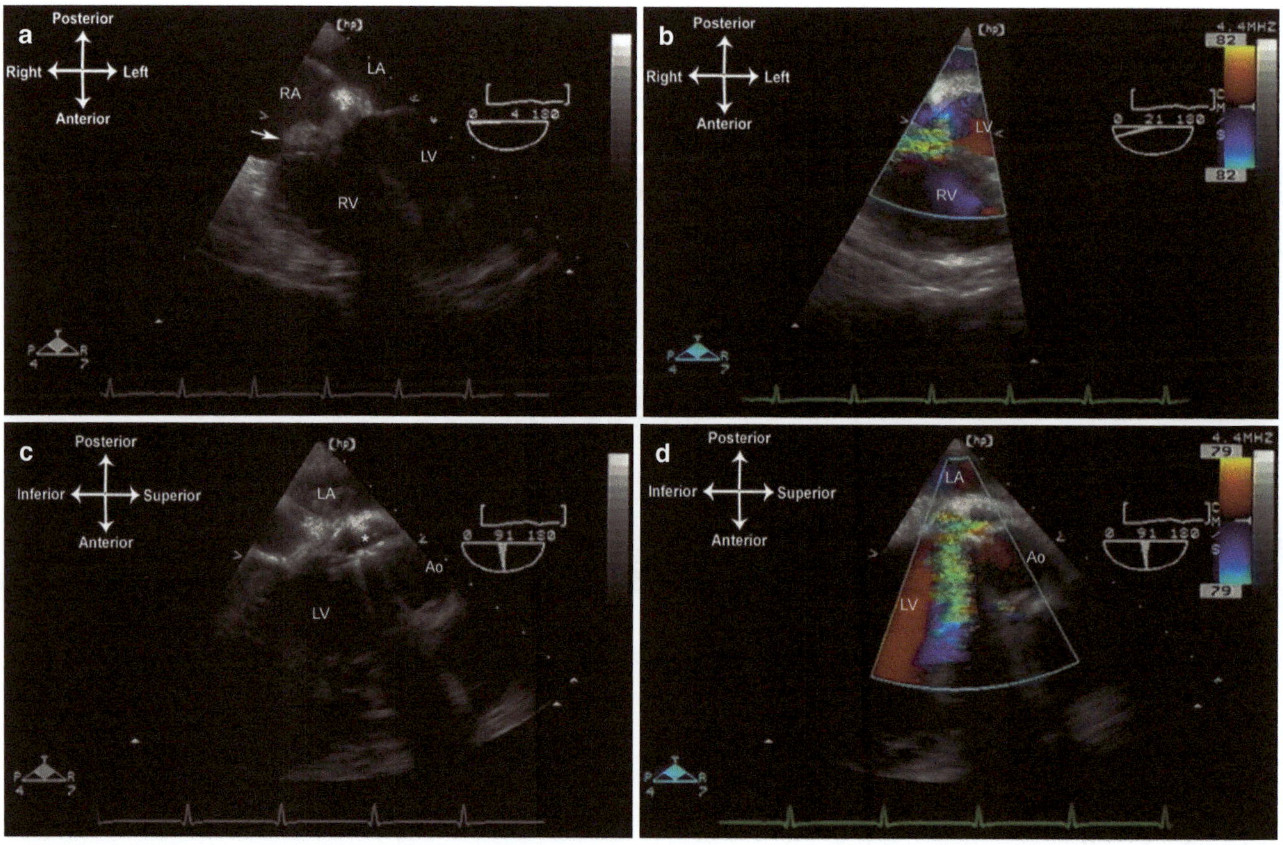

Fig. 16.3 Endocarditis in a patient with a prosthetic aortic valve (St. Jude bileaflet tilting disk valve). (**a**, **b**). The mid esophageal four chamber view demonstrates a perivalvar abscess that extends into the noncoronary cusp, causing a fistulous tract communicating with the right atrium. A large vegetation (*arrow*) has developed in this area and shunting is seen into the right atrium. (**c**, **d**). Mid esophageal aortic valve long axis view, angle about 90°. There is marked aortic regurgitation seen through an area of valve dehiscence (*). *Ao* aorta, *LA* left atrium, *LV* left ventricle, *RA* right atrium, *RV* right ventricle

more frequently with prosthetic valve IE, occurring in 56–100 % of patients [10, 27]. The characteristic echocardiographic appearance of abscess formation is as an echo-free space, representing purulent fluid, either within the wall surrounding the affected valve (e.g. the aortic root in aortic valve endocarditis), or extending into the adjacent tissue. In those patients with an abscess surrounding a prosthetic mitral valve, valve dehiscence is often seen. For the evaluation of abscesses, TEE has been shown to improve sensitivity dramatically compared to transthoracic echocardiography (TTE), and it is the preferred modality for diagnosis of perivalvar abscesses [28]. An example of an abscess that formed around a prosthetic aortic valve is shown in Fig. 16.3, Video 16.3.

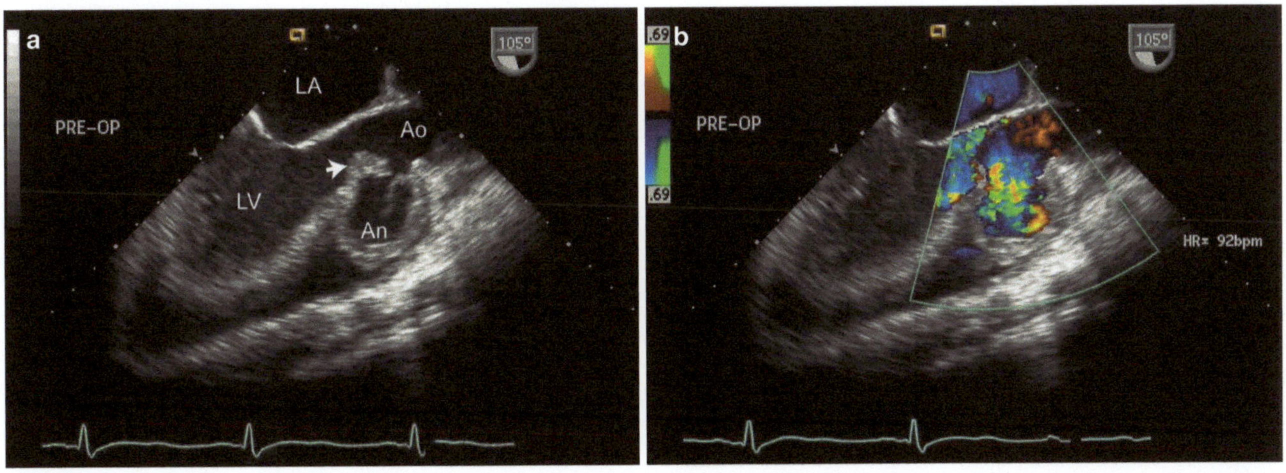

Fig. 16.4 Infected sinus of Valsalva aneurysm from aortic valve endocarditis, obtained from the mid esophageal aortic valve long axis view. Figure **a** shows a large vegetation of the aortic valve (*arrow*) and erosion of the right sinus of Valsalva, producing a large aneurysm (*An*). Figure **b** shows blood filling the aneurysm during diastole. *Ao* ascending aorta, *LA* left ventricle, *LV* left ventricle

Aneurysm Formation/Fistulous Tracts

If there is extension of the infection to the adjacent vessel wall, destruction of wall tissue can occur, leading to thinning and aneurysm formation. This can be seen especially with aortic valve IE, in which fistulous tracts can form between the sinus of Valsalva and an adjacent cardiac structure (i.e. an infected sinus of Valsalva aneurysm), or a fistulous tract can form into the pericardial space [29, 30]. In this setting, TEE will demonstrate the aneurysmal dilation of the vessel wall, and color flow Doppler will show systolic/diastolic (or continuous) flow between the aorta and the receiving chamber (Figs. 16.3 and 16.4, Videos 16.3 and 16.4). Infective endarteritis and pseudoaneurysm formation can also occur, particularly in areas of foreign material such as suture lines and biologic grafts [31, 32] (Fig. 16.5, Video 16.5).

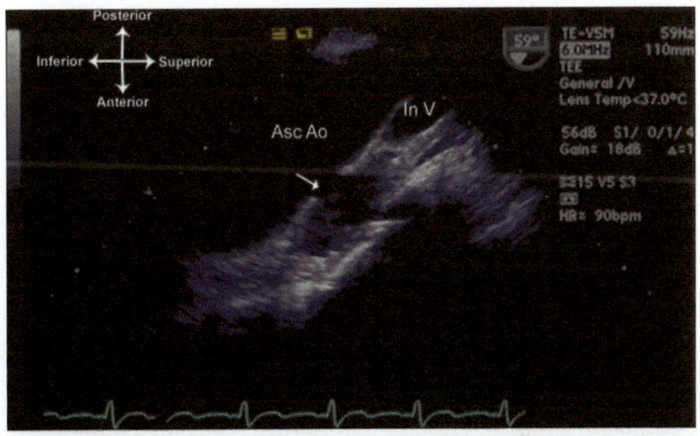

Fig. 16.5 Infected pseudoaneurysm off ascending aorta. This TEE was performed to evaluate the aortic valve in a patient with a previous aortic valve surgery and persistent fungemia. A large pseudoaneurysm (*arrow*) was discovered using an upper esophageal view, multiplane angle 60°. At surgery, the pseudoaneurysm was found to be infected and filled with fungus. Note that the superior portion of aorta and innominate vein can be seen well in this patient by TEE. *Asc Ao* ascending aorta, *In V* innominate vein

Congestive Heart Failure/Pericardial Effusion

Congestive heart failure (CHF) is a known complication of IE, and one associated with a poor prognosis [33–35]. It can occur as a result of several different complicating processes associated with IE: native valve destruction/perforation/chordal rupture, prosthetic valve dehiscence, abscess formation causing heart block, sudden intracardiac shunts due to fistulous tracts, and septic emboli to the coronaries causing myocardial ischemia/infarction [10, 19]. In addition, myocardial dysfunction can be seen with IE, either from myocardial toxicity due to the IE process (e.g. large abscess), ventricular decompensation from valvar regurgitation, or the overall septic process causing generalized depression of myocardial function (particularly with a virulent organism such as *Staphylococcus aureus*). In native valve IE, acute CHF is more frequently seen with left sided infections—aortic (29 %) and mitral (20 %)—than with tricuspid infections (8 %) [10]. A pericardial effusion can also be seen in patients with IE; it can be infectious, resulting from hematogenous seeding of the pericardium or as a direct extension from intracardiac IE (e.g. perforation of a perivalvar abscess). Rarely, it can occur as a reactive/serous effusion [36].

Use of TEE for Evaluation of Infective Endocarditis

As noted above, echocardiography is considered essential in the diagnosis and management of IE. The major question is whether to perform TTE or use TEE to evaluate for vegetations. In adults, a number of studies have confirmed the superior diagnostic sensitivity of TEE over TTE for IE [37–40]. This is particularly true in those patients with intracardiac abscesses and prosthetic valve endocarditis, in whom TEE appears clearly superior for diagnosis [28, 41]. In children, the advantages of TEE over TTE are less apparent, particularly with the infant and younger child, in whom TTE generally provides excellent imaging. For younger pediatric patients, TTE is usually adequate for the diagnostic evaluation of IE [42]. In most pediatric patients, particularly the younger age groups, the evidence suggests that TEE can be reserved for those patients in whom imaging quality is felt to be suboptimal. A recent study in pediatric patients ages 10 days to 17.5 years (over half of whom had CHD) showed that TTE, when used in conjunction with the Duke criteria, was useful for the diagnosis of IE; the authors recommended TEE only for an "inadequate" TTE study or when there was an organism with a high association of aortic root abscess [43].

The evaluation of IE by TEE can occur in several settings. It can be performed in the ICU or ambulatory setting, serving as either diagnostic evaluation for suspected IE or as a monitoring procedure for a patient receiving treatment for known IE. It also plays a vital role in the operating room. Preoperatively, TEE is used to assess not only the vegetation or abscess, but also valvar function and the surrounding cardiac structures. When applicable, prosthetic valve dehiscence and pseudoaneurysm formation can also be evaluated. Postoperatively, TEE is used to assess the results of operative repair or valve replacement, and to guide perioperative hemodynamic management [19, 36].

If TEE is performed to evaluate for IE, a complete study should be performed using all major TEE views/windows, as outlined in Chap. 4. Assessment should focus on a number of details. If a vegetation is present, its appearance and motion should be evaluated in multiple planes, and linear measurements can be obtained. The risk of embolic events appears to be greatest with vegetations >10 mm on the anterior leaflet of mitral valve [44]. Valve leaflet anatomy and motion should also be evaluated both by imaging and color flow Doppler, with attention paid to any valvar perforation or chordal disruption. In the case of aortic valve endocarditis, a careful evaluation should also be made for possible abscess or aneurysm formation. If a prosthetic valve is in place, a thorough assessment should be performed for vegetations, valve leaflet motion, and possible perivalvar abscess/dehiscence. Color flow Doppler is useful to determine valve competency and flow profile. A complete evaluation should be performed of other cardiac structures to rule out structural defects and/or other potential sites of IE, including the aorta and pulmonary artery (when the pulmonary artery can be visualized by TEE). Rarely, cases of endarteritis can also be found by TEE (Fig. 16.5, Video 16.5). Finally, myocardial function should also be assessed.

Three caveats are important to consider. First, even with TEE, not all vegetations will be visible, particularly if the vegetations are smaller than the resolution limits of the TEE probe and/or TEE imaging is suboptimal. This is an important consideration in patients with operated and unoperated CHD, who can have vegetations located in areas not readily visible by TEE (e.g. a Blalock-Taussig shunt). Studies have shown that—irrespective of whether TTE or TEE is used—patients with CHD and IE are less likely to have visible vegetations [5]. Thus, the echocardiographic data should be considered in the context of the entire clinical picture, as noted with the Duke criteria listed above. In some cases, if IE is still suspected, a TTE or TEE can be performed 7–10 days later to determine if a vegetation or abscess has appeared [10]. The second important caveat is that not all echogenic masses represent vegetations. Sterile thrombi, tumors, irregular valve excrescences, and foreign material (such as suture material) can sometimes resemble vegetations. Again, the echocardiogram should be reviewed in conjunction with the entire clinical picture. If previous echocardiograms are available (either transthoracic or transesophageal), these can be very useful to make direct comparisons to determine whether an abnormal finding is new or longstanding. New findings are much more suspicious for IE. The last important caveat is that not all vegetations are infectious. A number of medical conditions can produce sterile vegetations adherent to valvar surfaces. Examples of these include systemic lupus erythematosus (Libman-Sachs endocarditis), and nonbacterial thrombotic endocarditis (NBTE, also known as marantic endocarditis). The latter can occur as complication of malignancy, uremia, burns, hypercoagulable states, or autoimmune diseases, and it has been found in approximately 1.2 % of all autopsy patients, although the reported incidence is between 0.3–9.3 % [1, 45]. In fact, Libman-Sachs endocarditis is felt to be a form of NBTE [46]. These vegetations are usually seen on the valve closure contact line of the atrial surface of the atrioventricular (AV) valves and ventricular surface of the semilunar valves. In many cases, the vegetations are benign and clinically inapparent. However, systemic embolization has been described in up to 30–50 % of patients [45–47], with a tendency towards embolization to the brain, kidney, spleen, mesenteric bed, or extremities [46, 48].

Cardiac Masses

Aside from infective endocarditis, the most common pathologic cardiac masses are thrombus or tumors. The role of TEE in the diagnostic assessment of cardiac masses is generally complementary to TTE, particularly in pediatric patients. In most cases, TTE is more than adequate to evaluate the location and extent of a cardiac mass. However in older patients, and in those with poor echocardiographic windows, TEE might be called upon to assist in evaluation. For instance, TEE has become well established in adults as a requisite tool for evaluation of the etiology of ischemic strokes; approximately 15–20 % are caused by cardiogenic emboli (thrombi, tumors, vegetations, etc.) [49].

Cardiac Thrombi

Thrombi can vary considerably in their echocardiographic appearance and location. They are generally echogenic, relatively homogeneous in density, and irregular in shape. In some instances there can be calcification within the thrombus. They are generally attached to some structure in the heart, whether it is an endocardial surface, AV valve, or some type of foreign material. The attachment point is usually broad-based, but it can also be thin and pedunculated in appearance. In most clinical settings, thrombi are associated with an indwelling catheter, although in certain pathologic situations—e.g. where there is stasis of blood—they can arise spontaneously. An important example of this is dilated cardiomyopathy, in which reduced cardiac motion leads to stasis of blood flow and a propensity for thrombus formation, particularly near the apex of the left ventricle (Fig. 16.6, Video 16.6). In those situations in which a catheter is present, usually the superior vena cava (SVC) or right atrium, TEE can be used to evaluate the attachment point, size, and extent of the thrombus. Mid to upper esophageal views, with the probe rotated rightward and multiplane angle 80–95° (mid esophageal bicaval view), permit a sagittal visualization of the length of the SVC as it returns to the right atrium (Fig. 16.7, Video 16.7). If an indwelling catheter is present, it can be visualized and evaluated for a possible attached thrombus. It is important not to misinterpret normal structures or variants, such as the crista terminalis (the muscular ridge in the interior of the right atrium separating right atrial appendage from the remainder of the atrium), as an intracardiac thrombus. Color flow Doppler can evaluate the flow returning through the SVC to the right atrium. If there is obstruction to SVC return, a mean gradient can sometimes be obtained using the deep transgastric views (long axis and sagittal), rightward turning of the probe, and anteflexion to achieve posterior angulation (see Chap. 4). These maneuvers enable visualization of SVC flow as it enters the right atrium, and also provide an excellent angle of insonation for spectral Doppler interrogation.

Thrombi sometimes develop in the left (and less frequently, the right) atrial appendage in patients, particularly adults with severe mitral stenosis and/or atrial fibrillation [50, 51]. In adult studies, the incidence of left atrial thrombus in patients with atrial fibrillation ranges between 10–15 %, and right atrial thrombus 0.4–7.5 % [52]. These thrombi are often challenging to visualize by TTE [53]. It can also be difficult to distinguish these thrombi from pectinate muscles. In this setting, TEE proves invaluable because of the close proximity of the esophagus to both atria, providing excellent visualization of all atrial structures, including the atrial appendages [54, 55]. The left atrial appendage can be well visualized by TEE using the mid esophageal views and leftward rotation, with slight anteflexion to bring the appendage into view (Fig. 16.8, Video 16.8). Rotating the multiplane angle between 0° and 90° affords different views of the structure. The right atrial appendage is best seen from the mid esophageal bicaval view, multiplane angle 85–90°; it is seen anterior to the SVC/right atrial junction. The multiplane angle can also be rotated to 0° to visualize the right atrial appendage from a different plane. Again, it is important to inspect carefully both the right and left atrial appendages, and to distinguish pectinate muscles and multiple appendage lobations [56] from actual thrombus [54, 57].

There are certain normal anatomic structures that can resemble a thrombus, and must therefore be inspected carefully by TEE. As previously noted, the crista terminalis can occasionally be mistaken as a thrombus. A Chiari network can sometimes be confused for a thin thrombus or vegetation. This structure, an embryologic remnant of the right valve of the sinus venosus, is usually very mobile and can exhibit considerable

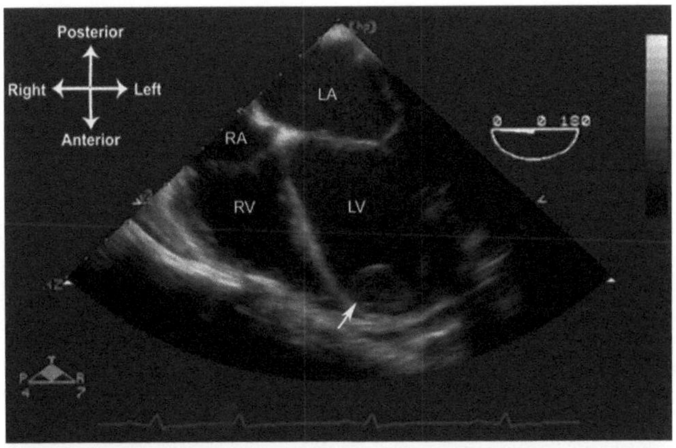

Fig. 16.6 Thrombus (*arrow*) in the left ventricular apex of a patient with Duchenne muscular dystrophy and dilated cardiomyopathy. Mid esophageal four chamber view, multiplane angle 0°. *LA* left atrium, *LV* left ventricle, *RA* right atrium, *RV* right ventricle

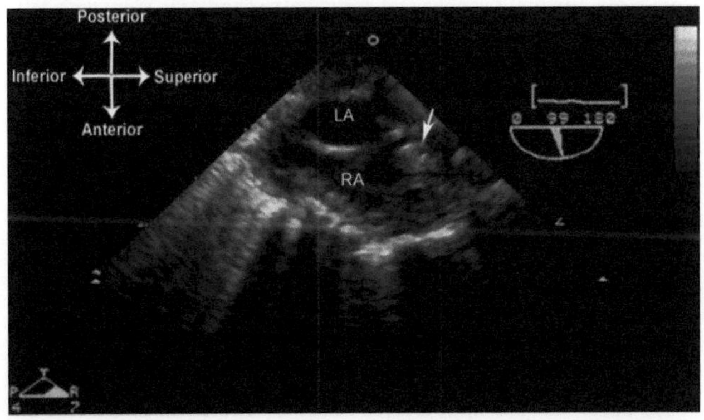

Fig. 16.7 Thrombus (*arrow*) in the superior vena cava, probably associated with a catheter. Seen from mid esophageal bicaval view, (multiplane angle 99°). *LA* left atrium, *RA* right atrium

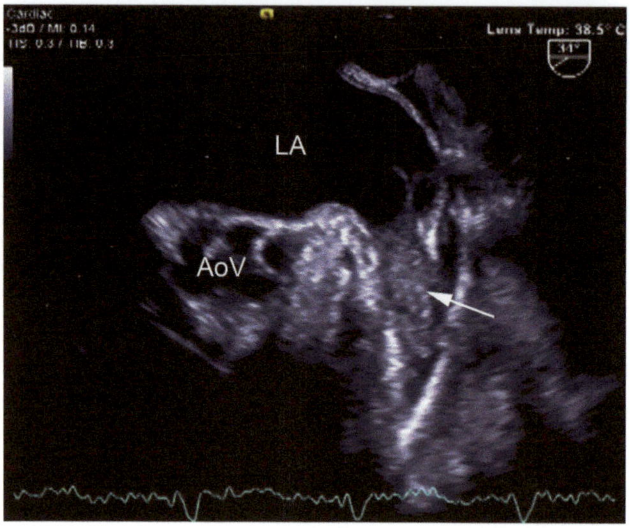

Fig. 16.8 Thrombus in the left atrial appendage (*arrow*), as viewed from a modified mid esophageal aortic valve short axis view with leftward rotation. There are mobile filamentous strands arising from the thrombus. *AoV* aortic valve, *LA* left atrium (Photograph courtesy of Siemens Medical Systems USA, Inc. © 2012–13 Siemens Medical Solutions USA, Inc. All Rights Reserved)

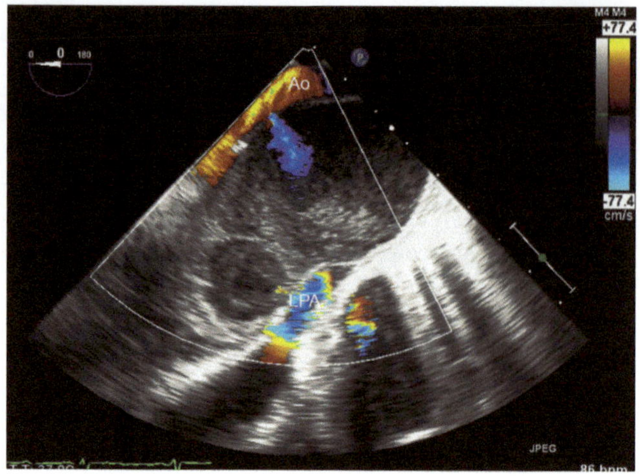

Fig. 16.9 Example of spontaneous echo contrast in a patient after repair of D-transposition of the great arteries, with a pseudoaneurysm arising from a previous cannulation site in the aorta. Image obtained from the upper esophageal aortic arch long axis view. Note the visible swirling of flow due to red cell aggregation. The left pulmonary artery (*LPA*) is compressed by the pseudoaneurysm. *Ao* ascending aorta

anatomic variation [58]. It is attached to the Eustachian and Thebesian valves; it is thin and redundant and often displays a porous, fenestrated or filamentous appearance. A related structure, a prominent Eustachian valve, can be very prominent and extend into the right atrium. It can also be very mobile, and in some cases has the appearance of long vegetation or thrombus. Both a Chiari network and Eustachian valve are well seen using the mid esophageal bicaval view, with multiplane angle approximately 80–90°. In the left atrium, a prominent ridge between left upper pulmonary vein and left atrial appendage (sometimes informally called the "coumadin ridge") can, on occasion, be mistaken for a thrombus. Another important artifact that may resemble an intracardiac thrombus is the presence of spontaneous echo contrast, or "smoke", in an atrial chamber [50, 59, 60]. This represents red cell aggregation from sluggish blood flow, such as that seen in a low-flow Fontan circuit (Chap. 10). When dense and echogenic, it can produce the appearance of thrombus. However, the swirling and circular movements differentiate this type of finding from a thrombus (Fig. 16.9, Video 16.9).

Cardiac Tumors

Cardiac tumors are divided into two categories: primary and secondary/metastatic. Primary cardiac tumors originate in the heart, and most of these are benign [61–64]. However despite their "benign" histopathology, some primary tumors can still cause significant clinical sequelae due to arrhythmias, mass effect (obstruction), or embolization. Rarely, primary cardiac tumors are malignant and, if so, they are usually sarcomas and are almost always associated with a poor outcome [62]. The other class of cardiac tumors comprises the secondary/metastatic tumors that are, by definition, malignant. Secondary cardiac tumors occur mostly as distant metastases, but they can also invade the heart by direct extension, for example via the inferior vena cava (IVC). Secondary malignant cardiac tumors are seen much more frequently than primary cardiac tumors, both in adults and children. Indeed, in the adult literature metastatic tumors outnumber primary cardiac tumors by a 20–30 to 1 ratio, and in children, by a 3–4 to 1 ratio [61, 62]. In adults, the most common primary sites for metastasis to the heart include lung, breast, lymphoma/leukemia, esophageal, uterine and melanoma. Most of these metastases are to the pericardium, and 90 % are clinically silent [63]. In children, the most common tumors with metastasis to the heart are non-Hodgkin's lymphoma, neuroblastoma, Wilms tumor, and soft tissue/bone sarcomas [61]. Direct extension of a tumor can occur from the IVC to the right atrium in patients with Wilms tumor [65], renal myosarcoma, or adrenal and hepatocellular carcinoma (Fig. 16.10, Video 16.10). As with adults, overt clinical signs and symptoms of secondary tumors are uncommon [61].

The echocardiographic presentation of cardiac tumors is highly variable, depending upon the type of tumor and the site of involvement. Cardiac tumors can involve only endocardium, only myocardium, only pericardium, or various combinations thereof [62]. There can be one or multiple foci, again depending on tumor type. An extensive discussion of cardiac tumors is beyond the scope of this chapter, and there are other excellent references available on the subject [62, 63, 66]. The remainder of this section will discuss a few of the more common primary cardiac tumors and

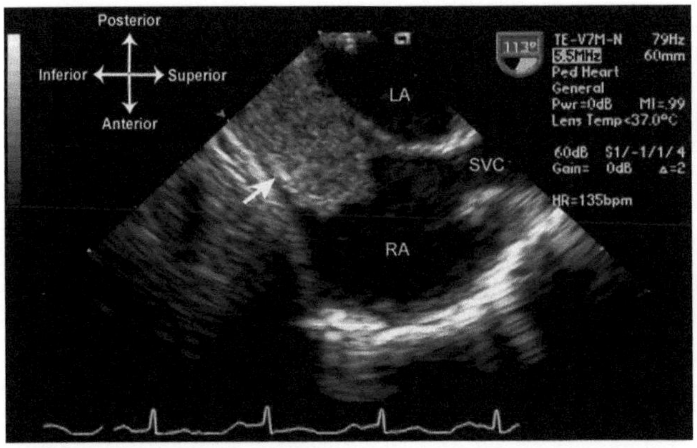

Fig. 16.10 Wilms tumor (*arrow*) invading the right atrium by direct extension from the inferior vena cava, as seen from the mid esophageal bicaval view, multiplane angle 113°. *LA* left atrium, *RA* right atrium, *SVC* superior vena cava

provide examples of their evaluation by TEE. The method of TEE evaluation for these particular tumors can be applied to the evaluation of cardiac tumors of any etiology.

Rhabdomyoma

Rhabdomyomas are the most commonly encountered primary cardiac tumors in the pediatric age group, comprising approximately 60–80 % [67, 68]. Typically, multiple tumors are located within the free wall of the right and left ventricle, as well as the interventricular septum. They can also be present in the right atrium. There is a strong association (at least 50 %) with tuberous sclerosis. These tumors are histologically benign but nevertheless patients can be clinically symptomatic in a number of different ways. Depending upon location, atrial or ventricular arrhythmias can occur. Tumors of sufficient size adjacent to an area of inflow or outflow can cause significant obstruction, which occasionally necessitates surgical resection. However with time, spontaneous regression of these tumors usually occurs, so surgery is not indicated in most patients unless the tumors cause significant mass effect.

Given the generally benign nature of cardiac rhabdomyomas, and the young age that these tumors are first diagnosed, it is very rare that a TEE is necessary for evaluation; TTE generally suffices. The major indication for TEE is in patients undergoing surgery for relief of inflow or outflow tract obstruction. Rhabdomyomas are characteristically homogenous, echogenic, and well circumscribed; they are easily distinguished from the surrounding myocardium. The mid esophageal four chamber (ME 4 Ch) view (multiplane angle 0°) is the best view from which to begin evaluation of the tumors, both ventricular and (if present) atrial. Once located, they can be visualized more closely with variations in multiplane angle, along with anteflexion and retroflexion to bring the tumor(s) into view. If a large tumor is causing possible obstruction to AV inflow, color flow and spectral Doppler should be used to evaluate for disturbed flow patterns around the tumor, and to determine a mean gradient across the area. If the tumor is causing possible outflow tract obstruction, mid esophageal views such as the ME 4 Ch, mid esophageal long axis (ME LAX), and mid esophageal right ventricular inflow-outflow (ME RV In-Out) with multiplane angles varying between 0° to 110° are best to evaluate the anatomic extent of the tumor and any turbulence as seen by color flow Doppler (Fig. 16.11, Video 16.11). Deep transgastric long axis (DTG LAX) and deep transgastric sagittal (DTG Sagittal) views with probe anteflexion/retroflexion provide the best angle of spectral Doppler interrogation of the ventricular outflow tracts. The transgastric views also provide other perspectives from which to visualize both right and left sided tumors. These views include the transgastric basal short axis (TG Basal SAX), mid short axis (TG Mid SAX), two chamber (TG 2 Ch), long axis (TG LAX), and right ventricular inflow (TG RV In).

Fibroma

Fibromas are the second most common cardiac tumor encountered in the pediatric age group (10–30 %) [69]. They are generally solitary and intramural, located within the ventricular septum or left ventricular free wall [62]. When large, they can impinge significantly upon the adjacent cardiac chamber (usually the left ventricle), causing symptomatology such as congestive heart failure and cyanosis. Rarely, they can be multiple and involve other parts of the heart including the ventricular conduction system, right ventricle and right ventricular free wall. They frequently cause ventricular arrhythmias [70]. Because these tumors do not regress spontaneously and sometimes can grow significantly, surgical resection is recommended.

The TEE evaluation of fibromas generally occurs in the operating room setting, and is similar to that involved with the evaluation of other cardiac tumors. The tumors are best seen using the mid esophageal views, with a combination of multiplane angles between 0° and 100°. Color flow and spectral Doppler should be employed to evaluate for potential compromise of ventricular inflow or outflow due to the tumor. The echocardiographic appearance of a fibroma is that of a single, bright, echo-dense intramural mass with calcifications and cystic areas within the tumor (Fig. 16.12, Video 16.12).

Myxoma

Myxomas represent the most common primary cardiac tumor in adults [62, 71]. On occasion, they can also be seen in children. They are most commonly located in the left atrial cavity (75–90 %), but can also be found in the right atrium [72], as well as the ventricles [62, 73]. Rarely, they can be present in more than one cavity [74]. Clinical

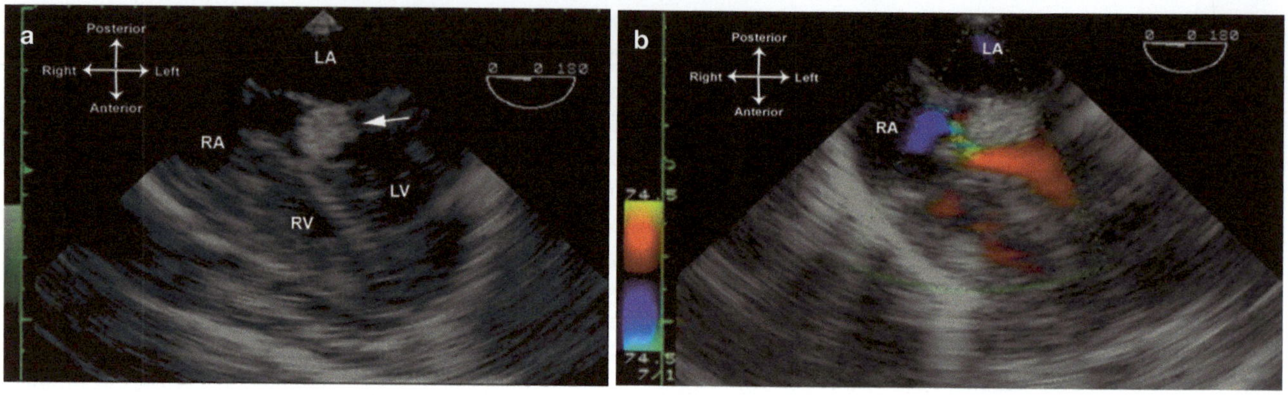

Fig. 16.11 Multiple rhabdomyomas in a patient with tuberous sclerosis, including one that caused near complete obstruction of the left ventricular outflow tract. Figure **a** is obtained from a mid esophageal four chamber view, multiplane angle 0°, showing a large tumor in the outflow tract (*arrow*). Turbulent color flow Doppler is seen in (**b**). This tumor was resected surgically. *LA* left atrium, *LV* left ventricle, *RA* right atrium, *RV* right ventricle

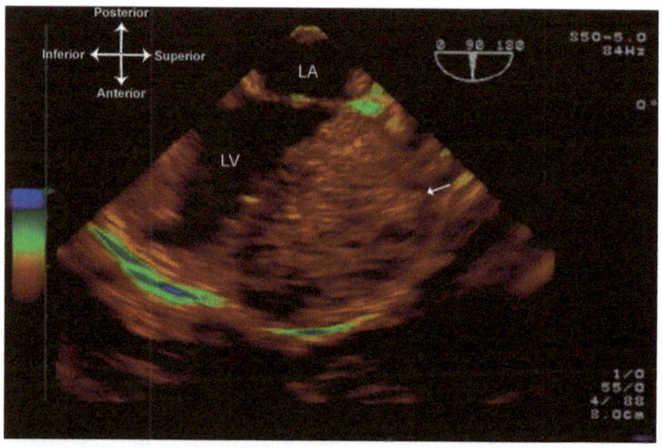

Fig. 16.12 Fibroma attached to the left ventricular free wall, visualized from mid esophageal long axis view, multiplane angle 90°. The fibroma (*arrow*) is very large, circumscribed, and has a heterogeneous appearance, studded with echolucent areas most likely representing cystic degeneration or necrosis. *LA* left atrium, *LV* left ventricle

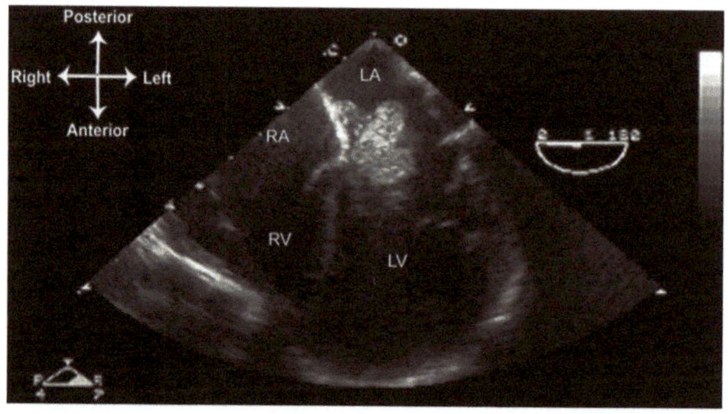

Fig. 16.13 Left atrial myxoma, seen from mid esophageal four chamber view, multiplane angle 0°. A large, lobulated myxoma is attached to the interatrial septum just posterior to the aortic root. *LA* left atrium, *LV* left ventricle, *RA* right atrium, *RV* right ventricle

manifestations of a left atrial myxoma are quite variable and can include embolic phenomena and/or obstruction to blood flow causing breathlessness, syncope, and congestive heart failure. Other constitutional symptoms such as fever, malaise, weight loss, and myalgias/arthralgias can also be present. Familial occurrence is reported in approximately 7–10 % of all myxomas, generally in younger patients. These are associated with multiple endocrine syndromes including LAMB (lentigines, atrial myxoma, mucocutaneous myxoma, and blue nevi) and NAME (nevi, atrial myxoma, neurofibromata, and ephelides).

Myxomas are gelatinous in consistency and they can be pedunculated. By echocardiography, they have a globular, lobulated, or fimbriated appearance, and a pedicle can be present. There may be small lucencies and calcifications in the tumor, resulting in an inhomogeneous appearance. Left atrial myxomas characteristically have attachments to the atrial septum, but they can also attach to other portions of the left atrium or to the mitral valve. If large enough, the myxoma can cause obstruction to mitral inflow. Given the numerous potential complications, including embolus, the treatment for atrial myxomas is surgery, and TEE plays an important role in the pre and postoperative assessment [75]. The attachment point, the extent of the tumor, the number of tumors, and relationship to surrounding structures, should all be evaluated carefully prior to surgical resection. Following surgery, it is important for TEE assessment to include evaluation of the left atrium and interatrial septum, in order to determine completeness of tumor resection as well as the integrity of the mitral valve. Atrial myxomas are best visualized by TEE with the mid esophageal views, using several multiplane angles to determine the location and extent of the tumor (Fig. 16.13, Video 16.13). Color flow and spectral Doppler should be used to evaluate any obstruction to mitral valve inflow, and/or mitral regurgitation resulting from damage to the mitral valve leaflets or valve interference by the tumor.

Other Cardiac Tumors

Hemangiomas and teratomas are two other primary tumors that are occasionally encountered in the pediatric population. Hemangiomas can be located anywhere within the heart, but have a predilection for the right atrium and ventricular septum [76]. By echocardiography, there are numerous echolucent spaces, and color flow Doppler often demonstrates multiple vascular channels (Fig. 16.14, Video 16.14). Teratomas are usually detected in the fetus and neonate. They most commonly occur in the pericardial space, but can also arise within the heart, attached to the atrial or ventricular wall. When in the pericardial space, they are often attached to the aortic root or pulmonary trunk, and they can grow to a large size. There may be an associated pericardial effusion. If sufficiently large, either the tumor or the effusion (or both) can compress the heart, leading to tamponade physiology. When intracardiac in location, these can cause clinical signs and symptoms similar to other intracardiac tumors. By echocardiography, the tumors appear heterogeneous and encapsulated [67].

Role of TEE in the Evaluation of Cardiac Tumors

Most cardiac tumors are well seen by TTE, particularly in younger patients, and therefore TTE serves as the principal modality for their evaluation and follow-up. Cardiac magnetic resonance imaging has become increasingly utilized for diagnostic evaluation of cardiac tumors [77–79]. The role of TEE is primarily for two settings: (a) for those patients in whom TTE imaging is poor or incomplete, and (b) for intraoperative assessment. Specifics of optimal TEE probe location and multiplane angles, along with methods of evaluation, will depend upon the type and location of the tumor (as detailed above). In adults, TEE has been reported to provide more precise depiction of tumor attachment sites and extent of myocardial/pericardial involvement [80, 81]. Intraoperatively, the preoperative TEE study is used to confirm the nature and extent of tumor involvement [82, 83]. The postoperative TEE study evaluates the results of cardiac surgery—focusing on completeness of tumor resection residual obstruction (if previously present), whether any adjacent cardiac structures (e.g. cardiac valves) might have been affected by the resection, and assessment of ventricular function [84, 85].

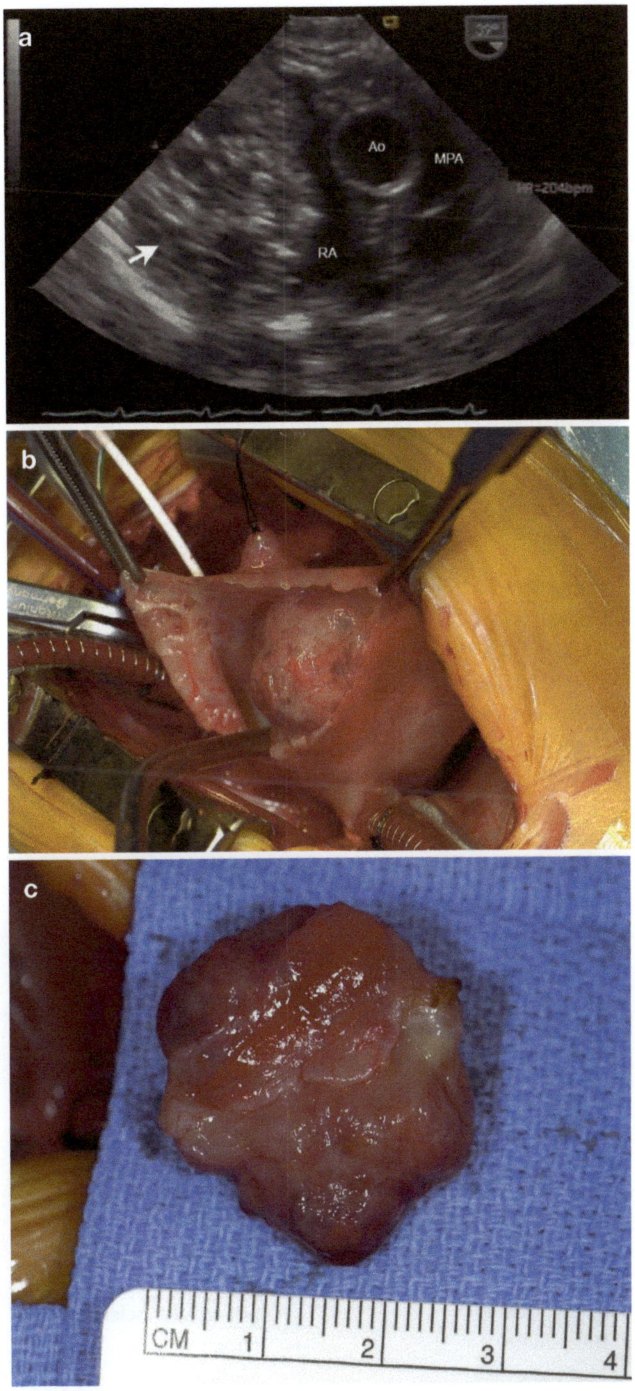

Fig. 16.14 Right atrial hemangioma as seen from a modified mid esophageal right ventricular inflow-outflow view. (**a**) Note the markedly heterogeneous nature of the large mass in the right atrium (*arrow*). The patient underwent surgery and the tumor was removed (**b** and **c**). *Ao* ascending aorta, *MPA* main pulmonary artery, *RA* right atrium

Evaluation of Prosthetic Valves

Prosthetic valves are integral to the medical and surgical management of pediatric and adult patients with CHD. These valves fall into two major categories—mechanical and biologic—based upon valve composition (Table 16.6).

Mechanical heart valves contain nonbiologic materials (polymers, metal, carbon) in all parts of the prosthesis: the valve ring, sewing cuff, and orifice occluder. A number of mechanical valves have been developed over the past 50 years, essentially of three major types. The first type to be developed was the caged ball valve, consisting of a silastic ball with a circular sewing ring and a cage formed by three metal arches. The most notable of these was the

Starr-Edwards valve (Fig. 16.15c), though similar valves have been produced including the Smeloff-Cutter valve. While these valves are no longer implanted, thousands of patients who received these valves are still alive, and continue to be followed regularly. The second type of mechanical valve is the monoleaflet valve, in which a single disk is secured by lateral or central metal struts, and surrounded by a sewing ring. The disk, generally made of extremely hard carbon (pyrolytic carbon), opens by tilting at an angle (about 60°–80°), resulting in two orifices of different sizes. Typical examples of this include the Bjork-Shiley (discontinued), and the Medtronic-Hall valve (Fig. 16.15b). The third major type of mechanical valve is the bileaflet tilting disk valve, made of two semicircular pyrolytic carbon disks attached by hinges to a rigid valve sewing ring. In the open position the valve leaflets tilt to an opening angle of 75°–90°, resulting in three orifices: a small slit-like orifice centrally between the two leaflets, and two semicircular orifices laterally. Of the three types of mechanical valves, the bileaflet tilting disk valve provides the most natural blood flow, greater effective orifice area for a given valve size, and it is also the least thrombogenic. Currently, they are the most commonly implanted mechanical valves, notably the St. Jude Medical (Fig. 16.15a) and Carbomedics bileaflet tilting disk valves. The latter two valves are available in a variety of sizes (from 16–33 mm) suitable for both pediatric and adult patients. The mechanical valves have a proven record of durability, however they require ongoing anticoagulation therapy, and there

Table 16.6 Typical biologic and mechanical valves

Valve name/type	Manufacturer	Valve type/origin
Biologic—Human		
Autograft		Pulmonary autograft
Allograft (Homograft)	Cryolife	Harvested cadaveric aortic, pulmonary homograft
Monocusp, bicuspid		Surgically handsewn valve using autologous pericardium
Biologic—Heterograft		
Stented		
Hancock II	Medtronic	Porcine
Mosaic	Medtronic	Porcine
Carpentier-Edwards	Edwards-Lifesciences	Porcine
Epic	St Jude	Porcine
Biocor	St Jude	Porcine
Trifecta	St Jude	Bovine pericardial
Carpentier-Edwards Perimount Magna	Edwards Lifesciences	Bovine pericardial
Mitroflow	Sorin Biomedica	Bovine pericardial
Soprano	Sorin Biomedica	Bovine pericardial
Stentless		
Freestyle	Medtronic	Porcine
Toronto SPV	St Jude	Porcine
Prima Plus	Edwards Lifesciences	Porcine
Pericarbon Freedom	Sorin Biomedica	Bovine pericardial
3 F Therapeutics Stentless Equine	3 F Therapeutics	Equine pericardial
Mechanical		
Starr-Edwards	Edwards Lifesciences	Ball-in-cage
Bjork-Shiley	Pfizer	Single leaflet tilting disk
Medtronic-Hall	Medtronic	Single leaflet tilting disk
St. Jude Medical	St Jude	Bileaflet tilting disk
CarboMedics	Sorin-CarboMedics	Bileaflet tilting disk
ATS Medical	ATS Medical	Bileaflet tilting disk
On-X	On-X Life Technologies	Bileaflet tilting disk
Percutaneous—Biologic		
Melody	Medtronic	Bovine jugular valve mounted on platinum-iridium stent
SAPIEN	Edwards Lifesciences	Bovine pericardium leaflets mounted on stainless steel or cobalt chromium alloy (SAPIEN XT)
CoreValve	Medtronic	Porcine pericardium leaflets mounted on self-expanding nitinol frame
Other		
SynerGraft	Cryolife	Tissue engineered decellularized allograft heart valve
Contegra	Medtronic	Valved conduit of bovine jugular vein

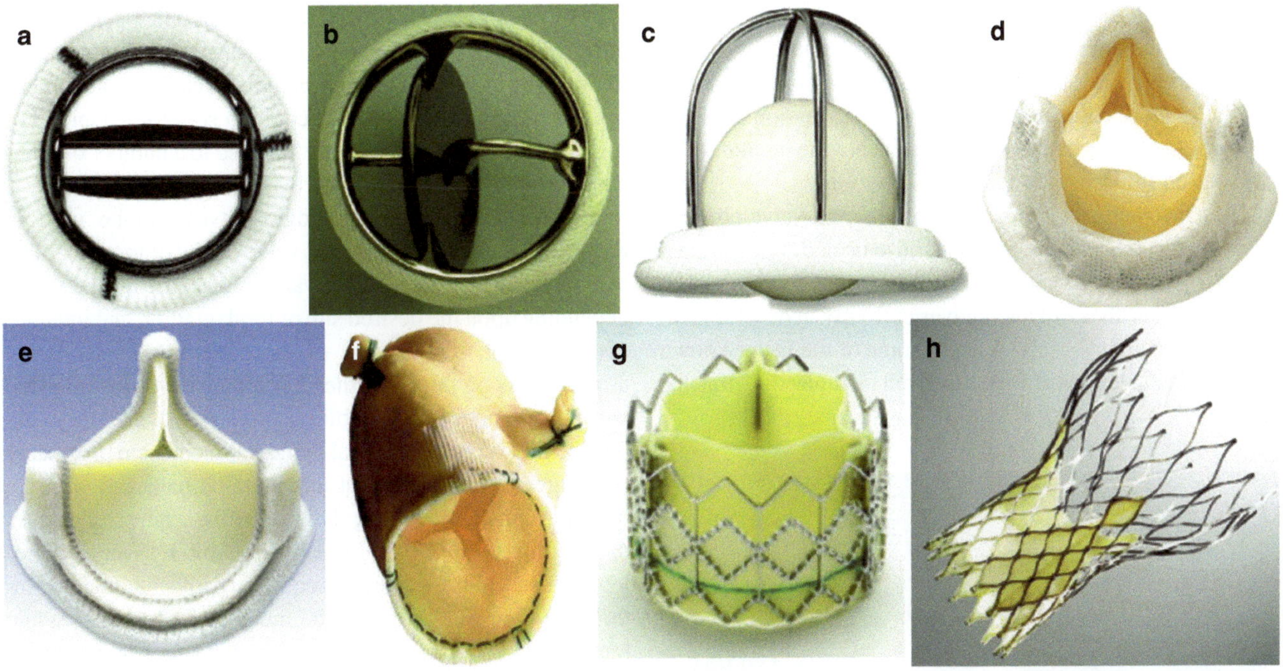

Fig. 16.15 Different types of prosthetic valves. (**a**) Bileaflet mechanical valve (St. Jude); (**b**) monoleaflet mechanical valve (Medtronic Hall); (**c**) caged ball valve (Starr-Edwards); (**d**) stented porcine bioprosthesis (Medtronic Mosaic); (**e**) stented pericardial bioprostheses (Carpentier-Edwards Magna); (**f**) stentless porcine bioprosthesis (Medtronic Freestyle); (**g**) percutaneous bioprosthesis expanded over a balloon (Edwards SAPIEN); (**h**) self-expandable percutaneous bioprosthesis (CoreValve). See text for details (*From Pibarot and Dumesnil* [95]*; with permission of Walters-Kluwer*)

are ever-present risks of thrombosis and endocarditis of the valve. In many types of mechanical valves, separate aortic and mitral versions are available; nonetheless for a number of the mechanical valves, implantation has been performed in any of the four valve positions.

Biologic heart valves are derived from human or animal tissue, and certain types contain nonbiologic material as well, such as metal and fabric. Human tissue valves fall into two categories: *homografts* (*allografts*) and *autografts*. Homograft valves are cryopreserved human cadaveric aortic and pulmonary valves, generally used as pulmonary or aortic valve replacements (Fig. 16.16). They come in a variety of sizes, depending upon donor availability. In contrast, an autograft represents the patient's own valve translocated from one site to another. Usually, the autograft is the patient's pulmonary valve translocated to the aortic position (Ross procedure) or rarely the mitral position (Ross II), with a homograft valve being placed in the original pulmonary position [86–88]. Biologic valves derived from animal tissue are known as *xenograft* (or *heterograft*) valves; the most commonly used animal tissues are porcine aortic valve and bovine pericardium, and the tissues are fixed with glutaraldehyde. These valves come in two major forms. *Stented* biologic valves contain a sewing ring and struts composed of nonbiologic material (metal, cloth), and valve tissue is sewn onto the fabric covering the struts. Both porcine valve (Fig. 16.15d) and bovine pericardium (Fig. 16.15e) are used with these types of valves. *Stentless* biologic valves contain no struts or sewing ring, which leaves more room for blood flow. Stentless xenograft valves derive primarily from harvested porcine aortic valves (Fig. 16.15f). Of note, human homograft and autograft valves also fall into the category of unstented biologic valves, since they contain no sewing ring or struts. This is because the entire homograft/allograft root (containing the valves) is harvested, thus the intrinsic structural support for the valve leaflets remains intact. Another category of bioprosthesis that has gained popularity is the Contegra pulmonary valve conduit. The Contegra conduit is a bovine jugular vein preserved in glutaraldehyde, and it contains a valve with three leaflets; the leaflets are similar to a human semilunar valve (Fig. 16.17). Since it is derived from a venous vascular structure, it is felt to be best suited for conditions of lower pressure such as the pulmonary circuit, and therefore it is used primarily for congenital heart surgeries in which a right ventricle to pulmonary artery conduit is needed such as the Ross procedure, tetralogy of Fallot, truncus arteriosus, etc. [89]. Thus it serves as an alternative to the homograft, and has achieved comparable short to intermediate term results [90–92]. Strictly speaking, it is a valved conduit (not solely a biologic valve), but it is used in a number of operations in which a valve is necessary. The Contegra conduit is available in both a supported and unsupported model;

the supported model contains two external cloth covered polypropylene rings that encircle the valve annulus and commissure to provide additional support (Fig. 16.17a), and is utilized in those cases in which sternal compression could be an issue. As will be discussed below, the bovine jugular valve is also used for transcatheter valve technology.

Over the years, a large number of different valve prostheses (both mechanical and biologic) have been developed, in a variety of valve sizes and profiles. Development continues at a rapid pace, with novel alternatives currently in development or advanced clinical trials. A list of some of the better-known biologic and mechanical valves is given in Table 16.6; this list is by no means exhaustive, and new models and types are periodically being introduced. A full discussion and elaboration of the many individual valves (including details about durability and complications) would require a separate chapter. For further information, the reader is referred to a number of references providing more detailed coverage of the topic [93–97].

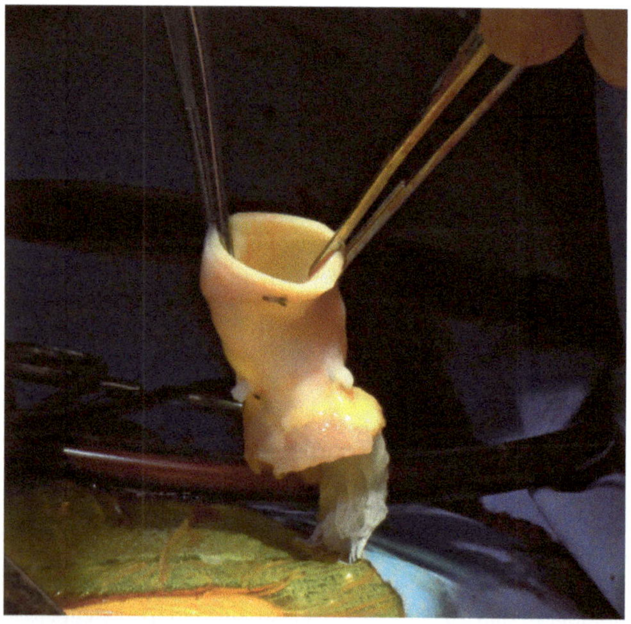

Fig. 16.16 Aortic homograft, following thawing and prior to implantation as a right ventricle to pulmonary artery conduit

Both mechanical and biologic valves can be used to replace a stenotic or regurgitant valve in any of the four valve positions. The preference for valve replacement type varies depending upon the desired site of implantation, and includes considerations such as age of the patient, evidence-based effectiveness of valve prosthesis alternatives for the intended valvar position, valve durability, valve size availability, and the need for ongoing medical therapy. Mechanical prostheses boast greater durability, but this must be balanced with the need for constant anticoagulation and the ever-present risks of bleeding, thrombosis, and endocarditis. Conversely, biologic valves do not generally require significant anticoagulation, but their durability can be much more variable. While there are multiple options for each valve site, some generalizations can be made [17]. For pulmonary valve replacement, biologic valves—notably homograft (allograft) and heterograft (porcine, bovine pericardial, contegra)—are generally preferred, though some investigators have advocated for mechanical valves [98]. For tricuspid, either a mechanical valve or stented porcine valve is generally used. For the aortic valve, both biologic (homograft, heterograft, pulmonary autograft) and mechanical prosthetic valves are utilized. A number of stented and unstented biosprosthetic xenograft valves have been developed for the aortic valve position. For the mitral valve, mechanical prostheses predominate in children and adults, although stented biologic valves (porcine and bovine pericardial) are selectively used in the adult group due to other important considerations (such as pregnancy and the risk of warfarin embryopathy) [17].

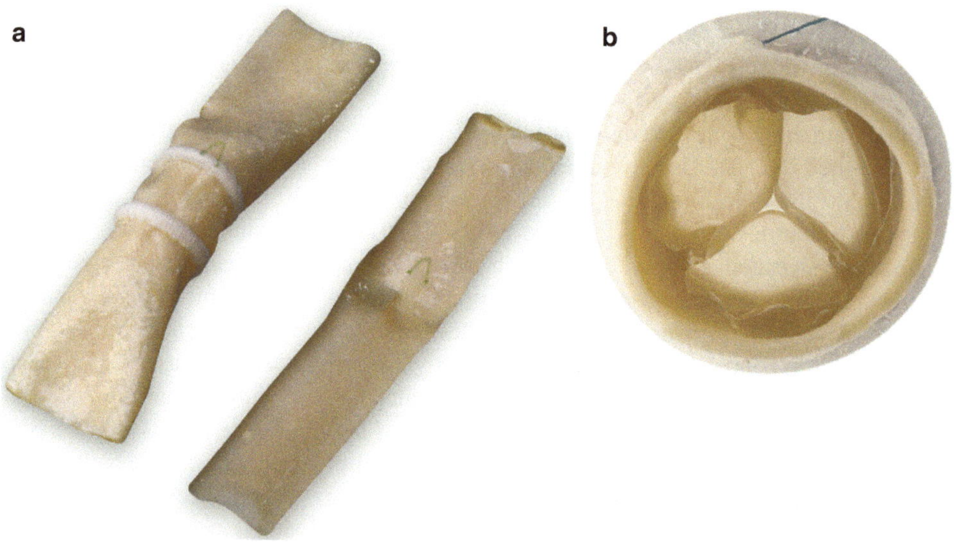

Fig. 16.17 Contegra pulmonary valve conduit. The Contegra conduit is a bovine jugular vein with a trileaflet valve that is similar to a human semilunar valve. (**a**) The conduit is available in supported and unsupported models. The supported model contains two external cloth covered polypropylene rings that encircle the valve annulus and commissure to provide additional support for the valve housed inside the conduit. (**b**) Cross-sectional *(en face)* view of the trileaflet bovine valve inside the conduit (Image published with permission from Medtronic, Inc)

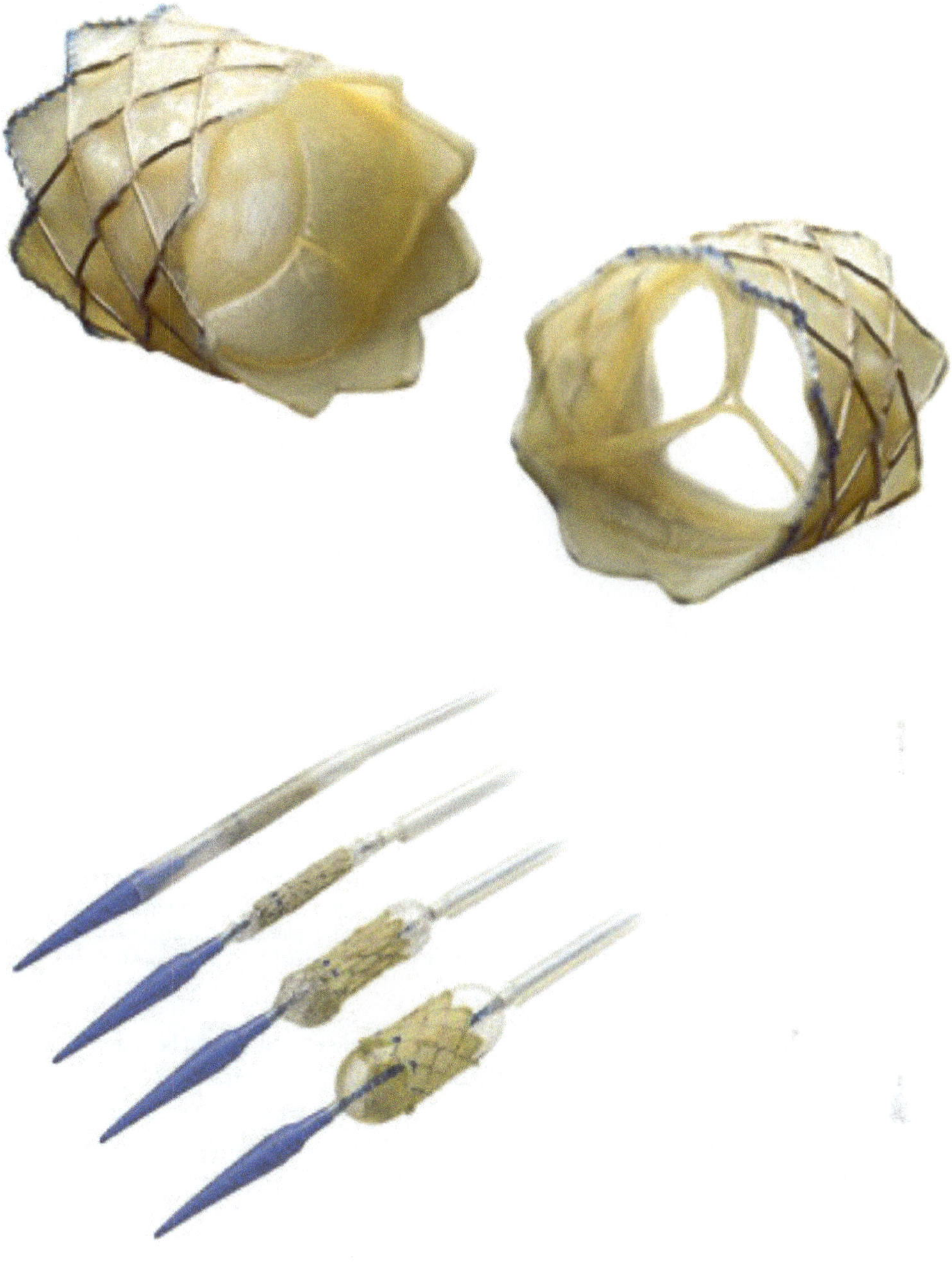

Fig. 16.18 The Medtronic Melody transcatheter pulmonary valve consists of bovine jugular vein sutured in a 28 mm platinum-iridium stent. The valve is inserted using a 22 French balloon in balloon catheter delivery system (Ensemble) with a retractable sheath that covers the Melody valve once it is front loaded and crimped over the balloon (Reprinted from Fleming et al [99]; with permission from Elsevier)

One of the most important and exciting new areas in prosthetic valve technology has been the development of catheter-based, implantable prosthetic valves, also known as transcatheter heart valves or THVs. Valve leaflets composed of biologic tissue are mounted in an expandable metal frame, which can then be delivered using various transcatheter techniques and precisely placed in the location of the diseased or absent valve. Several of these THVs are well known, having already gained a large clinical experience. The **Melody valve** (Fig. 16.18) is a bovine jugular valve mounted on a platinum iridium stent, and delivered by a 22 F balloon in balloon catheter delivery system [99]. It is primarily designed for pulmonary valve replacement, and in the United States it is currently used only in an existing right ventricular outflow conduit, though in Europe it has also been used in patients with tetralogy of Fallot and a right ventricular outflow tract patch (using pre-stenting techniques) [100]. It has also been used in other positions such as failed AV valve bioprostheses (also known as "valve-in-valve" replacement) [99, 101, 102], native aortic valve replacement [101], and in the branch pulmonary arteries [103]. For transcatheter aortic valve replacement/implantation (also known as TAVR, or TAVI), there are two major devices currently available. The **Edwards SAPIEN** valve contains bovine pericardial leaflets sewn inside a stainless steel or cobalt chromium alloy frame. The inflow of the frame is covered with fabric to provide an

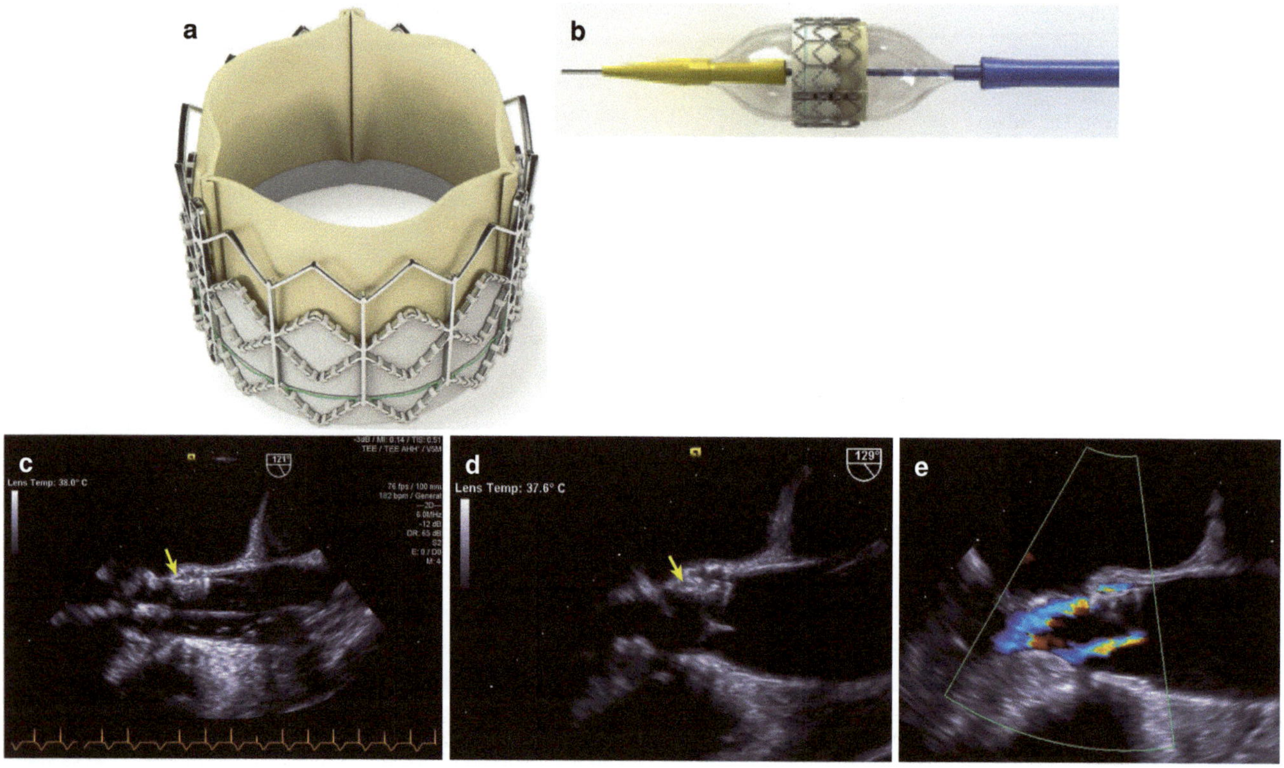

Fig. 16.19 Transcatheter aortic valve replacement/implantation (TAVR/TAVI). Figure **a** shows the Edwards SAPIEN valve (Edwards Lifesciences Inc., Irvine, California), a bovine pericardial valve mounted on a stainless steel frame. Figure **b** shows the same valve mounted on a balloon catheter that is used for valve delivery. Figure **c–e** are transesophageal echocardiographic images obtained from the mid esophageal aortic valve long axis view at 120°-130°. Figure **c** shows the balloon being inflated (device indicated with *arrow*), and figure **d** shows the valve (*arrow*) after implantation. In Figure **e**, following valve implantation color flow Doppler shows two small jets of regurgitation: one a central transvalvular jet, the other a peripheral paravalvular jet (Echocardiographic images were obtained from a Siemens SC 2000 platform and are courtesy of Siemens Medical Systems USA, Inc. © 2012–13 Siemens Medical Solutions USA, Inc. All Rights Reserved)

annulus seal (Figs. 16.15g and 16.19a, b). The valve is positioned through a sheath (22–24 F for the SAPIEN, 16–19 F for the SAPIEN XT) either from the femoral artery, ascending aorta, or through the left ventricular apex (the latter two methods utilizing a hybrid surgical approach). Once positioned, the frame and valve are balloon expanded within the diseased native aortic valve, displacing the native leaflets (Fig. 16.19). Rapid ventricular pacing is performed during implantation to reduce cardiac contraction during valve implantation [104]. This valve is also used for valve-in-valve replacement (mitral, tricuspid), and is undergoing trials for use in transcatheter pulmonary valve replacement (similar to the Melody valve) [99, 105]. The other major valve for TAVR/TAVI is the **Medtronic CoreValve** system. This valve is composed of porcine pericardial leaflets and annular seal, mounted in a self-expanding nitinol frame (Fig. 16.15h). It is delivered within an 18 F sheath, introduced percutaneously via femoral or subclavian artery access. Once the sheathed device is located in the desired position, the device expands (and becomes deployed) by retraction of the sheath. Deployment does not require rapid ventricular pacing. To date, it has limited utility for valve-in-valve therapy.

It should be noted that research and development in THVs continues at a very rapid pace; in the near future one can expect to see a number of new valves in various stages of clinical trials [106].

TEE Evaluation of Prosthetic Valves

Echocardiography is very important for the evaluation of both mechanical and biologic valves. This is particularly true in the intraoperative setting, in which TEE is used preoperatively to visualize the diseased valve location, size and pathology, and postoperatively to assess the function and anatomic appearance of the newly implanted prosthetic valve. However it is important to remember that the intraoperative setting presents unique challenges for valvar assessment due to physiologic alterations from changing preload/afterload, inotropic support, open sternum, positive pressure ventilation, and general anesthesia (also discussed in Chaps. 11 and 15).

The TEE evaluation of prosthetic valves utilizes the same principles applied to native valve pathology: one should perform a combination of careful 2D imaging, as well as color flow and spectral Doppler evaluation of flow across the valve. For imaging, a prosthetic valve should be examined from multiple views, with emphasis on valve occluder/leaflet motion, appearance of the sewing ring, and presence of an abnormal echo density attached to any part of the prosthesis. The examiner should establish that the valve is well seated, and without excessive movement or "rocking", which could be a sign of dehiscence [107]. The imaging findings should always be paired with color flow and spectral Doppler evaluation, which gives important information regarding valve function, including possible paravalvar leaks as well as areas of stenosis/abnormal flow. The examiner should understand the type of prosthetic valve implanted, and whether there are any unique imaging/flow characteristics expected with that particular prosthesis. For example, imaging artifacts produced by certain prosthetic valves can sometimes interfere with their assessment. In this case the use of multiple imaging planes and views can help to circumvent these artifacts, and this is particularly applicable to TEE.

For mechanical prosthetic valves, echocardiography (both TTE and TEE) serves as an essential tool for evaluation [107]. Normal flow across a mechanical valve will be different than that of the corresponding native valve; increased spectral Doppler velocities can be anticipated, depending upon valve manufacturer and valve location and size. These "normal" or expected Doppler velocities have been well documented for the different valve types and sizes (discussed below) [95, 107, 108]. Mechanical valves can be difficult to image by TTE due to their nonbiologic material composition (metal and pyrolytic carbon) that produces significant acoustic shadowing and reverberation, as well as side lobe artifacts. As such, limited information is available in those areas of the valve prosthesis distal to the ultrasound transducer. Thus for certain mechanical valves, TEE can play a very important role in their evaluation because of the proximity of the TEE probe to the heart, with a location proximal to the prosthesis, resulting in superior overall imaging (Fig. 16.20). Excellent visualization of mechanical valve motion, as well as color flow and spectral Doppler evaluation can be obtained. Mechanical valves generally have flow characteristics that differ markedly from native valves. For example, the typical bileaflet tilting disk valve (e.g. St. Jude), when open, has one major central orifice and two side orifices to allow forward flow [95, 107]. When closed, there are normally two small regurgitant ("washing") jets at the pivot points of the valve, angled centrally; these are intended to minimize thrombus formation [109] (Fig. 16.21, Video 16.15). Abnormalities of valve occluder/leaflet motion (such as a frozen leaflet), vegetations, thrombus, pannus formation (tissue ingrowth at the site of the valve prosthesis), and paravalvar leaks/valve dehiscence, can all be seen well by TEE [94, 109]. For mechanical prosthetic valve endocarditis, TEE has been shown to be clearly superior to TTE: vegetations and annular abscesses can be visualized much more readily [41, 110–112]. With mechanical prostheses, vegetations can significantly interfere with occluder motion, causing stenosis, regurgitation, or both [109].

With mechanical AV valve evaluation, TEE can very useful. This is especially true with mechanical mitral valves, in which the superiority of TEE imaging compared to TTE is most striking. The esophageal position of the TEE probe enables imaging of the important atrial surface of the valve—an area where pathology tends to occur, often obscured by standard TTE. Excellent valve detail is obtainable from the mid esophageal window: rotation of the multiplane angle can be performed between 0° and 90° to provide optimal visualization of the prosthesis leaflets and leaflet motion from an edge-on view (particularly for bileaflet tilting valves). Restricted leaflet motion and pannus/vegetations above the valve can be very well seen (Figs. 16.22 and 16.23, Videos 16.16 and 16.17). One other important issue to note is that the native papillary muscles and chordal tissue can sometimes be left in place following AV valve replacement, and the chordae can remain quite mobile during the cardiac cycle. These structures should not be confused with intracardiac masses or thrombi.

Mechanical aortic valves can be more challenging to evaluate, as the mid esophageal plane of imaging tends to be parallel to the plane of the valve, and therefore more perpendicular to the direction of valve flow. Depending upon valve leaflet orientation, it might be difficult to obtain an edge-on profile of leaflet motion. Instead, often the leaflets can be viewed from an *en face* perspective. They can be examined for any asymmetry of motion, and any paravalvar leaks can be viewed from a number of different multiplane angles between 0°–120° (Fig. 16.3, Video 16.3). If transgastric and deep transgastric views are available, these can be particularly useful to evaluate the proximal (subaortic) portion of the valve, visualize valve motion, evaluate for valvar regurgitation, and also obtain a spectral Doppler tracing across the valve [109] (Fig. 16.24, Video 16.18). These latter transducer positions help to avoid the shadowing artifacts associated with imaging from the mid esophageal position.

Biologic prosthetic valves—both stented and stentless—generally have much less acoustic shadowing, and are therefore seen more readily both by TTE and TEE (Fig. 16.25a, b). The struts of a stented valve are echogenic and easily seen arching above the plane of the valve ring; however the thin valve leaflets should be seen contained within the valve (Fig. 16.25a). Stentless valves (homograft, xenograft, autograft) often have an echocardiographic appearance similar to that of native valve tissue (Fig. 16.25b). Biologic prosthetic valve motion and valve characteristics are generally seen very well by echocardiography. Unlike mechanical valves, these valves do not incorporate valve regurgitation as part of their design. However, very minor degrees of regurgitation

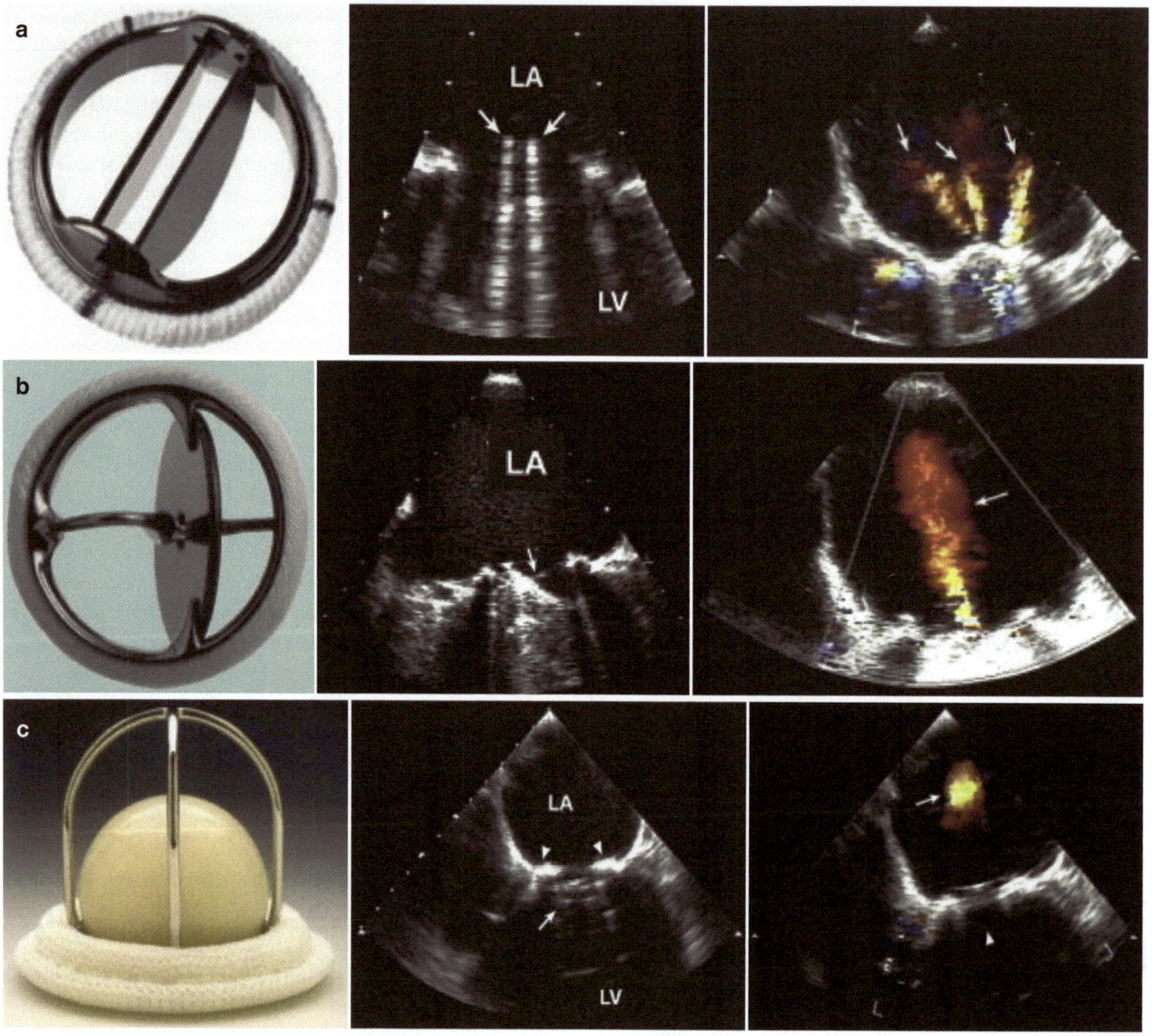

Fig. 16.20 Examples of bileaflet (St. Jude, **a**), single-leaflet (Medtronic-Hall, **b**), and caged-ball (Starr-Edwards, **c**) mechanical valves and their transesophageal echocardiographic characteristics taken in the mitral position in diastole (*middle*) and in systole (*right*). The *arrows* in diastole point to the occluder mechanism of the valve and in systole to the characteristic physiologic regurgitation observed with each valve. In Figure 16c, the *arrowheads* in the middle photograph indicate the valve sewing ring, and in the right photograph the caged ball occluding the valve. (Reprinted from: Zoghbi et al [107]; with permission from Elsevier)

are normally present in many patients [109]. Valve failure (stenosis and/or regurgitation) is readily seen and evaluated both by TTE and TEE, using imaging, color flow and spectral Doppler. Since TTE is adequate for most biologic valves, TEE is usually reserved for those patients in whom TTE imaging is suboptimal, in patients suspected of having endocarditis (see above), or in the intraoperative setting. One of the more useful aspects of the postoperative TEE study following prosthetic valve implantation (both biologic and mechanical) is to establish the flow profile across the new valve; this information (including velocities) can be used for subsequent comparisons.

Doppler Evaluation of Prosthetic Valves

For Doppler evaluation of prosthetic valves, the principles and techniques of valve interrogation and recording of flow velocity are similar to those used for evaluating native valve stenosis or regurgitation (see Chaps. 8 and 11) [113, 114]. However a few general comments are worth noting. Prosthetic valve regurgitation is primarily assessed with Doppler evaluation, mainly using color flow techniques, though spectral Doppler evaluation is helpful as well. It is important to differentiate between "normal" and pathologic prosthetic valve regurgitation. A mild degree of

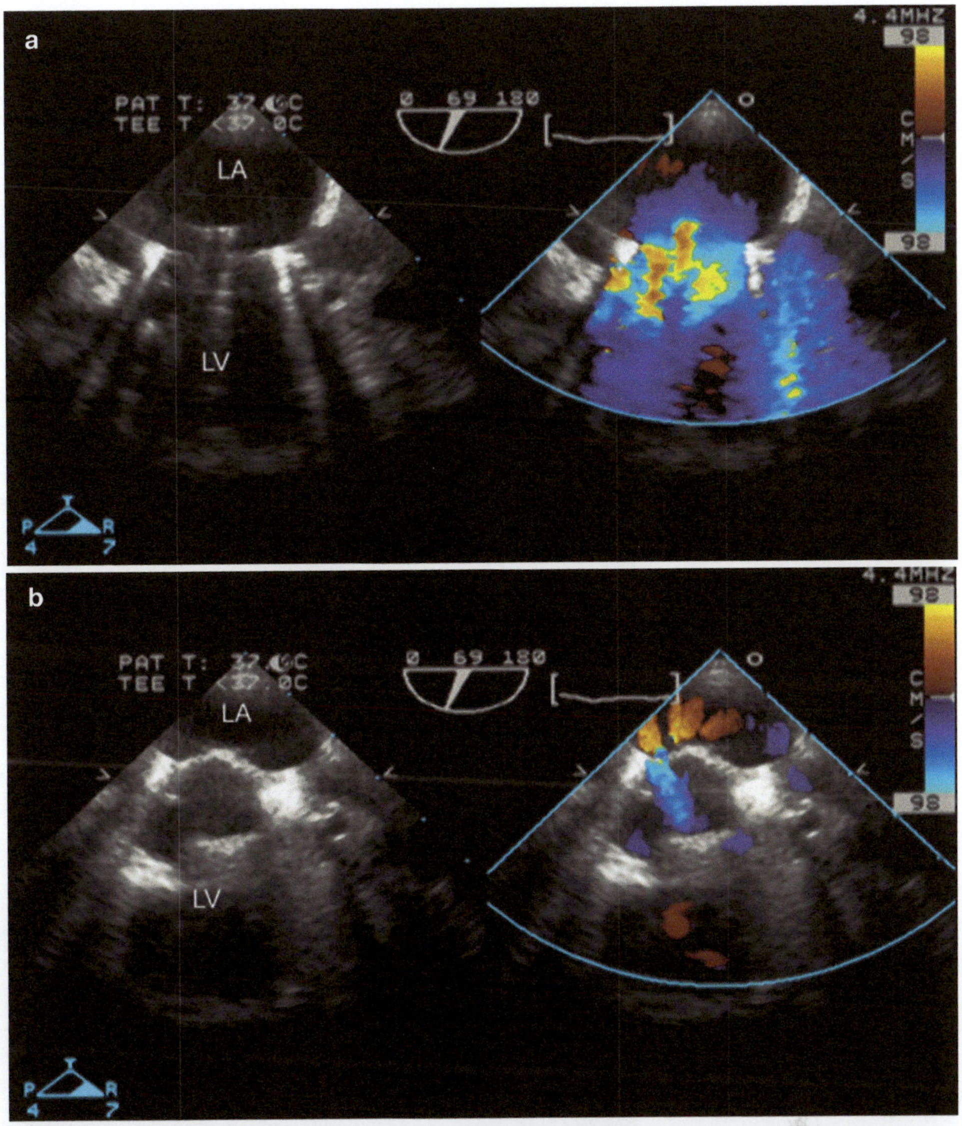

Fig. 16.21 Prosthetic mitral valve (St Jude bileaflet disk). Mid esophageal view mitral commissural view, multiplane angle 69°. The multiplane angle is rotated until both leaflets are profiled and open symmetrically in diastole (**a**) and systole (**b**). (**a**) There is the usual color flow Doppler profile across the valve (*see* text for details). (**b**) In systole, the "normal" pivot point washing jets are seen. *LA* left atrium, *LV* left ventricle

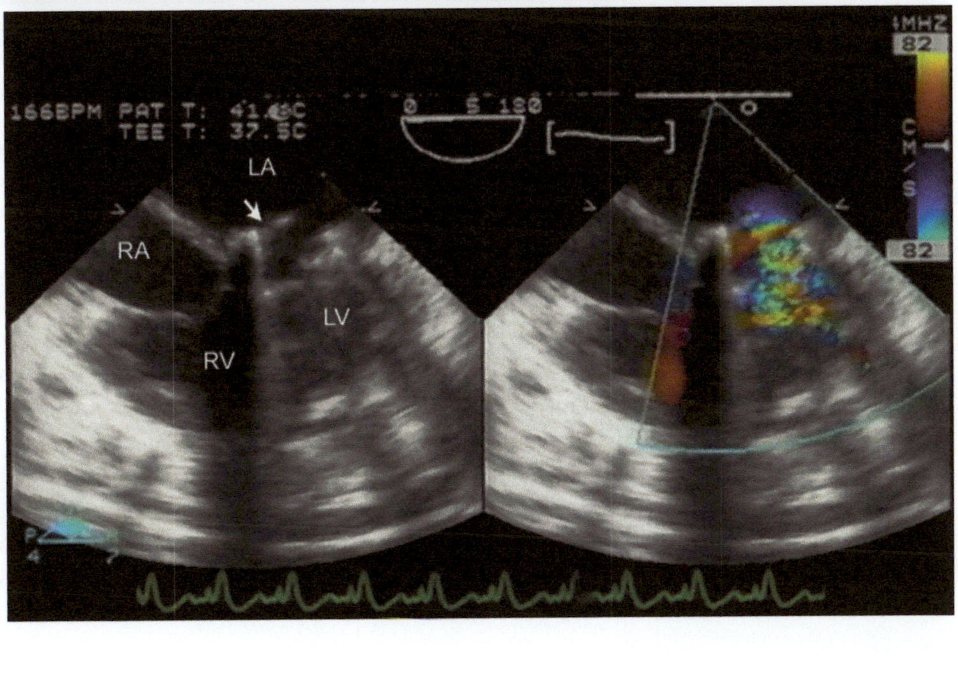

Fig. 16.22 Prosthetic mitral with a frozen leaflet (*arrow*), causing stenosis of the valve, seen as color flow Doppler aliasing in the right panel. Mid esophageal four chamber view, multiplane angle 0°. *LA* left atrium, *LV* left ventricle, *RA* right atrium, *RV* right ventricle

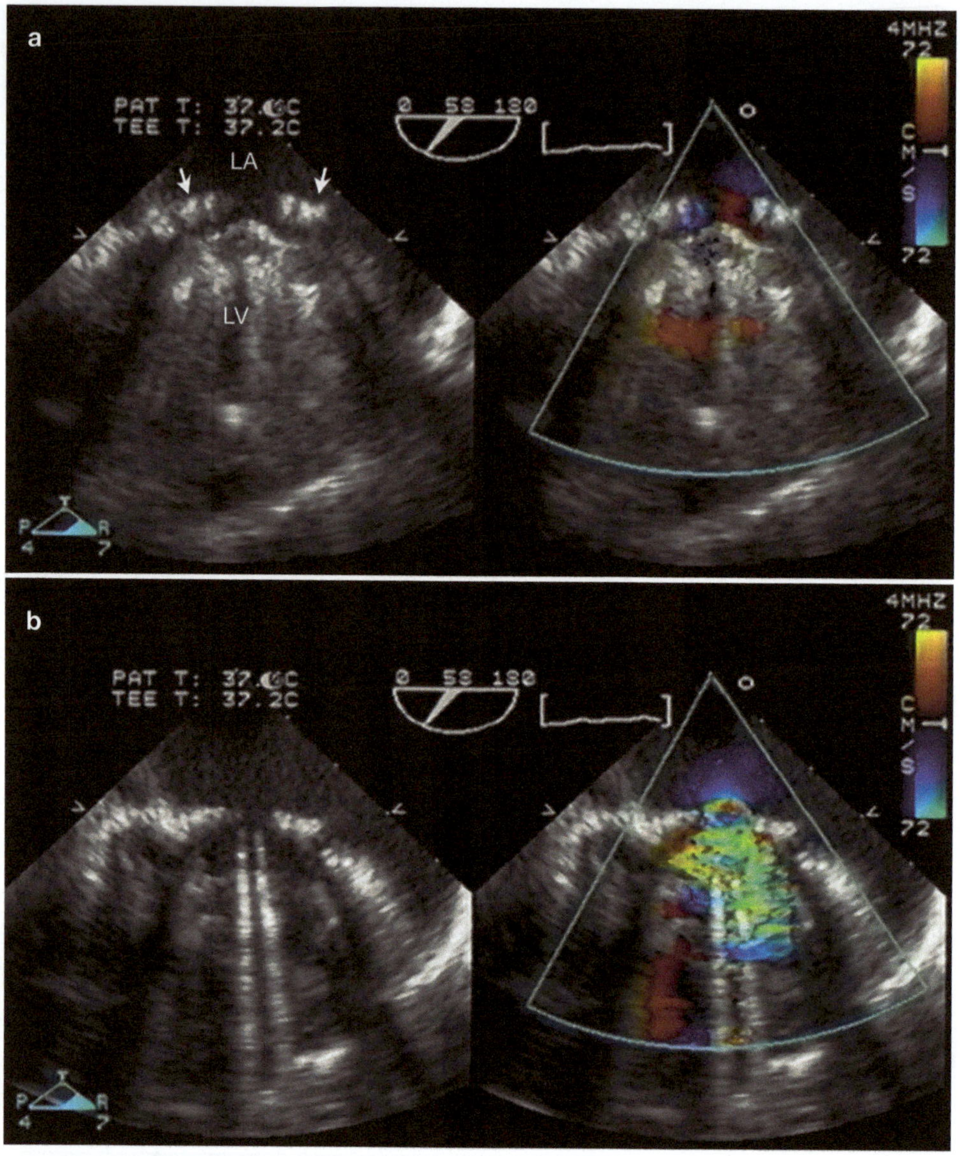

Fig. 16.23 Concentric pannus formation (*arrows*) above the mitral valve prosthesis (**a**), causing significant supravalvar narrowing, seen during diastole (**b**). In **b**, note the color flow Doppler aliasing that begins above the prosthetic valve, at the level of the pannus. Mid esophageal mitral commissural view, multiplane angle 58°. *LA* left atrium, *LV* left ventricle

regurgitation is normally seen in virtually all mechanical valves (Fig. 16.20); as noted above, this can be seen in the form of the "washing" jets seen with bileaflet valves (Fig. 16.21, Video 16.15). Minor regurgitant jets are also seen with biologic valves, including THVs. Pathologic regurgitation—characterized as one or more prominent areas of color flow Doppler regurgitation—can be either central or paravalvular (outside the valve sewing ring). Most pathologic central regurgitation is seen in biologic valves, but paravalvular regurgitation can occur with both biologic and mechanical valves. Paravalvular regurgitation is seen as jets outside the sewing ring of the prosthesis (Fig. 16.26, Video 16.19). The degree of regurgitation can be estimated using the methods for quantification of native valvular regurgitation [113], although these can be more challenging with the shadowing and reverberations caused by the prosthetic valves (particularly mechanical valves). Commonly used parameters for semilunar valves include color flow Doppler jet width, vena contracta, pressure half-time, and diastolic flow reversal in the distal great artery; for AV valves, parameters include vena contracta, color flow Doppler jet area, as well as reversal of flow in the pulmonary or systemic veins. A discussion of this evaluation is given in Chaps. 8 and 11. Regardless of valve type and position, when pathologic regurgitation is suspected, a careful evaluation must be made as to possible etiology. This includes location of the regurgitation (central vs. paravalvular), and possible mechanism of regurgitation (leaflet dysfunction, improper valve size/geometric mismatch, valve dehiscence, etc.).

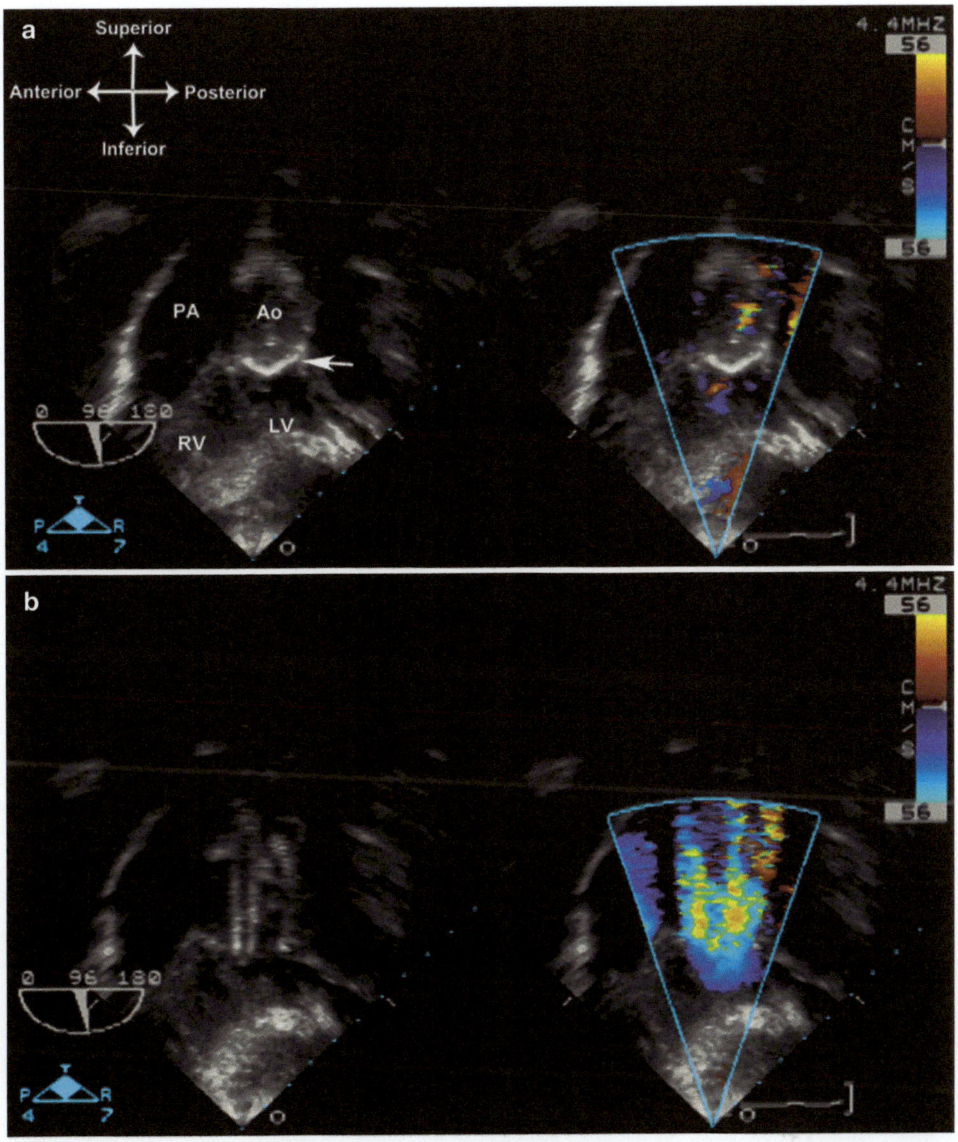

Fig. 16.24 Prosthetic aortic valve (bileaflet tilting disk) viewed from deep transgastric position, multiplane angle 96°. The multiplane angle has been rotated until both leaflets are profiled and symmetric leaflet motion is noted in diastole (**a**) and systole (**b**). The prosthetic valve position is marked by the *arrow*. This transducer position affords a good view of leaflet motion and flow across the valve, and also provides an excellent angle for spectral Doppler evaluation. *Ao* ascending aorta, *LV* left ventricle, *PA* pulmonary artery, *RV* right ventricle

When evaluating antegrade flow across prosthetic valves, it is important to remember that the flow characteristics and velocities across prosthetic valves (particularly mechanical valves) will often differ from comparably sized native valves. In general, the spectral Doppler velocities across these valves tend to be higher due to the phenomenon of pressure recovery [107]. As mentioned above, several studies have presented expected Doppler velocities, gradients and effective orifice area for a wide range of biologic and mechanical aortic and mitral valves [95, 107, 108]. Tables 16.7 and 16.8 show representative data abstracted from one of these studies [108] for several common prosthetic aortic and mitral valves. It should be noted that the labeled valve "size" (e.g. 21, 23 mm) represents the outer valve diameter in millimeters as given by the manufacturer. However this parameter should not be considered alone, because the flow characteristics and cross-sectional area between two identically sized valves might be completely different. Hence the effective orifice area (EOA) presented in these tables represents a better parameter for valve comparisons and overall prosthetic valve evaluation; it is an important parameter utilized in adult patients for clinical prosthetic valve assessment. The EOA is analogous to valve orifice area for a native valve, and is calculated in the same manner by the continuity equation (Chap. 1):

$$\mathbf{EOA = Stroke\ volume / VTI_{PrV}}$$

VTI_{PrV} = Velocity time integral (VTI) through the prosthesis, measured by continuous wave Doppler

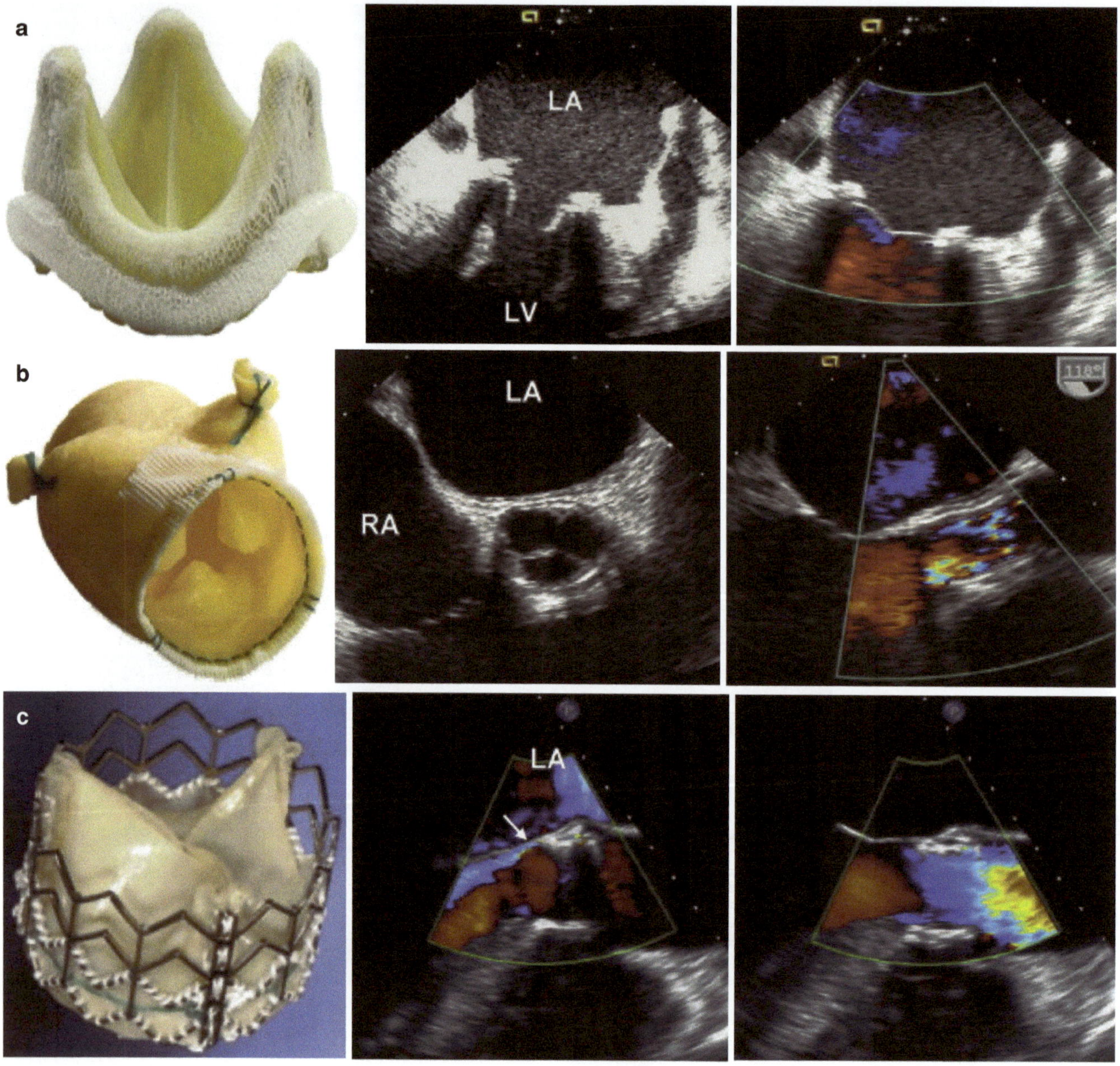

Fig. 16.25 Examples of stented (**a**), stentless (**b**), and percutaneous biologic valves (Edwards SAPIEN, **c**) and their echocardiographic features in diastole (*middle*) and in systole (*right*) as seen by TEE. The stentless valve is inserted by the root inclusion technique. Mild paravalvular aortic regurgitation in the percutaneous valve is shown by *arrow* (From: Zoghbi et al [107]; with permission from Elsevier)

Stroke volume = VTI of the left ventricular outflow tract (by pulsed wave Doppler) multiplied by the left ventricular outflow tract cross sectional area (with prosthetic mitral valves, this calculated stroke volume is valid assuming no significant aortic regurgitation exists).

The EOA is generally a better index of valve function than gradient alone, because it is will not vary with different flow states. An important concept for prosthetic valves is that the EOA must be appropriate for the flow requirements of the individual, otherwise *patient-prosthetic mismatch* (PPM) occurs. PPM is a term used to describe the clinical situation when the EOA of a prosthetic valve is too small in relation to a patient's body size, resulting in abnormally high postoperative gradients [95, 115]. Studies in adults have shown that aortic PPM is associated with worsening

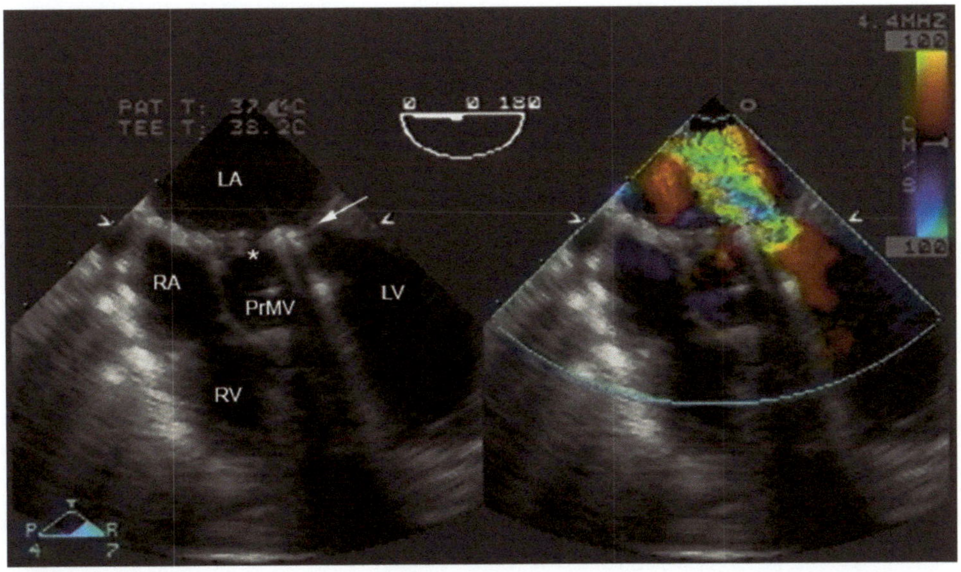

Fig. 16.26 Paravalvar regurgitation in a child who underwent mitral valve replacement with a mechanical bileaflet prosthesis (the patient previously underwent repair of an atrioventricular septal defect). This image was obtained from a mid esophageal four chamber view. The prosthesis was too large for the annulus and required insertion at an angle, which resulted both in a large area of paravalvular regurgitation (*arrow*) as well as a very small effective orifice (*asterisk*). *LA* left atrium, *LV* left ventricle, *PrMV* prosthetic mitral valve, *RA* right atrium, *RV* right ventricle

symptoms and impaired exercise capacity, as well as adverse cardiac events and long-term mortality [116–119]; mitral PPM is associated with persisting pulmonary hypertension and increased congestive heart failure as well as reduced survival [120]. When indexed to body surface area, the EOA is the only parameter found to be consistently related to postoperative gradients and/or adverse clinical outcomes [121–123]. Table 16.9 shows threshold values for indexed EOA generally used to identify and quantify the severity of PPM in adults [95].

As noted above, the information from Tables 16.7 and 16.8 are derived from studies in which data were compiled from a number of adult studies. The tables are voluminous and comprehensive, and the reader is referred to these for further reference regarding other prosthetic valves. Nonetheless, from these data, some simplified general guidelines can be formulated to assist in the assessment of possible prosthetic aortic and mitral valve stenosis, and these are summarized by Zoghbi et al [107] and presented in Table 16.10. These guidelines also utilize parameters such as Doppler velocity index (DVI) for prosthetic aortic valves, which is the ratio of velocities across the left ventricular outflow tract compared to the velocity across the prosthetic aortic valve, and the inverse relationship for mitral valves, the ratio of the prosthetic mitral valve VTI compared to the VTI across the left ventricular outflow tract. These dimensionless ratios—derived from the continuity equation—are much less dependent upon varying flow states. It should be noted that comparable data for prosthetic pulmonary and tricuspid valves is lacking, particularly regarding normal and abnormal EOAs and DVI/VTI. Therefore more general guidelines, also presented by Zoghbi et al, have been presented for these latter two valves as follows [107]:

- Findings suspicious for prosthetic pulmonary stenosis:
  - Cusp or leaflet thickening or immobility.
  - Narrowing of forward color map.
  - Peak velocity through the prosthesis >3 or >2 m/s through a homograft (suspicious but not diagnostic of stenosis).
  - Increase in peak velocity on serial studies (more reliable parameter).
  - Impaired right ventricular function or elevated right ventricular systolic pressure.
- Findings suspicious for tricuspid valve stenosis
  - Peak velocity >1.7 m/s (because of respiratory variation, average ≥5 cycles).
  - Mean gradient ≥6 mmHg (may be increased if there is valvular regurgitation).
  - Pressure half-time ≥230 ms.
  - Narrow inflow color map.
  - Nonspecific signs such as enlarged right atrium and engorged inferior vena cava.

In general, an integrated approach, using a combination of the criteria discussed above, works best when evaluating forward flow across any prosthetic valve.

For pediatric patients, there is a notable paucity of available published information regarding normal velocities and EOAs across prosthetic valves, particularly the smaller mitral and aortic valves. Much of the information used in the pediatric population originates from adult data. Fortunately many of the same principles can still be applied, though comparable values to those obtained in adults are still lacking, and it is unclear whether certain parameters are equivalent in this group of patients. For example, one study evaluating St. Jude and Carbomedics mitral prostheses in children found that peak early Doppler velocity—not EOA—correlated best with the manufacturer's geometric valve orifice area, and also pulmonary artery wedge pressure [124]. The use of the DVI and VTI ratios has not been established in the pediatric population. Also, PPM has not been evaluated closely in children, though it would seem evident that

Table 16.7 Doppler parameters across prosthetic aortic valves

Valve	Size (mm)	Peak gradient (mmHg)	Mean gradient (mmHg)	Peak velocity (m/s)	Effective orifice area (cm^2)
Stented biologic					
Hancock II (porcine)	21	20±0.4	14.8±4.1		1.23±0.3
	23	24.7±5.7	16.6±6.9		1.39±0.2
	25	20±2	10.7±3		1.47±0.2
	27	14±3			1.55±0.2
	29	15±3			1.6±0.2
Mosaic (porcine)	21		12.4±7.3		1.6±0.7
	23		12.5±7.4		2.1±0.8
	25		10.1±5.1		2.1±1.6
	27		9.0		1.8±0.4
	29		9.0		2.0±0.4
Carpentier-Edwards (pericardial)	19	32.1±3.4	24.2±8.6	2.8±0.1	
	21	25.7±9.9	20.3±9.1	2.6±0.4	1.2±0.3
	23	21.7±8.6	13.0±5.3	2.3±0.5	1.5±0.4
	25	16.5±5.4	9.0±2.3	2.0±0.3	1.8±0.3
	27	19.2±0	5.6	1.6	2.1±0.4
	29	17.6±0	11.6	2.1	2.2±0.4
Mitroflow (pericardial)	19	18.7±5.1	10.3±3		1.1±0.1
	21	20.2	15.4	2.3	1.3±0.1
	23	14.0±4.9	7.6±3.4	1.9±0.3	1.5±0.2
	25	17±11.3	10.8±6.5	2±0.7	1.8±0.2
	27	13±3	6.6±1.7	1.8±0.2	
Stentless biologic					
Medtronic Freestyle	19		13.0		
	21		8±2.6		1.6±0.3
	23		7.2±2.5		1.9±0.5
	25		5.4±1.5		2.0±0.4
	27		4.7±1.6		2.5±0.5
St. Jude Toronto SPV	21	18.6±11.8	7.6±4.4		1.2±0.7
	23	13.6±7.3	7.1±4.3		1.6±0.8
	25	12.2±5.8	6.2±3.1		1.6±0.4
	27	10±4.6	4.8±2.3		2±0.4
	29	7.9±4.2	3.9±2.2		2.4±0.7
Mechanical					
Medtronic-Hall	20	34.4±13.1	17.1±5.3	2.9±0.4	1.21±0.45
	21	26.9±10.5	14.1±5.9	2.4±0.4	1.08±0.17
	23	26.9±8.9	13.5±4.8	2.4±0.6	1.36±0.39
	25	17.1±7.0	9.5±4.3	2.3±0.5	1.9±0.47
	27	18.7±9.7	8.7±5.6	2.1±0.5	1.9±0.16
	29			1.6	
Carbomedics (bileaflet)	17	33.4±13.2	20.1±7.1	—	1.02±0.2
	19	33.3±11.2	11.6±5.1	3.1±0.4	1.25±0.4
	21	26.3±10.3	12.7±4.3	2.6±0.5	1.42±0.4
	23	24.6±6.9	11.3±3.8	2.4±0.4	1.69±0.3
	25	20.3±8.7	9.3±4.7	2.3±0.3	2.04±0.4
	27	19.1±7.0	8.4±2.8	2.2±0.4	2.55±0.3
	29	12.5±4.7	5.8±3.2	1.9±0.3	2.63±0.4

Table 16.7 (continued)

Valve	Size (mm)	Peak gradient (mmHg)	Mean gradient (mmHg)	Peak velocity (m/s)	Effective orifice area (cm²)
St. Jude (bileaflet)	19	35.2±11.2	19±6.2	2.9±0.5	1.01±0.2
	21	28.3±9.9	15.8±5.7	2.6±0.5	1.33±0.3
	23	25.3±7.9	13.8±5.3	2.6±0.4	1.6±0.4
	25	22.6±7.7	12.7±5.1	2.4±0.5	1.93±0.45
	27	19.9±7.6	11.2±4.8	2.2±0.4	2.35±0.6
	29	17.7±6.4	9.9±2.9	2±0.1	2.81±0.6
	31	16.0	10±6	2.1±0.6	3.08±1.1
On-X (bileaflet)	19	21.3±10.8	11.8±3.4	—	1.5±0.2
	21	16.4±5.9	9.9±3.6	—	1.7±0.4
	23	15.9±6.4	8.5±3.3	—	2.0±0.6
	25	16.5±10.2	9±5.3	—	2.4±0.8
	27–29	11.4±4.6	5.6±2.7	—	3.2±0.6
Starr-Edwards (Ball and Cage)	21	29			1.0
	23	32.6±12.8	22±8.8	4±0	
	24	34.1±10.3	22±7.5	3.5±0.5	1.1
	26	31.8±9.0	19.7±6.1	3.4±0.5	
	27	30.8±6.3	18.5±3.7	3.2±0.4	1.8
	29	29±9.3	16.3±5.5		

Table abstracted from Rosenhek et al [108]; with permission from Elsevier

Table 16.8 Doppler parameters across prosthetic mitral valves

Valve	Size (mm)	Peak gradient (mmHg)	Mean gradient (mmHg)	Peak velocity (m/s)	Pressure half-time (ms)	Effective orifice area (cm²)
Stented biologic						
Hancock II (porcine)	27					2.2±0.14
	29					2.8±0.11
	31					2.8±0.1
	33					3.2±0.2
Carpentier-Edwards (pericardial)	27		3.6	1.6		
	29		5.3 ±3.4	1.7±0.3		
	31		4±0.8	1.5±0.1		
	33		1.0	0.8		
Mitroflow (pericardial)	25		6.9	2.0	90	
	27		3.1±0.9	2.5	90±20	
	29		3.5±1.7	1.4±0.3	102±21	
	31		3.9±0.8	1.3±0.3	91±22	
Mechanical						
Carbomedics (bileaflet)	23			1.9±0.1	126±7	
	25	10.3±2.3	3.6±0.6	1.3±0.1	93±8	2.9±0.8
	27	8.8±3.5	3.5±1.0	1.6±0.3	89±20	2.9±0.8
	29	8.8±2.9	3.4±1.0	1.5±0.3	88±17	2.3±0.4
	31	8.9±2.3	3.3±0.9	1.6±0.3	92±24	2.8±1.1
	33	8.8±2.2	4.8±2.5	1.5±0.2	93±12	
St Jude (bileaflet)	23		4	1.5	160	1.0
	25		2.5±1	1.3±1.2	75±4	1.4±0.2
	27	11±4	5±1.8	1.6±0.3	75±10	1.7±0.2
	29	10±3	4.2±1.8	1.6±0.3	85±10	1.8±0.2
	31	12±6	4.5±2.2	1.6±0.3	74±13	2.0±0.3

(continued)

Table 16.8 (continued)

Valve	Size (mm)	Peak gradient (mmHg)	Mean gradient (mmHg)	Peak velocity (m/s)	Pressure half-time (ms)	Effective orifice area (cm^2)
On-X (bileaflet)	25	11.5±3.2	5.3±2.1			1.9±1.1
	27–29	10.3±4.5	4.5±1.6			2.2±0.5
	31–33	9.8±3.8	4.8±2.4			2.5±1.1
Starr-Edwards (Ball and Cage)	26		10			
	28		7±2.8			
	30	12.2±4.6	7±2.5	1.7±0.3	125±25	1.7±0.4
	32	11.5±4.2	5.1±2.5	1.7±0.3	110±25	2±0.4
	34		5			

Table abstracted from Rosenhek et al [108]; with permission from Elsevier.

this particular parameter has direct relevance in the pediatric population because of growth considerations. While the goal for valve replacement in children is to implant the largest possible prosthesis, patient growth will inevitably lead to some degree of PPM, even with a normally functioning prosthesis [107]. As noted above, the most widely accepted and validated parameter for identifying PPM in adult patients is the indexed EOA, and Table 16.9 shows threshold values for indexed EOA generally used to identify and quantify the severity of PPM in adults [95]. This table might also serve as useful guide in children, although the applicability of these values in pediatrics has yet to be fully determined.

Table 16.9 Threshold values of indexed prosthetic valve effective orifice area (EOA) for the identification and quantification of prosthesis-patient mismatch

	Mild or not clinically significant (cm^2/m^2)	Moderate (cm^2/m^2)	Severe (cm^2/m^2)
Aortic position	>0.85 (0.8–0.9)	≤0.85 (0.8–0.9)	≤0.65 (0.6–0.7)
Mitral position	>1.2 (1.2–1.3)	≤1.2 (1.2–1.3)	≤0.9 (0.9)

From Pibarot and Dumesnil [95]; with permission of Walters-Kluwer
Numbers in parentheses represent the range of threshold values that have been used in the literature

TEE Evaluation of Transcatheter Heart Valve Implantation

For catheter-based implantable heart valves, the role of TEE will vary based upon the type of THV and its position. With TAVR/TAVI (both SAPIEN and CoreValve), TEE plays an integral role in all three phases of the procedure: pre-procedural assessment of morphology and annular measurements, intraprocedural monitoring of all phases of the valve implantation (including guide wire and device positioning and valve deployment), and post-deployment assessment of possible paravalvular device leaks as well as ventricular function, mitral valve assessment, pericardial effusion, and aortic dissection [125, 126]. It is not uncommon to see some paravalvular regurgitation following valve implantation, particularly after TAVR/TAVI. An example of TEE monitoring during TAVR/TAVI (SAPIEN valve) is shown in Fig. 16.19, Video 16.20 (also in Chap. 11). For the Melody valve, TEE is generally not performed during valve implantation, though transthoracic imaging is routinely obtained after the procedure to assess valve function and competence. For valve-in-valve implantation, the role of TEE will vary depending upon the fluoroscopic visibility of the biologic valve. In most cases, when a stented bioprosthesis is readily visible on fluoroscopy, TEE might not be necessary. However in those cases in which the bioprostheses is not readily visible, or assessment of valve function is required, TEE can be very helpful [102].

Evaluation of Heart Transplantation/Ventricular Assist Devices

Management of heart transplant recipients requires ongoing cardiac assessment for rejection and cardiac function, and this necessitates both noninvasive and invasive surveillance using echocardiography and cardiac catheterization/myocardial biopsy. The bulk of noninvasive surveillance is provided primarily by TTE; the use of TEE for heart transplantation is generally confined to the immediate pre-transplant and post-transplant period. The specific applications for TEE in the setting of heart transplantation include the following:

- *Screening of cardiac transplant donors.* Echocardiography is an essential part of the evaluation of any prospective cardiac transplant donor. Cardiac function and segmental wall motion must be assessed, and any potential intracardiac abnormalities (congenital heart disease, valvar abnormalities) must be identified [127]. Most prospective donors are mechanically ventilated, which can lead to poor TTE imaging, particularly in older patients. Indeed, one study in adults showed technically inadequate TTE images in up to 29 % of mechanically ventilated brain-dead potential donors [128]. Thus when TTE assessment is inadequate, TEE evaluation must be performed.
- *Evaluation of ventricular assist device implantation.* The term ventricular assist device (VAD) refers to a broad range of mechanical circulatory devices designed to

Table 16.10 Doppler parameters across prosthetic aortic and mitral valves

Parameter	Normal	Possible stenosis	Suggests significant stenosis
Aortic mechanical, stented valves			
Peak velocity (m/s)	<3	3–4	>4
Mean gradient (mmHg)	<20	20–35	>35
DVI	≥0.30	0.29–0.25	<0.25
Effective Orifice Area (cm²)	>1.2	1.2–0.8	<0.8
Contour of jet velocity through prosthetic aortic valve	Triangular, early peaking	Triangular to intermediate	Rounded, symmetrical contour
Acceleration time (ms)	<80	80–100	>00
Other pertinent findings: left ventricular size, function, hypertrophy			
Mitral valve prostheses			
Peak velocity (m/s)	<1.9	1.9	≥2.5
Mean gradient (mmHg)	≤5	6–10	>10
VTI (PrMV)/VTI (LVOT)	<2.2	2.2–25.	>2.5
Effective Orifice Area (cm²)	≥2.0	1–2	<1
Pressure half-time (ms)	<130	130–200	>200
Other pertinent findings: left ventricular size and function, left atrial size, right ventricular size and function, estimation of pulmonary artery pressure			

From: Zoghbi et al [107]; with permission from Elsevier
DVI Doppler velocity index, equal to Velocity (Left ventricular outflow tract)/Velocity (Prosthetic aortic valve), *VTI* Velocity time integral, *PrMV* Prosthetic mitral valve, *LVOT* Left ventricular outflow tract

unload the failing heart, while at the same time provide adequate systemic (and in some cases pulmonary) perfusion [129]. These VADs are increasingly being utilized for patients with myocardial dysfunction, generally as a "bridge" to cardiac transplantation. Assist devices can be univentricular or biventricular, and there are two major types: pulsatile and continuous pumps. A number of VADs are currently available, and a full discussion of all these devices is beyond the scope of this chapter. Most of these devices are designed for the adult population; only a small number are available specifically for use in the pediatric population [130, 131], the most well-known being the Berlin Heart (EXCOR®), which will be the example used for the following discussion. The Berlin Heart is a paracorporeal pulsatile VAD that is connected to a pneumatically driven external pump to provide pulsatile flow into the aorta. For left sided assist, an inlet cannula is placed in the apex of the left ventricle (or rarely, the left atrium) (Fig. 16.27). Blood flows through this cannula to an extracorporeal pump. A pneumatic force from a separate driving unit is used to compress a membrane in the pump, expelling the blood into the systemic circulation through a separate arterial cannula connected to the ascending aorta, representing the device outflow [132]. The extracorporeal blood pump is available in a variety of volume sizes between 10–80 ml (Fig. 16.27), enabling use for the entire pediatric age range, including neonates [129] For right ventricular assist, a similar procedure is performed with the receiving cannula in the right atrium, and the arterial cannula in the pulmonary artery. A recent prospective multicenter study showed a clear survival advantage of the Berlin Heart (left or biventricular VAD) vs. extracorporeal membrane oxygenation as a bridge to heart transplantation [133].

For left sided VAD placement, intraoperative TEE serves several important roles. It is utilized to exclude important cardiac defects that could cause an intracardiac right to left shunt (e.g. patent foramen ovale) or compromise physiology after device placement (e.g. significant aortic regurgitation or mitral stenosis) [134]. In addition, TEE is used to evaluate the sites of device implantation within the heart, specifically the inflow connection to the atrium or ventricle, and the outflow connection to the aorta. Right and left ventricular size and function can also be assessed before and after device placement [135, 136]. Color flow and spectral Doppler are used to evaluate the flow characteristics into and out from the device. Thrombus in the cardiac chambers or attached to the inflow/outflow cannulae (if present) can also be evaluated. Monitoring for intracardiac air and appropriate de-airing also represent important applications of TEE in this setting. The type of cardiac connections, as well as the expected flow characteristics of a device, will vary by manufacturer, and these should be determined prior to performing the TEE [134]. An example of TEE evaluation of a Berlin Heart left sided VAD implantation is shown in Fig. 16.28, Video 16.21.

Following VAD implantation, echocardiography should be used for ongoing evaluation and monitoring while the patient is on support. Transthoracic echocar-

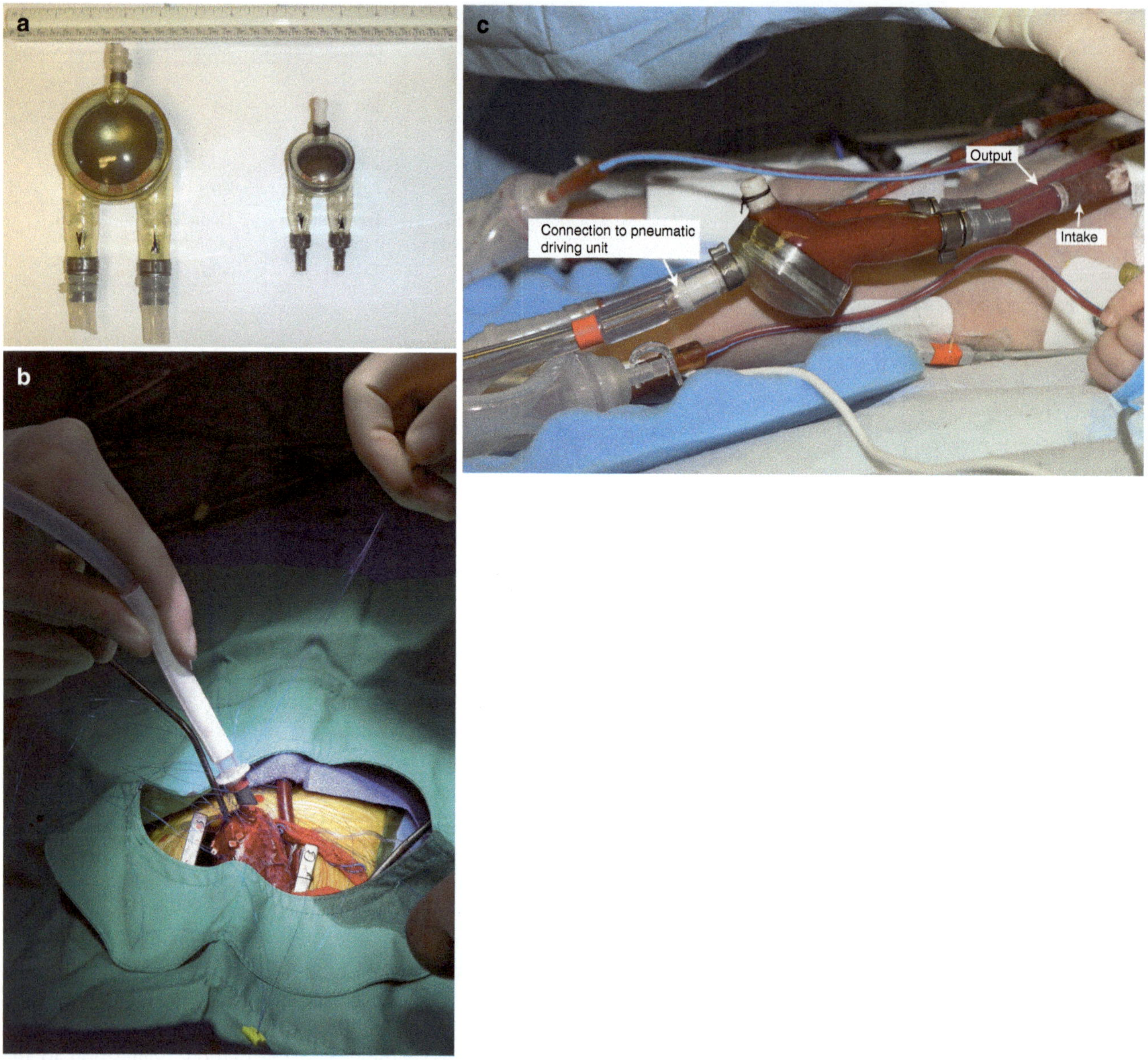

Fig. 16.27 Pictures of Berlin Heart. Figure **a** shows a pump for an older child (60 ml) on the *left*, next to an infant pump (10 ml) on the *right*. Figure **b** shows the intake cannula being implanted in the left ventricular apex. Figure **c** shows a pediatric pump that has been implanted. The intake and output cannulas enter the patient's thorax, as shown by the two tubes. The other tube is connected to the external pneumatic driving unit

diography generally suffices for these purposes, but TEE can also be used in selected patients in whom precordial echocardiographic windows are suboptimal or nonexistent. Ongoing evaluation should involve assessment of cannula position, and chamber size/function, as well as surveillance for possible valvular abnormalities, pericardial effusion/hematoma, intracardiac thrombus, endocarditis, and aortic dissection [137].

Note: The reader should be aware that an increasing number of new VAD designs are undergoing development for both adult and pediatric patients, so the variety of devices available for pediatric patients (pulsatile and continuous) is likely to widen considerably in the near future [138, 139]. The National Heart, Lung and Blood Institute (NHLBI) has been very active in this endeavor; in 2004 they initiated a 5 year program to develop a family of pediatric circulatory support devices [140]. Based on the results and progress made from this program, in 2010 the NHLBI created another support program—known as Pumps for Kids, Infants and Neonates (**PumpKIN**)—in which awards were granted to selected contractors (several of whom participated in the previous program) enabling them to begin the work necessary to receive Investigational Device Exemptions from the Food and Drug Administration for pediatric circulatory support devices. These devices will soon be ready for clinical trials [140, 141].

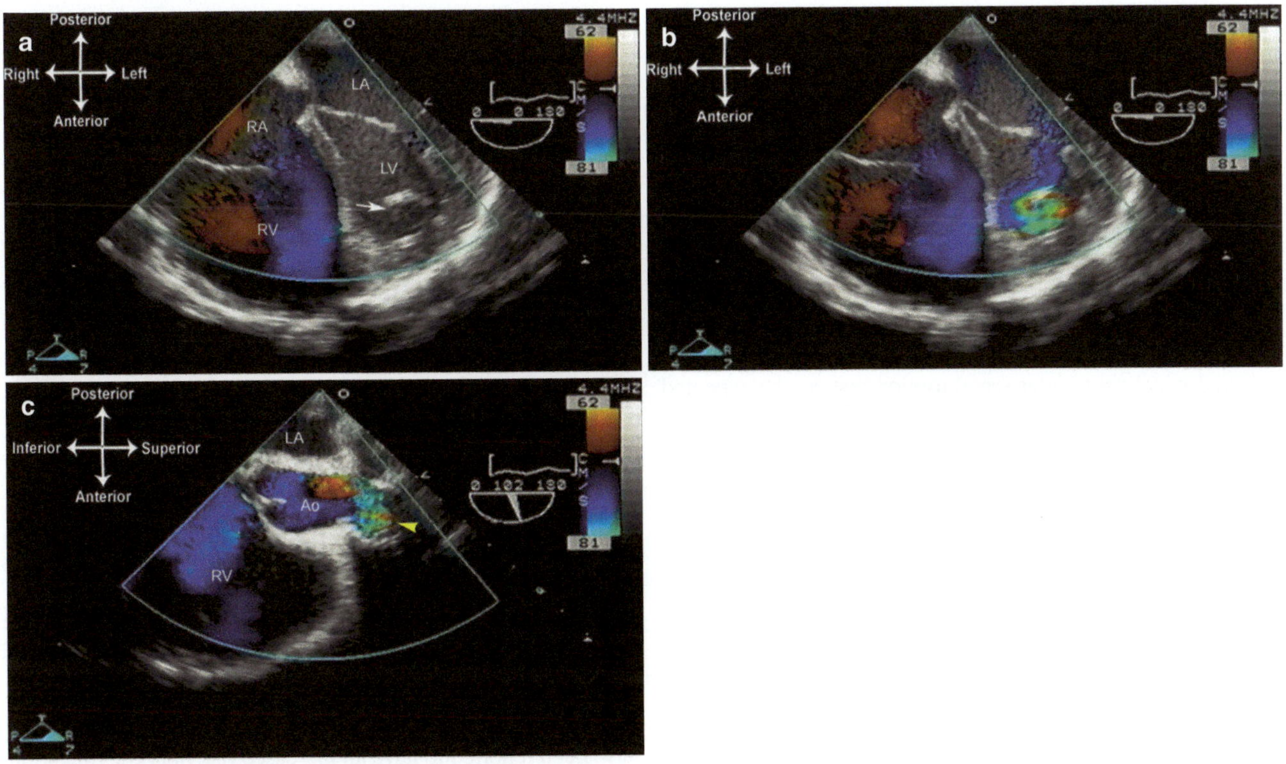

Fig. 16.28 Berlin Heart placement in a patient with dilated cardiomyopathy. Mid esophageal four chamber view, multiplane angle 0° (**a**, **b**) and 100° (**c**). The cannula (*arrow*) in the left ventricular apex withdraws blood returning from the left atrium. (**a**, **b**) When the blood has sufficiently filled the chamber in the device, it is pumped into the ascending aorta (*yellow arrowhead*), as shown from mid esophageal aortic valve long axis view, multiplane angle 102° (**c**). *Ao* aorta, *LA* left atrium, *LV* left ventricle, *RA* right atrium, *RV* right ventricle

- *Intraoperative monitoring/assessment of transplantation.* A preoperative TEE assessment during heart transplantation, if performed, is generally of limited utility. Since the recipient heart will be removed and replaced, most intracardiac anatomic and functional information regarding the recipient's native heart is irrelevant. However there could be some elements that have bearing upon the operative and postoperative course, particularly in patients with CHD. Specifically, abnormalities of cardiac position, systemic and pulmonary venous connections, and aortic/pulmonary artery anomalies (e.g. pulmonary atresia) need to be verified, as they could affect how an anatomically "normal" donor heart is implanted. Extra systemic venous or great artery length might need to be harvested for congenitally abnormal hearts. Additional useful information includes estimation of pulmonary arterial pressure (by tricuspid regurgitant jet velocity, if available).
- *Postoperative assessment of heart transplantation* requires an understanding of the current surgical technique, which enables the examiner to assess and recognize possible complications. Typically, the heart transplant procedure involves a systemic venous bicaval anastomosis (donor SVC/IVC to the recipient SVC/IVC), anastomosis of a recipient left atrial cuff to a cuff fashioned from the donor left atrium, and main pulmonary artery/aortic anastomoses between donor and recipient great arteries. The composite left atrial anastomosis gives the post-transplant left atrium a dilated and "hourglass" appearance with a prominent ridge that could be confused for thrombus [142] (Fig. 16.29, Video 16.22). The postoperative TEE assessment of heart transplantation is comprehensive, evaluating a number of different factors: any residual congenital cardiac defect (e.g. patent foramen ovale), possible retained intracardiac

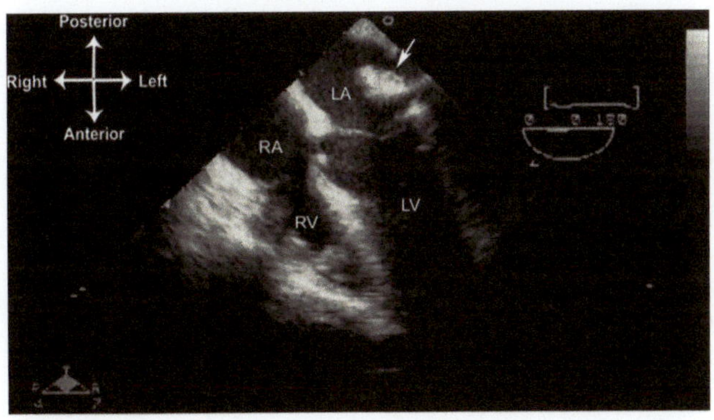

Fig. 16.29 Following heart transplantation, imaging in the mid esophageal four chamber view, multiplane angle 0°. The anastomosis of the donor left atrium to the cuff of the recipient left atrium creates an area of echogenicity (*arrow*) that can be mistaken for thrombus. *LA* left atrium, *LV* left ventricle, *RA* right atrium, *RV* right ventricle

air, intracardiac thrombus, right and left ventricular systolic function, AV and semilunar valve function, estimation of pulmonary artery pressure, and the patency of the donor-recipient anastomoses—aortic, pulmonary arterial, systemic and pulmonary veins [142, 143]. These assessments are particularly important when cardiac transplantation is performed in a patient with a complex form of CHD, e.g. dextrocardia or heterotaxy, and the possibility exists of kinking or torsion of these anastomoses [144]. Immediately following heart transplantation, overall biventricular systolic function is usually normal, although there can be paradoxical ventricular septal motion that can be expected to resolve with time. Also, right ventricular function can be affected if pulmonary vascular resistance is elevated [145].

- *Assessment of post-transplant cardiac allograft function in the intensive care unit.* Assessment of the transplanted heart essentially mirrors that of the postoperative TEE study discussed above. Other potential indications for TEE evaluation include surveillance for sources of systemic emboli, and also evaluation of possible pericardial effusion. Again, since TTE is usually sufficient, TEE is reserved for those patients with poor transthoracic acoustic images and/or when an open sternum prevents effective transthoracic imaging.

Evaluation of Lung Transplantation

In lung transplantation, cadaveric or living donor lungs are transplanted into a recipient with end-stage pulmonary or pulmonary vascular disease. For each lung (or lobe) transplanted, the donor mainstem (or lobar) bronchus, branch pulmonary artery, and pulmonary venous cuff are anastomosed to the corresponding structures in the recipient [146]. There are specific applications of TEE for lung transplant patients [147]. The preoperative TEE study is used to evaluate cardiac anatomy and exclude any potential intracardiac defects, e.g. small atrial septal defect, which should be addressed at the time of transplantation. Right and left heart function should also be assessed, because impaired cardiac function can have significant impact on the post-transplant outcome. The postoperative TEE study is used to assess the pulmonary arterial and venous anastomoses, as well as cardiac function and AV and semilunar valve function [148]. If tricuspid or pulmonary regurgitant jets are present, they can be used to estimate pulmonary arterial pressure. The evaluation of pulmonary venous return is one of the most important applications of TEE for post-lung transplant assessment. Because of its proximity to the left atrium and pulmonary veins, TEE provides superior imaging for pulmonary venous imaging and color flow/spectral Doppler evaluation (Chap. 4). Stenosis, kinking, or thrombosis of the pulmonary venous anastomosis—a very serious complication of lung transplantation—is readily detectable by TEE (Fig. 16.30, Video 16.23). In contrast, TTE imaging and color flow Doppler display of the pulmonary venous anastomoses is often inadequate, particularly in the immediate post-transplant period. Hence TEE evaluation should be strongly considered whenever there is a possibility of pulmonary venous obstruction in the lung transplant patient [149, 150].

Evaluation of Aortic Dissection

Aortic dissection is characterized by a separation in the ascending aortic wall between intima and media, resulting in a large intimal flap that separates a false from a true lumen in the ascending or descending aorta (or both). It is seen much more commonly in the adult age group (higher incidence of males than females, with a ratio between 2:1 to 5:1), with the most frequently associated condition being hypertension in approximately 80–90 % of patients [151, 152]. However, congenital abnormalities of aortic wall—notably Marfan syndrome, Loeys-Dietz syndrome, vascular Ehlers-Danlos, and other connective tissue abnormalities—are also associated with aortic dissection [153]. Recently, patients with Turner syndrome have also been reported to have an increased risk of aortic dilatation and aortic dissection [154]. Other congenital abnormalities that might predispose to an "aortopathy" and aortic dissection include bicuspid aortic valve, aortic coarctation, and iatrogenic causes such as cannula insertion or balloon dilation of coarctation [155]. The etiology is thought to be due to rupture of *vasa vasorum* but increased shear forces, and abnormalities of aortic media, can also result in intimal tears that ultimately lead to dissection. Left undiagnosed, aortic dissection can be a dangerous and potentially catastrophic condition, with complications including rupture, pericardial tamponade, aortic regurgitation, and coronary artery ischemia [152, 156].

Aortic dissection is commonly classified using either the Stanford or DeBakey classifications, both of which are based upon the location of the dissection. Stanford A involves the ascending aorta; Stanford B involves the descending aorta [157]. DeBakey I involves ascending and descending aorta, as well as the aortic arch; DeBakey II involves only the ascending aorta; DeBakey III involves only the descending aorta [158]. Typically, ascending aortic dissections (Stanford A, DeBakey II) carry much higher risk for complications compared to descending aortic dissections [152].

While other imaging modalities such as cardiac magnetic resonance imaging and computed tomography have assumed a primary role in the diagnosis of this condition, TEE provides an excellent imaging alternative, offering great sensitivity and specificity because of its superior spatial and temporal resolution [153, 159, 160]. Moreover, because of its portability and availability, TEE (when performed jointly with TTE imaging) is expeditious and can serve as rapid means to secure a diagnosis, particularly in an unstable patient. The advantage of TEE over static

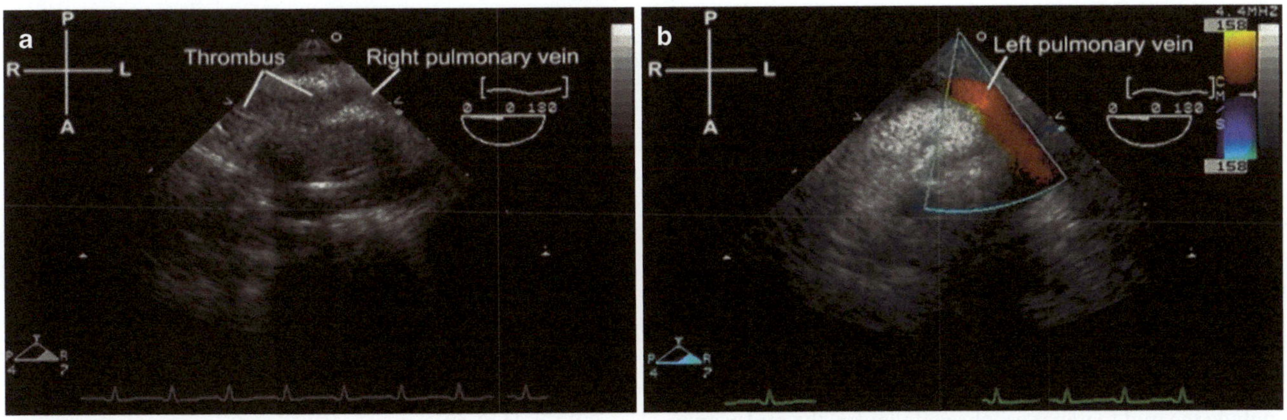

Fig. 16.30 Post-lung transplant, with thrombosis of the right pulmonary veins due to external compression by a large lymph node. Mid esophageal view, multiplane angle 0°. Figure **a** shows extensive thrombus in the right pulmonary veins. No flow was seen in the vessel by color flow Doppler. Figure **b** shows normal flow in the contralateral left pulmonary veins

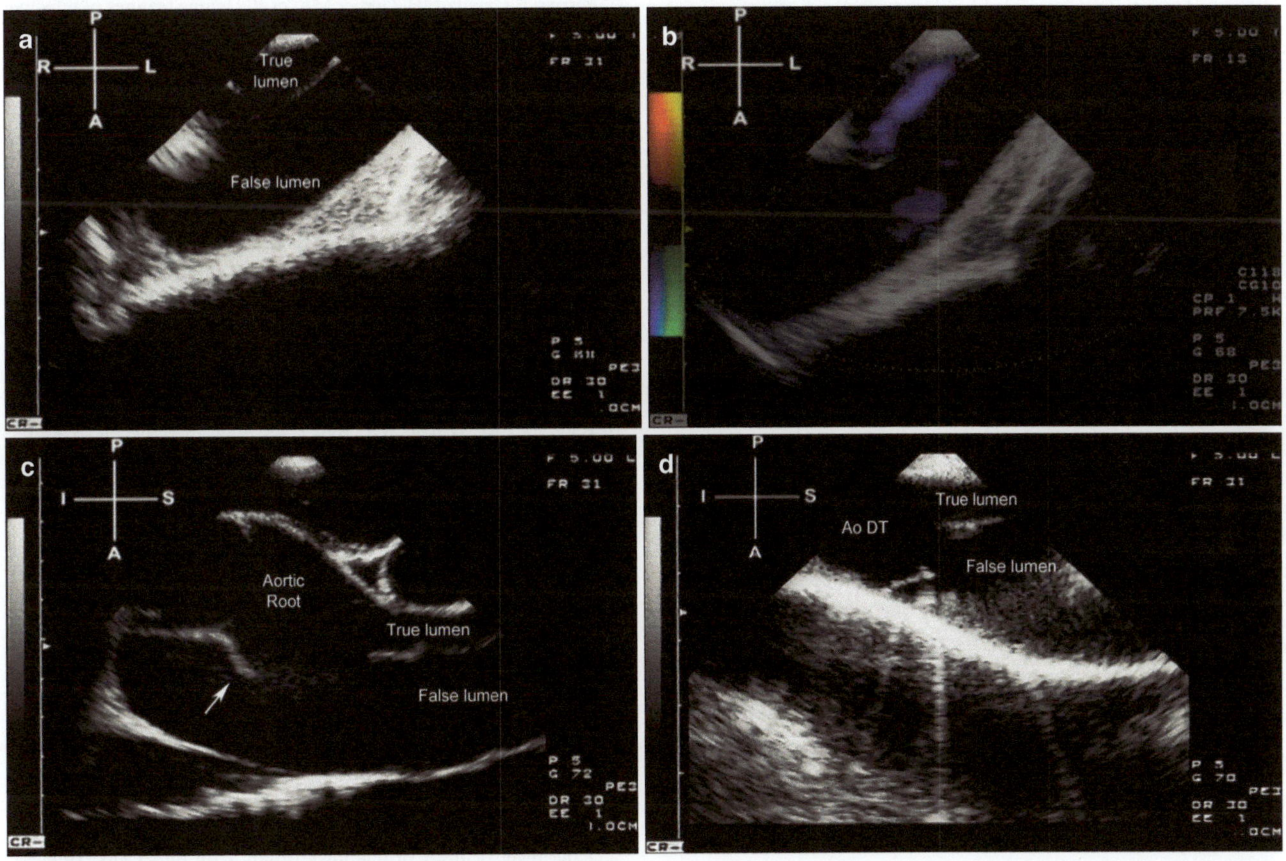

Fig. 16.31 Dissection of the ascending and descending aorta (DeBakey Type I) in a patient with Marfan syndrome. The patient also had a dilated aortic root and significant aortic valve regurgitation. (**a**) Upper esophageal aortic arch long axis view, multiplane angle 0°, shows true and false lumens. The false lumen is much larger than the true lumen in the ascending aorta and aortic arch. (**b**) Retrograde diastolic flow reversal is seen only in the true lumen by color flow mapping. (**c**) Mid esophageal aortic valve long axis view, multiplane angle 90°, shows the intimal flap (*arrow*) and true and false lumens. (**d**) Mid esophageal descending aortic long axis view, multiplane angle 90° (probe rotated leftward) shows the dissection extending into descending aorta. *AoDT* descending thoracic aorta

imaging modalities is that it readily detects and evaluates aortic regurgitation and pericardial effusion, and also assists in intraoperative assessment, although it cannot assess the abdominal aorta [161].

The aortic arch can be seen and evaluated by TEE, but the position of the esophagus in relation to the aortic arch presents some challenges. Unlike TTE, the entire aortic arch and descending aorta cannot be visualized in one plane, and instead must be evaluated in sections with a combination of multiplane angles, and rotation of the TEE probe. At the same time, the probe must be alternately advanced and withdrawn to visualize the more superior and inferior portions of the entire aorta. Because of the possibility of artifacts mimicking a dissection, an important practice in two-dimensional echocardiography is to visualize the abnormality in more than one plane. Therefore, several multiplane angles (preferably orthogonal) should be utilized to confirm the intra-luminal presence of the flap, and color flow Doppler can be used to show the flow patterns in and out of the false lumen. For ascending aortic evaluation, the most important views include the mid to upper esophageal views—the mid esophageal ascending aortic short and long axis views (ME Asc Ao SAX, ME Asc Ao LAX), as well as the upper esophageal ascending aortic arc long and short axis views (UE Ao Arch LAX, UE Ao Arch SAX). With the upper esophageal views, slow probe rotation from right to left will display the ascending aorta, then aortic arch, and finally descending aorta. The probe can be alternately advanced and withdrawn to visualize various portions of these structures. The descending aorta is best visualized by rotation of the probe so that faces posteriorly and away from the heart, using the descending aorta short and long axis views (Desc Ao SAX, Desc Ao LAX) to achieve orthogonal tomographic images, while withdrawing/advancing the probe to evaluate the different portions of the descending thoracic aorta [152].

Whether the dissection affects the ascending or descending aorta (or both), the characteristic echocardiographic feature of the dissection remains the same: intimal disruption that manifests as a thin, mobile intimal flap, separating the aorta into true and false lumens. In many instances, the false lumen is larger than the true lumen. There can be one or more re-entry sites between true and false lumens. Color flow Doppler will often show a difference in flow patterns between the true and false lumens; there can be much lower Doppler flow velocity in the false lumen, and spontaneous echo contrast or thrombus formation will sometimes be present [152]. In some cases, flow in the two lumens occurs in opposite directions, e.g. when aortic regurgitation is present (Fig. 16.31, Video 16.24). Because disruption of the aortic valve, aortic root, sinuses and coronary artery ostia may be associated with an aortic dissection, it is important to assess valve competence and global as well as segmental ventricular systolic function during the TEE evaluation.

Summary

This chapter reviewed a number of additional areas in which TEE has applications for the pediatric and young adult population. Some of these applications pertain equally to patients with and without congenital heart disease, and some have significant overlap with TEE as it is performed in adult patients with cardiac disease. These additional applications illustrate the wide applicability and important additive value that TEE can provide in cardiac patients of all ages.

References

1. Karchmer AW. Infective endocarditis. In: Bonow RO, Mann DL, Zipes DP, Libby P, editors. Braunwald's heart disease: a textbook of cardiovascular medicine. 9th ed. Philadelphia: Elsevier Saunders; 2012. p. 1540–60.
2. McDonald JR. Acute infective endocarditis. Infect Dis Clin North Am. 2009;23:643–64.
3. Bayer AS, Bolger AF, Taubert KA, et al. Diagnosis and management of infective endocarditis and its complications. Circulation. 1998;98:2936–48.
4. Ferrieri P, Gewitz MH, Gerber MA, et al. Unique features of infective endocarditis in childhood. Circulation. 2002;105:2115–26.
5. Saiman L, Prince A, Gersony WM. Pediatric infective endocarditis in the modern era. J Pediatr. 1993;122:847–53.
6. Morris CD, Reller MD, Menashe VD. Thirty-year incidence of infective endocarditis after surgery for congenital heart defect. JAMA. 1998;279:599–603.
7. Lin YT, Hsieh KS, Chen YS, Huang IF, Cheng MF. Infective endocarditis in children without underlying heart disease. J Microbiol Immunol Infect. 2012;46:121–8.
8. Durack DT, Lukes AS, Bright DK. New criteria for diagnosis of infective endocarditis: utilization of specific echocardiographic findings. Duke Endocarditis Service. Am J Med. 1994;96:200–9.
9. Li JS, Sexton DJ, Mick N, et al. Proposed modifications to the Duke criteria for the diagnosis of infective endocarditis. Clin Infect Dis. 2000;30:633–8.
10. Baddour LM, Wilson WR, Bayer AS, et al. Infective endocarditis: diagnosis, antimicrobial therapy, and management of complications: a statement for healthcare professionals from the Committee on Rheumatic Fever, Endocarditis, and Kawasaki Disease, Council on Cardiovascular Disease in the Young, and the Councils on Clinical Cardiology, Stroke, and Cardiovascular Surgery and Anesthesia, American Heart Association: endorsed by the Infectious Diseases Society of America. Circulation. 2005;111:e394–434.
11. Bayer AS, Ward JI, Ginzton LE, Shapiro SM. Evaluation of new clinical criteria for the diagnosis of infective endocarditis. Am J Med. 1994;96:211–9.
12. Del Pont JM, De Cicco LT, Vartalitis C, et al. Infective endocarditis in children: clinical analyses and evaluation of two diagnostic criteria. Pediatr Infect Dis J. 1995;14:1079–86.
13. Hoen B, Beguinot I, Rabaud C, et al. The Duke criteria for diagnosing infective endocarditis are specific: analysis of 100 patients with acute fever or fever of unknown origin. Clin Infect Dis. 1996;23:298–302.
14. Stockheim JA, Chadwick EG, Kessler S, et al. Are the Duke criteria superior to the Beth Israel criteria for the diagnosis of infective endocarditis in children? Clin Infect Dis. 1998;27:1451–6.
15. Tissieres P, Gervaix A, Beghetti M, Jaeggi ET. Value and limitations of the von Reyn, Duke, and modified Duke criteria for the diagnosis of infective endocarditis in children. Pediatrics. 2003;112:e467.
16. Prendergast BD. Diagnostic criteria and problems in infective endocarditis. Heart. 2004;90:611–3.
17. Bonow RO, Carabello BA, Chatterjee K, et al. 2008 Focused update incorporated into the ACC/AHA 2006 guidelines for the management of patients with valvular heart disease: a report of

the American College of Cardiology/American Heart Association Task Force on Practice Guidelines (Writing Committee to Revise the 1998 Guidelines for the Management of Patients With Valvular Heart Disease): endorsed by the Society of Cardiovascular Anesthesiologists, Society for Cardiovascular Angiography and Interventions, and Society of Thoracic Surgeons. Circulation. 2008;118:e523–661.
18. Tornos P, Iung B, Permanyer-Miralda G, et al. Infective endocarditis in Europe: lessons from the Euro heart survey. Heart. 2005;91:571–5.
19. Prendergast BD, Tornos P. Surgery for infective endocarditis: who and when? Circulation. 2010;121:1141–52.
20. Kang D-H, Kim Y-J, Kim S-H, et al. Early surgery versus conventional treatment for infective endocarditis. N Engl J Med. 2012;366: 2466–73.
21. Alexiou C, Langley SM, Monro JL. Surgery for infective valve endocarditis in children. Eur J Cardiothorac Surg. 1999;16: 653–9.
22. Karaci AR, Aydemir NA, Harmandar B, et al. Surgical treatment of infective valve endocarditis in children with congenital heart disease. J Card Surg. 2012;27:93–8.
23. Nomura F, Penny DJ, Menahem S, Pawade A, Karl TR. Surgical intervention for infective endocarditis in infancy and childhood. Ann Thorac Surg. 1995;60:90–5.
24. Martin JM, Neches WH, Wald ER. Infective endocarditis: 35 years of experience at a children's hospital. Clin Infect Dis. 1997;24:669–75.
25. Knirsch W, Nadal D. Infective endocarditis in congenital heart disease. Eur J Pediatr. 2011;170:1111–27.
26. Durack DT, Beeson PB. Experimental bacterial endocarditis. I. Colonization of a sterile vegetation. Br J Exp Pathol. 1972;53:44–9.
27. Fernicola DJ, Roberts WC. Frequency of ring abscess and cuspal infection in active infective endocarditis involving biologic valves. Am J Cardiol. 1993;72:314–23.
28. Daniel WG, Mugge A, Martin RP, et al. Improvement in the diagnosis of abscesses associated with endocarditis by transesophageal echocardiography. N Engl J Med. 1991;324:795–800.
29. Shaffer EM, Snider AR, Beekman RH, Behrendt DM, Peschiera AW. Sinus of Valsalva aneurysm complicating bacterial endocarditis in an infant: diagnosis with two-dimensional and Doppler echocardiography. J Am Coll Cardiol. 1987;9:588–91.
30. Anguera I, Miro JM, Vilacosta I, et al. Aorto-cavitary fistulous tract formation in infective endocarditis: clinical and echocardiographic features of 76 cases and risk factors for mortality. Eur Heart J. 2005;26:288–97.
31. Kearney RA, Eisen HJ, Wolf JE. Nonvalvular infections of the cardiovascular system. Ann Intern Med. 1994;121:219–30.
32. Sievers H-H, Stierle U, Charitos EI, et al. Major adverse cardiac and cerebrovascular events after the Ross procedure: a report from the German-Dutch Ross Registry. Circulation. 2010;122: S216–23.
33. Mills J, Utley J, Abbott J. Heart failure in infective endocarditis: predisposing factors, course, and treatment. Chest. 1974;66:151–7.
34. Pelletier LLJ, Petersdorf RG. Infective endocarditis: a review of 125 cases from the University of Washington Hospitals, 1963–72. Medicine (Baltimore). 1977;56:287–313.
35. Hasbun R, Vikram HR, Barakat LA, Buenconsejo J, Quagliarello VJ. Complicated left-sided native valve endocarditis in adults: risk classification for mortality. JAMA. 2003;289:1933–40.
36. Ryan EW, Bolger AF. Transesophageal echocardiography (TEE) in the evaluation of infective endocarditis. In: Foster E, editor. Cardiology clinics: transesophageal echocardiography. San Francisco; Division of Cardiology, Department of Medicine, University of California; 2000. p. 773–87.
37. Erbel R, Rohmann S, Drexler M, et al. Improved diagnostic value of echocardiography in patients with infective endocarditis by transoesophageal approach. A prospective study. Eur Heart J. 1988;9:43–53.
38. Shanewise JS, Martin RP. Assessment of endocarditis and associated complications with transesophageal echocardiography. Crit Care Clin. 1996;12:411–27.
39. Jacob S, Tong AT. Role of echocardiography in the diagnosis and management of infective endocarditis. Curr Opin Cardiol. 2002;17:478–85.
40. Reynolds HR, Jagen MA, Tunick PA, Kronzon I. Sensitivity of transthoracic versus transesophageal echocardiography for the detection of native valve vegetations in the modern era. J Am Soc Echocardiogr. 2003;16:67–70.
41. Daniel WG, Mugge A, Grote J, et al. Comparison of transthoracic and transesophageal echocardiography for detection of abnormalities of prosthetic and biologic valves in the mitral and aortic positions. Am J Cardiol. 1993;71:210–5.
42. Penk JS, Webb CL, Shulman ST, Anderson EJ. Echocardiography in pediatric infective endocarditis. Pediatr Infect Dis J. 2011;30: 1109–11.
43. Humpl T, McCrindle BW, Smallhorn JF. The relative roles of transthoracic compared with transesophageal echocardiography in children with suspected infective endocarditis. J Am Coll Cardiol. 2003;41:2068–71.
44. Steckelberg JM, Murphy JG, Ballard D, et al. Emboli in infective endocarditis: the prognostic value of echocardiography. Ann Intern Med. 1991;114:635–40.
45. Lopez JA, Ross RS, Fishbein MC, Siegel RJ. Nonbacterial thrombotic endocarditis: a review. Am Heart J. 1987;113:773–84.
46. Asopa S, Patel A, Khan OA, Sharma R, Ohri SK. Non-bacterial thrombotic endocarditis. Eur J Cardiothorac Surg. 2007;32:696–701.
47. González Quintela A, Candela MJ, Vidal C, Román J, Aramburo P. Non-bacterial thrombotic endocarditis in cancer patients. Acta Cardiol. 1991;46:1–9.
48. Beynon RP, Bahl VK, Prendergast BD. Infective endocarditis. BMJ. 2006;333:334–9.
49. Asinger RW, Dyken ML, Fisher M, Hart RG, Sherman DG. Cardiogenic brain embolism. The second report of the Cerebral Embolism Task Force. Arch Neurol. 1989;46:727–43.
50. Agmon Y, Khandheria BK, Gentile F, Seward JB. Echocardiographic assessment of the left atrial appendage. J Am Coll Cardiol. 1999;34: 1867–77.
51. de Divitiis M, Omran H, Rabahieh R, et al. Right atrial appendage thrombosis in atrial fibrillation: its frequency and its clinical predictors. Am J Cardiol. 1999;84:1023–8.
52. Ozer O, Sari I, Davutoglu V. Right atrial appendage: forgotten part of the heart in atrial fibrillation. Clin Appl Thromb Hemost. 2010;16:218–20.
53. Schweizer P, Bardos P, Erbel R, et al. Detection of left atrial thrombi by echocardiography. Br Heart J. 1981;45:148–56.
54. Aschenberg W, Schluter M, Kremer P, Schroder E, Siglow V, Bleifeld W. Transesophageal two-dimensional echocardiography for the detection of left atrial appendage thrombus. J Am Coll Cardiol. 1986;7:163–6.
55. Manning WJ, Weintraub RM, Waksmonski CA, et al. Accuracy of transesophageal echocardiography for identifying left atrial thrombi. A prospective, intraoperative study. Ann Intern Med. 1995;123:817–22.
56. Veinot JP, Harrity PJ, Gentile F, et al. Anatomy of the normal left atrial appendage: a quantitative study of age-related changes in 500 autopsy hearts: implications for echocardiographic examination. Circulation. 1997;96:3112–5.
57. Karakus G, Kodali V, Inamdar V, Nanda NC, Suwanjutah T, Pothineni KR. Comparative assessment of left atrial appendage by transesophageal and combined two- and three-dimensional transthoracic echocardiography. Echocardiography. 2008;25: 918–24.

58. Werner JA, Cheitlin MD, Gross BW, Speck SM, Ivey TD. Echocardiographic appearance of the Chiari network: differentiation from right-heart pathology. Circulation. 1981;63:1104–9.
59. Black IW. Spontaneous echo contrast: where there's smoke there's fire. Echocardiography. 2000;17:373–82.
60. Kwaan HC, Sakurai S, Wang J. Rheological abnormalities and thromboembolic complications in heart disease: spontaneous echo contrast and red cell aggregation. Semin Thromb Hemost. 2003;29: 529–34.
61. Chan HS, Sonley MJ, Moes CA, Daneman A, Smith CR, Martin DJ. Primary and secondary tumors of childhood involving the heart, pericardium, and great vessels. A report of 75 cases and review of the literature. Cancer. 1985;56:825–36.
62. Roberts WC. Primary and secondary neoplasms of the heart. Am J Cardiol. 1997;80:671–82.
63. Shapiro LM. Cardiac tumours: diagnosis and management. Heart. 2001;85:218–22.
64. Miyake CY, Del Nido PJ, Alexander ME, et al. Cardiac tumors and associated arrhythmias in pediatric patients, with observations on surgical therapy for ventricular tachycardia. J Am Coll Cardiol. 2011;58:1903–9.
65. Luck SR, DeLeon S, Shkolnik A, Morgan E, Labotka R. Intracardiac Wilms' tumor: diagnosis and management. J Pediatr Surg. 1982;17: 551–4.
66. Marx GR, Moran AM. Cardiac tumors. In: Allen HD, Dricoll DJ, Shaddy RE, Feltes TF, editors. Moss and Adams' heart disease in infants, children, and adolescents: including the fetus and young adult. 7th ed. Philadelphia: Lippincott Williams & Wilkins; 2008. p. 1479–95.
67. Uzun O, Wilson DG, Vujanic GM, Parsons JM, De Giovanni JV. Cardiac tumours in children. Orphanet J Rare Dis. 2007;2:11.
68. Günther T, Schreiber C, Noebauer C, Eicken A, Lange R. Treatment strategies for pediatric patients with primary cardiac and pericardial tumors: a 30-year review. Pediatr Cardiol. 2008;29:1071–6.
69. Becker AE. Primary heart tumors in the pediatric age group: a review of salient pathologic features relevant for clinicians. Pediatr Cardiol. 2000;21:317–23.
70. Burke AP, Rosado-de-Christenson M, Templeton PA, Virmani R. Cardiac fibroma: clinicopathologic correlates and surgical treatment. J Thorac Cardiovasc Surg. 1994;108:862–70.
71. Reynen K. Cardiac myxomas. N Engl J Med. 1995;333:1610–7.
72. Bulkley BH, Hutchins GM. Atrial myxomas: a fifty year review. Am Heart J. 1979;97:639–43.
73. Hada Y, Wolfe C, Murray GF, Craige E. Right ventricular myxoma. Case report and review of phonocardiographic and auscultatory manifestations. Am Heart J. 1980;100:871–7.
74. Leonhardt ET, Kullenberg KP. Bilateral atrial myxomas with multiple arterial aneurysms—a syndrome mimicking polyarteritis nodosa. Am J Med. 1977;62:792–4.
75. Perez de Isla L, de Castro R, Zamorano JL, et al. Diagnosis and treatment of cardiac myxomas by transesophageal echocardiography. Am J Cardiol. 2002;90:1419–21.
76. Burke A, Johns JP, Virmani R. Hemangiomas of the heart. A clinicopathologic study of ten cases. Am J Cardiovasc Pathol. 1990;3:283–90.
77. Niwa K, Tashima K, Terai M, Okajima Y, Nakajima H. Contrast-enhanced magnetic resonance imaging of cardiac tumors in children. Am Heart J. 1989;118:424–5.
78. Link KM, Lesko NM. MR evaluation of cardiac/juxtacardiac masses. Top Magn Reson Imaging. 1995;7:232–45.
79. Bardo DME. Cardiac magnetic resonance imaging signal characteristics of cardiac tumors in children. J Am Coll Cardiol. 2011;58: 1055–6.
80. Obeid AI, Marvasti M, Parker F, Rosenberg J. Comparison of transthoracic and transesophageal echocardiography in diagnosis of left atrial myxoma. Am J Cardiol. 1989;63:1006–8.
81. Geibel A, Kasper W, Keck A, Hofmann T, Konstantinides S, Just H. Diagnosis, localization and evaluation of malignancy of heart and mediastinal tumors by conventional and transesophageal echocardiography. Acta Cardiol. 1996;51:395–408.
82. Engberding R, Daniel WG, Erbel R, et al. Diagnosis of heart tumours by transoesophageal echocardiography: a multicentre study in 154 Patients. European Cooperative Study Group. Eur Heart J. 1993;14:1223–8.
83. Borges AC, Witt C, Bartel T, Muller S, Konertz W, Baumann G. Preoperative two- and three-dimensional transesophageal echocardiographic assessment of heart tumors. Ann Thorac Surg. 1996;61:1163–7.
84. Brown AS, Why H, Monaghan MJ. Value of multiplane transoesophageal echocardiography in recurrent atrial myxoma. Br Heart J. 1994;71:540.
85. Goldman JH, Foster E. Transesophageal echocardiographic (TEE) evaluation of intracardiac and pericardial masses. Cardiol Clin. 2000;18:849–60.
86. Ross DN. Replacement of aortic and mitral valves with a pulmonary autograft. Lancet. 1967;2:956–8.
87. Chambers JC, Somerville J, Stone S, Ross DN. Pulmonary autograft procedure for aortic valve disease: long-term results of the pioneer series. Circulation. 1997;96:2206–14.
88. Athanasiou T, Cherian A, Ross D. The Ross II procedure: pulmonary autograft in the mitral position. Ann Thorac Surg. 2004;78: 1489–95.
89. Protopapas AD, Athanasiou T. Contegra conduit for reconstruction of the right ventricular outflow tract: a review of published early and mid-time results. J Cardiothorac Surg. 2008;3:62.
90. Hickey EJ, McCrindle BW, Blackstone EH, et al. Jugular venous valved conduit (Contegra) matches allograft performance in infant truncus arteriosus repair. Eur J Cardiothorac Surg. 2008;33: 890–8.
91. Christenson JT, Sierra J, Colina Manzano NE, Jolou J, Beghetti M, Kalangos A. Homografts and xenografts for right ventricular outflow tract reconstruction: long-term results. Ann Thorac Surg. 2010;90:1287–93.
92. Dave H, Mueggler O, Comber M, et al. Risk factor analysis of 170 single-institutional contegra implantations in pulmonary position. Ann Thorac Surg. 2011;91:195–302; discussion 202–3.
93. Hopkins RA, editor. Tissue and bio-engineering for congenital cardiac disease. Prog Pediatr Cardiol. 2006;21(2):137–244.
94. Aslam AK, Aslam AF, Vasavada BC, Khan IA. Prosthetic heart valves: types and echocardiographic evaluation. Int J Cardiol. 2007;122:99–110.
95. Pibarot P, Dumesnil JG. Prosthetic heart valves: selection of the optimal prosthesis and long-term management. Circulation. 2009;119:1034–48.
96. Oosterhof T, Hazekamp MG, Mulder BJ. Opportunities in pulmonary valve replacement. Expert Rev Cardiovasc Ther. 2009;7:1117–22.
97. Kidane AG, Burriesci G, Cornejo P, et al. Current developments and future prospects for heart valve replacement therapy. J Biomed Mater Res B Appl Biomater. 2009;88:290–303.
98. Waterbolk TW, Hoendermis ES, den Hamer IJ, Ebels T. Pulmonary valve replacement with a mechanical prosthesis. Promising results of 28 procedures in patients with congenital heart disease. Eur J Cardiothorac Surg. 2006;30:28–32.
99. Fleming GA, Hill KD, Green AS, Rhodes JF. Percutaneous pulmonary valve replacement. Prog Pediatr Cardiol. 2012;33:143–50.
100. Momenah TS, El Oakley R, Al Najashi K, Khoshhal S, Al Qethamy H, Bonhoeffer P. Extended application of percutaneous pulmonary valve implantation. J Am Coll Cardiol. 2009;53:1859–63.
101. Hasan BS, McElhinney DB, Brown DW, et al. Short-term performance of the transcatheter Melody valve in high-pressure

hemodynamic environments in the pulmonary and systemic circulations. Circ Cardiovasc Interv. 2011;4:615–20.
102. Gurvitch R, Cheung A, Ye J, et al. Transcatheter valve-in-valve implantation for failed surgical biologic valves. J Am Coll Cardiol. 2011;58:2196–209.
103. Gillespie MJ, Dori Y, Harris MA, Sathanandam S, Glatz AC, Rome JJ. Bilateral branch pulmonary artery melody valve implantation for treatment of complex right ventricular outflow tract dysfunction in a high-risk patient. Circ Cardiovasc Interv. 2011; 4:e21–3.
104. Billings FT, Kodali SK, Shanewise JS. Transcatheter aortic valve implantation: anesthetic considerations. Anesth Analg. 2009;108:1453–62.
105. Kenny D, Hijazi ZM, Kar S, et al. Percutaneous implantation of the Edwards SAPIEN transcatheter heart valve for conduit failure in the pulmonary position: early phase 1 results from an international multicenter clinical trial. J Am Coll Cardiol. 2011;58:2248–56.
106. Webb JG, Wood DA. Current status of transcatheter aortic valve replacement. J Am Coll Cardiol. 2012;60:483–92.
107. Zoghbi WA, Chambers JB, Dumesnil JG, et al. Recommendations for evaluation of prosthetic valves with echocardiography and doppler ultrasound: a report From the American Society of Echocardiography's Guidelines and Standards Committee and the Task Force on Prosthetic Valves, developed in conjunction with the American College of Cardiology Cardiovascular Imaging Committee, Cardiac Imaging Committee of the American Heart Association, the European Association of Echocardiography, a registered branch of the European Society of Cardiology, the Japanese Society of Echocardiography and the Canadian Society of Echocardiography, endorsed by the American College of Cardiology Foundation, American Heart Association, European Association of Echocardiography, a registered branch of the European Society of Cardiology, the Japanese Society of Echocardiography, and Canadian Society of Echocardiography. J Am Soc Echocardiogr. 2009;22:975–1014.
108. Rosenhek R, Binder T, Maurer G, Baumgartner H. Normal values for Doppler echocardiographic assessment of heart valve prostheses. J Am Soc Echocardiogr. 2003;16:1116–27.
109. Bach DS. Transesophageal echocardiographic (TEE) evaluation of prosthetic valves. Cardiol Clin. 2000;18:751–71.
110. Morguet AJ, Werner GS, Andreas S, Kreuzer H. Diagnostic value of transesophageal compared with transthoracic echocardiography in suspected prosthetic valve endocarditis. Herz. 1995;20:390–8.
111. Schulz R, Werner GS, Fuchs JB, et al. Clinical outcome and echocardiographic findings of native and prosthetic valve endocarditis in the 1990's. Eur Heart J. 1996;17:281–8.
112. Lengyel M. The impact of transesophageal echocardiography on the management of prosthetic valve endocarditis: experience of 31 cases and review of the literature. J Heart Valve Dis. 1997;6:204–11.
113. Zoghbi WA, Enriquez-Sarano M, Foster E, et al. Recommendations for evaluation of the severity of native valvular regurgitation with two-dimensional and Doppler echocardiography. J Am Soc Echocardiogr. 2003;16:777–802.
114. Quiñones M. Echocardiographic assessment of valve stenosis: EAE/ASE recommendations for clinical practice. J Am Soc Echocardiogr. 2009;22:1–23.
115. Rahimtoola SH. The problem of valve prosthesis-patient mismatch. Circulation. 1978;58:20–4.
116. Pibarot P, Dumesnil JG. Hemodynamic and clinical impact of prosthesis-patient mismatch in the aortic valve position and its prevention. J Am Coll Cardiol. 2000;36:1131–41.
117. Mohty D, Mohty-Echahidi D, Malouf JF, et al. Impact of prosthesis-patient mismatch on long-term survival in patients with small St Jude Medical mechanical prostheses in the aortic position. Circulation. 2006;113:420–6.
118. Walther T, Rastan A, Falk V, et al. Patient prosthesis mismatch affects short- and long-term outcomes after aortic valve replacement. Eur J Cardiothorac Surg. 2006;30:15–9.
119. Rahimtoola SH. Choice of prosthetic heart valve in adults an update. J Am Coll Cardiol. 2010;55:2413–26.
120. Lam B-K, Chan V, Hendry P, et al. The impact of patient-prosthesis mismatch on late outcomes after mitral valve replacement. J Thorac Cardiovasc Surg. 2007;133:1464–73.
121. Blackstone EH, Cosgrove DM, Jamieson WR, et al. Prosthesis size and long-term survival after aortic valve replacement. J Thorac Cardiovasc Surg. 2003;126:783–96.
122. Koch CG, Khandwala F, Estafanous FG, Loop FD, Blackstone EH. Impact of prosthesis-patient size on functional recovery after aortic valve replacement. Circulation. 2005;111:3221–9.
123. Pibarot P, Dumesnil JG. Prosthesis-patient mismatch: definition, clinical impact, and prevention. Heart. 2006;92:1022–9.
124. Masuda M, Kado H, Tatewaki H, Shiokawa Y, Yasui H. Late results after mitral valve replacement with bileaflet mechanical prosthesis in children: evaluation of prosthesis-patient mismatch. Ann Thorac Surg. 2004;77:913–7.
125. Zamorano JL, Badano LP, Bruce C, et al. EAE/ASE recommendations for the use of echocardiography in new transcatheter interventions for valvular heart disease. J Am Soc Echocardiogr. 2011;24:937–65.
126. Holmes DR, Mack MJ, Kaul S, et al. 2012 ACCF/AATS/SCAI/STS expert consensus document on transcatheter aortic valve replacement. J Am Coll Cardiol. 2012;59:1200–54.
127. Zaroff J. Echocardiographic evaluation of the potential cardiac donor. J Heart Lung Transplant. 2004;23:S250–2.
128. Stoddard MF, Longaker RA. The role of transesophageal echocardiography in cardiac donor screening. Am Heart J. 1993;125:1676–81.
129. Hetzer R, Potapov EV, Alexi-Meskishvili V, et al. Single-center experience with treatment of cardiogenic shock in children by pediatric ventricular assist devices. J Thorac Cardiovasc Surg. 2011;141:616–23, 623.e1.
130. Cooper DS, Jacobs JP, Moore L, et al. Cardiac extracorporeal life support: state of the art in 2007. Cardiol Young. 2007;17 Suppl 2:104–15.
131. Potapov EV, Stiller B, Hetzer R. Ventricular assist devices in children: current achievements and future perspectives. Pediatr Transplant. 2007;11:241–55.
132. Hetzer R, Potapov EV, Stiller B, et al. Improvement in survival after mechanical circulatory support with pneumatic pulsatile ventricular assist devices in pediatric patients. Ann Thorac Surg. 2006;82:917–24; discussion 924–5.
133. Fraser CD, Jaquiss RDB, Rosenthal DN, et al. Prospective trial of a pediatric ventricular assist device. N Engl J Med. 2012; 367:532–41.
134. Chumnanvej S, Wood MJ, MacGillivray TE, Melo MFV. Perioperative echocardiographic examination for ventricular assist device implantation. Anesth Analg. 2007;105:583–601.
135. Davila-Roman VG, Barzilai B. Transesophageal echocardiographic evaluation of patients receiving mechanical assistance from ventricular assist devices. Echocardiography. 1997;14:505–12.
136. Scohy TV, Gommers D, Maat APWM, Dejong PL, Bogers AJJC, Hofland J. Intraoperative transesophageal echocardiography is beneficial for hemodynamic stabilization during left ventricular assist device implantation in children. Paediatr Anaesth. 2009; 19:390–5.
137. Sachdeva R, Frazier EA, Jaquiss RDB, Imamura M, Swearingen CJ, Vyas HV. Echocardiographic evaluation of ventricular assist devices in pediatric patients. J Am Soc Echocardiogr. 2013;26:41–9.

138. Baldwin JT, Duncan BW. Ventricular assist devices for children. Prog Pediatr Cardiol. 2006;21:173–84.
139. Miera O, Potapov EV, Redlin M, et al. First experiences with the HeartWare ventricular assist system in children. Ann Thorac Surg. 2011;91:1256–60.
140. Baldwin JT, Borovetz HS, Duncan BW, Gartner MJ, Jarvik RK, Weiss WJ. The national heart, lung, and blood institute pediatric circulatory support program: a summary of the 5-year experience. Circulation. 2011;123:1233–40.
141. Addonizio LJ. Pediatric ventricular assist devices—first steps for babies. N Engl J Med. 2012;367:567–8.
142. Romano P, Mangion JM. The role of intraoperative transesophageal echocardiography in heart transplantation. Echocardiography. 2002;19:599–604.
143. Ishizuka N, Nakamura K, Fujita Y, et al. Transesophageal echocardiographic findings in patients after heart transplantation. J Cardiol. 1997;29:163–70.
144. del Rio MJ. Transplantation in complex congenital heart disease. Prog Pediatr Cardiol. 2000;11:107–13.
145. Kirklin JK, Naftel DC, Kirklin JW, Blackstone EH, White-Williams C, Bourge RC. Pulmonary vascular resistance and the risk of heart transplantation. J Heart Transplant. 1988;7:331–6.
146. Meyers BF, Lynch J, Trulock EP, Guthrie TJ, Cooper JD, Patterson GA. Lung transplantation: a decade of experience. Ann Surg. 1999;230:362–70; discussion 370–1.
147. Serra E, Feltracco P, Barbieri S, Forti A, Ori C. Transesophageal echocardiography during lung transplantation. Transplant Proc. 2007;39:1981–2.
148. Hausmann D, Daniel WG, Mugge A, et al. Imaging of pulmonary artery and vein anastomoses by transesophageal echocardiography after lung transplantation. Circulation. 1992;86:II251–8.
149. Gonzalez-Fernandez C, Gonzalez-Castro A, Rodriguez-Borregan JC, et al. Pulmonary venous obstruction after lung transplantation. Diagnostic advantages of transesophageal echocardiography. Clin Transplant. 2009;23:975–80.
150. McIlroy DR, Sesto AC, Buckland MR. Pulmonary vein thrombosis, lung transplantation, and intraoperative transesophageal echocardiography. J Cardiothorac Vasc Anesth. 2006;20:712–5.
151. Asfoura JY, Vidt DG. Acute aortic dissection. Chest. 1991;99:724–9.
152. Flachskampf FA, Daniel WG. Aortic dissection. In: Foster E, editor. Cardiology Clinics: Transesophageal Echocardiography. 18(4) ed. Medizinische Klinik II, Universitat Erlangen-Nurnberg, Germany. frank.flachskampf@rzmail.uni-erlangen.de: United States; 2000. p. 807–17.
153. Nienaber CA, Spielmann RP, von Kodolitsch Y, et al. Diagnosis of thoracic aortic dissection. Magnetic resonance imaging versus transesophageal echocardiography. Circulation. 1992;85:434–47.
154. Matura LA, Ho VB, Rosing DR, Bondy CA. Aortic dilatation and dissection in Turner syndrome. Circulation. 2007;116:1663–70.
155. Erbel R, Bednarczyk I, Pop T, et al. Detection of dissection of the aortic intima and media after angioplasty of coarctation of the aorta. An angiographic, computer tomographic, and echocardiographic comparative study. Circulation. 1990;81:805–14.
156. Kouchoukos NT, Blackstone EH, Hanley FL, Doty DB, Karp RB. Acute aortic dissection. In: Kirklin/Barratt-Boyes cardiac surgery. 3rd ed. Philadelphia: Churchill Livingstone; 2003. p. 1820–49.
157. Miller DC, Mitchell RS, Oyer PE, Stinson EB, Jamieson SW, Shumway NE. Independent determinants of operative mortality for patients with aortic dissections. Circulation. 1984;70:I153–64.
158. DeBakey ME, McCollum CH, Crawford ES, et al. Dissection and dissecting aneurysms of the aorta: twenty-year follow-up of five hundred twenty-seven patients treated surgically. Surgery. 1982;92:1118–34.
159. Keren A, Kim CB, Hu BS, et al. Accuracy of biplane and multiplane transesophageal echocardiography in diagnosis of typical acute aortic dissection and intramural hematoma. J Am Coll Cardiol. 1996;28:627–36.
160. Penco M, Paparoni S, Dagianti A, et al. Usefulness of transesophageal echocardiography in the assessment of aortic dissection. Am J Cardiol. 2000;86:53G–6.
161. Thrumurthy SG, Karthikesalingam A, Patterson BO, Holt PJE, Thompson MM. The diagnosis and management of aortic dissection. BMJ. 2012;344:d8290.

Applications of Transesophageal Echocardiography in the Cardiac Catheterization Laboratory

17

Peter R. Koenig, Qi-Ling Cao, and Ziyad M. Hijazi

Abstract

Transesophageal echocardiography (TEE) has proven to be of significant benefit in the cardiac catheterization laboratory. This modality enables continuous, noninvasive monitoring of an entire interventional procedure, while at the same time allowing maintenance of a sterile field without interfering with fluoroscopy or the interventional procedure itself. Moreover, the superior intracardiac imaging offered by TEE provides unparalleled real-time visualization of intracardiac anatomy, thus TEE has become indispensable for many catheter-based interventions such as closure of atrial and ventricular septal defects. Currently, the availability of pediatric multiplane TEE probes permits TEE monitoring of procedures even in infants and very young children. This chapter discusses the use and applications of TEE in the cardiac catheterization setting, specifically as regards its utility for interventional procedures.

Keywords

Transesophageal echocardiography • Congenital heart disease • Cardiac catheterization • Catheter-based interventions • Interventional catheterization • Transcatheter device occlusion • Fontan fenestration closure

Introduction

The techniques and advantages of transesophageal echocardiography (TEE), as outlined in this textbook, have proven to be of significant benefit during cardiac catheterization. The advantages of TEE have been clearly shown in allowing maintenance of a sterile field without interfering with fluoroscopy or the interventional procedure [1, 2]. In addition, the use of TEE may reduce fluoroscopy time and minimize the amount of contrast used, especially in multi-interventional procedures [2, 3].

Improvements in TEE technology have seen single plane imaging progress to biplane and then multiplane imaging. Probe miniaturization has enabled TEE imaging in pediatric

P.R. Koenig, MD, FACC, FASE (✉)
Department of Pediatric Cardiology,
Ann & Robert H. Lurie Children's Hospital of Chicago,
Northwestern University Feinberg School of Medicine,
225 East Chicago Ave. Box 21,
Chicago, IL 60611-2605, USA
e-mail: pkoenig@luriechildrens.org

Q.-L. Cao, MD • Z.M. Hijazi, MD, MPH, FSCAI, FACC, FAAP
Departments of Pediatrics and Internal Medicine,
Rush Center for Congenital and Structural Heart Disease,
Rush University Medical Center,
1653 W. Congress Parkway,
Chicago, IL 60612, USA
e-mail: zhijazi@rush.edu

The online version of this chapter (doi:10.1007/978-1-84800-064-3_17) contains supplementary material, which is available to authorized users.

P.C. Wong, W.C. Miller-Hance (eds.), *Transesophageal Echocardiography for Congenital Heart Disease*, DOI 10.1007/978-1-84800-064-3_17, © Springer-Verlag London 2014

patients. With this, the use of TEE in children and in the diagnosis of congenital heart disease (CHD) has greatly increased. The applications and benefits of TEE during congenital heart surgery have been well described [4–7], particularly in the intraoperative setting. Similarly, this imaging modality can be incorporated into the interventional cardiac catheterization laboratory without significant additional risk. The information gained can be used to further define the cardiac anatomy; in turn, this information may change the conduct of the cardiac catheterization (e.g., may demonstrate that the intended intervention is not necessary or needs modification). TEE has the additional unique role of being able to guide cardiac interventions in a continuous fashion [8]. Guidance may include facilitating placement of catheters, wires or pacing catheters [1, 9]. It may also include the guidance for creation or enlargement of an interatrial communication [10–13], balloon angioplasty [9, 11], dilation or stent insertion of a narrowed area [1, 3, 9–11, 14], or for closure of defects in the interatrial or interventricular septum [2, 14–19].

This chapter describes the applications of TEE during these procedures. Most of the descriptions of the particular techniques are those incorporated at our own center; however, these have also been applied at other institutions, as referenced at the end of this chapter. Applications of TEE related to transcatheter valve implantation are addressed in Chap. 16.

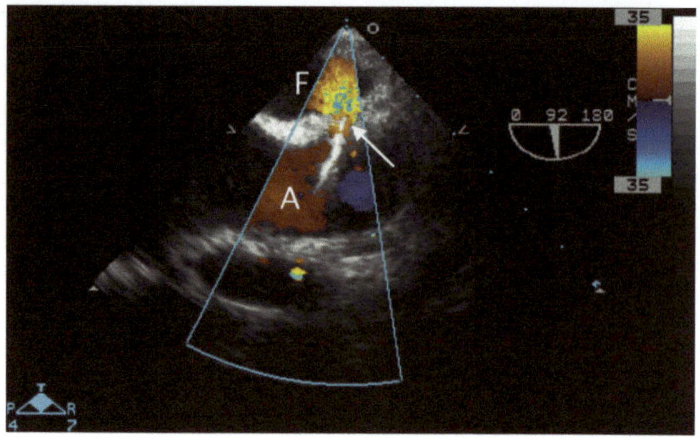

Fig. 17.1 Radiofrequency ablation procedure facilitated by TEE. Mid esophageal bicaval view with color Doppler imaging demonstrating puncture (*arrow*) of a Fontan baffle (*F*) in a patient with complex heart disease consisting of dextrocardia, double inlet left ventricle and pulmonary atresia to facilitate an electrophysiologic procedure . (*A*) Atrium

Specific Applications of TEE During Interventions for Congenital Heart Disease

Electrophysiologic Studies

Given its superb imaging of the posterior anatomy, TEE may be called upon to guide procedures during electrophysiologic studies. Applications include guidance during pacing catheter placement, especially in the coronary sinus [20, 21], as well as transseptal puncture [21, 22]. These TEE applications are similar in the pediatric and adult population undergoing invasive electrophysiologic evaluation. However, in patients with congenital heart lesions and altered anatomy, placement of catheters may require unusual locations which can be imaged well via the transesophageal approach as shown in Fig. 17.1 [23, 24].

Valve Dilation Procedures

TEE has been utilized during valvuloplasty of stenotic valves. Although it has been applied to procedures involving all cardiac valves, most of the experience in children relates to mitral [25], aortic, and pulmonary valves [11, 14]. Its use may be more important in describing the anatomy of the valvar structures, measuring the valve annulus, and assessing associated subvalvar or supravalvar obstruction [11, 14]. In addition, TEE facilitates the evaluation of associated lesions. During a valve intervention, TEE allows for guidance of proper wire, catheter, and balloon position to prevent entanglement with valvar apparatus or important surrounding structures [3, 9]. In cases of radiofrequency perforation of the pulmonary valve, TEE, in conjunction with fluoroscopy, facilitates the procedure by confirming wire/catheter position, documenting when valve perforation occurs, and monitoring the catheter as it is successfully advanced across the perforation of the atretic pulmonary valve.

TEE is extremely valuable in the assessment of the results of the intervention and exclusion of potential complications such as pericardial effusion or injury to other valves [3, 9]. The main issues to be addressed following an intervention are residual valvar obstruction and the presence and severity of regurgitation. TEE is particularly helpful in this assessment.

The imaging views used before, during, and after valve procedure are similar to those described for a diagnostic TEE study (Chap. 4) and as noted throughout this textbook. The focus of the examination should be on the relevant pathology. Hemodynamics should be evaluated in imaging planes able to achieve Doppler alignment parallel to blood flow, and balloon dilation observed in views perpendicular to the valve or other modified views to demonstrate the entire length of the balloon as it is being distended.

Transcatheter Closure of Atrial Septal Defects

Transesophageal imaging of atrial septal defects (ASD) is described in Chap. 7. Currently, only secundum ASDs are amenable to transcatheter closure. Two devices are approved for ASD closure in the United States: the Amplatzer septal occluder (St. Jude Medical, St. Paul, MN) and the Helex device (W.L. Gore & Associates, Flagstaff, AZ). The Amplatzer® septal occluder represents the most commonly utilized device. This is a self-expanding, double-disc device composed of braided nitinol mesh enclosing polyester fabric, available in various sizes ranging from 4 to 38 mm. The Helex septal occluder is a double-disk device composed of an expanded polytetrafluoroethylene membrane bonded to a single nitinol wire frame.

In most cases, TEE is performed under general endotracheal anesthesia for transcatheter closure of intracardiac communications. A complete TEE study is undertaken including the standard TEE imaging locations: upper, mid and lower esophageal, transgastric, and deep transgastric windows. Views are obtained in multiple imaging planes. The atrioventricular valves are interrogated at baseline for evidence of regurgitation as these can potentially be altered during device placement.

In order to understand the manner in which TEE may help guide transcatheter ASD closure, a review of the procedure for Amplatzer® ASD device placement is described. After the baseline study is obtained, the size of the ASD is determined. The defect is measured in multiple planes including the mid esophageal four chamber (ME 4 Ch), mid esophageal aortic valve short axis (ME AV SAX), and mid esophageal bicaval (ME Bicaval) views. Tissue rims (anterior, posterior, superior, inferior, basal, apical) are also measured in the above views as shown in Fig. 17.2. This is a crucial step in the selection of the proper device size. Sizing balloons may be utilized. In this case, the balloon is positioned across the defect and inflated with diluted contrast until cessation of flow is documented by color Doppler. At that point, a still TEE image is obtained to measure the size of the balloon at the sites of indentation by the rims of the surrounding atrial septal tissue. The imaging plane used is usually modified such that the balloon is profiled longitudinally and the waist created by the rims of the ASD is well seen. The measurements can be confirmed by fluoroscopic imaging.

The proper size device is selected to be ±2 mm of the stop flow balloon diameter. The balloon is then removed leaving the guide wire in place. An appropriate size sheath is positioned over the wire into a pulmonary vein or left atrium. A cable with the occluder device is advanced to the distal tip of the sheath. The tip of the delivery sheath is positioned in the mid left atrium, which is confirmed best by TEE imaging in the ME AV SAX view. The sheath is retracted over the cable to open the left atrial disc of the device. TEE confirms that the disc indeed is in the left atrium and has not opened in a pulmonary vein [26]. The cable and sheath are then withdrawn so that the left atrial disc is pulled closer to the atrial septum. The connecting waist is then partially deployed within the left atrium and then pulled back into the ASD to stent the defect. The right atrial disc is then deployed and the device stability is assessed as the arms of the device straddle the defect. Color Doppler assists in the determination of appropriate occlusion of the interatrial communication.

It is essential to have continuous TEE monitoring of the deployment at this stage to demonstrate capture of the rims of the ASD within the two discs of the occluder. Multiple TEE views, as described above, should be utilized to confirm this. If the device is not well positioned it can be retrieved and repositioned. When the device is confirmed to be in good position, the patency of the right upper pulmonary vein, superior vena cava, inferior vena cava, and coronary sinus are assessed by TEE, as is the presence of any mitral or tricuspid valve regurgitation using appropriate multiplane imaging for each structure as described throughout this textbook. The device is then released. Due to slight tension of the delivery cable, there is often a notable change in the angle of the device as it is released and self-centers within the defect and aligns with the interatrial septum. After deployment, TEE is used to image the device and a repeat assessment for residual shunts, vessel patency and valve competency is performed. Frequently, there is flow detected by color Doppler due to "foaming" within the device disks immediately after release. This does not represent significant shunting and should not be considered abnormal. The steps involved in transcatheter ASD occlusion with corresponding TEE imaging are summarized in Table 17.1, and imaging sequences are shown in Fig. 17.3.

Although intracardiac echocardiography may be utilized during ASD occlusion [27], TEE remains the main imaging approach for guiding these procedures at many institutions.

Transcather Occlusion of Ventricular Septal Defects

Transesophageal imaging of ventricular septal defects (VSDs) is described in Chap. 9. Transcatheter closure of VSDs has been well described [14, 17, 18]. Currently, only muscular and perimembranous VSDs are amenable to transcatheter device closure. At the time of this writing, the only device approved in the United States for closure of muscular VSDs is the Amplatzer® muscular VSD occluder (St. Jude Medical, St. Paul, MN). As described in the previous section regarding transcatheter closure of ASDs, in order to understand the manner in which TEE may guide VSD closure procedures, it is appropriate to review the steps involved. The description that follows applies to the use of the Amplatzer® device.

The Amplatzer® muscular VSD occluder is designed specifically for the muscular septum. The waist of the device, which centers and fills the defect, measures 7 mm in length. The left and right ventricular disks are 8 mm larger than the connecting waist in all but the smallest size device. Various occluder sizes are available, ranging from device size/waist diameter of 4 mm (corresponding disk diameter of 9 mm) to device size/waist diameter of 18 mm (corresponding disk diameter of 26 mm). These muscular defects can be closed using percutaneous or perventricular techniques.

Although percutaneous closure of a single muscular VSD is feasible without TEE guidance, many centers consider that TEE provides information not readily available by

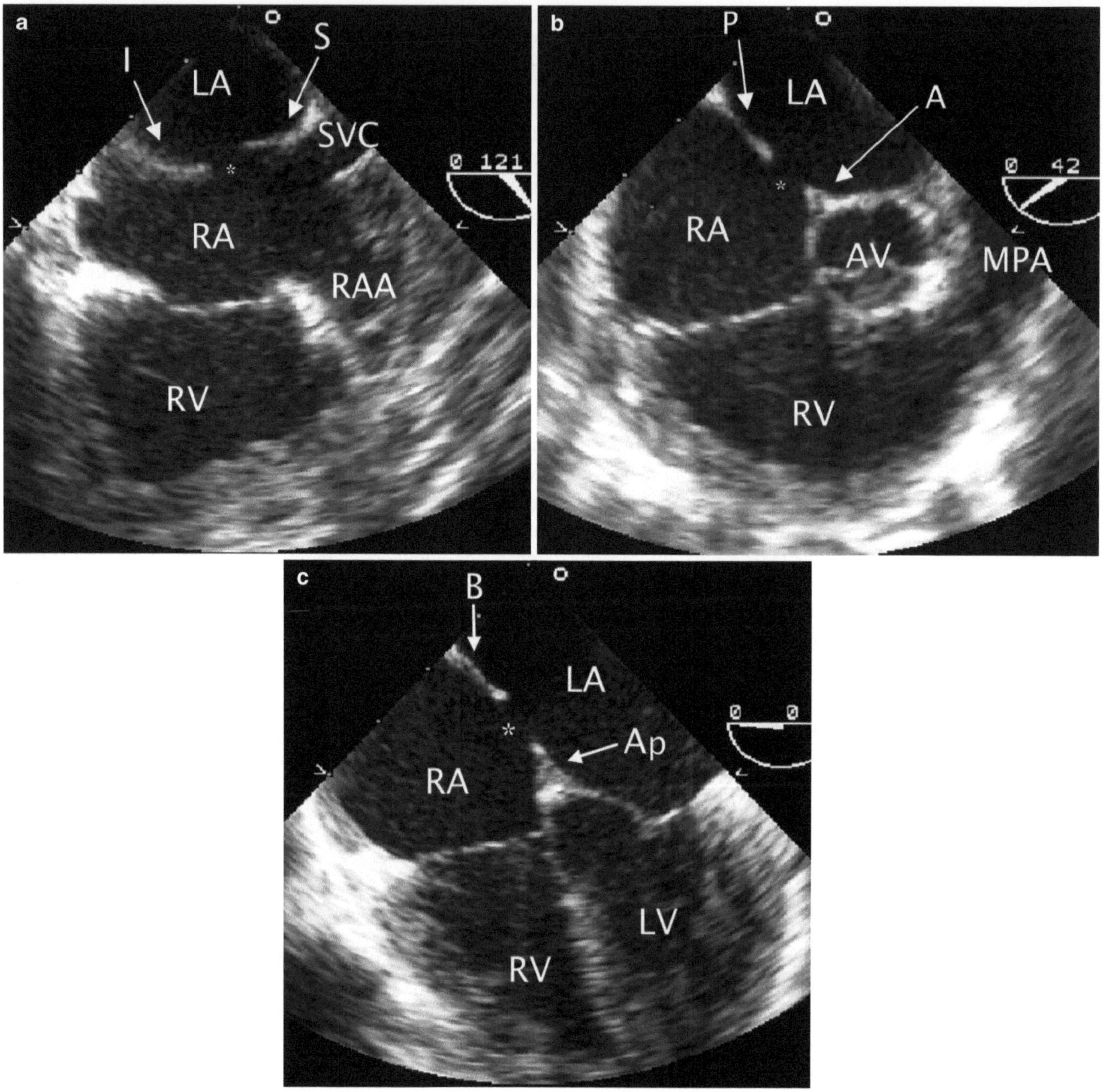

Fig. 17.2 Rims of secundum atrial septal defect (ASD). The rims of a secundum ASD are characterized in multiple TEE views. (**a**) Mid esophageal bicaval view with leftwards probe shaft rotation to display the superior (*S*) and inferior (*I*) rims of a secundum ASD (*asterisk*). (**b**) In a mid esophageal aortic valve short axis view, the anterior (*A*) and posterior (*P*) rims of the defect (*asterisk*) are seen. (**c**) Mid esophageal four chamber view is shown demonstrating the basal (*B*) and apical (*Ap*) rims of the defect (*asterisk*). *AV* aortic valve, *LA* Left atrium, *LV* left ventricle, *MPA* main pulmonary artery, *RA* right atrium, *RAA* right atrial appendage, *RV* right ventricle, *SVC* superior vena cava

Table 17.1 Transesophageal echocardiography during trancatheter occlusion of atrial septal defect

Baseline complete TEE study to survey the defect and exclude additional lesions. Specifically, locate the defect, size and surrounding rims, most importantly the inferior, superior, and posterior rims.
Demonstrate successive guidewire, catheter, sheath, and occluder delivery within the sheath. Suggested imaging planes: mid esophageal four chamber and mid esophageal bicaval views. Additional mid esophageal and deep transgastric views can also be used for complementary imaging.
Demonstrate the deployment, in succession, of the left disc, waist, and right disc with capture of interatrial septum between the right and left discs. Suggested imaging planes: mid esophageal four chamber and mid esophageal bicaval views. Additional mid esophageal views can also be used for complementary imaging.
Two-dimensional and color flow Doppler assessment for any residual shunt or valve injury/encroachment prior to device release.
Repeat of the above after device release to demonstrate adequate device position, absence of residual shunt, venous obstruction, or valve injury.

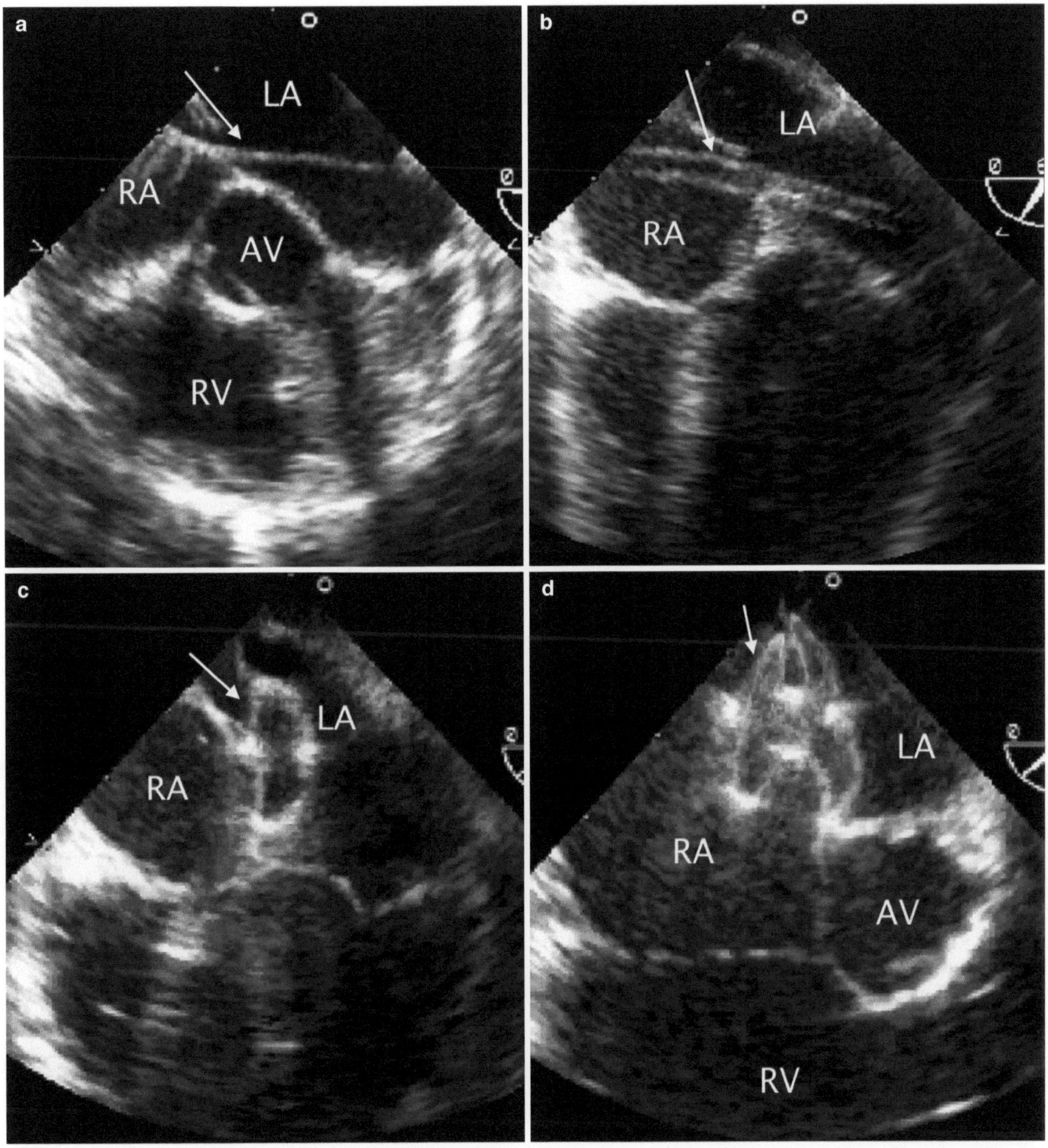

Fig. 17.3 Sequence of transcatheter occlusion of secundum atrial septal defect (ASD). (**a**) TEE image in the mid esophageal aortic valve short axis view demonstrating a guide wire (*arrow*) crossing the interatrial septum through an ASD during transcatheter device occlusion. (**b**) Following guidewire placement across the ASD, well into the left atrium/pulmonary vein, a sheath (*arrow*) is advanced across the ASD as shown in this mid esophageal view. (**c**) After deployment of the left atrial disc of occluder device (*arrow*), (**d**) the right disk (*arrow*) is opened. Note the appearance of the waist between the two discs. (**e**) After the occluder has been released, the position of the device relative to surrounding structures should be evaluated. As demonstrated in this mid esophageal four chamber view, there should be no impingement of the device on the atrioventricular valves. *AV* aortic valve, *LA* Left atrium, *LV* left ventricle, *RA* right atrium, *RV* right ventricle

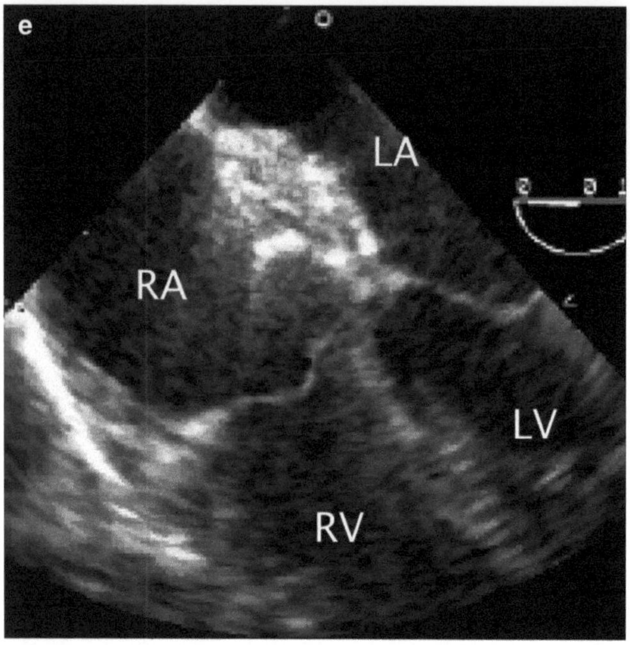

Fig. 17.3 (continued)

fluoroscopy, such as the relationship between the device and the mitral and tricuspid valve leaflets, and thus the use of this imaging modality is beneficial. For multiple defects ("Swiss cheese septum") it is considered that TEE is mandatory to identify the location of the defects, the relationship of these to surrounding structures, and to enhance the overall safety and success of the intervention.

Routine right and left heart catheterization is performed to assess the degree of shunting, evaluate the pulmonary vascular resistance, and to perform angiography to define the location, size, and number of ventricular communications. A complete TEE study is undertaken from the standard imaging locations. The views that allow for assessment of the ventricular septum represent the focus of the examination as described in Chap. 9. Any associated cardiovascular abnormalities should be characterized and gross assessment of chamber size and ventricular function should be made. Specific attention is then paid to the VSD(s) and nearby structures, including the aortic and atrioventricular valves, papillary muscles, moderator band, and chordae tendineae. The atrioventricular valves are interrogated at baseline for any degree of regurgitation.

The appropriate device size is chosen to be 1–2 mm larger than the VSD size as assessed by TEE or angiography at end-diastole (the larger of the two diameter estimates). The next step in the closure sequence is to place a sheath across the defect. This is accomplished in a variety of ways. The most common approach used for mid muscular VSD device closure is to advance a catheter via retrograde catheterization from the left ventricle (LV) across the VSD into the right ventricle (RV). An exchange wire is advanced through the VSD and the RV into either branch pulmonary artery or retrograde through the tricuspid valve into the superior vena cava. In the latter case the wire is then snared and exteriorized through the right internal jugular vein. This provides a stable arteriovenous loop and allows a sheath to be advanced over the wire, from the right jugular vein to the RV and positioned into the LV across the VSD.

Larger mid muscular or apical VSDs can be easily crossed from the RV. However, there is an increased risk of entrapment in the trabeculae of the RV. Once the catheter crosses into the LV, an exchange guide wire is positioned into the LV apex and a delivery sheath is advanced over this wire and positioned into the body of the chamber. TEE and angiography are helpful in guiding device position. The LV disk is deployed in the middle of the LV cavity. Then, the entire assembly (cable/sheath) is pulled towards the interventricular septum with further retraction of the sheath to expand the waist within the VSD. Repeat TEE and angiography confirms device position. Assessment of mitral valve function is essential prior to deployment of the RV disk. It is important to assess the device position in multiple planes. Once proper position is confirmed, further retraction of the sheath to expand the RV disk is performed. Again, prior to device release, repeat TEE and angiography are performed. After deployment, TEE imaging allows for confirmation of device placement, assessment of residual shunting and/or any obstruction or regurgitation induced by the device. With release of the device and elimination of all tension, the device orientation frequently changes, which allows it to align with the ventricular septum. If there are any additional defects, they are occluded in similar fashion. A summary of the steps for transcatheter muscular VSD occlusion with suggested TEE imaging is provided in Table 17.2. Corresponding TEE images are shown in Fig. 17.4.

In some cases, due to patient size and associated safety concerns related to percutaneous closure or if the muscular VSD is within the context of additional malformations requiring surgical repair, device closure of the ventricular communication can be achieved in the operating room [28]. An initial complete TEE assessment of the ventricular septum is performed. If the muscular VSD is the only defect, the procedure can be performed even without placement of the cardiopulmonary bypass cannulae; if there are associated malformations requiring cardiopulmonary bypass, cannulation may be performed however bypass is not initiated until after occlusion of the VSD. TEE images for a typical procedure are shown in Fig. 17.5. An 18-gauge needle is used to puncture the right ventricular free wall aiming towards the VSD, as assessed by TEE, which may also be used to demonstrate the indentation over the right ventricular free wall by the needle prior to puncture. A short guide wire is passed through the needle to the VSD into the LV. Over this wire, a proper size sheath and dilator are advanced into the LV. After dilator removal, a proper size device is advanced inside the delivery

Table 17.2 Transesophageal echocardiography during trancatheter occlusion of ventricular septal defect

Baseline complete TEE study to survey the ventricular septal defect and exclude additional lesions. Specifically, locate the defect, size, surrounding rims and whether or not the rims are in close proximity to valves or other structures that may cause potential injury.
Demonstrate successive guidewire, catheter, sheath, and occluder delivery within the sheath. Suggested imaging planes: mid esophageal four chamber, transgastric short axis and occasionally, mid esophageal long axis view.
Demonstrate the deployment, in succession, of the left disc, waist, and right disc with capture of interventricular septum between the right and left discs. Suggested imaging planes: mid esophageal four chamber and transgastric short axis, and occasionally, transgastric long axis and mid esophageal long axis view views.
Two-dimensional and color flow Doppler assessment for any residual shunt or valve injury/encroachment prior to device release.
Repeat the above after device release to demonstrate adequate device position, and absence of residual shunt, venous obstruction, or valve injury.

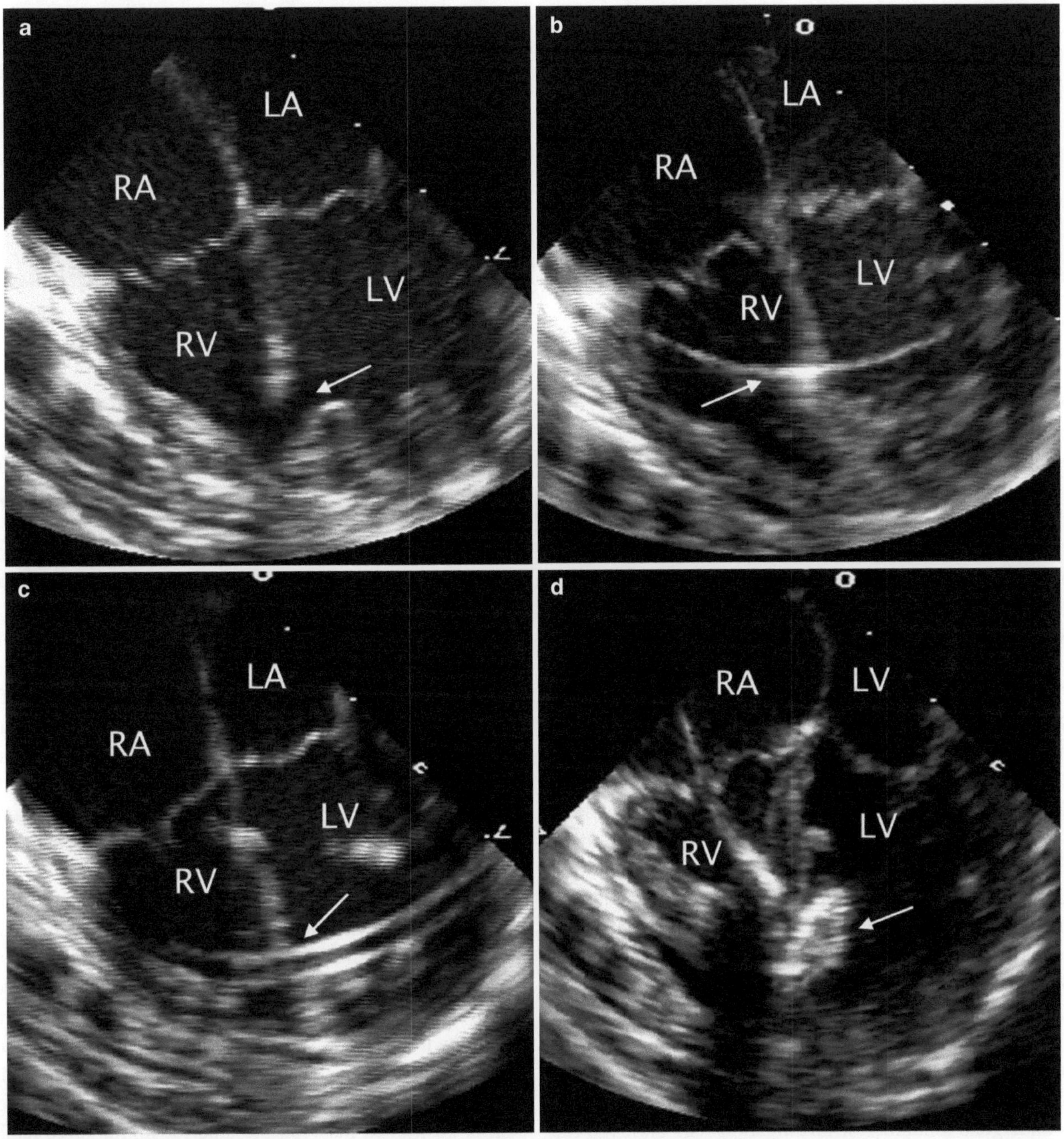

Fig. 17.4 Sequence of transcatheter occlusion of muscular ventricular septal defect (VSD). (**a**) TEE image in the mid esophageal four chamber view demonstrating a muscular VSD (*arrow*) near the apex of the heart. During transcatheter occlusion of the defect the intervention is facilitated by TEE monitoring. The sequential steps in the procedure include: (**b**) guidewire placement across the defect (*arrow*), (**c**) sheath positioning (*arrow*), (**d**) opening of the left disc (*arrow*) of the occluder, and (**e**) subsequent opening of the right disc (*arrow*) followed by release of the device. (**f**) The position of the device after deployment is then assessed. *LA* left atrium, *LV* left ventricle, *RA* right atrium, *RV* right ventricle

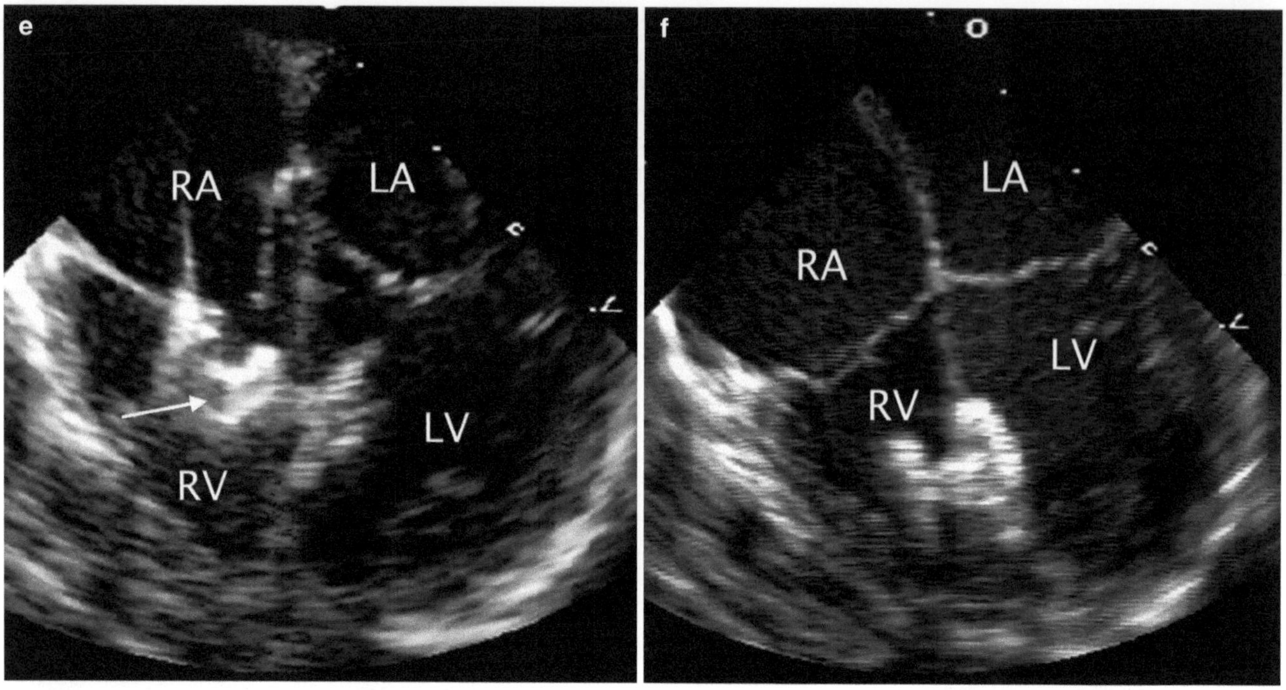

Fig. 17.4 (continued)

sheath under TEE guidance until the left disk is deployed in the LV. The entire assembly (cable and sheath) is then pulled towards the septum, followed by retraction of the sheath over the cable in order to deploy the connecting waist and right disk. If satisfactory position is achieved as documented by TEE, the device is released. The same procedure can be repeated for multiple VSDs. As in the case of closure in the cardiac catheterization laboratory, TEE imaging is performed post device placement to ensure closure of the intracardiac communication. Color Doppler is essential in this assessment for evaluation of residual shunting around the device and for any potential procedural complications. During these interventions, TEE allows for continuous monitoring of cardiac volume and function, and optimization of hemodynamics. It is important to consider that moderate to large defects and co-existent pathology may result in elevated pulmonary artery and right ventricular pressures. Therefore, the post device placement exam should explore not only the potential for residual left-to-right shunting but also right-to-left ventricular level shunting either around the device or through additional VSDs. In some cases, closure of a larger interventricular communication may unmask additional smaller defects.

A device developed specifically for transcatheter membranous VSD closure (Amplatzer membranous VSD occluder; AGA Medical Corporation, Golden Valley, MN) has undergone a number of investigations and although the initial clinical experience was very encouraging [29], this device has been associated with an increased risk of complications, including complete atrioventricular block. A redesigned device has been developed to prevent conduction abnormalities (Amplatzer® membranous VSD occluder 2; St. Jude Medical, St. Paul, MN) and is currently undergoing investigation. As of this writing, this device is not yet approved for clinical use.

In the initial evaluation of the original device, patients weighing more than 8 kg with moderate size and somewhat restrictive perimembranous VSDs (PMVSDs) with indications for closure were considered potential candidates. The presence of a 2 mm or more rim of tissue between the aortic valve and the defect was also considered a prerequisite for device closure as documented by transthoracic echocardiography (TTE) and confirmed by TEE. It is emphasized that echocardiography plays an essential role in delineating the exact location of the VSD and suitability for device closure.

Similar to the closure of muscular VSDs, the procedure is performed under general endotracheal anesthesia with continuous TEE guidance. Using a catheter over a wire technique, the VSD is crossed in a retrograde fashion from the aorta to the LV to the RV. The wire is then brought down and exteriorized out the femoral vein. A sheath is then advanced over the wire from the femoral vein into the ascending aorta, traversing the VSD. This is then pulled back until the sheath tip is in the LV apex aided by a catheter. The VSD occluder is then advanced into the sheath and out into the LV. The left disk is positioned between the anterior mitral valve leaflet and the left ventricular outflow tract. TEE is essential in this procedure to ensure that the mitral valve apparatus is not entangled with the left disk. The entire assembly is withdrawn

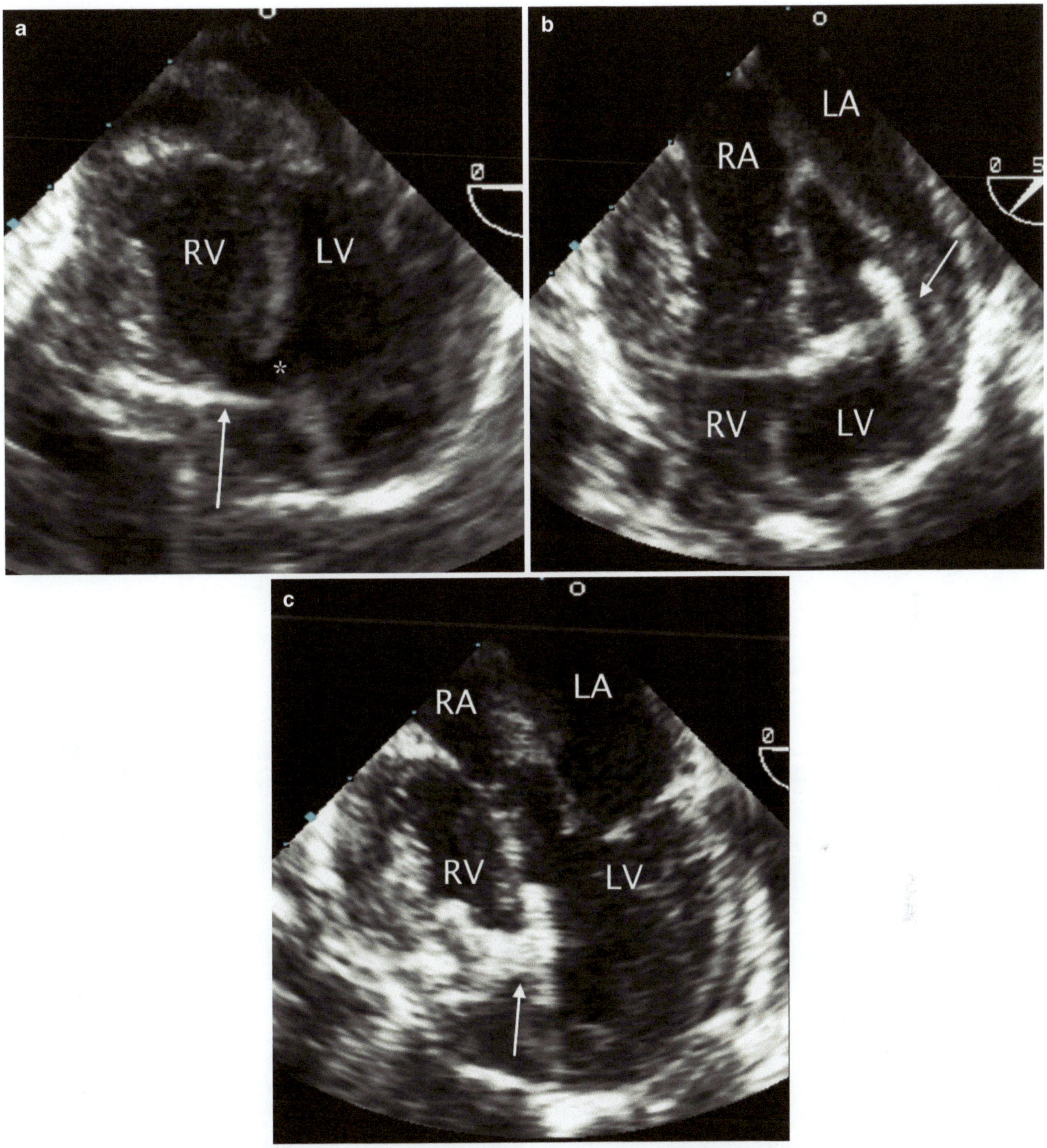

Fig. 17.5 Perventricular, hybrid closure of ventricular septal defect (VSD). Mid esophageal four chamber view demonstrating the sequence of events associated with perventricular closure of a muscular VSD in the operating room as a hybrid approach by the interventionalist and surgeon. Following sternotomy, the right ventricular free wall is exposed. (**a**) Indentation of the RV free wall and needle puncture (*arrow*) near a muscular VSD (*asterisk*). (**b**) Following wire and sheath placement into the left ventricle the occluder device is advanced and the left disc of the occluder (*arrow*) is delivered. (**c**) After opening of the right ventricular disk the position of the device is documented and the device is released. Note the appearance of the occluder waist (*arrow*) at the defect and the minimal space for the right ventricular disc. *LA* left atrium, *LV* left ventricle, *RA* right atrium, *RV* right ventricle

towards the septum. This can be monitored by TEE and confirmed by left ventricular angiography. The waist of the device is then deployed while also aligning the left disk appropriately by fluoroscopy. The right disk can then be deployed after confirmation of adequate device position. Prior to disengagement, proper device position is again verified. The final step is to release the device. TEE is important to exclude entrapment of the device by the atrioventricular valve apparatus, aortic valve injury or encroachment. Once the device is released, repeat TEE and angiography are performed to assess the final result in terms of device position, residual shunting, and to evaluate atrioventricular and aortic valve function. Serial TEE imaging during transcatheter closure of a PMVSD is shown in Fig. 17.6.

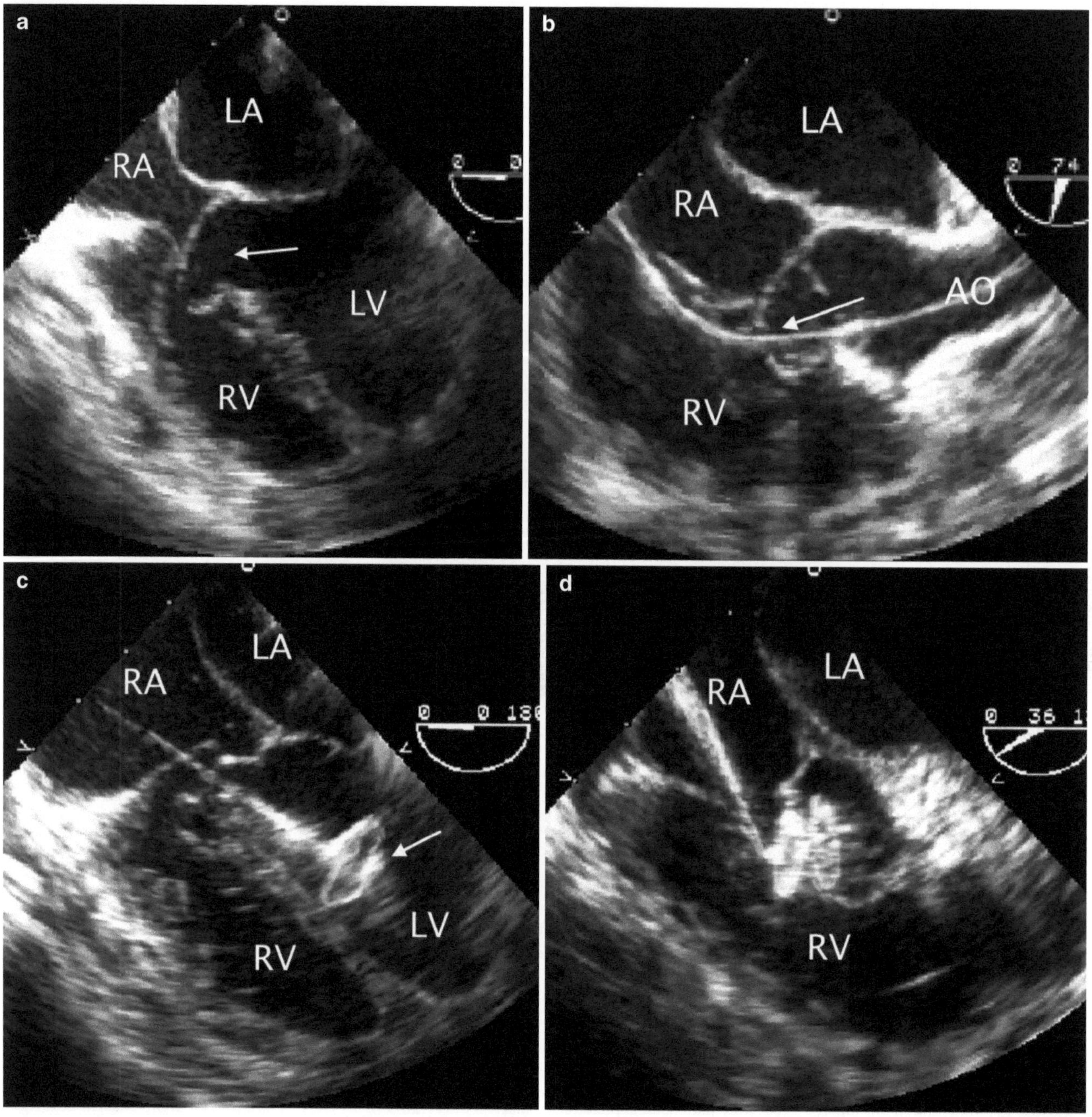

Fig. 17.6 Transcatheter perimembranous ventricular septal defect (VSD) occlusion. (**a**) Mid esophageal four chamber view of a perimembranous VSD (*arrow*). Note the tricuspid valve pouch formation (tricuspid valve aneurysmal tissue) surrounding the VSD. (**b**) Mid esophageal right ventricular inflow-outflow view (composite image) showing a guidewire crossing the VSD (*arrow*) during transcatheter device occlusion. (**c**) Mid esophageal four chamber view with probe anteflexion displaying opening of the left-sided disc (*arrow*) of the VSD device at the mid left ventricular region. (**d**) The device has been pulled towards the defect and the right ventricular disc has been opened. (**e**) Mid esophageal four chamber view (with anteflexion to view portions of the left ventricular outflow tract) after release of the VSD occluder (*arrow*). It may appear in this still frame as if the occluder is entrapping the septal leaflet of the tricuspid valve, however, this represents tricuspid pouch (tricuspid valve tissue) that was partially occluding the VSD as shown in Fig. 17.6a. *AO* aorta, *LA* left atrium, *LV* left ventricle, *RA* right atrium, *RV* right ventricle

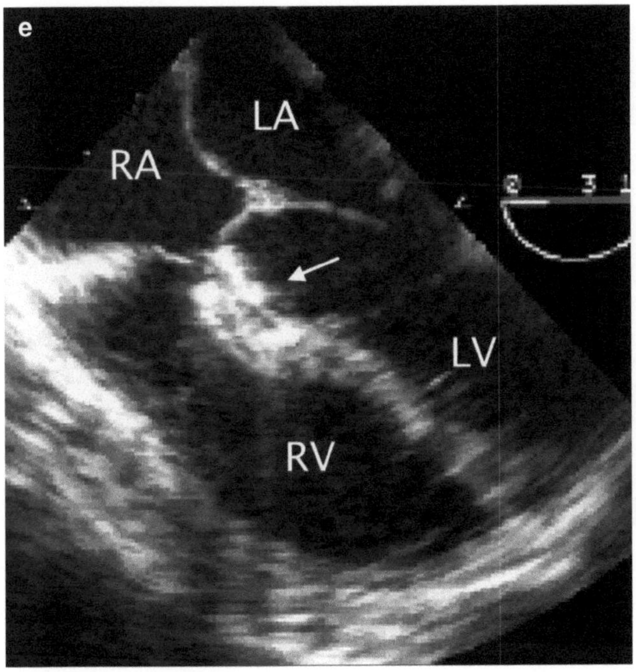

Fig. 17.6 (continued)

Creation or Enlargement of Atrial Communication

Creation or enlargement of an interatrial communication may be required in patients with the following: transposition physiology (to enhance mixing), severe inflow restriction to one of the ventricles (either due to inflow obstruction, ventricular hypoplasia, or outflow obstruction not amenable to relief), severe left ventricular dysfunction, or in patients with severe pulmonary vascular disease [14, 30–33]. Balloon atrial septostomy has been traditionally performed under fluoroscopic guidance [34]. However, echocardiographic monitoring has offered the ability to display pertinent anatomic structures, and this in principle should decrease the risk of the procedure. Bedside balloon atrial septostomy using TTE has been well described [30, 31]. Most centers use fluoroscopy, TTE, or both for procedural guidance. TEE has also been applied in this setting and offers the benefit of continuous monitoring while maintaining a sterile field and avoiding interference with the intervention [1, 2, 9]. TEE may be particularly useful when attempting to create or enlarge an interatrial communication in individuals with unusual anatomy or small atria [14].

Similar to closure of ASDs, TEE is initially utilized to confirm the anatomy and disclose any new anatomic, hemodynamic or other important findings (e.g., thrombus in a patient with severe myocardial dysfunction). After this assessment, it is used to guide wire and catheter placement, demonstrate balloon position and the appearance of the latter prior to the septostomy. It can then be used to monitor the actual procedure and adequacy of the result. Based on the information acquired it can be determined whether or not the procedure needs to be repeated, modified, or abandoned.

The typical views used include the ME 4 Ch view (to image the atrial septum, atria and atrioventricular valves), as well as the ME Bicaval view to demonstrate the interatrial septum, caval veins, and atrial appendages in an orthogonal plane. Rapid, frequent alternations amongst these two planes, as well as modified planes, are usually required to maintain visualization of the catheter and septostomy balloon. Excellent communication between the echocardiographer and interventionalist is also necessary throughout the procedure to help avoid inadvertent injury to nearby structures or hemodynamic compromise.

In infants with hypoplastic left heart syndrome and an intact atrial septum, an emergent procedure to decompress the left atrium may be undertaken in the cardiac catheterization laboratory under combined TEE and fluoroscopic guidance. Echocardiographic imaging is particularly helpful to document when the radiofrequency catheter creates a perforation across the interatrial septum (Chap. 7). The remainder of the intervention is aimed at creating an adequate outlet for the left atrium by balloon/blade atrial septostomy or balloon dilation of the perforation.

In cases where a septostomy procedure is (a) unsuccessful, (b) determined likely to be so, or (c) not considered the most favorable approach, a stent may be placed across the interatrial septum and balloon dilated to achieve a similar result. This might be necessary, for example, in young infants with a thick interatrial septum or small atria, who are felt to be at significant high risk for blade septostomy. The procedure is similar to that described above for creation of an ASD, with similar imaging planes. In the case of stent deployment, followed by balloon dilation of the stent, these procedures are monitored instead (Fig. 17.7).

Figure 17.8 displays another application of TEE related to the atrial septum. The representative images illustrate transseptal catheterization during placement of a left ventricular vent.

Closure of Fontan Fenestrations or Baffle Leaks

The use of transcatheter occlusion techniques to close fenestrations or baffle leaks in a Fontan connection has been well described [19]. Representative TEE images of this sequence are demonstrated in Fig. 17.9. Although TEE has been shown to be of benefit during these interventions, in some cases the procedures have been performed only with fluoroscopy and angiography. However patients with unusual or complicated cardiac anatomy can present unique challenges, making TEE a requirement for procedural guidance. This may also be the case in settings in which precise intracardiac anatomic information

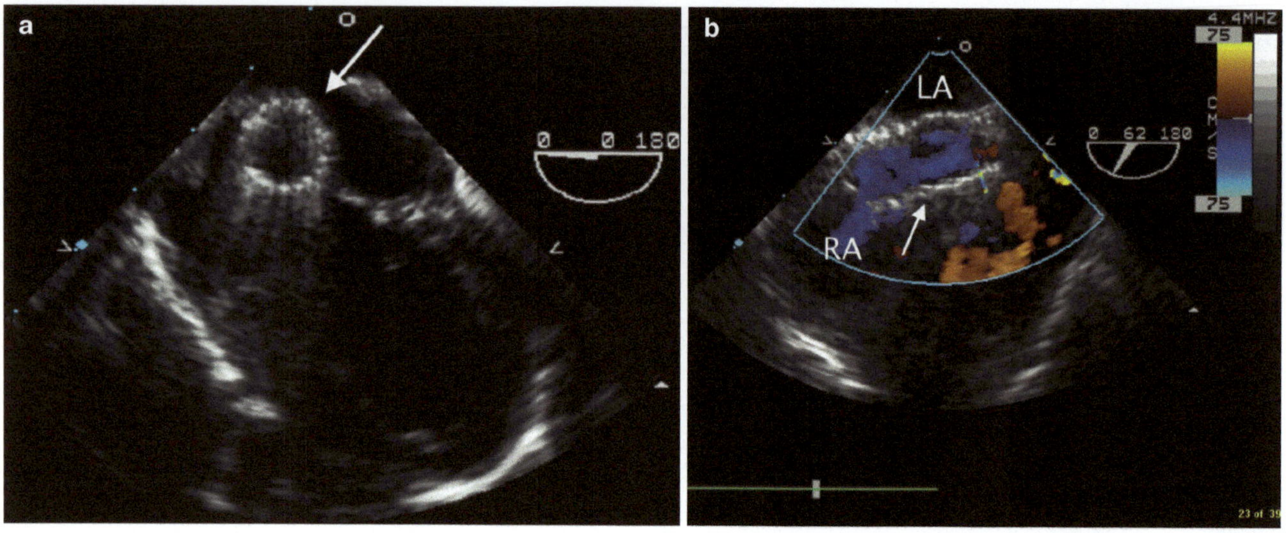

Fig. 17.7 Placement of interatrial septal stent. Mid esophageal four chamber view demonstrating a stent (*arrow*) across the interatrial septum in a patient with mitral atresia and an intact atrial septum. In this view, the appropriate position of the stent cannot be fully confirmed (**a**). By using a complementary view at an angle of 62° (**b**), the stent is seen in its long axis (*arrow*) crossing the interatrial septum and color Doppler confirms flow across the stent from the left atrium (*LA*) into the right atrium (*RA*)

is necessary (for example, if the leak is near a margin of the patch closure of an atrioventricular valve) [19].

TEE has also been useful in guiding pre and post operative hemodynamics with purse string closure of a Fontan fenestration [1]. For both leaks and fenestrations, the use of a biplane or multiplane TEE probe has allowed visualization of the anatomy in two or more planes to provide the interventionist a better understanding of the three-dimensional anatomical relation and how to conduct the procedure. The primary imaging planes used are the ME 4 Ch and ME Bicaval views. Frequent alternation between these two views allows the echocardiographer to visualize the structures of interest and help guide the procedure. Modifications of these planes are frequently required with varying locations of the defect. The goal of TEE imaging is to display the defect perpendicular to the imaging plane in two different viewing angles, to ensure appropriate deployment of an occluder device.

Other intra-atrial baffle leaks, namely, those involving Senning and Mustard connections can be approached in a similar fashion using views such as those shown in Fig. 17.10.

TEE for Guidance of Dilation of Other Congenital Heart Lesions

Pathology associated with intracardiac baffles (Fontan, Senning, Mustard, Rastelli) is adequately visualized by angiography (similar to valve dilation procedures). However, TEE allows for continuous monitoring of interventions associated with baffle obstruction to help guide wire, balloon, and/or stent to the appropriate area. This has been described in cases of Mustard baffle obstruction [1, 9, 10] as well as obstruction of the left ventricular to aortic pathway in an individual with a history of a prior Rastelli procedure [14]. In addition, because of its excellent imaging of the pulmonary veins, TEE can guide pulmonary vein dilation as has been described previously [34].

Suitable TEE views for enlargement of baffle narrowing are similar to those used for closure of fenestrations and/or leaks, namely the ME 4 Ch and ME Bicaval views, with appropriate use and modification of additional planes as required. These modifications are made to obtain the optimal imaging plane(s), which ideally should longitudinally demonstrate the area of narrowing. Complementary deep transgastric views may be helpful.

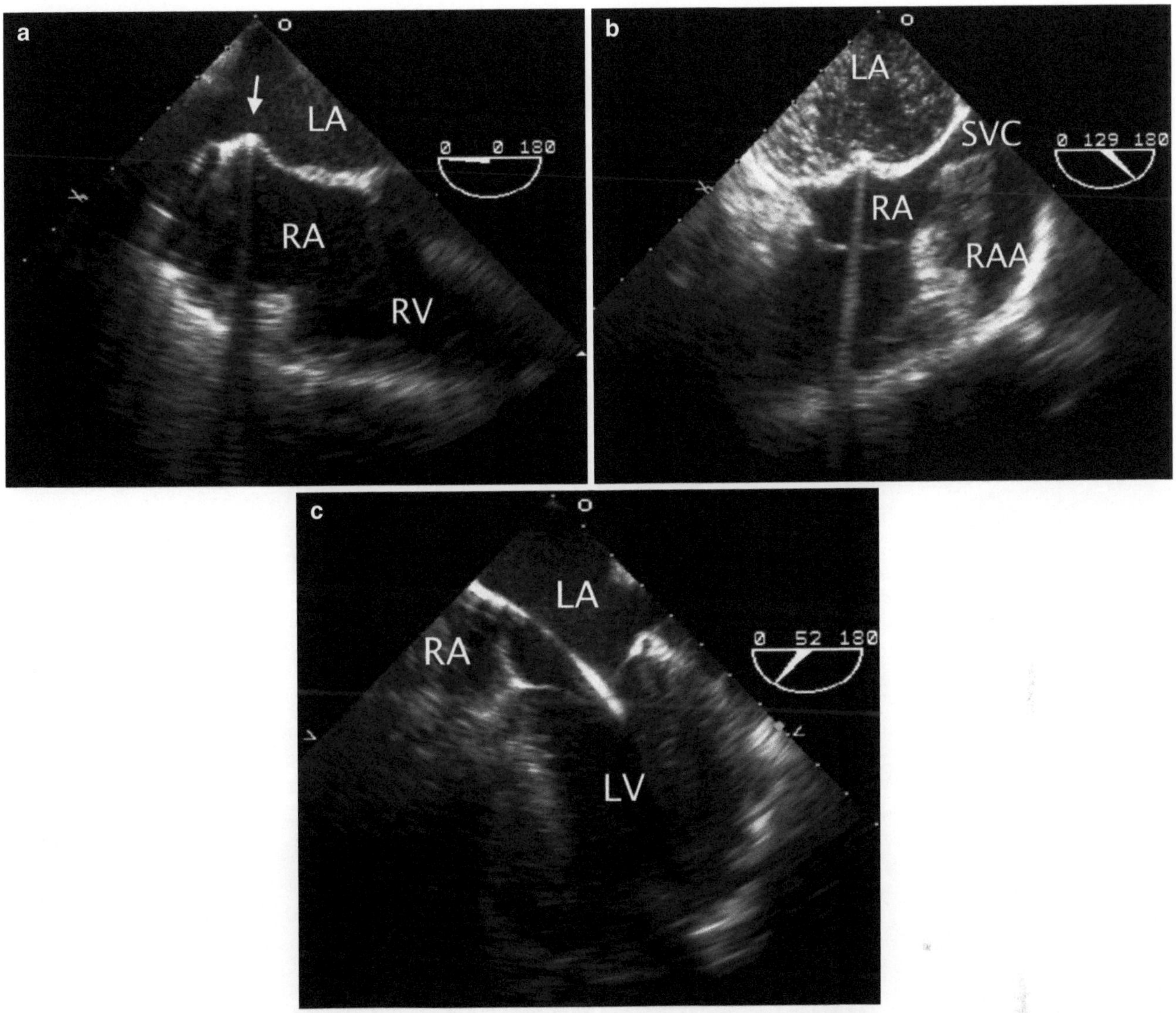

Fig. 17.8 Placement of left ventricular venting catheter. (**a**) Mid esophageal four chamber view with attention to the interatrial septum to demonstrate indentation of the interatrial septum (*arrow*) towards the left atrium by a needle prior to transseptal puncture. (**b**) In a modified mid esophageal bicaval view, injection of agitated saline creates a "bubble" contrast to confirm position of a catheter tip within the left atrium prior to further interventions. (**c**) Mid esophageal view demonstrating placement of a left ventricular venting catheter through the interatrial septum and across the mitral valve into the left ventricle. *LA* left atrium, *LV* left ventricle, RA right atrium, *RAA* right atrial appendage, *RV* right ventricle, *SVC* superior vena cava

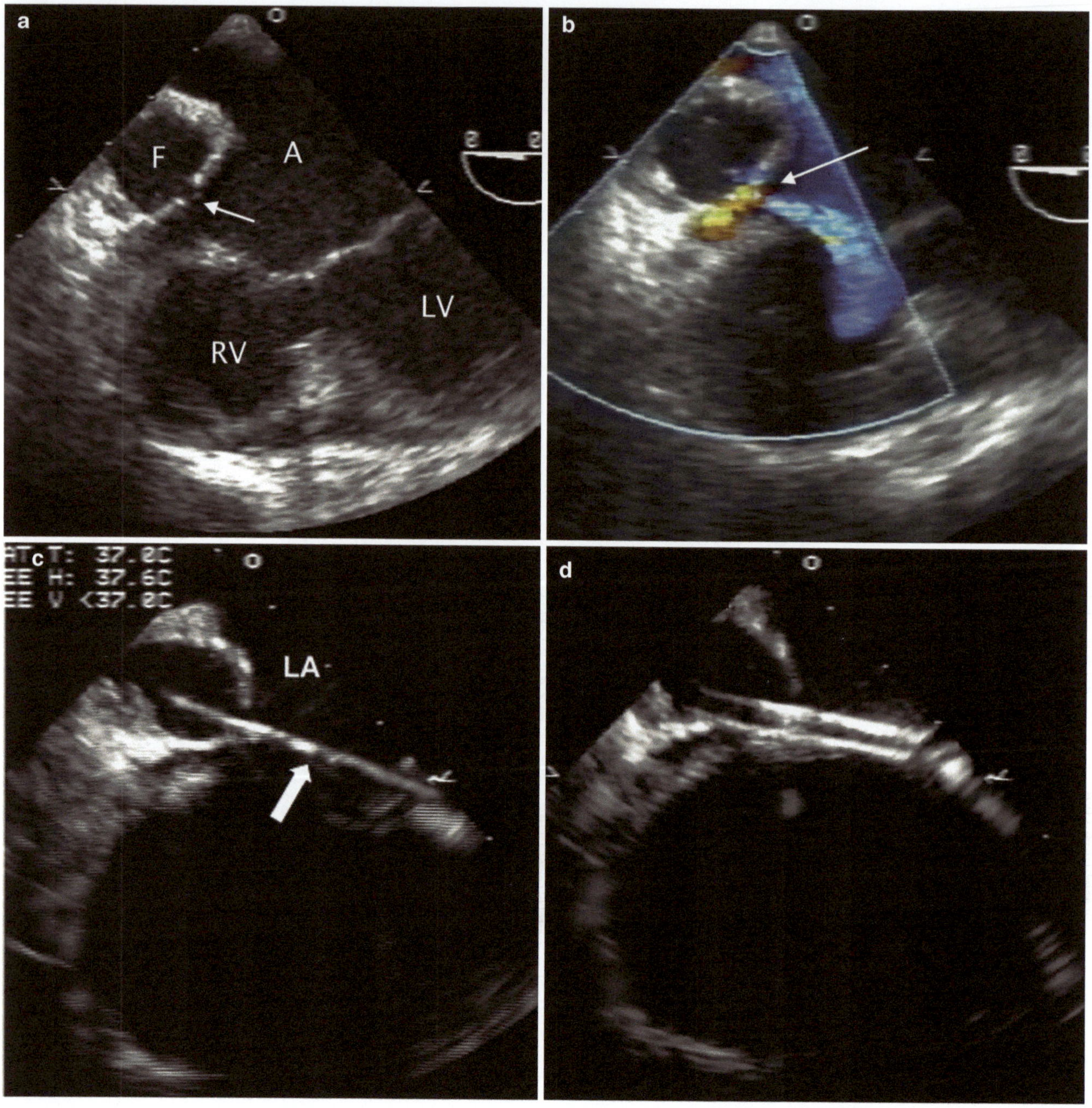

Fig. 17.9 Occlusion of Fontan fenestration. (**a**) Mid esophageal four chamber two-dimensional imaging demonstrating a Fontan fenestration (*arrow*) in a patient with an unbalanced atrioventricular septal defect, status post lateral tunnel Fontan (*F*) procedure. (**b**) Corresponding color Doppler interrogation demonstrates right-to-left shunting across the fenestration (blue jet noted by *arrow*) allowing for egress of blood from the systemic venous side of the Fontan baffle to the pulmonary venous circulation as blood enters the common atrium. The steps during Amplatzer® device occlusion of the Fontan fenestration as monitored by transesophageal imaging are illustrated as follows: (**c**) guide wire across fenestration in the lateral tunnel (*arrow*); (**d**) sheath across the defect; (**e**) device being advanced over fenestration; (**f**) post device release; (**g**) color Doppler interrogation post Amplatzer® occluder device placement demonstrating no residual shunting across the fenestration. *A* pulmonary venous atrium (functional left atrium, *LA*), *LV* left ventricle, *RV* right ventricle

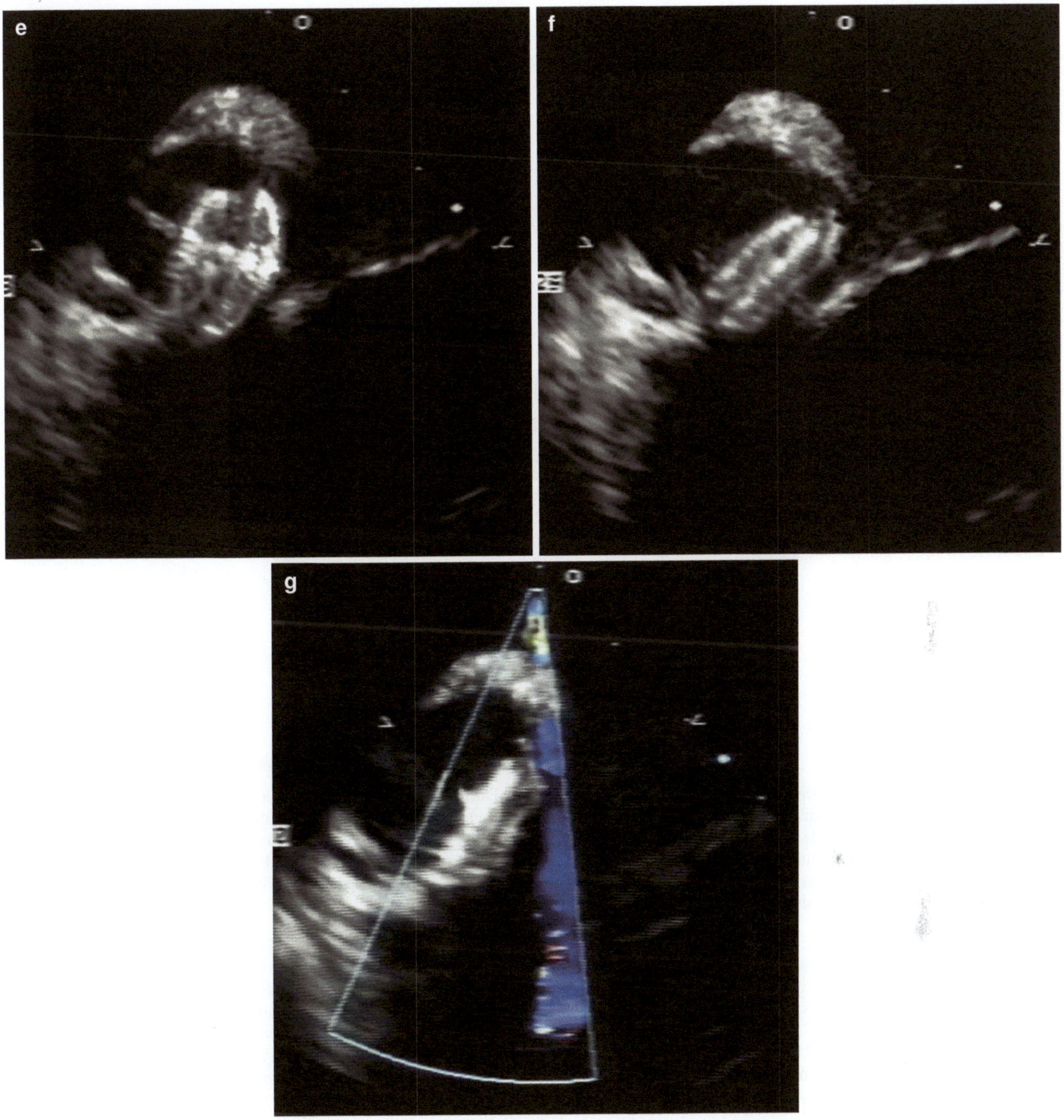

Fig. 17.9 (continued)

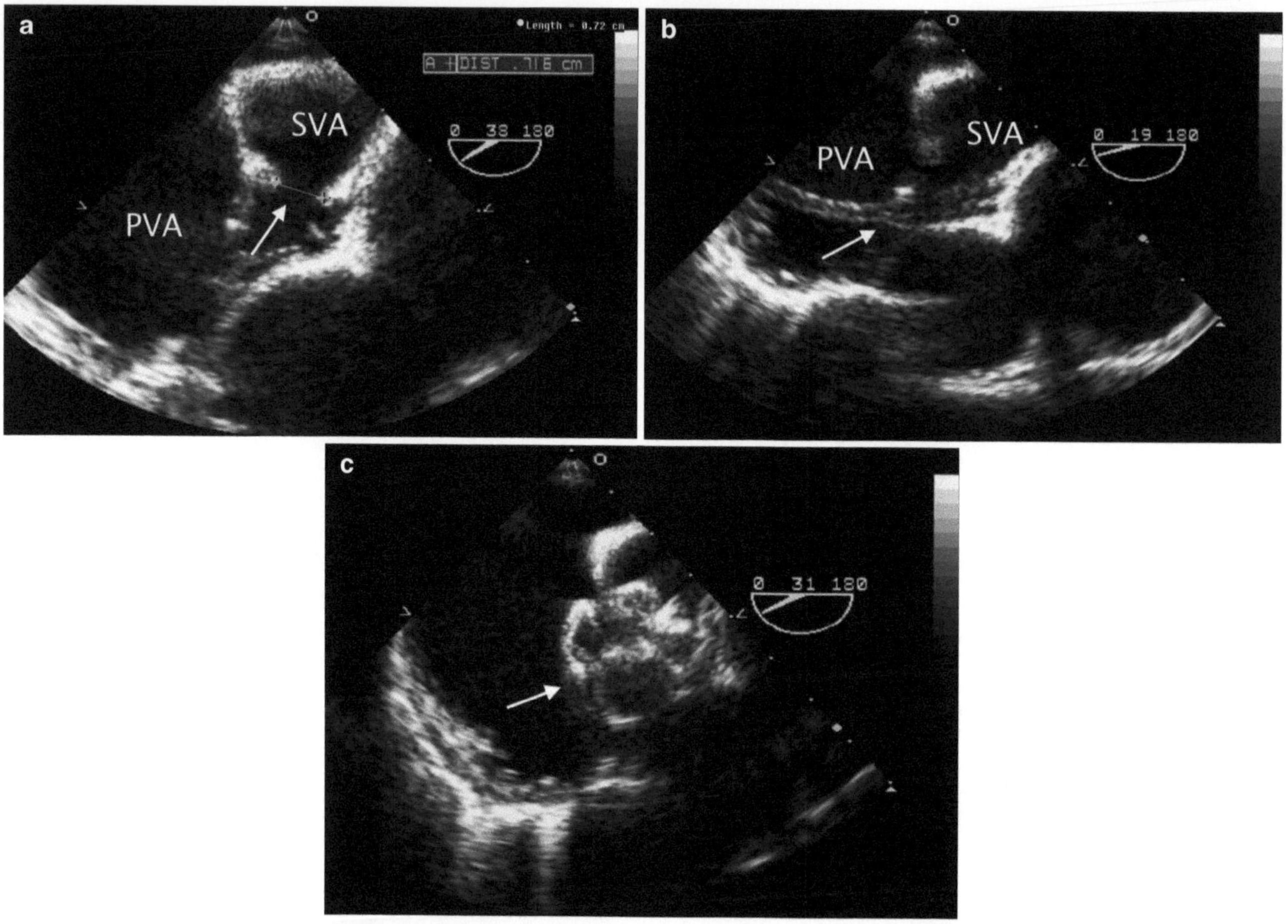

Fig. 17.10 Occlusion of baffle leak following Mustard atrial baffle procedure. (**a**) TEE imaging in a mid esophageal modified view demonstrating a defect in the atrial baffle (*arrow*) that divides the systemic venous atrium (*SVA*) from the pulmonary venous atrium (*PVA*) in a patient with d-transposition of the great arteries following a prior Mustard operation. The defect measures approximately 7.2 mm. (**b**) During occlusion of the defect a sheath is placed across this region (*arrow*), to allow for the delivery shaft that carries the occluder to be advanced into the pulmonary venous atrium. (**c**) Following occlusion of the leak using an Amplatzer® atrial septal defect occluder (*arrow*) the position of the device is documented

Summary

This chapter has provided an overview of the use of TEE during catheter-based interventions in the cardiac catheterization laboratory, operating room setting, and electrophysiologic studies. The benefits of TEE in providing procedural guidance, assessing the success of interventions, identifying complications, and overall enhancing the safety of the procedures, have been highlighted to document the applications of this imaging approach during interventions for CHD.

References

1. Douglas DE, Fyfe DA. Use of miniature biplane transesophageal echocardiography during pediatric atrial catheter interventional procedures. Am Heart J. 1996;132:179–86.
2. van der Velde ME, Perry SB, Sanders SP. Transesophageal echocardiography with color Doppler during interventional catheterization. Echocardiography. 1991;8:721–30.
3. Tumbarello R, Sanna A, Cardu G, et al. Usefulness of transesophageal echocardiography in the pediatric catheterization laboratory. Am J Cardiol. 1993;71:1321–5.
4. Ayres NA, Miller-Hance W, Fyfe DA, et al. Indications and guidelines for performance of transesophageal echocardiography in the patient with pediatric acquired or congenital heart disease: report from the task force of the Pediatric Council of the American Society of Echocardiography. J Am Soc Echocardiogr. 2005;18:91–8.
5. Bengur AR, Li JS, Herlong JR, et al. Intraoperative transesophageal echocardiography in congenital heart disease. Semin Thorac Cardiovasc Surg. 1998;10:255–64.
6. Stevenson JG. Role of intraoperative transesophageal echocardiography during repair of congenital cardiac defects. Acta Paediatr Suppl. 1995;410:23–33.
7. Randolph GR, Hagler DJ, Connolly HM, et al. Intraoperative transesophageal echocardiography during surgery for congenital heart defects. J Thorac Cardiovasc Surg. 2002;124:1176–82.
8. Khalid O, Koenig P. The use of echocardiography in congenital heart surgery and intervention. Expert Rev Cardiovasc Ther. 2006;4:263–71.

9. Stumper O, Witsenburg M, Sutherland GR, et al. Transesophageal echocardiographic monitoring of interventional cardiac catheterization in children. J Am Coll Cardiol. 1991;18:1506–14.
10. Tong AD, Rothman A, Shiota T, et al. Interventional cardiac catheterization under transesophageal echocardiographic guidance. Am Heart J. 1995;129:827–31.
11. Cheung YF, Leung MP, Lee J, et al. An evolving role of transesophageal echocardiography for the monitoring of interventional catheterization in children. Clin Cardiol. 1999;22:804–10.
12. Walayat M, Cooper SG, Sholler GF. Transesophageal echocardiographic guidance of blade atrial septostomy in children. Catheter Cardiovasc Interv. 2001;52:200–2.
13. Mahajan A, Shabanie A, Laks H. Interatrial septostomy under transesophageal echocardiography guidance: a novel approach. J Thorac Cardiovasc Surg. 2002;123:824–6.
14. van der Velde ME, Perry SB. Transesophageal echocardiography during interventional catheterization in congenital heart disease. Echocardiography. 1997;14:513–28.
15. Rigby ML. Transoesophageal echocardiography during interventional cardiac catheterisation in congenital heart disease. Heart. 2001;86 Suppl 2:II23–9.
16. Mazic U, Gavora P, Masura J. The role of transesophageal echocardiography in transcatheter closure of secundum atrial septal defects by the Amplatzer septal occluder. Am Heart J. 2001;142:482–8.
17. van der Velde ME, Sanders SP, Keane JF, et al. Transesophageal echocardiographic guidance of transcatheter ventricular septal defect closure. J Am Coll Cardiol. 1994;23:1660–5.
18. Carminati M, Butera G, Chessa M, et al. Transcatheter closure of congenital ventricular septal defect with Amplatzer septal occluders. Am J Cardiol. 2005;96:52L–8.
19. Moore JW, Murdison KA, Baffa GM, et al. Transcatheter closure of fenestrations and excluded hepatic veins after fontan: versatility of the Amplatzer device. Am Heart J. 2000;140:534–40.
20. Goldman AP, Irwin JM, Glover MU, et al. Transesophageal echocardiography to improve positioning of radiofrequency ablation catheters in left-sided Wolff-Parkinson-White syndrome. Pacing Clin Electrophysiol. 1991;14:1245–50.
21. Kantoch MJ, Frost GF. Robertson MA Use of transesophageal echocardiography in radiofrequency catheter ablation in children and adolescents. Can J Cardiol. 1998;14(4):519–23.
22. Tucker KJ, Curtis AB, Murphy J, et al. Transesophageal echocardiographic guidance of transseptal left heart catheterization during radiofrequency ablation of left-sided accessory pathways in humans. Pacing Clin Electrophysiol. 1996;19:272–81.
23. Drant SE, Klitzner TS, Shannon KM, et al. Guidance of radiofrequency catheter ablation by transesophageal echocardiography in children with palliated single ventricle. Am J Cardiol. 1995;76:1311–2.
24. Hatala R, Weiss C, Koschyk DH, et al. Radiofrequency catheter ablation of left atrial tachycardia originating within the pulmonary vein in a patient with dextrocardia. Pacing Clin Electrophysiol. 1996;19:999–1002.
25. Spevak PJ, Bass JL, Ben-Shachar G, et al. Balloon angioplasty for congenital mitral stenosis. Am J Cardiol. 1990;66:472–6.
26. Ludomirsky A. The use of echocardiography in pediatric interventional cardiac catheterization procedures. J Interv Cardiol. 1995;8:569–78.
27. Koenig PR, Abdulla RI, Cao QL, et al. Use of intracardiac echocardiography to guide catheter closure of atrial communications. Echocardiography. 2003;20:781–7.
28. Diab KA, Hijazi ZM, Cao QL, et al. A truly hybrid approach to perventricular closure of multiple muscular ventricular septal defects. J Thorac Cardiovasc Surg. 2005;130:892–3.
29. Holzer R, de Giovanni J, Walsh KP, et al. Transcatheter closure of perimembranous ventricular septal defects using the amplatzer membranous VSD occluder: immediate and midterm results of an international registry. Catheter Cardiovasc Interv. 2006;68:620–8.
30. Perry LW, Ruckman RN, Galioto Jr FM, Shapiro SR, Potter BM, Scott 3rd LP. Echocardiographically assisted balloon atrial septostomy. Pediatrics. 1982;70(3):403–8.
31. Koenig PR, Ralston MA, Kimball TR, et al. Balloon atrial septostomy for left ventricular decompression in patients receiving extracorporeal membrane oxygenation for myocardial failure. J Pediatr. 1993;122:S95–9.
32. Seib PM, Faulkner SC, Erickson CC, et al. Blade and balloon atrial septostomy for left heart decompression in patients with severe ventricular dysfunction on extracorporeal membrane oxygenation. Catheter Cardiovasc Interv. 1999;46:179–86.
33. Johnston TA, Jaggers J, McGovern JJ, et al. Bedside transseptal balloon dilation atrial septostomy for decompression of the left heart during extracorporeal membrane oxygenation. Catheter Cardiovasc Interv. 1999;46:197–9.
34. Yoshii S, Matsukawa T, Nishida K, et al. Transesophageal echo-guided balloon dilatation for postoperative pulmonary venous obstruction. Surg Today. 1994;24:666–8.

Transesophageal Echocardiography in Adults with Congenital Heart Disease

18

Jamil A. Aboulhosn and John S. Child

Abstract

Significant medical and surgical advances over the past several decades have dramatically altered the care of patients with congenital heart disease (CHD). In the current era, most affected children survive into adulthood. This has resulted in a growing population of adults or "grown-up" patients with CHD, while this patient group continues to increase further. Transesophageal echocardiography (TEE) represents an important diagnostic tool in the management of adults with CHD. In addition, this modality plays an important role during catheter-based and surgical interventions in this patient group. With continuous evolution of and further refinements in technologies applicable to the cardiovascular system, TEE is likely to remain a key imaging modality in the adult patient with CHD.

Keywords

Adult congenital heart disease • Grown-up congenital heart disease • Transesophageal echocardiography • Imaging in the adult with structural heart disease

Introduction

Surgical and medical advances over the past 60 years have dramatically altered the care of patients with congenital heart disease (CHD). In the current era, over 85 % of patients with CHD survive to reach adulthood [1]. From 1940 to 2002, nearly 1.5 million patients with CHD were born in the United States, of these, it is estimated that over 800,000 individuals have survived to reach adulthood [2, 3]. Adults with CHD are more likely than the general population to give birth to infants with CHD, therefore, the number of affected individuals is expected to further increase. Many patients have undergone surgical interventions that were thought to be curative. However, the concept of a surgical 'cure' for CHD is a common misconception as it has been pointed out that with the exception of early ligation of a patent ductus arteriosus, there is no surgical 'cure' for CHD without operative sequelae or possible need for reoperation [4]. This chapter addresses the applications of transesophageal echocardiographic imaging in the adult population with CHD.

Echocardiographic Imaging in the Adult with Congenital Heart Disease

Transthoracic (TTE) and transesophageal (TEE) echocardiography are important diagnostic modalities in the management of adults with CHD [5, 6]. For an adequate

J.A. Aboulhosn, MD (✉)
Departments of Medicine and Pediatrics, David Geffen School of Medicine at UCLA, 650 Charles Young Drive, Los Angeles, CA 90095, USA
e-mail: jaboulhosn@mednet.ucla.edu

J.S. Child, MD
Department of Medicine, David Geffen School of Medicine at UCLA, 650 Charles Young Drive, Los Angeles, CA 90095, USA

The online version of this chapter (doi:10.1007/978-1-84800-064-3_18) contains supplementary material, which is available to authorized users.

P.C. Wong, W.C. Miller-Hance (eds.), *Transesophageal Echocardiography for Congenital Heart Disease*, DOI 10.1007/978-1-84800-064-3_18, © Springer-Verlag London 2014

Table 18.1 Cognitive skills required for the transesophageal echocardiographic evaluation of adults with congenital heart disease

Knowledge and application of the segmental anatomic approach
Knowledge of the spectrum of individual congenital cardiovascular lesions, including common and unusual associated abnormalities
Understanding of the natural history of congenital heart disease, residua, and expected sequelae
Understanding of the dynamic nature of cardiovascular defects
Familiarity with the various surgical and transcatheter interventions available for patient management
Understanding of the effect of adult acquired heart disease on congenital pathology

assessment of the patient with CHD the echocardiographer must understand the following (Table 18.1) [7]:

1. native anatomy and physiology
2. how these change over time
3. types of surgical or transcatheter intervention(s) that may have been performed or for which the patient may be considered a candidate
4. expected postoperative sequelae and residua
5. potential postoperative short and long-term changes and complications
6. influence of adult acquired diseases on underlying congenital malformation or postoperative anatomy and function

A systematic segmental analysis as discussed in Chap. 4 is essential for the echocardiographic evaluation of CHD. This analysis, in most cases performed during childhood, involves determination of atrial and ventricular situs, atrioventricular and ventriculoarterial connections, and the relationship of the great arteries to each other.

The advent and widespread availability of multiplane probes has improved the efficiency and ease of TEE in patients with CHD in general, but particularly those with complex malformations [7]. Imaging the adult with repaired or unrepaired complex CHD is often challenging given the often unusual location and orientation of the heart and extracardiac vessels. The examiner must locate pertinent anatomical structures and align the imaging plane to obtain optimal visualization of anatomy and flow. Needless to say, this requires an in-depth knowledge of the panoply of operated and unoperated congenital malformations prior to performing the study. Review of prior imaging data, including TTE, chest radiography, cardiac-computed tomography, cardiac angiography, and magnetic resonance imaging, is imperative to understanding the underlying anatomy prior to undertaking TEE.

An operator's innate ability to form a three-dimensional construct of the cardiovascular anatomy in his/her mind and effectively manipulate the TEE probe is essential to acquire the most important images. The full use of two- and three-dimensional echocardiography, color and spectral Doppler, and tissue Doppler facilitates the gathering of important data. It is imperative that "high risk" patients are recognized and managed appropriately when performing TEE (Table 18.2).

Table 18.2 Conditions of increased risk during transesophageal imaging in adult patients

History of cyanotic heart disease with right-to-left shunting *Concerns related to sedatives*: Hypoventilation and increased arterial desaturation Central nervous system/respiratory depression resulting from faster onset of action of intravenous agents Potential acute decreases in systemic vascular resistance leading to hypotension, increased right-to-left shunting, and worsening cyanosis Withdrawal of sympathetic tone augmenting myocardial depression
Hemodynamically unstable patients
Acute myocardial ischemia or infarction
Congestive heart failure
Trauma, if airway, esophagus, neck or oropharynx are involved
History of radiation to the neck and/or chest
History of rheumatoid or juvenile rheumatoid arthritis with cervical spinal involvement
History of scleroderma with esophageal involvement
Large esophageal varices
Elderly patients *Concerns*: Less tolerance for sedatives Cervical spurs may impinge on esophagus Esophageal diverticulum Potential for arrhythmias Coronary artery disease
Obstructive and/or restrictive lung disease
Intubated patients *Concerns*: Endotracheal tube dislodgment Mainstem or endobronchial intubation Probe manipulation may impact mechanical ventilation

Applications of TEE in adults with CHD include the use in the operating room, cardiac catheterization laboratory, electrophysiology laboratory, intensive care units, and other settings [8, 9]. In the operating room, prior to cardiopulmonary bypass, TEE helps refine anatomic diagnosis and may detect previously unsuspected pathology that may require modification of the operative approach (refer to Chap. 15). Once cardiopulmonary bypass is weaned, TEE can be used to evaluate the anatomic, functional, and hemodynamic consequences of the surgical intervention(s). If the initial result

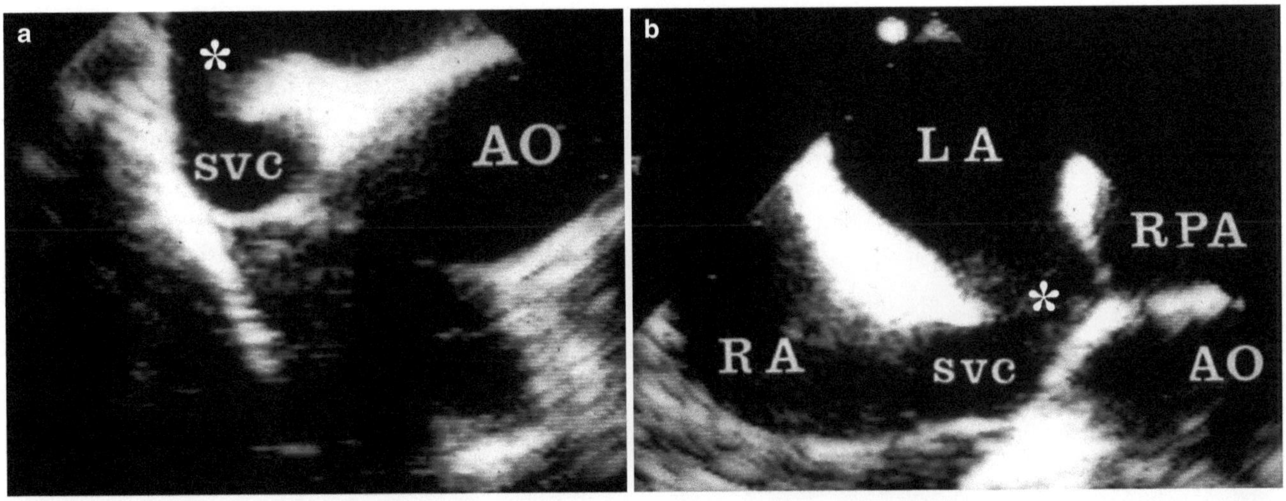

Fig. 18.1 (**a**) Sinus venosus atrial septal defect (*) imaged in the mid esophageal four chamber view with rightwards transducer rotation. (**b**) Mid esophageal bicaval view demonstrates the communication (*) between the right atrium (*RA*) and the left atrium (*LA*) at the superior vena cava (*SVC*) and RA junction. *AO* ascending aorta, *RPA* right pulmonary artery

is deemed unsatisfactory, return to cardiopulmonary bypass and revision of the repair can be undertaken.

In the cardiac catheterization laboratory, TEE is helpful in guiding transeptal puncture as well as a variety of transcatheter interventional procedures including balloon mitral valvuloplasty or septal defect closure (also refer to Chap. 17) [10, 11]. TEE in adult patients is particularly useful in the identification of thrombus formation and the assessment of findings related to infective endocarditis [12, 13]. This particular patient population may also benefit from transesophageal imaging as this approach overcomes limitations related to suboptimal TTE windows due to prior cardiothoracic interventions or body habitus.

Cardiovascular Malformations in Adults with Congenital Heart Disease and Applications of Transesophageal Imaging

Atrial Septal Defects

Atrial septal defects (ASDs) can go undiagnosed in childhood and in some cases may first come to medical attention during adolescence or adulthood. In such instances, patients commonly present with palpitations and exercise intolerance. The initial echocardiographic examination focuses on diagnosis and hemodynamic assessment of the defect. Precise definition of atrial septal anatomy, identification of coexisting anomalies, quantification of shunt size and right ventricular systolic pressure, are important aspects of the assessment (also refer to Chap. 7). In the adult population, TEE is more sensitive than TTE in detecting atrial communications, especially sinus venosus defects located near the junction of the superior vena cava and right atrium (Fig. 18.1). In general, all ASDs should be imaged in multiple planes in order to determine location and defect size. Determination of adequate rims is important in the case of a secundum ASD for consideration regarding transcatheter device closure (Videos 18.1 and 18.2). Three-dimensional imaging may offer additional benefits in this regard [14]. In general, secundum defects under 40 mm in balloon stretched diameter (Fig. 18.2, Video 18.3) and those with adequate rims are considered potentially suitable for percutaneous device closure [15]. TEE also plays an important role in guiding transcatheter device placement, evaluating residual shunting, and determining device stability (Fig. 18.3, Video 18.4). TEE following transcatheter device closure can identify complications related to the occluder such as thrombus formation [16].

Ventricular Septal Defects

Ventricular septal defects (VSDs) may be classified as muscular or non-muscular, aligned or malaligned, and restrictive or non-restrictive. The most common site for an unrepaired VSD in the adult is in the membranous septum, followed by muscular, inlet, and outlet septum.

The ventricular septum cannot be fully imaged in any one or a single plane because it is a curved structure (refer to Chap. 9). Communications in the region of the membranous septum are best seen in the mid esophageal four chamber (ME 4 Ch) view with probe anteflexion. Additional views to define this type of defect include the mid esophageal right ventricular inflow-outflow (ME RV In-Out) and mid esophageal long axis (ME LAX) views (Fig. 18.4, Video 18.5). Continuous wave Doppler allows estimation of shunt velocity and classification into a restrictive versus non-restrictive defect, if the peak velocity across the defect is high or low

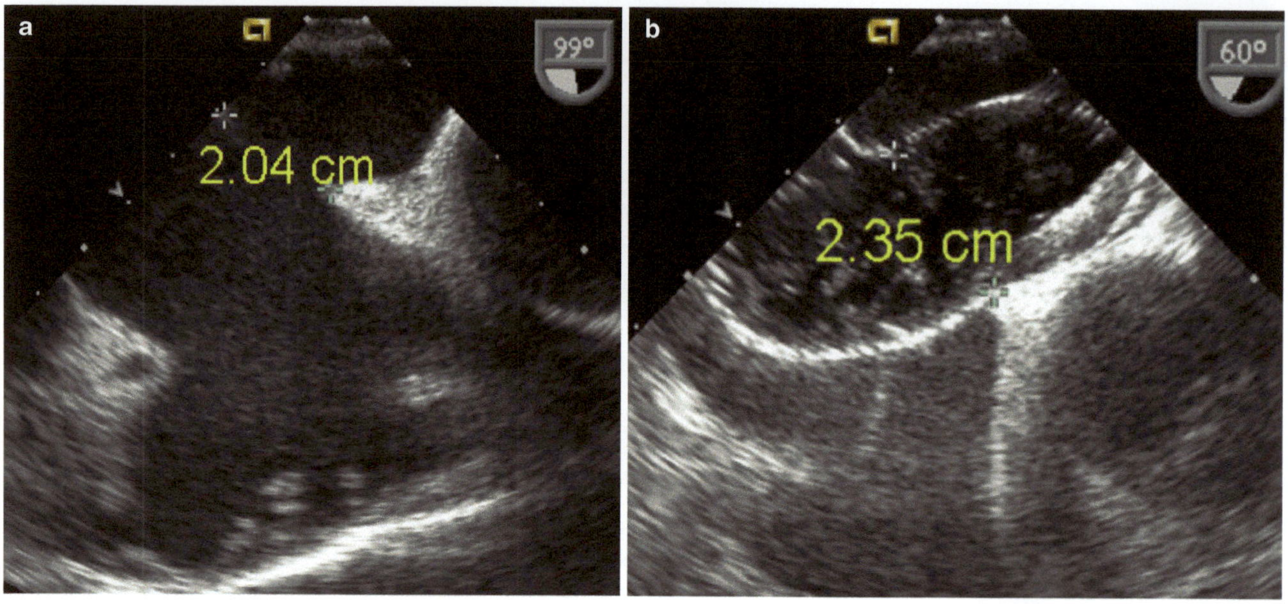

Fig. 18.2 (**a**) Mid esophageal bicaval view of secundum atrial septal defect measuring 2 cm (unstretched diameter). (**b**) 60° view of the same defect after balloon sizing during transcatheter device placement. The stretched defect diameter measures 2.35 cm in this plane

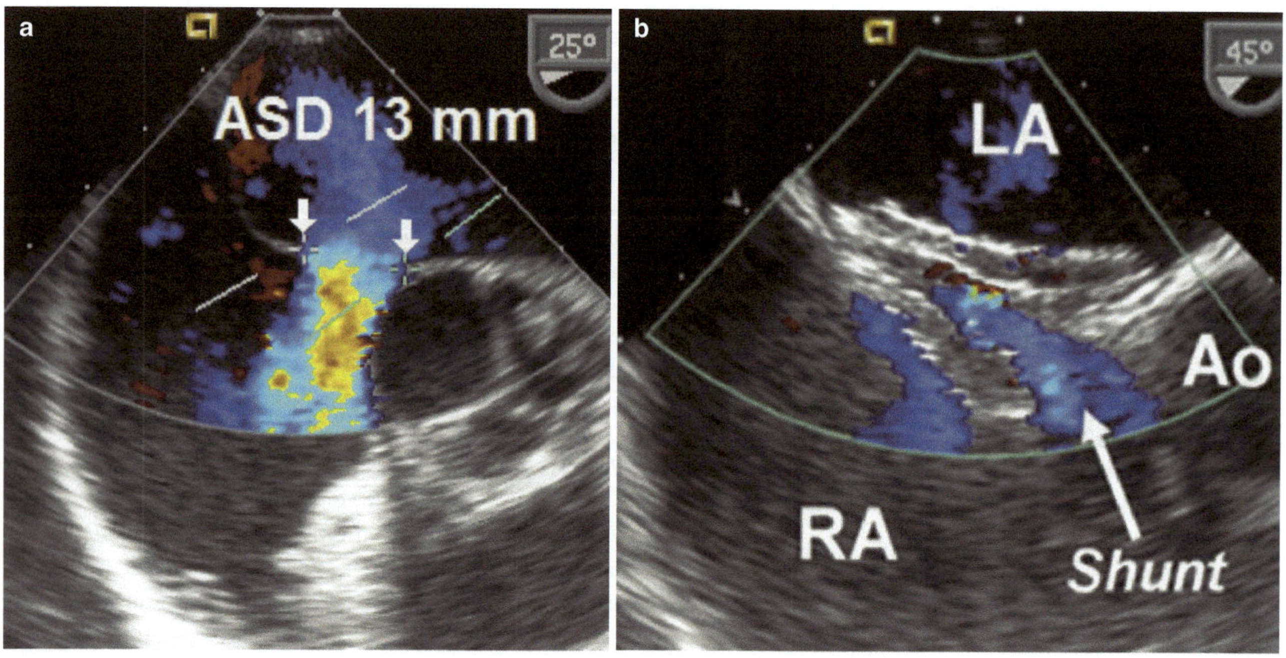

Fig. 18.3 (**a**) Secundum atrial septal defect (*ASD*) measuring 13 mm (unstretched diameter) with thin posterior rim and deficient anterior rim as seen in a mid esophageal view. Color flow Doppler demonstrates left-to-right shunting across the defect. (**b**) Immediately following successful deployment of an Amplatzer septal occluder device a small amount of left-to-right shunting is noted through the device. Because of the deficient anterior (retro-aortic) rim, the septal occluder is filleted over the posterior portion of the aortic root (*Ao*). *LA* left atrium, *RA* right atrium

respectively. Spontaneous closure of a membranous VSD usually occurs by adherence of a redundant aneurysmal tricuspid septal leaflet to the membranous septum. This may be seen in several planes but is best imaged in the 30–60° mid esophageal aortic valve short axis (ME AV SAX) view.

Imaging and Doppler interrogation of the right ventricle may identify anomalous muscle bundles resulting in a high-pressure proximal chamber and a low-pressure distal chamber characteristic of double-chambered right ventricle (DCRV) (Fig. 18.5, Video 18.6). It has been proposed that

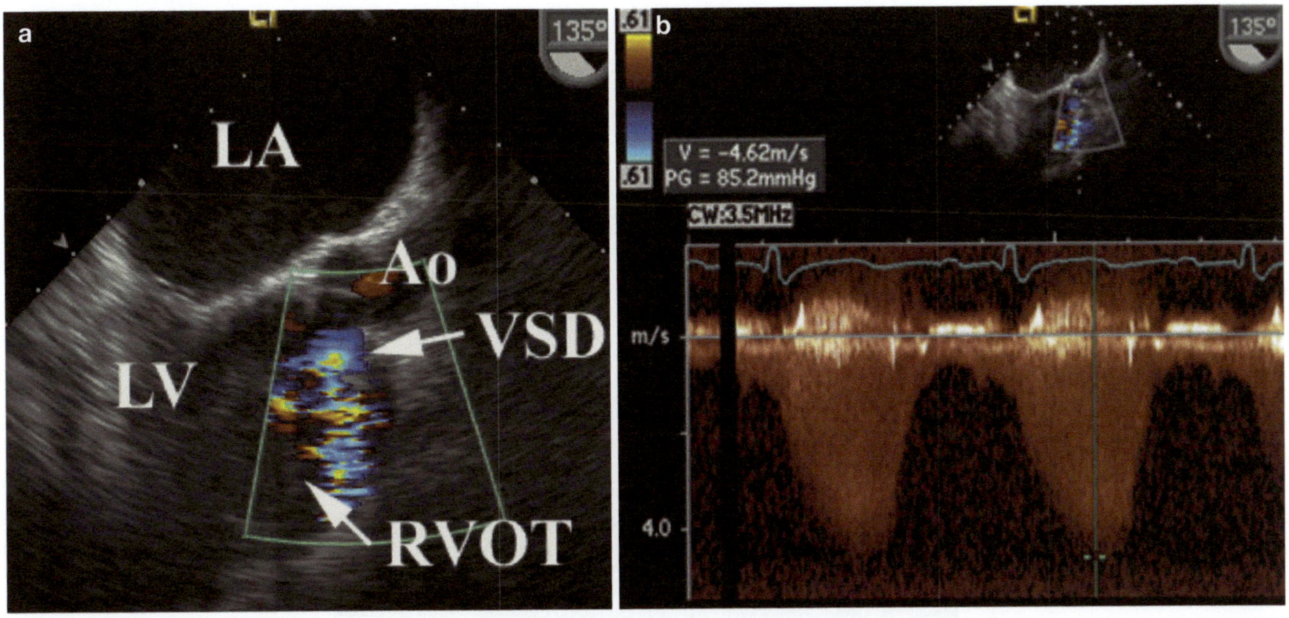

Fig. 18.4 (**a**) Mid esophageal long axis view in a 135° plane demonstrating shunting across a membranous ventricular septal defect (*VSD*) into to the right ventricular outflow tract (*RVOT*) by color flow Doppler. (**b**) Continuous wave Doppler demonstrates high velocity flow consistent with a restrictive defect. *Ao* aorta, *LA* left atrium, *LV* left ventricle

this is an acquired lesion potentially related to chronic high velocity VSD flow impacting the right ventricle, however, some controversy still remains regarding this notion. This anomaly is best assessed in the mid esophageal position in the ME RV In-Out view (between 30° and 60°) or from the deep transgastric sagittal (DTG Sagittal) view [17]. Isolated DCRV without a VSD is exceedingly rare.

Occasionally, a patient with a repaired or unrepaired membranous VSD may have a left ventricular-to-right atrial shunt known as a "Gerbode defect". This is usually a high velocity shunt that may be confused with a jet of high pressure tricuspid regurgitation. This is best seen in the ME 4 Ch and ME RV In-Out views.

A malaligned VSD is associated with great artery annular overriding; typically the aorta overrides the septum as seen in patients with tetralogy of Fallot. The ventriculoarterial connections and malaligned VSD are often best seen in the mid esophageal aortic valve long axis (ME AV LAX) or ME LAX views. Prolapse of the aortic valve (usually the right coronary cusp) into the VSD may cause partial closure of the defect and/or aortic regurgitation. This is seen in outlet (conal or supracristal) defects and is best appreciated in the ME LAX or ME RV In-Out views.

Following surgical or transcatheter VSD closure, interrogation of the septal patch or device for leaks and position as well as assessment of nearby structures is important, preferably done in the operating room or catheterization laboratory at the time of defect closure [18, 19]. In addition, color flow Doppler interrogation of the entire septum in multiple planes may reveal previously undetected small muscular VSDs. TEE plays an important role in transcatheter device occlusion by providing monitoring and guidance during the procedure, decreasing radiation exposure and allowing for detections of complications (refer to Chap. 17).

Atrioventricular Canal Defects

Atrioventricular canal defects, also known as atrioventricular septal defects (AVSDs) or endocardial cushion defects, are a group of malformations that share a common embryologic defect related to the endocardial cushions (refer to Chap. 8). This region influences the development of the atrioventricular septum and the atrioventricular valves.

In the "partial" form, a primum ASD is present with either a restrictive ventricular septal defect (VSD) or intact ventricular septum. This is frequently associated with a commissure or cleft in the anterior mitral leaflet (Fig. 18.6, Video 18.7). The "complete" form of the AVSD is characterized by the presence of a common atrioventricular valve, primum ASD and inlet VSD. The deficiency of the inlet ventricular septum along with abnormalities of the atrioventricular valves (overriding, straddling, and/or cleft) produces an elongated left ventricular outflow tract that has characteristically been described as having a "goose neck" appearance on left ventriculography. Subaortic stenosis is a common association often caused by chordal attachments of the left atrioventricular valve (mitral valve) to the left ventricular outflow septum (Fig. 18.6, Video 18.8).

Patients with complete defects frequently undergo definitive surgical repair in infancy. Palliated or unrepaired defects

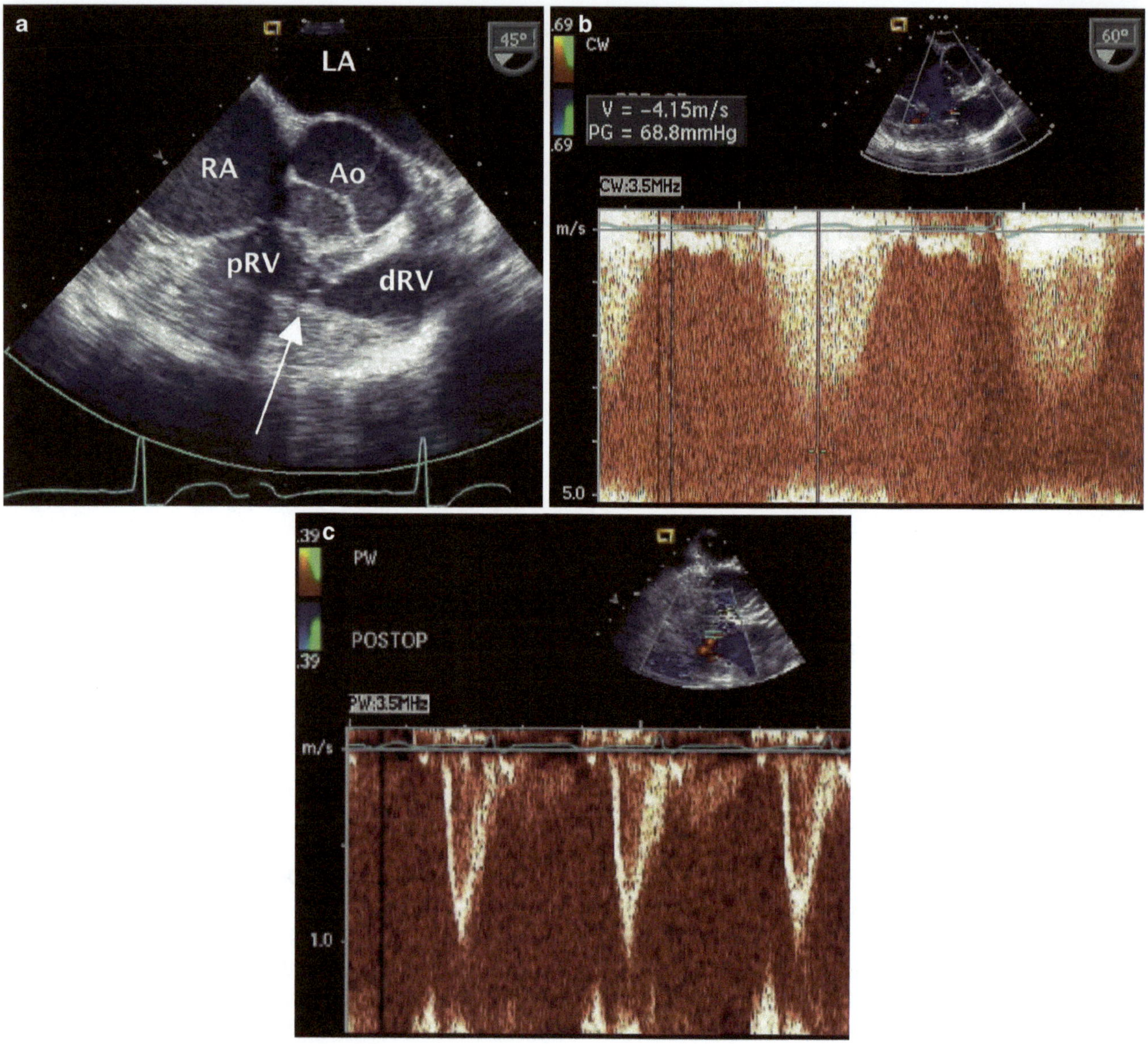

Fig. 18.5 (**a**) Right ventricular inflow-outflow view at the level of the mid esophagus displaying the typical echocardiographic features in an adult with double-chambered right ventricle. There is mid-cavitary narrowing resulting from a fibromuscular diaphragm (*arrow*) that partitions the right ventricle into proximal (*pRV*) and distal (*dRV*) portions. Note the associated severe right ventricular free wall muscular hypertrophy. (**b**) Continuous wave Doppler interrogation across the narrowed mid right ventricular region demonstrates a peak velocity of 4.1 m/s consistent with severe obstruction. (**c**) Following resection of the obstruction pulsed wave Doppler assessment demonstrates low velocity flow across this region confirming the adequacy of the surgical intervention. *Ao* aorta, *LA* left atrium, *RA* right atrium

are now rarely seen in adulthood. Palliation is usually in the form of a pulmonary artery band aimed at restricting pulmonary blood flow. Unrepaired defects in adulthood are likely associated with severely elevated pulmonary vascular resistance (Eisenmenger syndrome) and cyanosis related to reversal in the direction of the shunt.

Presentation of an AVSD in the adult patient is most frequently in the form of a partial defect and associated mitral regurgitation. Chordal attachments to the ventricular septum may account for subaortic stenosis and symptomatology. In patients who have undergone a prior repair, TEE is predominantly utilized to evaluate the reconstructed atrioventricular valve(s), with special attention to the degree, etiology, and progression of regurgitation, iatrogenic stenosis, and presence/degree of subaortic stenosis.

TEE evaluation of the mitral apparatus is best done in the mid esophageal and transgastric locations. The various planes that display the mitral valve apparatus are essential for comprehensive visualization of the base and tips of the leaflets with dedicated imaging of the valve scallops from 0° to 180° (refer to Chaps. 4 and 8). The transgastric basal short axis view (TG Basal SAX) that displays the mitral valve in short axis is helpful

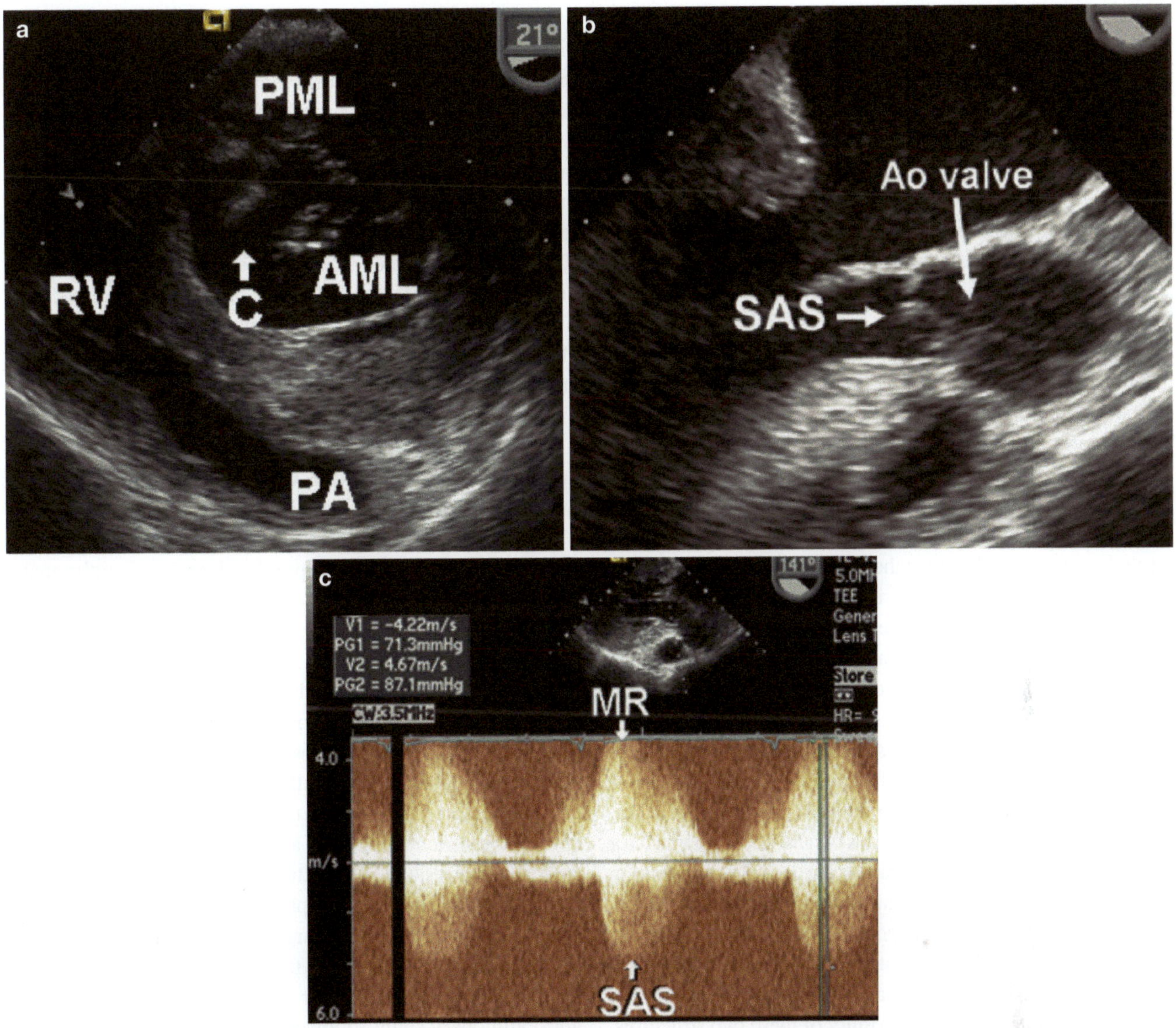

Fig. 18.6 (**a**) Transgastric basal short axis view of the left ventricle in diastole displays a cleft (*C*) in the anterior mitral leaflet (*AML*). The posterior mitral leaflet (*PML*) is well developed. (**b**) Mid esophageal aortic valve long axis view demonstrating chordal attachments from the anterior mitral leaflet into the outflow septum causing subaortic stenosis (*SAS*). (**c**) Continuous wave Doppler interrogation acquired from a transgastric 141° plane through the region of the mitral leaflet tips and left ventricular outflow tract. Note the jet of mitral regurgitation (*MR*) directed inferiorly towards the transducer through the cleft in the AML. High velocity systolic antegrade flow away from the transducer is noted, consistent with SAS. *Ao* aortic, *PA* pulmonary artery, *RV* right ventricle

for direct visualization of the commissure or cleft in the anterior leaflet and all of the scallops of the posterior leaflet (Fig. 18.6, Video 18.7). Color flow Doppler interrogation in this view demonstrates the location and etiology of mitral regurgitation. Short axis views at the level of the mid left ventricular cavity—known as the transgastric mid short axis (TG Mid SAX) views—define papillary muscle anatomy and chordal attachments. In the deep transgastric long axis (DTG LAX) view, flow acceleration in the region of the chordae should arouse the suspicion of subaortic stenosis. The tricuspid valve is also well seen in the ME RV In-Out view and from the transgastric location in the transgastric right ventricular inflow (TG RV In) view.

Interrogation of residual intracardiac shunts, particularly in the case of defects that involve a ventricular level communication or ventriculoatrial shunt, requires the use of multiple planes and is assisted by color flow Doppler imaging.

Anomalous Pulmonary Venous Connections

Pulmonary venous connections are well imaged by TEE (also refer to Chap. 6). In the normal heart, the right and left upper pulmonary veins are usually identified draining into the left atrium at the level of the mid esophagus in the horizontal or transverse plane from zero to 30° with movement of the probe towards the right and left respectively. The left upper pulmonary vein courses into the left atrium posterolateral to the left atrial appendage. The vertical or longitudinal plane at approximately 90° allows visualization of the left and right lower pulmonary veins as they enter the left atrium but modifications of the interrogating plane maybe necessary.

Determination of pulmonary venous anatomy is imperative in patients with ASDs because anomalous pulmonary venous drainage may necessitate surgical intervention as opposed to simple percutaneous closure of an interatrial communication. The most common malformation in this setting is the presence of an anomalous right upper pulmonary vein entering at the junction of the superior vena cava and right atrium in the presence of a superior sinus venosus ASD. Anomalous pulmonary venous connections to the low superior vena cava (between the azygous vein and right atrium) can be visualized by TEE imaging. The probe is positioned at the level of the superior vena cava-right atrial junction with imaging of this area performed in the ME 4 Ch and in the mid esophageal bicaval (ME Bicaval) views. A comprehensive assessment of this defect can be challenging solely on the basis of TEE. In many cases preoperative imaging with modalities such as chest-computed tomography, magnetic resonance imaging, or cardiac catheterization and angiography may be undertaken.

Uncorrected total anomalous pulmonary venous return is an unusual presentation in the adult but may be seen in patients who have received limited or no medical attention, for example, those in third world countries where the resources for appropriate diagnosis and therapies are lacking. A common form of total anomalous pulmonary venous connection seen in adults is the presence of a posteriorly located pulmonary venous confluence chamber into which all four pulmonary veins drain (Fig. 18.7). This chamber is not connected to the left atrium despite the close proximity of these two structures. The confluence typically drains into a greatly dilated coronary sinus that thereafter drains into a dilated right atrium. The presence of a patent foramen ovale or atrial septal defect is necessary to allow venous admixture. In some cases this condition may be confused with cor triatriatum because the close proximity of the venous confluence to the left atrium gives the appearance of a dividing membrane in the left atrium. Less frequently, a vertical vein or other venous structure connects the pulmonary venous confluence to the innominate vein, superior vena cava or travels below the level of the diaphragm to anastomose with the portal vein or a hepatic vein.

Right Ventricular Outflow Tract Lesions

Pulmonary Stenosis

Pulmonary stenosis (PS) may occur at the valvar, supravalvar, or subvalvar level (or any combination of the three levels). Management requires elucidation of the location(s) and severity of the stenosis as well as presence of any associated abnormalities (ASD or VSD). TTE with Doppler interrogation is usually sufficient for the assessment of the adult with PS. However, in patients with supravalvar PS with involvement of the branch pulmonary arteries, TEE provides better visualization of the proximal branch pulmonary arteries, usually best seen at a high esophageal level in the upper esophageal pulmonary artery long axis (UE PA LAX) view. A comprehensive evaluation of the pulmonary vascular tree may not be feasible by TEE, particularly if pathology is suspected distally. In this case alternate diagnostic modalities may be required such as cardiac catheterization, chest tomography or magnetic resonance imaging.

In cases of isolated non-dysplastic pulmonary valve stenosis, transcatheter balloon valvuloplasty is the treatment of choice if the obstruction is considered significant [20, 21]. Transcatheter balloon valvuloplasty provides sufficient relief with an acceptable degree of pulmonary regurgitation.

Tetralogy of Fallot

Tetralogy of Fallot (TOF) is the most common cyanotic congenital heart malformation and one of the first moderately complex lesions to be successfully palliated and repaired. Anterior deviation of the outlet septum results in the four classic characteristic findings of TOF: (1) a malaligned VSD; (2) right ventricular outflow and/or pulmonary valve/artery stenosis or atresia; (3) a dextroposed overriding aorta; and (4) right ventricular hypertrophy.

In the modern era, early surgical repair consisting of VSD closure and alleviation of the right ventricular outflow obstruction has gained favor over early palliation with an aortopulmonary shunt followed by a second stage, definitive repair. The site and degree of right ventricular outflow obstruction, malalignment of the VSD, and aortic override are best assessed with a combination of mid esophageal, transgastric and deep transgastric views. Aortopulmonary collaterals, if present, may be imaged with the aid of color flow imaging and should be sought at multiple levels and locations by rotation of the probe to visualize the descending aorta (descending aorta long axis, Desc Ao LAX view) and slowly withdrawing the probe to fully image the aortic arch and arch vessels in the upper esophageal views. In most cases, the detailed assessment of aortopulmonary collaterals requires additional imaging modalities.

The surgical techniques utilized in the definitive repair of TOF have changed significantly over the past 40 years. The deleterious hemodynamic and electrophysiologic effects of pulmonary regurgitation and a ventriculotomy scar are now well recognized. Thus current approaches aim at limiting pulmonary valve regurgitation and minimizing the extent of the ventricular incision.

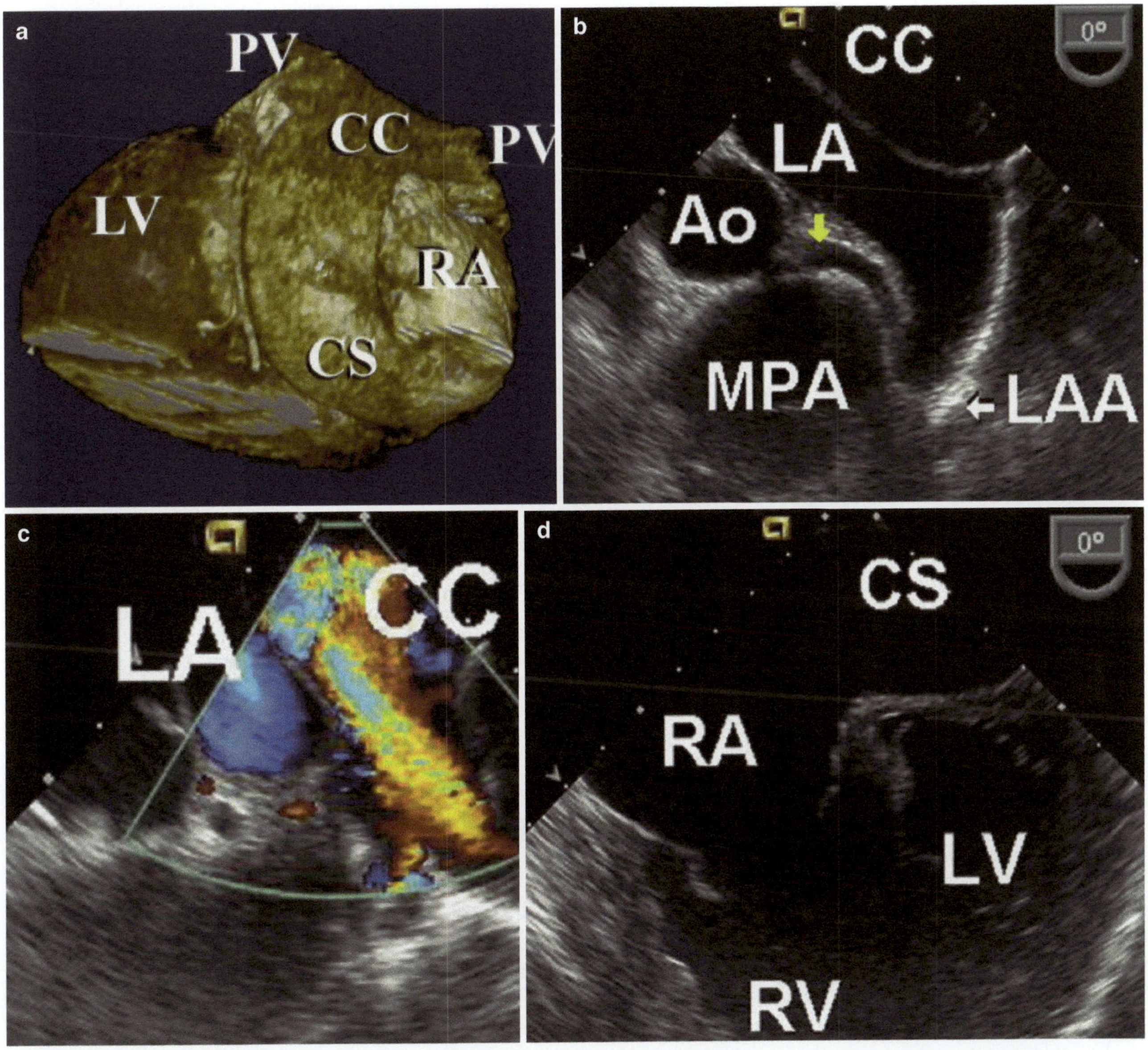

Fig. 18.7 (**a**) Three-dimensional reconstruction of ECG gated CT angiogram in a 27 year-old cyanotic patient with uncorrected total anomalous pulmonary venous return. Two pulmonary veins (*PV*) connect to a posterior confluence chamber (*CC*) that courses inferiorly behind the left atrium (*LA*) into a dilated coronary sinus (*CS*) that in turn connects to the right atrium (*RA*). (**b**) TEE in the same patient, in the mid esophageal aortic valve short axis view with leftward probe position. Note the posterior CC closely apposing but not connected to the LA. The left main coronary artery (*yellow arrow*) is seen emerging from the aortic root (*Ao*) and coursing anterior to the left atrial appendage (*LAA*) and posterior to a dilated main pulmonary artery (*MPA*). (**c**) Color flow Doppler imaging demonstrating low velocity flow towards the transducer from the left sided pulmonary veins to the *CC*. Note the absence of flow between the *CC* and *LA*. (**d**) Mid esophageal four chamber view with the transducer in a more inferior position at the level of entry of the dilated *CS* into an enlarged *RA*. The right ventricle (*RV*) is also dilated, in comparison to the left ventricle (*LV*)

Advancements in surgical repair now confer for survival into adulthood in most patients with CHD in the United States and many other countries [22]. In the case of TOF, the technique used for complete repair depends on many factors but to a significant degree on the level and extent of the outflow obstruction. At one end of the spectrum the repair may require VSD patch closure and pulmonary valvotomy/commissurotomy. More severe or complex outflow tract obstruction may necessitate more extensive reconstruction of the right ventricular outflow tract or complete bypass of the right ventricular outflow tract by placement of a conduit. The first generation of intracardiac repairs were performed via a large anterior ventriculotomy and frequently included incision of the pulmonary valve annulus and placement of a trans-annular patch made of pericardium or synthetic material. This technique successfully relieved the outflow tract obstruction

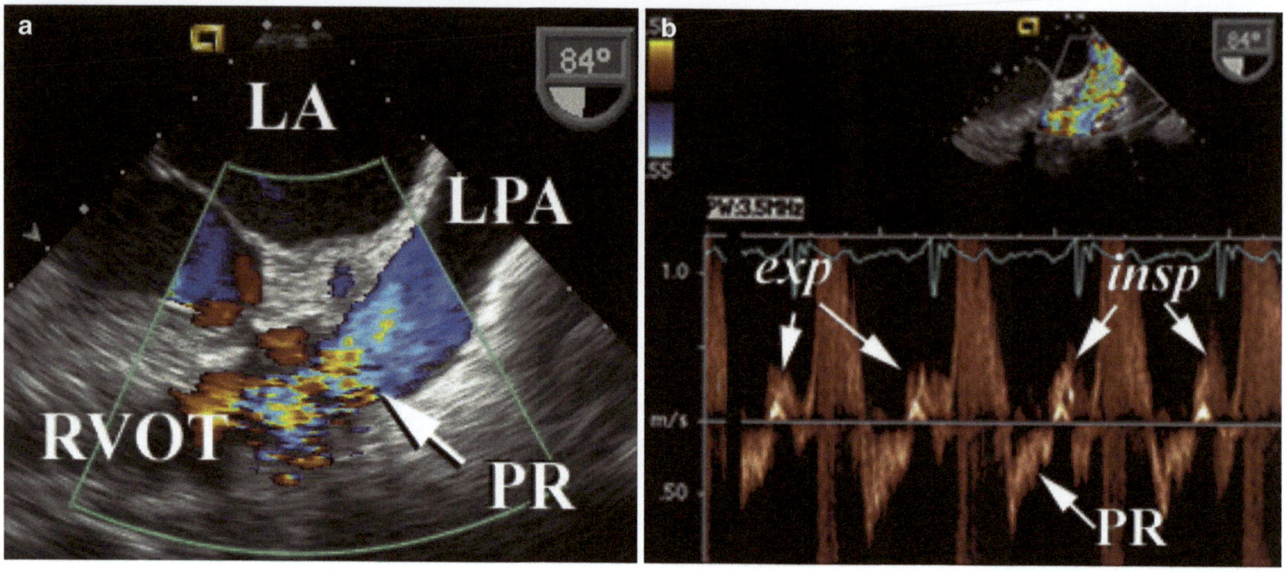

Fig. 18.8 (**a**) Color flow mapping of the pulmonary outflow tract in a modified mid esophageal long axis view (84°), demonstrating severe pulmonary regurgitation (*PR*) in a patient with tetralogy of Fallot previously repaired with a transannular patch. (**b**) Pulsed wave Doppler interrogation within the main pulmonary artery depicts some of the hallmarks of significant PR, early deceleration of retrograde flow (pressure half time <100 ms) and PR duration less than 77 % of diastole (PR index <0.77), both indicative of a rapid rise of right ventricular filling pressure [23, 24]. Note the end-diastolic forward flow with atrial contraction that increases in volume and velocity during inspiration (*insp*) when right heart volume increases compared with expiration (*exp*); this finding is indicative of restrictive right ventricular physiology. *LA* left atrium, *LPA* left pulmonary artery, *RVOT* right ventricular outflow tract

but inevitably resulted in severe pulmonary regurgitation (Fig. 18.8, Video 18.9) [23, 24]. Pulmonary regurgitation was thought to have minimal adverse clinical consequences, which may be true for the first two decades following transannular patch repair. However, with time, the adverse hemodynamic effects of severe low-pressure pulmonary regurgitation become problematic with right ventricular dilation, functional deterioration, and increased risk of arrhythmias. The tricuspid annulus frequently dilates and tricuspid regurgitation often occurs. Additionally, the right ventricle develops 'restrictive' diastolic properties that further compromise energy efficient hemodynamics (Fig. 18.8) [25]. Thus, the desire to limit the extent of the transannular patch, preserve pulmonary valve competence and infundibular function as much as possible.

Residual shunting may occur anywhere along the VSD patch. Comprehensive assessment requires multiple probe positions and TEE planes in addition to color flow interrogation for accurate detection (refer to Chaps. 9 and 12). Continuous wave Doppler determines shunt velocity from which pressure gradient estimates may be derived and a determination of pressure restriction. Transgastric and deep transgastric imaging with multiplane angles from 0° to 90° allow visualization of the inferior portion of the VSD patch. This is a crucial view because a small leak may be masked or shadowed by the patch if imaging the superior portion of the patch from the mid and lower esophageal positions. Residual shunts should be identified by intraoperative TEE so as to allow immediate reinstitution of cardiopulmonary bypass if these are considered hemodynamically significant.

Left Ventricular Outflow Tract Lesions

Bicuspid Aortic Valve

Bicuspid aortic valve (BAV) is the most common congenital cardiac malformation and is the most common cause of aortic valve stenosis and/or regurgitation in adults that are less than 60 years of age (refer to Chap. 11) [26]. A BAV is best imaged in a 30–60° "short axis" plane, also known as the ME AV SAX (Fig. 18.9, Video 18.10). Systolic doming is best seen in the 110–130° plane or ME AV LAX view. The transgastric long axis (TG LAX) and DTG LAX views allow for coaxial Doppler alignment with the direction of flow providing for assessment of flow velocities and estimation of gradients. Associated lesions include coarctation of the aorta and aortic root dilation. Although TEE has not been fully evaluated in the assessment of distal aortic arch obstruction, this area can be interrogated by turning the probe posteriorly and slowly withdrawing it in the Desc Ao LAX view.

Aortic root dilation is commonly encountered in patients with BAV and is thought to be secondary to medial degeneration of the aortic wall [27]. These patients may also develop complications such as endocarditis.

Patients with a BAV may require interventions such as balloon valvuloplasty or surgery to alleviate the obstruction. TEE is very useful in guiding transcatheter procedures and assessing changes in the degree of aortic stenosis and/or regurgitation following balloon dilation (Fig. 18.10, Videos 18.11 and 18.12). Many patients ultimately require aortic valve replacement with a bioprosthetic or mechanical valve, or a pulmonary autograft (Ross procedure). During these procedures various measurements of the valvar annulus and root dimensions are routinely obtained. For the aortic valve this is accomplished in the ME AV LAX and ME LAX views. In the Ross procedure the pulmonary valve is examined to exclude significant stenosis/regurgitation. The pulmonary valve/outflow in the long axis is best seen in the ME RV In-Out view. In most cases with anteflexion of the TEE imaging probe in the upper and mid esophageal windows, a short axis view of the pulmonary valve can be obtained thus allowing for comparison of these dimensions to those of the aortic valve to ensure parity. Following the Ross procedure, parameters to be examined include autograft function, right ventricular to pulmonary artery conduit patency, and segmental/global left ventricular function. Coronary reimplantation sites should be evaluated for position, patency, and presence of normal color flow (mostly diastolic).

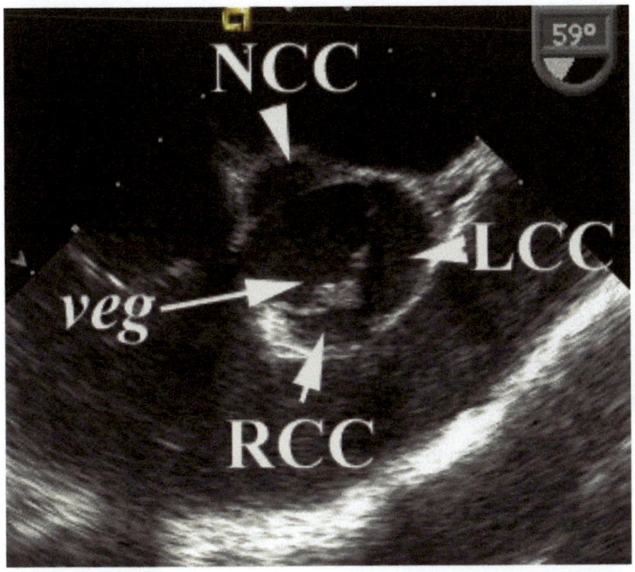

Fig. 18.9 Mid esophageal aortic valve short axis view of a bicuspid aortic valve during systole. There is fusion of the right (*RCC*) and left (*LCC*) coronary cusps. This previously undiagnosed 36 year-old female was admitted with fever and rigors three weeks following dental cleaning. A small aortic valve vegetation (*veg*) is clearly visualized. Blood cultures were positive for *Streptococcus epidermidis*. *NCC* non coronary cusp

Subaortic Stenosis

Subaortic stenosis (SAS) is most commonly due to a discrete fibromuscular ridge or membrane directly below the aortic valve that results in left ventricular outflow tract obstruction (Fig. 18.11, Video 18.13). Typically there is flow accelera-

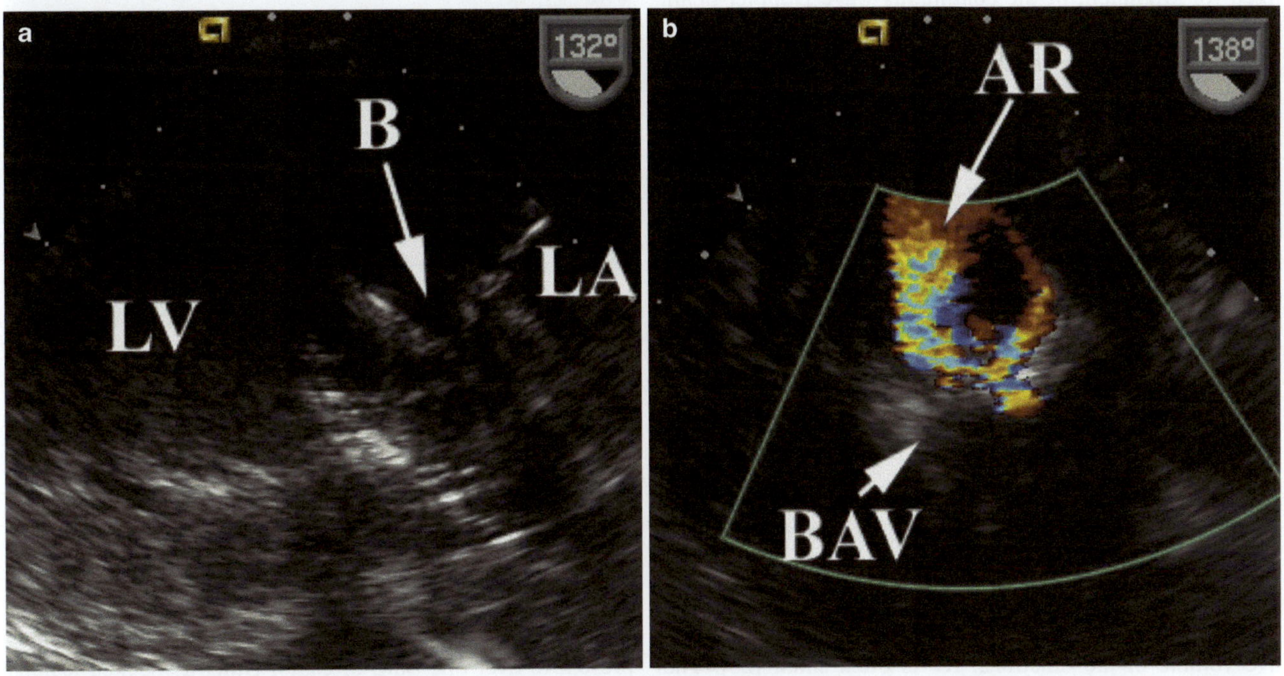

Fig. 18.10 (**a**) Transgastric long axis left ventricular view at a plane of 132° during transcatheter balloon valvuloplasty (*B*) of a bicuspid aortic valve (*BAV*). (**b**) Color flow Doppler interrogation post-balloon dilation of the BAV demonstrates moderate aortic regurgitation (AR). *LA* left atrium, *LV* left ventricle

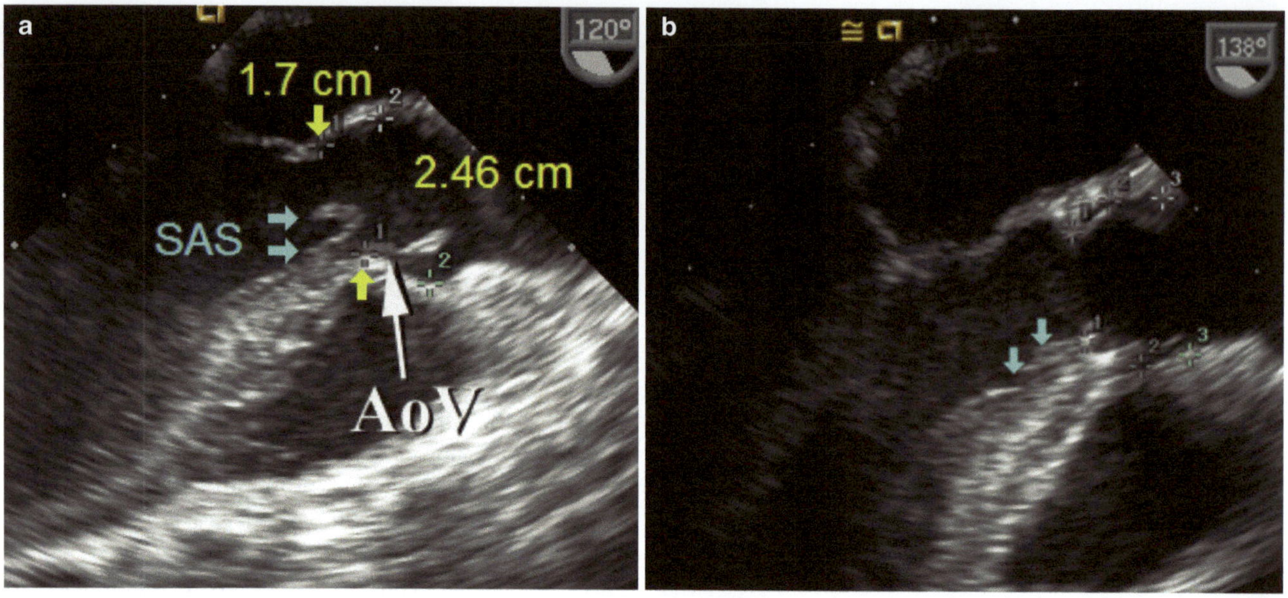

Fig. 18.11 (**a**) Mid esophageal aortic valve long axis view at a 120° plane demonstrating a membrane directly below the aortic valve (*AoV*) causing subaortic stenosis (*SAS*). The AoV annulus measures 1.7 cm and the aortic root at the level of the sinuses, 2.46 cm. (**b**) Two dimensional image post-surgical resection of subaortic membrane and septal myomectomy (*vertical arrows*)

tion across this region that may lead to damage to the aortic valve and subsequent regurgitation [26].

The left ventricular outflow tract should be evaluated in the long axis plane in multiple views (ME AV LAX, TG LAX, DTG LAX) to identify the location, type, and extent of SAS. Transgastric and deep transgastric views are utilized for alignment of the continuous wave Doppler beam for determination of flow velocity and gradient quantification. Excision of the membrane or fibromuscular ridge is the treatment of choice if significant, often accompanied by focal septal myomyectomy to reduce likelihood of recurrence. Intraoperative TEE verifies complete excision of the subaortic membrane, relief of obstruction, degree of aortic regurgitation, absence of iatrogenic VSD or injury to the anterior mitral leaflet. Occasionally, SAS is secondary to mitral valve chordal attachments to the outflow septum (Fig. 18.6).

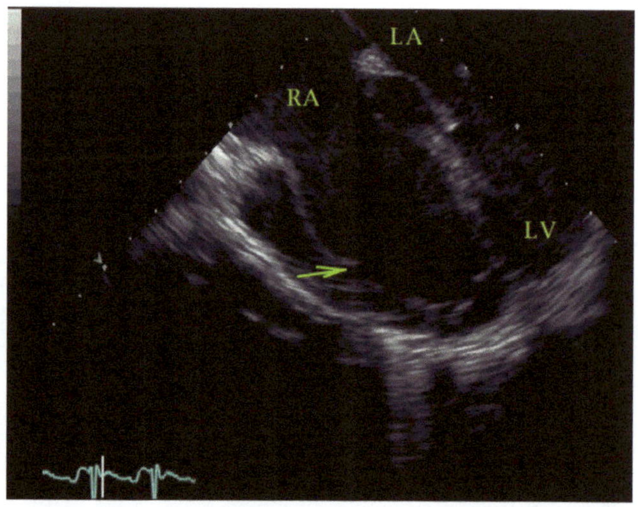

Fig. 18.12 Mid esophageal four chamber view displaying the redundant, 'sail-like' anterior leaflet (*arrow*) in Ebstein malformation of the tricuspid valve. *LA* left atrium, *LV* left ventricle, *RA* right atrium

Ebstein Anomaly

Ebstein anomaly is characterized by apical displacement of the septal (and often the posterior) leaflet(s) of the tricuspid valve into the right ventricular cavity (also refer to Chap. 8). The right ventricle (RV) is therefore divided into a basal "atrialized" portion and an apical "functional" portion. The effective volume of the functional RV is often small [28]. The anterior leaflet is elongated and often has attachments to the right ventricular free wall (Fig. 18.12, Video 18.14). Various degrees of valvar dysplasia may be seen. The mobility of the anterior leaflet is an important determinant when considering "repair" versus "replacement" of the tricuspid valve.

The "atrialized" portion of the RV is usually thin due to congenital absence of myocardium. The effective right atrium (including the atrialized portion of the RV) is dilated and becomes more so in the presence of tricuspid regurgitation, a frequent finding. An ASD or patent foramen ovale is present in over one third of cases. Other associated lesions are less commonly encountered in the adult and portend a poor prognosis, they can include PS, VSD, and patent ductus arteriosus [29].

An "Ebsteinoid" malformation of the tricuspid valve is commonly found in patients with congenitally corrected transposition of the great arteries. In most cases this is associated with systemic atrioventricular valve (tricuspid valve) regurgitation (see below).

Echocardiographic definition in Ebstein malformation, if comprehensive, is sufficient for diagnosis and prediction of suitability of valve repair. Cardiac catheterization is usually not performed unless obstructive coronary artery disease is suspected due to risk factors or non-invasive stress testing demonstrates evidence of ischemia. Associated abnormalities as described above must be characterized. Suitable TEE views for a comprehensive assessment include the ME 4 Ch, ME RV In-Out, TG RV In, DTG LAX, and DTG sagittal views. It is important to consider that the origin of tricuspid regurgitation in typically below the level of the annulus. The functional state of the right and left ventricles should be evaluated as this may have implications for perioperative care.

Tricuspid valve repair and annuloplasty along with atrial plication are preferable to valve replacement. An anterior leaflet that is long, mobile, with minimal adhesions to the right ventricular free wall is necessary for adequate repair. Intraoperative TEE is widely utilized to verify satisfactory reduction in tricuspid regurgitation severity with minimal or absent stenosis and acceptable repair of any associated lesions. In some cases, during the valve repair a concomitant cavopulmonary or Glenn connection (see below) may be performed in hopes to decrease right ventricular preload. This is known as a 'one and a half ventricle strategy [30]. The patency of this connection may also be confirmed by TEE.

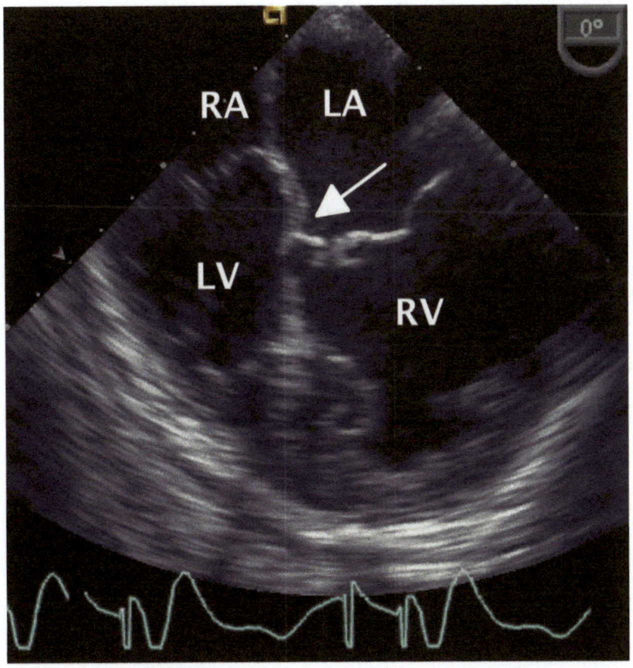

Fig. 18.13 Four chamber view at the level of the mid esophagus in a patient with congenitally corrected transposition of the great arteries (atrioventricular and ventriculoarterial discordance). In this anomaly the right atrium (*RA*) empties into a smooth-walled left ventricle (*LV*) whereas the left atrium (*LA*) drains into a trabeculated, left-sided right ventricle (*RV*). Note the apical displacement (*arrow*) of the tricuspid or left-sided (systemic) atrioventricular valve (Ebsteinoid tricuspid valve) and the rolled valve edges

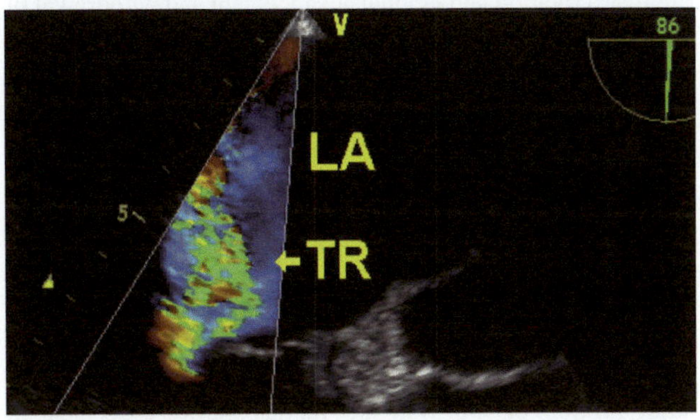

Fig. 18.14 Mid esophageal cross-section (86° plane) demonstrating tricuspid regurgitation (*TR*) in a patient with congenitally corrected transposition of the great arteries. *LA* left atrium

Transposition Complexes

Transposition complexes are defined by ventriculoarterial discordance. In patients with *d*-transposition of the great arteries (*d*-TGA), the atrioventricular connections are concordant, however, the ventriculoarterial connections are discordant. Congenitally corrected or *l*-transposition (*l*-TGA) is characterized by atrioventricular and ventriculoarterial discordance, also know as double discordance (Fig. 18.13, Video 18.15). The atrioventricular valves are associated with their respective ventricles; therefore, the tricuspid valve and right ventricle are in the systemic position both in *d*-TGA and *l*-TGA.

In the minority of patients with corrected transposition without associated defects, unoperated survival into adulthood is common and survival into the eighth and ninth decade has been reported [31]. Progressive morphologic (systemic) right ventricular dysfunction and congestive heart failure occur in over 50 % of patients with associated lesions by the time they reach 45 years of age [32]. As previously mentioned, tricuspid (systemic atrioventricular valve) abnormalities are common and regurgitation occurs in over 80 % of adults with this lesion (Fig. 18.14, Videos 18.15 and 18.16) [33]. Morphologic left ventricular dysfunction occurs less often but may be present in up to 20 % of patients.

Mustard/Senning Atrial Switch Operations

The atrial switch procedures utilize atrial tissue, pericardial tissue, and/or synthetic material to fashion 'baffles' to redirect systemic and pulmonary venous returns to the ventricles in patients with *d*-TGA and less frequently in "double switch" procedures for congenitally corrected transposition of the great arteries (*l*-TGA) (also refer to Chap. 12). The atria are therefore effectively divided as follows: a) an anterior chamber receiving systemic venous return (systemic venous atrium) and emptying into the subpulmonic left ventricle, and b) a posterior chamber receiving pulmonary venous return and draining into the systemic right ventricle (Fig. 18.15, Video 18.17). Between the 1960s to the 1980s, the atrial switch procedures served as the corrective operation of choice for patients with *d*-TGA. Since then, over the past two decades the atrial switch operations have been largely supplanted by the arterial switch or "Jatene" procedure in patients with *d*-TGA where anatomic correction is achieved restoring ventriculoarterial concordance. However, given the relatively 'new' status of the arterial switch procedure, the majority of adults currently living with *d*-TGA have likely undergone an atrial switch operation. With this procedure, baffle stenoses and/or leaks are not infrequently encountered [34]. When present, obstruction in most cases affects the systemic venous baffle. This pathology may be difficult to fully characterize by transthoracic imaging and is a well know indication for TEE. This imaging approach can also be useful to guide percutaneous interventions involving atrial baffles. In order to adequately image the caval-atrial baffle junctions, a vertical plane equivalent to approximately 90° is required with rightward rotation and gradual advancement and withdrawal of the probe (Fig. 18.15, Video 18.17). Color flow and pulsed wave Doppler are used to determine the functional significance and severity of a baffle narrowing. Color flow mapping can identify baffle leaks (Fig. 18.16, Video 18.18), however, it may be difficult to do so if the leak is small and the pressures in the pulmonary and systemic venous baffles are similar. In this case, peripheral venous injection with agitated saline or albumin may be necessary to identify small baffle leaks. Contrast echocardiography is also helpful for confirmation of baffle leaks identified by color mapping (Fig. 18.17, Video 18.19). The atrial portion of the systemic venous baffle, especially in patients with permanent pacemaker leads, is another potential site of obstruction. The pulmonary venous baffle is less commonly obstructed, however, it should be assessed to ensure the absence of stenosis. These structures should be interrogated in multiple planes with transducer tip positions within the esophagus and stomach.

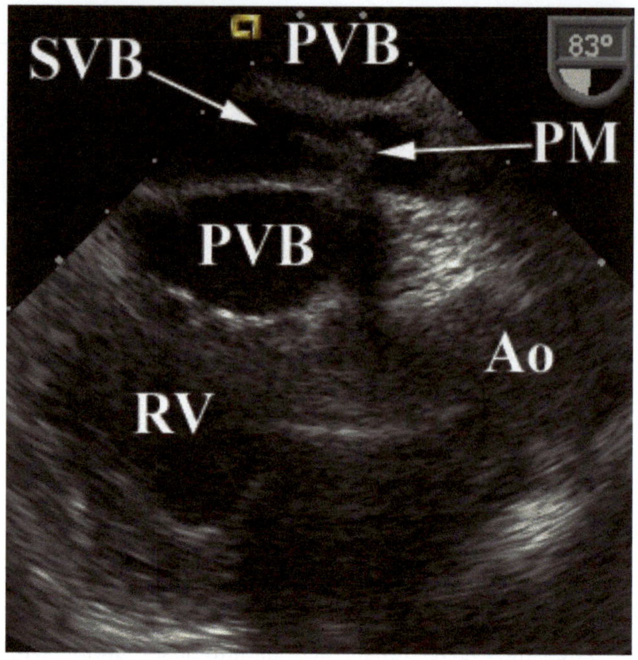

Fig. 18.15 Mid esophageal long axis view in a patient with *d-transposition* of the great arteries status post Senning atrial baffle procedure. The systemic venous baffle (*SVB*) is visualized at the caval-atrial junction. Two pacemaker leads (*PM*) traverse the *SVB*. The pulmonary venous baffle (*PVB*) encircles the *SVB* antero-posteriorly and connects to the right ventricle (*RV*), the systemic chamber ejecting into the aorta (*Ao*)

Glenn Shunt

First performed in 1954, this superior vena cava to pulmonary artery connection paved the way for more extensive cavopulmonary Fontan connections [35]. The initial Glenn shunt consisted of an end to side anastomosis of the superior vena cava to the right pulmonary artery. In its classic "unidirectional" form, the right pulmonary artery was divided to allow for the superior vena caval return to enter only the right lung. This surgical procedure has largely been abandoned in favor of the "bidirectional" Glenn cavopulmonary connection in which the pulmonary artery is not divided but rather an anastomosis is created typically between the superior vena cava and right pulmonary artery allowing for blood flow into both branch pulmonary arteries (hence the appellation "bidirectional"). This operation has been widely used as either a definitive palliation or as an important staging procedure prior to Fontan completion. In cases where bilateral superior vena cavae are present, bilateral bidirectional Glenn connections are performed as indicated.

A more recent application of the Glenn shunt is in the surgical management of cases where the right ventricle is unable to tolerate the entire systemic venous return as previously discussed. Therefore a portion of the systemic venous return is routed directly to the pulmonary arteries via the Glenn shunt, thereby bypassing the heart. This may be the case in patients with a severe form of Ebstein anomaly or other conditions characterized by right ventricular hypoplasia. In this setting, as well as others where there are concerns regarding right ventricular size/function, the cavopulmonary connection is part of a so-called "one and a half ventricle approach".

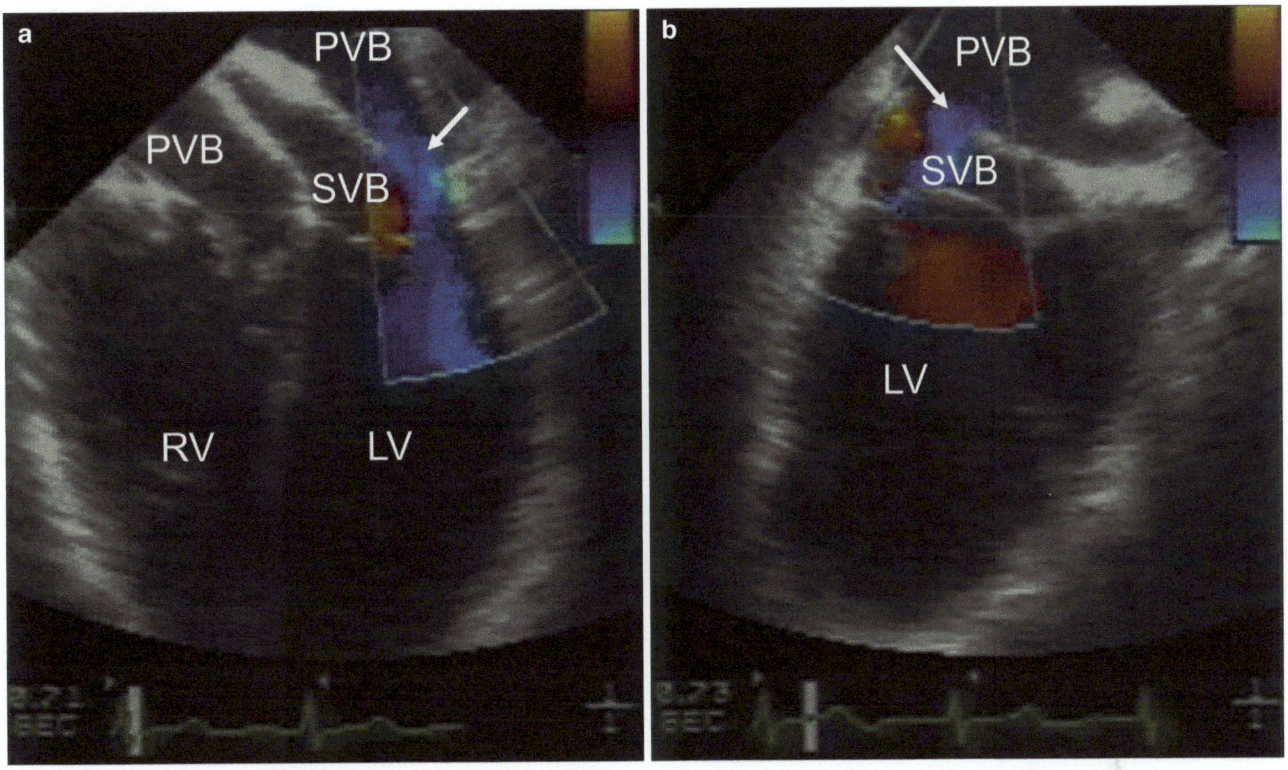

Fig. 18.16 Color flow Doppler imaging in orthogonal planes obtained in a patient with *d*-transposition of the great arteries several years post Senning procedure demonstrating a communication (*arrow*) between the pulmonary (*PVB*) and systemic venous baffle (*SVB*) baffles resulting in left-to-right shunting (*PVB* to *SVB*). *LV* left ventricle, *RV* right ventricle

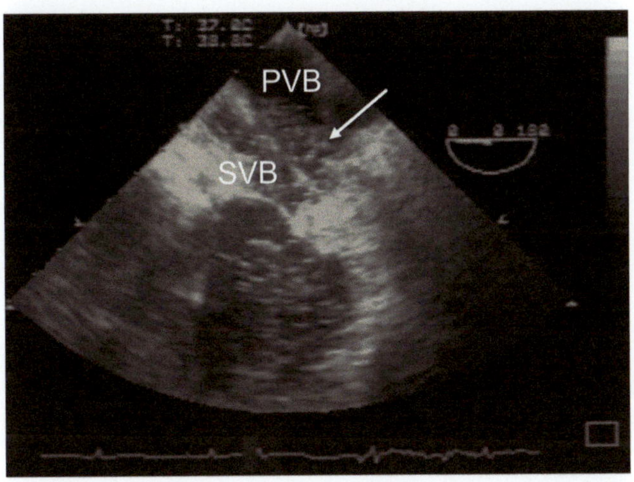

Fig. 18.17 Contrast injection into a central venous catheter in the patient shown in Fig. 18.16 results in opacification of the systemic (*SVB*) and pulmonary venous (*PVB*) portions of the atrial baffle confirming the presence of the baffle leak (*arrow*)

TEE imaging in the 90–100° multiplane alignment, also known as the ME Bicaval view, identifies the right atrium and the lower stump of the superior vena cava. With further rotation of the probe rightwards, the Glenn cavopulmonary anastomosis can be seen. A combination of color flow and pulsed wave Doppler interrogation can be use to assess this connection. Worsening cyanosis in patients following a Glenn operation may be attributed to the development of bypassing venous collaterals including the azygous vein, and/or pulmonary arteriovenous malformations that develop in a circulation deprived of a yet uncharacterized "hepatic factor" [36]. In the latter case, administration of agitated saline into an arm vein or internal jugular vein will demonstrate contrast entering the atria via the pulmonary veins that drain the involved lung segment(s). On the other hand, appearance of agitated saline in the inferior vena cava suggests bypassing collaterals and/or a patent azygous vein with reversed flow. TEE may be utilized during cardiac catheterization with selective injections of agitated saline to help localize the source(s) of desaturation and guide transcatheter interventions.

Fontan Connection

Since Fontan and Baudet's original description in 1971, the Fontan operation for patients with single ventricle physiology has undergone a great number of modifications and improvements [37–39]. In the current era, the extracardiac total cavopulmonary connection and the lateral or intra-atrial tunnel Fontan are widely utilized. The right atrial to pulmonary artery Fontan (atriopulmonary connection) was widely

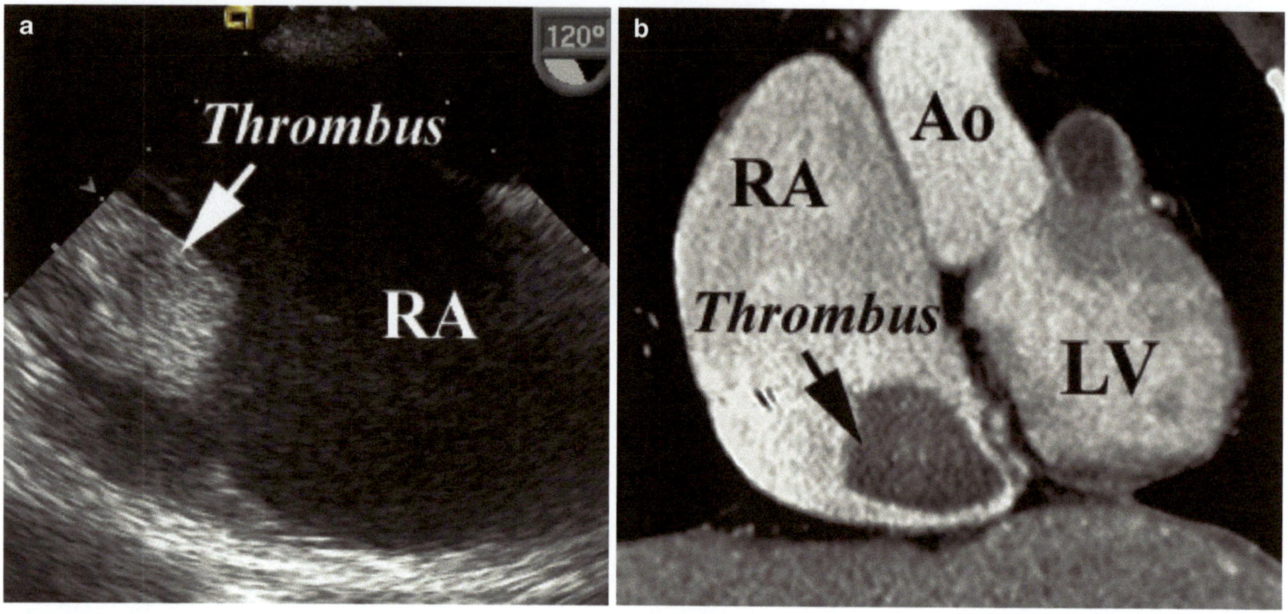

Fig. 18.18 (**a**) Mid esophageal 120° view in a patient with an atriopulmonary Fontan connection and history of intra-atrial reentrant tachycardia. Note the large thrombus in the inferior portion of the dilated right atrium (*RA*). (**b**) Chest computed tomography in the coronal projection, demonstrates the large thrombus in the severely dilated *RA*. *Ao* aorta, *LV* left ventricle

performed in the 1970s and 1980s but has been abandoned because of the high incidence of atrial arrhythmias, atrial dilation, and other complications. The majority of adults now in their late 20s and older patients likely underwent an atriopulmonary Fontan connection. Many of these patients are plagued by atrial arrhythmias and are at increased risk of thromboembolic complications (Fig. 18.18, Video 18.20).

The Bjork modification of the Fontan operation was performed in patients with tricuspid atresia and adequate right ventricular function. A non-valved conduit was typically placed from the right atrium to the right ventricular outflow tract (Fig. 18.19, Video 18.21). These patients also develop atrial arrhythmias and elevated right sided filling pressures leading to right-to-left shunting and cyanosis if a residual ASD or patent foramen ovale is present (Fig. 18.19, Video 18.22). It has been the current practice of many congenital heart centers that manage these patients to perform a Fontan conversion to either an extracardiac or lateral tunnel connection. In most cases concomitant atrial Maze/Cox III arrhythmia surgery is undertaken to decrease the risk of atrial arrhythmias [40]. This is combined with implantation of a dual chamber epicardial pacemaker to either restore atrioventricular synchrony or be able to medically manage arrhythmias safely in case of drug-related side effects such as bradycardia.

TEE is indicated and shown to be of benefit in the detection of atrial thrombi, evaluation of Fontan patency, and identification of shunts in this patient group (also refer to Chap. 10). The classic right atrial to pulmonary artery connection is best seen at the level of the mid esophagus, in the longitudinal (90°) plane in patients with malposed great arteries and in the 0–45° plane in those with normally related great arteries. In patients with the Bjork modification, the right atrial to right ventricular conduit is best evaluated at the mid esophagus in views from 0° to 60° (Fig. 18.19, Video 18.21). Imaging of the lateral tunnel or intra-atrial tunnel Fontan requires a combination of cross-sections for complete evaluation, however, these Fontan variations are usually best visualized throughout their course in the 50–90° planes (Fig. 18.20, Videos 18.23 and 18.24). Extracardiac connections may be difficult to image because of shadowing from the Gore-tex material used to fashion the conduit. Intraoperative TEE is used to assess patency of the cavopulmonary connection, flow across a fenestration if present, and leaks along the lateral tunnel Fontan pathway. This imaging modality is also very valuable in the cardiac catheterization laboratory when Fontan fenestrations need either to be created or obliterated.

Coronary Artery Anomalies

Anomalies of the coronary arteries refer to a wide variety of malformations characterized by abnormal origin and/or course of coronary arteries [41], abnormal connections to other vessels or chambers (e.g. anomalous origin of the left coronary artery from the pulmonary trunk or arteriovenous fistulae), or coronary artery ectasia/aneurysms (Fig. 18.21, Video 18.25). Many of these abnormalities are benign but others may result in myocardial ischemia, infarction, ven-

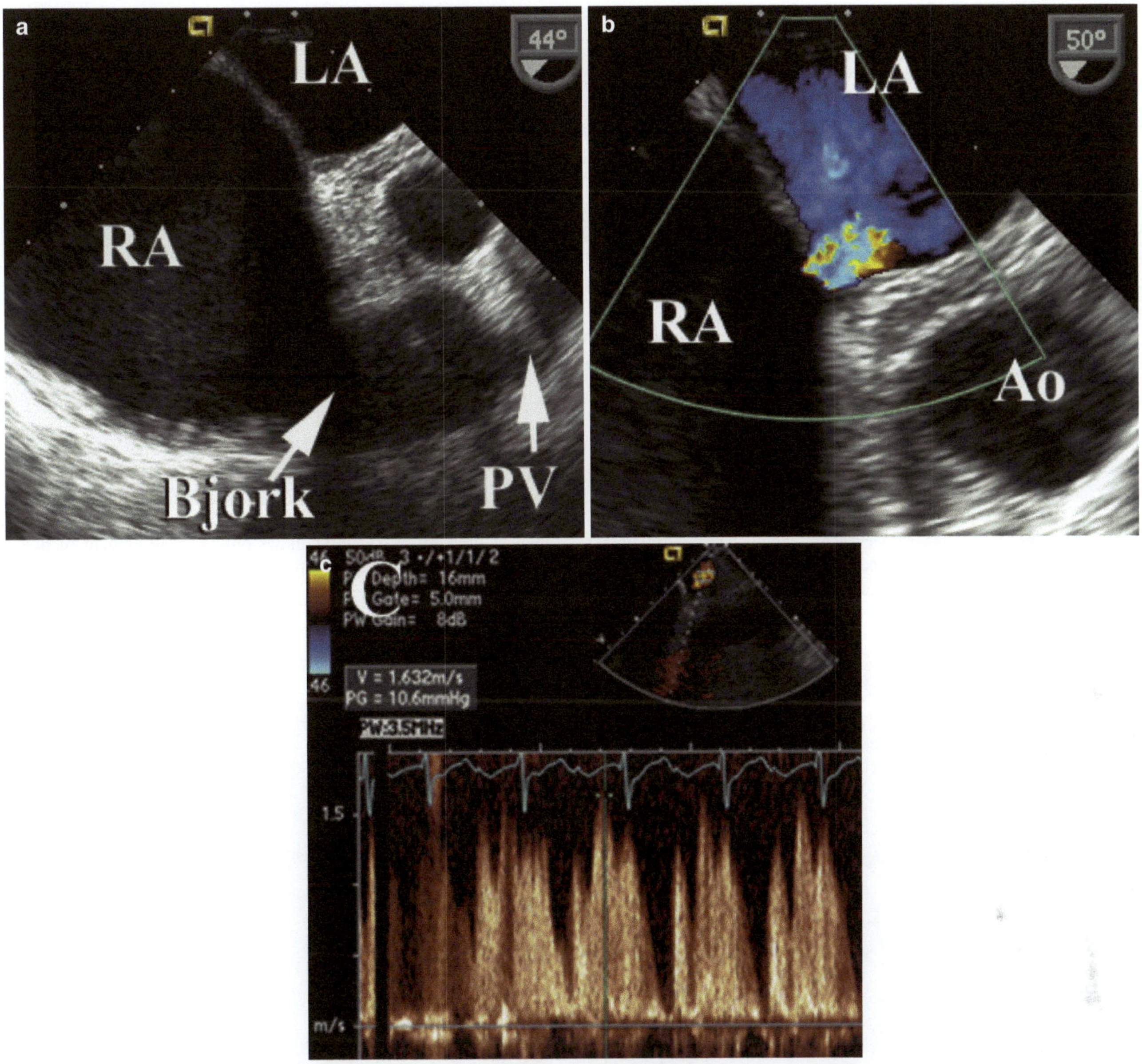

Fig. 18.19 (**a**) Mid esophageal view (44°) of a Bjork Fontan or right atrial (*RA*) to right ventricular outflow tract connection in a patient with tricuspid atresia. The Bjork connection has been fashioned from the right atrial appendage and pericardium and inserts below the pulmonary valve (*PV*). (**b**) Note the right-to-left shunt across the interatrial septum by color Doppler, consistent with a pressure gradient between the atria. (**c**) Pulsed wave Doppler interrogation demonstrates atrial flutter and an estimated peak pressure gradient of 10.6 mmHg between the atria. *Ao* aorta, *LA* left atrium

tricular dysfunction, arrhythmias, volume overload, coronary rupture, chamber compression, and sudden death. TEE readily identifies the coronary artery origins and their initial course, as well as the size and patency of the proximal vessels (also refer to Chap. 14). Abnormal fistulous communications can also be assessed by TEE. During surgical interventions color flow mapping is helpful in the characterization of vessel patency. Catheter interventions applied to the obliteration of fistulous coronary artery to cameral connections may be guided by transesophageal imaging.

Summary

TEE has become an essential imaging modality in the evaluation of adults with CHD. The ability to perform a comprehensive anatomic and hemodynamic assessment in these patients has reduced the need for diagnostic catheterization and other studies. Importantly, TEE has evolved into a complementary tool that is integral to the guidance of interventional procedures and surgical interventions in this challenging patient group.

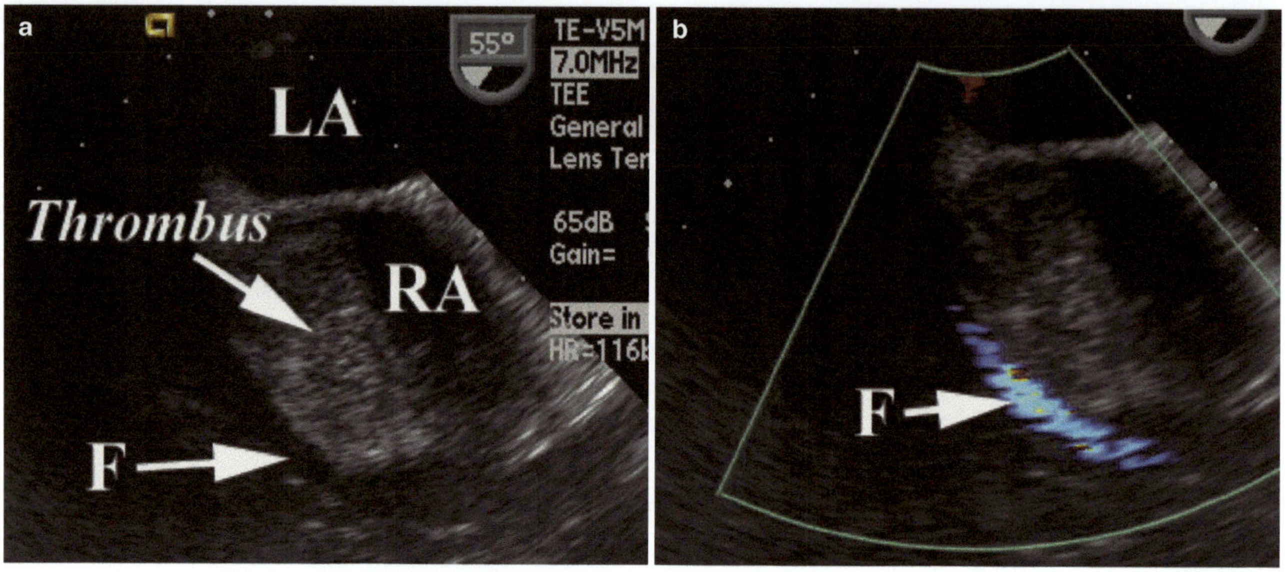

Fig. 18.20 (**a**) Mid esophageal view at 55° shows an intra-atrial tunnel Fontan (*F*) connection with evidence of a large thrombus (*arrow*) in its mid-portion within the right atrium (*RA*). (**b**) Color flow Doppler (Nyquist limit set at 28 cm/s) shows only a small amount of blood flowing past the thrombus. *LA* left atrium

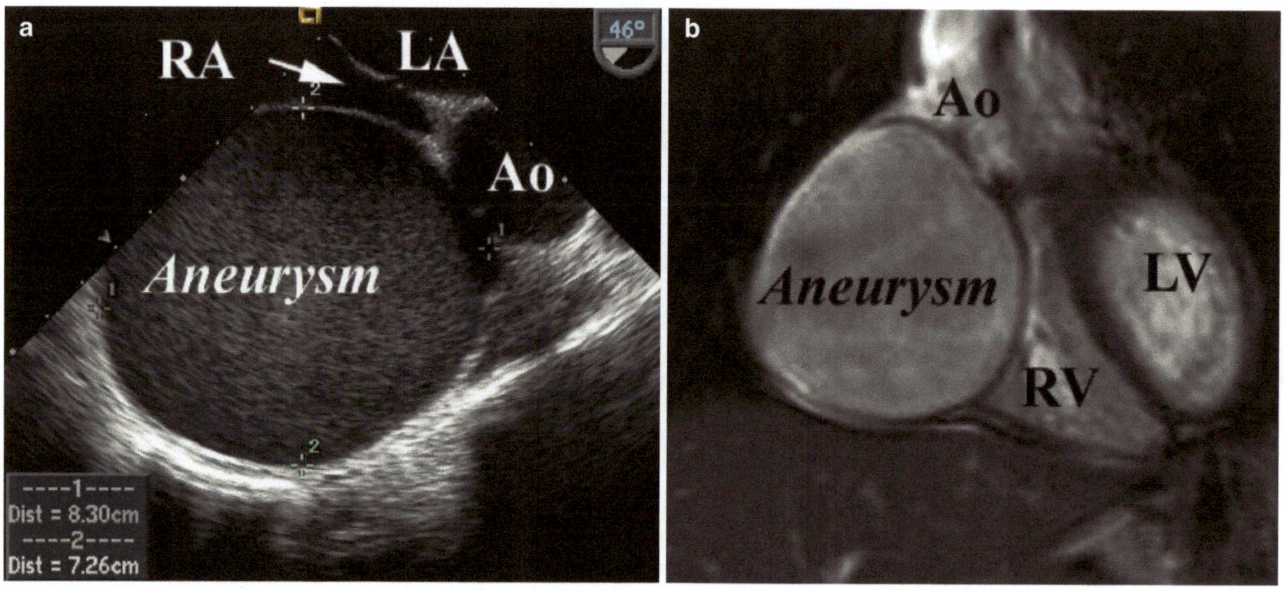

Fig. 18.21 (**a**) Mid esophageal aortic valve short axis view with rightward probe rotation and multiplane angle of 46° demonstrating a gigantic right coronary artery aneurysm in a patient with congenital coronary artery ectasia. The aneurysm compresses the right atrium (*RA*). (**b**) Gradient echo cine magnetic resonance imaging in a coronal projection showing the gigantic aneurysm also compressing the right ventricle (*RV*). *Ao* aorta, *LA* left atrium, *LV* left ventricle

To fully evaluate adults with structural heart disease, the echocardiographer must have an in-depth anatomic, spatial, and functional understanding of the various simple and complex defects and detailed knowledge of anatomy and pathophysiology as well as the many types of surgical and transcatheter interventions, their residua, sequelae, and complications. Acquired diseases of adulthood must be taken into account and their potential interaction with the congenital abnormalities considered. In summary, TEE represents an invaluable tool for the adult CHD specialist and with further refinements and evolution of the technology, promises to remain a key imaging modality in this patient population.

References

1. Warnes CA, Liberthson R, Danielson GK, et al. Task force 1: the changing profile of congenital heart disease in adult life. J Am Coll Cardiol. 2001;37:1170–5.
2. Hoffman JI, Kaplan S, Liberthson RR. Prevalence of congenital heart disease. Am Heart J. 2004;147:425–39.
3. Rhodes LA, Gustafson RA, Phillips JP, et al. The adult with congenital heart disease. W V Med J. 2006;102:310–3.
4. Stark J. Do we really correct congenital heart defects? J Thorac Cardiovasc Surg. 1989;97:1–9.
5. Miller-Hance WC, Silverman NH. Transesophageal echocardiography (TEE) in congenital heart disease with focus on the adult. Cardiol Clin. 2000;18:861–92.
6. Russell IA, Rouine-Rapp K, Stratmann G, et al. Congenital heart disease in the adult: a review with internet-accessible transesophageal echocardiographic images. Anesth Analg. 2006;102:694–723.
7. Marelli AJ, Child JS, Perloff JK. Transesophageal echocardiography in congenital heart disease in the adult. Cardiol Clin. 1993;11:505–20.
8. Tucker KJ, Curtis AB, Murphy J, et al. Transesophageal echocardiographic guidance of transseptal left heart catheterization during radiofrequency ablation of left-sided accessory pathways in humans. Pacing Clin Electrophysiol. 1996;19:272–81.
9. Bettex DA, Pretre R, Jenni R, et al. Cost-effectiveness of routine intraoperative transesophageal echocardiography in pediatric cardiac surgery: a 10-year experience. Anesth Analg. 2005;100: 1271–5.
10. Omeish A, Hijazi ZM. Transcatheter closure of atrial septal defects in children & adults using the Amplatzer Septal Occluder. J Interv Cardiol. 2001;14:37–44.
11. Srinivasa KH, Manjunath CN, Dhanalakshmi C, et al. Transesophageal Doppler echocardiographic study of pulmonary venous flow pattern in severe mitral stenosis and the changes following balloon mitral valvuloplasty. Echocardiography. 2000;17:151–7.
12. Krumsdorf U, Ostermayer S, Billinger K, et al. Incidence and clinical course of thrombus formation on atrial septal defect and patient foramen ovale closure devices in 1,000 consecutive patients. J Am Coll Cardiol. 2004;43:302–9.
13. Daniel WG, Mugge A, Martin RP. Improvement in the diagnosis of abscesses associated with endocarditis by transesophageal echocardiography. N Engl J Med. 1991;324:795–800.
14. Abdel-Massih T, Dulac Y, Taktak A, et al. Assessment of atrial septal defect size with 3D-transesophageal echocardiography: comparison with balloon method. Echocardiography. 2005;22:121–7.
15. Mazic U, Gavora P, Masura J. The role of transesophageal echocardiography in transcatheter closure of secundum atrial septal defects by the Amplatzer septal occluder. Am Heart J. 2001;142:482–8.
16. Franke A, Kuhl HP. The role of antiplatelet agents in the management of patients receiving intracardiac closure devices. Curr Pharm Des. 2006;12:1287–91.
17. Hoffman P, Wojcik AW, Rozanski J, et al. The role of echocardiography in diagnosing double chambered right ventricle in adults. Heart. 2004;90:789–93.
18. Trehan V, Ramakrishnan S, Goyal NK. Successful device closure of an acquired Gerbode defect. Catheter Cardiovasc Interv. 2006;68:942–5.
19. Perez-David E, Garcia Fernandez MA, Garcia E, et al. Successful transcatheter closure of a postmyocardial infarction ventricular septal rupture in a patient rejected for cardiac surgery: usefulness of transesophageal echocardiography. J Am Soc Echocardiogr. 2007;20:1417–12.
20. Allen HD, Beekman III RH, Garson Jr A, et al. Pediatric therapeutic cardiac catheterization: a statement for healthcare professionals from the Council on Cardiovascular Disease in the Young, American Heart Association. Circulation. 1998;97:609–25.
21. Hayes CJ, Gersony WM, Driscoll DJ, et al. Second natural history study of congenital heart defects. Results of treatment of patients with pulmonary valvar stenosis. Circulation. 1993;87:I28–37.
22. Murphy JG, Gersh BJ, Mair DD, et al. Long-term outcome in patients undergoing surgical repair of tetralogy of Fallot. N Engl J Med. 1993;329:593–9.
23. Silversides CK, Veldtman GR, Crossin J, et al. Pressure half-time predicts hemodynamically significant pulmonary regurgitation in adult patients with repaired tetralogy of fallot. J Am Soc Echocardiogr. 2003;16:1057–62.
24. Li W, Davlouros PA, Kilner PJ, et al. Doppler-echocardiographic assessment of pulmonary regurgitation in adults with repaired tetralogy of Fallot: comparison with cardiovascular magnetic resonance imaging. Am Heart J. 2004;147:165–72.
25. Sachdev MS, Bhagyavathy A, Varghese R, et al. Right ventricular diastolic function after repair of tetralogy of Fallot. Pediatr Cardiol. 2006;27:250–5.
26. Aboulhosn J, Child JS. Left ventricular outflow obstruction: subaortic stenosis, bicuspid aortic valve, supravalvar aortic stenosis, and coarctation of the aorta. Circulation. 2006;114:2412–22.
27. Niwa K, Perloff JK, Bhuta SM, et al. Structural abnormalities of great arterial walls in congenital heart disease: light and electron microscopic analyses. Circulation. 2001;103:393–400.
28. Frescura C, Angelini A, Daliento L, et al. Morphological aspects of Ebstein's anomaly in adults. Thorac Cardiovasc Surg. 2000;48: 203–8.
29. Pavlova M, Fouron JC, Drblik SP, et al. Factors affecting the prognosis of Ebstein's anomaly during fetal life. Am Heart J. 1998; 135:1081–5.
30. Chowdhury UK, Airan B, Talwar S, et al. One and one-half ventricle repair: results and concerns. Ann Thorac Surg. 2005; 80:2293–300.
31. Lundstrom U, Bull C, Wyse RK, et al. The natural and "unnatural" history of congenitally corrected transposition. Am J Cardiol. 1990;65:1222–9.
32. Graham Jr TP, Bernard YD, Mellen BG, et al. Long-term outcome in congenitally corrected transposition of the great arteries: a multi-institutional study. J Am Coll Cardiol. 2000;36:255–61.
33. Caso P, Ascione L, Lange A, et al. Diagnostic value of transesophageal echocardiography in the assessment of congenitally corrected transposition of the great arteries in adult patients. Am Heart J. 1998;135:43–50.
34. Kaulitz R, Stumper OF, Geuskens R, et al. Comparative values of the precordial and transesophageal approaches in the echocardiographic evaluation of atrial baffle function after an atrial correction procedure. J Am Coll Cardiol. 1990;16(3):686–94.
35. Glenn WW, Patino JF. Circulatory by-pass of the right heart. I. Preliminary observations on the direct delivery of vena caval blood into the pulmonary arterial circulation; azygos vein-pulmonary artery shunt. Yale J Biol Med. 1954;27:147–51.
36. Aboulhosn J, Danon S, Levi D, et al. Regression of pulmonary arteriovenous malformations after transcatheter reconnection of the pulmonary arteries in patients with unidirectional Fontan. Congenit Heart Dis. 2007;2:179–84.
37. Fontan F, Baudet E. Surgical repair of tricuspid atresia. Thorax. 1971;26:240–8.
38. Aboulhosn J, Child JS. The adult with a Fontan operation. Curr Cardiol Rep. 2007;9:331–5.
39. Aboulhosn JA, Shavelle DM, Castellon Y, et al. Fontan operation and the single ventricle. Congenit Heart Dis. 2007;2:2–11.
40. Mavroudis C, Deal BJ, Backer CL. The beneficial effects of total cavopulmonary conversion and arrhythmia surgery for the failed Fontan. Semin Thorac Cardiovasc Surg Pediatr Card Surg Annu. 2002;5:12–24.
41. Angelini P. Coronary artery anomalies: an entity in search of an identity. Circulation. 2007;115:1296–305.

Transesophageal Three-Dimensional Echocardiography in Congenital Heart Disease

19

Gerald Ross Marx

Abstract

In the past 10 years, real-time three-dimensional echocardiography has emerged as an important new technique in echocardiography for the diagnosis and evaluation of both acquired and congenital heart disease. In recent years, three-dimensional transesophageal echocardiography (3D TEE) probes have become available. While these probes were designed primarily for use in the adult age group, they have also been utilized effectively in older children and adolescents. These probes are capable of real-time 3D TEE imaging and color flow Doppler, providing excellent spatial detail of selected acquired and congenital heart defects. Thus 3D TEE serves an important and ever-increasing role during cardiac surgery as well as interventional cardiology procedures. This chapter describes the technique of 3D TEE imaging as well as some of its most common applications for congenital heart disease evaluation.

Keywords

Transesophageal echocardiography • Three-dimensional echocardiography • Atrial septal defect • Subaortic stenosis • Atrial septal defects, transcatheter closure • Ebstein anomaly of the tricuspid valve

History and Development

With the advent of matrix array transducers and sophisticated computer analysis, three-dimensional (3D) echocardiography is now widely applied in the diagnostic imaging domain for congenital heart disease (CHD). In particular, congenital heart surgeons, in the operative management of complex CHD, will sometimes request 3D imaging to provide additional information about cardiac anatomy and spatial relationships. This also applies for repair of valve dysfunction, in which the anatomic substrate can be difficult to discern with standard two-dimensional (2D) imaging.

In the initial development of 3D echocardiography, a reconstructive approach was first utilized. This consisted of sequential acquisition of multiple transesophageal 2D echocardiographic images, followed by offline reconstruction and 3D rendering of the collected image dataset [1–6]. During image acquisition, the probe was moved in a linear or rotational format, and was advanced to subsequent imaging planes, based on electrocardiographic (ECG) and respiratory gating. Excellent 3D gray scale and color flow studies were obtained. However, this technology was time consuming and cumbersome. Depending on the heart rate, the acquisition would last at least 3–5 min. Significant arrhythmias would interfere with the acquisition. Moreover, to maintain spatial integrity, the heart had to be stationary from a positional standpoint. Furthermore, the formatting of the 2D images into a 3D construct consumed additional valuable time. Although certain dedicated and cooperative surgeons would participate, this form of 3D imaging was not widely applied in the operative suite.

G.R. Marx, MD
Department of Cardiology, Boston Children's Hospital, Harvard School of Medicine, 300 Longwood Ave., Boston, MA 02115, USA
e-mail: gerald.marx@cardio.chboston.org

The online version of this chapter (doi:10.1007/978-1-84800-064-3_19) contains supplementary material, which is available to authorized users.

P.C. Wong, W.C. Miller-Hance (eds.), *Transesophageal Echocardiography for Congenital Heart Disease*,
DOI 10.1007/978-1-84800-064-3_19, © Springer-Verlag London 2014

With advancements in probe design, and sophisticated, efficient and fast computers, nearly simultaneous imaging of volumetric echocardiographic 3D data sets became available for transthoracic echocardiography transducers. These advanced matrix array transducers were relatively smaller. Hence, epicardial 3D echocardiography evolved as these matrix array probes could be held and manipulated comfortably on the heart by the surgeon [7]. The surgeon could investigate the anatomy in the "live" 3D display. Similar to 2D imaging, immediate anatomic "feedback" was available, but in a 3D spatial orientation. Even full volume acquisitions could be obtained, and the specific anatomy segmented and displayed to the surgeon in minutes.

Although excellent 3D images could be shown in the operating room, available for surgical planning, certain disadvantages with epicardial 3D echocardiography were apparent. First, imaging in the near field was sub-optimal due to the very short focal distance. Second, in the vigorously beating heart, stable contact of the transducer with the cardiac structures was difficult to maintain. Third, this type of image acquisition occupied and usurped the time and concentration of the operating surgeon [8]. These important limitations, coupled with the development of a real-time 3D transesophageal echocardiography (TEE) probe in 2007 (X7-2t, Philips Medical Systems, Andover, Massachusetts) [9], have led to the use of 3D TEE as the preferred 3D technique in the operative setting (for patients of adequate size). Despite this important achievement, epicardial 3D echocardiography can still be used: (1) for young and small pediatric patients in whom the 3D TEE probe is too large; (2) for those pediatric or adult patients with specific contraindications to TEE.

3D TEE has readily become accepted for adult patients undergoing cardiothoracic surgery or catheter-based interventions [9–12]. This technological advancement has also been applied to adult patients with congenital heart defects. However, with careful patient selection, and collaboration between the cardiologist and anesthesiologist, 3D TEE can be used safely in selected children and adolescents [13]. As opposed to epicardial imaging, 3D TEE can be undertaken without interfering with the surgical field. Additionally, this imaging can provide a more comprehensive and larger field of view. This latter advantage probably arises from the offset of the transducer from the heart. Still, 3D TEE imaging can be difficult in the near field, especially for visualization of the atria and pulmonary veins.

The following chapter will provide a methodological description of real time 3D TEE in CHD based on the experience to date. Emphasis will be focused on specific clinical examples in which intraoperative 3D TEE imaging can provide additional important information to guide either catheter-based or surgical planning. Additional applications of 3D technology will also be presented.

A note regarding terminology: In the medical literature, both "3D" and "4D" (four-dimensional) are used when referring to 3D echocardiography. The use of the term 4D is meant to describe the 3D depiction of a moving object (such as the heart), with 3D rendering displayed using real-time motion—thus time represents the fourth dimension. In current ultrasound parlance, the two terms are used synonymously and interchangeably. For simplicity, in this chapter "3D" will used to represent both terms.

General Concepts

3D TEE Probe Technology

The technology of the current real-time 3D TEE probes was discussed in Chaps. 1 and 2, but will be detailed again in this chapter. The following discussion applies specifically to one device (the Philips X7-2t 3D TEE probe); however, many of the same principles apply to other 3D systems utilizing matrix array technology.

Physically, the 3D TEE probe looks very similar to a standard 2D TEE probe. The same standard TEE handle controls are available—antero-posterior and left-right flexion, as well as a multiplane angle control which rotates the 2D tomographic plane from 0° to 180° (Fig. 19.1a). The 3D TEE probe tip is shaped similar to its 2D counterpart, although it is slightly larger in size (Fig. 19.1b). This larger tip is designed to accommodate the highly advanced, miniaturized technology that makes possible real-time 3D TEE imaging.

The typical 2D multiplane TEE probe consists of a phased array transducer containing 64 piezoelectric crystals (elements) placed side by side in a rectangular row (Fig. 19.2a). As described in Chap. 1, sequential activation of these crystals produces a beam that is steered to obtain a flat, pie-shaped scanning plane. This creates the standard tomographic 2D images customarily seen with the TEE systems currently in use. In a 2D multiplane TEE probe, the rectangular array of elements is physically rotated (electronically or mechanically) in a semicircular manner between 0° and 180° (Fig. 19.2a), thereby obtaining the various 2D TEE tomographic images commonly seen in this and other sources. In contrast, the 3D TEE probe contains a matrix array of 2,500+ piezoelectric crystals arranged in a square 10 × 10 mm grid (Figs. 19.1b and 19.2b). The individual elements are electrically independent, allowing for generation of scan lines than can vary both azimuthally (laterally) and elevationally (Fig. 19.2b). Thus a pyramidal 3D "wedge" of acoustic raw data information can be obtained and subsequently processed into Cartesian coordinates using a 3D scan converter; each discrete point in the scan converter is known as a voxel ("volumetric pixel"), which is cubic in shape and carries a discrete coordinate in 3D space as well as a value for echo intensity [14–16]. This is analogous to the pixels (picture elements) used to form a 2D image. Voxels therefore constitute the basic components used to construct a 3D dataset [5]. Since voxels represent discrete data points,

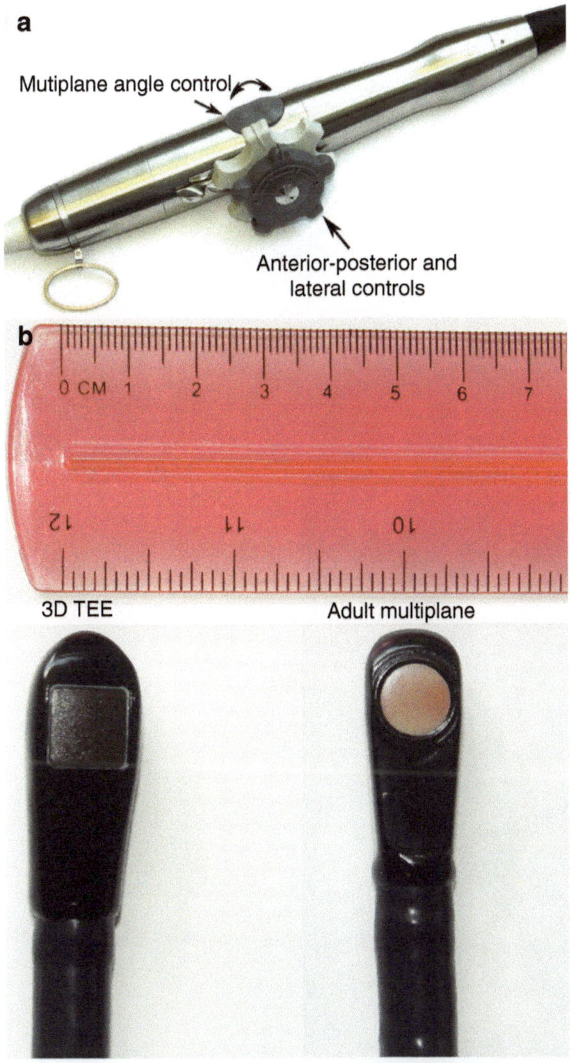

Fig. 19.1 The Philips X7-2t 3D TEE probe. (**a**) Shows the handle of the probe; it has identical controls as a standard 2D TEE probe. When used for 2D TEE imaging, the multiplane angle control (shown) rotates the imaging plane between 0° and 180°. (**b**) Is a photo of the Philips adult transesophageal (TEE) 3D and 2D probes side by side. Note that the 3D TEE probe is slightly larger than its 2D counterpart

interpolation is used to fill in the gaps between the voxels, using adjacent data of similar characteristics [15].The resultant 3D image depends upon the size and density of the voxels. Analogous to 2D imaging, smaller voxels and increased number of scan lines lead to a higher voxel count and less data interpolation, which in turn enhances the spatial resolution of the 3D image. However the tradeoff is temporal resolution. There is a large volume of data (several thousand scan lines) that needs to be collected and processed for a single 3D volume dataset, and if the processing of this dataset were performed in a manner akin to standard 2D echocardiography, the time required would result in unacceptably low frame rates. To address this, parallel beamforming (parallel processing) is utilized. In this technique, the system transmits one wide beam and receives multiple narrow beams in parallel [17], which enables much faster 3D image processing, thereby permitting the motion of the 3D images to be displayed at clinically acceptable frame rates. Nonetheless as a result of the greater data processing requirements, the current frame rates for live 3D imaging are still much less than those achievable by conventional 2D imaging. Also, parallel beamforming comes at a cost: there is an accompanying increase in the amount of electronics, as well as size, cost, and power consumption of the system [17].

The process of displaying a 3D data set on a 2D computer screen is known as *rendering*, and can be performed by one of several different methods. The first method, known as *wireframe rendering*, shows the surface of a structure as a series of lines connected together to form a mesh of interconnected polygons that altogether form a cage-like, wireframe 3D model of the surface of the heart (Fig. 19.3a). This method was originally designed for computer-assisted design and manufacturing (CAD/CAM), and is well suited for ventricular wall motion although it cannot display more complex internal structures such as valvular structures [5]. The second method is known as *surface rendering*. Similar to wireframe rendering, surface rendering displays the details

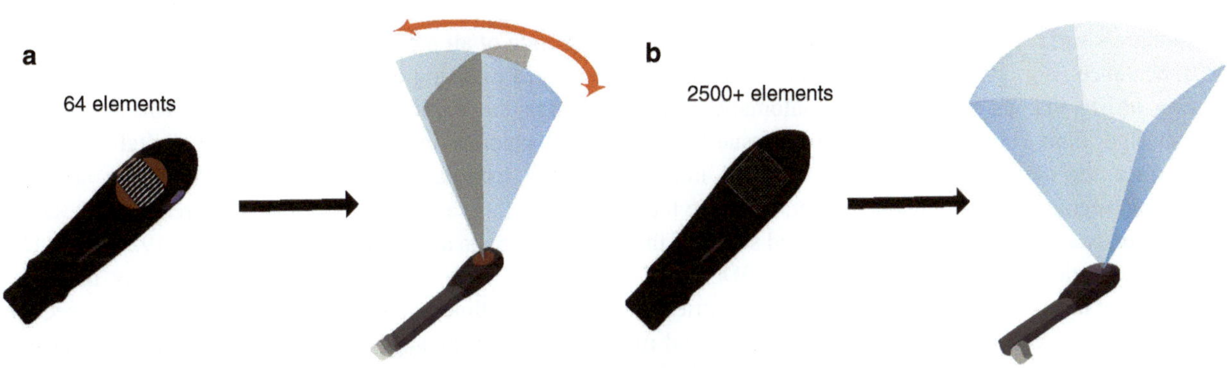

Fig. 19.2 Diagram of adult transesophageal (TEE) 2D and 3D probes. (**a**) Illustrates a standard multiplane 2D TEE probe, which uses a linear phased array containing 64 piezoelectric elements. Using a control on the TEE probe handle, the array is physically rotated either electronically or mechanically to obtain a multiplane angle between 0° and 180°. (**b**) Illustrates a 3D TEE matrix array probe with over 2,500 elements arranged in a square grid. Scan lines are generated both azimuthally (laterally) and elevationally, thus a pyramidal volume can be obtained, enabling the acquisition of a 3D volume dataset

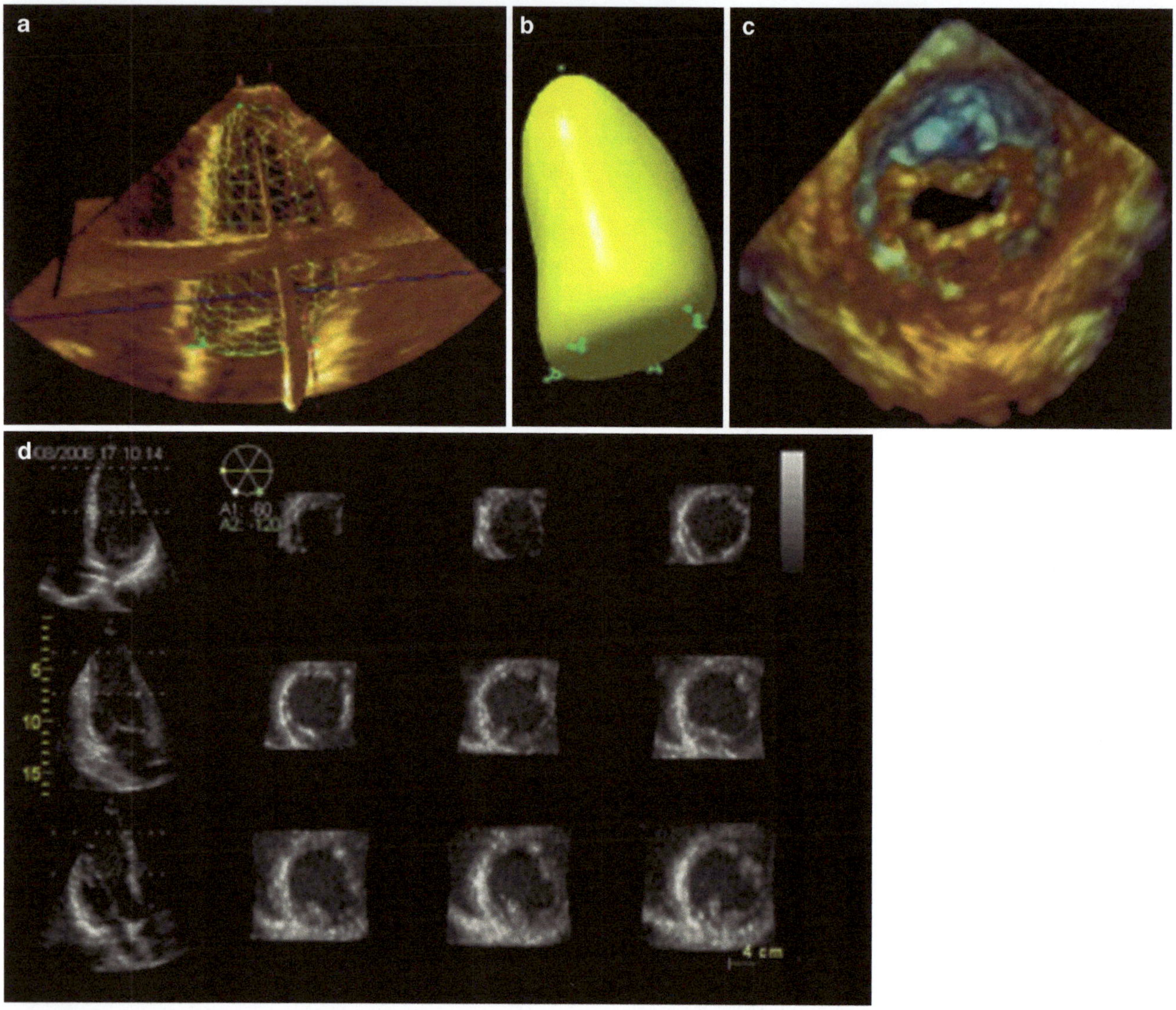

Fig. 19.3 Examples of different modes in which 3D echocardiographic data sets can be visualized and rendered. The techniques used to display the images can be divided into four broad categories: wireframe (**a**), surface rendering (**b**), volume rendering (**c**), and 2D tomographic slicing (**d**). These displays were obtained from transthoracic 3D imaging, but the principles of image rendering and display apply equally with 3D transesophageal imaging (Reprinted from Lang et al. [18]; with permission from Elsevier)

of a structure's surface but defines more points to present a solid appearance (Fig. 19.3b). Both wireframe and surface rendering utilize manual tracing or semiautomatic border detection algorithms (identification of blood-tissue boundary) to trace the endocardium in cross-sectional images derived from segmentation of the 3D dataset; these are then used to generate a 3D model of the surface and shape of the structure in question (usually a ventricle). This 3D/4D volume "cast" can then be used for quantification of ventricular volume, synchrony and function [14]. The third method of rendering, known as *volume rendering*, is the method used most frequently in real-time 3D imaging, particularly for the evaluation of structural abnormalities such as those seen in CHD. This method preserves all 3D information within the dataset, and rendering is performed to provide a realistic 3D depiction of all the anatomic details within the heart. This is achieved by using different algorithms to cast a light beam through the voxels, and weighting the voxels to obtain a voxel gradient intensity. A variety of digital shading and lighting techniques (perspective, light casting, and depth color-coding) are used to achieve the perception of 3D depth and texture on a 2D computer screen (Fig. 19.3c) [18]. Using tools available both on the echocardiography machine as well as offline, these volume datasets can be sectioned (cropped) from any number of different viewpoints, and rotated to reveal the spatial relationships of atrioventricular/semilunar valves and complex intracardiac anatomy. Also, the source of the light beam (and therefore shading/lighting) is projected to maintain a sense of depth and three dimensionality, even while the 3D volume dataset is rotated and sectioned. Volume rendered datasets can be displayed in four principal modes:

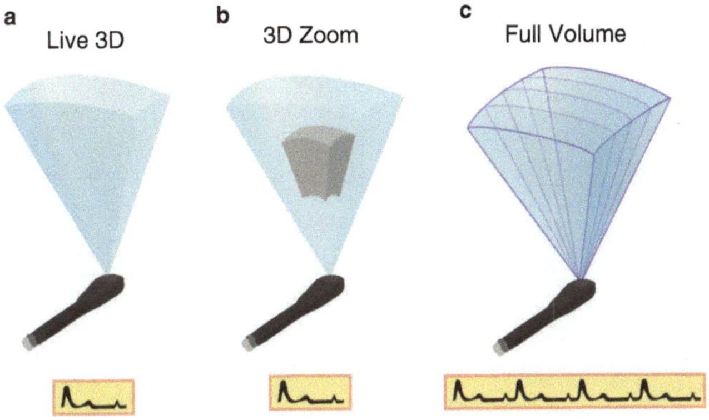

Fig. 19.4 The different modes of volume rendering. (**a**) Is an illustration showing a Live 3D volume, acquired in one beat and without the need for gating. (**b**) Shows 3D zoom mode: only data within a small region of interest are acquired, the data are collected in one beat, and no gating is required. (**c**) Shows a full volume dataset in which four subvolumes that have been sequentially acquired and "stitched" together to form one large volume. Creation of a full volume requires gating to the electrocardiogram

- **Real-time** (**Live**) **3D**. This mode, activated by a single button, provides true live, real-time 3D imaging of the beating heart. However only a portion of the heart is contained in 3D dataset. It is obtained in such a manner that the "front" portion of the dataset (nearest the observer) automatically displays a tomographic slice identical to the 2D image that was shown prior to 3D activation, but with rendered volumetric imaging behind the slice to provide additional information and a 3D perspective (Figs. 19.4a and 19.5, Video 19.1). This 3D mode yields a narrow pyramidal volume with dimensions 30° × 60°. Since the "live" format is truly real-time, no gating to respiration or electrocardiogram (ECG) is necessary. However because the structure(s) in question has been "sectioned" to mimic the 2D tomographic image for visualization and orientation, the resultant 3D dataset will not include the entire structure. This mode has a temporal resolution (frame rate) of 20–30 Hz, which is sufficient for monitoring real-time motion and guiding interventional procedures.

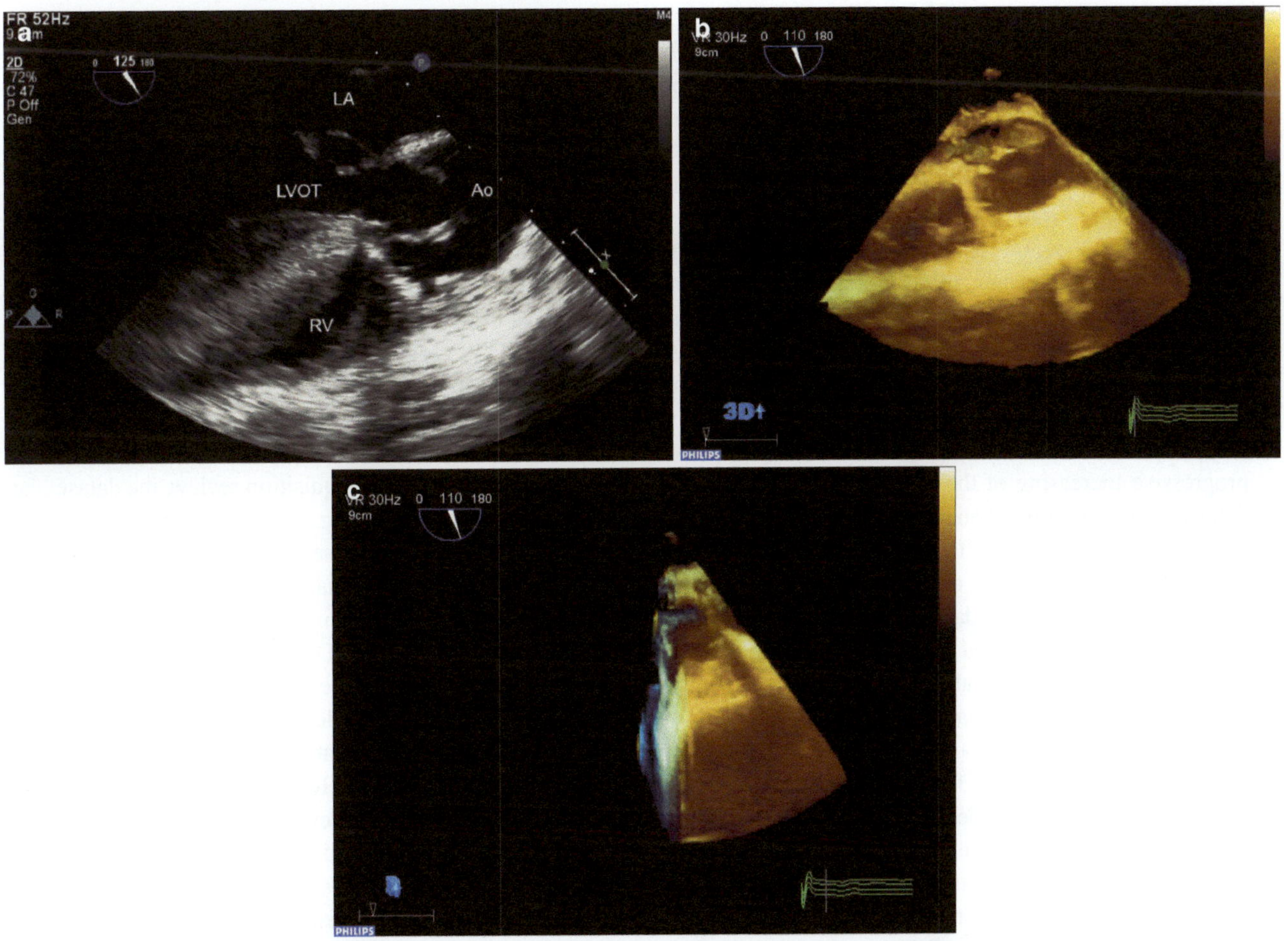

Fig. 19.5 Example of three-dimensional "Live 3D" format in a patient with repaired tetralogy of Fallot and an abnormal aortic valve. A standard mid esophageal aortic valve long axis view (**a**) was used to position and orient the probe. (**b**) Shows the "Live 3D" mode volume dataset. Note that the front portion of the dataset displays the tomographic image similar to the standard 2D image, which helps to orient the echocardiographer. (**c**) Shows the dataset rotated to show the thickness of the volume. Note that volumetric data is obtained behind the image, but the entire aortic valve is not contained in the dataset. *Ao* aorta, *LA* left atrium, *LVOT* left ventricular outflow tract, *RV* right ventricle

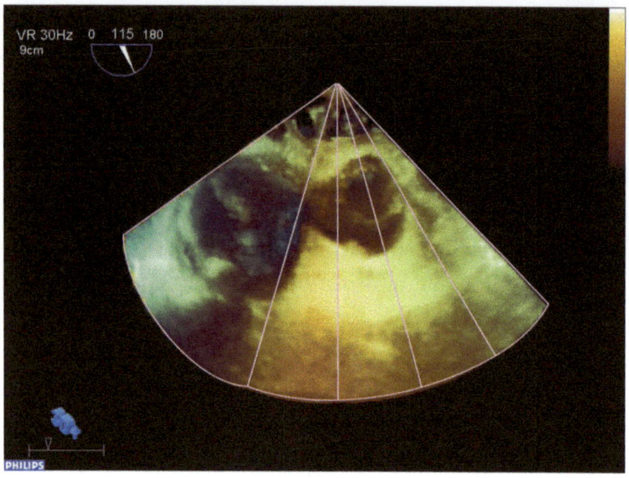

Fig. 19.6 Example of the three-dimensional full volume dataset acquired in the patient from Fig. 19.4. Four subvolumes were collected and rapidly stitched together to form a pyramidal dataset. Now a significant portion of the heart, including the whole aortic valve, is contained in this dataset. The volume has been rotated from its initial acquisition display, and lines have been drawn to illustrate the manner in which the subvolumes are collected and stitched together

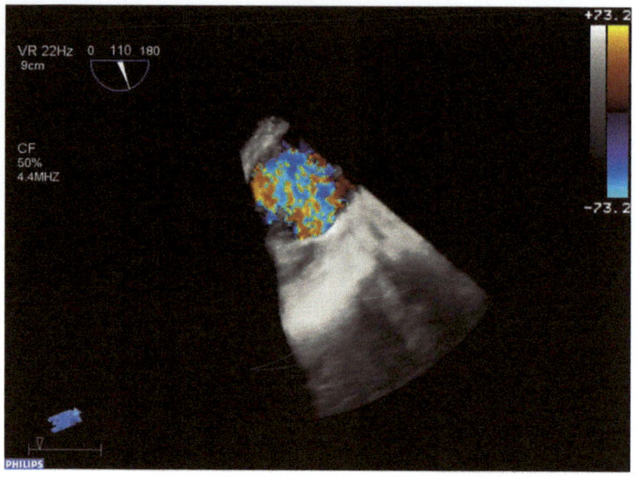

Fig. 19.7 Example of a three-dimensional color flow dataset in the same patient in Figs. 19.5 and 19.6. Turbulent systolic flow is noted across the aortic valve

- **3D Zoom**. This mode is also a "live" mode. A specific region of interest (e.g. the mitral valve) is identified, and a smaller volume dataset positioned to provide a focused, magnified, complete 3D visualization of the region as a smaller and narrower pyramid (Fig. 19.4b). The pyramid angles can vary from 20° × 20° to 90° × 90°, with a dimension of 30° × 30° commonly used. By reducing the volume size and focusing solely upon the structure of interest, the entire structure can be contained in the dataset, and the lateral resolution can be improved by increasing the number of scan lines, while still maintaining acceptable frame rates. The live images can still be cropped and rotated in multiple orientations. However progressive increasing of the magnification can produce deterioration in both spatial and temporal resolution (sometimes down to 5–10 Hz) [18].
- **3D Full Volume**. This is a gated acquisition mode in which a large 3D volume dataset is assembled from several adjacent wedge-shaped 3D subvolumes that are collected rapidly and sequentially using ECG-gating. A total of 4–7 subvolumes are obtained and then digitally reassembled or "stitched" into a large pyramidal digital dataset, which is then available for viewing and manipulation (Figs. 19.4c and 19.6, Video 19.2). Strictly speaking, a full volume dataset is not real-time since it represents an ECG-gated assemblage of subvolumes collected sequentially over a matter of seconds, but for all practical purposes it is nearly so because of the very short acquisition and display time. This mode provides excellent spatial and temporal resolution (20–50 Hz, depending upon number of beats captured), and because of the wide dimensions of the volume dataset (90° × 90°), entire structures can be completely captured within the dataset. However due to the gating, full volume datasets can be subject to "stitch" artifact (imperfect alignment of subvolumes) if there is significant respiratory motion or any ECG abnormality.
- **3D Color Doppler**. 3D color flow Doppler volume datasets can also be obtained, with the 3D color Doppler information superimposed upon the 3D image information (Fig. 19.7, Video 19.3). These 3D color flow volume datasets are assembled from 7 to 14 thin ECG-gated subvolumes in the same manner as the full volume datasets described above, although they smaller than the full volume datasets. Due to the many subvolumes required, some degree of stitch artifact is not uncommon with these datasets. Also, temporal resolution tends to be reduced (<10 Hz). During post-acquisition review, the dataset can be viewed as only imaging, only color Doppler, and with color Doppler superimposed upon the image, similar to standard 2D/color flow imaging.

Newer 3D software now enables a larger volume of scanning while performing live 3D imaging; often the size of the volume approaches that of the stitched full volumes detailed above. This is termed "single beat" full volume scanning, and does not require ECG-gating; hence it is not subject to artifacts from arrhythmias. However there is a tradeoff, as less information (due to lower frame rates) is available for this single beat. For improved resolution, more data must be obtained over several successive ECG-gated beats (2, 4, or 6), thus replicating the process of the stitched full volume acquisition. The newer software also allows real time 3D color Doppler scanning to be performed, though frame rate decreases appreciably. Again, this can be improved with acquisition over multiple ECG-gated beats. With both the

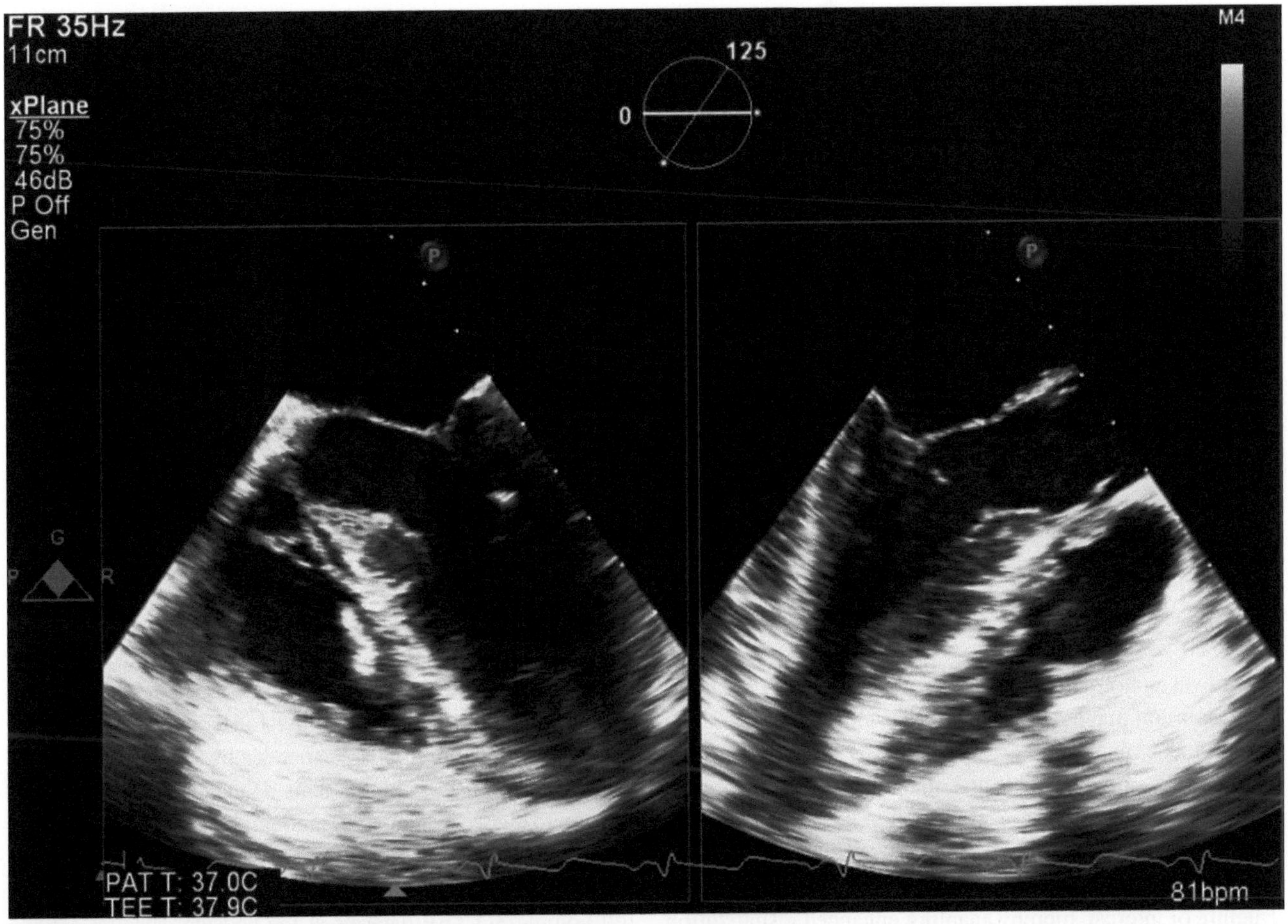

Fig. 19.8 xPlane mode from the Philips X7-2t 3D TEE probe. Two different 2D planes are shown simultaneously in this patient with mild subaortic stenosis. On the left is a mid esophageal four chamber view, on the right a mid esophageal long axis view. The circle on the display indicates the relationship of the two planes

single beat full volume imaging as well as color flow Doppler modes, the selection of an increasing number of ECG-gated beats produces incremental improvements in frame rates, but the potential for stitch artifact also increases.

In addition to its 3D capabilities, the 3D TEE matrix transducer can also function as a standalone 2D multiplane probe, with full 2D, color flow and spectral pulse/continuous Doppler as well as M-mode capabilities (tissue Doppler imaging is available in later software releases). Like a standard 2D TEE probe, the tomographic plane position can be steered between 0° and 180° using a control on the probe handle (Fig. 19.1a). However, unlike a 2D TEE probe, no physical motion of the elements actually occurs at the probe tip—instead the tomographic plane is electrically steered by coordinated activation of the matrix elements to vary scan lines and obtain a multiplane angle between 0° and 180°. Moreover, one of the unique features of the matrix array is that several different 2D tomographic planes can be displayed simultaneously from the same volume dataset, a feature variously known as biplane, triplane, or multiplane imaging (Fig. 19.3d). These can be displayed as equidistant parallel slices (as shown in Fig. 19.3d), three orthogonal planes together, or slices rotated around a common axis. For example, with the Philips 3D TEE system, two different live 2D images can be displayed next to each other using the xPlane mode, as shown in Fig. 19.8, Video 19.4. In this example, mid esophageal four chamber and long axis views are shown simultaneously. Multiplane imaging from a 3D volume dataset has been shown to be useful when evaluating CHD [19].

Advantages of Real-Time 3D TEE

With conventional 2D imaging, the tomographic planes, once acquired, cannot undergo further alteration of the views. Instead, further images must be collected by various TEE probe maneuvers and multiplane angles (Chap. 4) to provide additional visualization of a structure in question. The advantage of real time 3D TEE is the immediate manner in which the volume datasets are available for analysis, and the multiple ways in which a dataset can be manipulated to

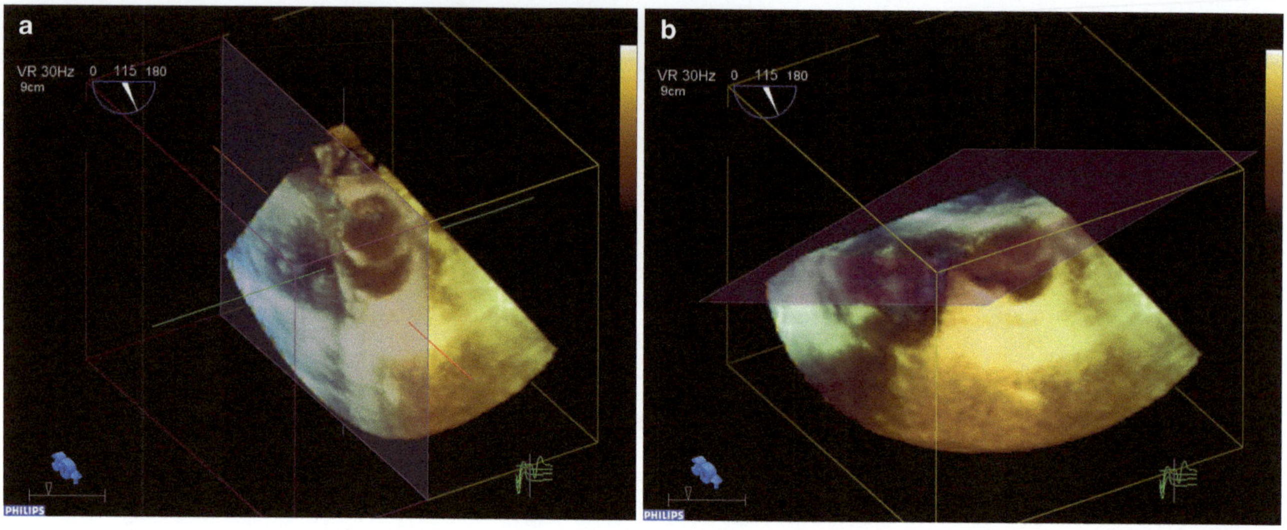

Fig. 19.9 Example of cropping of a full volume dataset in the patient from Figs. 19.4 and 19.5. (**a, b**) Show the full volume dataset cropped in different planes: one of the standard perpendicular (x,y,z) cropping planes (**a**), and an "anyplane" cropping mode that can be performed from any angle (**b**). The latter can be used to visualize the intracardiac anatomy from a multitude of different perspectives

yield novel anatomic perspectives not visible by 2D imaging. Two important maneuvers are used to evaluate a rendered 3D dataset; these maneuvers are unique to 3D imaging, and not used for 2D imaging. The first maneuver is **cropping**, in which a flat plane can be used to section the heart from any desired angle or perspective (Fig. 19.9, Video 19.5). This maneuver "crops away" a portion of the heart adjacent to the structure of interest, thereby enabling enhanced visualization of the structure, often in a manner or from a vantage point that cannot be provided by conventional 2D imaging. Examples of this include an *en face* view of the atrioventricular valves, or an *en face* view of an atrial or ventricular septal defect. The second maneuver is **rotation**: the dataset can be rotated (cropped or uncropped) in any direction to provide different views of the structure in question from a number of perspectives, e.g. visualization of an atrial septal defect, first from right atrium, then from the left atrium. Rotation enhances the understanding and appreciation of the 3D layout of the cardiac structures. Together, cropping and rotation enable the examiner to perform a "virtual dissection" of the heart. For those observers less familiar with the more unconventional cropped views, a 3D volume dataset can also be cropped and rotated to provide images that resemble their analogous (and more recognizable) standard 2D TEE images. Moreover, the multiplane 2D mode allows production of simultaneous high quality 2D TEE images, which are sometimes more familiar to viewers (Fig. 19.8, Video 19.4). Dataset viewing and manipulation can be performed directly on the echocardiography machine, or subsequently offline on a computer workstation equipped with 3D rendering/analysis software.

At our center, we first evaluate the area of interest in a "live" 3D TEE format. This mode allows for changes in threshold and gain settings with immediate feedback. Using the live data sets for transducer orientation, the full volume data sets are then obtained. Respiration is suspended by the anesthesiologist during the acquisition phase. This acquisition phase is short, i.e. four to eight cardiac cycles, and does not create respiratory/cardiac compromise. With experience, the echocardiographer can perform rapid manipulation and analysis of both live and full volume 3D TEE datasets at the bedside; specific cardiac abnormalities can be immediately segmented and displayed for the surgeon. The full volume acquisitions in particular provide a broad, encompassing display of large portions of the heart. This can enable an excellent display of the anatomy and spatial relationships of the various cardiac structures.

3D Image Display

At our center we have developed specific anatomic displays of the 3D images. We have found this to be important for several reasons. First, this establishes the underpinnings of the anatomic display to enhance understanding and communication between the surgeon, cardiologist and anesthesiologist. In particular, we strive to portray the 3D images similar to the view or perspective of the cardiovascular surgeon. Second, with experience we have learned the specific cut planes that best depict the optimal imaging information for the specific defects. Third, with time, we believe this will establish a more universal or ubiquitous imaging display orientation to enhance understanding and communication with other imaging centers, cardiologists and surgeons.

As mentioned above, the imaging planes have been established to simulate the surgeon's perspective of the anatomic defect. For example, if displaying the mitral valve from

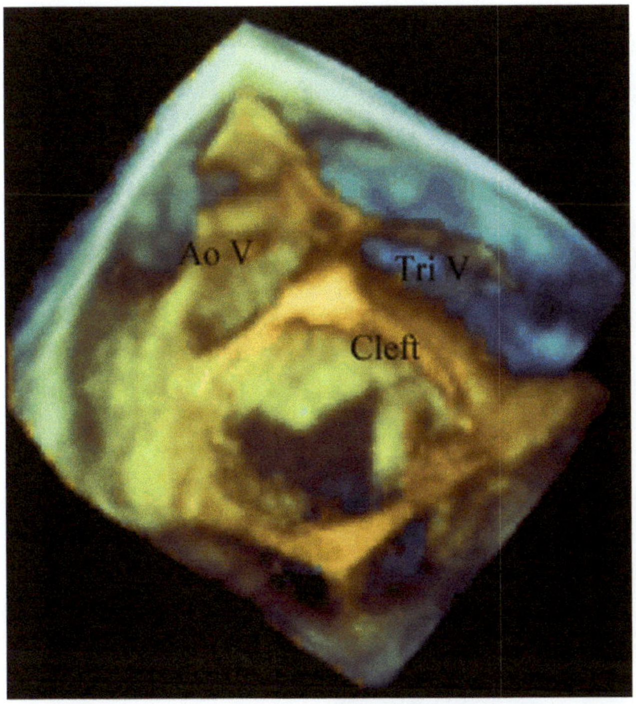

Fig. 19.10 Left atrial view imaging the superior surfaces of the left atrioventricular valve in a 23 year old woman who had previous closure of a primum atrial septal defect and had progressive left atrioventricular valve regurgitation. The aortic valve or superior aspect of the heart is to the left, and the anterior aspect, tricuspid valve, is to the top of the screen. During diastole a significant residual cleft in the anterior leaflet is easily seen, with thickened leaflet edges. *Ao V* aortic valve, *Tri V* tricuspid valve

above, i.e. atria, the anterior aspect is to the top of the screen and the more superior aspect to the left. This will place the anterior leaflet to the superior/leftward aspect of the monitor screen, and the mural or posterior leaflet to the right/inferior aspect of the monitor, (Fig. 19.10, Video 19.6).

Again, to establish conventional imaging planes, the aortic valve is displayed similar to the surgeon's view as if looking from the aortic root onto the superior aspects of the valve (Fig. 19.11, Video 19.7a and 19.7b). Thus, the right coronary leaflet is to the top, and the left coronary leaflet is to the left and inferior. The non-coronary cusp is to the right and inferior. Creating these specific-anatomic orientations is essential for optimal communication with the surgeon.

The transducer orientation depends on the specific anatomic abnormality. Naturally for the aortic valve the transesophageal imaging plane is set to obtain good short and long axis views. Both live and full volume gray scales, as well as color flow full volume acquisitions, are obtained in both the short axis and corresponding orthogonal imaging planes. One might argue that orthogonal image acquisitions would not seem to be necessary in that all the information should be within the full volume data set. If optimal temporal and spatial gating is met, imaging artifacts should not be present regardless of the segmentation planes. Nonetheless spatial artifacts can be present, and some will be more apparent depending upon the acquisition orientation.

3D TEE for CHD Evaluation

Considerations for 3D TEE in the Evaluation of CHD

One of the most often asked questions is: which patients should get a 3D echocardiographic study, in addition to standard 2D imaging? This is especially germane to 3D TEE imaging, which requires some additional effort compared to 2D TEE imaging. At our center, the surgeon most often requests 3D echocardiographic imaging especially for valve repairs [20–23]. Beyond this straightforward answer, 3D imaging is applied to particular congenital heart abnormalities in which a 3D perspective would provide important additional information in addition to 2D imaging. Another 3D TEE application includes imaging in certain congenital defects that have often required multiple re-operations. Hence any imaging that might be useful in providing information to the surgeon to enhance the repair and prevent re-operation would be advantageous. This certainly would apply to congenital heart defects such as complex atrioventricular canal defects [6], complex left ventricular (LV) outflow tract obstructive lesions [24], or repair of Ebstein anomaly of the tricuspid valve [25]. As discussed below, 3D TEE has proven application for catheterization closure of atrial and ventricular septal defects [26–29]. It provides important spatial imaging that can significantly enhance anatomic assessment of these defects. Furthermore, it can provide real-time information during the device deployment procedure, thereby guiding more precise device placement, and helping to reduce fluoroscopic imaging time.

The currently available real-time 3D TEE probes are relatively large, and their use in pediatric patients is limited by patient size. They are suitable primarily for older children and adolescents >25–30 kg, although successful probe insertion down to 15.5 kg has been reported [13]. Nonetheless even in older patients with CHD, 3D TEE has found widespread utility in a number of different clinical settings. For example, 3D TEE imaging is readily applicable in the catheterization laboratory. This applies not only for visualization of the atrial and ventricular septal defects for device closure, but also for detection of thrombus formation for patients considered for electrical cardioversion. In the ambulatory setting, 3D TEE can be used for the adolescent or adult patient in whom surgery is contemplated, when transthoracic imaging is suboptimal and cardiac MRI imaging either not feasible or contraindicated. Thus, a patient may undergo a 3D TEE study to determine the feasibility of either catheterization or surgical based intervention. Naturally, 3D TEE is also

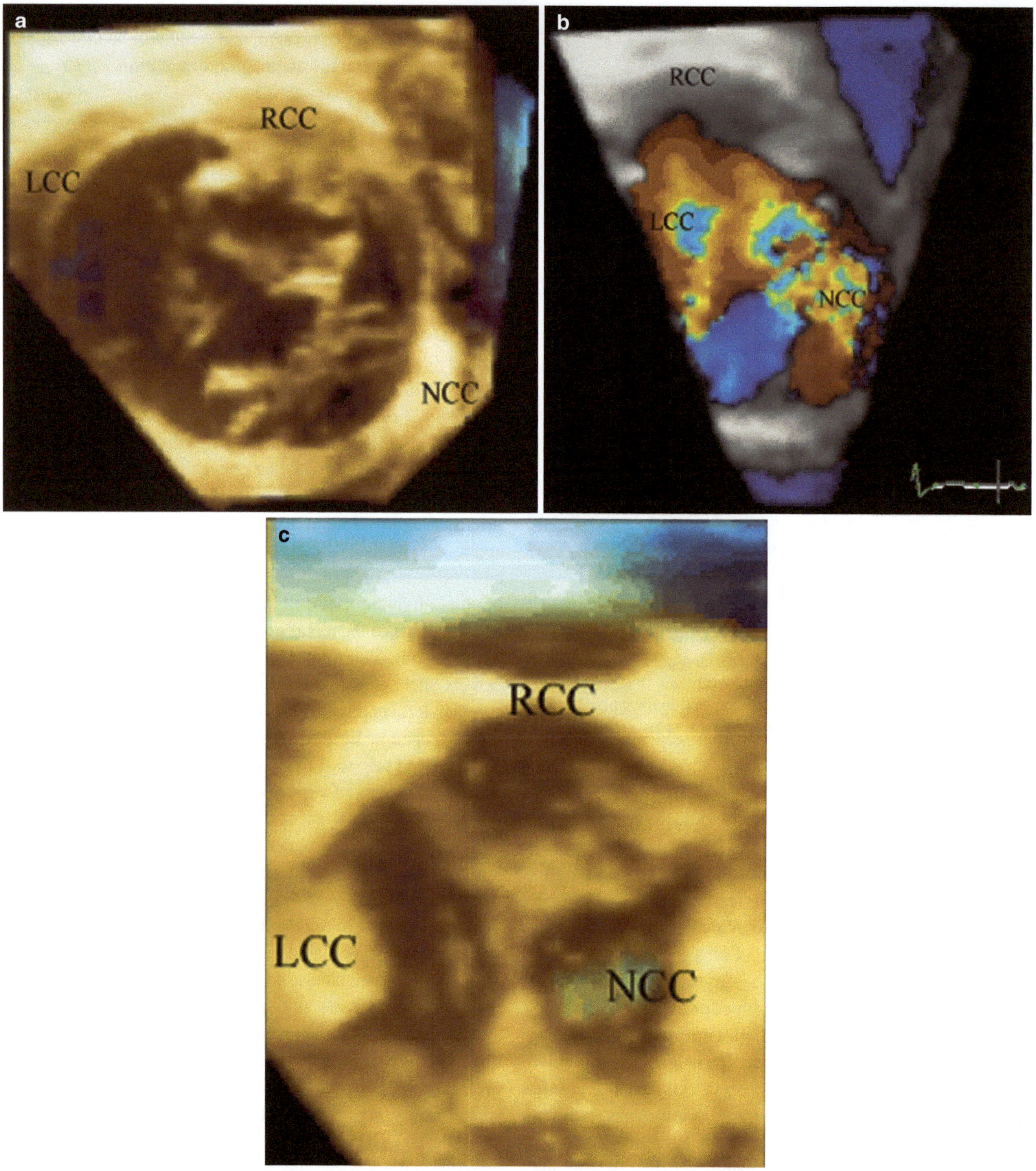

Fig. 19.11 A 12 year old with severe aortic regurgitation. Images are constructed to view the superior surface of the aortic valve as if looking from the aorta down on to the leaflets. To the top is the right coronary cusp, to the left the left coronary cusp, and to the right is the non-coronary cusp. (**a**) Is obtained during the pre-bypass period and shows the marked lack of coaptation and resulting area of regurgitation due to the retracted, scarred non-coronary cusp. (**b**) Verifies color protruding through the region on the regurgitant orifice area of the non-coronary cusp. The patient had pericardial replacement of the non-coronary cusp, and pericardial extension of the right and left coronary cusps. The resultant post bypass 3D echo, (**c**) shows excellent coaptation of all three leaflets. *LCC* left coronary cusp, *NCC* non-coronary cusp, *RCC* right coronary cusp

used in the operative setting. Often 3D TEE has better imaging resolution than transthoracic 3D echocardiography, hence the preoperative study serves a vital role by providing important imaging planes for the surgeon to aid in the planning of the operation. Postoperatively, this imaging can be applied during separation from bypass to evaluate the success of the surgery.

Clinical Application for 3D TEE in the Evaluation of CHD

Much of the published literature on the subject of 3D echocardiography for CHD evaluation is based upon extensive experience with real-time transthoracic (and even fetal) 3D echocardiography [30–36]. However, the matrix array technologies for real-time transthoracic and transesophageal 3D echocardiography are very similar, and therefore one can expect considerable overlap between the two modalities in terms of clinical applications. The major advantage of 3D TEE is the enhanced resolution of the 3D images, particularly in larger patients with poor transthoracic windows. Furthermore TEE is typically performed in more controlled clinical settings (often intubated patients undergoing general anesthesia), thus permitting better acquisition of full volume datasets. Thus there is a growing body of literature documenting the expanding clinical applications of 3D TEE for CHD evaluation [13, 36–39]. Up to the present time, most of these applications focus upon structural/morphologic evaluation of CHD, primarily in the intraoperative and interventional catheterization settings (as befits the most common venues for TEE in this setting). In this section, some of the more common clinical applications will be discussed. Not all applications of 3D TEE can be presented; however, examples of specific CHD abnormalities most commonly evaluated will be discussed below.

Evaluation of Atrioventricular Valves

Evaluation of the atrioventricular valves represents one of the most well-established indications for 3D echocardiography in adults and children. A number of studies have documented the utility of both transthoracic and transesophageal 3D echocardiography, especially for mitral valve disease in adults [18, 20, 40, 41]. In particular, 3D echocardiography enhances the anatomic visualization of all levels of the atrioventricular valve—leaflets, chordae, and papillary muscles. Moreover 3D echocardiography is able to display the valve in a manner unavailable by 2D echocardiography, including the *en face* "surgeon's view" as described above. In adults, 3D TEE provides a realistic and detailed *en face* visualization of the individual mitral valve anterior leaflet segments and posterior leaflet scallops [40]. The same holds true for congenital atrioventricular valve abnormalities, in which 3D echocardiography (primarily transthoracic, but also TEE) has proven very useful, particularly for endocardial cushion defects (atrioventricular septal defects) and Ebstein anomaly of the tricuspid valve [6, 25, 42, 43]. A number of studies have also discussed the use of 3D echocardiography for evaluation of mitral valve disease due to parachute mitral valve [44], double orifice mitral valve [45, 46], mitral valve arcade [47], and congenital mitral regurgitation as well as other mitral valve anomalies. There have also been some recently published studies evaluating the utility 3D echocardiography (both transthoracic and TEE) for more precise evaluation of the pathology of congenital atrioventricular valve abnormalities, specifically in regard to mechanisms and sites of valve regurgitation [32, 47]. Some examples of 3D TEE for assessment of congenital atrioventricular valve abnormalities will be discussed below.

Despite excellent surgical results for endocardial cushion defects, a disquieting number of patients require re-operation for left atrioventricular valve stenosis or regurgitation. In patients that require re-operation for valve regurgitation, 3D imaging provides an excellent perspective of residual regurgitation via clefts in the anterior leaflet, (Fig. 19.10, Video 19.6). The length and position of the residual cleft can be depicted, as well as the precise zones of leaflet prolapse. Intraoperative 3D TEE imaging is used pre and post bypass to evaluate the anatomic extent of residual cleft and associated potential stenosis or regurgitation. Figure 19.10 shows the 3D display, similar to the surgeons viewing, i.e. imaging the superior surfaces of the left atrioventricular valve from the left atrium.

Our center has recently embarked on the "Cone" procedure to improve surgical repair of Ebstein malformation of the tricuspid valve [48]. Previous types of valve repair for this anomaly have been associated with variable success [49, 50]. In part, this has been predicated on preoperative imaging that has, to date, not clearly depicted the anatomic abnormalities. The very complex and variable anatomy of Ebstein malformation does not allow for optimal imaging in a standard 2D display. For example, in the most severe form of Ebstein malformation the leaflet structures are displaced anterior and superiorly towards the right ventricular (RV) outflow tract. The long and ample anterior leaflet envelops the RV as it attaches to the infundibulum. This is often unappreciated by 2D imaging, but can readily be appreciated from full volume 3D echocardiographic data sets obtained

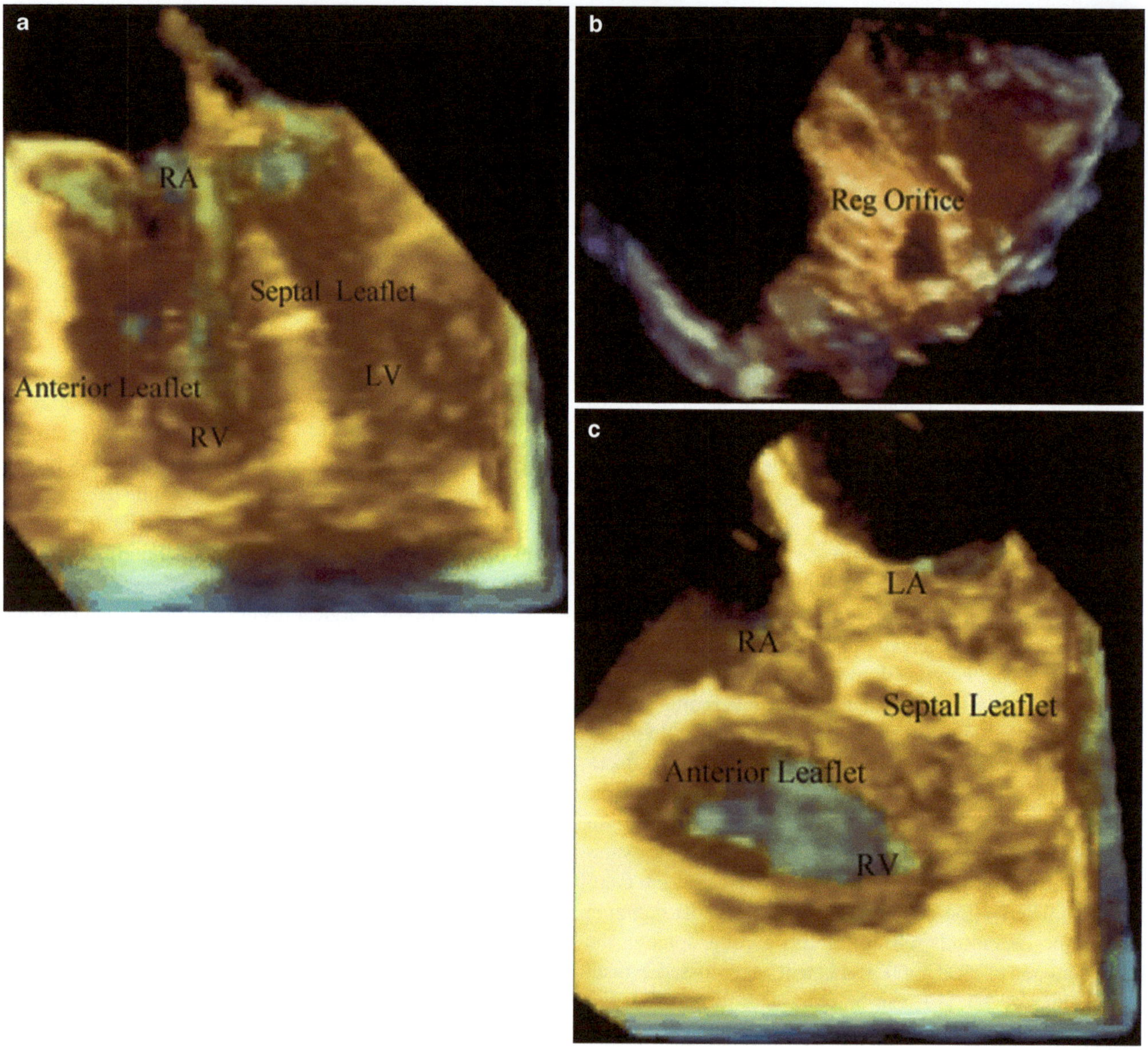

Fig. 19.12 Ebstein malformation of the tricuspid valve. (**a**) Is a four chamber view of the heart oriented anteriorly and shows a very large anterior leaflet and severely tethered septal leaflet. (**b**) Is a short axis plane oriented from the RV apex to base of the heart demonstrating a very large zone of non-coaptation (*Reg Orifice*). (**c**) Is a post-bypass image in the same patient in (**a**) after the cone operation. The entire leaflet structure now folds together during systole without a region of non-coaptation. *LA* left atrium, *LV* left ventricle, *RA* right atrium, *Reg Orifice* regurgitant orifice, *RV* right ventricle

from 3D TEE studies (Fig. 19.12, Video 19.8a and 19.8b) [25]. Moreover, unusual clefts, and attachments from the RV free wall to the anterior leaflet are well appreciated with 3D TEE (Fig. 19.12a, Video 19.8a). Often a large zone of the regurgitant orifice area can readily be depicted from short axis planes oriented from apex to base (Fig. 19.12b, Video 19.8a). Similar to aortic and mitral valve repairs, a more dynamic and complete depiction of tricuspid valve leaflet structure and coaptation can readily be seen from 3D TEE after separation from bypass in the operating room (Fig. 19.12c, Video 19.8b).

In addition to native atrioventricular valve pathology, 3D TEE has been found to be useful for the evaluation of prosthetic atrioventricular valves (primarily prosthetic mitral valves) [51]. It allows detailed assessment of valve dehiscence and clot formation. 3D color is especially helpful when evaluating for perivalvar leaks [15, 52].

Evaluation of Semilunar Valves

Aortic valve repair rather than replacement is often preferred in the pediatric patient for obvious reasons. Transesophageal and epicardial 3D echocardiography have become useful for the pre-operative assessment of the pediatric or adolescent patient with aortic valve disease being considered for valve repair [7, 13]. 3D TEE provides important information to determine the precise etiology of valve regurgitation (Fig. 19.11a, Video 19.7a). The specific anatomic defect can be seen, and 3D color flow can be applied to further confirm the abnormality (Fig. 19.11b, Video 19.7a). 3D imaging provides not only for more precise depiction of commissural fusion, but also the more exact site and extent of lack of leaflet coaptation. More importantly, 3D imaging can provide a perspective as to the depth of the valve leaflet, and hence effective areas of leaflet coaptation. 3D TEE can be immediately applied during separation from cardiopulmonary bypass to analyze the integrity of the aortic valve repair (Fig. 19.11c, Video 19.7b). This modality demonstrates the effectiveness of leaflet coaptation and opening, visualizing the depth of leaflet integrity. As seen in Fig. 19.11a–c and Video 19.7a and 19.7b, the 3D echocardiographic images were oriented to simulate the surgeons view, depicting the valve as looking inferiorly (from the examiner's perspective) onto the superior surfaces of the aortic valve leaflets as if viewed from the aorta.

In adult patients with aortic valve stenosis and/or regurgitation, 3D TEE has been shown to provide anatomic detail regarding valve leaflet morphology and function [41, 53, 54]. Furthermore, the ability to obtain *en face* views of the valve (both above and below the valve) enables the direct planimetry of the aortic valve orifice area [55] in cases of stenosis, or vena contracta/regurgitant orifice area in aortic valve regurgitation [56]. The information from 3D TEE can be used to complement that from 2D TEE imaging, 2D color flow, and spectral Doppler assessment of the aortic valve (Chap. 11). Combining Doppler velocities of the LV outflow tract (obtained from transgastric or deep transgastric views) with the cross-sectional area of the outflow tract obtained by direct planimetry of the 3D TEE image enables a more accurate calculation of aortic valve area when using the continuity equation. A number of investigators have found the LV outflow tract to be ellipsoid rather than circular in shape, when directly measured by 3D echocardiography (transthoracic or TEE) [18, 57–59]. Thus the use of 3D echocardiography likely results in a more accurate calculation of aortic valve area than the method commonly used with 2D echocardiography [60].

There is little information currently available in either the pediatric or adult literature on the use of 3D echocardiography (transthoracic or TEE) for the evaluation of congenital pulmonary valve pathology. One report using transthoracic 3D echocardiography in adult patients with congenital RV outflow tract abnormalities demonstrated that the pulmonary valve could be visualized in 70 % of patients, but the RV outflow tract in only 40 %. However the anatomic findings, when visible, were useful [61].

Evaluation of Atrial and Ventricular Septal Defects

Evaluation of atrial and ventricular septal defects represents a very important clinical application for 3D echocardiography. This is especially true because of the unique *en face* views of the atrial and ventricular septa that are provided by cropping the 3D datasets; these views can greatly enhance the understanding of the morphology and extent of the cardiac defects [29, 62–67]. This information is invaluable when planning and performing (monitoring) interventional catheterization procedures [11, 28, 68, 69]. Because of the proximity of the TEE probe to the atrial and ventricular septa, 3D TEE often provides a significantly greater amount of detail compared to transthoracic 3D imaging. Thus 3D TEE is a natural "fit" for interventional catheterization procedures involving the atrial and ventricular septa. As mentioned, 3D TEE imaging can be applied to atrial septal defect closure in the catheterization laboratory. The full circumference of the atrial septal defect can be imaged from the left and right atrium. These *en face* views allow for depiction of the defect, surrounding rims, as well as the spatial orientation to other anatomic structures (Fig. 19.13a, b; Video 19.9a and 19.9b). In conjunction with live transesophageal imaging, the procedure of closing the defect can be seen from a 3D perspective. This includes the placement of the sheath in the left atrium as well as unfolding of the device in the left atrium. Under simultaneous visualization, the orientation of the disc to the left atrial surface can be seen in a 3D perspective as the device is maneuvered to the left atrial surface (Fig. 19.13c, Video 19.9c). The surface of the disc to the left atrial surface can be depicted prior to deployment. After the left and right atrial discs are deployed, a direct *en face* view of the disc can be seen to verify the appropriate position (Fig. 19.13d, Video 19.9d).

The advantages that 3D TEE confers to atrial septal defect closure also apply to device closure of ventricular septal defects (both percutaneous and perventricular). 3D TEE assists in all phases of the intervention: from pre-procedure evaluation of defect morphology, to catheter positioning and monitoring of device delivery, to relationship of the deployed device to ventricular septum prior to release, and finally device evaluation following complete release. Only a few studies have yet been published on the use of 3D echocardiography (transthoracic and TEE) for ventricular septal defect device closure [33, 70, 71]. However, given that standard 2D TEE is already an integral part of these procedures [72–78], it seems likely that 3D TEE can only serve to provide additive value in those patients of sufficient size to accommodate the larger probe.

In the intraoperative setting, 3D TEE can provide incremental value in the preoperative assessment of ventricular septal defects prior to surgery. As noted above, 3D TEE

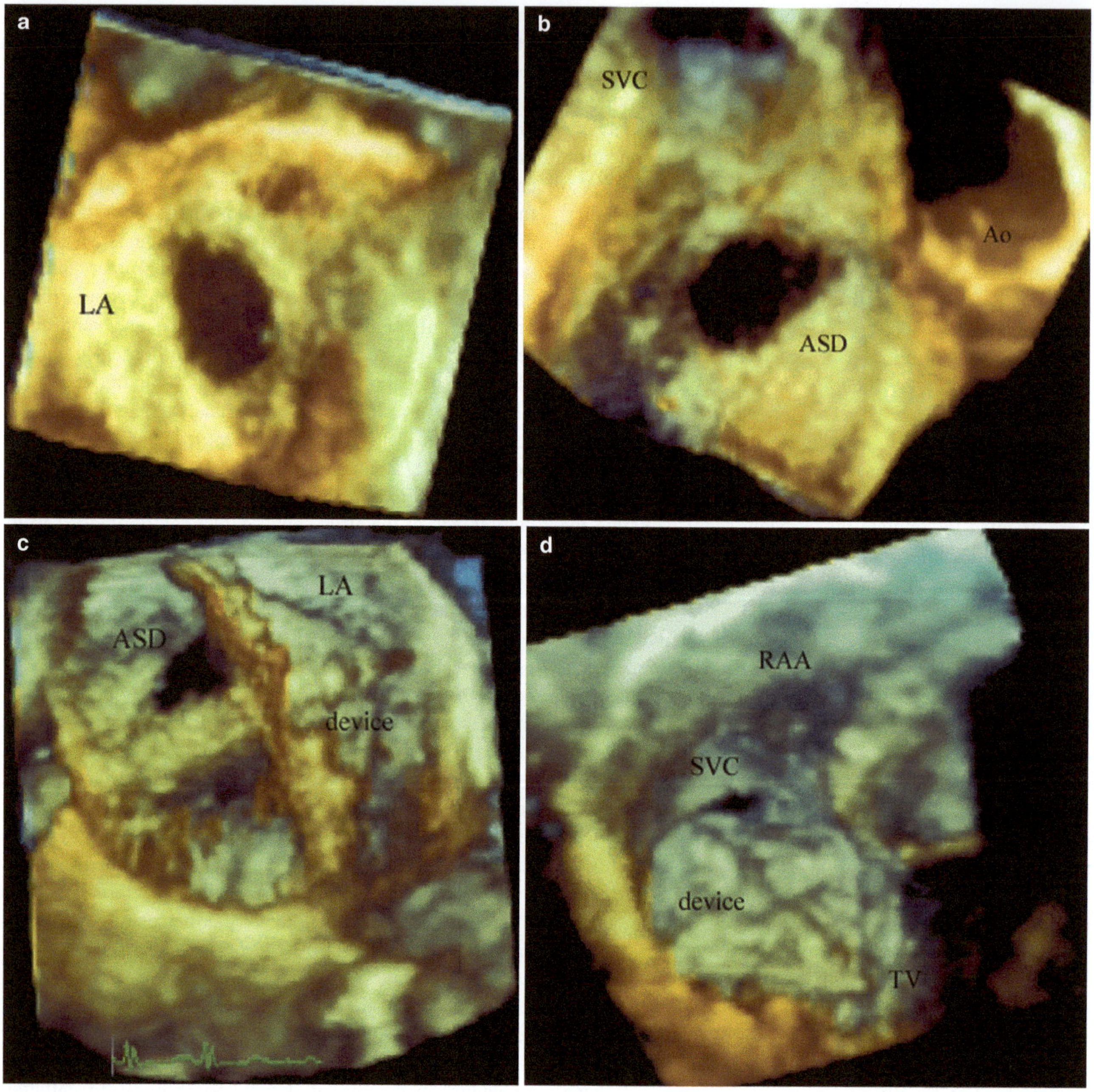

Fig. 19.13 Catheterization device closure of a secundum atrial septal defect. (**a**) Is a Full volume acquisition displaying an *en face* view of a secundum atrial septal defect from the left atrium. (**b**) Is a Full Volume acquisition of the atrial septal defect from the right atrial side demonstrating the relationship to the aorta and superior vena cava. (**c**) Is a live acquisition from the left atrial view demonstrating the sheath placed through the defect and the left atrial disc deployed within the left atrium. (**d**) Is an *en face* view of the right atrial disc after being deployed. *ASD* atrial septal defect, *Ao* aorta, *LA* left atrium, *RAA* right atrial appendage, *SVC* superior vena cava, *TV* tricuspid valve

enables visualization of ventricular septal defects in unique *en face* imaging planes not available by standard 2D imaging (Fig. 19.14, Video 19.10). Although 3D TEE might not seem to add significant additional clinical information for surgical closure, certain unusual defects may need a better definition of the spatial relations of the defect to other anatomic structures. Figure 19.15 is taken from a young adolescent followed for many years with a restrictive ventricular septal defect. Although suspected by 2D imaging, 3D TEE provided additional imaging projections to improve understanding of the hemodynamic abnormalities. Figure 19.15 and Video 19.11 show the 3D TEE aspects of severe prolapse of the right coronary cusp of the aortic valve through a doubly committed subarterial ventricular septal defect. The prolapse was so severe that it created moderate RV outflow tract obstruction.

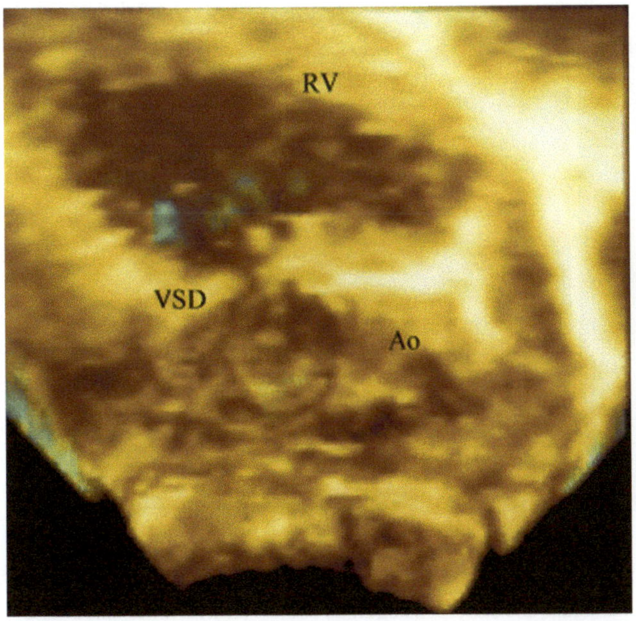

Fig. 19.14 *En face* view of large membranous ventricular septal defect from the left ventricle. *Ao* aorta, *RV* right ventricle, *VSD* ventricular septal defect

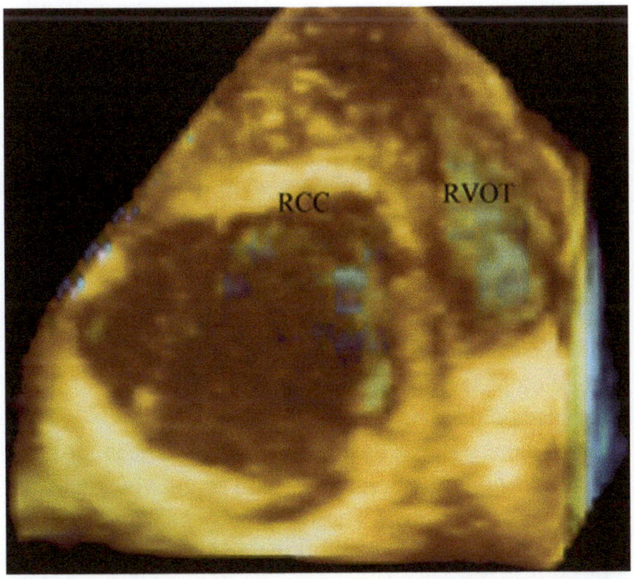

Fig. 19.15 Cross sectional view of doubly committed subarterial ventricular septal defect with prolapse of the right coronary cusp through the defect causing right ventricular outflow tract obstruction. *RCC* right coronary cusp, *RVOT* right ventricular outflow tract

Evaluation of Other Congenital Cardiac Defects

Another conundrum in CHD is complex sub-aortic stenosis. The anatomic substrate is often difficult to define and delineate from associated aortic valve disease. Moreover, an important incidence of re-operation for sub-aortic stenosis persists [79, 80]. Much of this difficulty certainly seems to be related to less than optimal understanding of this complex anatomy from standard 2D imaging planes. Again, 3D TEE can image the sub-aortic obstruction, in a plane from the LV apex towards the aortic valve (Fig. 19.16, Video 19.12). This view is unavailable to the surgeons unless a left ventriculotomy is performed. The concentric nature of the obstruction, as well as the juxtaposition to the mitral and aortic valve and ventricular septum can be better appreciated in a 3D domain. In older adolescents and young adults who have undergone a myriad of prior surgeries, standard transthoracic imaging may not provide information of sufficient quality to help guide surgical management (due to larger patient size, poorer transthoracic imaging windows, etc.). In such situations, 3D TEE can be employed either as an outpatient procedure, or in the intraoperative setting (before cardiopulmonary bypass) to assist in surgical planning and enhance the success of the surgical intervention [81, 82].

The application of 3D TEE to other congenital cardiac defects is still being developed. A number of case reports have described the use of this modality for evaluation of cor triatriatum [83], aortico LV tunnel [38], corrected and uncorrected transposition of the great arteries [84], and postoperative Fontan [39]. Most of these studies were performed in adult patients with CHD. Interestingly, however, all patients in the Fontan study were 7 years of age or less, underlining the growing use of 3D TEE in the pediatric population.

Further Applications and Development of 3D TEE

The introduction in 2007 of the first commercially available 3D TEE probe (Philips X7-2t 3D TEE probe), along with the large probe size, have limited its widespread applicability in the pediatric population. Nonetheless as discussed above, the published applications of 3D TEE for CHD have steadily grown, both for use in the operating room and interventional catheterization laboratory, as well as a separate diagnostic modality by itself [4, 26–30, 37, 39, 66, 85–87]. In adults, impressive work has already been performed that explores and extends the use of 3D TEE in a number of settings, including those pertinent to adult CHD patients. This includes its use during cardiac surgery [86, 87] and adult transcatheter procedures, along with diagnostic evaluation of atrioventricular and semilunar valve anatomic pathology [15, 20, 86, 88]. Similar to the pediatric population, 3D TEE is used in adults to guide closure of atrial and ventricular septal defects [11, 28, 69, 70, 85]. In addition 3D TEE has proven integral to a number of transcatheter interventional procedures specific to adult cardiology patients including the following: percutaneous mitral valve edge to edge clip technique [11, 89], mitral balloon valvuloplasty [85], left atrial appendage obliteration [90, 91], transcatheter aortic valve implantation (TAVI) [11, 85, 92], and occlu-

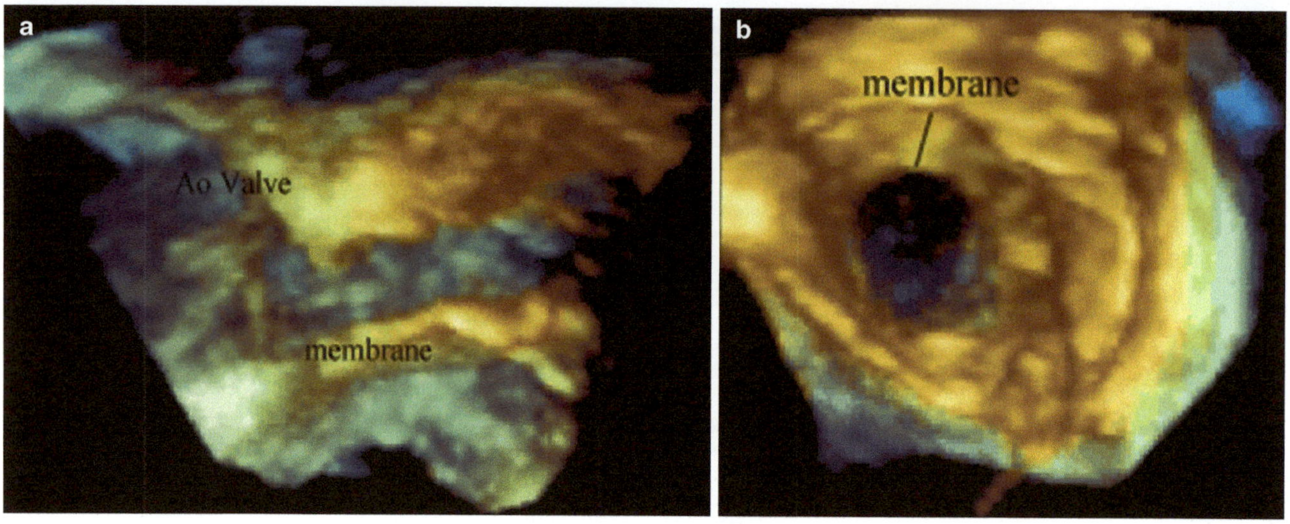

Fig. 19.16 A 7 year old male with severe sub-aortic stenosis. (**a**) Is a slightly oblique long axis view showing the thickened sub-aortic membrane immediately below the aortic valve. (**b**) Is a short axis view oriented from the left ventricular apex to the aorta, and viewed from the left ventricular perspective, demonstrating the concentric nature of the sub-aortic membrane and corresponding small outflow area. *Ao Valve* aortic valve

sion of mitral valve perivalvar leaks [11, 21, 93]. The list of these applications is likely to grow significantly in the near future.

There is considerable potential for the use of 3D TEE in the quantitative analysis of cardiac anatomy, mechanics and function. Similar to cardiac magnetic resonance imaging (CMR), the use of a 3D dataset enables volumetric analysis that avoids the geometric assumptions used with 2D methods such as Simpson's method of LV volume calculation. To date, most studies evaluating the assessment of left and right ventricular volumes have been performed using transthoracic 3D echocardiography, and have shown promising results. For the left ventricle, a surface rendered cast chamber is obtained generally by semi-automated border detection of the LV endocardial-blood interface, although manual tracing is sometimes used. The volume is then calculated by direct voxel count and followed throughout the cardiac cycle (Fig. 19.17, Video 19.13). The volumes obtained by 3D echocardiography have been shown to correlate well with CMR, although 3D echocardiography tends to underestimate LV volumes, probably due to its inability to distinguish the trabeculations from myocardium [94–96]. Nonetheless, 3D echocardiographic-measured volumes have better reproducibility than 2D echocardiography [94], and therefore would appear to be a better alternative for the volumetric assessment of the LV. Assessment of RV volumes/function can also be performed by generation of a surface-rendered cast of the RV, usually by semiautomated border quantification using specialized offline software (TomTec 4D echo analysis software, Tom Tec Imaging Systems GmbH, Munich, Germany) (Fig. 19.18, Video 19.14). This analysis can be more involved because of the unusual geometry and shape of the RV. Using this method, published studies have shown a good correlation between 3D echocardiography and CMR with respect to RV volumes and function [97–99]. However like the 3D evaluation of LV, there appears to be an underestimation of RV volume by 3D echocardiography compared to CMR [100]. Studies evaluating 3D TEE assessment of LV and RV volumes have yet to be performed extensively with 3D TEE [15], but it seems likely that similar results can be obtained with this modality as well. In fact, the superior imaging quality of TEE might actually enhance volume and function assessment in larger patients. Several recent studies have demonstrated the ability of intraoperative 3D TEE to obtain adequate images for subsequent offline measurement of LV/RV volume and function, using images obtained from the mid esophageal window and the same methods of semi-automated border detection [101, 102].

Even more sophisticated evaluations of cardiac mechanics and function have been reported in adults with the use of 3D echocardiography. These evaluations are valuable because they can be difficult to obtain by 2D methods. 3D echocardiography has been shown to be useful for evaluation of LV segmental wall motion analysis and dyssynchrony (Fig. 19.19). Using either a 16 segment model (American Society of Echocardiography) or 17 segment model (American Heart Association) [103], a systolic dyssynchrony index (SDI) can be calculated as the standard deviation of the time required to reach minimum systolic volume for each segment as a percentage of the cardiac cycle (Fig. 19.17b). For normal subjects, the mean SDI (16 segment model) is 3.5 ± 1.8 % [104]. This 3D model of dyssynchrony can be used as one of the measures to evaluate the results of cardiac resynchronization therapy [105–110].

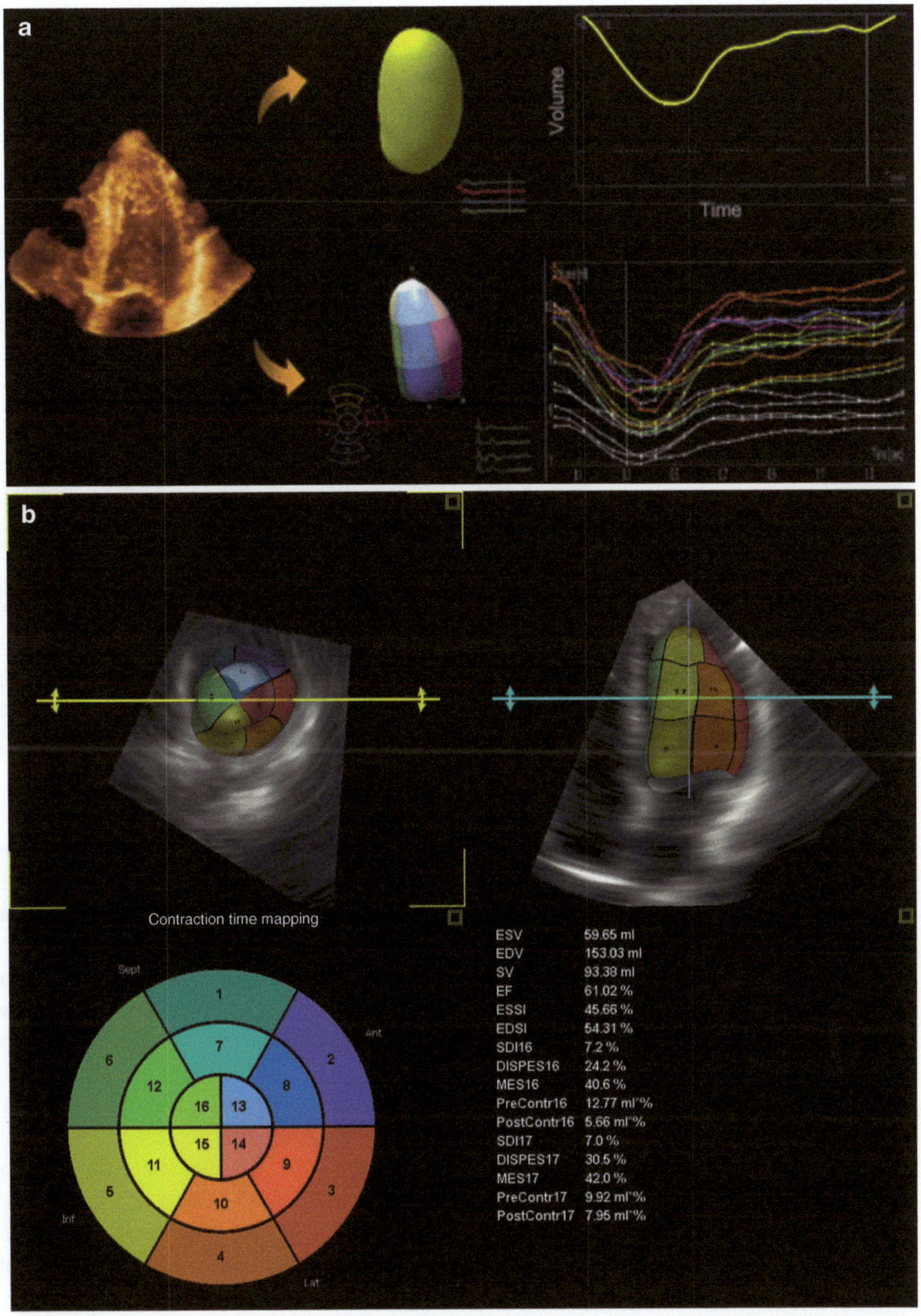

Fig. 19.17 Quantitative assessment of left ventricle (LV) volume and systolic function using three-dimensional (3D) echocardiography. (**a**) From a transthoracic 3D echocardiographic data set of the LV (*left panel*), the LV endocardium can be traced (*middle panel, top*) to obtain the LV volume throughout the cardiac cycle (*right panel, top*). Using the maximum and minimum volumes obtained from this curve, an ejection fraction can be calculated. As well, the LV endocardium can be divided according to the 17-segment mode l (*middle panel, bottom*), and the time each segment requires to attain minimal volume in the cardiac cycle can be identified (*right panel, bottom*) (Reprinted from Lang et al. [18]; with permission from Elsevier). (**b**) Evaluation of LV systolic function and dyssynchrony. The upper left and right panels show the 3D surface-rendered LV volume from two views. The *bottom left panel* shows an example of the 16 segment model. Calculation of systolic dyssynchrony index (SDI) can automatically be performed using the 16 segment (SDI 16) and 17 segment (SDI 17) models (*bottom right panel*). See text for details

Several 3D echocardiographic systems provide the ability for offline calculation of myocardial strain, strain rate, rotation, torsion and twist, and some preliminary studies in adults (using transthoracic 3D echocardiography) have already been published that evaluate these parameters [111–114]. Using readily available offline 3D software, quantitative assessment of linear and area measurements can be performed on 3D transthoracic and TEE datasets, along with detailed mitral and aortic valve analysis. The latter allows for evaluation of noncircular vena contracta (Fig. 19.20) [115] and planimetry of anatomic regurgitant orifice area in mitral regurgitation stenotic orifice area in mitral stenosis [116, 117]. Recently, 3D TEE has enabled sophisticated evaluation of mitral valve parametric mapping [118] and volumetric quantification (Fig. 19.21) [18], aortic valve dynamic motion (Fig. 19.22) [18, 22], and mitral-aortic valve coupling [119]. An important disadvantage of most of the aforementioned analyses (including volume/function

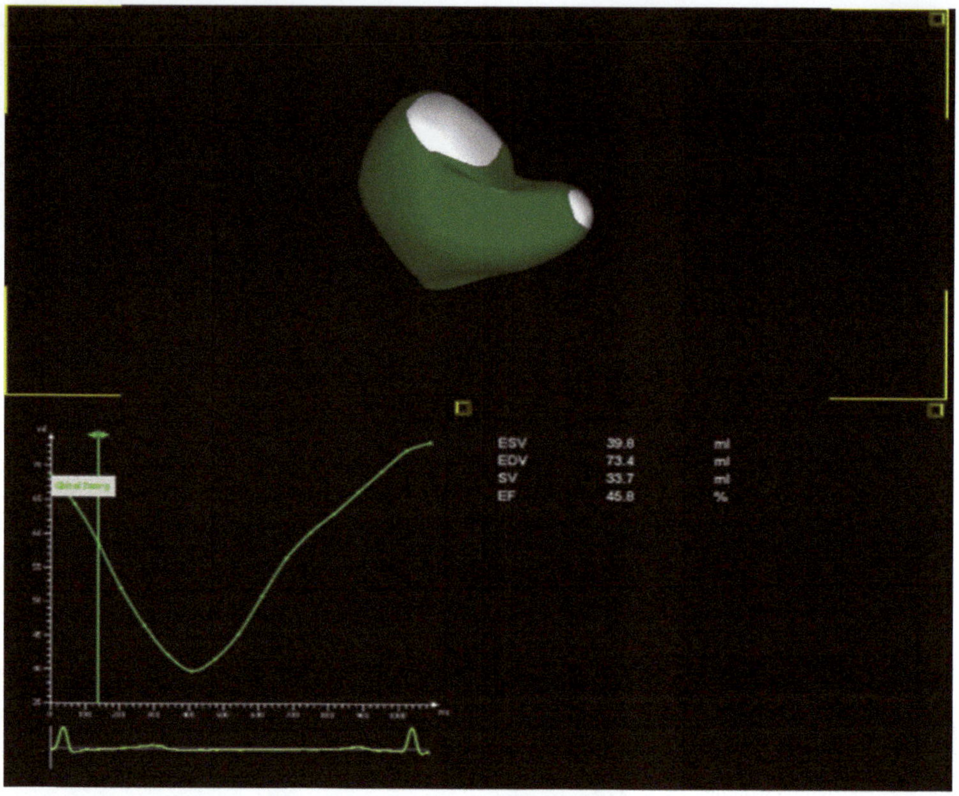

Fig. 19.18 Quantitative assessment of right ventricular (RV) volume and systolic function using three-dimensional (3D) echocardiography, using software from TomTec (4D RV-function©). From a full volume transthoracic 3D echocardiographic data set of the RV, the endocardium is manually traced in three orthogonal planes. The software utilizes a semi-automated border detection method to generate a dynamic model of the RV, which is displayed in the *top panel*. RV volume is displayed on a curve of volume over time throughout the cardiac cycle in the *lower left panel*. The RV stroke volume (*SV*) and ejection fraction (*EF*) are automatically calculated and displayed in the *lower right panel*

quantification) is that they must be performed offline and the analysis can be rather time-consuming, thus limiting their immediate utility in the intraoperative and interventional cardiology settings where rapid access to information is essential [120]. However 3D echocardiography systems are rapidly evolving, and future advances in semi-automated quantification, as well as on-cart availability of analysis tools, could make many of the quantitative 3D TEE analyses readily accessible at the time of the study. One previous report of 3D TEE during a Ross procedure demonstrated the use of 3D volumetric and function quantification before and after cardiopulmonary bypass (using techniques described above); the authors were able to quantify LV function and identify wall motion abnormalities following bypass [53]. A 3–5 min time period was needed for quantification, and this short period of time allowed it to be performed contemporaneously with the operation.

The other important consideration pertains to the use of 3D TEE for quantitative analysis of cardiac mechanics and function in patients with CHD. The evaluations of right and single ventricle volumes and function are currently some of the most important and active areas of investigation among CHD specialists. These type of evaluations are pertinent for a number of important and topical issues in CHD: RV function in postoperative tetralogy of Fallot patients with chronic pulmonary regurgitation, ventricular function in various forms of single ventricle/Fontan patients, function of the systemic RV in congenitally corrected transposition of the great arteries, and other clinically challenging conditions. Currently CMR is the gold standard for quantification of ventricular volumes and function in these settings, but a number of pediatric studies have shown a reasonably good correlation between 3D echocardiography and CMR in volumes and function for the LV [121–126], RV [99, 101, 127–129], and even single ventricles [130, 131]. These studies were performed primarily with transthoracic 3D echocardiography, and it remains to be seen how useful and effective 3D TEE will be in this setting. This represents one of the many interesting areas of future research in 3D echocardiography.

Another interesting area for future development is the use of 3D color flow Doppler (3D CFD) for evaluation of CHD. As noted earlier in this chapter, 3D CFD is used qualitatively for assessment of atrioventricular and semilunar valve pathology, to localize and display sites of stenosis or regurgitation. In addition, 3D CFD has been utilized in CHD as an "echocardiographic angiogram" to assess vascular structures such as coarctation, vascular ring, and systemic to pulmonary artery shunts [132]. Quantitative use of 3D CFD also holds some promise as a method of volumetric flow assessment [133]. A recent study by Poh et al. evaluated cardiac output in sheep with experimentally distorted ventricular septal geometry, and found that, using flow-probe data as a reference standard, a much better correlation was obtained when calculated by 3D CFD as compared to 2D-derived methods [134]. Lu et al. have compared the use of 3D CFD to 3D ventricular volumetric calculations as a method for measurement of valvar volumetric flow in children. These

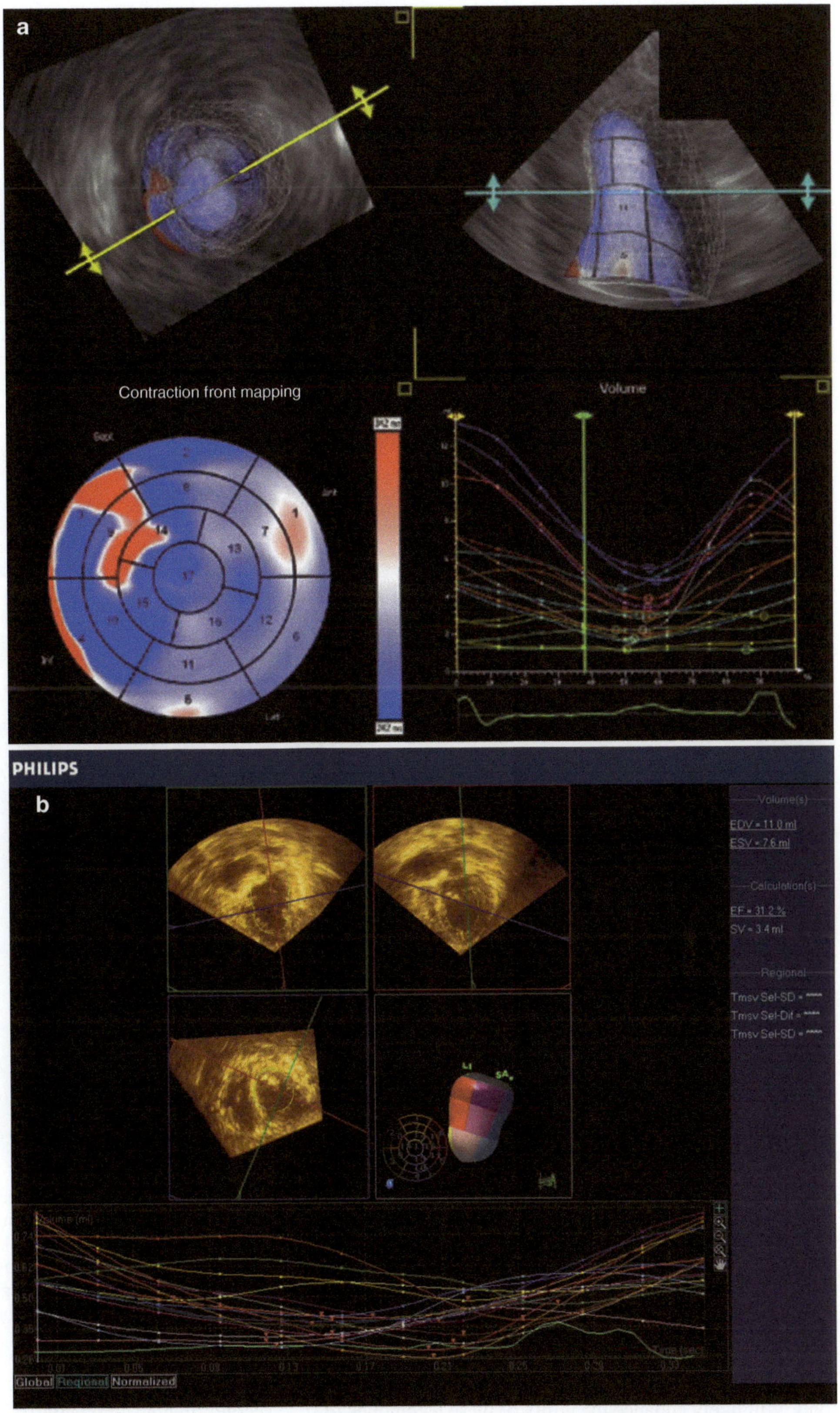

Fig. 19.19 Evaluation of left ventricle (LV) segmental wall motion. (**a**) Shows a three-dimensional transthoracic echocardiogram data set of the LV as viewed from the apex (*left, top*) or anteriorly (*right, top*), with dynamic tracking of the LV endocardium. The end-diastolic LV endocardium is visualized as a mesh shell and the end-systolic endocardium as a solid shell. *Lower left*: a 17-segment, bull's-eye map of contraction front mapping demonstrating the time required for each segment to reach minimal LV volume (*left, bottom*). *Lower right*: Graph, with time along the x axis and volume along the y axis, demonstrating the time for each segment to reach minimal volume. *Ant* anterior, *Inf* inferior, *Lat* lateral, *Sept* septum (Reprinted from Lang et al. [18]; with permission from Elsevier). (**b**) Is taken from a patient with dilated cardiomyopathy and dyssynchronous LV contraction; note the marked lack of synchrony of the individual cardiac segments as compared to Fig. 19.17a

investigators found the best correlation with the mitral valve, good correlations for aortic and pulmonary valves, and a poor correlation with the tricuspid valve [135]. Nonetheless despite the encouraging data from these studies, more investigation will need to be performed to verify the utility of 3D CFD, especially given the potentially limiting factors of smaller volume datasets, stitch artifact, and marginal spatial/temporal resolution. Improvements in 3D CFD technology,

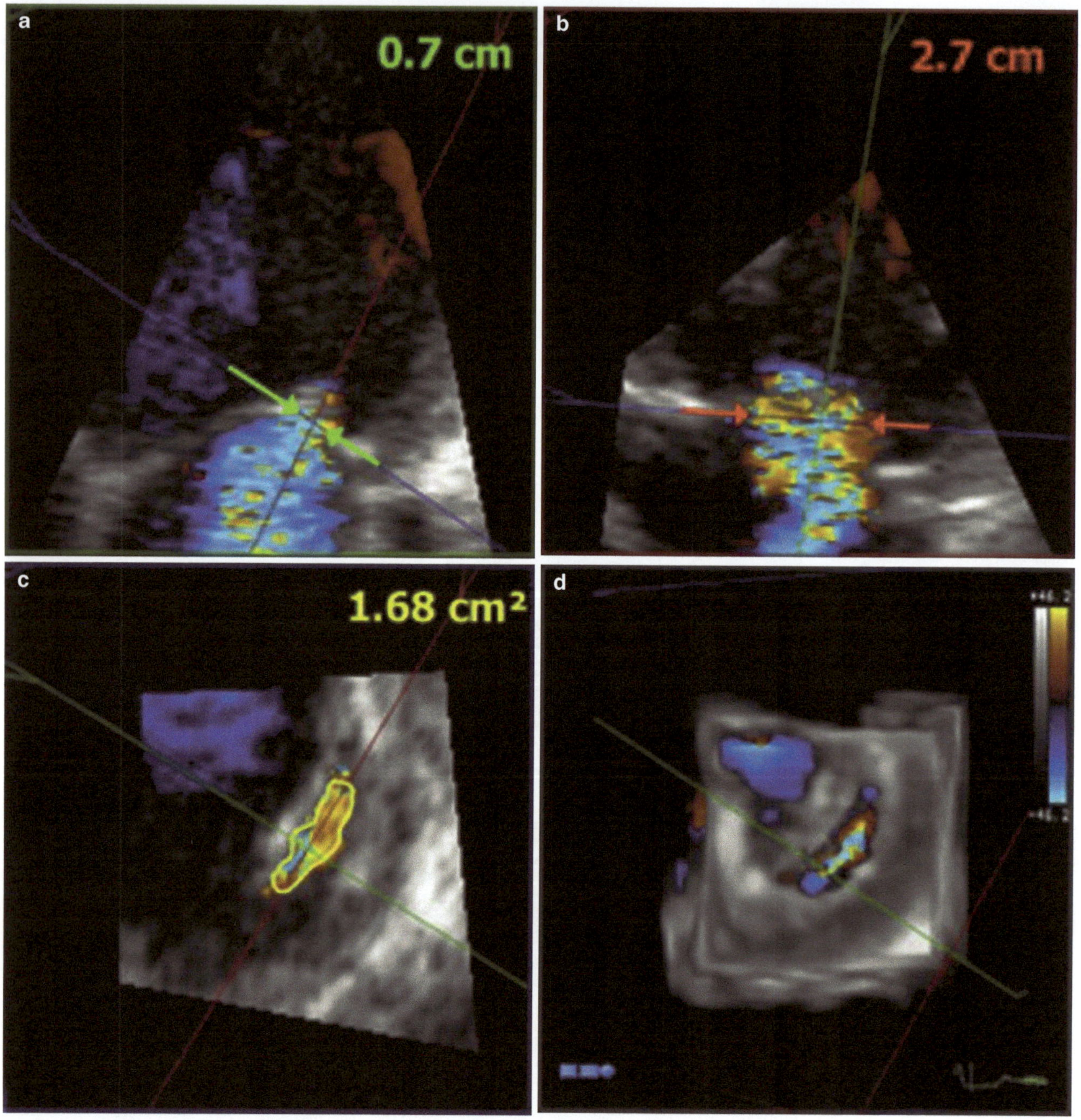

Fig. 19.20 Example of measurement of vena contracta (VC) dimensions in a cross-sectional plane through the VC in a patient with functional mitral regurgitation caused by leaflet tethering. Panel **a** shows a four-chamber view with measurement of a narrow VC width. Panel **b** shows a two chamber view with measurement of a broad VC width. Panel **c** shows a cross-sectional plane through the VC with direct planimetry of vena contracta area. The *green* and the *red lines* indicate the orientation of the four chamber plane (panel **a**, *green frame*) and the two chamber plane (panel **b**, *red frame*). Panel **d** shows a 3D *en face* view of VC area. Note that the significant asymmetry of the VC area makes difficult the accurate assessment of regurgitation from a single plane (From Kahlert et al. [115]; with permission from Elsevier)

along with more robust semi-automated flow quantification tools, will likely enhance the utility of these techniques [43].

Until recently, the availability of 3D TEE from only one company also provided some limitation, as it was necessary for practitioners to purchase or already own the echocardiographic system that accommodated this probe. However, another 3D TEE probe is now commercially available from a second major company (BT-12 3D/4D TEE probe, GE Medical Systems), and it is anticipated that other companies will follow. This should stimulate further adoption of 3D TEE in a number of clinical settings, including that of CHD evaluation.

3D Imaging: Limitations, Artifacts, and Pitfalls

Despite its growing popularity, 3D imaging still has important potential limitations with which the examiner should be aware. First, despite the dramatic advances in 3D technology, both spatial and temporal resolutions are still inferior to that of comparable 2D imaging. The 3D TEE probe images at the same high frequency (7 MHz) as many adult TEE probes as well as some pediatric transthoracic probes, but some degree of fine gray scale and tissue detail are lost when imaging in 3D. Temporal resolution is also reduced (sometimes significantly) when compared to 2D imaging, and this can impair the ability to visualize precise motion of structures such as atrioventricular and semilunar valves. It can also be a potential issue in younger patients with faster heart rates; the lower frame rates can result in cardiac motion that appears less smooth.

Since 3D echocardiography is still a form of ultrasound, it will be subject to the same artifacts as those encountered with 2D echocardiography, such as reverberations and shadowing. In addition, there are some artifacts particular to 3D imaging. Such artifacts include false dropout of certain areas due to lack of 3D data collected by the matrix transducer. This can also occur because of reduced gain settings that lead to data loss. The result is transparency or apparent absence of tissue in certain structures such as the atrioventricular and semilunar valves. In some cases, the dropout can mimic an anatomic defect. It can also become apparent when nonstandard cropping planes are used, due to the data loss that can occur from objects oriented more parallel to the ultrasound beam(s) [136]. To compensate, gain settings can be increased but too much gain will lead to speckling artifacts and worsened 3D rendering that can obscure cardiac structures. Another important artifact is the "stitch artifact" (described above) that can occur with full volume imaging, due to irregularities in ECG gating and/or movement of the cardiac position from respiration or other external factors (Fig. 19.23, Video 19.15). This can introduce errors in the depiction of real-time motion [18].

The other important point is that the 3D images actually represent 2D renderings of 3D structures, with color shading used to give the perception of depth. While 3D TEE images provide excellent detail, it can be difficult to determine the precise front to back spatial orientation of cardiac structures in a given 3D image. These 3D relationships can be particularly important with CHD. Thus it is important to perform both cropping and rotation of a 3D rendering, and to visualize a cardiac structure in several different views [18].

Summary

3D TEE has become an integral part in the evaluation of patients with complex CHD at our medical center and other facilities that care for these patients. Such imaging provides

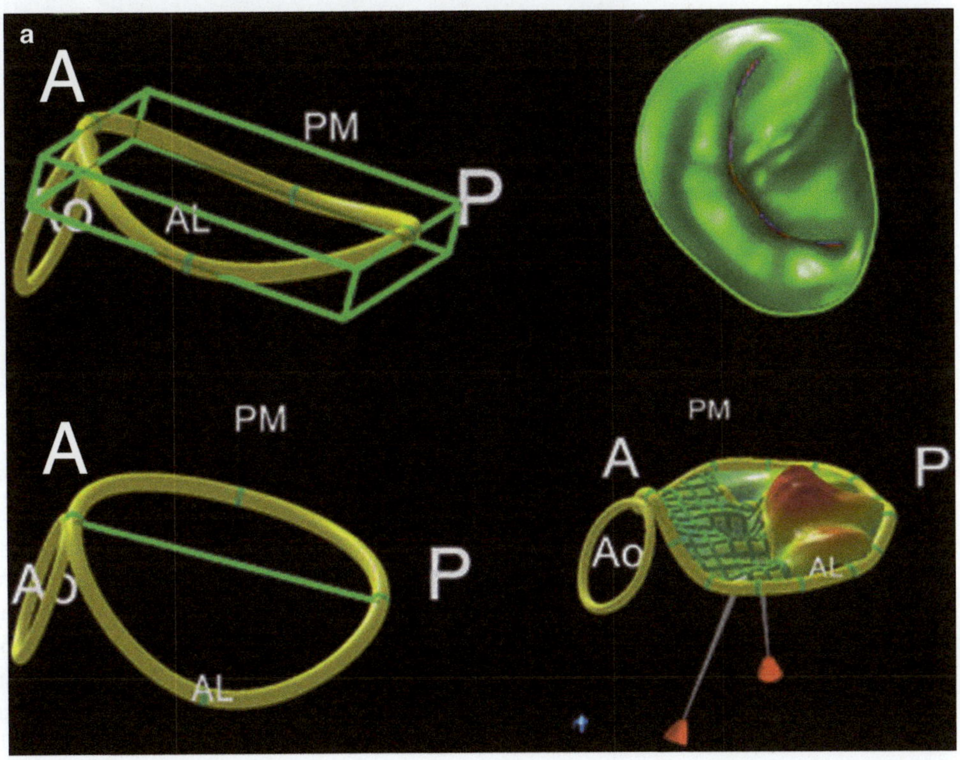

Fig. 19.21 Quantitative evaluation of the mitral valve. (**a**) Volumetric quantification of the mitral valve allows accurate measurements of the height of the saddle-shaped mitral valve (*top left*), commissure-to-commissure diameter measurements of the mitral annulus (*bottom left*), mitral annular surface area (*top right*), and the angle between the aortic root and the mitral annulus (*bottom right*). *A* Anterior, *AL* anterolateral, *Ao* aorta, *P* posterior, *PM* posteromedial (Reprinted from Lang et al. [18]; with permission from Elsevier). (**b**) Mitral valve evaluation using TomTec 4D MV-Assessment© software. *Top panel* shows dynamic 3D depiction of mitral valve P2 scallop prolapse. *Bottom panel* shows various quantitative measurements available for mitral valve assessment. (Reprinted with permission of TomTec Imaging Systems GmbH, Munich, Germany)

Fig. 19.21 (continued)

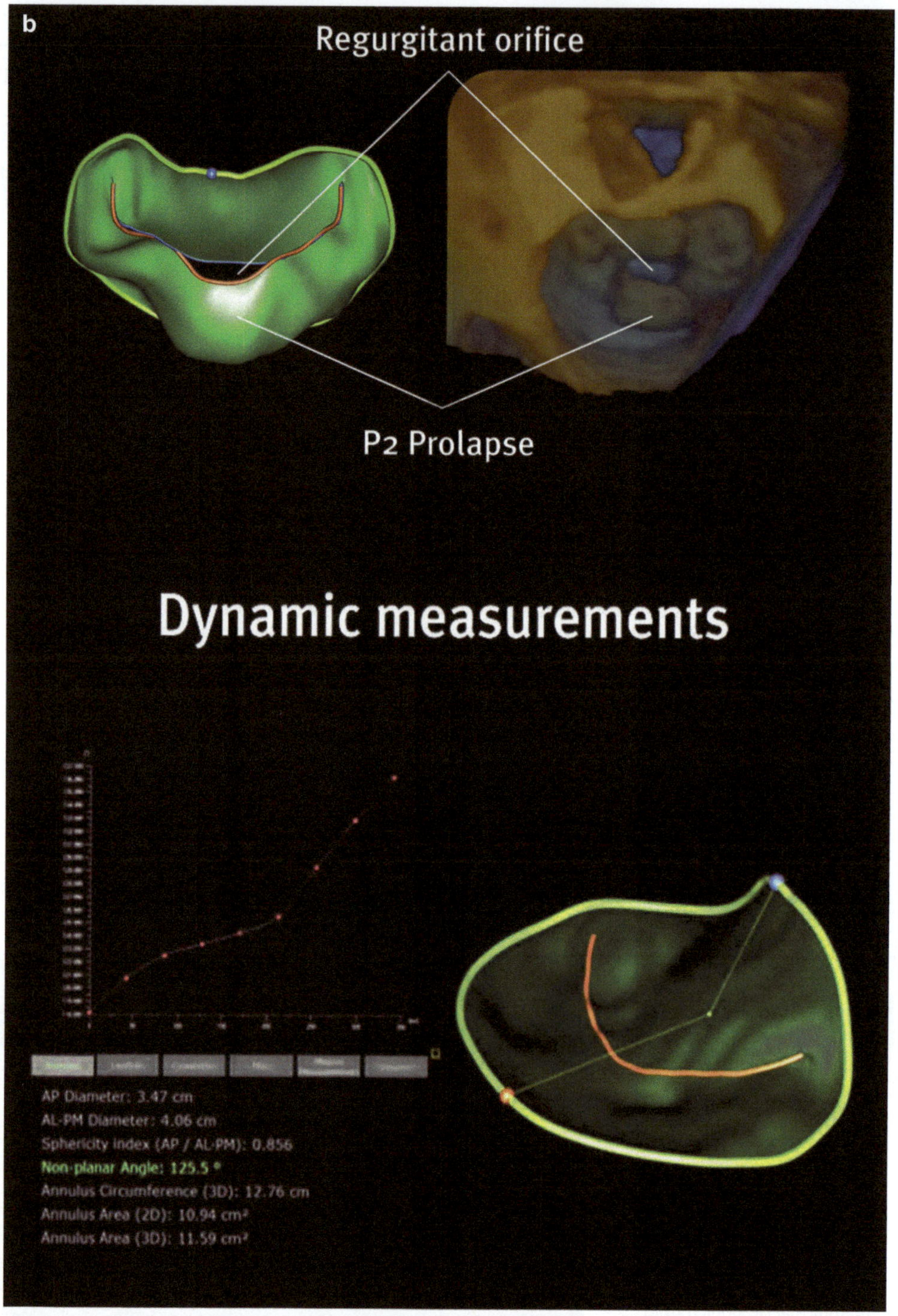

unique planes and projections that are unavailable with standard 2D display. Moreover, in pre and post bypass patients the heart and corresponding anatomy is depicted in dynamic motion, rather than the surgeon's perspective of the non-beating heart.

Certain aspects will need to continue to evolve, for example improved imaging in the near field is necessary. Transesophageal probes need to be reduced in size, with higher transmit frequencies for the smaller pediatric patients. Live full volume imaging will be more advantageous with improved temporal resolution (for the faster heart rates in children) and overall improved spatial resolution. Also, the ability to perform online linear, area and volume measurements directly on the echocardiography machine will facilitate the ability to provide timely important information to surgeons and interventional cardiologists. This will be further enhanced by automated quantification tools that are beginning to appear on the advanced 3D echocardiography platforms.

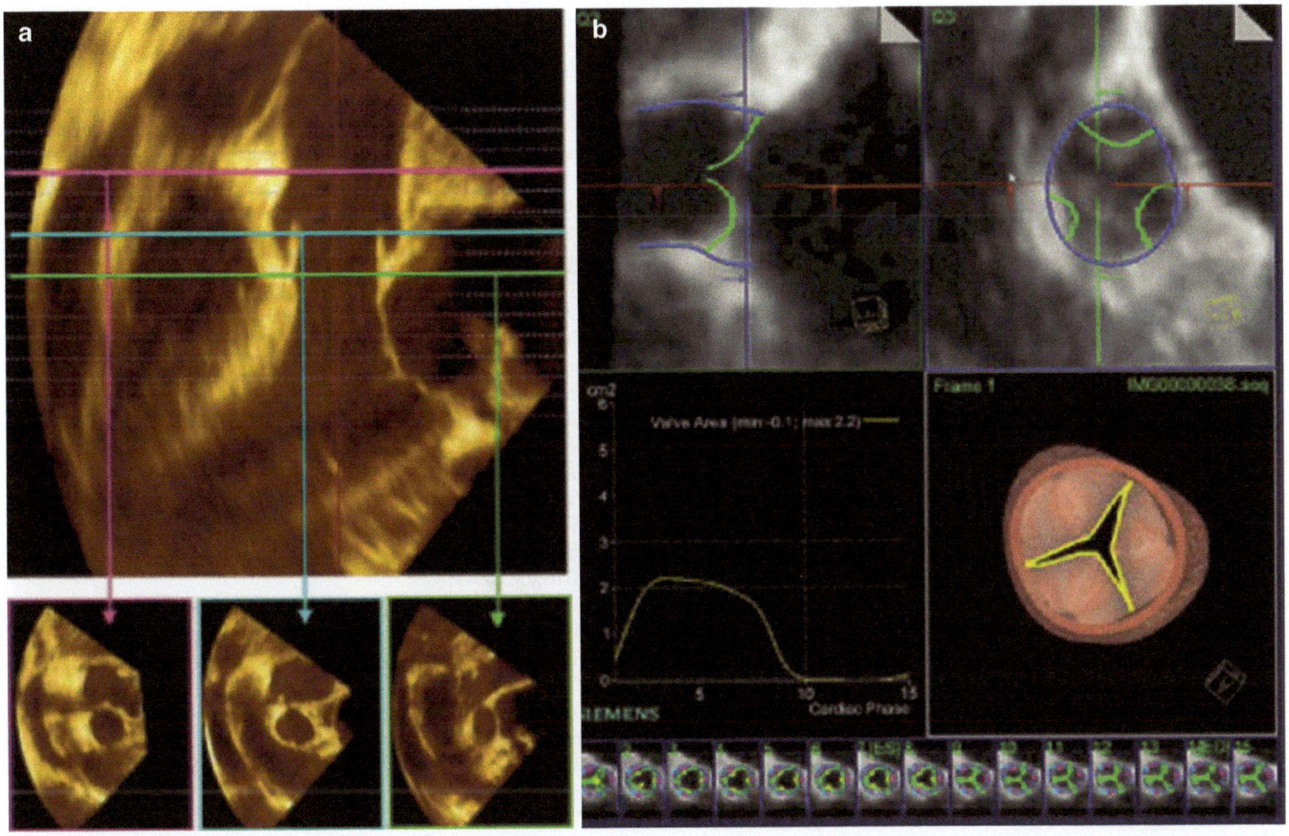

Fig. 19.22 Three-dimensional transesophageal data set cropped to demonstrate the aorta in long axis (**a**, *top*). Using this image, *en face* views of the sinotubular junction (**a**, *bottom left*), sinus of Valsalva (**a**, *bottom middle*), and aortic annulus (**a**, *bottom right*) can be obtained for assessment. Dynamic, automatic tracking of the aortic valve leaflets (**b**, *top left*) and annulus (**b**, *top right*) can be performed, providing aortic valve area throughout the cardiac cycle (**b**, *middle left* and *bottom strip*). A model derived from the automated tracking is also produced (*middle right*) (Reprinted from Lang et al. [18]; with permission from Elsevier)

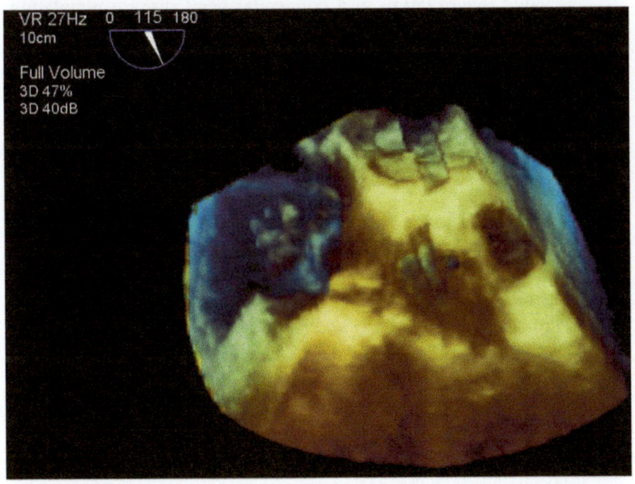

Fig. 19.23 Example of stitch artifact with a full volume dataset. This can occur as a result of irregularities in cardiac rhythm, or respiratory/ patient movement

Equally important for successful development of 3D TEE imaging are the interactions between the cardiologist and surgeon in trying to comprehend and display this complex anatomy. Intraoperative 3D TEE imaging is still early in development, and cooperation between surgeons, anesthesiologists, and cardiologists will hasten this progress.

References

1. Belohlavek M, Foley DA, Gerber TC, Greenleaf JF, Seward JB. Three-dimensional ultrasound imaging of the atrial septum: normal and pathologic anatomy. J Am Coll Cardiol. 1993;22:1673–8.
2. Marx GR, Fulton DR, Pandian NG, et al. Delineation of site, relative size and dynamic geometry of atrial septal defects by real-time three-dimensional echocardiography. J Am Coll Cardiol. 1995;25:482–90.
3. Franke A, Kühl HP, Rulands D, et al. Quantitative analysis of the morphology of secundum-type atrial septal defects and their dynamic change using transesophageal three-dimensional echocardiography. Circulation. 1997;96:II-323-7.
4. Cao Q, Radtke W, Berger F, Zhu W, Hijazi ZM. Transcatheter closure of multiple atrial septal defects. Initial results and value of two- and three-dimensional transoesophageal echocardiography. Eur Heart J. 2000;21:941–7.
5. Mumm B, Nanda NC, Sorrell VL, et al. Technical background and current & future aspects of three-dimensional echocardiography. In: Nanda NC, Sorrell VL, editors. Atlas of three-dimensional

echocardiography. Armonk: Futura Publishing Company, Inc.; 2002. p. 1–20.
6. Miller AP, Nanda NC, Aaluri S, et al. Three-dimensional transesophageal echocardiographic demonstration of anatomical defects in AV septal defect patients presenting for reoperation. Echocardiography. 2003;20:105–9.
7. Vida VL, Hoehn R, Larrazabal LA, Gauvreau K, Marx GR, del Nido PJ. Usefulness of intra-operative epicardial three-dimensional echocardiography to guide aortic valve repair in children. Am J Cardiol. 2009;103:852–6.
8. Salandin V, De Castro S, Cavarretta E, et al. Epicardial real-time 3-dimensional echocardiography with the use of a pediatric transthoracic probe: a technical approach. J Cardiothorac Vasc Anesth. 2010;24:43–50.
9. Sugeng L, Shernan SK, Salgo IS, et al. Live 3-dimensional transesophageal echocardiography initial experience using the fully-sampled matrix array probe. J Am Coll Cardiol. 2008;52: 446–9.
10. Sugeng L, Weinert L, Lang RM. Left ventricular assessment using real time three dimensional echocardiography. Heart. 2003;89 Suppl 3:iii29–36.
11. Perk G, Lang RM, Garcia-Fernandez MA, et al. Use of real time three-dimensional transesophageal echocardiography in intracardiac catheter based interventions. J Am Soc Echocardiogr. 2009;22:865–82.
12. Mackensen GB, Swaminathan M, Mathew JP. PRO editorial: PRO: three-dimensional transesophageal echocardiography is a major advance for intraoperative clinical management of patients undergoing cardiac surgery. Anesth Analg. 2010;110:1574–8.
13. Baker GH, Shirali G, Ringewald JM, Hsia TY, Bandisode V. Usefulness of live three-dimensional transesophageal echocardiography in a congenital heart disease center. Am J Cardiol. 2009;103:1025–8.
14. Salgo IS. Three-dimensional echocardiographic technology. Cardiol Clin. 2007;25:231–9.
15. Vegas A, Meineri M. Core review: three-dimensional transesophageal echocardiography is a major advance for intraoperative clinical management of patients undergoing cardiac surgery: a core review. Anesth Analg. 2010;110:1548–73.
16. Salgo IS. 3D transesophageal echocardiographic technologies. In: Badano LP, Lang RM, Zamorano JL, editors. Textbook of real-time three dimensional echocardiography. London: Springer; 2011. p. 25–32.
17. Rabben SI. Technical principles of transthoracic three-dinensional echocardiography. In: Badano LP, Lang RM, Zamorano JL, editors. Textbook of real-time three dimensional echocardiography. London: Springer; 2011. p. 9–24.
18. Lang RM, Badano LP, Tsang W, et al. EAE/ASE recommendations for image acquisition and display using three-dimensional echocardiography. J Am Soc Echocardiogr. 2012;25:3–46.
19. Bharucha T, Roman KS, Anderson RH, Vettukattil JJ. Impact of multiplanar review of three-dimensional echocardiographic data on management of congenital heart disease. Ann Thorac Surg. 2008;86:875–81.
20. Grewal J, Mankad S, Freeman WK, et al. Real-time three-dimensional transesophageal echocardiography in the intraoperative assessment of mitral valve disease. J Am Soc Echocardiogr. 2009;22:34–41.
21. Kronzon I, Sugeng L, Perk G, et al. Real-time 3-dimensional transesophageal echocardiography in the evaluation of post-operative mitral annuloplasty ring and prosthetic valve dehiscence. J Am Coll Cardiol. 2009;53:1543–7.
22. Mahmood F, Subramaniam B, Gorman JH, et al. Three-dimensional echocardiographic assessment of changes in mitral valve geometry after valve repair. Ann Thorac Surg. 2009;88: 1838–44.
23. Scohy TV, Soliman OII, Lecomte PVEL, et al. Intraoperative real time three-dimensional transesophageal echocardiographic measurement of hemodynamic, anatomic and functional changes after aortic valve replacement. Echocardiography. 2009;26:96–9.
24. Kelpis TG, Ninios VN, Dardas PS, Pitsis AA. Subaortic stenosis in an adult caused by two discrete membranes: a three-dimensional transesophageal echocardiographic visualization. Ann Thorac Surg. 2009;88:1703.
25. van Noord PT, Scohy TV, McGhie J, Bogers AJJC. Three-dimensional transesophageal echocardiography in Ebstein's anomaly. Interact Cardiovasc Thorac Surg. 2010;10:836–7.
26. Acar P, Dulac Y, Roux D, Rougé P, Duterque D, Aggoun Y. Comparison of transthoracic and transesophageal three-dimensional echocardiography for assessment of atrial septal defect diameter in children. Am J Cardiol. 2003;91:500–2.
27. Georgakis A, Radtke WAK, Lopez C, et al. Complex atrial septal defect: percutaneous repair guided by three-dimensional echocardiography. Echocardiography. 2010;27:590–3.
28. Price MJ, Smith MR, Rubenson DS. Utility of on-line three-dimensional transesophageal echocardiography during percutaneous atrial septal defect closure. Catheter Cardiovasc Interv. 2010;75:570–7.
29. Saric M, Perk G, Purgess JR, Kronzon I. Imaging atrial septal defects by real-time three-dimensional transesophageal echocardiography: step-by-step approach. J Am Soc Echocardiogr. 2010; 23:1128–35.
30. Dall'Agata A, Cromme-Dijkhuis AH, Meijboom FJ, et al. Use of three-dimensional echocardiography for analysis of outflow obstruction in congenital heart disease. Am J Cardiol. 1999;83: 921–5.
31. Chan K-L, Liu X, Ascah KJ, Beauchesne LM, Burwash IG. Comparison of real-time 3-dimensional echocardiography with conventional 2-dimensional echocardiography in the assessment of structural heart disease. J Am Soc Echocardiogr. 2004;17: 976–80.
32. Takahashi K, Mackie AS, Rebeyka IM, et al. Two-dimensional versus transthoracic real-time three-dimensional echocardiography in the evaluation of the mechanisms and sites of atrioventricular valve regurgitation in a congenital heart disease population. J Am Soc Echocardiogr. 2010;23:726–34.
33. Simpson JM, Miller O. Three-dimensional echocardiography in congenital heart disease. Arch Cardiovasc Dis. 2011;104:45–56.
34. Yagel S, Cohen SM, Rosenak D, et al. Added value of three-/four-dimensional ultrasound in offline analysis and diagnosis of congenital heart disease. Ultrasound Obstet Gynecol. 2011;37: 432–7.
35. Shirali GS. Three-dimensional echocardiography in congenital heart disease. Echocardiography. 2012;29:242–8.
36. Vettukattil JJ. Three dimensional echocardiography in congenital heart disease. Heart. 2012;98:79–88.
37. Magni G, Hijazi ZM, Pandian NG, et al. Two- and three-dimensional transesophageal echocardiography in patient selection and assessment of atrial septal defect closure by the new DAS-Angel Wings device: initial clinical experience. Circulation. 1997;96:1722–8.
38. Chang C-Y, Hsiung MC, Tsai SK, et al. Live three-dimensional transesophageal echocardiography in an unusual case of aorto-left ventricular tunnel with a large interventricular septal aneurysm. Echocardiography. 2011;28:E12–5.
39. Mart CR. Three-dimensional echocardiographic evaluation of the Fontan conduit for thrombus. Echocardiography. 2012;29: 363–8.
40. Salcedo EE, Quaife RA, Seres T, Carroll JD. A framework for systematic characterization of the mitral valve by real-time three-dimensional transesophageal echocardiography. J Am Soc Echocardiogr. 2009;22:1087–99.

41. Lang RM, Tsang W, Weinert L, Mor-Avi V, Chandra S. Valvular heart disease the value of 3-dimensional echocardiography. J Am Coll Cardiol. 2011;58:1933–44.
42. Vettukattil JJ, Bharucha T, Anderson RH. Defining Ebstein's malformation using three-dimensional echocardiography. Interact Cardiovasc Thorac Surg. 2007;6:685–90.
43. Zhang L, Xie M, Balluz R, Ge S. Real time three-dimensional echocardiography for evaluation of congenital heart defects: state of the art. Echocardiography. 2012;29:232–41.
44. Valverde I, Rawlins D, Austin C, Simpson JM. Three-dimensional echocardiography in the management of parachute mitral valve. Eur Heart J Cardiovasc Imaging. 2012;13:446.
45. Anwar AM, McGhie JS, Meijboom FJ, Ten Cate FJ. Double orifice mitral valve by real-time three-dimensional echocardiography. Eur J Echocardiogr. 2008;9:731–2.
46. Han J, He Y, Li Z, et al. Isolated double-orifice mitral valve anomaly on 3-dimensional transesophageal echocardiography. J Ultrasound Med. 2009;28:1589–92.
47. Seliem MA, Fedec A, Szwast A, et al. Atrioventricular valve morphology and dynamics in congenital heart disease as imaged with real-time 3-dimensional matrix-array echocardiography: comparison with 2-dimensional imaging and surgical findings. J Am Soc Echocardiogr. 2007;20:869–76.
48. da Silva JP, Baumgratz JF, da Fonseca L, et al. The cone reconstruction of the tricuspid valve in Ebstein's anomaly. The operation: early and midterm results. J Thorac Cardiovasc Surg. 2007; 133:215–23.
49. Kiziltan HT, Theodoro DA, Warnes CA, O'Leary PW, Anderson BJ, Danielson GK. Late results of bioprosthetic tricuspid valve replacement in Ebstein's anomaly. Ann Thorac Surg. 1998;66: 1539–45.
50. Dearani JA, Danielson GK. Surgical management of Ebstein's anomaly in the adult. Semin Thorac Cardiovasc Surg. 2005;17: 148–54.
51. Sugeng L, Shernan SK, Weinert L, et al. Real-time three-dimensional transesophageal echocardiography in valve disease: comparison with surgical findings and evaluation of prosthetic valves. J Am Soc Echocardiogr. 2008;21:1347–54.
52. Kwak J, Andrawes M, Garvin S, D'Ambra MN. 3D transesophageal echocardiography: a review of recent literature 2007-2009. Curr Opin Anaesthesiol. 2010;23:80–8.
53. Weitzel N, Salcedo E, Puskas F, Nasrallah F, Fullerton D, Seres T. Using real time three-dimensional transesophageal echocardiography during Ross procedure in the operating room. Echocardiography. 2009;26:1278–83.
54. Brantley HP, Nekkanti R, Anderson CA, Kypson AP. Three-dimensional echocardiographic features of unicuspid aortic valve stenosis correlate with surgical findings. Echocardiography. 2012;29:E204–7.
55. Bharucha T, Fernandes F, Slorach C, Mertens L, Friedberg MK. Measurement of effective aortic valve area using three-dimensional echocardiography in children undergoing aortic balloon valvuloplasty for aortic stenosis. Echocardiography. 2012;29:484–91.
56. Chin C-H, Chen C-H, Lo H-S. The correlation between three-dimensional vena contracta area and aortic regurgitation index in patients with aortic regurgitation. Echocardiography. 2010;27: 161–6.
57. Khaw AV, Bardeleben RSV, Strasser C, et al. Direct measurement of left ventricular outflow tract by transthoracic real-time 3D-echocardiography increases accuracy in assessment of aortic valve stenosis. Int J Cardiol. 2009;136:64–71.
58. Gaspar T, Adawi S, Sachner R, et al. Three-dimensional imaging of the left ventricular outflow tract: impact on aortic valve area estimation by the continuity equation. J Am Soc Echocardiogr. 2012;25:749–57.
59. Saitoh T, Shiota M, Izumo M, et al. Comparison of left ventricular outflow geometry and aortic valve area in patients with aortic stenosis by 2-dimensional versus 3-dimensional echocardiography. Am J Cardiol. 2012;109:1626–31.
60. Baumgartner H, Hung J, Bermejo J, et al. Echocardiographic assessment of valve stenosis: EAE/ASE recommendations for clinical practice. J Am Soc Echocardiogr. 2009;22:1–23; quiz 101–2.
61. Anwar AM, Soliman O, van den Bosch AE, et al. Assessment of pulmonary valve and right ventricular outflow tract with real-time three-dimensional echocardiography. Int J Cardiovasc Imaging. 2007;23:167–75.
62. Cheng TO, Xie M-X, Wang X-F, Wang Y, Lu Q. Real-time 3-dimensional echocardiography in assessing atrial and ventricular septal defects: an echocardiographic-surgical correlative study. Am Heart J. 2004;148:1091–5.
63. Chen FL, Hsiung MC, Nanda N, Hsieh KS, Chou MC. Real time three-dimensional echocardiography in assessing ventricular septal defects: an echocardiographic-surgical correlative study. Echocardiography. 2006;23:562–8.
64. Mercer-Rosa L, Seliem MA, Fedec A, Rome J, Rychik J, Gaynor JW. Illustration of the additional value of real-time 3-dimensional echocardiography to conventional transthoracic and transesophageal 2-dimensional echocardiography in imaging muscular ventricular septal defects: does this have any impact on individual patient treatment? J Am Soc Echocardiogr. 2006;19:1511–9.
65. van den Bosch AE, Ten Harkel D-J, McGhie JS, et al. Feasibility and accuracy of real-time 3-dimensional echocardiographic assessment of ventricular septal defects. J Am Soc Echocardiogr. 2006;19:7–13.
66. Acar P, Abadir S, Aggoun Y. Transcatheter closure of perimembranous ventricular septal defects with Amplatzer occluder assessed by real-time three-dimensional echocardiography. Eur J Echocardiogr. 2007;8:110–5.
67. Huang X, Shen J, Huang Y, et al. En face view of atrial septal defect by two-dimensional transthoracic echocardiography: comparison to real-time three-dimensional transesophageal echocardiography. J Am Soc Echocardiogr. 2010;23:714–21.
68. Morgan GJ, Casey F, Craig B, Sands A. Assessing ASDs prior to device closure using 3D echocardiography. Just pretty pictures or a useful clinical tool? Eur J Echocardiogr. 2008;9:478–82.
69. Taniguchi M, Akagi T, Watanabe N, et al. Application of real-time three-dimensional transesophageal echocardiography using a matrix array probe for transcatheter closure of atrial septal defect. J Am Soc Echocardiogr. 2009;22:1114–20.
70. Halpern DG, Perk G, Ruiz C, Marino N, Kronzon I. Percutaneous closure of a post-myocardial infarction ventricular septal defect guided by real-time three-dimensional echocardiography. Eur J Echocardiogr. 2009;10:569–71.
71. Zhu D, Tao K-Y, Liu B. Successful repair of a traumatic ventricular septal defect using an amplatzer occluder guided by three-dimensional transesophageal echocardiography. J Card Surg. 2010;25:685–9.
72. Van der Velde ME, Sanders SP, Keane JF, Perry SB, Lock JE. Transesophageal echocardiographic guidance of transcatheter ventricular septal defect closure. J Am Coll Cardiol. 1994;23: 1660–5.
73. Holzer R, Balzer D, Cao Q-L, Lock K, Hijazi ZM, Amplatzer Muscular Ventricular Septal Defect Investigators. Device closure of muscular ventricular septal defects using the Amplatzer muscular ventricular septal defect occluder: immediate and mid-term results of a U.S. registry. J Am Coll Cardiol. 2004;43:1257–63.
74. Bacha EA, Cao QL, Galantowicz ME, et al. Multicenter experience with perventricular device closure of muscular ventricular septal defects. Pediatr Cardiol. 2005;26:169–75.

75. Butera G, Chessa M, Carminati M. Percutaneous closure of ventricular septal defects. Cardiol Young. 2007;17:243–53.
76. Gan C, An Q, Lin K, et al. Perventricular device closure of ventricular septal defects: six months results in 30 young children. Ann Thorac Surg. 2008;86:142–6.
77. Pedra CAC, Pedra SRF, Chaccur P, et al. Perventricular device closure of congenital muscular ventricular septal defects. Expert Rev Cardiovasc Ther. 2010;8:663–74.
78. Bendaly EA, Hoyer MH, Breinholt JP. Mid-term follow up of perventricular device closure of muscular ventricular septal defects. Catheter Cardiovasc Interv. 2011;78:577–82.
79. Geva A, McMahon CJ, Gauvreau K, Mohammed L, del Nido PJ, Geva T. Risk factors for reoperation after repair of discrete subaortic stenosis in children. J Am Coll Cardiol. 2007;50:1498–504.
80. Valeske K, Huber C, Mueller M, et al. The dilemma of subaortic stenosis—a single center experience of 15 years with a review of the literature. Thorac Cardiovasc Surg. 2011;59:293–7.
81. Miyamoto K, Nakatani S, Kanzaki H, Tagusari O, Kobayashi J. Detection of discrete subaortic stenosis by 3-dimensional transesophageal echocardiography. Echocardiography. 2005;22:783–4.
82. Maréchaux S, Juthier F, Banfi C, Vincentelli A, Prat A, Ennezat P-V. Illustration of the echocardiographic diagnosis of subaortic membrane stenosis in adults: surgical and live three-dimensional transoesophageal findings. Eur J Echocardiogr. 2011;12:E2.
83. Hanna R, Chen MA, Gill EA. Cor triatriatum evaluated by real time 3D TEE. Echocardiography. 2011;28:E125–8.
84. Enar S, Singh P, Douglas C, et al. Live/real time three-dimensional transthoracic echocardiographic assessment of transposition of the great arteries in the adult. Echocardiography. 2009;26:1095–104.
85. Balzer J, Kühl H, Rassaf T, et al. Real-time transesophageal three-dimensional echocardiography for guidance of percutaneous cardiac interventions: first experience. Clin Res Cardiol. 2008;97:565–74.
86. Gripari P, Tamborini G, Barbier P, et al. Real-time three-dimensional transoesophageal echocardiography: a new intraoperative feasible and useful technology in cardiac surgery. Int J Cardiovasc Imaging. 2010;26:651–60.
87. Scohy TV, Ten Cate FJ, Lecomte PVEL, et al. Usefulness of intraoperative real-time 3D transesophageal echocardiography in cardiac surgery. J Card Surg. 2008;23:784–6.
88. La Canna G, Arendar I, Maisano F, et al. Real-time three-dimensional transesophageal echocardiography for assessment of mitral valve functional anatomy in patients with prolapse-related regurgitation. Am J Cardiol. 2011;107:1365–74.
89. Swaans MJ, Van den Branden BJL, Van der Heyden JAS, et al. Three-dimensional transoesophageal echocardiography in a patient undergoing percutaneous mitral valve repair using the edge-to-edge clip technique. Eur J Echocardiogr. 2009;10:982–3.
90. Brinkman V, Kalbfleisch S, Auseon A, Pu M. Real time three-dimensional transesophageal echocardiography-guided placement of left atrial appendage occlusion device. Echocardiography. 2009;26:855–8.
91. Perk G, Biner S, Kronzon I, et al. Catheter-based left atrial appendage occlusion procedure: role of echocardiography. Eur Heart J Cardiovasc Imaging. 2012;13:132–8.
92. Jánosi RA, Kahlert P, Plicht B, et al. Guidance of percutaneous transcatheter aortic valve implantation by real-time three-dimensional transesophageal echocardiography—A single-center experience. Minim Invasive Ther Allied Technol. 2009;18:142–8.
93. Horton KD, Whisenant B, Horton S. Percutaneous closure of a mitral perivalvular leak using three dimensional real time and color flow imaging. J Am Soc Echocardiogr. 2010;23:903.e5–7.
94. Jenkins C, Bricknell K, Chan J, Hanekom L, Marwick TH. Comparison of two- and three-dimensional echocardiography with sequential magnetic resonance imaging for evaluating left ventricular volume and ejection fraction over time in patients with healed myocardial infarction. Am J Cardiol. 2007;99:300–6.
95. Mor-Avi V, Jenkins C, Kühl HP, et al. Real-time 3-dimensional echocardiographic quantification of left ventricular volumes: multicenter study for validation with magnetic resonance imaging and investigation of sources of error. JACC Cardiovasc Imaging. 2008;1:413–23.
96. Sugeng L, Mor-Avi V, Weinert L, et al. Quantitative assessment of left ventricular size and function: side-by-side comparison of real-time three-dimensional echocardiography and computed tomography with magnetic resonance reference. Circulation. 2006;114:654–61.
97. Leibundgut G, Rohner A, Grize L, et al. Dynamic assessment of right ventricular volumes and function by real-time three-dimensional echocardiography: a comparison study with magnetic resonance imaging in 100 adult patients. J Am Soc Echocardiogr. 2010;23:116–26.
98. Sugeng L, Mor-Avi V, Weinert L, et al. Multimodality comparison of quantitative volumetric analysis of the right ventricle. JACC Cardiovasc Imaging. 2010;3:10–8.
99. Tamborini G, Marsan NA, Gripari P, et al. Reference values for right ventricular volumes and ejection fraction with real-time three-dimensional echocardiography: evaluation in a large series of normal subjects. J Am Soc Echocardiogr. 2010;23:109–15.
100. Shimada YJ, Shiota M, Siegel RJ, Shiota T. Accuracy of right ventricular volumes and function determined by three-dimensional echocardiography in comparison with magnetic resonance imaging: a meta-analysis study. J Am Soc Echocardiogr. 2010;23:943–53.
101. Fusini L, Tamborini G, Gripari P, et al. Feasibility of intraoperative three-dimensional transesophageal echocardiography in the evaluation of right ventricular volumes and function in patients undergoing cardiac surgery. J Am Soc Echocardiogr. 2011;24:868–77.
102. Karhausen J, Dudaryk R, Phillips-Bute B, et al. Three-dimensional transesophageal echocardiography for perioperative right ventricular assessment. Ann Thorac Surg. 2012;94:468–74.
103. Lang RM, Bierig M, Devereux RB, et al. Recommendations for chamber quantification. Eur J Echocardiogr. 2006;7:79–108.
104. Kapetanakis S, Kearney MT, Siva A, Gall N, Cooklin M, Monaghan MJ. Real-time three-dimensional echocardiography: a novel technique to quantify global left ventricular mechanical dyssynchrony. Circulation. 2005;112:992–1000.
105. Gorcsan III J, Abraham T, Agler DA, et al. Echocardiography for cardiac resynchronization therapy: recommendations for performance and reporting–a report from the American Society of Echocardiography Dyssynchrony Writing Group endorsed by the Heart Rhythm Society. J Am Soc Echocardiogr. 2008;21:191–213.
106. Tanaka H, Hara H, Adelstein EC, Schwartzman D, Saba S, Gorcsan J. Comparative mechanical activation mapping of RV pacing to LBBB by 2D and 3D speckle tracking and association with response to resynchronization therapy. JACC Cardiovasc Imaging. 2010;3:461–71.
107. Soliman OII, Geleijnse ML, Theuns DAMJ, et al. Usefulness of left ventricular systolic dyssynchrony by real-time three-dimensional echocardiography to predict long-term response to cardiac resynchronization therapy. Am J Cardiol. 2009;103:1586–91.
108. Kapetanakis S, Bhan A, Murgatroyd F, et al. Real-time 3D echo in patient selection for cardiac resynchronization therapy. JACC Cardiovasc Imaging. 2011;4:16–26.
109. Kleijn SA, Aly MF, Knol DL, et al. A meta-analysis of left ventricular dyssynchrony assessment and prediction of response to

cardiac resynchronization therapy by three-dimensional echocardiography. Eur Heart J Cardiovasc Imaging. 2012;13:763–75.
110. Wang H, Shuraih M, Ahmad M. Real time three-dimensional echocardiography in assessment of left ventricular dyssynchrony and cardiac resynchronization therapy. Echocardiography. 2012; 29:192–9.
111. Seo Y, Ishizu T, Enomoto Y, et al. Validation of 3-dimensional speckle tracking imaging to quantify regional myocardial deformation. Circ Cardiovasc Imaging. 2009;2:451–9.
112. Ashraf M, Myronenko A, Nguyen T, et al. Defining left ventricular apex-to-base twist mechanics computed from high-resolution 3D echocardiography: validation against sonomicrometry. JACC Cardiovasc Imaging. 2010;3:227–34.
113. Andrade J, Cortez LD, Campos O, et al. Left ventricular twist: comparison between two- and three-dimensional speckle-tracking echocardiography in healthy volunteers. Eur J Echocardiogr. 2011;12:76–9.
114. Kleijn SA, Aly MFA, Terwee CB, van Rossum AC, Kamp O. Three-dimensional speckle tracking echocardiography for automatic assessment of global and regional left ventricular function based on area strain. J Am Soc Echocardiogr. 2011;24:314–21.
115. Kahlert P, Plicht B, Schenk IM, Janosi R-A, Erbel R, Buck T. Direct assessment of size and shape of noncircular vena contracta area in functional versus organic mitral regurgitation using real-time three-dimensional echocardiography. J Am Soc Echocardiogr. 2008;21:912–21.
116. Pérez de Isla L, Casanova C, Almería C, et al. Which method should be the reference method to evaluate the severity of rheumatic mitral stenosis? Gorlin's method versus 3D-echo. Eur J Echocardiogr. 2007;8:470–3.
117. Altiok E, Hamada S, van Hall S, et al. Comparison of direct planimetry of mitral valve regurgitation orifice area by three-dimensional transesophageal echocardiography to effective regurgitant orifice area obtained by proximal flow convergence method and vena contracta area determined by color Doppler echocardiography. Am J Cardiol. 2011;107:452–8.
118. Tsang W, Weinert L, Sugeng L, et al. The value of three-dimensional echocardiography derived mitral valve parametric maps and the role of experience in the diagnosis of pathology. J Am Soc Echocardiogr. 2011;24:860–7.
119. Veronesi F, Caiani EG, Sugeng L, et al. Effect of mitral valve repair on mitral-aortic coupling: a real-time three-dimensional transesophageal echocardiography study. J Am Soc Echocardiogr. 2012;25:524–31.
120. Badano LP, Muraru D. Towards an integrated echocardiographic assessment of valvular mechanics by three-dimensional volumetric imaging. J Am Soc Echocardiogr. 2012;25:532–4.
121. Lu X, Xie M, Tomberlin D, et al. How accurately, reproducibly, and efficiently can we measure left ventricular indices using M-mode, 2-dimensional, and 3-dimensional echocardiography in children? Am Heart J. 2008;155:946–53.
122. Riehle TJ, Mahle WT, Parks WJ, Sallee D, Fyfe DA. Real-time three-dimensional echocardiographic acquisition and quantification of left ventricular indices in children and young adults with congenital heart disease: comparison with magnetic resonance imaging. J Am Soc Echocardiogr. 2008;21:78–83.
123. Raedle-Hurst TM, Mueller M, Rentzsch A, Schaefers H-J, Herrmann E, Abdul-Khaliq H. Assessment of left ventricular dyssynchrony and function using real-time 3-dimensional echocardiography in patients with congenital right heart disease. Am Heart J. 2009;157:791–8.
124. Friedberg MK, Su X, Tworetzky W, Soriano BD, Powell AJ, Marx GR. Validation of 3D echocardiographic assessment of left ventricular volumes, mass, and ejection fraction in neonates and infants with congenital heart disease: a comparison study with cardiac MRI. Circ Cardiovasc Imaging. 2010;3:735–42.
125. Hascoët S, Brierre G, Caudron G, Cardin C, Bongard V, Acar P. Assessment of left ventricular volumes and function by real time three-dimensional echocardiography in a pediatric population: a TomTec versus QLAB comparison. Echocardiography. 2010;27: 1263–73.
126. Laser KT, Bunge M, Hauffe P, et al. Left ventricular volumetry in healthy children and adolescents: comparison of two different real-time three-dimensional matrix transducers with cardiovascular magnetic resonance. Eur J Echocardiogr. 2010;11:138–48.
127. Iriart X, Montaudon M, Lafitte S, et al. Right ventricle three-dimensional echography in corrected tetralogy of fallot: accuracy and variability. Eur J Echocardiogr. 2009;10:784–92.
128. Khoo NS, Young A, Occleshaw C, Cowan B, Zeng ISL, Gentles TL. Assessments of right ventricular volume and function using three-dimensional echocardiography in older children and adults with congenital heart disease: comparison with cardiac magnetic resonance imaging. J Am Soc Echocardiogr. 2009;22: 1279–88.
129. van der Zwaan HB, Helbing WA, McGhie JS, et al. Clinical value of real-time three-dimensional echocardiography for right ventricular quantification in congenital heart disease: validation with cardiac magnetic resonance imaging. J Am Soc Echocardiogr. 2010;23:134–40.
130. Soriano BD, Hoch M, Ithuralde A, et al. Matrix-array 3-dimensional echocardiographic assessment of volumes, mass, and ejection fraction in young pediatric patients with a functional single ventricle: a comparison study with cardiac magnetic resonance. Circulation. 2008;117:1842–8.
131. Kutty S, Graney BA, Khoo NS, et al. Serial assessment of right ventricular volume and function in surgically palliated hypoplastic left heart syndrome using real-time transthoracic three-dimensional echocardiography. J Am Soc Echocardiogr. 2012;25: 682–9.
132. Hlavacek A, Lucas J, Baker H, Chessa K, Shirali G. Feasibility and utility of three-dimensional color flow echocardiography of the aortic arch: the "echocardiographic angiogram". Echocardiography. 2006;23:860–4.
133. Pemberton J, Ge S, Thiele K, Jerosch-Herold M, Sahn DJ. Real-time three-dimensional color Doppler echocardiography overcomes the inaccuracies of spectral Doppler for stroke volume calculation. J Am Soc Echocardiogr. 2006;19:1403–10.
134. Poh KK, Levine RA, Solis J, et al. Assessing aortic valve area in aortic stenosis by continuity equation: a novel approach using real-time three-dimensional echocardiography. Eur Heart J. 2008; 29:2526–35.
135. Lu X, Nadvoretskiy V, Klas B, et al. Measurement of volumetric flow by real-time 3-dimensional doppler echocardiography in children. J Am Soc Echocardiogr. 2007;20:915–20.
136. Rajpoot K, Grau V, Noble JA, Szmigielski C, Becher H. Multiview fusion 3-D echocardiography: improving the information and quality of real-time 3-D echocardiography. Ultrasound Med Biol. 2011;37:1056–72.

Clinical Applications of Three-Dimensional Transesophageal Echocardiography in Congenital Heart Disease

20

Vivian Wei Cui and David A. Roberson

Abstract

In this chapter we present a collection of three-dimensional (3D) transesophageal echocardiographic images from scenarios and cases that constitute representative examples of the useful clinical application of this technique to patients with congenital heart disease (CHD). Four general areas of discussion include: (1) 3D anatomic assessment; (2) use during interventional catheterization; (3) imaging of representative surgical treatments; and (4) applications related to electrophysiologic issues. Acquisitions using live 3D, 3D zoom, full volume 3D, X-plane and 3D color modalities are included. Suggestions for the choice of acquisition modality and image optimization are made for various imaging scenarios. The recommendations in this chapter are based largely on personal experience and preferences gained from performing 3D TEE in over 400 patients with CHD. We hope the reader will find this information useful and prompt further training, practice, more widespread use, and investigation of the applications of 3D TEE in CHD.

Keywords

Three-dimensional echocardiography • 3D Transesophageal echocardiography • Real-time 3D transesophageal echocardiography • 3D Image acquisition modalities • 3D Full volume • 3D Live • 3D Zoom • X-Plane • 3D Color mode • Congenital heart disease

Introduction

Since the time that three-dimensional transesophageal echocardiography (3D TEE) first became available in 2008, its adoption and application as an essential imaging modality in adult cardiology have been substantial, particularly for aortic and mitral valve interventions [1–12]. Notwithstanding this progress, the use of 3D TEE in patients with congenital heart disease (CHD) has developed at a considerably slower rate. This may be due in part to the limitation of the use of 3D TEE for those patients with a body weight greater than 20 kg because the lack of suitable probes for smaller children. However there are other factors, including (a) limited information on protocols for usage, (b) lack of widespread communication about the best practices for image acquisition and optimization, and (c) limited demonstration in the literature of the clinical utility of 3D TEE for CHD evaluation. All of these have contributed to the relatively slow proliferation of 3D TEE as a commonly applied, useful, and valuable clinical imaging tool for those with CHD.

In this chapter we present images from various clinical scenarios that, in our opinion, clearly demonstrate the benefits of 3D TEE in CHD. Images from both simple and complex

Note on the figures used in this chapter: An orientation icon is provided for each figure in this chapter. This icon contains abbreviations for the different planes and directions used to orient the reader. Figure 20.1 displays the standard orientation used in the figures and the corresponding abbreviations noted by the markers.

The online version of this chapter (doi:10.1007/978-1-84800-064-3_20) contains supplementary material, which is available to authorized users.

V.W. Cui, MD • D.A. Roberson, MD (✉)
Division of Pediatric Cardiology, Department of Pediatrics,
Advocate Children's Hospital Heart Institute,
4440 W. 95th St, Oak Lawn, IL 60453, USA
e-mail: david.roberson@advocatehealth.com

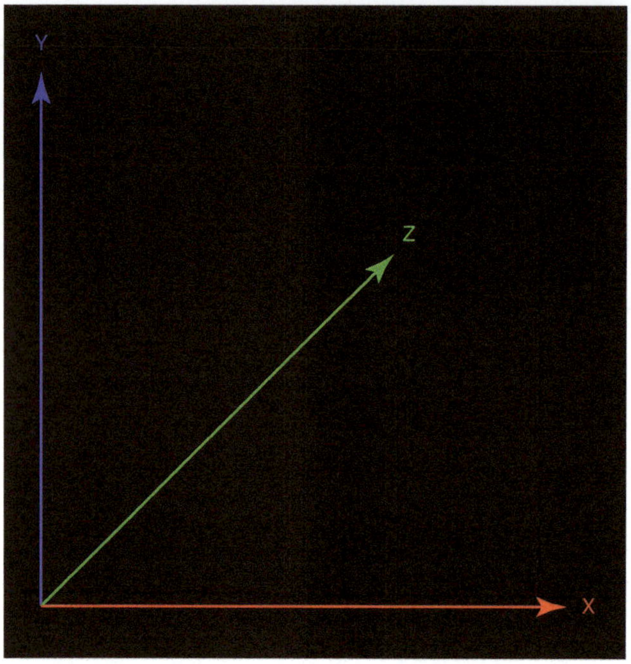

Fig. 20.1 Three-dimensional orientation icon displayed in the figures. *Abbreviations* for orientation markers used in the figures throughout this chapter: *A* anterior, *I* inferior, *L* left, *P* posterior, *R* right, *S* superior

congenital cardiac anomalies are presented. Representative applications in the interventional catheterization laboratory are provided. Selected examples of surgical repairs and palliations are displayed. Lastly, images useful during the treatment of patients undergoing electrophysiologic procedures are illustrated.

We also offer suggestions, based on our experience, of ways to optimize 3D TEE capabilities. These include the acquisition modality that might best be applied for a particular structure of interest, cropping methods that are most useful, and other methods to optimize image display.

Our entire case collection for 3D TEE and the examples presented in this chapter are based solely upon our experience using the Philips iE33 echocardiographic system and X7–2t 3D TEE transducer (Philips Medical Systems, Andover, Massachusetts). Nonetheless we believe the principles embodied in this chapter will have widespread applicability to all forms of 3D TEE evaluation of CHD, irrespective of ultrasound platform or manufacturer. The reader is also referred to Chap. 19 for an overview of general concepts regarding 3D imaging.

Defining Three-Dimensional Cardiac Anatomy

The ability of 3D echocardiography to demonstrate surfaces, volumes, and spatial relationships allows the echocardiographer to acquire and display views of the heart and great vessels that are analogous to viewing a cardiac pathology specimen [13–24]. Valve leaflets, septal structures, and the real time depiction of spatial relationships provide clearer anatomic definition and better understanding of the actual cardiac anatomy as compared to Two-dimensional (2D) echocardiography [25–27].

Case Examples

Congenitally Corrected Transposition (*L*-Transposition of the Great Arteries)

Figure 20.2 was obtained from a patient with congenitally corrected transposition, illustrating the four cardiac chambers and valves, imaged from the mid esophageal four chamber (ME 4 Ch) view. These images were obtained using a *full volume 3D acquisition mode*. This 3D echocardiographic modality is most useful for obtaining the entire cardiac echocardiographic (echo) volume in one cine loop. Once acquired, this echo volume can be cropped and rotated from any or all directions in order to display the relevant anatomy. As this 3D echo modality can be prone to stitch artifact (refer to Chap. 19), breath holding, maximizing 3D echo volume rate, using multiplanar reconstruction mode (MPR), and editing out cine loops in which artifact is present, are important skills to master. Figure 20.2a is cropped with one touch by using the auto crop button, which removes the anterior 50 % of the echo volume. Figure 20.2b is not cropped at all, but is merely a full volume acquisition with the superior plane tilted towards the viewer. Relatively low gain and compression settings, as well as slight angulation or tilting of the 3D cardiac image, should be used in order to enhance the depth shading. Figure 20.3 is a deep transgastric sagittal (DTG Sagittal) view obtained from the same patient with inverted ventricles shown in Fig. 20.2 depicting the three leaflets of the tricuspid valve in the morphologic right ventricle. This image was obtained using the *live 3D mode*, which maximizes volume rate at the expense of requiring a smaller 3D echo sample volume. This modality has an additional advantage of minimizing stitch artifact and is therefore quite useful for patients with faster heart rates or for viewing rapidly moving structures such as semilunar valves. Especially when learning 3D echo, as well as in cases in which imaging time is limited, such as during surgery and interventional catheterization procedures, we have found it most effective to have two echocardiographers involved: one manipulates the transducer while the other operates the controls on the echocardiography machine. Both roles must be learned and coordinated by both operators in order to achieve the full potential of 3D TEE.

Cor Triatriatum

Images from a patient with dextrocardia, multiple ventricular septal defects (VSDs) and cor triatriatum undergoing surgical resection of the obstructive membrane are shown in Fig. 20.4. Note the clearly defined anatomic details including the depth, orifices, and surfaces of the cardiac structures in this complex lesion. Also note that, as in the prior case example, we applied 3D full volume to obtain the entire cardiac

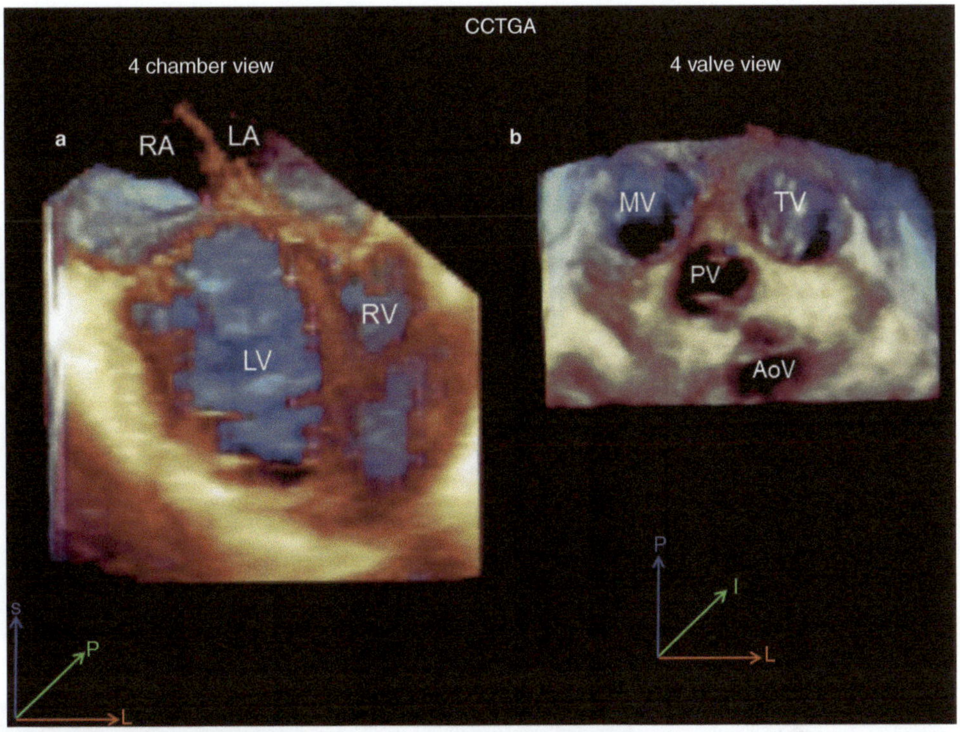

Fig. 20.2 Full volume 3D acquisitions of congenitally corrected transposition (*CCTGA*). (**a**) Mid esophageal four chamber view. (**b**) Four valve upper esophageal view. *AoV* aortic valve, *LA* left atrium, *LV* left ventricle, *MV* mitral valve, *PV* pulmonary valve, *RA* right atrium, *RV* right ventricle, *TV* tricuspid valve

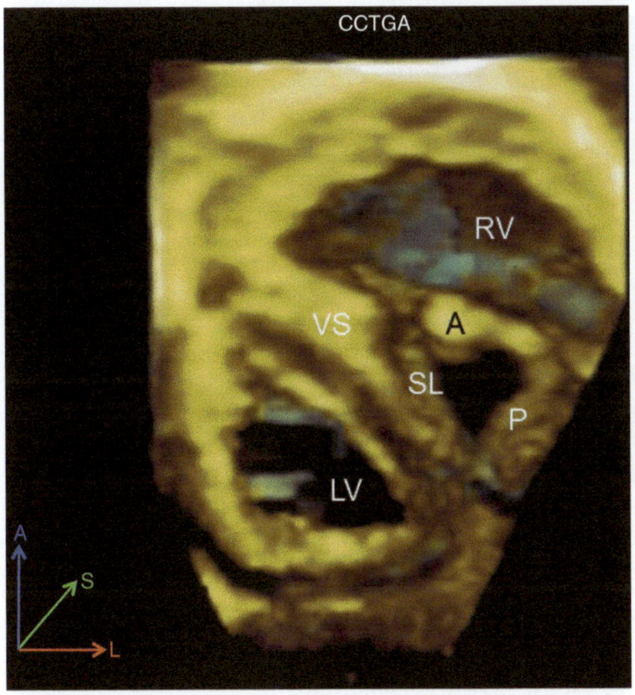

Fig. 20.3 Live 3D deep transgastric sagittal axis view obtained in the same patient presented in Fig. 20.2 with congenitally corrected transposition (*CCTGA*). Note the *en face* view of the tricuspid valve in the left-sided, anteriorly positioned right ventricle (*RV*). *A* anterior leaflet of tricuspid valve, *LV* left ventricle, *P* posterior leaflet of tricuspid valve, *SL* septal leaflet of the tricuspid valve, *VS* ventricular septum

3D volume as a first step as illustrated in Fig. 20.4a and Video 20.1. Subsequently we used live 3D to focus on specific details in real time as seen in Fig. 20.4b. The actual obstructive orifice of the cor triatriatum membrane is seen in this figure as if one were viewing a pathology specimen from above. In Fig. 20.5a we applied *X-plane color Doppler flow mapping* consisting of live biplane echocardiography, analogous to biplane angiography, which provides simultaneous live imaging of the frontal and lateral planes. Using any of the 3D echo modalities one can rotate the cardiac images 180° in order to provide unique views of the heart from its posterior aspect. This is depicted in the 3D color Doppler flow map in Fig. 20.5b and Video 20.2, demonstrating flow through the obstructive membrane orifice in this case.

Bicuspid Aortic Valve

Live 3D images of the two most common types of bicuspid aortic valve, namely left–right commissural fusion and right non-coronary commissure fusion, are presented in Fig. 20.6. The valve leaflet surface and depth can be clearly displayed by 3D imaging (Fig. 20.6, Videos 20.3 and 20.4). The blue depth shading provided by using the H tissue algorithm (3D tissue display), along with lower gain settings, are essential to provide the optimal 3D effect. Also, the anatomic details of leaflet thickening, raphe thickness and orientation, and the valve orifice shape, size, and location are viewed in greater detail. We consider live 3D acquired from the mid esophageal aortic valve short axis (ME AV SAX) view to be the best currently available modality to obtain these anatomic details of the aortic valve.

Parachute Mitral Valve

Parachute mitral valve deformities from two patients are presented on Figs. 20.7 and 20.8 respectively. Figure. 20.7a is a

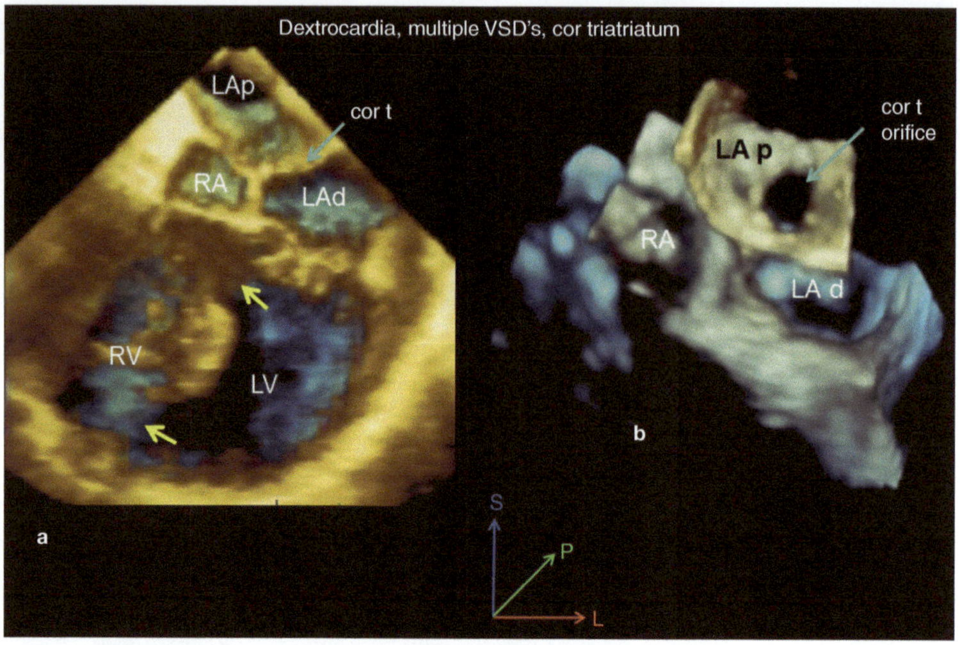

Fig. 20.4 A case of cor triatriatum, dextrocardia and multiple ventricular septal defects (*yellow arrows*) as seen from the mid esophageal four chamber view, using full volume 3D acquisition. (**a**) The cor triatriatum membrane (*cor t*; *green arrow*) divides the left atrium into proximal (*LAp*) and distal (*LAd*) chambers. (**b**) The image has been cropped from above and tilted forward to demonstrate the cor triatriatum orifice. *LV* left ventricle, *RA* right atrium, *RV* right ventricle

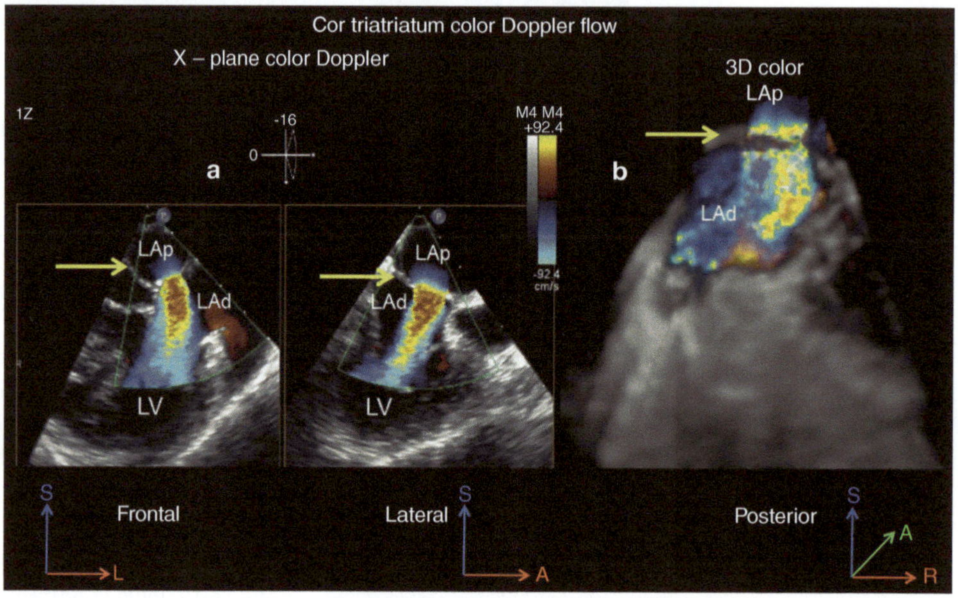

Fig. 20.5 Color Doppler flow analysis is presented from the same case shown in Fig. 20.4. (**a**) X-plane color Doppler display of the turbulent flow through the cor triatriatum orifice as seen from orthogonal views (*frontal* and *lateral*). The cor triatriatum membrane is indicated by the arrow. (**b**) 3D color Doppler flow map as seen from a *posterior* view is shown. *LAp* proximal chamber, *LAd* distal chamber, *LV* left ventricle

3D zoom acquisition of the mitral valve in which the hypoplastic mitral valve orifice is viewed from the left atrium. 3D zoom mode is our preferred method to visualize the mitral valve because it is live, rapid and very easy to perform. It has the drawback of having a slow volume rate, although this problem can be mitigated by using the high volume rate (HVR) imaging modality. This modality is chosen on the control knobs of the echocardiographic platform. It provides for increased volume rate at the expense of slightly decreased resolution and limited quantitative capabilities. Figure 20.7b and Video 20.5 are from a frontal cropped 3D full volume of the hypoplastic stenotic parachute mitral valve, obtained from the ME 4 Ch view. Live 3D was used to acquire Fig. 20.8, which demonstrates a parachute mitral valve in a patient with double inlet left ventricle. Note from these three examples that after the image has been acquired and appropriately cropped and displayed, it is not always easy to determine which acquisition modality—3D zoom vs. full volume 3D vs. live 3D—was employed.

Ventricular Septal Defects

The advantages of 3D TEE to demonstrate the anatomy of VSDs are apparent in Figs. 20.9 and 20.10. *En face* views of the ventricular septum from either the right or left ventricular aspect demonstrate the size, shape, location, and orientation of the defect as well as its relationship to surrounding structures. An interesting aspect of VSD imaging we have noted is that the majority of defects we have examined have

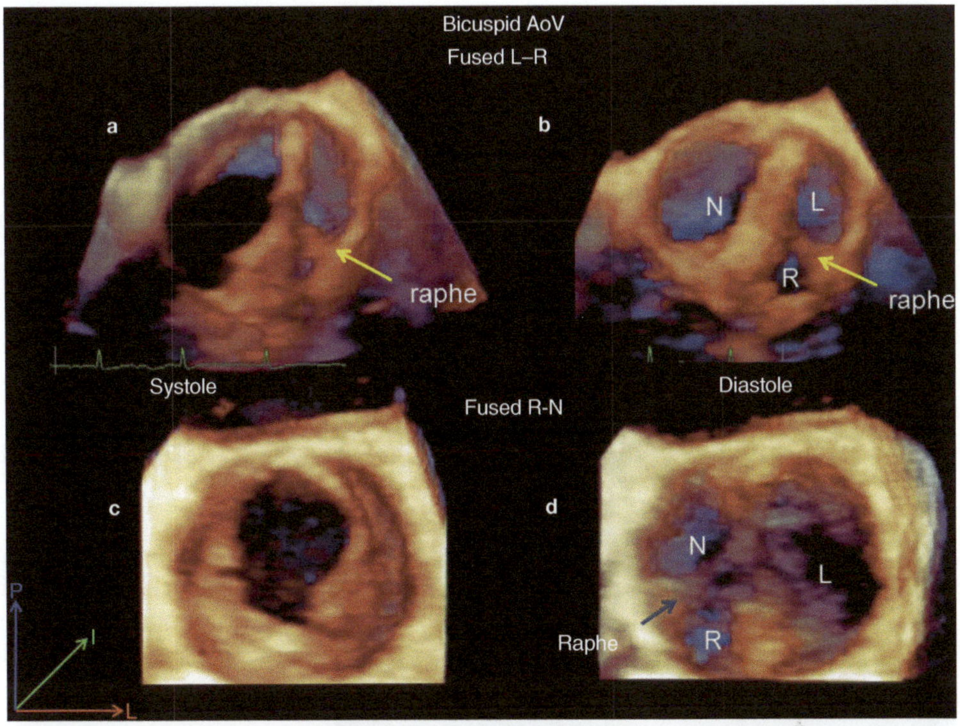

Fig. 20.6 Live 3D mid esophageal aortic valve short axis acquisitions of the two most common variants of the bicuspid aortic valve. Images in the *top row* are from a patient with left and right leaflet fusion (*fused L-R*). The view during systole is labeled (**a**) and the view during diastole is labeled (**b**). Images in the *bottom row* are from a patient with right and non-coronary leaflet fusion (*fused R-N*). The view during systole is labeled (**c**) and the view during diastole is labeled (**d**)

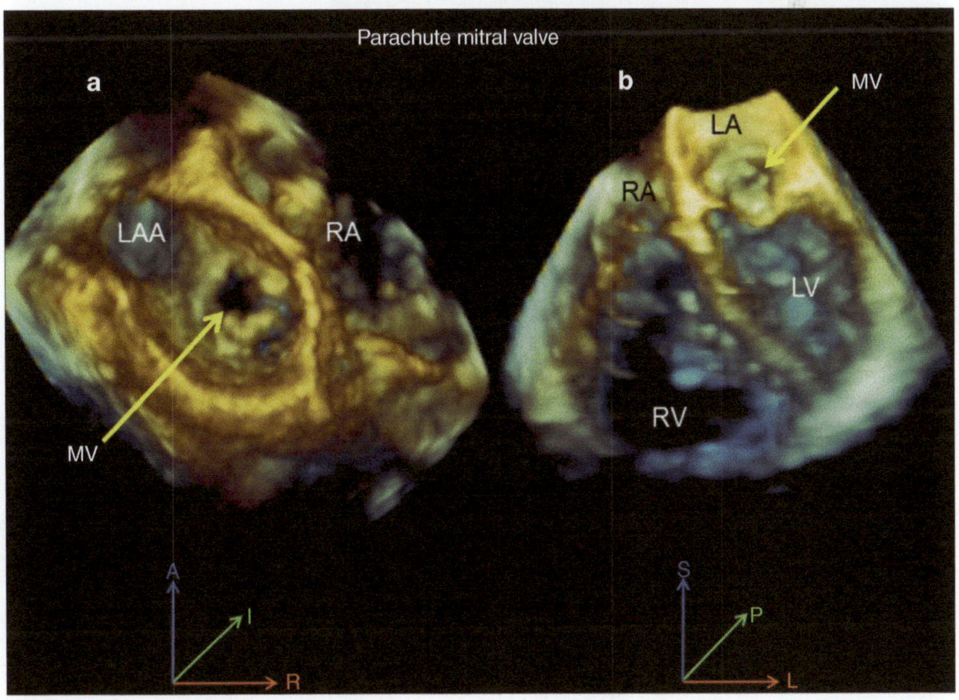

Fig. 20.7 Views of a parachute mitral valve. (**a**) 3D zoom mode acquisition viewed from the left atrium shows the hypoplastic mitral valve (*MV*) orifice (*yellow arrow*). (**b**) Full volume 3D mid esophageal four chamber view displays the hypoplastic and doming mitral valve (*yellow arrow*). *LA* left atrium, *LAA* left atrial appendage, *LV* left ventricle, *RA* right atrium, *RV* right ventricle

the longest dimension in the Z plane (anterior-posterior), a plane unique to 3D echocardiography. Therefore the actual largest dimension and overall size of the VSD may be better depicted using 3D versus 2D echocardiography in many cases. Figure 20.9 represents live 3D color Doppler flow maps of a muscular VSD from a slightly oblique ME 4 Ch view (Fig. 20.9a) and a mid esophageal long axis (ME LAX) view (Fig. 20.9b, Video 20.6). The images in Fig. 20.10 are cropped full volume 3D acquisitions of a perimembranous VSD. The right (Fig. 20.10a) and left ventricular *en face* views (Fig. 20.10c) are obtained by cropping from the respective right or left sides and rotating the images to face the viewer. Obtaining *en face* views of septal structures is one of the basic 3D echo skills that must be mastered in the assessment of congenital heart defects. The center Fig. 20.10b and Video 20.7 are the frontal cropped full volume images obtained from the ME 4 Ch view, as previously discussed.

Double Inlet Left Ventricle

Images from a patient with double inlet left ventricle, acquired from the ME 4 Ch view using full volume 3D TEE are presented in Fig. 20.11. By cropping the image from the superior direction and tilting the cardiac base toward the viewer, the atrioventricular (AV) valves are seen from the atrial view (Fig. 20.11a). By cropping from the inferior direction and tilting the apex toward the viewer, the AV valves are seen from the ventricular view (Fig. 20.11b). Finally, another example of a frontal cropped ME 4 Ch view is demonstrated (Fig. 20.11c). This view functions as a good home base view from which to proceed with more involved 3D cropping and views.

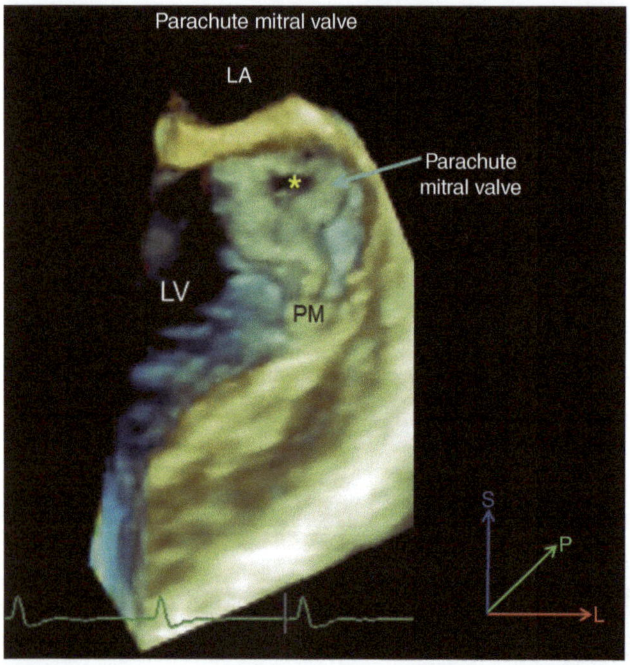

Fig. 20.8 Live 3D acquisition in a patient with double inlet left ventricle and parachute left sided atrioventricular valve obtained from the mid esophageal four chamber view. The very small mitral orifice (*), single small papillary muscle (*PM*) and parachute or funnel shape deformity of the mitral valve are apparent. *LA* left atrium, *LV* left ventricle

Atrial Septal Defects

Analogous to 3D imaging of VSDs, imaging of atrial septal defects (ASDs) using 3D TEE employs *en face* and long axis views. In Fig. 20.12a, a 3D zoom *en face* view of a large inferior sinus venosus ASD is shown from the right atrial aspect. A superior type sinus venosus ASD with partial anomalous pulmonary veins is presented in Fig. 20.12b. This image was obtained from a modified mid esophageal bicaval view (probe has been withdrawn), using a cropped full volume 3D image.

Applications During Interventional Cardiac Catheterization

The closure of secundum ASDs and muscular VSDs using interventional catheterization techniques has become commonplace at busy CHD treatment centers. The *en face* views of the septal anatomy and surrounding structures, as

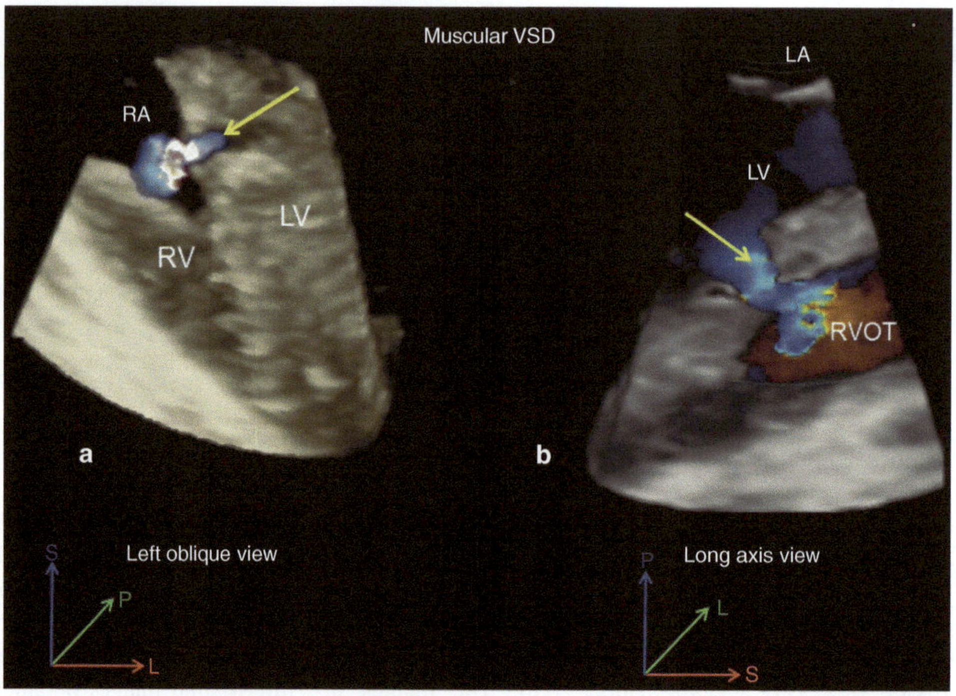

Fig. 20.9 Live 3D color Doppler flow mapping images of a muscular ventricular septal defect (*VSD*). (**a**) Mid esophageal four chamber view showing the VSD with a left oblique rotation. (**b**) Demonstration of the defect using a mid esophageal long axis view, the *left* to *right* shunt is indicated by the *arrow*

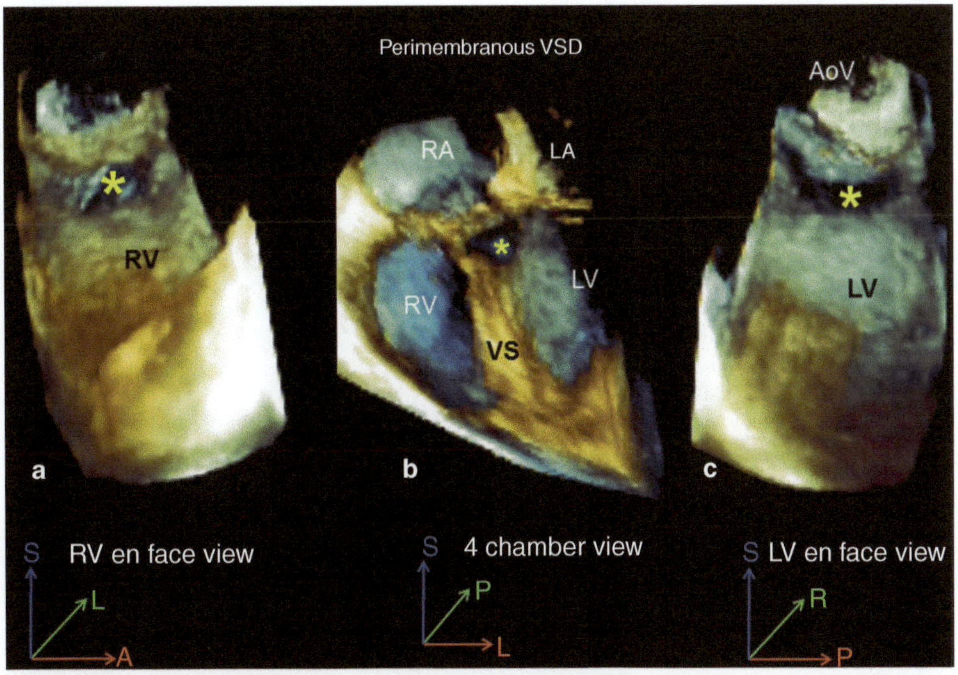

Fig. 20.10 A perimembranous ventricular septal defect (*VSD*; *asterisk*) as seen from a mid esophageal four chamber view using full volume 3D acquisition. (**a**) Right-sided *en face* view. (**b**) Four chamber view with slight rightward probe rotation. (**c**) Left-sided *en face* view. *AoV* aortic valve, *LA* left atrium, *LV* left ventricle, *RA* right atrium, *RV* right ventricle, *VS* ventricular septum

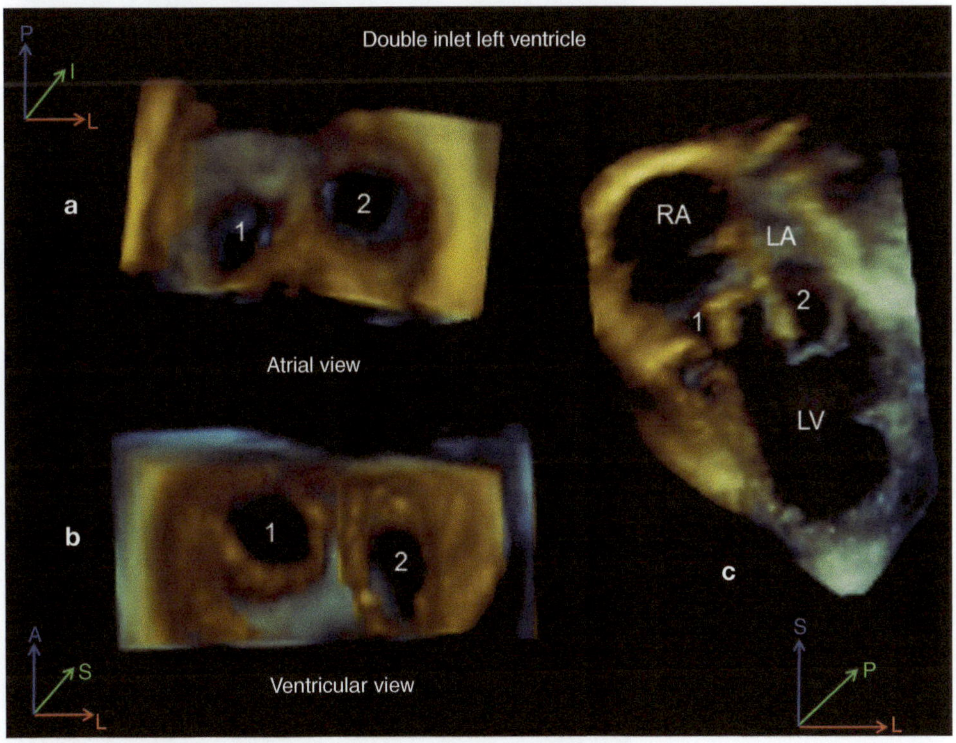

Fig. 20.11 Full volume 3D acquisition from a mid esophageal four chamber view in a patient with double inlet left ventricle. (**a**) View of both atrioventricular valves from the atrium. The right-sided atrioventricular valve is labeled (*1*) and the left-sided valve is labeled (*2*). (**b**) View of both atrioventricular valves from the ventricular aspect. (**c**) The mid esophageal four chamber view is depicted. *LA* left atrium, *LV* left ventricle, *RA* right atrium

well as the ability of 3D TEE to visualize interventional procedure hardware rapidly and in rendered 3D detail, are quite helpful to guide the performance of these procedures. Currently, our interventional cardiology colleagues expect that we perform this analysis on a routine basis during these procedures. The 3D TEE acquisition modalities most useful during these tasks include 3D zoom and live 3D, both of which are live 3D modalities.

Case Examples

Transcatheter Closure of Secundum Atrial Septal Defect

The *en face* views of the atrial septum acquired at the mid esophageal level using the 3D zoom mode are most useful during transcatheter ASD device closure. In a single view the dimensions, location, shape, rims, number of orifices,

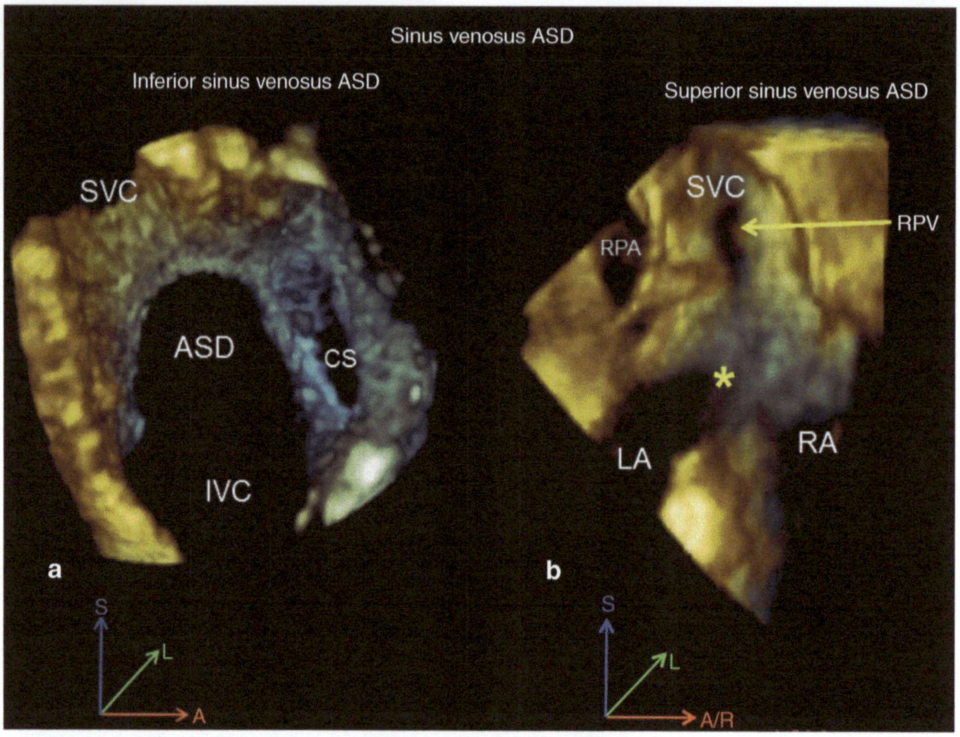

Fig. 20.12 Sinus venosus atrial septal defects. (**a**) A 3D zoom acquisition view of inferior sinus venosus atrial septal defect (*ASD*) is shown. (**b**) 3D full volume acquisition from a modified mid esophageal bicaval view (with probe withdrawal) of a superior sinus venosus ASD with anomalous drainage of the right pulmonary veins (*RPV*) into the superior vena cava (*SVC*). The inter-atrial communication is indicated by the asterisk (*). *CS* coronary sinus, *IVC* inferior vena cava, *LA* left atrium, *RA* right atrium, *RPA* right pulmonary artery

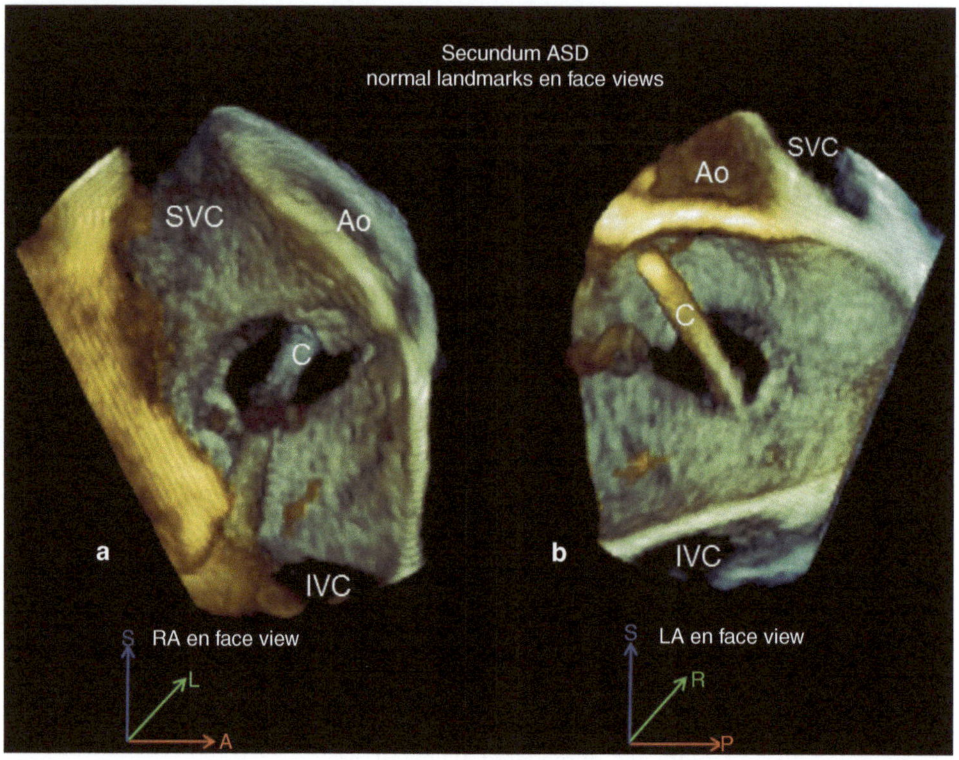

Fig. 20.13 Anatomic landmarks obtained from views in the mid esophagus using 3D zoom mode during secundum atrial septal defect (ASD) device closure. (**a**) Right atrial (*RA*) *en face* view. (**b**) Left atrial (*LA*) *en face* view. A catheter *C* passes through the ASD. *Ao* aorta, *IVC* inferior vena cava, *SVC* superior vena cava

and important surrounding structures are demonstrated. This is illustrated in Fig. 20.13. This view is also very useful to monitor wire, catheter, and device manipulations. The common ASD rim deficiencies that can make device deployment challenging or impossible are presented in Fig. 20.14. Figure 20.14a, b display the usual 3D zoom *en face* views from a right atrial perspective. Figure 20.14c shows another very useful 3D TEE view used during transcatheter ASD device closure. This is a live 3D DTG Sagittal view that provides the best view possible of the inferior rim of the ASD. Multiple orifice secundum ASDs are not rare, therefore a collection of these is presented in

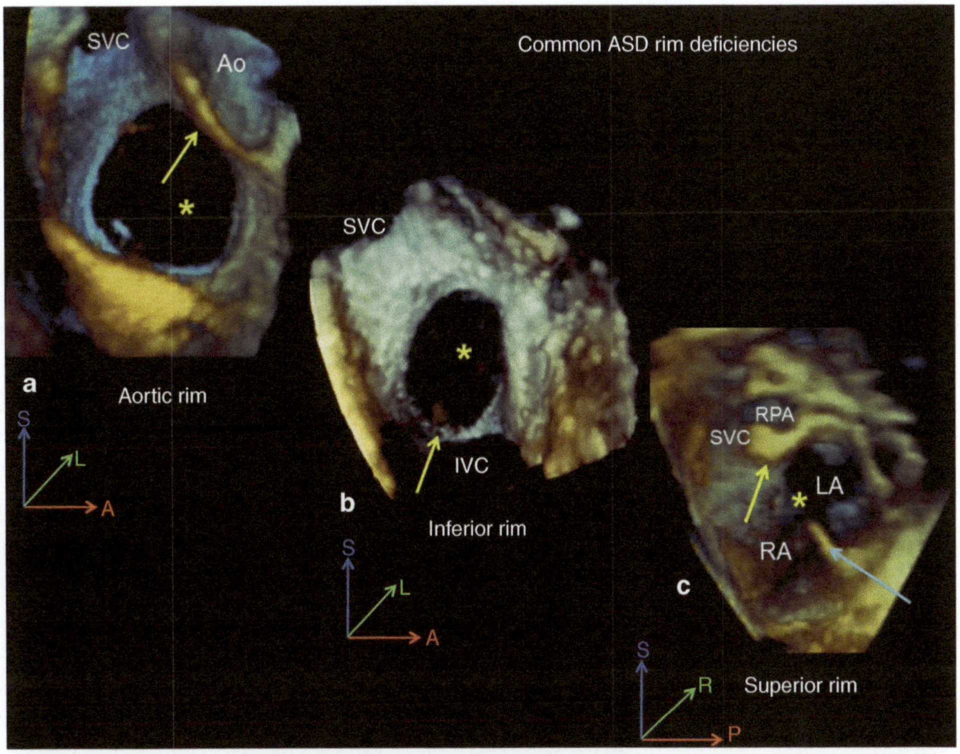

Fig. 20.14 Common secundum atrial septal defect (*ASD*) rim deficiencies are presented. In each figure the deficient rim is indicated by the *yellow arrow* and the ASD is marked by an asterisk (*). (**a**) Aortic rim deficiency as seen from a mid esophageal right atrial (*RA*) *en face* 3D zoom view. (**b**) Inferior rim deficiency as seen from a mid esophageal RA *en face* 3D zoom view. (**c**) Superior rim deficiency as seen from a deep transgastric sagittal live 3D view. The *blue arrow* indicates the inferior rim of the defect, typically optimally seen in this view. *Ao* aorta, *IVC* inferior vena cava, *LA* left atrium, *RPA* right pulmonary artery, *SVC* superior vena cava

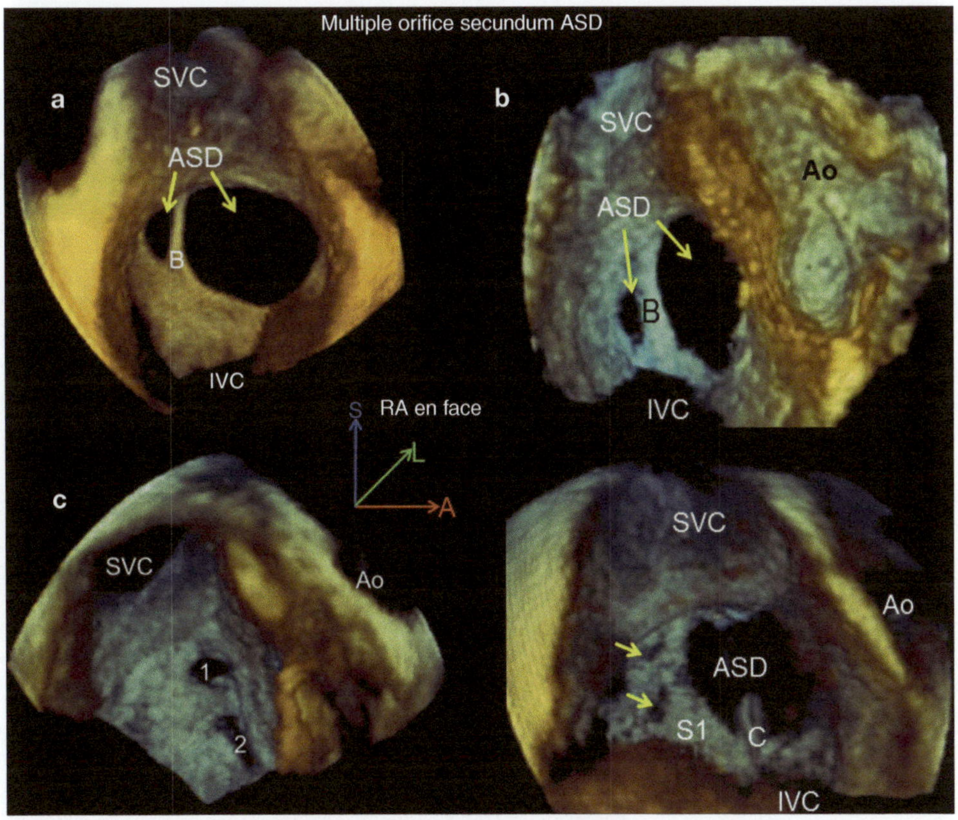

Fig. 20.15 Examples of four patients with multiple orifice secundum atrial septal defect (*ASD*). All images were obtained from the mid esophageal level using 3D zoom mode. (**a**) A thin vertical band (*B*) of septum primum divides the ASD (*arrows*) into two orifices (large anterior and small posterior orifices). (**b**) Similar findings from a different patient. (**c**) Two small defects are demonstrated (identified as *1* and *2*). (**d**) Two small defects (*arrows*) and a larger defect are present. *Ao* aorta, *C* catheter, *IVC* inferior vena cava, *S1* septum primum, *SVC* superior vena cava

Fig. 20.15 and Video 20.8. Lastly, views of the two most commonly used contemporary ASD closure devices are presented in Fig. 20.16, namely the Amplatzer (Video 20.9) and Helex devices.

Transcatheter Closure of Muscular Septal Defect

The use of 3D TEE during device closure of muscular VSDs is illustrated in Figs. 20.17 and 20.18, Video 20.10. All images in the two figures are obtained from ME 4 Ch full volume

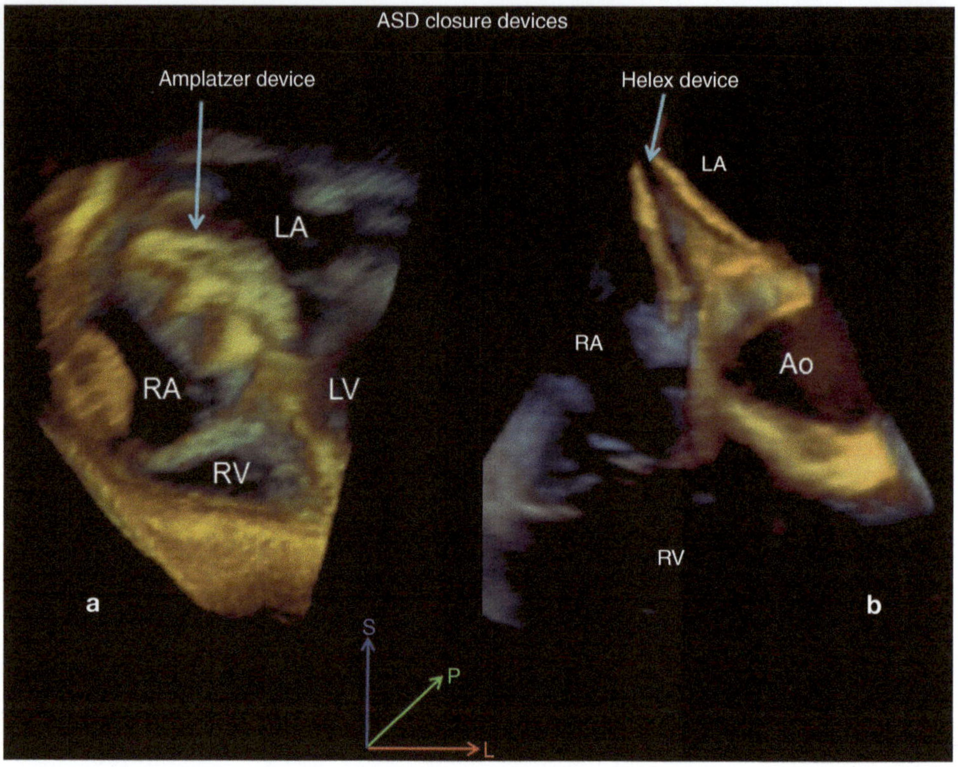

Fig. 20.16 Four chamber views of the most commonly used transcatheter atrial septal defect (ASD) closure devices. These appear to be in good position. (**a**) Amplatzer device as seen from a modified deep transgastric view using live 3D. (**b**) Full volume 3D acquisition of a Helex device as seen from a mid esophageal four chamber view with transducer anteflexion. *Ao* aorta, *LA* left atrium, *LV* left ventricle, *RA* right atrium, *RV* right ventricle

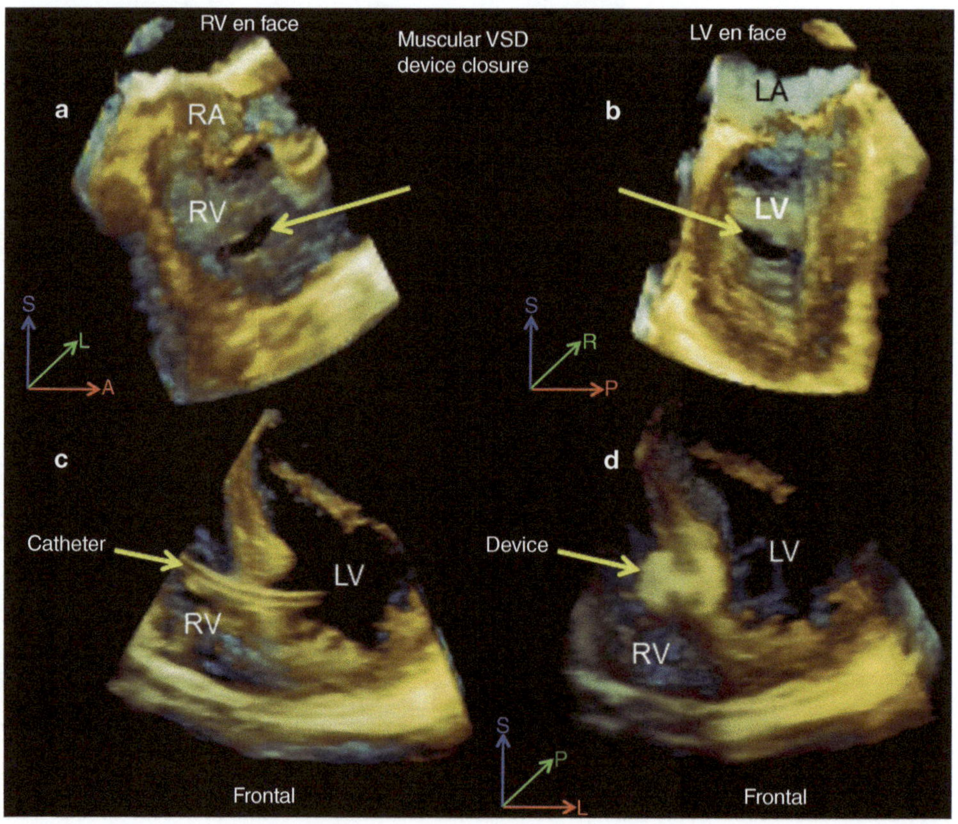

Fig. 20.17 Full volume 3D acquisitions showing a muscular ventricular septal defect (VSD) before and after transcatheter device closure. The images were obtained from the mid esophageal four chamber view. (**a**) Right *en face* view of the VSD (shown by *arrow*). (**b**) Left *en face* view of the VSD (*arrow*). (**c**) The delivery catheter is through the VSD. (**d**) The closure device is in place. *LA* left atrium, *LV* left ventricle, *RA* right atrium, *RV* right ventricle

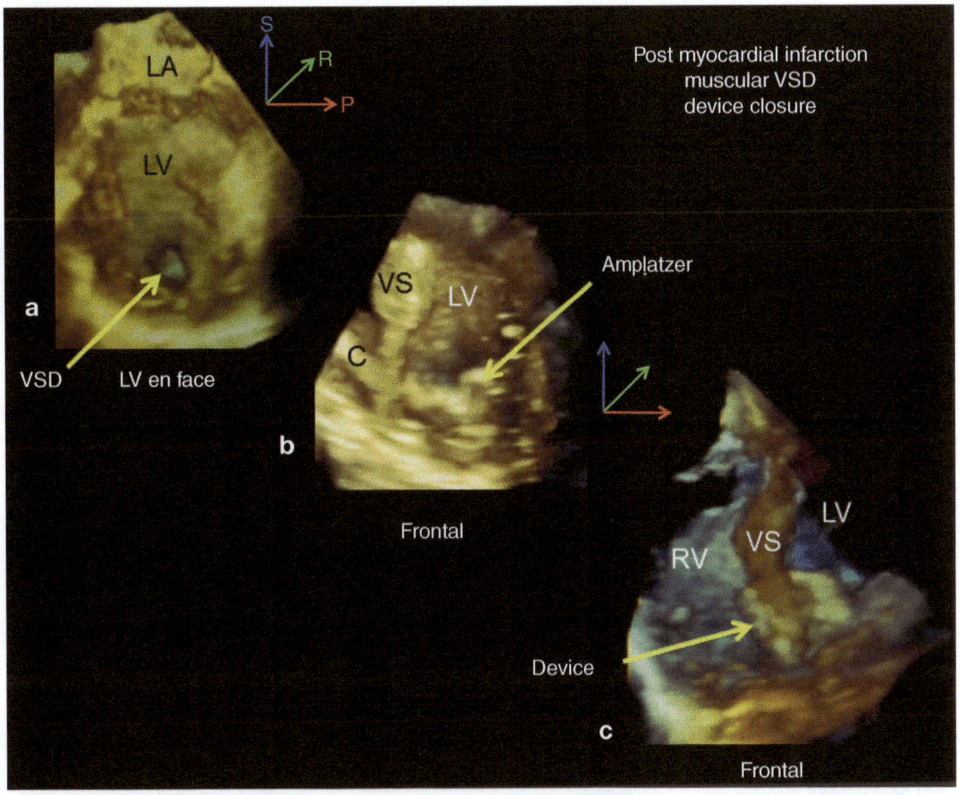

Fig. 20.18 Live 3D views of a ventricular septal defect (*VSD*) caused by a myocardial infarction, located in the apical muscular ventricular septum. Images were obtained from the mid esophageal four chamber view during device closure. (**a**) Left sided *en face* view of the VSD (*arrow*). (**b**) Left side of the device deployed in the left ventricle. The delivery catheter is labeled (*C*). (**c**) The device is in good position. *LA* left atrium, *LV* left ventricle, *RV* right ventricle, *VS* ventricular septum

acquisitions with side cropping to show *en face* views or frontal cropping to demonstrate the VSD and the device. Figure 20.17 is from a patient with a congenital VSD and Fig. 20.18 is from a case with post-myocardial infarction VSD.

Assessment of the Surgical Intervention

The outstanding advances accomplished over the years have resulted in survival into adulthood for most children with CHD. The plethora of surgical procedures and their myriad variations available today can sometimes be challenging to the echocardiographer. As is the case of the preoperative assessment, postoperative 3D TEE provides unique detailed views as well as information complementary to 2D echocardiographic findings that are clinically useful as well as educational. A representative collection of such images is presented in this section.

Case Examples

Surgery for Left-Sided Obstructive Lesions

Representative 3D images of several different surgical procedures applied in the management of left-sided obstructive lesions are presented in Figs. 20.19, 20.20, and 20.21. In Fig. 20.19 and Video 20.11, dehiscence of aortic valve leaflet augmentation material is demonstrated in a mid esophageal aortic valve long axis (ME AV LAX) full volume 3D view with frontal cropping. A Konno procedure with bioprosthetic valve is shown using live 3D mode acquisitions from the ME AV LAX (Fig. 20.20a, Video 20.12) and ME AV SAX (Fig. 20.20b, Video 20.13) views. Figure 20.21 is a DTG Sagittal live 3D view of a Damus-Kaye-Stansel procedure.

Surgery for Atrioventricular Valves

En face views of the AV valves are most often obtained using 3D zoom mode. The valves may be viewed from either the atrial or ventricular aspect. Despite the slow volume rate of this modality, fine anatomic details can be demonstrated. The newly developed high volume rate (HVR) software adjustment mitigates the slow volume rate to a significant degree. Fig. 20.22 displays dehiscence of a tricuspid valve ring repair in a patient with Ebstein anomaly. Subsequent successfully repair is shown in Fig. 20.23.

Right Ventricular to Pulmonary Artery Conduit

The right ventricular to pulmonary artery conduit in a Rastelli operation is sometimes difficult to image clearly by TEE due to its anterior and superior position relative to the esophagus. In Fig. 20.24, live 3D anatomic and live 3D color flow Doppler mapping views of a Rastelli conduit are demonstrated.

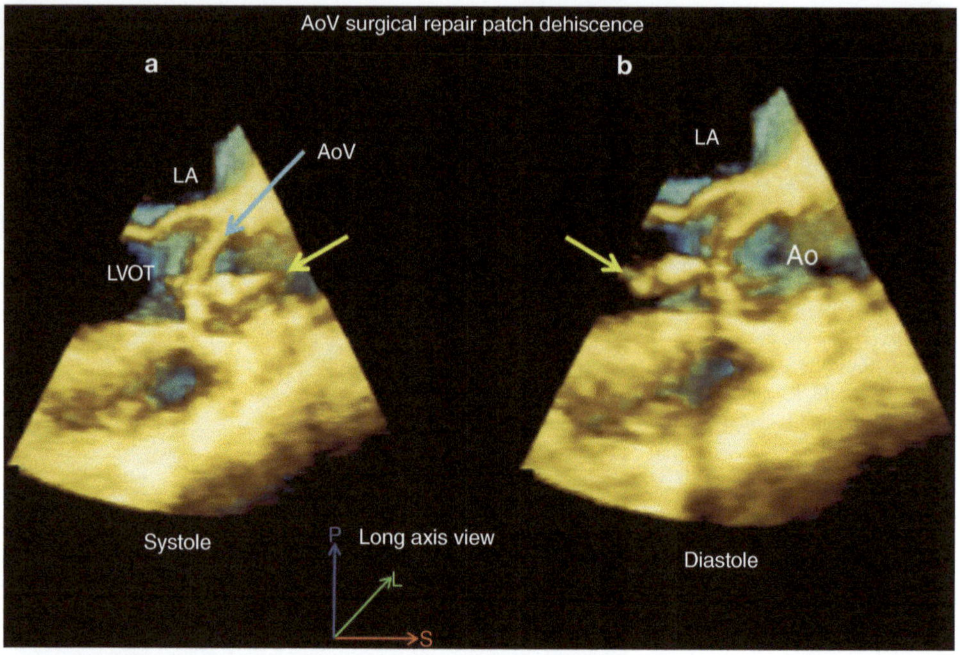

Fig. 20.19 Live 3D acquisition in mid esophageal aortic valve long axis view displaying dehiscence of a bicuspid aortic valve leaflet augmentation repair in a patient with endocarditis. (**a**) The leaflet augmentation flap of Goretex (*yellow arrow*) is within the aorta during systole. The aortic valve is noted by a *blue arrow*. (**b**) The flap is within the left ventricle during diastole. *Ao* aorta, *AoV* aortic valve, *LA* left atrium, *LVOT* left ventricular outflow tract

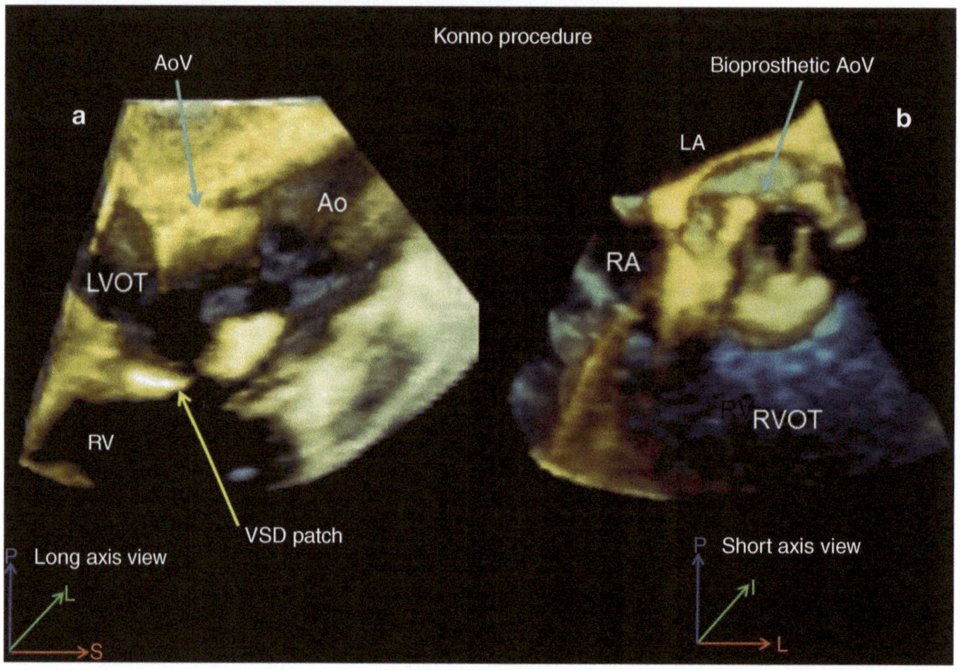

Fig. 20.20 Mid esophageal aortic valve long axis (**a**) and short axis (**b**) full volume 3D acquisitions of a Konno procedure are displayed. The ventricular septal defect (*VSD*) patch and bioprosthetic aortic valve are demonstrated. *Ao* aorta, *AoV* aortic valve, *LVOT* left ventricular outflow tract, *RA* right atrium, *RV* right ventricle, *RVOT* right ventricular outflow tract

Atrial Switch Procedures

The atrial switch procedures (Mustard and Senning), formerly first line surgical therapies for *D*-transposition of the great arteries, are compatible with long term survival, albeit a number of complications can occur over time including baffle obstruction, baffle leak, and arrhythmias. Because of these issues, follow up interventions are often required. The use of 3D TEE guidance is frequently very useful to visualize the complex systemic and pulmonary venous baffles. A collection of the most useful mid esophageal full volume 3D long and short axis views, X-plane long and short axis views, and live 3D DTG sagittal views in this setting are presented in Figs. 20.25, 20.26, 20.27, and 20.28, Videos 20.14 and 20.15.

Imaging Related to Electrophysiologic Issues

Successful treatment of the majority of patients with CHD, and their resultant prolonged survival, has resulted in a sizeable population of individuals who develop arrhythmias that might require cardioversion, a cardiac defibrillator, and/or pacemaker implantation. Illustrative cases in which 3D TEE can be utilized are presented in this section.

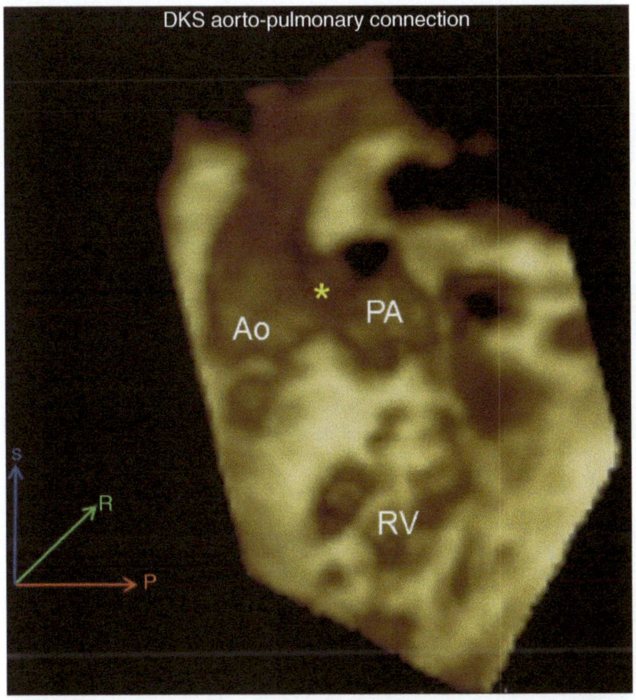

Fig. 20.21 Demonstration of the Damus-Kaye-Stansel (*DKS*) procedure (*asterisk*) performed in a patient with univentricular heart, subaortic stenosis and *D*-malposed aorta. This is a deep transgastric sagittal live 3D acquisition. *Ao* aorta, *PA* pulmonary artery, *RV* right ventricle

Case Examples

Atrial Flutter

The ever expanding and aging population of patients surviving with CHD has resulted in the increasing incidence of atrial flutter. Prior to cardioversion in these patients, it is important to exclude the presence of an intracardiac thrombus, particularly, within the left atrial appendage (Fig. 20.29). This is best imaged using X-plane and live 3D modes. Similarly, patients who have undergone the Fontan procedure are prone to thrombus formation within the Fontan pathway, particularly those with a classic atriopulmonary connection (see Chap. 10) and/or if arrhythmias develop. Most often, X-plane (Fig. 20.30) and live 3D (Fig. 20.31, Video 20.16 and 20.17) are the best modalities to search for thrombi within the Fontan pathway.

Implantable Cardioverter-Defibrillator

Implantable defibrillator devices have proven to be successful treatment for the prevention of sudden death in patients with hypertrophic cardiomyopathy. However the device leads are somewhat stiff, the hearts hyperdynamic, and patients with these implanted devices are often physically active. Therefore lead problems such as fracture and rarely perforation can occur (Fig. 20.32, Video 20.18). Live 3D mode is often very useful to analyze the position of intracardiac hardware and assess the size of a pericardial effusion.

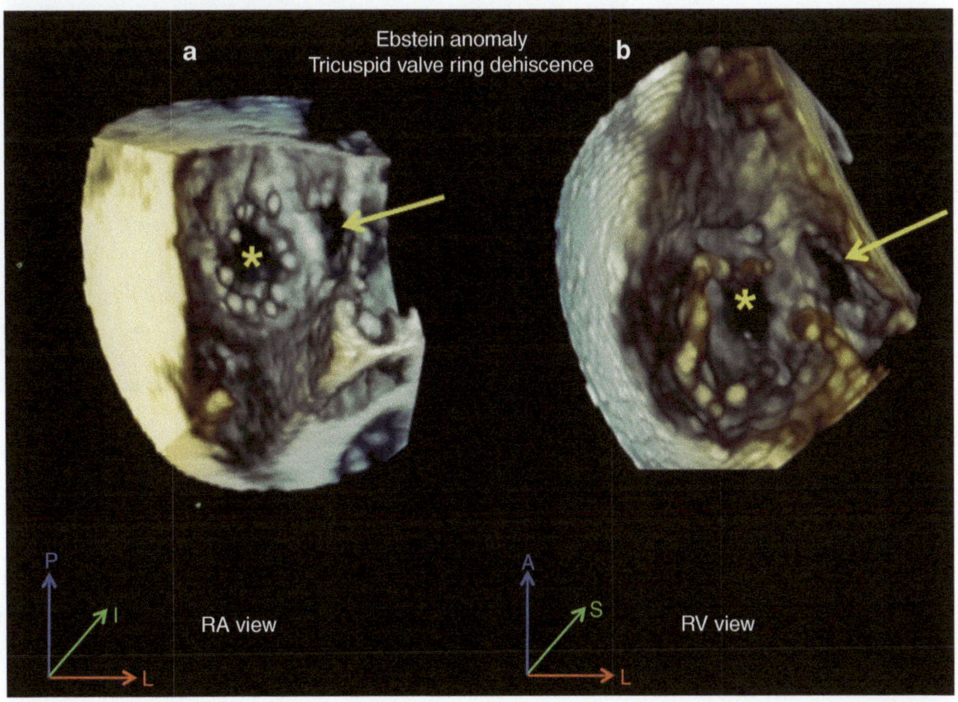

Fig. 20.22 3D zoom mode views of a tricuspid valve ring dehiscence (*arrow*) after repair of Ebstein anomaly as viewed from the right atrium (*RA*, **a**) and the right ventricle (*RV*, **b**). The tricuspid valve orifice is marked with an *asterisk* (*)

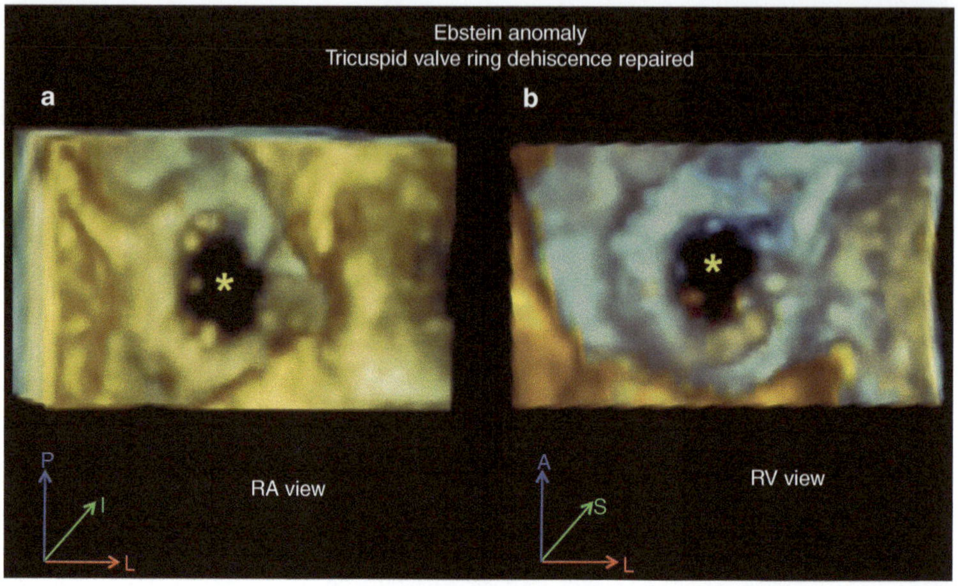

Fig. 20.23 3D zoom mode views from the same patient as shown in Fig. 20.22, following repair of the tricuspid valve ring dehiscence as viewed from the right atrium (*RA*, **a**) and the right ventricle (*RV*, **b**). The tricuspid valve orifice is marked with an *asterisk* (*)

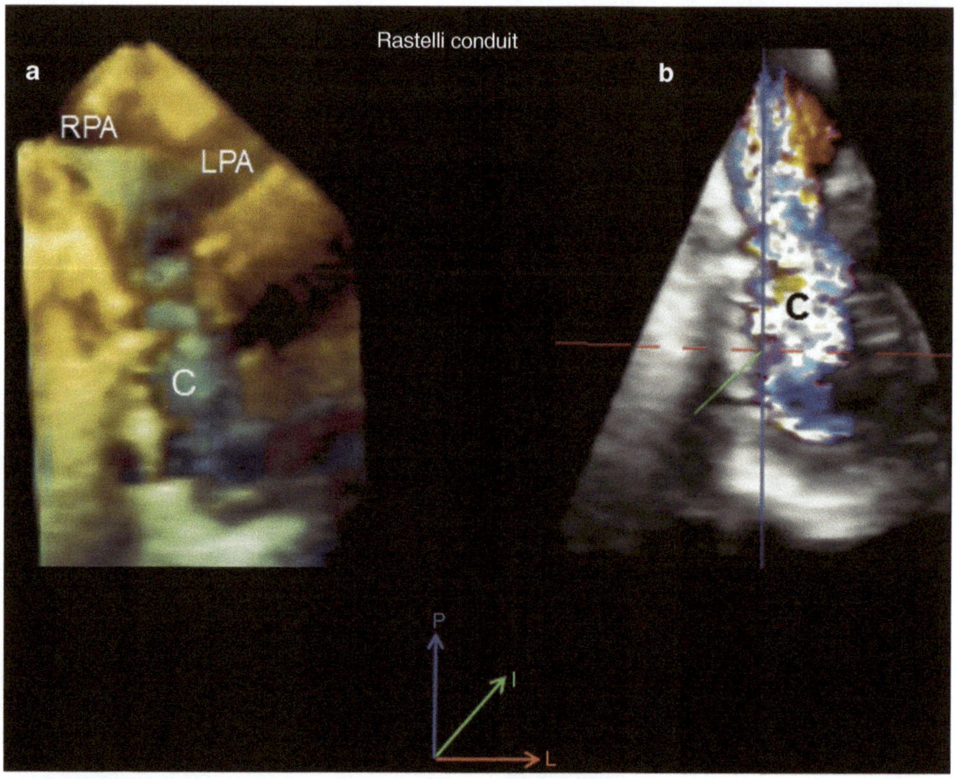

Fig. 20.24 Live 3D anatomic (**a**) and color Doppler flow mapping (**b**) views of a right ventricular to pulmonary artery conduit in a Rastelli operation imaged from the upper esophageal level. *C* conduit, *LPA* left pulmonary artery, *RPA* right pulmonary artery

Resynchronization Therapy

In patients with ventricular systolic dysfunction and dyssynchrony, the use of multi-lead ventricular pacing may result in improved function and synchrony [28–30]. Using 3D TEE quantitative function and synchrony software, the measurement of ejection fraction, synchrony index, and determination of the site of most delayed contraction can be performed during the procedure in order to appropriately place the ventricular leads. This information can be used to optimize lead placement and the adjustment of V-V intervals in order to enhance ventricular performance as illustrated in Fig. 20.33.

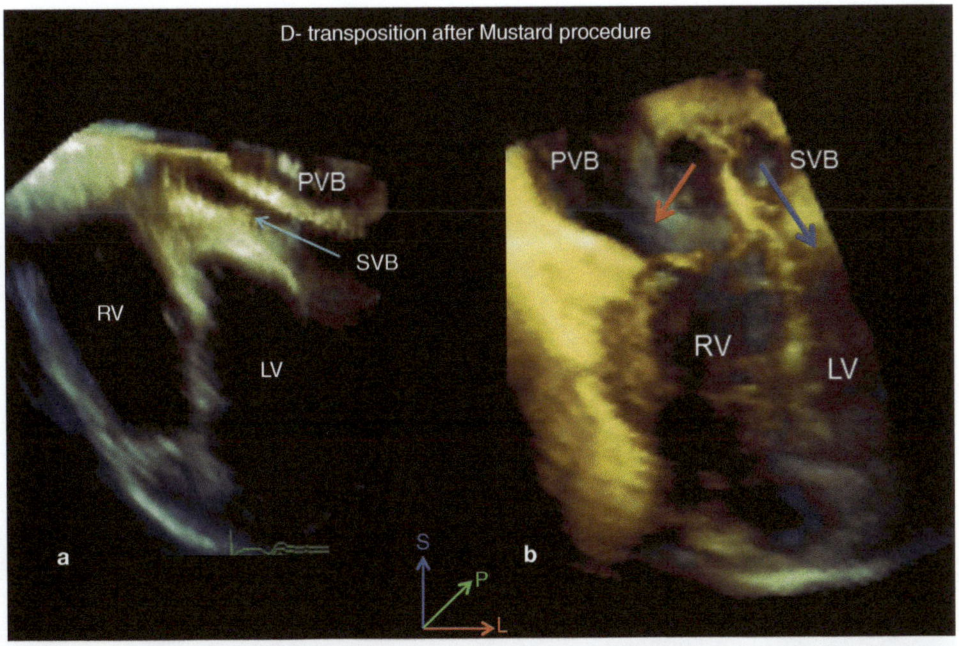

Fig. 20.25 Mid esophageal four chamber views acquired using full volume 3D in patients with *D*-transposition of the great arteries, after a Mustard procedure. (**a**) There is narrowing within the systemic venous baffle in this case (*SVB*). (**b**) In an image from a different patient the systemic venous baffle and the pulmonary venous baffle (*PVB*) appear unobstructed. *LV* left ventricle, *RV* right ventricle

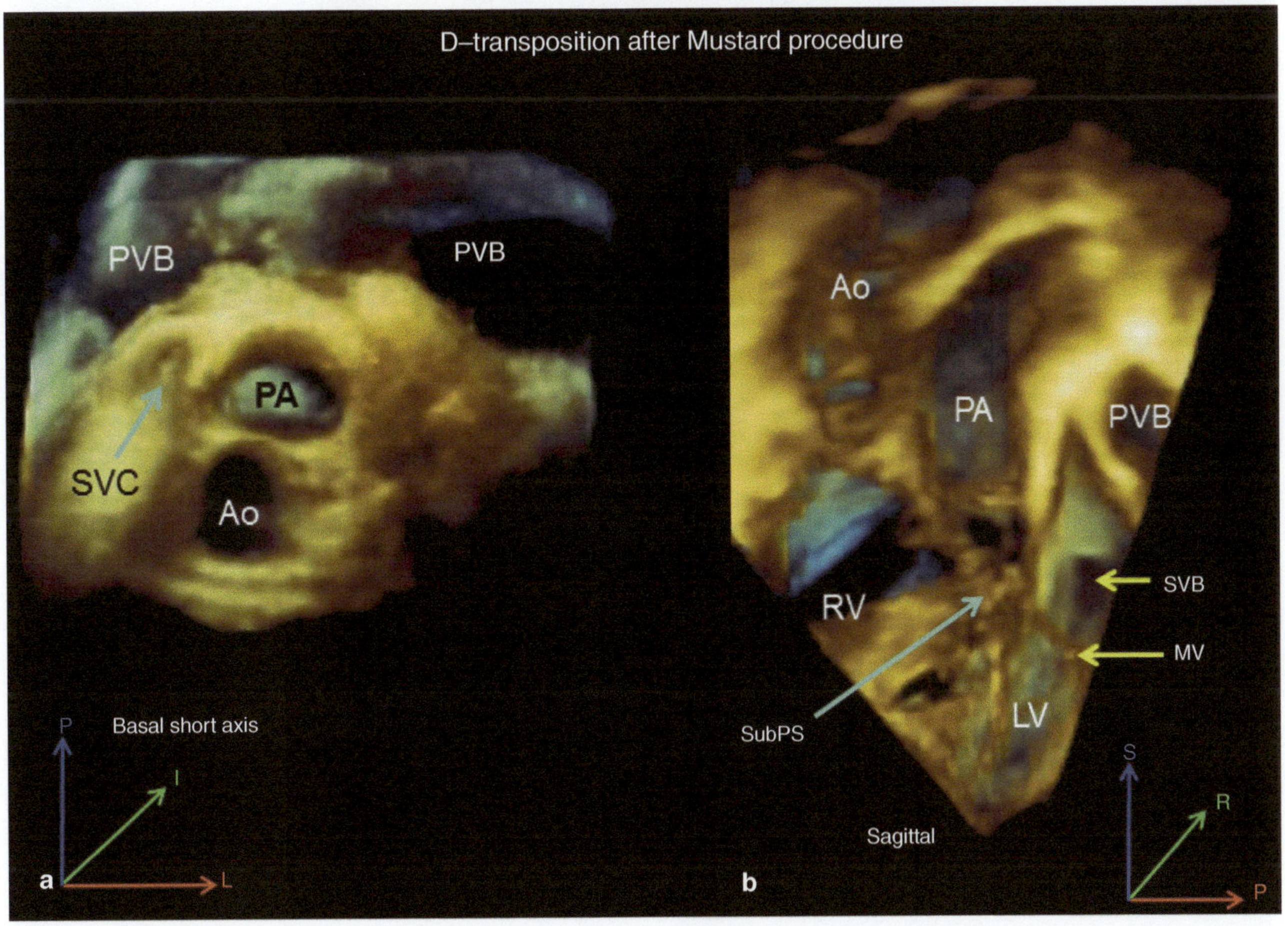

Fig. 20.26 Images from a patient with *D*–transposition of the great arteries after Mustard procedure. (**a**) Mid esophageal aortic valve short axis equivalent view with full volume 3D acquisition showing narrowing of the superior vena cava (*SVC*) limb of the systemic venous baffle. The aorta (*Ao*) is positioned anterior and rightward with respect to the pulmonary artery (*PA*). The pulmonary venous baffle (*PVB*) is located posteriorly and is unobstructed. (**b**) Deep transgastric sagittal view live 3D acquisition demonstrating stenosis in the left ventricular outflow tract beneath the pulmonary valve (subPS). *LV* left ventricle, *MV* mitral valve, *RV* right ventricle, *SVB* systemic venous baffle

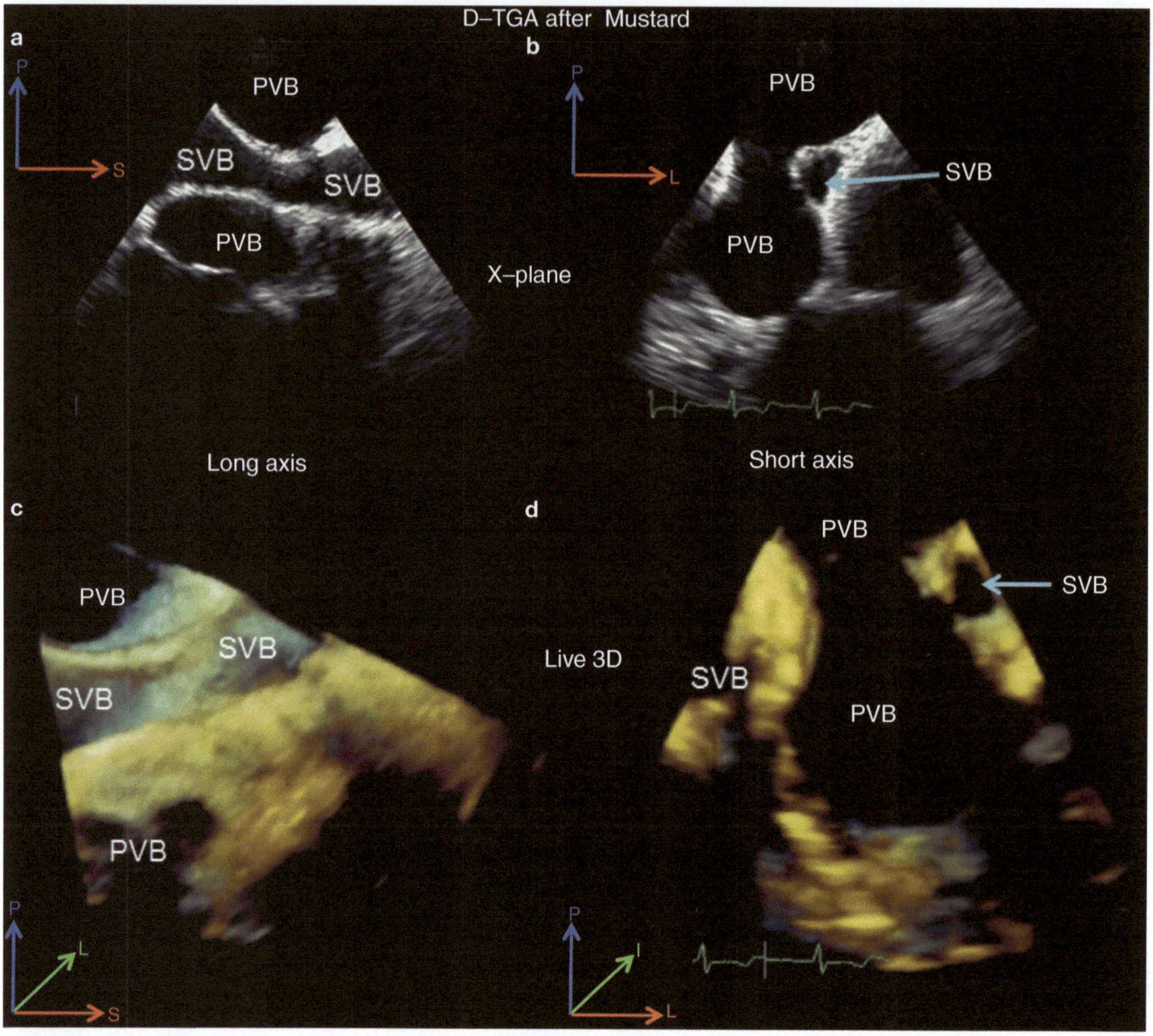

Fig. 20.27 Mid esophageal long and short axis views of the systemic venous baffle (*SVB*) and pulmonary venous baffle (*PVB*) in *D*-transposition of the great arteries (*D*-TGA) after a Mustard procedure. (**a**) Long axis X-plane view of the Mustard baffles. (**b**) Short axis X-plane view of the Mustard baffles. (**c**) Live 3D long axis view of the Mustard baffles. (**d**) Live 3D short axis view of the Mustard baffles

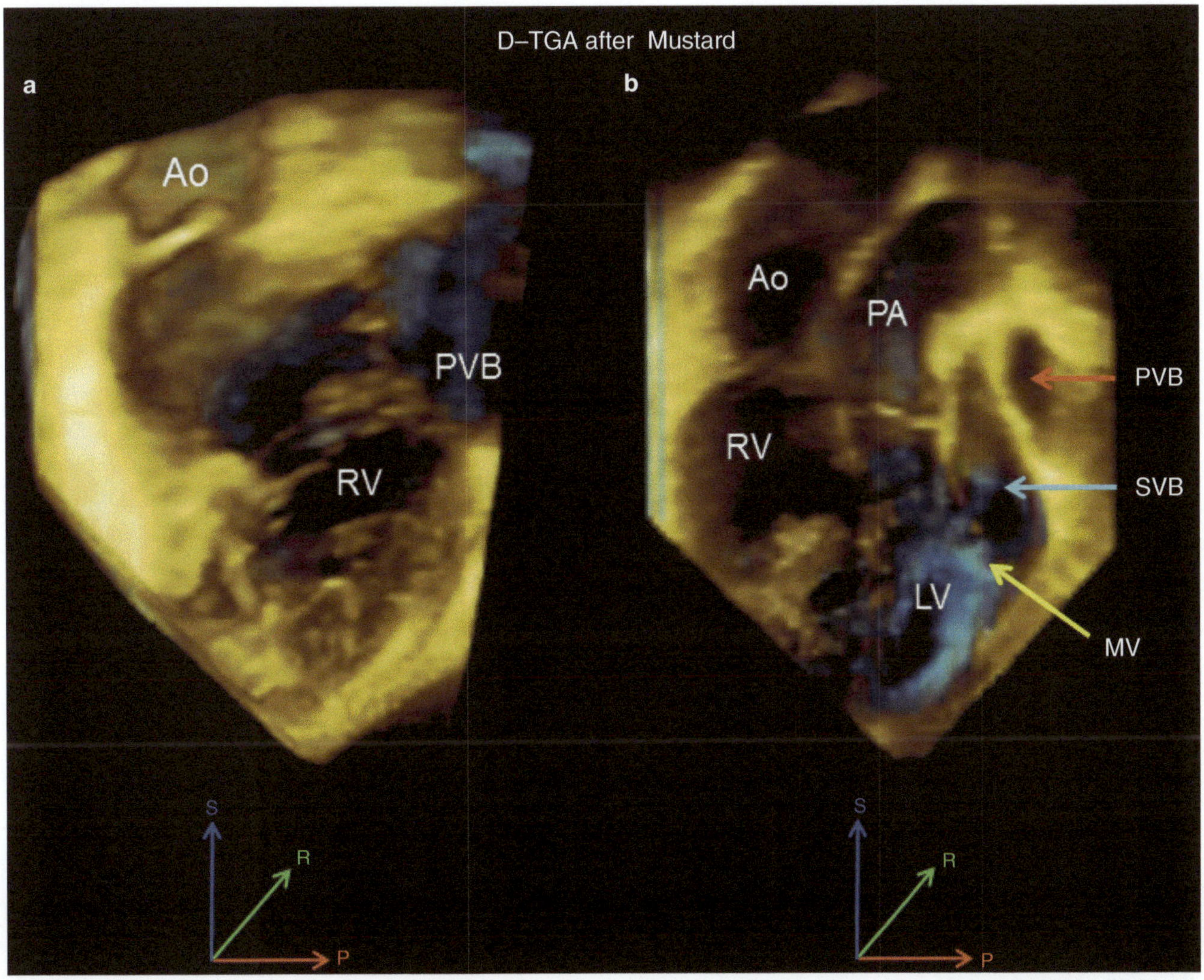

Fig. 20.28 Live 3D acquisition deep transgastric views of *D*-transposition of the great arteries (*D*-TGA) after the Mustard procedure. (**a**) The pulmonary venous baffle (*PVB*) connects to the right ventricle (*RV*) in unobstructed fashion. The right ventricle is enlarged and connects to the anterior positioned aorta (*Ao*). (**b**) The systemic venous baffle (*SVB*) connects to the left ventricle (*LV*) through the mitral valve (*MV*). The left ventricle connects to the pulmonary artery (*PA*), positioned posterior to the aorta. The most posterior structure seen in this figure corresponds to a portion of the pulmonary venous baffle

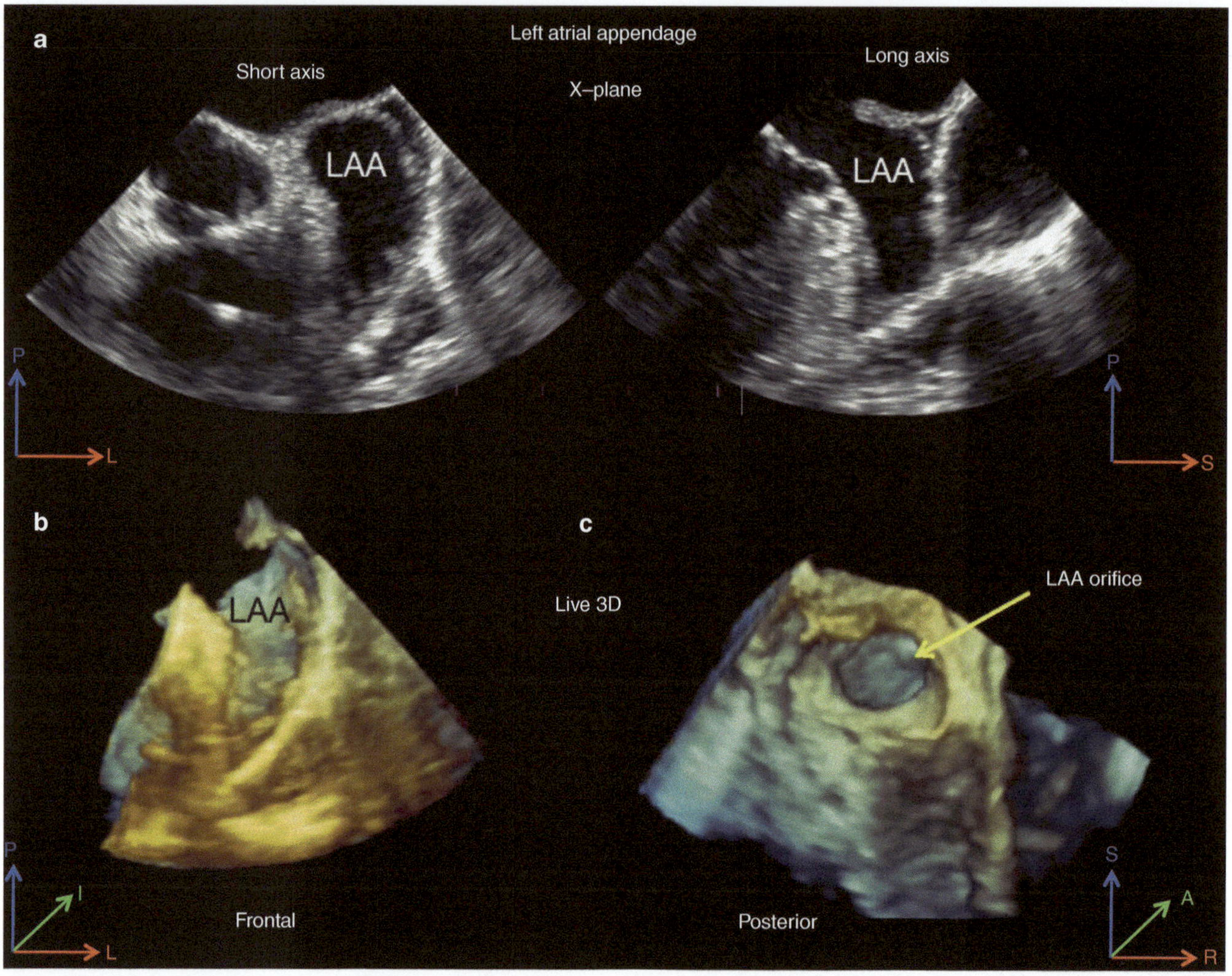

Fig. 20.29 Views of the left atrial appendage (*LAA*) obtained in a patient with atrial flutter prior to cardioversion. (**a**) Case example of simultaneous biplane 2D imaging referred to as X-plane echocardiography, showing a mid esophageal short and long axis views depicting a normal LAA that is free of thrombus. (**b**) Live 3D frontal view of the same normal LAA. (**c**) The orifice of the appendage is demonstrated using live 3D

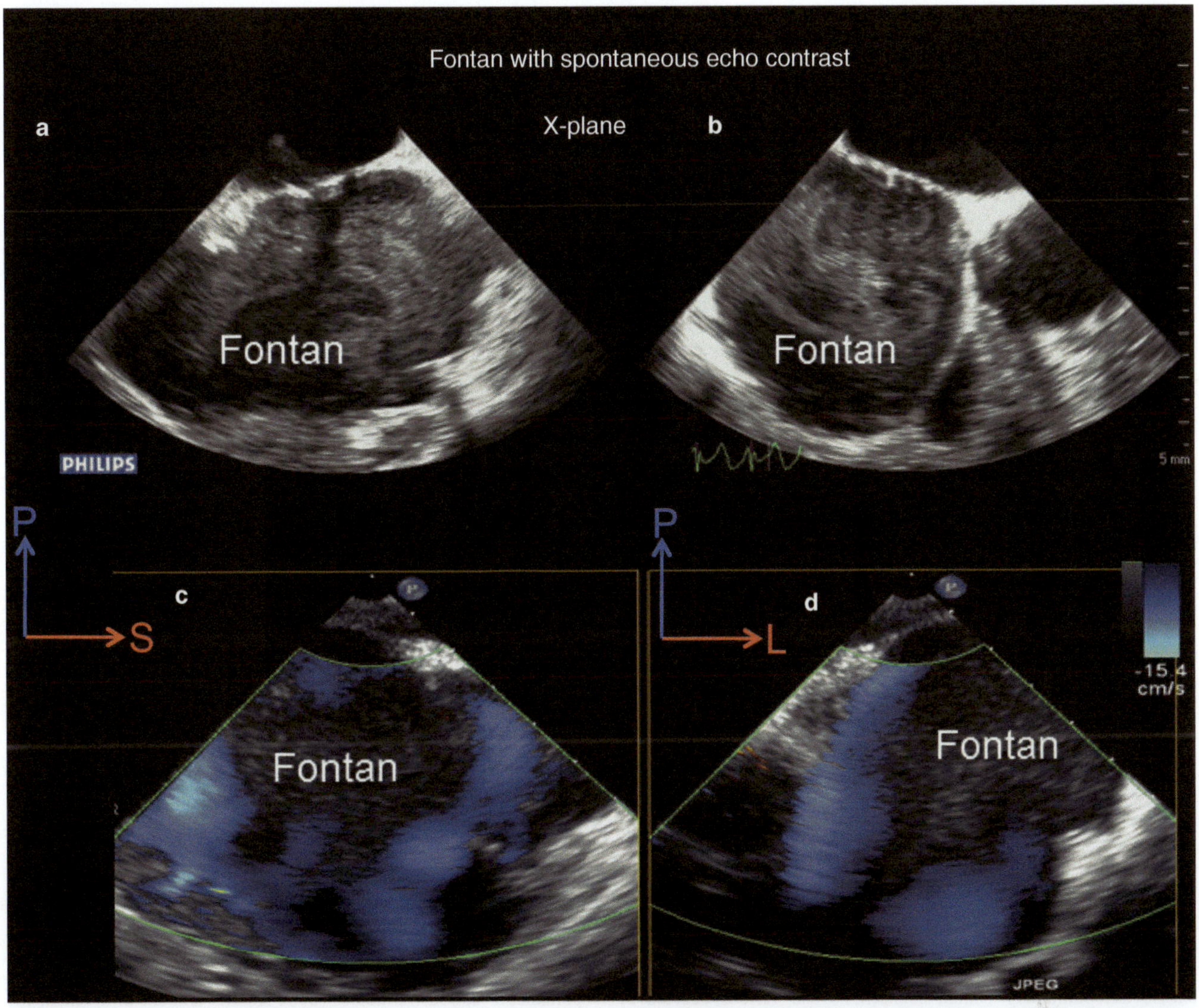

Fig. 20.30 Simultaneous biplane echocardiograms (X-plane imaging) of a classic Fontan connection with very slow flow velocity apparent as spontaneous echocardiographic contrast. In the *top row* is the simultaneous biplane 2D echo depiction with a mid esophageal bicaval view (**a**) and mid esophageal aortic valve short axis view (**b**) focusing on this region. In the *bottom row* the corresponding color Doppler flow mapping bicaval (**c**) and short axis views (**d**) are demonstrated

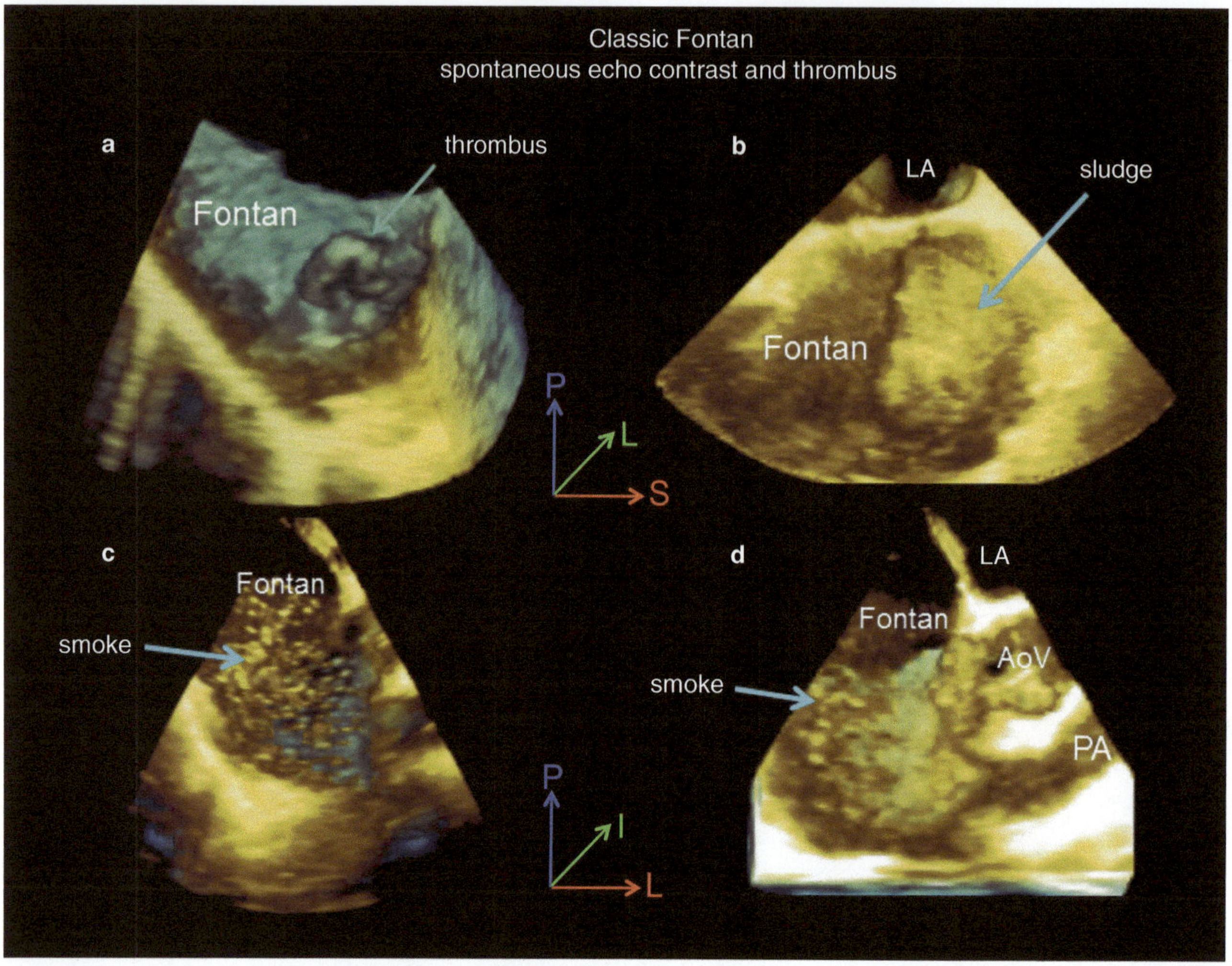

Fig. 20.31 Figure depicts images from four different patients with classic atriopulmonary Fontan connections and various degrees of spontaneous echocardiographic contrast, sludge, and a thrombus as seen is various views. (**a**) An organized thrombus is present. (**b**) There is very dense spontaneous contrast (sludge). (**c**) A moderate amount of spontaneous contrast is noted. (**d**) A smaller amount of spontaneous contrast (smoke) is seen. *AoV* aortic valve, *LA* left atrium, *PA* pulmonary artery

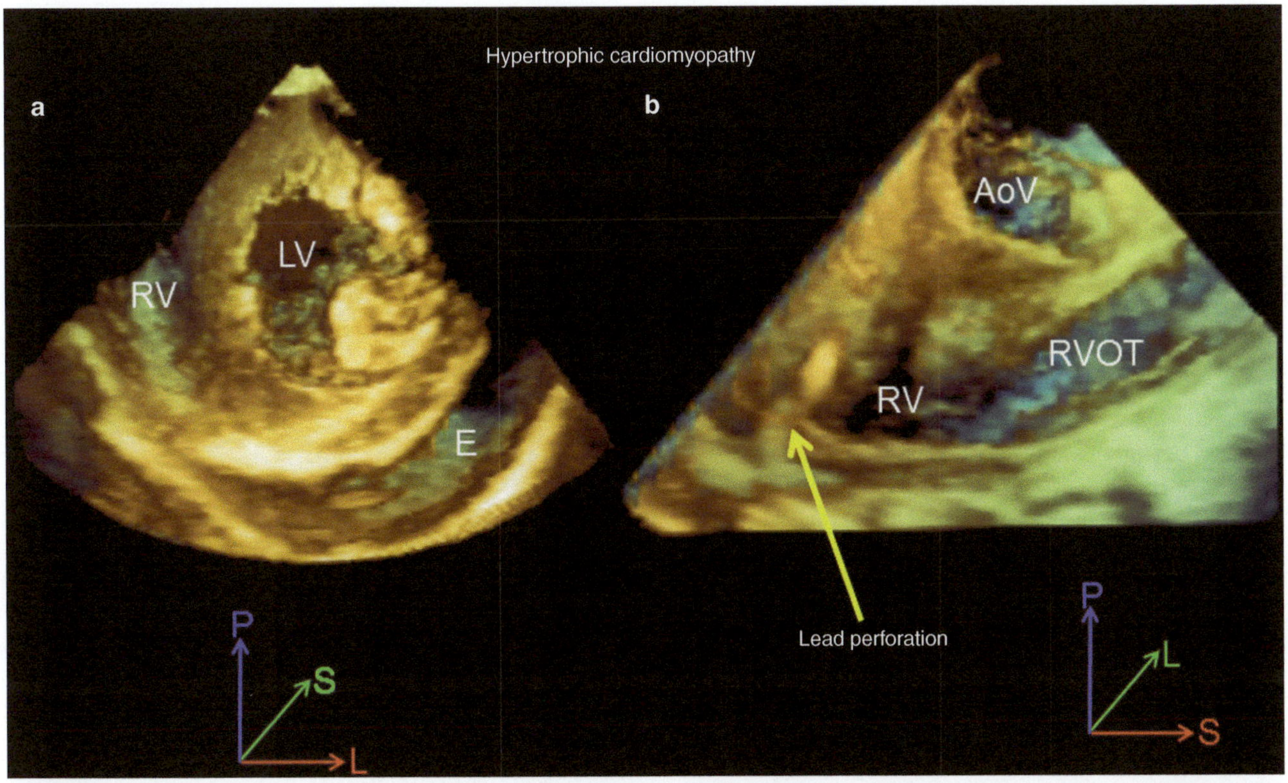

Fig. 20.32 Hypertrophic cardiomyopathy with defibrillator lead perforation of the right ventricle (*RV*) and pericardial effusion. (**a**) Transgastric mid left ventricular short axis live 3D view demonstrating the hypertrophied left ventricle (*LV*) and a pericardial effusion (*E*). (**b**) Mid esophageal right ventricular inflow-outflow view with live 3D acquisition demonstrating the defibrillator lead perforating (*arrow*) the RV anterior wall near the apex. *AoV* aortic valve, *RVOT* right ventricular outflow tract

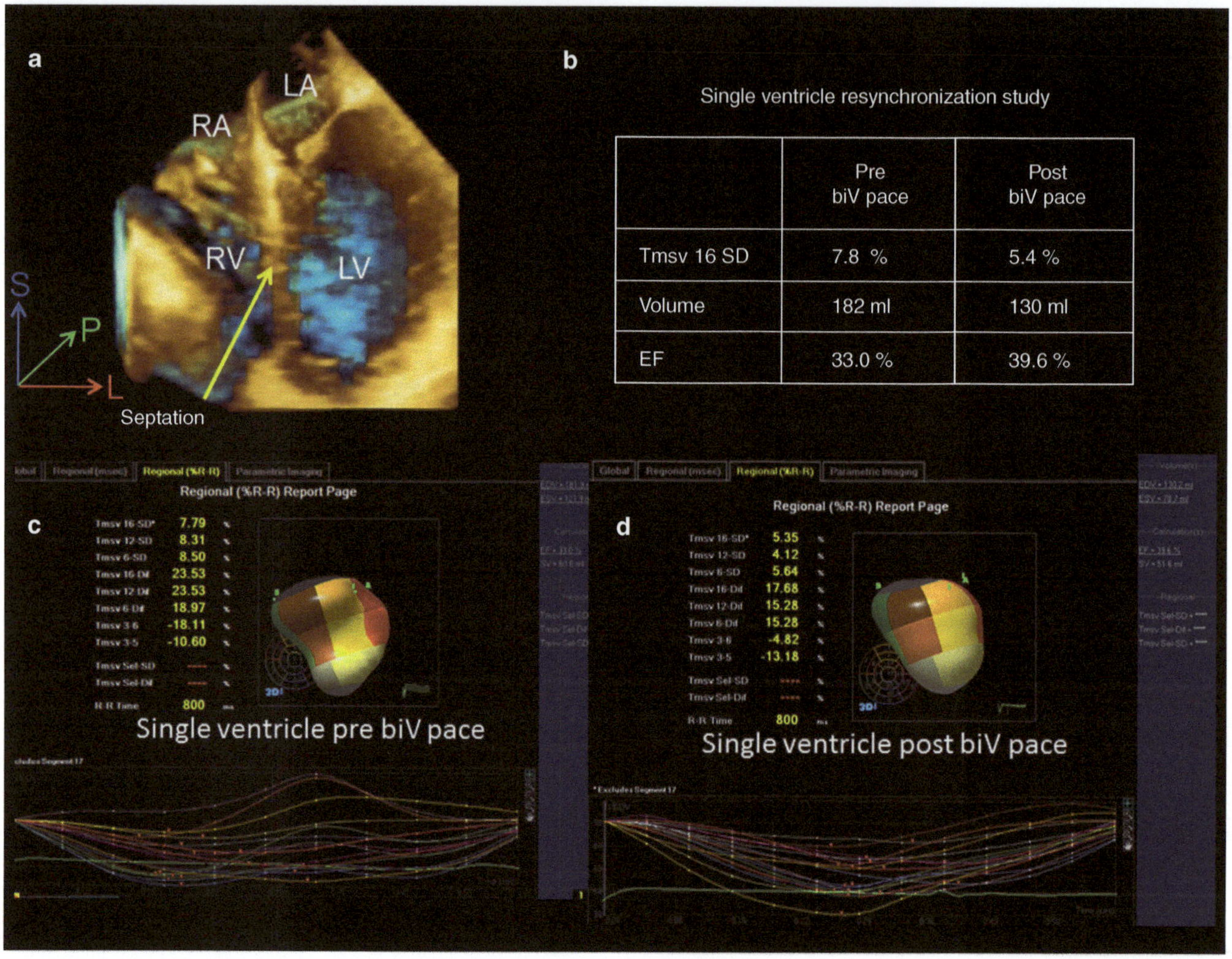

Fig. 20.33 Patient with double inlet left ventricle after septation procedure and bidirectional Glenn undergoing resynchronization therapy with multi-lead pacing (biV pace) to improve ventricular systolic function. Quantitative data was obtained using commercially available software able to measure 3D derived ejection fraction (*EF*) and dyssynchrony index (Tmsv 16 SD) before and after pacing with two ventricular leads (biV-pace). (**a**) The mid esophageal four chamber full volume view is seen. (**b**) The quantitative 3D data for left ventricular systolic function and synchrony are presented. (**c**) Dyssynchronous regional time volume curves are seen prior to biV pacing. (**d**) Improved but still mildly abnormal regional time volume curves are depicted post biV pacing. *LA* left atrium, *LV* left ventricle, *ml* milliliters, *RA* right atrium, *RV* right ventricle

Summary

It is clear from these illustrative cases that 3D TEE in its current form has important and very useful clinical applications. Unique cross sections, as well as complementary views, can be obtained that enhance the assessment of anatomy, assist interventional device placement, and facilitate surgical interventions and electrophysiologic procedures. With practice, these images can be obtained rapidly, consistently, and reproducibly. Further revisions of 3D TEE hardware and software will likely continue to improve the ease of application and image quality of 3D TEE for the evaluation of CHD and related issues.

References

1. Lang RM, Badano LP, Tsang W, et al. EAE/ASE recommendations for image acquisition and display using three-dimensional echocardiography. J Am Soc Echocardiogr. 2012;25:3–46.
2. Lang RM, Tsang W, Weinert L, et al. Valvular heart disease. The value of 3-dimensional echocardiongraphy. J Am Coll Cardiol. 2011;58:1933–44.
3. Perk G, Lang RM, Garcia-Fernandez MA, et al. Use of real time three-dimensional transesophageal echocardiography in intracardiac catheter based interventions. J Am Soc Echocardiogr. 2009; 22:865–82.
4. Sugeng L, Shernan SK, Weinert L, et al. Real-time three-dimensional transesophageal echocardiography in valve disease: comparison with surgical findings and evaluation of prosthetic valves. J Am Soc Echocardiogr. 2008;21:1347–54.

5. Swaans MJ, Van den Branden BJL, Van der Heyden JAS, et al. Three-dimensional transoesophageal echocardiography in a patient undergoing percutaneous mitral valve repair using the edge-to-edge clip technique. Eur J Echocardiogr. 2009;10:982–3.
6. Mackensen GB, Swaminathan M, Mathew JP. PRO Three-dimensional transesophageal echocardiography is a major advance for intraoperative clinical management of patients undergoing cardiac surgery. Anesth Analg. 2010;110:1574–8.
7. Vegas A, Meineri M. Core review: three-dimensional transesophageal echocardiography is a major advance for intraoperative clinical management of patients undergoing cardiac surgery: a core review. Anesth Analg. 2010;110:1548–73.
8. Gripari P, Tamborini G, Barbier P, et al. Real-time three-dimensional transoesophageal echocardiography: a new intraoperative feasible and useful technology in cardiac surgery. Int J Cardiovasc Imaging. 2010;26:651–60.
9. Lang RM, Mor-Avi V, Sugeng L, et al. Three-dimensional echocardiography: the benefits of the additional dimension. J Am Coll Cardiol. 2006;48:2053–69.
10. Tsang W, Bateman MG, Weinert L, et al. Accuracy of aortic annular measurements obtained from three-dimensional echocardiography, CT and MRI: human in vitro and in vivo studies. Heart. 2012;98:1146–52.
11. Tsang W, Lang RM, Kronzon I. Role of real-time three dimensional echocardiography in cardiovascular interventions. Heart. 2011;97:850–7.
12. Lee AP, Lam YY, Yip GW, et al. Role of real time three-dimensional transesophageal echocardiography in guidance of interventional procedures in cardiology. Heart. 2010;96:1485.
13. Roberson DA, Cui W, Patel D, et al. Three-dimensional transesophageal echocardiography of atrial septal defect: a qualitative and quantitative anatomic study. J Am Soc Echocardiogr. 2011; 24:600–10.
14. Marx GR, Fulton DR, Pandian NG, et al. Delineation of site, relative size and dynamic geometry of atrial septal defects by real-time three-dimensional echocardiography. J Am Coll Cardiol. 1995; 25:482–90.
15. Taniguchi M, Akagi T, Watanabe N, et al. Application of real time three-dimensional transesophageal echocardiography using a matrix array probe for trans-catheter closure of atrial septal defect. J Am Soc Echocardiogr. 2009;22:1114–20.
16. Faletra FF, Ho SY, Auricchio A. Anatomy of right atrial structures by real-time 3D transesophageal echocardiography. J Am Coll Cardiol Img. 2010;3:966–75.
17. Pushparajah K, Miller OI, Simpson JM. 3D Echocardiography of the atrial septum: anatomical features and landmarks for the echocardiographer. J Am Coll Cardiol Img. 2010;3:981–4.
18. Saric M, Perk G, Purgess JR, Kronzon I. Imaging atrial septal defects by real-time three-dimensional transesophageal echocardiography: step-by-step approach. J Am Soc Echocardiogr. 2010;23:1128–35.
19. Roberson DA, Cui W. Evaluation of atrial and ventricular septal defects with real-time three-dimensional echocardiography. Curr Cardiovasc Imaging Rep. 2011;4:349–60.
20. Van den Bosch AE, Ten Harkel DJ, McGhie JS, et al. Feasibility and accuracy of real-time 3-dimensional echocardiographic assessment of ventricular septal defects. J Am Soc Echocardiogr. 2006;19:7–13.
21. Acar P, Abadir S, Aggoun Y. Transcatheter closure of perimembranous ventricular septal defects with Amplatzer occluder assessed by real-time three-dimensional echocardiography. Eur J Echocardiogr. 2007;8:110–5.
22. Takahashi K, Guerra V, Roman KS, et al. Three-dimensional echocardiography improves the understanding of the mechanisms and site of left atrioventricular valve regurgitation in atrioventricular septal defect. J Am Soc Echocardiogr. 2006;19:1502–10.
23. Seliem MA, Fedec A, Szwast A, et al. Atrioventricular valve morphology and dynamics in congenital heart disease as imaged with real-time 3-dimensional matrix-array echocardiography: comparison with 2-dimensional imaging and surgical findings. J Am Soc Echocardiogr. 2007;20:869–76.
24. Kutty S, Smallhorn JF. Evaluation of atrioventricular septal defects by three-dimensional echocardiography: benefits of navigating the third dimension. J Am Soc Echocardiogr. 2012;25:932–44.
25. Marx GR, Su X. Three-dimensional echocardiography in congenital heart disease. Cardiol Clin. 2007;25:357–65.
26. Baker GH, Shirali G, Ringewald JM, et al. Usefulness of live three-dimensional transesophageal echocardiography in a congenital heart disease center. Am J Cardiol. 2009; 103(7):1025–8.
27. Shirali GS. Three-dimensional echocardiography in congenital heart disease. Echocardiography. 2012;29:242–8.
28. Gorcsan III J, Abraham T, Agler DA, et al. Echocardiography for cardiac resynchronization therapy: recommendations for performance and reporting–a report from the American Society of Echocardiography Dyssynchrony Writing Group endorsed by the Heart Rhythm Society. J Am Soc Echocardiogr. 2008; 21:191–213.
29. Tanaka H, Hara H, Adelstein EC, Schwartzman D, Saba S, Gorcsan J. Comparative mechanical activation mapping of RV pacing to LBBB by 2D and 3D speckle tracking and association with response to resynchronization therapy. JACC Cardiovasc Imaging. 2010; 3:461–71.
30. Cui W, Gambetta K, Zimmerman F, et al. Real-time three-dimensional echocardiographic assessment of left ventricular systolic dyssynchrony in healthy children. J Am Soc Echocardiogr. 2010;23:1153–9.

Index

P.C. Wong, W.C. Miller-Hance (eds.), *Transesophageal Echocardiography for Congenital Heart Disease*,
DOI 10.1007/978-1-84800-064-3, © Springer-Verlag London 2014

O

P

FSC
www.fsc.org
MIX
Papier | Fördert gute Waldnutzung
FSC® C083411

Kolibri 360 GmbH
Ferdinand-Jühlke-Straße 7
99095 Erfurt, Deutschland
produktsicherheit@kolibri360.de